Myles Textbook for Midwives

Sixteenth Edition

Content Strategist: Mairi McCubbin
Content Development Specialist: Carole McMurray
Project Manager: Caroline Jones
Designer/Design Direction: Miles Hitchen
Illustration Manager: Jennifer Rose
Illustrator: Antbits

Myles Textbook for Midwives

Sixteenth Edition

Edited by

Jayne E Marshall PhD MA PGCEA ADM RM RGN

Head of School of Midwifery and Child Health, Faculty of Health, Social Care and Education, St Georges, University of London/Kingston University, UK

Former Associate Professor in Midwifery, Director for Postgraduate Taught Studies in Midwifery University of Nottingham, Academic Division of Midwifery, School of Health Sciences, Faculty of Medicine and Health Sciences, Postgraduate Education Centre, Nottingham, UK

Maureen D Raynor MA PGCEA ADM RMN RM RM

Lecturer and Supervisor of Midwives, University of Nottingham, Academic Division of Midwifery, School of Health Sciences, Faculty of Medicine and Health Sciences, Postgraduate Education Centre, Nottingham, UK

Foreword by

Emeritus Professor Diane M Fraser

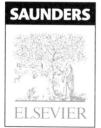

SAUNDERS

ELSEVIER

Edinburgh   London   New York   Oxford   Philadelphia   St Louis   Sydney   Toronto   2014

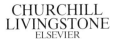

CHURCHILL
LIVINGSTONE
ELSEVIER

First edition 1953
Second edition 1956
Third edition 1958
Fourth edition 1961
Fifth edition 1964
Sixth edition 1968
Seventh edition 1971
Eighth edition 1975

Ninth edition 1981
Tenth edition 1985
Eleventh edition 1989
Twelfth edition 1993
Thirteenth edition 1999
Fourteenth edition 2003
Fifteenth edition 2009
Sixteenth edition 2014

ISBN 9780702051456
International ISBN 9780702051463

2   **British Library Cataloguing in Publication Data**
A catalogue record for this book is available from the British Library

3   **Library of Congress Cataloging in Publication Data**
A catalog record for this book is available from the Library of Congress

Notices
Knowledge and best practice in this field are constantly changing. As new research and experience broaden our understanding, changes in research methods, professional practices, or medical treatment may become necessary.

Practitioners and researchers must always rely on their own experience and knowledge in evaluating and using any information, methods, compounds, or experiments described herein. In using such information or methods they should be mindful of their own safety and the safety of others, including parties for whom they have a professional responsibility.

With respect to any drug or pharmaceutical products identified, readers are advised to check the most current information provided (i) on procedures featured or (ii) by the manufacturer of each product to be administered, to verify the recommended dose or formula, the method and duration of administration, and contraindications. It is the responsibility of practitioners, relying on their own experience and knowledge of their patients, to make diagnoses, to determine dosages and the best treatment for each individual patient, and to take all appropriate safety precautions.

To the fullest extent of the law, neither the Publisher nor the authors, contributors, or editors, assume any liability for any injury and/or damage to persons or property as a matter of products liability, negligence or otherwise, or from any use or operation of any methods, products, instructions, or ideas contained in the material herein.

 your source for books, journals and multimedia in the health sciences
www.elsevierhealth.com

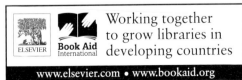

The publisher's policy is to use **paper manufactured from sustainable forests**

Printed in Scotland

Last digit is the print number: 10   9   8

Contents

Evolve online resources: http://evolve.elsevier.com/Marshall/Myles/

Contents

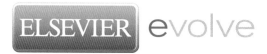 ELSEVIER | evolve

Additional online resources

To access your Student Resources, visit:

http://evolve.elsevier.com/Marshall/Myles/

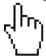

Register today and gain access to:

- **Over 500 multiple-choice questions** enable students to test their knowledge.
- **Full image bank of illustrations** to make study more visual and assist with projects.

Contributors

Jenny Bailey, BN MedSci/ClinEd DANS RM RGN
Midwife Teacher, University of Nottingham, Faculty of
Medicine and Health Sciences, School of Health Sciences,
Academic Division of Midwifery, Nottingham, UK
*Chapter 5 Hormonal cycles: fertilization and early
development*
Chapter 6 The placenta
Chapter 7 The fetus

Helen Baston, BA(Hons) MMEdSci PhD ADM RN RM
Consultant Midwife, Public Health, Supervisor of Midwives,
Sheffield Teaching Hospitals NHS Foundation Trust, Sheffield,
UK
Chapter 10 Antenatal care

Cecily Begley, MSc MA PhD RGN RM RNT FFNRCSI FTCD
Professor of Nursing and Midwifery, School of Nursing and
Midwifery, Trinity College Dublin, Dublin, Ireland
*Chapter 18 Physiology and care during the third stage
of labour*

Jenny Brewster, MEd(Open) BSc(Hons) PGCert RM RN
Senior Lecturer in Midwifery, College of Nursing, Midwifery
and Health Care, University of West London, Brentford, UK
*Chapter 12 Common problems associated with early
and advanced pregnancy*

Susan Brydon, BSc(Hons) MSc PGDip(Mid) DipApSsc,
CertHP RN RM
Supervisor of Midwives, Nottingham University Hospitals NHS
Trust, Nottingham, UK
*Chapter 16 Physiology and care during the first stage
of labour*

Kinsi Clarke
Advocacy Worker, Nottingham, UK
*Chapter 15 Care of the perineum, repair and female genital
mutilation*

Terri Coates, MSc ADM DipEd RN RM
Freelance Lecturer and Writer; Clinical Midwife, Salisbury
NHS Trust, Salisbury, UK
Chapter 20 Malpositions of the occiput and malpresentations
Chapter 22 Midwifery and obstetric emergencies

Helen Crafter, MSc ADM PGCEA FPCert RGN RM
Senior Lecturer in Midwifery/Course Leader, College of
Nursing, Midwifery and Health Care, University of West
London, Brentford, UK
*Chapter 12 Common problems associated with early
and advanced pregnancy*

Margie Davies, RGN RM
Midwifery Advisor, Multiple Births Foundation, Queen
Charlotte's and Chelsea Hospital, London, UK
Chapter 14 Multiple pregnancy

Rowena Doughty, PGDE BA(Hons) MSc ADM RM RN
Senior Lecturer – Midwifery, School of Nursing and
Midwifery, De Montfort University, Leicester, UK
*Chapter 13 Medical conditions of significance to midwifery
practice*

Soo Downe, BA(Hons) MSc PhD RM
University of Central Lancashire, School of Health, Research
in Childbirth and Health (ReaCH group), Preston, Lancashire,
UK
*Chapter 17 Physiology and care during the transition and
second stage phases of labour*

Carole England, BSc(Hons) ENB405 CertEd(FE) RGN RM
Midwife Teacher, Academic Division of Midwifery, School of
Health Sciences, University of Nottingham, Derby, UK
*Chapter 28 Recognizing the healthy baby at term through
examination of the newborn screening*
*Chapter 29 Resuscitation of the healthy baby at birth: the
importance of drying, airway management and establishment
of breathing*
Chapter 30 The healthy low birth weight baby
Chapter 33 Significant problems in the newborn baby

Angie Godfrey, BSc(Hons) RM RN
Midwife/Antenatal and NewbornScreening Coordinator,
Nottingham University Hospitals NHS Trust, Nottingham, UK
Chapter 11 Antenatal screening of the mother and fetus

Contributors

Claire Greig, ADM MTD Neonatal Certificate BN MSc PhD RGN SCM
Senior Lecturer (retired), Lecturer (part time), Edinburgh Napier University, Edinburgh, UK
Chapter 31 Trauma during birth, haemorrhages and convulsions

Jenny Hassall, BSc(Hons) MSc MPhil RN RM
School of Nursing and Midwifery, University of Brighton, Eastbourne, UK
Chapter 9 Change and adaptation in pregnancy

Richard Hayman, BSc MB BS DFFP DM FRCOG
Consultant Obstetrician and Gynaecologist, Gloucestershire Hospitals NHS Trust, Gloucester, UK
Chapter 21 Operative births

Sally Inch, RN RM
Honorary Research Fellow, Applied Research Centre Health and Lifestyles Interventions, Coventry University, Coventry, UK
Chapter 34 Infant feeding

Karen Jackson, BSc (Hons) MPhil ADM RN RM
Midwife Lecturer, University of Nottingham, Faculty of Medicine and Health Sciences, School of Health Sciences, Academic Division of Midwifery, University of Nottingham, UK
Chapter 16 Physiology and care during the first stage of labour
Chapter 27 Contraception and sexual health in a global society

Lucy Kean, BM BCh MD FRCOG
Consultant Obstetrician, Subspecialist in Fetal Medicine, Nottingham University Hospitals NHS Trust, Nottingham, UK
Chapter 11 Antenatal screening of the mother and fetus

Rosemary Mander, MSc PhD MTD RGN SCM
Emeritus Professor of Midwifery, School of Health in Social Science, University of Edinburgh, Edinburgh, UK
Chapter 1 The midwife in contemporary midwifery practice
Chapter 26 Bereavement and loss in maternity care

Jayne E Marshall, PhD MA PGCEA ADM RM RGN
Head of School of Midwifery and Child Health, Faculty of Health, Social Care and Education, St Georges, University of London/Kingston University, UK
Chapter 1 The midwife in contemporary midwifery practice
Chapter 2 Professional issues concerning the midwife and midwifery practice
Chapter 13 Medical conditions of significance to midwifery practice
Chapter 16 Physiology and care during the first stage of labour
Chapter 17 Physiology and care during the transition and second stage phases of labour

Carol McCormick, BSc(Hons) PGDL ADM RN RM
Specialist Midwife (FGM), Nottingham University Hospitals NHS Trust (City Campus), Hucknall Road, Nottingham, UK
Chapter 15 Care of the perineum, repair and female genital mutilation

Moira McLean, RGN RM ADM PGCEA PGDIP SOM
Senior Lecturer – Midwifery and Supervisor of Midwives, School of Nursing and Midwifery, De Montfort University, Leicester, UK
Chapter 13 Medical conditions of significance to midwifery practice

Irene Murray, BSc(Hons) MTD RN RM
Teaching Fellow (Midwifery), Department of Nursing and Midwifery, University of Stirling, Centre for Health Science, Inverness, UK
Chapter 9 Change and adaptation in pregnancy

Mary Louise Nolan, BA(Hons) MA PhD RGN
Professor of Perinatal Education, Institute of Health and Society, University of Worcester, Worcester, UK
Chapter 8 Antenatal education for birth and parenting

Margaret R Oates, OBE MB ChB FRCPsych FRCOG
Consultant Perinatal Psychiatrist and Clinical Lead, Strategic Clinical Network for Mental Health, Dementia and Neurological Conditions, NHS England, Nottingham, UK
Chapter 25 Perinatal mental health

Kathleen O'Reilly, MB ChB MA MRCPCH
Consultant Neonatologist, Neonatal Intensive Care Unit, Royal Hospital for Sick Children, Glasgow, UK
Chapter 32 Congenital malformations

Jean Rankin, BSc(Hons) MSc PhD PGCert LTHE RN RSCN RM
Senior Lecturer in Research (Maternal, Child and Family Health)/Supervisor of Midwives, University of the West of Scotland, Paisley, UK
Chapter 4 The female urinary tract

Maureen D Raynor, MA PGCEA ADM RMN RN RM
Lecturer and Supervisor of Midwives, Academic Division of Midwifery, School of Health Sciences, Faculty of Medicine and Health Sciences, University of Nottingham, Nottingham, UK
Chapter 1 The midwife in contemporary midwifery practice
Chapter 2 Professional issues concerning the midwife and midwifery practice
Chapter 15 Care of the perineum, repair and genital mutilation
Chapter 25 Perinatal mental health

Annie Rimmer, BEd(Hons) ADM RM RN
Senior Lecturer – Midwifery, School of Nursing and
Midwifery, University of Brighton, Eastbourne, UK
*Chapter 19 Prolonged pregnancy and disorders of uterine
action*

S. Elizabeth Robson, MSc ADM Cert(A)Ed MTD RGN
RM FHEA
Principal Lecturer – Midwifery, School of Nursing and
Midwifery, De Montfort University, Leicester, UK
*Chapter 13 Medical conditions of significance to midwifery
practice*

Judith Simpson, MB ChB MD MRCPCH
Consultant Neonatologist, Neonatal Intensive Care Unit,
Royal Hospital for Sick Children, Glasgow, UK
Chapter 32 Congenital malformations

Mary Steen, BSc PhD MCGI PGDipHE PGCRM
RM RGN
Professional Editor, *RCM Journal*, Professor of Midwifery,
University of Chester, Chester, UK, Adjunct Professor of
Midwifery, University of South Australia (UniSA), Adelaide,
Australia
Chapter 23 Physiology and care during the puerperium
*Chapter 24 Physical health problems and complications in
the puerperium*

Amanda Sullivan, BA(Hons) PGDip PhD RM RGN
Director of Quality and Governance for NHS Nottinghamshire
County, NHS Nottinghamshire County, Mansfield,
Nottinghamshire, UK
Chapter 11 Antenatal screening of the mother and fetus

Abdul H Sultan, MD FRCOG
Consultant Obstetrician and Gynaecologist, Croydon
University Hospital, Croydon, UK
Chapter 3 The female pelvis and the reproductive organs
*Chapter 15 Care of the perineum, repair and female genital
mutilation*

Ranee Thakar, MD MRCOG
Consultant Obstetrician and Urogynaecologist, Department
of Obstetrics and Gynaecology, Croydon University Hospital,
Croydon, UK
Chapter 3 The female pelvis and the reproductive organs
*Chapter 15 Care of the perineum, repair and female genital
mutilation*

Mary Vance, MPhil PGCert TLT BSc(Hons) RM RGN
LSA Midwifery Officer, North of Scotland LSA Consortium,
Inverness, UK
*Chapter 2 Professional issues concerning the midwife and
midwifery practice*

Stephen P Wardle, MB ChB MD FRCPCH
Consultant Neonatologist, Neonatal Intensive Care Unit,
Nottingham University Hospitals NHS Trust, Nottingham, UK
Chapter 33 Significant problems in the newborn baby

Julie Wray, ONC MSc PhD PGCHE ADM RM RN
Joint Editor, *The Practising Midwife Journal;* Senior Lecturer,
User and Carer Lead, School of Nursing, Midwifery and
Social Work, University of Salford, Salford, UK
Chapter 23 Physiology and care during the puerperium
*Chapter 24 Physical health problems and complications in
the puerperium*

Foreword

The strength and longevity of *Myles Textbook for Midwives* lies in its ability to juxtapose continuity and change from the first edition in 1953 to this sixteenth edition, over 60 years later. In continuity, some of the excellent early illustrations have been replicated throughout the editions. These provide clarity of understanding of essential anatomy for students. Changes of and additional colours in this edition have made a dramatic improvement to this clarity. In addition the clearly set out sections, chapter titles and index, aid systematic learning as well as facilitating easy reference when a new situation is encountered in practice. Of equal importance is how this text demonstrates the changes that have taken place in midwifery practice.

Unlike the early editions, when midwives relied on one textbook and teachers alone, this sixteenth edition draws together theory, current practices, research and best evidence. In contrast to the first edition where Myles, in the Preface, wrote: *'No bibliographical references have been given because of the vast number of sources which have been tapped in compiling the text* (by Margaret Myles herself) *and because pupil midwives become confused when they study from more than one or two textbooks'*, this edition signposts students to further resources to increase their depth and breadth of knowledge. This is essential as no textbook can capture all the information needed for contemporary midwifery practice.

In all editions the needs of women and their families have been central and this edition continues to emphasize the emotional, socio-economic, educational and physical needs of women during the life changing experience of pregnancy and parenthood, or bereavement. These events have a lasting impact on women's lives. Of importance is always how well women are listened to and involved in making decisions about their or their babies' care. Running through this edition is an emphasis on the need for midwives to be emotionally aware and develop good communication and interpersonal relationships with women, their partners and colleagues in the interdisciplinary team. The midwife has a key role to play in assisting women to make choices and feel in control, even when presented with difficult options and dilemmas. This text demonstrates the midwife's role as lead professional when pregnancy is straightforward and co-ordinator of care when others need to be involved.

The maternity services have seen major changes in recent years, in particular the massive increase in the birth rate, the changing demographics of women who become pregnant and the politics surrounding childbirth. Section One effectively brings together the issues that midwives need to understand, not just during their education programme, but also as part of their future responsibility in helping to bring about improvements in maternity care both in the UK and internationally. The vision for UK midwifery set out in Midwifery 2020 (Midwifery 2020 UK Programme, 2010) and the global initiatives of the International Confederation of Midwives are well summarized.

Whilst Margaret Myles in her first 10 editions drew upon the knowledge of obstetricians and paediatricians in England and Scotland, she wrote the entire book herself. Recent edited editions demonstrate the need to draw upon the expertise of other midwives and health professionals in chapter writing. Thakar's and Sultan's inclusion of diagrams and photographs of perineal anatomy and trauma in chapter three are very timely given the increasing number of students who now learn to suture. These will help understanding of the importance of accurate diagnosis and effective perineal repair to aid women's physical and emotional recovery.

The value of antenatal education has been emphasized since the inception of this textbook, yet today not all women or their partners attend. Mary Nolan stresses the importance of sessions to be women-centred and expertly facilitated, not lecture based. She reminds readers that many women are not being provided with sufficient opportunity to attend, yet classes can make a big difference to women's experiences of birth and parenting. In addition she draws attention to the value they have in giving women social networks. This has been evident in my daughter's experience of classes in Germany. Whilst she was critical of some of the content of the classes, she and four other women who birthed one to 10 days apart, have supported each other in parenting. Two years on they remain good friends.

Chapter 13 skilfully draws together the most significant medical conditions a midwife is likely to encounter in her practice. Much attention is given to obesity. The authors qualify that although obesity is not in itself a disease it is considered abnormal in western cultures and is now a key health concern affecting society. They discuss the additional risks to pregnant women who are obese and the association of obesity with poor socioeconomic status. Midwives have a key role in educating these women and their families to develop healthier life styles, but the women will only be receptive if they do not experience judgemental attitudes.

Myles advice to midwives in the 1960s that, *nature is capable of performing her function without aid in most instances; meddlesome midwifery increases the hazards of birth'*, is still as relevant today. In this edition, given all the technological advances in the maternity services, Section 4 on labour begins by reminding students that: *'birth is a physiological process characterized by non-intervention, a supportive environment and empowerment of the woman'*. However, an appropriate reflection of multi-cultural changes in UK society is the inclusion of female genital mutilation in chapter 15. Whilst many students will not be involved in the care of women who have undergone such a procedure, it is essential that all midwives understand the mutilation some young women have undergone and the special care they will need in childbirth. The inclusion of Kinsi's poignant and brave story of her own experiences should help midwives develop the empathy they will need when caring for women who have been subject to similar mutilation.

Perinatal mental health has figured since the early days of the textbook but only in recent editions have students been provided with the necessary information to understand the complexity of the psychology of childbearing and psychiatric disorders. A useful inclusion in this edition is tocophobia, fear of giving birth. Students need to take this fear seriously in supporting women and they cannot afford to trivialize these very real phobias.

As ever this textbook includes a comprehensive section on the newborn baby, often neglected in other general texts for midwives. This is so important when parents turn to midwives for advice and reassurance or explanations. With many midwifery curricula including a module on the specialist education for the Newborn and Infant Physical Examination, chapter 28 clearly differentiates between the midwife's and the doctor's responsibilities when undertaking this examination. The publishers have brought about major improvements also, through locating the colour photographs in these newborn baby chapters close to where they are described in the text rather than as a separate colour plate section.

Midwifery is the best career you can have. It is a privilege to work with women and their families as they experience pregnancy, birth and parenting. The knowledge, skills and attitudes that students need to be competent midwives and professional friends to women have been skilfully interwoven in this sixteenth edition. The chapter authors and editors have summarized where appropriate, elaborated when needed, referenced liberally and used illustrations effectively to enhance understanding. Given the infinite depth and breadth of information available in written and electronic forms, they have succeeded in producing a textbook that remains invaluable for the next generation of midwives.

Diane M Fraser
Bed MPhil PhD MTD RM RGN
Emeritus Professor of Midwifery
University of Nottingham

REFERENCE

Midwifery 2020 UK Programme, 2010. Midwifery 2020: Delivering expectations. Edinburgh: Midwifery 2020 UK Programme

Preface

It is a great privilege to have been approached by Elsevier to undertake the editorship of the sixteenth edition of *Myles Textbook for Midwives*. It is over 60 years since the Scottish midwife Margaret Myles wrote the first edition and this book remains highly regarded as the seminal text for student midwives and practising midwives alike throughout the world. Over the ensuing decades, many changes have taken place in the education and training of future midwives alongside increasing demands and complexities associated with the health and wellbeing of childbearing women, their babies and families within a global context. Furthermore, the development of evidence-based practice and advances in technology have also contributed to major reviews of how undergraduate midwifery curricula are delivered to ensure that today's graduate midwives are able to rise to the many challenges of the midwife's multi-faceted role: being *fit for both practice and purpose*. It is with these issues in mind that the sixteenth edition of *Myles* has been developed as, without a doubt, women expect midwives to provide safe and competent care that is tailored to their individual needs, with a professional and compassionate attitude.

The content and format of this edition of *Myles* has been developed in response to the collated views from students and midwives regarding the fifteenth edition. Midwifery practice clearly should always be informed by the best possible up-to-date evidence and, whilst it is acknowledged that it is impossible to expect any new text to contain the most contemporary of research and systematic reviews, this edition provides the reader with annotated further reading and appropriate websites in addition to comprehensive reference lists.

There has been a major revision of chapters, which have been streamlined and structured into reflect similar themes and content. Throughout its history, *Myles Textbook for Midwives* has always included clear and comprehensible illustrations to compliment the text. In this sixteenth edition, full colour has been used throughout the book, and new diagrams have been added where appropriate.

It is pleasing that a number of chapter authors have continued their contribution to successive editions of this pivotal text and we also welcome the invaluable contributions from new authors. Whilst it is vital to retain the ethos of the text being a *textbook for midwives* that is *written by midwives* with the appropriate expertise, it is also imperative that it reflects the eclectic nature of maternity care and thus, some of the chapters have been written in collaboration with members of the multi-professional team. This clearly demonstrates the importance of health professionals working and learning together in order to enhance the quality of care women and their families receive, especially when complications develop in the physiological process throughout the childbirth continuum. The presence of the midwife is integral to all clinical situations and the role is significant in ensuring the woman always receives the additional care required from the most-appropriate health professional at the most-appropriate time.

A significant change has been to the first section of the text where content from the final section has been included. From an international perspective, we believe that issues such as the globalization of midwifery education and practice, best depicted by the Millennium Development Goals, professional regulation and midwifery supervision, legal and ethical issues as well as risk management and clinical governance are fundamental to every midwife practising in the twenty-first century and should therefore be given more prominence. We acknowledge that medicalization and the consequential effect of a risk culture in the maternity services have eroded some aspects of the midwife's role over time. It is our aim to challenge midwives into thinking outside the box and to have the confidence to empower women into making choices appropriate for them and their personal situation. An example is the decision to incorporate breech presentation and vaginal breech birth at term into the first and second stage of labour chapters rather than within the malpresentations chapter.

Recognizing that midwives increasingly care for women with complex health needs within a multicultural society and taking on specialist or extended roles, significant topics have been added to make the text more contemporary. Chapter 13 incorporates the dilemmas faced by midwives when caring for women who have a raised body mass index and chapter 15 is a new chapter that addresses how care of the perineum can be optimized alongside the physiological and psychosocial challenges when women present with some degree of female genital mutilation. Furthermore, as an increasing number of midwives are undertaking further training to carry out the neonatal physiological examination and neonatal life support, specific details have been included in chapter 28 and a new chapter 29 dedicated to basic neonatal resuscitation respectively, to provide a foundation for students to build upon.

Additional online multiple-choice questions have been updated and revised to reflect the focus of the chapters in this edition, as readers appreciate their use in aiding self-assessment of learning.

We hope that this new edition of *Myles Textbook for Midwives* will provide midwives with the foundation of the physiological theory and underpinning care principles to inform their clinical practice and support appropriate decision-making in partnership with childbearing women and members of the multi-professional team. We recognize that knowledge is boundless and that this text alone cannot provide everything midwives should know when undertaking their multi-faceted roles, however, it can afford the means to stimulate further enquiry and enthusiasm for continuing professional development.

London and Nottingham, 2014

Jayne E Marshall
Maureen D Raynor

Acknowledgements

The editors of the sixteenth edition are indebted to the many authors of earlier editions whose work has provided the foundations from which this current volume has evolved. From the fifteenth edition, these contributors include the volume editors, Diane M Fraser and Margaret A Cooper, and chapter authors:

Robina Aslam
Jean E Bain
Diane Barrowclough
Kuldip Kaur Bharj OBE
Susan Dapaah
Victor E Dapaah
Jean Duerden
Philomena Farrell
Alison Gibbs
Adela Hamilton
Pauline Hudson
Billie Hunter
Beverley Kirk
Judith Lee
Carmel Lloyd
Sally Marchant
Christine McCourt
Sue McDonald

Christina McKenzie
Alison Miller
Salmon Omokanye
Lesley Page
Patricia Percival
Lindsay Reid
Nancy Riddick-Thomas
Jane M Rutherford
Iolanda G J Serci
Della Sherratt
Norma Sittlington
Nina Smith
Ian M Symonds
Ros Thomas
Denise Tiran
Tom Turner
Anne Viccars

Whilst the support and guidance from the production team at Elsevier has been invaluable in the culmination of an exciting and much improved illustrated text, the editors must also acknowledge the support of family, friends and colleagues in enabling them to accomplish the task amidst their full-time academic roles.

Section | 1 |

The midwife in context

Chapter | 1 |

The midwife in contemporary midwifery practice

Maureen D Raynor, Rosemary Mander, Jayne E Marshall

In the United Kingdom (UK) midwives are encouraged to broaden their toolkit of skills and knowledge in an effort to strengthen their public health remit and leadership potential in order to work collaboratively with women as equal partners in their care. Midwifery 2020 (Department of Health [DH] 2010a) outlines the future vision for midwifery. This initiative is a unique UK-wide collaborative programme where the four countries of Great Britain share a common purpose and ideology that can benchmark their midwifery planning and provision. It is envisaged that each country will be able to identify their own priorities to deliver care that is woman-centred, safe and fulfilling within existing resources. There are parallels here to be drawn with wider global initiatives such as the United Nations [UN] (2010, 2013) Millennium Development Goals (MDGs) and the International Confederation of Midwives (ICM 2011) international definition of the midwife.

THE CHAPTER AIMS TO:

- explore the midwife in context, taking a number of influential social and global issues into consideration; the key factors are –
- globalization and internationalization with due consideration of the Millennium Development Goals, the European (EU) Directives and International Confederation of Midwives Education Standards
- the emotional context of midwifery
- working with women from socially disadvantaged groups
- evidence-based practice.

INTERNATIONALIZATION/ GLOBALIZATION

Globalization and internationalization against the background of midwifery practice are difficult terms to define, compounded by the fact that the terms are often used interchangeably and synonymously, even though they are construed as distinctly separate entities. Globalization is not a new phenomenon (Baumann and Blythe 2008) with a number of varying definitions evident in the literature. The definition with the greatest resonance for midwives is that provided by the World Health Organization (2013), who states that *globalization* is:

> *the increased interconnectedness and interdependence of people and countries, is generally understood to include two interrelated elements: the opening of borders to increasingly fast flows of goods, services, finance, people and ideas across international borders; and the changes in institutional and policy regimes at the international and national levels that facilitates or promote such flows.*

Globalization is not without its critics but it is acknowledged that the consequences of globalization are not predetermined and can have both positive and negative outcomes (Baumann and Blythe 2008). It is essential therefore to have an awareness of both the good and harm globalization may impose on a society.

Conversely, *internationalization* has no agreed definition but from a midwifery perspective it can be defined as the international process of planning and implementing midwifery education and services in order that there is a shared vision that can easily be translated or adapted to meet the local and national needs of individual nations in both resource-rich and resource-poor countries.

Internationalization is important for the midwifery profession because in a global society midwives are required to have a broad understanding of cross-cultural issues. They need to be flexible and adaptable in order to provide care that is sensitive and responsive to women's dynamic healthcare needs. This requires the midwife to be an effective change agent, and the onus is very much on the midwife to keep pace with change. This means having a good comprehension of internationalization, learning to deal with uncertainty, embracing the ethos of life-long learning as well as the gains and challenges of interprofessional or multidisciplinary collaboration, contributing to quality assurance issues such as audit, research, risk assessment and the wider clinical governance agenda. Even though skills of problem-solving, clinical judgement, decision-making and clinical competence in the practical

assessment, planning, implementation, evaluation and documentation of care are all crucial for midwifery practice, human factors also matter. In England, the Francis Report (Mid Staffordshire NHS Foundation Trust Public Inquiry 2013) was the outcome of a public inquiry into failings at Mid Staffordshire and relevant regulatory bodies. It represents a watershed moment in the history of the UK National Health Service (NHS). The scale of the problems highlighted by the report relates to the unusually high death rates amongst the sick and vulnerable at Mid Staffordshire in the late 2000s. The key lessons learnt convey the importance of transparent, compassionate, committed, competent and confident caring premised on strong leadership. It can be argued therefore that common standards and a shared vision established through global initiatives such as the MDGs and the ICM definition of a midwife are essential for midwives working within a global community. Not least because there is a strong correlation between outcomes for mothers and babies and the specific professional competencies the midwife possesses.

Definition and scope of the midwife

Midwives should be informed about the legal framework in which their role and scope of practice are enshrined. A definition of the midwife was developed by the ICM in 1972, which was later adopted by the International Federation of Gynaecology and Obstetrics (FIGO) followed by the World Health Organization (WHO). In 1990, at the Kobe Council meeting, the ICM amended the definition, later ratified in 1991 and 1992 by FIGO and WHO respectively. In 2005 and 2011 it was amended slightly by the ICM Council (Box 1.1).

At the European level, member states of the EU (known at the time as the European Community [EC]) prepared a list of activities (Box 1.2) that midwives should be entitled to take up within its territory (EC Midwives Directive 1980; WHO 2009). Although midwives must learn about all of these activities, in the UK, where there is skilled medical care available to all pregnant women, it is recognized that it is highly unlikely that midwives would be expected to be proficient in all the activities identified by the EU. The manual removal of the placenta, for example, would routinely be carried out by a doctor unless no doctor is available and the mother's life is at risk.

The ICM Global Midwifery Education Standards

The ICM acknowledges that all midwifery programmes should be accountable to the public, mothers and their families, the profession, employers, students as well as one another. It is therefore the responsibility of the provider education institution to ensure that the undergraduate or

Box 1.1 **An International definition of the midwife**

A midwife is a person who has successfully completed a midwifery education programme that is duly recognized in the country where it is located and that is based on the ICM Essential Competencies for Basic Midwifery Practice and the framework of the ICM Global Standards for Midwifery Education; who has acquired the requisite qualifications to be registered and/or legally licensed to practice midwifery and use the title 'midwife'; and who demonstrates competency in the practice of midwifery.

Scope of practice

The midwife is recognized as a responsible and accountable professional who works in partnership with women to give the necessary support, care and advice during pregnancy, labour and the postpartum period, to conduct births on the midwife's own responsibility and to provide care for the newborn and the infant. This care includes preventative measures, the promotion of normal birth, the detection of complications in mother and child, the accessing of medical care or other appropriate assistance and the carrying out of emergency measures. The midwife has an important task in health counselling and education, not only for the woman, but also within the family and the community. This work should involve antenatal education and preparation for parenthood and may extend to women's health, sexual or reproductive health and child care. A midwife may practice in any setting including the home, community, hospitals, clinics or health units.

Revised and adopted by ICM Council 15 June 2011; due for review 2017 www.internationalmidwives.org

Box 1.2 **European Union Standards for Nursing and Midwifery: Article 42 – Pursuit of the professional activities of a midwife**

The provisions of this section shall apply to the activities of midwives as defined by each Member State, without prejudice to paragraph 2, and pursued under the professional titles set out in Annex V, point 5.5.2.

The Member States shall ensure that midwives are able to gain access to and pursue at least the following activities:

(a) provision of sound family planning information and advice;

(b) diagnosis of pregnancies and monitoring normal pregnancies; carrying out the examinations necessary for the monitoring of the development of normal pregnancies;

(c) prescribing or advising on the examinations necessary for the earliest possible diagnosis of pregnancies at risk;

(d) provision of programmes of parenthood preparation and complete preparation for childbirth including advice on hygiene and nutrition;

(e) caring for and assisting the mother during labour and monitoring the condition of the fetus in utero by the appropriate clinical and technical means;

(f) conducting spontaneous deliveries including where required episiotomies and in urgent cases breech deliveries;

(g) recognizing the warning signs of abnormality in the mother or infant which necessitate referral to a doctor and assisting the latter where appropriate; taking the necessary emergency measures in the doctor's absence, in particular the manual removal of the placenta, possibly followed by manual examination of the uterus;

(h) examining and caring for the newborn infant; taking all initiatives which are necessary in case of need and carrying out where necessary immediate resuscitation;

(i) caring for and monitoring the progress of the mother in the postnatal period and giving all necessary advice to the mother on infant care to enable her to ensure the optimum progress of the new-born infant;

(j) carrying out treatment prescribed by doctors;

(k) drawing up the necessary written reports.

Source: WHO (World Health Organization) 2009 European Union Standards for Nursing and Midwifery: information for accession countries, 2nd edn. www.euro.who.int/__data/assets/pdf_file/0005/102200/E92852.pdf

preregistration curricula they provide have a stated philosophy, transparent, realistic, achievable goals and outcomes that prepare students to be fully qualified competent and autonomous midwives. The Global Standards for Midwifery Education 2010 as developed, outlined and amended by the ICM (2013) are deemed as the mainstays to strengthen midwifery education and practice. These standards, outlined in Box 1.3, were developed alongside two further documents: *Companion Guidelines* and *Glossary*, which are all available on the ICM website. In order to meet the needs of childbearing women and their families, the ICM (2013) highlights that these publications are 'living' documents subjected to continual scrutiny, evaluation and amendment as new evidence regarding midwifery education and practice unfolds. Therefore it is recommended by the ICM (2013) that all three documents should be reviewed together in the following order: the *Glossary* followed by the *Global Standards for Education* and concluding with the *Companion Guidelines*.

Box 1.3 **Global Standards for Midwifery Education 2010**

I Organization and administration

1. The host institution/agency/branch of government supports the philosophy, aims and objectives of the midwifery education programme.

2. The host institution helps to ensure that financial and public/policy support for the midwifery education programme are sufficient to prepare competent midwives.

3. The midwifery school/programme has a designated budget and budget control that meets programme needs.

4. The midwifery faculty is self-governing and responsible for developing and leading the policies and curriculum of the midwifery education programme.

5. The head of the midwifery programme is a qualified midwife teacher with experience in management/administration.

6. The midwifery programme takes into account national and international policies and standards to meet maternity workforce needs.

II Midwifery faculty

1. The midwifery faculty includes predominantly midwives (teachers and clinical preceptors/clinical teachers) who work with experts from other disciplines as needed.

2. The midwife teacher
   a. has formal preparation in midwifery;
   b. demonstrates competency in midwifery practice, generally accomplished with 2 years full scope practice;
   c. holds a current licence/registration or other form of legal recognition to practise midwifery;
   d. has formal preparation for teaching, or undertakes such preparation as a condition of continuing to hold the position; and
   e. maintains competence in midwifery practice and education.

3. The midwife clinical preceptor/clinical teacher
   a. is qualified according to the ICM definition of a midwife;
   b. demonstrates competency in midwifery practice, generally accomplished with 2 years full scope practice;
   c. maintains competency in midwifery practice and clinical education;
   d. holds a current licence/registration or other form of legal recognition to practice midwifery; and
   e. has formal preparation for clinical teaching or undertakes such preparation.

4. Individuals from other disciplines who teach in the midwifery programme are competent in the content they teach.

5. Midwife teachers provide education, support and supervision of individuals who teach students in practical learning sites.

6. Midwife teachers and midwife clinical preceptors/clinical teachers work together to support (facilitate), directly observe and evaluate students' practical learning.

7. The ratio of students to teachers and clinical preceptors/clinical teachers in classroom and practical sites is determined by the midwifery programme and the requirements of regulatory authorities.

8. The effectiveness of midwifery faculty members is assessed on a regular basis following an established process.

III Student body

1. The midwifery programme has clearly written admission policies that are accessible to potential applicants. These policies include:
   a. entry requirements, including minimum requirement of completion of secondary education;
   b. a transparent recruitment process;
   c. selection process and criteria for acceptance; and
   d. mechanisms for taking account of prior learning.

2. Eligible midwifery candidates are admitted without prejudice or discrimination (e.g., gender, age, national origin, religion).

3. Eligible midwifery candidates are admitted in keeping with national health care policies and maternity workforce plans.

4. The midwifery programme has clearly written student policies that include:
   a. expectations of students in classroom and practical areas;
   b. statements about students' rights and responsibilities and an established process for addressing student appeals and/or grievances;
   c. mechanisms for students to provide feedback and ongoing evaluation of the midwifery curriculum, midwifery faculty, and the midwifery programme; and
   d. requirements for successful completion of the midwifery programme.

5. Mechanisms exist for the student's active participation in midwifery programme governance and committees.

6. Students have sufficient midwifery practical experience in a variety of settings to attain, at a minimum, the current ICM Essential Competencies for basic midwifery practice.

Box 1.3 Continued

7. Students provide midwifery care primarily under the supervision of a midwife teacher or midwifery clinical preceptor/clinical teacher.

IV Curriculum

1. The philosophy of the midwifery education programme is consistent with the ICM philosophy and model of care.
2. The purpose of the midwifery education is to produce a competent midwife who:
   a. has attained/demonstrated, at a minimum, the current ICM Essential Competencies for basic midwifery practice;
   b. meets the criteria of the ICM Definition of a Midwife and regulatory body standards leading to licensure or registration as a midwife;
   c. is eligible to apply for advanced education; and
   d. is a knowledgeable, autonomous practitioner who adheres to the ICM International Code of Ethics for Midwives, standards of the profession and established scope of practice within the jurisdiction where legally recognized.
3. The sequence and content of the midwifery curriculum enables the student to acquire essential competencies for midwifery practice in accord with ICM core documents.
4. The midwifery curriculum includes both theory and practice elements with a minimum of 40% theory and a minimum of 50% practice.
   a. Minimum length of a direct-entry midwifery education programme is 3 years;
   b. Minimum length of a post-nursing/health care provider (post-registration) midwifery education programme is 18 months.
5. The midwifery programme uses evidence-based approaches to teaching and learning that promote adult learning and competency based education.
6. The midwifery programme offers opportunities for multidisciplinary content and learning experiences that complement the midwifery content.

V Resources, facilities and services

1. The midwifery programme implements written policies that address student and teacher safety and wellbeing in teaching and learning environments.
2. The midwifery programme has sufficient teaching and learning resources to meet programme needs.
3. The midwifery programme has adequate human resources to support both classroom/theoretical and practical learning.
4. The midwifery programme has access to sufficient midwifery practical experiences in a variety of settings to meet the learning needs of each student.
5. Selection criteria for appropriate midwifery practical learning sites are clearly written and implemented.

VI Assessment strategies

1. Midwifery faculty uses valid and reliable formative and summative evaluation/assessment methods to measure student performance and progress in learning related to:
   a. knowledge;
   b. behaviours;
   c. practice skills;
   d. critical thinking and decision-making; and
   e. interpersonal relationships/communication skills.
2. The means and criteria for assessment/evaluation of midwifery student performance and progression, including identification of learning difficulties, are written and shared with students.
3. Midwifery faculty conducts regular review of the curriculum as a part of quality improvement, including input from students, programme graduates, midwife practitioners, clients of midwives and other stakeholders.
4. Midwifery faculty conducts ongoing review of practical learning sites and their suitability for student learning/experience in relation to expected learning outcomes.
5. Periodic external review of programme effectiveness takes place.

Source: ICM 2013

The purpose of the ICM (2013) global education standards is to establish benchmarks so that internationally all countries, with or without such standards, can educate and train midwives to be competent and autonomous practitioners who are equipped to work within global norms. Additionally, it is envisaged that not only can the standards be expanded to meet the needs of individual countries but they can be achieved within the context of these individual countries' norms and cultural mores, thus embracing the whole ethos of globalization previously outlined. The core aims of the ICM (2013) Global Standards for Midwifery Education are three-fold:

1. Essentially, to assist countries that do not have robust training programme(s) but are striving to meet the country's needs for outputs of qualified midwives to establish basic midwifery.

2. To support countries striving to improve and/or standardize the quality of their midwifery programme(s), ensuring that midwives are fit for both practice and purpose.
3. Offer a framework to countries with established programme(s) for midwifery education who may wish to compare the quality of their existing standards of midwifery education against the ICM minimum standards. This can be achieved during the design, implementation and evaluation of the ongoing quality of the midwifery programme.

The ICM expects that the global standards for midwifery education outlined in Box 1.3 will be adopted by all those with a vested interest in the health and wellbeing of mothers, babies and their families. This requires engagement from policy-makers, governments/health ministers, midwives and wider healthcare systems. The standards not only promote an education process that prepares midwives with all the essential ICM competencies, it also supports the philosophy of life-long learning through continuing education. This approach it is hoped will foster and promote safe midwifery practice alongside quality and evidence-based care. A further goal is to strengthen and reinforce the autonomy of the midwifery profession as well as uphold the virtue of midwives as well-informed, reflective and autonomous practitioners.

To ensure students are educated and prepared to be responsible global citizens, Tuckett and Crompton (2013) stress that undergraduate programmes for student nurses and midwives should expose learners to global health systems within a culturally diverse society. Maclean (2013) concurs with this view, highlighting that global health issues are much more mainstream in contemporary midwifery practice as a direct consequence of elective placements abroad. Elective placements enable students from high-income countries to gain an invaluable insight into the health challenges faced by resource-poor countries. Furthermore, the importance of global strides to reduce disadvantages and health inequalities, such as Millennium Development Goals 4 and 5 (see below), and the principles on which the safe motherhood initiative is based, have greater significance when students have first-hand experience of the struggles encountered on a daily basis by those who are socially and economically disadvantaged.

The ERASMUS programme

ERASMUS is an acronym for EuRopean Action Scheme for the Mobility of University Students. Salient aspects of globalization have led to this initiative in Europe, incepted in 1987 to allow international mobility for university student exchange between European countries (Papatsiba 2006). Milne and Cowie (2013) extol the virtues of the ERASMUS scheme in preparing the future generation of healthcare professionals to provide culturally diverse and competent care. However, for a multiplicity of reasons, only a minority of students undertake the ERASMUS exchange.

The Millennium Development Goals (MDGs)

Despite its detractors, globalization has resulted in a rich tapestry of skills, knowledge and research to inform midwifery practice and help deliver culturally sensitive and responsive care to mothers, babies and their families. Having undertaken global travel as a consultant with the WHO to promote safer childbirth through the safe motherhood initiative, Maclean (2013) acknowledges the importance of both globalization and internationalization for midwives. She states that this is pivotal in developing a shared philosophy and building a strong alliance, especially from a cross-cultural perspective in the quest to achieve the MDGs by 2015.

Although the MDGs have placed poverty reduction, gender and wider social inequalities on the international agenda, some would argue that the blueprint or framework has its flaws (Waage et al 2010; Subramanian et al 2011) given that the goals must be achieved by 2015 and much work is still needed as the deadline looms. However, the targets outlined in Fig. 1.1 have assisted in the cooperation and collaboration of international agencies and government in addressing many of the major moral challenges of modern day society and healthcare provision for mothers and babies in the quest to realize a healthier nation.

THE EMOTIONAL CONTEXT OF MIDWIFERY

In a dynamic health service, midwives need to have an emotional awareness in order to deliver care sensitively, as well as to ensure that these feelings are acknowledged and responded to. To do this effectively, midwives should be aware not only of their own feelings but of how the delivery of the care meted out to women may impact on women's affective state (see Chapter 25). Much of midwifery work is emotionally demanding, thus an understanding by midwives of why this is so, and exploration of ways to manage feelings, can only benefit women and midwives. How midwives 'feel' about their work and the women they care for is important. It has significant implications for communication and interpersonal relationships with not only women and families but also colleagues. It also has much wider implications for the quality of maternity services in general.

By its very nature, midwifery work involves a range of emotions. Activities that midwives perform in their day-to-day role are rarely dull, spanning a vast spectrum. What may appear routine and mundane acts to midwives are often far from ordinary experiences for women – the

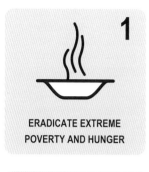

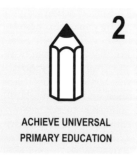

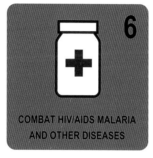

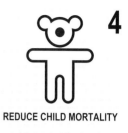

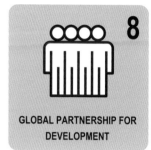

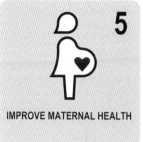

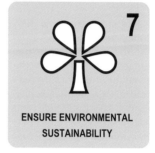

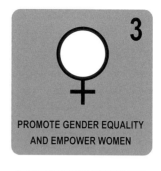

1 ERADICATE EXTREME POVERTY AND HUNGER

2 ACHIEVE UNIVERSAL PRIMARY EDUCATION

3 PROMOTE GENDER EQUALITY AND EMPOWER WOMEN

4 REDUCE CHILD MORTALITY

5 IMPROVE MATERNAL HEALTH

6 COMBAT HIV/AIDS MALARIA AND OTHER DISEASES

7 ENSURE ENVIRONMENTAL SUSTAINABILITY

8 GLOBAL PARTNERSHIP FOR DEVELOPMENT

Fig. 1.1 The eight Millennium Development Goals.
Reproduced with permission from www.un.org/millenniumgoals/.

recipients of maternity care. While birth is often construed as a highly charged emotional event, it may be less obvious to appreciate why a routine antenatal 'booking' history or postnatal visit can generate emotions. However, women's experience of maternity care conveys a different picture (Goleman 2005; Redshaw and Heikkila 2010). There is clear evidence from research studies that women do not always receive the emotional support from midwives that they would wish (Beech and Phipps 2008; Redshaw and Heikkila 2010).

What is 'emotion work'?

Over the past three decades there has been increased interest in how emotions affect the work professionals do (Fineman 2003). This interest was stimulated by an American study undertaken by Hochschild (1983), which drew attention to the importance of emotion in the workplace, and to the work that needs be done when managing emotions. This study focused on American flight attendants, who identified that a significant aspect of their work was to create a safe and secure environment for passengers, and in order to do so they needed to manage the emotions of their customers and themselves.

Consequently, emotional labour can be defined as the work that is undertaken to manage feelings so that they are appropriate for a particular situation (Hochschild 1983; Hunter and Deery 2009). This is done in accordance with 'feeling rules', social norms regarding which emotions it is considered appropriate to feel and to display. This is best depicted by Hunter and Deery (2005), who note how midwives describe suppressing their feelings in order to maintain a reassuring atmosphere for women and their partners.

Hochschild (1983) used the term 'emotional labour' to mean management of emotion within the public domain, as part of the employment contract between employer and employee; 'emotion work' referred to management of emotion in the private domain, i.e. the home. The research focused particularly on commercial organizations, where workers are required to provide a veneer of hospitality in order to present a corporate image, with the ultimate aim of profit-making (e.g. the 'switch-on smile' of the flight attendants or the superficial enjoinders to 'have a nice day' from shop assistants). This requires the use of 'acting' techniques, which Hochschild (1983) argues may be incongruent with what workers are really feeling. Hunter (2004a) suggests that the emotion management of midwives is different to this. Midwives are more able to exercise autonomy in how they control emotions, and emotion management is driven by a desire to 'make a difference', based on ideals of caring and service.

Sources of emotion work in midwifery practice

Research studies suggest that there are various sources of emotion work in midwifery (Hunter 2004a, 2004b;

Hunter and Deery 2005, 2009). These can be grouped into three key themes, which are discussed in turn:

1. Midwife–woman relationships
2. Collegial relationships
3. The organization of maternity care.

It is important to note that these themes are often interlinked. For example, the organization of maternity care impacts on both midwife–woman relationships and on collegial relationships.

Midwife-woman relationships

The nature of pregnancy and childbirth means that midwives work with women and their families during some of the most emotionally charged times of human life. The excited anticipation that generally surrounds the announcement of a pregnancy and the birth of a baby may be tempered with anxieties about changes in role identity, altered sexual relationships and fears about pain and altered body image (Raphael-Leff 2005). Thus it is important to remember that even the most delighted of new mothers may experience a wide range of feelings about their experiences (see Chapter 25).

Pregnancy and birth are not always joyful experiences: for example, midwives work with women who have unplanned or unwanted pregnancies, who are in unhappy or abusive relationships, and where fetal abnormalities or antenatal problems are detected. In these cases, midwives need to support women and their partners with great sensitivity and emotional awareness. This requires excellent interpersonal skills, particularly the ability to listen. It is easy in such distressing situations to try to help by giving advice and adopting a problem-solving approach. However, the evidence suggests that this is often inappropriate, and that what is much more beneficial is a non-judgemental listening ear (Turner et al 2010).

Childbirth itself is a time of heightened emotion, and brings with it exposure to pain, bodily fluids and issues of sexuality, all of which may prove challenging to the woman, her partner and also to those caring for her. Attending a woman in childbirth is highly intimate work, and the feelings that this engenders may come as a surprise to new students. For example, undertaking vaginal examinations is an intimate activity, and needs to be acknowledged as such (Stewart 2005). In the past, the emotional aspects of these issues have tended to be ignored within the education of midwives.

Relationships between midwives and women may vary considerably in their quality, level of intimacy and sense of personal connection. Some relationships may be intense and short-lived (e.g. when a midwife and woman meet on the labour suite or birth centre for the first time); intense and long-lived (e.g. when a midwife provides continuity of care throughout pregnancy, birth and the postnatal period via models of care such as caseholding). They may also be relatively superficial, whether the contact is short-lived or longer-standing. There is evidence that a key issue in midwife–woman relationships is the level of 'reciprocity' that is experienced (Hunter 2006; McCourt and Stevens 2009; Pairman et al 2010; Raynor and England 2010). Reciprocity is defined as 'exchanging things with others for mutual benefit' (Oxford English Dictionary 2013). When relationships are experienced as 'reciprocal' or 'balanced', the midwife and woman are in a harmonious situation. Both are able to give to the other and to receive what is given, such as when the midwife can give support and advice, and the woman is happy to accept this, and in return affirm the value of the midwife's care. Achieving partnership with women requires reciprocity. Pairman et al (2010: viii) defines partnership as a relationship of trust and equity 'through which both partners are strengthened'. This implies that the power in the mother–midwife relationship is diffused. There is no imposition of ideas, values and beliefs, but rather the midwife uses skills of negotiation and effective communication to ensure the woman remains firmly in the driving seat of all decision-making relating to her care.

In contrast, relationships may become unbalanced, and in these situations emotion work is needed by the midwife. For example, a woman may be hostile to the information provided by the midwife, or alternatively, she may expect more in terms of personal friendship than the midwife feels it is appropriate or feasible to offer. Some midwives working in continuity of care schemes have expressed concerns about 'getting the balance right' in their relationships with women, so that they can offer authentic support without overstepping personal boundaries and becoming burnt out (Hunter 2006; McCourt and Stevens 2009; Pairman et al 2010). However, establishing and maintaining reciprocal relationships can prove challenging at times.

Intelligent kindness

In their thought-provoking book, Ballatt and Campling (2011) assert that in the modern NHS that has undergone relentless structural and regulatory reforms, healthcare professionals need to find a way to return to a way of working and being based on 'intelligent kindness', kinship and compassion. 'Intelligent kindness', they claim, is being kind while acting intelligently. This approach not only results in individual acts of kindness but it promotes a sense of wellbeing, helps to reduce stress and leads to increased satisfaction with care. It is also liberating to the individual, team and organization as it promotes a harmonious way of working and being. Thus the interest of the individual woman, the midwife and the maternity care organization are inextricably bound together. Measures should be in place to mitigate against inhibiting factors such as a culture of negativity and blame. However, kindness alone is not sufficient. Women want care from a midwife that is not only kind but is also attentive, intelligent and competent in her clinical skills to make the woman feels safe. Equally, Ballatt and Campling (2011) state that kindness should be genuine and not contrived, which results in congruence.

Collegial relationships

Relationships between midwives and their colleagues, both within midwifery and the wider multidisciplinary and multiagency teams are also key sources of emotion work. Much of the existing evidence attests to relationships between midwifery colleagues, which may be positive or negative experiences.

Positive collegial relationships provide both practical and emotional support (Sandall 1997). Walsh (2007) provides an excellent example of these in his ethnography of a free-standing birth centre. He observed a strong 'communitarian ideal' (Walsh 2007: 77), whereby midwives provided each other with mutual support built on trust, compassion and solidarity. He attributes this to the birth centre model, with its emphasis on relationships, facilitation and cooperation.

Sadly, however, such experiences are not always universal. There is also evidence that intimidation and bullying exists within contemporary UK midwifery (Leap 1997; Kirkham 1999; Hadikin and O'Driscoll 2000; Hunter and Deery 2005). The concept of 'horizontal violence' (Leap 1997) is often used to explain this problem. Kirkham (1999) explains how groups who have been oppressed internalize the values of powerful groups, thereby rejecting their own values. As a result, criticism is directed within the group (hence the term 'horizontal violence'), particularly towards those who are considered to have different views from the norm. This type of workplace conflict inevitably affects the emotional wellbeing of the midwifery workforce (Hunter and Deery 2005).

The organization of maternity care

In the UK the way in which maternity care is organized may also be a source of emotion work for midwives. The fragmented, task-orientated nature of much hospital-based maternity care creates emotionally difficult situations for midwives (Ball et al 2002; Deery 2005; Dykes 2005; Hunter 2004a, 2005; Kirkham 1999), as it reduces opportunities for establishing meaningful relationships with women and colleagues, and for doing 'real midwifery'. The study by Ball et al (2002) identified frustration with the organization of maternity care as one of the key reasons why midwives leave the profession. A study by Lavender and Chapple (2004) explored the views of midwives working in different settings. They found that

all participants shared a common model of ideal practice, which included autonomy, equity of care for women and job satisfaction. However, midwives varied in how successful they were in achieving this. Strong midwifery leadership and a workplace culture that promoted normality are deemed to be facilitative rather than inhibiting factors. Free-standing birth centres were usually described as being more satisfying and supportive environments, which facilitated the establishing of rewarding relationships with women and their families. Conversely, consultant-led units were often experienced negatively; this was partly the result of a dominant medicalized model of childbirth, a task-orientated approach to care and a culture of 'lots of criticism and no praise' (Lavender and Chapple 2004: 9).

In general, it would appear that midwives working in community-based practice, continuity of care schemes or in birth centre settings are more emotionally satisfied with their work (Sandall 1997; Hunter 2004a; Walsh 2007; Sandall et al 2013). Although there is the potential for continuity of care schemes to increase emotion work as a result of altered boundaries in the midwife–woman relationship, there is also evidence to suggest that when these schemes are organized and managed effectively, they provide emotional rewards for women and midwives.

A key reason underpinning these differing emotion work experiences appears to be the co-existence of conflicting models of midwifery practice (Hunter 2004a). Although midwifery as a profession has a strong commitment to providing woman-centred care, this is frequently not achievable in practice, particularly within large institutions. An approach to care that focuses on the needs of individual women may be at odds with an approach that is driven by institutional demands to provide efficient and equitable care to large numbers of women and babies 24 hours a day, 7 days a week. When midwives are able to work in a 'with woman' way, there is congruence between ideals and reality, and work is experienced as being emotionally rewarding. When it is impossible for midwives to work in this way, as is often the case, midwives experience a sense of disharmony. This may lead to anger, distress and frustration, all of which require emotion work (Hunter 2004a).

Managing emotions in midwifery

Hunter (2004a) and Hunter and Deery (2005) found that midwives described two different approaches to emotion management: *affective neutrality* and *affective awareness*. These different approaches were often in conflict and presented mixed messages to student midwives.

Affective neutrality

Affective neutrality, described as 'professional detachment', suggests that emotion must be suppressed in order to get the work done efficiently. By minimizing the emotional content of work, its emotional 'messiness' is reduced and work becomes an emotion-free zone. This approach fits well within a culture that values efficiency, hierarchical relationships, standardization of care and completion of tasks. Personal emotions are managed by the individual, in order to hide them as much as possible from women and colleagues. Coping strategies, such as distancing, 'toughening up' and impression management are used in order to present an appropriate 'professional performance', i.e. a professional who is neutral and objective. When dealing with women, there is avoidance of discussing emotional issues and a focus on practical tasks. This is clearly not in the best interests of women.

Although this may appear to be an outdated approach to dealing with emotion in contemporary maternity care, there is ample evidence that this approach continues, particularly within hospital settings. This can be problematic for midwives who wish to work in more emotionally aware ways, and can detract from the quality of care.

Affective awareness

In contrast, affective awareness fits well with a 'new midwifery' approach to practice (Page and McCandlish 2006). In this approach it is considered important to be aware of feelings and express them when possible. This may be in relation to women's emotional experiences, or when dealing with personal emotions. Sharing feelings enables them to be explored and named. It also provides opportunities for developing supportive and nurturing relationships between midwives and women, and between midwives and colleagues.

Affective awareness fits within a wider contemporary Western culture, which emphasizes the benefits of the 'talking cure', that is the therapeutic value of talking things through (e.g. via counselling or psychotherapy). However, it is important that midwives recognize the limits of their own expertise, so they do not find themselves out of their depth. Working in partnership with women, particularly in continuity of care schemes, means that midwives are more likely to develop close connections with women and their families. If emotionally difficult events occur, midwives 'feel' more.

Challenges

It is also important not to be overly critical of midwives who adopt an 'affectively neutral' approach, but to try to understand why this may be occurring. In Hunter and Deery's (2005) study, most participants did not consider this to be the best way of dealing with emotion, believing that 'affective awareness' was the ideal way to practise. But when they felt 'stressed out', they described 'retreating' emotionally and 'putting on an act' to get through the day. Stress may be the result of unsustainable workloads, staff shortages, conflicts with colleagues or difficulties in personal lives. In order to understand emotion work in midwifery, midwives need to be aware of the broader social and political context in which maternity care is provided. Understanding emotion work requires careful thought and reflection, not just about individual midwives, but also about the complexities of the maternity services. In order to move away from a blame culture in midwifery, we need to work at developing empathy, in order to better understand each others' behaviour.

It is also important to ensure cultural sensitivity in relation to emotion. The ways that emotions are displayed, and the types of emotion that are considered appropriate for display will vary from culture to culture, as well as within cultures (Fineman 2003). Midwives need to develop skills in reading the emotional language of a situation and avoid ethnocentricity.

Developing emotional awareness

It is possible to develop emotional skills in the same way as it is possible to develop any skills. In other words, individuals can develop 'emotional awareness' (Hunter 2004b) or 'emotional intelligence', according to (Goleman 2005). He claims that emotionally intelligent people: know their emotions, manage their emotions, motivate themselves, recognize the emotions of others and handle relationships effectively. Goleman (2005) suggests ways that emotional intelligence can be developed, so that an individual can have a high 'EQ' (emotional intelligence quotient) in the way that they may have a high IQ (intelligence quotient).

The idea of emotional intelligence has caught the public imagination, although some would argue that Goleman's ideas are rather simplistic and lack a substantive research base (e.g. Fineman 2003: 52). Instead, Fineman (2003: 54) prefers the notion of 'emotional sensitivity', which he claims can be developed through 'processes of feminization, emotionally responsive leadership styles, valuing intuition, and tolerance for a wide range of emotional expression and candour'. Whatever the preferred terminology, it would seem that these ideas have particular relevance to midwifery, given the emotionally demanding nature of this work. Midwives need to develop emotional awareness so that they know what it is they are feeling, why they are feeling it, and how others may be feeling. They also need to develop a language to articulate these feelings, in a manner that is authentic.

So how can midwives develop their emotional awareness? There are a number of options that may be helpful. Attendance on counselling and assertiveness courses can help to develop insights into personal feelings, which by extension provide insights into the possible feelings of others. Supervision may also provide opportunities for exploration of the emotions of both self and others, with the aim of recognizing and responding appropriately to these.

It is particularly important that emotional issues are given careful and sensitive attention during pre-registration education. This could take the form of role-play, or by making use of participative theatre. Drama workshops have been used effectively with student midwives (Baker 2000) to explore various aspects of their clinical experience, including a range of emotional issues, in a safe and supportive environment. One advantage of such an approach is that participants realize that they are not alone in their experiences. With a skilled workshop facilitator, difficult situations can be considered in a broader context, so that they are understood as shared rather than personal problems. These methods could also be beneficial for qualified midwives, especially clinical mentors, as part of their continuing professional development.

Emotional issues also need attention within clinical practice, if they are not to be seen as something that is explored only 'in the classroom'. As previously discussed, there may be 'mixed messages' about what emotions should be felt and displayed. These mixed messages are not helpful in creating an emotionally attuned environment. Supervision could have a role to play here, having the potential to provide a supportive environment for understanding emotion, particularly if a 'clinical supervision' approach is taken. This is a method of peer support and review aimed at creating a safe and non-judgemental space in which the emotional support needs of midwives can be considered (Kirkham and Stapleton 2000; Deery 2005). The importance of 'caring for the carers' is crucial, but often underestimated.

Finally, as Fineman (2003) recommends, those in leadership positions within midwifery need to set the scene by adopting leadership styles that are emotionally responsive. In this way, a ripple effect through the whole workforce could be created.

THE SOCIAL CONTEXT OF PREGNANCY, CHILDBIRTH AND MOTHERHOOD

A number of influential social policies have resulted in radical reforms of the maternity services in the UK over many years. Consequently, the twenty-first century has heralded the transformation of the NHS at systems and at organizational level to provide better care, enhanced experience for mothers and their families and improved value for money. The reforms are to deliver excellence and equity in the NHS (DH 2010b). Since 2009, the policy reforms have ensured that women and their families are provided with a greater choice in the services they want and need, and guaranteed a wider choice in the type

and place of maternity care, including birth (DH 2007a, 2007b).

As key public health agents midwives are at the forefront of social change and act as the cornerstone to the delivery of maternity service reforms. Their roles and responsibilities will increasingly focus to deliver greater productivity and best value for money, offering real choice and improvement in women's maternity experiences. These reforms are creating opportunities for midwives to work in new ways and undertake new and different roles. Midwives are required to be much more oriented towards public health and the reforms provide increased opportunities to work in more diverse teams to provide integrated services. The working environment is changing where midwives are increasingly accountable for the care they provide, creating a new form of ownership.

Disadvantaged groups

Many of the reasons given by women for dissatisfaction with maternity services include fragmented care, long waiting times, insensitive care, lack of emotional support, inadequate explanations, lack of information, medical control, inflexibility of hospital routines and poor communication (Redshaw and Heikkila 2010).

Universally, there is no agreed definition of vulnerability, however, the term 'vulnerable groups' is often used to refer to groups of people who are at risk of being socially excluded and marginalized in accessing maternity services. These groups of people or communities are more likely to experience social marginalization as a result of a number of interrelated factors such as unemployment, poor or limited skills, low income, poor housing, poverty, high crime environment, poor or ill health and family breakdown. Women from these vulnerable groups may experience disadvantage either due to mental or physical impairment, or particular characteristics no longer attributed to mental or physical impairment but that have historically led to individuals experiencing prejudice and discrimination, for example ethnicity or disability. Box 1.4 provides examples of some of the groups of women who may be disadvantaged in the maternity service.

Providing woman-centred care is a complex issue, particularly in a diverse society where individual's and families' health needs are varied and not homogeneous. Listening and responding to women's views and respecting their ethnic, cultural, social and family backgrounds is critical to developing responsive maternity services. Persistent concerns have been expressed about the poor neonatal and maternal health outcomes among disadvantaged and socially excluded groups (Lewis and Drife 2001, 2004; Lewis 2007; CMACE [Centre for Maternal and Child Enquiries] 2011), suggesting not all groups in society enjoy equal access to maternity services (Redshaw and Heikkila 2010).

There is strong evidence that disadvantaged groups have poorer health and poorer access to healthcare, with clear links between inequality in social life and inequality in health, demonstrating that inequality exists in both mortality and morbidity (Marmot 2010). The WHO (2008) refers to the social determinants of health as conditions in which people are born, live, develop, work and age. This includes the healthcare system, which paradoxically is formulated and influenced by the distribution of wealth, power and resources at all levels. Moreover, the social determinants of health are largely responsible for health inequalities, i.e. the unfair and avoidable differences in health status seen within and between countries (WHO 2008).

To facilitate care that is responsive to the needs of women, health professionals need to understand women's social, cultural and historical backgrounds so that care is tailored to meet their individual needs. A number of models of care have been introduced to deliver culturally congruent care, including some examples of midwifery-led caseloading teams developed around the needs of vulnerable groups, e.g. Blackburn Midwifery Group Practice (Byrom 2006) and the Wirral one-to-one care scheme (McGarrity Dodd 2012).

Women from disadvantaged groups

Young mothers

Previously the UK had the unenviable reputation for the highest rate of teenage pregnancy and teenage parenthood in Europe. However, recent figures from the Office of National Statistics (ONS 2013) reveal that in England and Wales the tide is finally changing: teenage pregnancy rates are actually declining. Recent statistical data from ONS (2013) reveals that pregnancies in young women <18 years old in 2011 was 31 051 compared to 45 495 in 1969 when records began, a decrease of 32%. In contrast, the figure for conceptions to all women in 2011 was 909 109

compared to 832 700 in 1969, signalling an overall increase of 9.2%

Why teenage pregnancy matters

It is important to acknowledge that some young mothers do achieve a successful outcome to their pregnancy and parenting with appropriate social support (Olds 2002). Nonetheless, it is widely understood that there is a strong association between teenage pregnancy resulting in early motherhood and poor educational achievement and wider health inequalities and social deprivation, e.g. poor physical and mental health, social isolation, and poverty and wider related factors (Arai 2009). It should also be recognized that mortality and morbidity among babies born to these mothers is increased and that the mothers show a higher risk of developing complications, such as hypertensive disorders and intrapartum complications (Lewis and Drife 2004). Many young teenage mothers tend to present late for antenatal care and are disproportionately likely to have some risk factors associated with poor antenatal health (e.g. poverty and smoking). Moreover, there is a growing recognition that socioeconomic disadvantage can be both a cause and effect of teenage parenthood. Consequently, in the UK the former government led by the Labour party established a target to half the teenage pregnancy rate by 2010, when compared with 1998. This signified a radical shift in the position of local authorities, who set a 10-year target that aimed to reduce the local teenage conception rate between 40% and 60%. Such an ambitious goal was meant to contribute to the national 50% reduction target. However, although the Teenage Pregnancy Strategy ended in 2010, the actual teenage pregnancy rate has remained an area of policy interest and contentious debate. The current Coalition government (Conservatives and Liberal Democrats) places teenage pregnancy rate to young women <18 as one of its three sexual health indicators in its Public Health Outcomes Framework 2013–2016 (DH 2013). In fact this emboldened approach is one of the national measures of progress on child poverty, which aims to ensure a continued focus on preventing teenage conceptions as well as the social impact upon teenage mothers (ONS 2013).

With appropriate support, young mothers and young fathers can make an effective transition to parenthood. They can be assisted to develop good parenting and life skills to prevent a potential downward spiral and break the cycle of social deprivation and health inequalities by early intervention schemes such as the Family Nurse Partnership developed by Olds (2002).

Women with disability

Women with disability are increasingly engaged with the maternity services as they seek to live full and autonomous lives. A UK national survey on disabled women's experiences of pregnancy, labour and postpartum care compared to non-disabled women was conducted by Redshaw et al (2013). The study found that while in many areas there were no differences in the quality of care disabled women received there was evidence for areas of improvement. This includes infant feeding and better communication if women are to experience truly individualized care. Thus the midwife needs to allow sufficient time to assess how the disability may impact on the woman's experience of childbirth and parenting and to work with her in identifying helpful ways to make reasonable adjustment, including the assistance of multiagency departments as required.

The woman will probably be better informed about her disability than the midwife. However, she may need the midwife to provide information and guidance on the impact that the physiological changes of pregnancy and labour may have on her, for example the increased weight and change in posture. Some women and their partners may raise concerns regarding the inheritance pattern of a genetic condition, and may need referral to specialist services such as a genetic counsellor. Midwives and other healthcare professionals should recognize the need to approach antenatal screening in a sensitive manner (see Chapter 11). Midwives need to be aware of local information pertaining to professional and voluntary organizations and networks and adopt a multidisciplinary approach to planning and provision of services. The Common Assessment Framework may be an appropriate tool for the midwife to use to ensure a coordinated multiagency approach to care (DfES 2006).

A birth plan is a useful communication tool providing the woman with scope to identify her specific needs alongside the issues that most pregnant women are concerned with, such as coping strategies for labour and birth and views on any medical intervention that might be deemed necessary. Assisting women with a disability to make informed choices about all aspects of their antenatal, intrapartum and postnatal care (Royal College of Midwives [RCM] 2008) is empowering. If the woman is to give birth in hospital it may be helpful for her to visit the unit, meet some of the staff and assess the environment and resources in relation to her special needs, e.g. if she is planning to have a waterbirth a thorough risk assessment of the environment will be needed. A single room should be offered to her to facilitate the woman's control over her immediate environment and, where appropriate, to adapt it to accommodate any equipment that she may wish to bring with her. A woman who is blind or partially sighted may prefer to give birth at home where she is familiar with the environment. If she has a guide dog then consideration needs to be given to its presence in the hospital environment.

Women with learning difficulties may need a friend or carer to help with the birth plan but the midwife should remember that the woman must remain at the centre of care. Midwives need to understand the worldview of women with disabilities in order to shape the maternity services to meet the individual needs of these women, and work within an ethical framework that values key principles of rights, independence, choice and inclusion (Chapter 2).

Women living in poverty

It is well documented that women living in poverty are more likely to suffer health inequalities and have a higher rate of maternal and perinatal mortality (Lewis 2007; Marmot 2010; CMACE 2011; UN 2013). Tackling inequality is high on the public health agenda and the midwife has an important role in targeting women in need.

Women from black and minority ethnic (BME) communities

The UK has continued to see major demographic changes in the profile of its population and is more ethnically diverse now than ever before (ONS 2012). According to the 2011 census, England and Wales are more ethnically diverse, with rising numbers of people identifying with minority ethnic groups. Nevertheless, although the white ethnic group is decreasing in size, it remains the majority ethnic group that people identify with. Furthermore, there are regional variations for ethnic diversity. London has the most concentrated and rich ethnic mix while Wales remains largely white, despite pockets of minority ethnic groups (ONS 2012).

When referring to multiethnic societies, a basic understanding of the culture is often assumed to mean the way of life of a society or a group of people and is used to express social life, food, clothing, music and behaviours. The concept of culture has been defined by many, such as Helman (2007), providing a variety of insights into the concept. However, the commonalities are that culture is learned, it is shared and it is passed on from generation to generation. Members of the society learn a set of guidelines through which they attain concepts of role expectancies, values and attitudes of society; it is therefore not genetically inherited but is socially constructed and the behaviour of individuals is shaped by the values and attitudes they hold as well as the physical and geographical surroundings in which they interact. Individuals perceive and respond to stimuli from economic, social and political factors in different ways and they will be affected differently according to age, gender, social class, occupation and many other factors. Culture is very much a dynamic state, it is not a group phenomenon, and to treat it as homogeneous is foolhardy as it can lead to generalizations and negative stereotypes. Some aspects can be true for some and not for others belonging to the same cultural group.

An understanding of some of the cultural differences between social groups is essential in ensuring that professional practice is closely matched to meet the needs of individual women, promoting the delivery of culturally congruent care. An understanding of the role culture plays in determining health, health behaviours and illness is essential when planning and delivering services that meet the health needs of the local population. However, caution is needed as the role of culture in explaining patterns of health and health-related behavior is somewhat simplistic. Placing emphasis on culture diverts attention away from the role of broad structural process in discrimination and the role that racism plays in health status (Ahmad 1993, 1996; Stubbs 1993).

Ethnic diversity in the UK has created major challenges for maternity services (Lewis 2007; CMACE 2011). Successive reports of the Confidential Enquiries into Maternal Deaths in the UK have demonstrated that the inability to respond appropriately to the individual needs of women from different backgrounds is reflected in persistent poor communication practice and ineffective care culminating in poor health outcomes for both mother and baby (Lewis and Drife 2001, 2004; Lewis 2007; CMACE 2011).

Women from the BME population experience disadvantage and are socially excluded for two main reasons. First, some women are more likely to be categorized into lower socioeconomic status; they are predominantly residents of deprived inner city areas, have poor housing, are at risk of high unemployment, and have low-paid occupations, poor working conditions, poor social security rights and low income, all of which lead to poverty. Often factors such as lifestyle, environmental factors and genetic determinants are cited as indicators of poor health outcomes, dismissing key social determinants of poverty, poor housing and poor education (Nazroo 1997; Platt 2007).

Second, because their skin colour and ethnic origin make them visible minorities, they are more likely to experience racial harassment, discrimination and social inequalities (Nazroo 2001). Institutionalized racism and general reluctance by organizations and individuals to address the sensitive issue of ethnicity are likely contributors to inequalities of health and access to maternity services (RCM 2003). It is important to understand concepts of discrimination and racism and how this can marginalize women.

Ethnicity has largely replaced the term 'race', encompassing all of the ways in which people from one group seek to differentiate themselves from other groups. 'Ethnicity is an indicator of the process by which people create and maintain a sense of group identity and solidarity which they use to distinguish themselves from "others"' (Smaje 1995: 16). Ethnicity is a self-claimed identity and is socially constructed; people of a particular group have a common sense of belonging, and have shared beliefs, values and cultural traditions as well as biological characteristics. In general, people use these terms to identify the 'other' groups but it must be remembered that all people have a culture and ethnicity.

When people value their own culture more highly, perceiving their cultural ways to be the best, they devalue and belittle other ethnic groups, perceiving 'others' culture as bizarre and strange; this is referred to as *ethnocentrism*. Ethnocentric behaviour, in particular when other individuals' cultural requirements may be ignored or dismissed as unimportant, would do very little to meet the tenets of woman-centred care and hinders the delivery of responsive care. Many maternity services are still based on an ethnocentric model, e.g. education for parenthood is not culturally sensitive where women and their partners are positively encouraged to attend jointly (Katbamna 2000).

BME groups as users of the maternity service: The majority of women from BME groups express satisfaction with maternity services. While some argue that ethnicity is not a marker for good or poor quality (Hirst and Hewison 2001, 2002), others have reported a plausible relationship between ethnicity and women's proficiency in speaking and reading English with poor quality of care (Bharj 2007). Many women assert that their ability to access maternity services is impaired because they are offered little or no information regarding options of care during pregnancy, childbirth and the postnatal period (Katbamna 2000; Bharj 2007). Women are therefore not aware of the range of maternity services and choices available to them.

Evidence indicates that lack of proficiency to speak and read English adversely impacts on women's experience and their ability to access and utilize maternity services, also adversely affecting the quality of maternity services and maternity outcomes (Lewis 2007; CMACE 2011). Often lack of interventions to overcome communication and language barriers, such as qualified interpreters, is cited as a major challenge in accessing maternity services (Lewis 2007; CMACE 2011). Furthermore, use of relatives or friends as interpreters during sensitive consultations is not recommended (Lewis 2007) and is viewed by women as inappropriate. In some studies, women reported that their requests to see a female doctor were dismissed and they were distressed when treated by a male doctor, particularly when they observed purdah (Sivagnanam 2004).

Women seeking refuge/asylum

Midwives need to be aware of the complex needs of this group of vulnerable women who, in addition to the problems described above, have often experienced traumatic events in their home country, may be isolated from their family and friends and face uncertainty regarding their future domicile.

Women from travelling families

Travelling families are not a homogeneous group. Travellers may belong to a distinct social group such as the Romanies, their origins may lie in the UK or elsewhere such as Ireland or Eastern Europe, or they may be part of the social grouping loosely termed 'New Age' travellers or part of the Showman's Guild travelling community. As with all social groups, their cultural background will influence their beliefs about and experience of health and childbearing.

A common factor, which may apply to all, is the likelihood of prejudice and marginalization. Midwives need to examine their own beliefs and values in order to develop their knowledge to address the needs of travelling families with respect, plus provide a caring and non-judgemental service. An informed approach to lifestyle interpretation may stop the midwife identifying the woman as an antenatal defaulter with the negative connotations that accompany that label. Moving on may be through choice related to lifestyle, but equally it may be the result of eviction from unofficial sites.

Some health authorities have designated services for travelling families that contribute to uptake and continuity of care. These carers understand the culture and are aware of specific health needs; they can also access appropriate resources, for example a general practitioner (GP) who is receptive to travellers' needs. A trusting relationship is important to people who are frequently subjected to discrimination. Handheld records contribute to continuity of care and communication between care providers, but the maternity service also needs to address communication challenges for individuals who do not have a postal address or who have low levels of literacy.

Women who are lesbian

Evidence suggests that an increasing number of women are seeking motherhood within a lesbian relationship. The exact numbers are unclear as it is the woman's choice as to whether she makes her sexual orientation known. The midwife can, however, create an environment in which she feels safe to do so. Communication and careful framing of questions can reduce the risk of causing offence and assist the midwife in the provision of woman-centred care.

Wilton and Kaufmann (2001) identify the booking interview as the first time, as a user of the maternity service, that the woman must consider how she will respond to questions such as 'when did you last have sex?' or 'what is the father's name?' Issues such as parenting, sex and contraception may have different meanings for the midwife and the woman and therefore careful use of non-heterosexist language by the midwife will help to promote a climate for open communication (Hastie 2000). She argues that the 'realities of lesbian experiences are hidden from the mainstream heterosexist society and

so stereotypes are rife among health practitioners'; Hastie (2000) also states that oppression and invisibility damage health. The RCM (2000) suggest that midwives should take a lead in challenging discriminatory language and behaviour, both positively and constructively.

Midwives meeting the needs of women from disadvantaged groups

Midwives are in a unique position to exploit the opportunities created by the NHS reforms to deliver equitable services, and to create responsive organizations and practices. They have a moral, ethical, legal and professional responsibility to provide individualized care and to develop equitable service provision and delivery (Nursing and Midwifery Council [NMC] 2008). They play a key role in bringing about change. They also have a responsibility to facilitate an environment that provides all women and their families with appropriate information and encourages more active participation in the decision-making process, including ensuring 'informed consent'.

Meeting information needs

Women from disadvantaged backgrounds often lack knowledge and understanding of the maternity services. They are not always given adequate information about the full range of maternity services and options of care available to them during pregnancy, labour and the postnatal period. Often information is not available in appropriate formats to reach women who have visual or hearing impairment or who lack proficiency in speaking and reading English. Therefore, they are unaware of the range of maternity services and choices available to them. Midwives can play an important role in facilitating two-way communication to enable women to participate in making decisions about the care they want, need and receive.

Midwives recognize that communication and language difficulties may be addressed by making use of professional qualified interpreters or liaison workers or signers. In practice, the use of qualified interpreters is intermittent and fragmented. Financial resources, midwives' beliefs and attitudes, time constraints and the nature of employment of qualified interpreters determine the availability of qualified interpreters (Bharj 2007).

Advocacy

In circumstances where women cannot effectively communicate with their midwives, they are unable to fully participate in decisions made about their care. These women feel that professionals and hospitals 'take over' and make decisions about them without first discussing all the options, or informing them of their rights. Having a strong advocate is therefore important.

Working in partnership

As identified earlier in the chapter, for midwives to work in partnership with women, they need to cultivate a meaningful relationship with them. Partnership working and its impact in promoting woman-centred care should take account of trust and power (Calvert 2002; Kirkham 2010). A relationship based on trust builds confidence and makes women feel safe and respected.

Stereotyping and discrimination on the other hand play a major role in hindering the development of meaningful relationships. There is well-documented evidence illustrating the detrimental effect of discrimination and racism on people's health (Virdee 1997). Several studies confirm that midwives commonly use stereotypes of women in determining their needs and preferences and utilize these to make judgements about the kind of care women deserve, as well as what a particular woman is likely to want during labour and birth (Kirkham and Stapleton 2004). Often these stereotypes and prejudices have detrimental effect on women's maternity experiences (Redshaw and Heikkla 2010).

Discriminatory attitudes and hostility coupled with their adverse impact on women will do little towards the development of a meaningful relationship. Consequently, partnership working will be rhetoric for women from disadvantaged background as will issues of continuity, choice and control. Midwives need to consider such issues and where possible draw upon transcultural models to provide anti-oppressive care promoting the tenets of woman-centred care for women from disadvantaged groups.

RESEARCH

When she provides care during childbearing, the midwife does so by virtue of her expert knowledge. This knowledge distinguishes her from all the people who offer opinions to the childbearing woman. The midwife's unique knowledge which determines her practice derives from many sources. Traditionally, the midwife drew on her personal experience of childbearing. More recently, the midwife's occupational experience has assumed greater significance. Precedent has been quoted as an important influence (Thomson 2000), which may have been enforced by authority figures. Ritual has also influenced midwifery practice (Rodgers 2000). Relatively recently research and research evidence have been required to determine midwifery practice.

The term 'research' carries many implications, so a dictionary definition is useful: 'systematic investigation towards increasing the sum of knowledge' (Macdonald 1981: 1148).

Clearly, research is about asking questions, but not haphazardly. Systematic questioning is crucial, making planning, in the form of the 'research process', the basis of research activity. The purpose of this activity is encompassed in the dictionary definition, as research into the improvement or increase in knowledge in midwifery is intended to ensure more effective care.

EVIDENCE

The term 'evidence' refers to a particular form of research, which is considered by some to be particularly strong and crucial to effective practice (Chalmers 1993: 3). The need for 'evidence' began with observations by Cochrane (1972). He identified the lack of scientific rigour in medical decisions, and singled out obstetricians for withering criticism of their want of rigour. Some obstetricians, with other maternity practitioners, responded by attempting to correct the deficiency. To develop material for practitioners who lacked inclination, ability and opportunities to search and evaluate the literature, this group began reviewing research systematically. This resulted, first, in the publication of two significant volumes (Chalmers et al 1989) and later, the ongoing development of the Cochrane database. Unsurprisingly, evidence is intended to facilitate evidence-based practice, defined as:

> *The conscientious, explicit and judicious use of current best evidence in making decisions about the care of individual patients.*
> *(Sackett et al 1996: 71)*

As well as evidence, other forms of research are used in healthcare, such as audit.

The stated rationale for evidence-based practice (EBP)

Research-based practice has long been said to ensure high-quality care. Additionally, professions' status may be enhanced by such intellectual activity. EBP has been advocated by many UK policy documents which have argued that it may facilitate more appropriate resource allocation, by increasing effectiveness and efficiency. While midwifery has long benefited from strong evidence relating to episiotomy (Sleep 1991), other aspects of care are seriously deficient; these include contentious issues such as the location of uncomplicated childbirth (Olsen and Clausen 2012), continuous electronic fetal monitoring (CEFM) in labour (Alfirevic et al 2013) and routine ultrasound examination in pregnancy (Bricker and Neilson 2007; Bricker et al 2008).

The randomized controlled trial (RCT)

The research design usually regarded as most likely to ensure good quality evidence is the RCT. The RCT overcomes bias inherent in using other approaches without comparison groups to decide between alternative forms of care (Donnan 2000). The power of the RCT lies in its objectivity or freedom from bias, possibly arising from the sampling or selection of subjects for the experimental treatment and control (no/usual treatment) group, who receive a placebo or standard care. Implemented conscientiously, the RCT is regarded as 'the gold standard for comparing alternative forms of care' (Enkin et al 2000: 10). The data collected are analysed statistically to assess whether differences in outcomes are due to chance, rather than the experimental intervention. Despite the RCT's power, the practitioner should scrutinize research reports to ensure relevance. In maternity care, where systems of care differ and culture matters, scrutiny takes account of the context, the woman, her personal and clinical experience and her intuition.

DISCUSSION

As with other forms of quantitative research, RCTs have been criticized as being reductionist. This is because, to make sense of the subjects' behaviour or responses, the researcher must simplify or reduce events to their basic component parts. Those who undertake or use research should consider carefully the effect of reductionism in a field such as childbearing. It is possible that some important aspect of the phenomenon may be neglected because the researcher is unaware of it, or it is too complicated, or challenging, to address.

The midwifery evidence base has been criticized for its lack of completeness; as evidence, obviously, exists only on aspects of care already subjected to research. The result is that the evidence base is inadequate to permit comprehensive evidence-based midwifery care. This incomplete evidence base is being addressed by ongoing research, to produce new evidence which may conflict with or contradict existing knowledge. To utilize current best evidence, the practitioner should assess or critique the research, which means its careful examination or criticism. Critique, though, carries no negative overtones, comprising a fair, balanced judgement, seeking strengths and limitations.

The appropriateness of EBP in an activity as uniquely human as childbearing deserves attention. EBP may reduce the humanity of care, not only through reductionism, but also through 'routinization' or even 'cookbook care' (Kim 2000). This argument about reducing care's humanity has been extended to include the effects of EBP on midwifery *per se*. These effects are reflected in concerns that have been expressed regarding the relevance of RCT-based evidence to the care decisions made by midwives (Page 1996; Clarke 1999). The possibility has been raised of EBP constituting a threat to midwifery through its prescriptive medical orientation (Bogdan-Lovis and Sousa 2006).

EBP's relevance to midwifery continues to be questioned. This applies particularly to the widely accepted need for the active input of the childbearing woman in any decisions about her care (Munro and Spiby 2010). The likelihood exists that research evidence that is RCT-based may be less than appropriate to midwifery practice; this likelihood has also cast doubt on the EBP agenda more generally (McCourt 2005).

These concerns about the uncertain relevance of EBP to midwifery have resulted in the need for a more woman-centred framework to inform decision-making (Wickham 1999). What may be a compromise position, termed 'evidence-informed practice' (EIP), is intended to utilize the strengths of EBP at the same time as avoiding dogmatic and prescriptive approaches. While interventions based solely on prejudice or superstition are unacceptable, the knowledge and judgement of the midwife practitioner and the childbearing woman form an equal triangular foundation with research-based evidence (Nevo and Slonim-Nevo 2011). Thus, the woman and the midwife enjoy a dynamic relationship which is recognized and encouraged in EIP. The dialogue into which they enter through this caring relationship becomes constructively transparent.

The pressure on midwives to adhere to the EBP agenda, though, has been both profound and enduring. This has been demonstrated by the early and ongoing efforts by medical practitioners to direct midwives along the path of EBP. Such direction came from authorities such as Chalmers (1993: 3) in his requirement that midwives use only 'strong research'. Direction of midwives towards EBP, however, has brought with it an element of medical hypocrisy which has taken the form of 'do as I say and not as I do'. While there may be many examples of such hypocrisy, a familiar one would be the continuing, and possibly increasing, medical reliance on routine ultrasound during pregnancy, the benefits of which have yet to be established (Bricker and Neilson 2007; Bricker et al 2008).

The issue that underpins the adherence of the midwife to EBP is the question of knowledge or knowledges. Knowledge of theory must precede practice, in a relationship that ideally develops as a virtuous and escalating cycle; but a cycle which is affected by a range of factors. Such influence means that practice enhances not just knowledge, but knowledges. These differing knowledges arise out of a multiplicity of belief systems within one health culture. The result is that the authority or dominant nature of a certain set of beliefs may serve to limit, threaten or undermine other belief systems which, though equally legitimate, are accepted to the same extent and do not carry equal kudos. The dominant knowledge system in maternity has been identified as the 'medical model', as characterized by EBP, and the other knowledges as midwifery, social or woman-centred. The existence of these discrete knowledges may give rise to tension and conflict between different disciplines, practitioners and the childbearing woman.

REFERENCES

Ahmad W I U (ed) 1993 'Race' and health in contemporary Britain. Open University Press, Buckingham

Ahmad W I U 1996 The trouble with culture. In: Kelleher D, Hillier S (eds) Researching cultural differences in health. Routledge, London, p 190–219

Alfirevic Z, Devane D, Gyte G M L 2013 Continuous cardiotocography (CTG) as a form of electronic fetal monitoring (EFM) for fetal assessment during labour. Cochrane Database of Systematic Reviews 2013, Issue 5. Art. No. CD006066. doi: 10.1002/14651858.CD006066. pub2

Arai L 2009 Teenage pregnancy: the making and unmaking of a problem. Policy Press, Bristol

Baker K 2000 Acting the part: using drama to empower student midwives. Practising Midwife 3(1):20–1

Ball L, Curtis P, Kirkham M 2002 Why do midwives leave? Women's Informed Childbearing and Health Research Group, University of Sheffield

Ballatt J, Campling P 2011 Intelligent kindness: reforming the culture of the NHS. Royal College of Psychiatrists, London

Baumann A, Blythe J 2008 Globalization of higher education in nursing. Online Journal of Issues in Nursing. doi 10.3912/OJIN vol 13 no. 02 Man4. Accessed at www .nursingworld.org 20 August 2013

Beech BL, Phipps B 2008 Normal birth: women's stories. In: Downe S (ed) Normal childbirth: evidence and debate. Churchill Livingstone, Edinburgh, p 67–80

Bharj K K 2007 Pakistani Muslim women birthing in northern England; exploration of experiences and context. Doctoral Thesis. Sheffield Hallam University, Sheffield

Bogdan-Lovis E A, Sousa A 2006 The contextual influence of professional culture: certified nurse-midwives' knowledge of and reliance on evidence-based practice. Social Science and Medicine 62(11):2681–93

Bricker L, Neilson JP 2007 Routine Doppler ultrasound in pregnancy. Cochrane Database of Systematic Reviews 2007, Issue 2. Art. No. CD001450. doi:10.1002/14651858. CD001450.pub2

Bricker L, Neilson J P, Dowswell T 2008 Routine ultrasound in late pregnancy (after 24 weeks' gestation). Cochrane Database of Systematic Reviews 2008, Issue 4. Art. No. CD001451. doi: 10.1002/14651858.CD001451. pub3

Byrom S (2006) Antenatal care in children's centres – making it happen. Midwives 9(11):446–7

Calvert S 2002 Being with women: the midwife–woman relationship. In: Mander R, Fleming V (eds) Failure to progress, the contraction of the midwifery profession. Routledge, London

CMACE (Centre for Maternal and Child Enquiries) 2011 Saving mothers' lives: reviewing maternal deaths to make motherhood safer: 2006–08. The Eighth Report on Confidential Enquiries into Maternal Deaths in the United Kingdom. BJOG: An International Journal of Obstetrics and Gynaecology 118(Suppl 1):1–203

Chalmers I 1993 Effective care in midwifery: research, the professions and the public. Midwives Chronicle 106(1260):3–12

Chalmers I, Enkin M, Keirse M J N C (eds) 1989 Effective care in pregnancy and childbirth, vols I and II. Oxford University Press, Oxford

Clarke J B 1999 Evidence-based practice: a retrograde step? The importance of pluralism in evidence generation for the practice of health care. Journal of Clinical Nursing 8(1):89–94

Cochrane A L 1972 Effectiveness and efficiency. Nuffield Provincial Hospitals Trust, London

Deery R 2005 An action research study exploring midwives' support needs and the effect of group clinical supervision. Midwifery 21(2):161–76

DfES (Department for Education and Skills) 2006 Working together to safeguard children. TSO, London

DH (Department of Health) 2007a Maternity matters: choice, access and continuity of care in a safe service. DH, London

DH (Department of Health) 2007b Choice matters: 2007–8: putting patients in control. DH, London

DH (Department of Health) 2010a Midwifery 2020: delivering expectations. DH, London

DH (Department of Health) 2010b Equity and excellence: liberating the NHS. DH, London

DH (Department of Health) 2013 Introduction to the public health outcomes framework 2013–2016. www.gov.uk (accessed 20 August 2013)

Donnan P T 2000 Experimental research. In: Cormack D F S (ed) The research process in nursing, 4th edn. Blackwell Science, Oxford, p 175

Dykes F 2005 A critical ethnographic study of encounters between midwives and breastfeeding women in postnatal wards in England. Midwifery 21(3):241–52 Bantam Books, London

EC Midwives Directive 1980 EC Council Directive 80/155/EEC Article 4. Official Journal of the European Communities L33/28

Enkin M, Keirse M, Renfrew M et al 2000 A guide to effective care in pregnancy and childbirth, 3rd edn. Oxford University Press, Oxford

Fineman S 2003 Understanding emotion at work. Sage, London

Goleman D 2005 Emotional intelligence. Bantam Books, London

Hadikin R, O'Driscoll M 2000 The bullying culture: cause, effect, harm reduction. Books for Midwives Press, Oxford

Hastie N 2000 Cultural conceptions. In: Fraser D (ed) Professional studies for midwifery practice. Churchill Livingstone, Edinburgh, p 63–75

Helman C G 2007 Culture, health and illness, 5th edn. Hodder Arnold, London

Hirst J, Hewison J 2001 Pakistani and indigenous 'white' women's views and the Donabedian–Maxwell grid: a consumer-focused template for assessing the quality of maternity care. International Journal of Healthcare Quality Assurance 14(7):308–16

Hirst J, Hewison J 2002 Hospital postnatal care: obtaining the views of Pakistani and indigenous 'white' women. Clinical Effectiveness in Nursing 6(1):10–18

Hochschild A R 1983 The managed heart. Commercialization of human feeling. University of California Press, Berkeley, CA

Hunter B 2004a Conflicting ideologies as a source of emotion work in midwifery. Midwifery 20:261–72

Hunter B 2004b The importance of emotional intelligence in midwifery. Editorial. British Journal of Midwifery 12(10):1–2

Hunter B 2006 The importance of reciprocity in relationships between community-based midwives and mothers. Midwifery 22(4):308–22

Hunter B, Deery R 2005 Emotion work and boundary maintenance in hospital-based midwifery. Evidence Based Midwifery 3(1):10–15

Hunter B, Deery R (eds.) 2009 Emotions in midwifery and reproduction. Palgrave Macmillan, Basingstoke

ICM (International Confederation of Midwives) 2011 Definition of the midwife. www.internationalmidwives .org (accessed 20 August 2013)

ICM (International Confederation of Midwives) 2013 Global Standards for Midwifery Education 2010, amended 2013. www .internationalmidwives.org (accessed 22 August 2013)

Katbamna S 2000 'Race' and childbirth. Open University Press, Buckingham

Kim M 2000 Evidence-based nursing: connecting knowledge to practice. Chart 97(9):1, 4–6

Kirkham M 1999 The culture of midwifery in the National Health Service in England. Journal of Advanced Nursing 30(3):732–9

Kirkham M (ed) 2010 The midwife–mother relationship, 2nd edn. Macmillan, Basingstoke

Kirkham M, Stapleton H 2000 Midwives' support needs as childbirth changes. Journal of Advanced Nursing 32(2):465–72

Kirkham MJ, Stapleton H 2004 The culture of maternity services in Wales

and England as a barrier to informed choice. In: Kirkham M (ed) Informed choice in maternity care. Basingstoke, Palgrave, p 117–45

Lavender T, Chapple J 2004 An exploration of midwives' views of the current system of maternity care in England. Midwifery 20(4):324–34

Leap N 1997 Making sense of 'horizontal violence' in midwifery. British Journal of Midwifery 5(11):689

Lewis G (ed) 2007 Confidential Enquiry into Maternal and Child Health (CEMACH) Saving mothers' lives: reviewing maternal deaths to make motherhood safer – 2003–2005. The Seventh Report on Confidential Enquiries into Maternal Deaths in the United Kingdom. CEMACH, London

Lewis G, Drife J (eds) 2001 Confidential Enquiry into Maternal and Child Health (CEMACH) Why mothers die 1997–1999. The Fifth Report of the Confidential Enquiries into Maternal Deaths in the United Kingdom. The National Institute of Clinical Excellence. RCOG Press, London

Lewis G, Drife J (eds) 2004 Confidential Enquiry into Maternal and Child Health (CEMACH) Why mothers die 2000–2002. The Sixth Report of the Confidential Enquiries into Maternal Deaths in the United Kingdom. RCOG Press, London

Macdonald A M 1981 Chambers' twentieth century dictionary. Chambers, Edinburgh, p 1148

Maclean G D 2013 Electives and international midwifery consultancy: a resource for students, midwives and other healthcare professionals. London: Quay Books

Marmot M 2010 Fair society, health lives: strategic review of health inequalities in England post-2010. The Marmot Review, London

McCourt C 2005 Research and theory for nursing and midwifery: rethinking the nature of evidence. Worldviews on Evidence-Based Nursing 2(2):75–83

McCourt C, Stevens T 2009 Relationship and reciprocity in caseload midwifery. In: Hunter B, Deery R (eds) Emotions in midwifery and reproduction. Palgrave Macmillan, Basingstoke, p 17–35

McGarrity Dodd L 2012 NHS Wirrall maternity services evaluation 2012. www.info.wirral.nhs.uk (accessed 20 August 2013)

Mid Staffordshire NHS Foundation Trust Public Inquiry(chair R Francis) 2013 Report of the Mid Staffordshire NHS Foundation Trust Public Inquiry. Executive Summary. HC 947. TSO, London. Available at www.midstaffspublicinquiry.com (accessed 20 August 2013)

Milne A, Cowie J 2013 Promoting culturally competent care: the ERASMUS exchange programme. Nursing Standard 27(30):42–6

Munro J, Spiby H 2010 The nature and use of evidence in midwifery care. In: Spiby H, Munro H (eds) Evidence-based midwifery: applications in context. Wiley–Blackwell, Oxford, p 1–16

Nazroo J 1997 The health of Britain's ethnic minorities: findings from a national survey. Policies Studies Institute, London

Nazroo J 2001 Ethnicity, class and health. Policy Studies Institute, London

Nevo I, Slonim-Nevo V 2011 The myth of evidence-based practice: towards evidence-informed practice. British Journal of Social Work 41(6):1176–97

NMC (Nursing and Midwifery Council) 2008 The Code. Standards of conduct, performance and ethics for nurses and midwives. NMC, London

ONS (Office for National Statistics) 2012 Ethnicity and national identity in England and Wales 2011. www .ons.gov.uk (accessed 20 August 2013)

ONS (Office of National Statistics) 2013 Conceptions in England and Wales 2011. www.ons.gov.uk (accessed 20 August 2013)

Olds L D 2002 Prenatal and infancy home visiting by nurses: from randomized trials to community replication. Prevention Science 3(3):153–72

Olsen O, Clausen J A 2012 Planned hospital birth versus planned home birth. Cochrane Database of Systematic Reviews 2012, Issue 9. Art. No.: CD000352. doi: 10.1002/14651858.CD000352.pub2

Oxford English Dictionary 2013 http://oxforddictionaries.com/definition/english/reciprocity (accessed 20 August 2013)

Page L 1996 The backlash against evidence-based care. Birth 23(4):191–2

Page L A, McCandlish R (eds) 2006 The new midwifery. Science and sensitivity in practice, 2nd edn. Churchill Livingstone, Edinburgh

Pairman S, Tracy S K, Horogood C et al 2010 Midwifery: preparation for practice, 2nd edn. Churchill Livingstone, Edinburgh

Papatsiba V 2006 Making higher education more European through student mobility? Revisiting EU initiatives in the context of the Bologna process. Comparative Education 42(1):93–111

Platt L 2007 Poverty and ethnicity in the UK. The Policy Press, Bristol

Raphael-Leff J 2005 Psychological processes of childbearing. Centre for Psychoanalytic Studies, London

Raynor M D, England C 2010 Psychology for midwives: pregnancy, childbirth and puerperium. Open University Press, Maidenhead

Redshaw M, Heikkila K 2010 Delivered with care: a national survey of women's experience of maternity care 2010. National Perinatal Epidemiology Unit (NPEU), Oxford

Redshaw M, Malouf R, Gao H et al 2013 Women with disability: the experience of maternity care during pregnancy, labour and birth and the postnatal period. BMC Pregnancy and Childbirth 13:174

Rodgers S E 2000 The extent of nursing research utilization in general medical and surgical wards. Journal of Advanced Nursing 32(1):182–93

RCM (Royal College of Midwives) 2000 Maternity care for lesbian mothers. Position Paper No. 22. RCM, London

RCM (Royal College of Midwives) 2003 Evidence provided for the House of Commons Health Committee. Inequalities in access to maternity services. Eighth Report of Session 2002–2003. TSO, London, p 17

RCM (Royal College of Midwives) 2008 Maternity care for disabled women: guidance paper. www.rcm.org.uk (accessed 20 August 2013)

Sackett D, Rosenburg W, Gray J A et al 1996 Evidence-based medicine: what it is and what it isn't. British Medical Journal 312(7023):71–2

Sandall J 1997 Midwives' burnout and continuity of care. British Journal of Midwifery 5(2):106–11

Sandall J, Soltani H, Gates S et al 2013 Midwife-led continuity models versus other models of care for childbearing women. Cochrane Database of Systematic Reviews 2013, Issue 8. Art. No. CD004667. doi: 10.1002/14651858.CD004667.pub3

Sivagnanam R (ed) 2004 Experiences of maternity services: Muslim women's perspectives. The Maternity Alliance, London

Sleep J 1991 Perineal care: a series of five randomised controlled trials. In: Robinson S, Thomson AM (eds) Midwives' research and childbirth. Chapman & Hall, London, p 199–251

Smaje C 1995 Health, race and ethnicity: making sense of the evidence. King's Fund Institute, London, p 16

Stewart M 2005 'I'm just going to wash you down': sanitizing the vaginal examination. Journal of Advanced Nursing 51(6):587–94

Stubbs P 1993 'Ethnically sensitive' or 'anti-racist'? Models for health research and service delivery. In: Ahmad W I U (ed), Race and health in contemporary Britain. Open University Press, Buckingham, p 34–47

Subramanian S, Naimoli J, Matsubayashi T et al 2011 Do we have the right models for scaling up health services to achieve the millennium development goals? BMC Health Research 11(36): doi: 10.1186/1472-6963-11-336

Thomson A 2000 Is there evidence for the medicalisation of maternity care? MIDIRS Midwifery Digest 10(4):416–20

Tuckett A, Crompton P 2013 Qualitative understanding of an international learning experience: what Australian undergraduate nurses and midwives said about Cambodia. International Journal of Nursing Practice doi: 10.1111/ijn.12142 (accessed at www.onlinelibrary.wiley.com 220813)

Turner K M, Chew-Graham C, Folkes L et al 2010 Women's experiences of health visitor delivered listening visits as a treatment for postnatal depression: a qualitative study. Patient Education and Counselling 78(2):234–9.

United Nations (UN) 2013 We can end poverty 2015: Millennium Development Goals. www.un.org/millenniumgoals/ (accessed 23 March 2013)

United Nations Development Programme (UNDP) 2010 Beyond the midpoint: achieving the Millennium Development Goals. UNDP, New York. www.un.org (accessed 23 March 2013)

Virdee S 1997 Racial harassment. In: Mohood T, Berthoud R, Lakey J et al (eds) Ethnic minorities in Britain: diversity and disadvantage. Fourth National Survey of Ethnic Minorities. Policies Studies Institute, London, ch 8: 259–89

Waage J, Banerji R, Campbell O et al 2010 The millennium development goals: a cross-sectional analysis and principles for goal setting after 2015. The Lancet 376(9745):991–1023

Walsh D 2007 Improving maternity services. Small is beautiful – lessons from a birth centre. Radcliffe Publishing, Oxford

Wickham S 1999 Evidence-informed midwifery (1). What is evidence-informed midwifery? Midwifery Today 51: 42–3

Wilton T, Kaufmann T 2001 Lesbian mothers' experiences of maternity care in the UK. Midwifery 17: 203–11

WHO (World Health Organization) 2008 Social determinants of health. www.who.int/social_determinants/en/index.html (accessed 20 August 2013)

WHO (World Health Organization) 2009 European Union Standards for Nursing and Midwifery: information for accession countries, 2nd edn (revised and updated by Thomas Keighley). www.euro.who.int/__data/assets/pdf_file/0005/102200/E92852.pdf (accessed 20 August 2013)

WHO (World Health Organization) 2013 Glossary of globalization, trade and health terms. www.who.int/trade/glossary/en/ (accessed 22 August 2013)

FURTHER READING

Association of Radical Midwives 2013 New vision for maternity care. www.midwifery.org.uk
Acknowledges the centrality of the mother–midwife relationship and identifies *some of the policy and cultural changes needed to protect and support this dyad.*

Heath I 2012 Kindness in health care: what goes around. BMJ 344: e1171
A thought-provoking review in how simple acts of kindness can be healing for both recipients of care and caregivers.

USEFUL WEBSITES

Association of Radical Midwives: www.midwifery.org.uk

Department of Health: www.gov.uk

International Confederation of Midwives: www.internationalmidwives.org

National Perinatal Epidemiology Unit: www.npeu.ox.ac.uk

Office of National Statistics: www.ons.gov.uk

Royal College of Midwives: www.rcm.org.uk

United Nations: www.un.org

World Health Organization: www.who.int

Chapter | 2 |

Professional issues concerning the midwife and midwifery practice

Jayne E Marshall, Mary Vance, Maureen D Raynor

This chapter affords the student with the frameworks governing the midwifery profession and underpinning the professional practice of the midwife. It emphasizes how the statutory supervision of midwives framework is a vital element of leadership and clinical governance supporting risk management by monitoring the development of maternity services and standards of midwifery practice. Having knowledge of these various frameworks is essential to every midwife so they are able to function effectively as autonomous, accountable practitioners and provide care to all childbearing women and their families that follows legal and ethical principles and is also contemporary, safe and of a high quality.

THE CHAPTER AIMS TO:

- identify the purpose of regulation of healthcare professionals in protecting public safety
- explain the role and functions of the regulatory body governing midwifery practice within the United Kingdom – the Nursing and Midwifery Council
- review the legal framework midwives should work within to maximize safety and minimize risk to women, their babies and families
- raise awareness of ethical frameworks and principles in supporting midwifery practice and empowering childbearing women
- describe the statutory supervision of midwives
- promote the supervision of midwives as a mechanism for quality assurance, sensitive to the needs of mothers and babies
- review the various aspects of clinical governance and demonstrate how statutory supervision supports the clinical governance framework.

STATUTORY MIDWIFERY REGULATION

Statutory regulation provides structure and boundaries that can be understood and interpreted by both professionals and the public: it is the basis of a contract of trust between the public and the profession. Although the primary purpose of regulation is protection and safety of the public, the same mechanism also protects and supports midwives in their practice.

Regulation of midwifery should play a key part in helping to improve women's experiences of the maternity services and preventing harm from occurring in midwifery practice. It is essential that women and their families can be assured they are being cared for by competent and skilled midwives who are effectively educated and knowledgeable in contemporary midwifery practice. Consequently, midwifery regulation should *not* be viewed as an abstract concept but from how it is perceived in ordinary everyday healthcare terms, that is: *supporting the standard of care that women want* or *what midwives would want for themselves and their families.*

Midwife is a title protected in statute in the United Kingdom (UK). This means that no one can call themselves a midwife or practise as a midwife unless they are registered on the Nursing and Midwifery Council's (NMC) Register. This registration must be *active*, in that the midwife has met the continuing professional development and practice requirements to remain on the Register and has paid the renewal of registration fee (every three years supported by a signed notification of practice form [NOP]) or a retainer fee (every interim first and second year of active registration). There are over 35 000 midwives on the NMC Midwives Register (NMC 2013).

SELF-REGULATION

In the UK, midwives are members of a self-regulating profession. This is a privilege in that the standards for education and practice of any midwife are set by midwives themselves. Self-regulating professions have regulatory bodies that are funded by their own professionals. In the case of midwives and nurses, their initial and subsequent retaining/renewal of registration payments is the sole funding that pays for all the functions of their regulatory body, the NMC.

Self-regulation of midwives is achieved through a statutory Midwifery Committee of the NMC which advises the Nursing and Midwifery Council (The Council) about what is required to ensure safe and competent midwives. The powers of the Midwifery Committee are defined under Section 41 of The Nursing and Midwifery Order (2001). The term *statutory* means that the role and scope of the committee is enshrined in law and cannot be reduced or disbanded unless there is a change in the legislation to allow it to happen. Any rule or standards for midwifery education or practice set by the Midwifery Committee are subsequently approved by the Council before they can come into effect.

Self-regulation of midwifery, however, does not exist in all countries and consequently regulations for midwifery education or practice are set by the national government or by another professional group who may be perceived as senior/superior. However, it is acknowledged that the midwifery profession, as other health professions in the UK, is affected to varying degrees by national regulations that are set by others who are not part of the profession: for example, legislation for safeguarding vulnerable children or adults (Safeguarding Vulnerable Groups Act 2006; Department of Health [DH] 2011; HM Government 2013); medicines legislation (Human Medicines Regulations 2012); health and safety in the workplace regulations (Health and Safety at Work Act 1974). All midwives are bound by these national laws in the same way as others.

Protection of the public cannot be achieved by the regulatory body alone and thus it involves a combination of statutory regulation, personal self-regulation, employment practices, professional organizations, education and working in an effective and collaborative way with others. It can, however, be difficult for individuals to act ethically and escalate concerns about practices within their organizations. It is here where the regulator and regulation can support the midwife by offering appropriate guidance. The NMC can also work actively with other service regulators such as the Care Quality Commission (CQC) in England, Healthcare Improvement Scotland, the Regulator and Quality Improvement Authority in Northern Ireland and Healthcare Inspectorate Wales, to ensure early action is taken to prevent unnecessary harm to women and their families.

Overseeing the NMC and other healthcare regulators and working with them to improve the way the professions are regulated is the Professional Standards Authority (PSA), which was previously known as the Council for Healthcare Regulatory Excellence (CHRE). This organization is accountable to Parliament for the health, safety and wellbeing of patients and other members of the public. The PSA is also required to undertake research, develop policy and provide advice to the four governments of the UK on regulating healthcare professionals and consequently provides an annual review of each of the healthcare regulators.

There has been, and still remains, a degree of public concern in the UK about self-regulation of the healthcare professions as a result of some high profile media cases where patient care was severely compromised (Bristol Royal Infirmary Inquiry 2001; Clothier et al 1994; HM Government 2007; Mid Staffordshire NHS Foundation Trust Public Inquiry 2013). Consequently, a number of reviews of professional regulation have been undertaken to improve safety and quality of care, the maintenance of professional standards and public assurance that poor practice or bad behaviour will be identified and promptly dealt with (DH 2007; CHRE 2008). The outcome of these reports and the introduction of the Health and Social Care Act 2012 have led to a major reorganization of the structure and function of the NMC.

HISTORICAL CONTEXT

Whilst it is appreciated that the establishment of legislation governing the practice of midwifery had been taken by the governments in Austria, Norway and Sweden as early as 1801, it was not until a century later, in 1902, that the first Midwives Act sanctioned the establishment of a statutory body – the Central Midwives Board (CMB) in England and Wales, followed by the Midwives (Scotland) Act 1915 and the Midwives (Ireland) Act 1918. The first Act in 1902 was promoted by individual members of Parliament through Private Members' Bills in the House of Lords and by others who supported midwife registration rather than being initiated by the government of the time. All three Acts of the UK prescribed the constitution and function of the CMBs in each of the four countries and laid down their statutory powers that included the development of systems for licensing midwives and prohibiting

unqualified practice. The CMB had the responsibility for regulating the issue of certificates, keeping a central roll of midwives and providing a means for the suspension of practitioners through Local Supervising Authorities (LSA) and the supervision of midwives. It also had the responsibility for regulating any courses of training and examinations and generally supervising the effective running of the profession. A series of further Acts of Parliament in 1926, 1934, 1936 and 1950 amended this initial legislation and were consolidated in the Midwives Act 1951 and Midwives (Scotland) Act 1951. However all midwifery statutory bodies of the UK were dominated by doctors who also held the chairmanships and there was no requirement for even one midwife to be included on the Council of any CMB. This remained the case until the dissolution of the CMBs in 1983.

The Nurses, Midwives and Health Visitors Act 1979 established the framework of the United Kingdom Central Council for Nursing, Midwifery and Health Visiting (UKCC) and the National Boards for England, Scotland, Northern Ireland and Wales to regulate education and practice, leading to the abolition of the CMBs in 1983. This was the first time that midwives had been amalgamated in law with other professional groups as up to this point midwifery had remained independent of any nursing infrastructure with the regulation of the nursing profession being undertaken by the General Nursing Councils (GNC). However, a separate Midwifery Committee was set up in Statute after much campaigning by the Royal College of Midwives (RCM) and the Association of Radical Midwives (ARM) who feared that the voice of midwifery would be over-ruled by that of nursing. Nevertheless, in 1987, the profession-specific education officers were replaced by generic education officers, over-ruling the Midwifery Committee and protests from members of the midwifery profession at the time.

A decade later, an external review of the Nurses, Midwives and Health Visitors Act 1979 was commissioned by the DH which resulted in a smaller, directly elected central council with smaller national boards. Regional Health Authorities (RHA) were assigned the responsibility of funding nursing and midwifery education, whilst the national boards retained responsibility for course validation and accreditation. This in essence established the *purchaser–provider model*, where hospitals were expected to contract with education providers for a requisite number of training places for nurses and midwives to fulfil their local workforce planning. These arrangements and the new streamlined structure of the UKCC and national boards were incorporated into the 1992 Nurses, Midwives and Health Visitors Act. Further consolidation of the 1979 and 1992 Acts incorporating all the reforms, resulted in the 1997 Nurses, Midwives and Health Visitors Act.

During the 1990s, the government devolved power away from the UK Parliament based in Westminster to the other three countries of the UK to enable them to establish their own parliaments or assemblies. This devolution has not impacted greatly on the regulation of midwives as midwifery is one of the established professions of which the power to regulate remains with the UK Parliament at Westminster, advised by the Department of Health England. Only new health-related professions that are established in the future will be exempt from this approach.

Further reform of the health professions was included in the Health Act 1999 that repealed the Nurses, Midwives and Health Visitors Act 1997. This resulted in replacing primary legislation with a Statutory Instrument by Order, which meant a departure from the normal practice of parliamentary procedure experienced during the previous century, involving professional scrutiny through all the earlier stages, including the publication of Green and White Papers. Section 62 (9) of the Health Act 1999 set out the Order for the establishment of the Nursing and Midwifery Council (NMC) which commenced operating in 2002. The NMC took over the quality assurance functions of the UKCC and the four national boards, although some of the functions of the national boards in Scotland, Northern Ireland and Wales are provided by NHS Education Scotland, the Northern Ireland Practice and Education Council for Nursing and Midwifery, and Healthcare Inspectorate Wales. This development reunited standards for education with standards for practice and supervision of midwives on a UK basis. However, the creation of this UK-wide regulatory body, the NMC, was contrary to the trend of devolution.

Statutory Instruments (SI)

The Nursing and Midwifery Order 2001: SI 2002 No: 253

This is the main legislation that established the NMC and was made under Section 60 of the Health Act 1999: it is generally known as The Order. The Order sets out what the Council is required to do (*shall*) and provides permissive powers for things that it can choose to do (*may*). The numbered paragraphs within The Order are referred to as Articles.

The structure of registration was set up according to Part III of The Order, resulting in three parts of the Register being opened from August 2004:

- Nurses
- Midwives
- Specialist Community Public Health Nurses: namely health visitors, school nurses, occupational health nurses, health promotion nurses and sexual health nurses.

Part IV set up Education and Training; Part V set up Fitness to Practise; Part VIII relates to Midwifery.

Midwifery-specific Articles established the following:

- Article 41: The Midwifery Committee
- Article 42: Rules specific to midwifery practice
- Article 43: Regulation of the LSA and supervisors of midwives
- Article 45: Regulation of attendance in childbirth.

The Order has been subject to a number of amendments, which are detailed in Box 2.1.

Box 2.1 **Notable amendments to the Nursing and Midwifery Order SI 2001: No. 253**

Statutory instrument	Title
SI 2006 No. 1914 *Part 16: Paragraph 82*	The Medical Act 1983 (Amendment) and Miscellaneous Amendments Order 2006
SI 2007 No. 3101 *Part 10: Paragraphs 155–173*	The European Qualifications (Health and Social Care Professions) Regulations 2007
SI 2008 No. 1485	The Nursing and Midwifery (Amendment) Order 2008
SI 2009 No. 1182 *Schedule 4: Part 2 Paragraph 22* *Part 6 Paragraphs 38, 41* *Schedule 5: Part 2 Paragraph 12*	The Healthcare and Associated Professions (Miscellaneous Amendments) and Practitioner Psychologists Order 2009
SI 2009 No. 2894	The Nursing and Midwifery Council (Midwifery and Practice Committees) (Constitution) (Amendment) Rules 2009
SI 2011 No. 17	Nursing and Midwifery Council (Fitness to Practise) (Amendment) Rules 2011
SI 2011 No. 2297	The Nursing and Midwifery Council (Fees and Education, Registration and Registration Appeals) (Amendment) Rules 2011
SI 2012 No. 2754	The Nursing and Midwifery Council (Education, Registration and Registration Appeals) (Amendment) Rules 2012
SI 2012 No. 3025	The Nursing and Midwifery Council (Midwives) Rules 2012
SI 2013 No. 235 *Schedule 2: Part 1 Paragraphs 51, 177*	The National Treatment Agency (Abolition) and the Health and Social Care Act 2012 (Consequential, Transitional and Savings Provisions) Order 2013

THE NURSING AND MIDWIFERY COUNCIL

Being the UK-wide regulator for two professions, namely nursing and midwifery, the Nursing and Midwifery Council (NMC) has two key functions: setting the strategic direction for the NMC and overseeing the work of senior NMC staff. The Council ensures that the NMC complies with all relevant legislation governing nursing and midwifery practice, including the Nursing and Midwifery Order 2001 (The Order) and adheres to the Charities Act 1993. Having charitable status, the NMC should use all funds received from its registrants purely for the benefit of the public, i.e. in the regulation of nursing and midwifery to safeguard the public's health and wellbeing.

Functions of the NMC

The powers of the NMC are specified within The Order and, as was the case with the CMB and UKCC, its primary function is to establish and improve standards of midwifery and nursing care in order to safeguard the public by:

- Establishing and maintaining a Register of all qualified nurses, midwives and specialist community public health nurses
- Setting standards for the education and practice of all nurses, midwives and specialist community public health nurses to ensure they have the right skills and qualities at the point of registration which continue to develop throughout their professional careers
- Regulating fitness to practise, conduct and performance through rules, codes and statutory supervision of midwives.

Where a registrant does not meet the standards for skills, education and behaviour, the NMC has the power to remove them from the Register permanently or for a set period of time.

Membership

The NMC comprises of 12 lay and registrant members, including one member from each of the four UK countries who are appointed by the Privy Council. Each registrant member is from either a nursing or midwifery background with the lay members selected for their expertise in various areas and strategic experience. These members also sit on various Committees within the framework of the NMC.

Committees

Following the NMC Governance review (NMC 2013), a number of the Council Committees were disbanded: the Appointments Board, the Education Committee, the Finance and Information Technology Committee and the Fitness to Practise Committee. As a result only three main Council Committees remain: the Audit Committee, the Midwifery Committee and the Remuneration Committee. There are, however, three further statutory committees: the Investigating Committee, the Conduct and Competence Committee and the Health Committee, known collectively as the Practice Committees, which are responsible for considering allegations under Part 5 of the Order.

The Audit Committee

This committee is responsible for ensuring that Council business is conducted with the highest integrity, probity and efficiency in addition to guaranteeing that there are appropriate systems in place for managing risk.

The Midwifery Committee

The role of the Midwifery Committee is to advise Council on any matter affecting midwifery, such as policy issues and standards influencing midwifery practice, education and statutory supervision of midwives, responding to policy trends, research and ethical issues concerning all registrants. The Midwifery Committee recommendations and subsequent Council decisions influence midwifery developments in the UK affecting the lives of individual women and their families for whom the midwife provides care.

The Remuneration Committee

The responsibility of this Committee is to determine and agree with Council the framework for the remuneration of the NMC's Chief Executive and Registrar, directors and other such members of the executive team as it is designated to consider.

Practice Committees

Any allegations of impaired Fitness to Practise referred to the NMC are considered by Panels of the Investigating Committee, with a possible referral to the Conduct and Competence Committee or the Health Committee, depending on the outcome of the Panel's decision. In 2014 a system of professional case examiners is to be introduced to make decisions at the investigation stage of the process as to whether cases should proceed to a final public hearing stage. The NMC expects this will improve the consistency of decisions and develop a faster and more cost-effective process. Furthermore, the introduction of a new power to review decisions to close cases at the investigation stage is also being considered. The final stage of a Fitness to Practise case, however, will still be heard by an independent panel, comprising of at least one nurse or midwife and at least one lay member advised by a legal expert.

The Investigating Committee

The responsibility of the panels of the Investigating Committee is to consider any allegations of a registrant being *unfit to practise*. If the registrant's health is in question, it is usual for a medical practitioner to be present. These hearings take place in private and the Panel decides if there is a case to answer. If there is, then a referral is made to either the Conduct and Competence Committee or the Health Committee. However, if the registrant is thought to be an immediate risk to the public, the Panel may refer the case immediately to an Interim Orders hearing. The Panel can then impose the following:

- *An interim suspension order:* registration is suspended to prevent the registrant from working during investigation of the case. This can be imposed for up to 18 months, but must be reviewed after 6 months and every 3 months thereafter.
- *An interim conditions of practice order:* the panel imposes conditions on the registrant for up to 18 months. According to the situation, this order can be revoked, modified or replaced with a different order.
- *Removal from the Register:* can be authorized by the Investigating Committee should there be fraudulent or incorrect entries in the register (NMC 2012a).

The Conduct and Competence Committee

This committee considers cases where a registrant's fitness to practise is alleged to be impaired due to:

- misconduct
- lack of competence
- a criminal offence
- a finding by any other health or social care regulator or licensing body that fitness to practise is impaired, or
- a barring under the arrangements provided by the Safeguarding Vulnerable Groups Act 2006 (Controlled Activity and Miscellaneous Provisions) Regulations 2010, the Safeguarding Vulnerable Groups (Northern Ireland) Order 2007 or the Protection of Vulnerable Groups (Scotland) Act 2007.

Panel hearings are held in public, reflecting the NMC's public accountability, although the Panel may agree to hold parts of the case in private, to protect the anonymity of the alleged victim, or if disclosure of confidential medical evidence is involved.

The Health Committee

This committee decides whether a registrant's fitness to practise is impaired by physical or mental ill health and, if so, determines the appropriate sanction required to protect the public. Because of the confidential nature of the medical evidence considered, Panel hearings are held in private.

Decisions made by the Practice Committees

Hearings follow a four stage process:

- establishing whether the facts are proved
- establishing whether the person's fitness to practise is impaired
- receiving information about the person's previous professional and employment history and in mitigation, and
- deciding the sanction.

Since 2008, Panels have used the Civil Standard of Proof to decide whether the facts of an allegation are proved (Health and Social Care Act 2007, 2008). Evidence is therefore based on the *balance of probabilities*, rather than the Criminal Standard of Proof where facts previously needed to be proved *beyond reasonable doubt*. When deciding on impairment, panels look for the level of conduct and competence expected of the *average registrant*, not for the highest possible level of practice. Even if there has been a breach of a standard set out in The Code (NMC 2008), it does not automatically follow that a registrant's fitness to practise is impaired. That is a judgement for the Panel to make.

A range of sanctions is available and the Panel uses the Council's *indicative sanctions* guidance to determine the one that is most appropriate for the particular case. The Panel must first consider whether, taking account of all the circumstances of the case, it is appropriate to take no further action. If the Panel decides this option is not appropriate, the following sanctions are available:

- to issue a *caution order* for a specified period of between one and five years
- to impose a *conditions of practice order* for a specified period up to three years
- to impose a *suspension order* for up to one year
- to impose *a striking off* order of the nurse or midwife from the Register (in lack of competence cases, this option is available only if the registrant has been continuously suspended or under conditions of practice for the previous two years).

Consensual panel determination

From 2013, the NMC have introduced consensual panel determination, which enables a registrant who is subject to a fitness to practise allegation to agree a provisional sanction with the NMC before it is put before a panel for consideration. This option is offered to a registrant following a full investigation and who has readily admitted all the charges against them in that their fitness to practise is impaired and a sanction is then provisionally agreed. The agreement is then put before a Conduct and Competence Committee or Health Committee Panel who will decide to accept or reject it. If rejected, the case is put before a new panel to conduct a full hearing and decide an appropriate outcome. This new arrangement reduces the need for witnesses to attend hearings, the length of hearings and enables the NMC to concentrate their resources on cases where there are significant matters in dispute.

Voluntary removal from the Register

Voluntary removal allows a registrant who admits that their fitness to practise is impaired, and who does not intend to continue practising, to apply to be permanently removed from the NMC Register without a full public hearing. This development was introduced in January 2013 to enable the NMC to take swift action in protecting the public following its investigation and liberating resources that can be used in more significant cases.

Voluntary removal is allowed in only limited circumstances where there is no public interest in holding a full hearing and where the public is best protected by a nurse or midwife's immediate removal from the Register. Such registrants would be those who accept that they are no longer fit to practise due to a serious or long-term health condition or are near retirement age. Voluntary removal will not be allowed where the allegations are so serious that public confidence in professional standards would suffer if they were not dealt with at a public hearing. This includes cases where the actions of a registrant have caused the death of a patient or other significant harm, including sexual misconduct.

While an application for voluntary removal can be made at any time, it is not allowed until a full investigation into the allegation has been completed. Where possible, the Registrar should consider the views of the person who made the initial allegation before making a decision. If an application is allowed, the registrant will appear on the NMC website with the status 'Voluntarily removed' adjacent to their name. The admissions made by the registrant may be made available to relevant enquirers, including potential employers, other regulators and overseas medical authorities.

Restoration to the Register following a striking off order

A registrant's name is removed from the NMC Register for five years during which time they are not allowed to work as a nurse or midwife in the UK. The application process to be restored to the Register can be made five years after the striking off order was made, as this is not done automatically. The process is as follows:

- The nurse or midwife must make an application to the NMC Registrar for the process to begin.

- A NMC committee will then decide at a hearing whether or not to allow the former nurse or midwife to be readmitted to the Register.
- They will take into consideration the initial charge, the nurse or midwife's understanding and insight into their past behaviour, and any action they may have taken with regard to the reasons for which they were struck off.

If the registrant can demonstrate they have achieved the additional education, training and experience required and once the registration fee has been paid, their name can be restored to the Register. However, if the application is unsuccessful, an appeal may be made within 28 days of the decision date. The individual may be suspended indefinitely should subsequent applications be made while the striking off order is in place and they are also unsuccessful.

Responsibility and accountability

Although midwives practise in a wide range of settings, they are all unified by underlying values and *responsibilities*. Each midwife has a *personal responsibility* for their own practice by being aware of their personal strengths and limitations and is therefore required to continually develop their knowledge and skills to maintain competence. Self-regulation and professional freedom are based on the assumption that each professional can be trusted to work without supervision and, where necessary, take action against colleagues should their practice not be up to the appropriate standards. Furthermore midwives share a *collective responsibility* in how women and their families are treated and cared for. This means that each midwife should highlight instances where individual practices or where the systems or processes within organizations providing maternity services, are compromising safe and appropriate care to women and their babies.

Accountability is more than having responsibility, although the concepts are used interchangeably and means that midwives are answerable for their actions and omissions, regardless of advice or directions by another professional. To be accountable, a midwife is required to have the ability, responsibility and authority for their actions (Bergman 1981). Each registrant is *professionally accountable* for their actions and omissions to the NMC, *legally accountable* to the law and *contractually accountable* to their employer. They must always act in the best interests of the individuals to whom they are providing care. In the case of midwives this would be the childbearing woman, her baby and family. There may be occasions when midwives have difficulty appreciating their own accountability, especially when carrying out the instructions of medical staff, but it is clear from The Code (NMC 2008) that registrants' accountability cannot be delegated to or borne by others. Midwives can gain greater clarity and understanding of their accountability through discussions with their supervisor of midwives.

Different levels of individual and corporate accountability exist in relation to professional practice and management structures. *Duty of care* and the advice contained in The Code (NMC 2008) provide further clarity around a registrant's professional accountability.

LEGAL ISSUES AND THE MIDWIFE

Contemporary midwifery practice is characterized by increasing complexities in respect of the health needs of childbearing women, their babies and families as well as increasing uncertainties about what is right and wrong. Midwives can find themselves faced with dilemmas and have to make decisions where there may not be evidence of any robust clinical evidence. It is therefore important each midwife is fully aware of the legislation and legal framework in which they should practise as accountable practitioners within the context of normal midwifery for which they have been duly trained and have the appropriate expertise.

Legislation

The Nursing and Midwifery Order 2001 (SI 2002 No: 253) is the statutory legislation that currently governs the midwifery profession and endorsed the formation of the regulatory body, the NMC.

Primary legislation is enshrined in Acts of Parliament, which have been debated in the House of Commons and House of Lords before receiving Royal Assent. Such legislation is expected to last at least a couple of decades before being revised. With the pressure on Parliamentary time, Acts of Parliament are frequently designed as *enabling legislation* in that they provide a framework from which statutory rules may be derived: known as *secondary* or *subordinate legislation*. All secondary legislation is published in Statutory Instruments.

Statutory rules/secondary legislation can in theory be implemented or amended much more quickly as it is the Privy Council which lays the rules before the House of Commons for formal and generally automatic approval rather than is the case for primary legislation that requires endorsement by the Secretary of State. However, this may still take several weeks or months to occur.

The Human Rights Act 1998

The European Convention for the Protection of Human Rights and Fundamental Freedoms (1951) set out to protect basic human rights and the UK was the first signatory to the Convention. The Convention is enforced through the European Court of Human Rights in Strasbourg. The Human Rights Act was passed in 1998 and

came into force on 2 October 2000, since when most of the articles of the convention have been directly enforceable in the UK courts in relation to public authorities and organizations, such as the National Health Service (NHS). It is important that midwives are aware of, and encouraged to work within, the boundaries of this Act. Of particular importance to midwives and those working in health care are the following Articles of the Act:

- Article 2: The right to life (e.g. continuing treatment of the life of a severely disabled baby).
- Article 3: The right not to be tortured or subjected to inhumane or degrading treatment (e.g. chaining a pregnant prisoner to a bed during labour would contravene this Article).
- Article 5: The right to liberty and security (e.g. safe and competent care during childbirth).
- Article 6: The right to a fair trial (e.g. civil hearings and tribunals as well as criminal proceedings).
- Article 8: The right to respect privacy and family life (e.g. supports a woman's right to give birth at home).
- Article 12: The right to marry (e.g. found a family, including fertility and assisted fertility).
- Article 14: The right not to be discriminated against (e.g. women with a disability, from a different ethnic/cultural background).

One benefit of this Act is that it has placed the public at the centre of health care. The individual's experience has become an important measure of quality and effectiveness in health care and as a consequence of this Act the NHS complaints system has been reviewed. Midwives should be aware that when someone has a right to something, there is usually a corresponding duty on someone else to facilitate the right (Beauchamp and Childress 2012). It could be said that women have a *right to safe and competent care during childbirth*, fitting in with Article 5. It would therefore follow that as midwives are educated to provide midwifery care, they have an obligation that the care is both *safe and competent*. Similarly, the UK Government via the NMC has an obligation in regulating its practitioners to ensure they practise safely and competently. The NMC does this by setting the *Midwives Rules and Standards* (NMC 2012b), via the *Post Registration Education and Practice (PREP) Standards* (NMC 2011) and the statutory supervision of midwives framework.

Legal frameworks: rules and standards

Each midwife must meet Standard 17 of the Standards for Pre-registration Midwifery Education (NMC 2009a), which stipulate the competencies and Essential Skills Clusters (ESCs) required of all midwives and which also comply with Article 42 of the European Union Directive on professional qualifications (2005/36/EC). In addition, the role and sphere of a midwife's practice are clearly defined in the Midwives Rules and Standards (NMC 2012b), the latter of which supplement the standards set out in The Code (NMC 2008) and thus provides the midwife with the legal frameworks in which to practise. Furthermore, the midwife's role is also embodied in the International Confederation of Midwives (ICM) Definition of the Midwife (ICM 2011) (see Chapter 1).

Midwives Rules and Standards

The Midwives Rules and Standards (NMC 2012b) are specific to the midwifery profession and relate to midwifery practice and the supervision of midwives. They are developed through the Midwifery Committee and approved by the Council. The current Midwives Rules and Standards are organized into five parts: *preliminaries, requirements for practice, obligations and scope of practice, supervision and reporting* and *action by the local supervising authority*. They provide detail about the specific rule, the LSA standard and the midwifery standard. Details of the rules contained within these parts can be seen in Box 2.2. Midwives need to be mindful that as the Midwives *Rules* are established by legislation set out in The Order, they are a legal requirement for midwifery registration and practice, whereas the *Standards* provide each midwife with guidance as to how each rule can be met in practice.

Rule 5: Scope of practice

Rule 5 (NMC 2012b) clarifies the midwife's responsibility in that she should refer to other appropriately qualified

---

Box 2.2 Midwives Rules and Standards

Part 1: Preliminaries	Rule 1: Citation and commencement	Cites the authority by which the rules are made and the date they come into effect
	Rule 2: Interpretation	Provides statutory definitions of key terms and titles used in the midwives rules in order to leave no doubt as to the intent of the term
Part 2: Requirements for practice	Rule 3: Notification of intention to practise	States that all midwives must notify the LSA when intending to practise in its area and explains the process for doing this
	Rule 4: Notifications by Local Supervising Authority (LSA)	States what the LSA must publish in relation to the intention to practise process
Part 3: Obligations and scope of practice	Rule 5: Scope of practice	States the standards expected of a practising midwife
	Rule 6: Records	Sets the requirements for the transfer and storage of midwifery records
Part 4: Supervision and reporting	Rule 7: The Local Supervising Authority Midwifery Officer (LSAMO)	States the standards required for the appointment, role and remit of the LSAMO
	Rule 8: Supervisors of midwives (SoM)	States the standards required for the appointment of SoMs
	Rule 9: LSA's responsibilities for supervision of midwives	Prescribes the requirements for the provision of supervision to all practising midwives
	Rule 10: Publication of LSA procedures	States the requirement for the LSA to publish its procedures in relation to adverse incidents, supervisory investigations and complaints. It also gives detailed guidance on the investigation process and potential outcomes
	Rule 11: Visits and inspections	Prescribes the ways that visits and inspections may be carried out by the NMC, LSA and SoM. This includes the requirement for the inspection of a midwife's place of work
	Rule 12: Exercise by a LSA of its functions	Requires the reporting of complaints/concerns about a LSAMO or SoM to be reported to the NMC
	Rule 13: LSA reports	States the requirement for the LSA to submit reports to the NMC
Part 5 Action by the Local Supervising Authority	Rule 14: Suspension from practice by a LSA	Prescribes the process for the suspension of a midwife by the LSA

Source: Midwives Rules and Standards (NMC 2012b)

health or social care professionals whenever any emergency or deviation from the norm occurs in a woman or baby which is outside of her current scope of practice. It is imperative that a midwife is fully aware that Rule 5 also states that a midwife should *not permit* anyone else or arrange for anyone else to act as *their substitute* other than another practising midwife or a registered medical practitioner. Permitting maternity support workers (MSW) to undertake activities associated with the role of the midwife would therefore be contravening Rule 5 and the midwife would be fully accountable for the consequences of the actions or omissions of the MSW. Similarly, the midwife remains professionally accountable for what a student midwife does or fails to do in clinical practice, but the subtle difference is that this delegation *is permitted* as the student is training to become a midwife and thus will be developing the underpinning knowledge and skills expected of a practising midwife.

Rule 6: Records

Rule 6 (NMC 2012b) outlines the midwife's responsibilities in respect of the safe storage of records relating to the advice and care provided to women and babies following their discharge from that care, including situations where the midwife is self-employed and when a midwife ceases to be registered with the NMC. The LSA standard relates to guidance concerning transfer of midwifery records from self-employed midwives. The midwife standards specify that all records relating to the care of a woman and baby should be kept securely for 25 years, including work diaries. Self-employed midwives should also ensure that women are able to access their records and inform them of the location of the records if they are transferred to the LSA. Claims can arise up to 25–30 years after a baby's birth and, if the documentation is lost, it is difficult for the case to be successfully defended. The guidance for storage and access to records is in accordance with the Data Protection Act 1998 that covers both computerised and manually held records.

In addition, the NMC guidance on *record keeping* (NMC 2009b) provides the principles that support good record keeping that should be integral to the practice of every registrant and includes details relating to confidentiality, access to records and information disclosure. It also stresses the importance of registrants keeping up to date with relevant legislation, case law and national and local policies relating to information and record keeping as well as undertaking audits to assess the quality and standard of the record keeping and communications.

The Code: Standards of Conduct, Performance and Ethics for Nurses and Midwives

The Code (NMC 2008) provides the registrant with the foundation of good nursing and midwifery practice and is

---

Box 2.3 **NMC Code: Public trust**

The people in your care must be able to trust you with their health and wellbeing. To justify that trust you must:
- Make the care of people your first concern, treating them as individuals and respecting their dignity
- Work with others to protect and promote the health and wellbeing of those in your care, their families and carers, and the wider community
- Provide a high standard of practice and care at all times
- Be open and honest, act with integrity and uphold the reputation of your profession

Source: The Code: standards of conduct, performance and ethics for nurses and midwives (NMC 2008)

---

a vital mechanism in safeguarding the health and wellbeing of the public. It highlights four standards that each registrant must clearly demonstrate through their professional practice in order to meet public trust. These are identified in Box 2.3.

These four standards are further expanded upon in The Code and include gaining consent, adhering to professional boundaries, working effectively as part of a team and delegation appropriately to others, keeping knowledge and skills up to date, maintaining clear and accurate records and upholding the reputation of the profession at all times. The Code reaffirms the registrant's personal accountability for their actions and omissions and being able to justify their decisions. Furthermore, the registrant's actions should always be lawful whether these relate to their professional or personal life. A registrant who does not practise according to these standards could find themselves before the NMC's Practice Committees with a possible suspension from practice and/or removal from the professional Register.

The increase in social networking has necessitated further guidance from the NMC (2012c) in that conduct online should be judged in the same way as conduct in the real world. The consequences of improper action or behaviour when posting information on such sites could put a nurse's or midwife's registration at risk or could jeopardize a student from being eligible to join the professional Register.

The Post Registration Education and Practice (PREP) Standards

In order for all registrants to retain their name on the professional Register, they have to fulfil the requirements of the Post Registration Education and Practice Standards (NMC 2011), which are as follows:

- undertake a minimum of 450 hours in clinical practice during the previous three years (*practice standard*)
- undertake a minimum of 35 hours study relevant to their practice every three years (*continuing professional development standard*)
- maintain a professional portfolio of their learning activity
- complete a notification of practice (NOP) form every three years
- undertake a *return to practice programme* if they have been out of practice for three years or more.

From a legal perspective it is every midwife's responsibility to ensure they remain professionally up to date with developments in practice, are clinically competent to fulfil their role and their practice is evidence-based. It is no defence for the midwife to disregard developments in practice and continue to use out-of-date policies, protocols and guidelines. All employers are required to provide regular education and training programmes either within the workplace or alternative educational institutions to support midwives in meeting their professional development needs. The supervisor of midwives can also support midwives in this respect through the annual supervisory meetings with each supervisee.

Standards for Medicines Management

Medicines management and prescribing in the UK are governed by a complex framework of legislation, policy and standards of which the NMC standards are only one part. However, the Human Medicines Regulations 2012 have attempted to simplify medicines legislation while maintaining effective safeguards for public health. The regulations replaced much of the Medicines Act 1968, repealing most of the obsolete law in the process to ensure the legislation is fit for purpose. In the Standards for Medicines Management (NMC 2007a) there are 26 standards detailed that stress the importance of the responsibility all nurses and midwives should have towards safe administration of medicines, including being conversant with local and national policies to maximize public protection. A useful source in providing information about medicines legislation and regulation in the UK that midwives can access is the Medicines Healthcare Products Regulatory Agency (MHRA). The NMC has also published guidance for those registrants who have undertaken further training to become nurse or midwife prescribers (NMC 2006a).

Litigation

This is the term used for the process of taking a case through the courts, where a claimant brings a charge against a defendant to seek some form of redress. In healthcare terms, this may be as a consequence of the claimant experiencing an *act of trespass* to their person by the defendant or suffering harm from the defendant's actions/omissions that could be proven as *negligence*. The National Health Service Litigation Authority (NHSLA) manages litigation and other claims against the NHS in England on behalf of member organizations and is responsible for providing advice on human rights case law and handling equal pay claims.

Consent

The concept of consent is complex and this section is intended as only a brief introduction. It is important the midwife or doctor obtains consent from a woman before undertaking any procedure to avoid any future allegations of *trespass to the person* that may be made against them. Obtaining consent is therefore the legal defence to trespass to the person.

Informed consent is taken to mean the *reasonable person standard* or the *Bolam standard* (*Bolam* v *Friern Hospital Management Committee* 1957) whereby an individual is given as much information as any *reasonable person* could be expected to understand in order to make a decision about their care/treatment (DH 2009a). This implies that the person is mentally competent to make such a decision (is legally an adult: 18 years or over) or is not mentally incapacitated in any way. The purpose and significance or potential complication of any procedure or treatment should also be discussed with the childbearing woman by the midwife or doctor. Where possible, the woman should be given time to consider her options before making a decision. This should be done voluntarily and without any duress or undue influence from health professionals, family or friends for it to be *valid*. Only the woman can give consent for treatment or intervention and although it is desirable if the partner or other relatives are in agreement, ultimately the woman's views are the only ones that should be taken into consideration (DH 2009a).

Incapacity may be temporary, for example as a result of shock, pain, fatigue, confusion, or panic induced by fear. However, it would not usually be reasonable to consider that a woman in labour, experiencing the pain of contractions, would be so affected that she lacked capacity. If a healthcare professional fears that a woman's decision-making (capacity) is impaired they should seek assistance in assessing capacity, which is usually provided by the courts. If a woman requires emergency treatment to save her life, and she is unable to give consent due to being unconscious, treatment can be carried out if it is in her best interests and according to the reasonable standard of the profession (Mental Capacity Act 2005). Once the woman has recovered, the reasons why treatment was necessary must be fully explained to her.

In the case of minors (children under 16 years), it is important to carefully assess whether there is evidence that they have sufficient understanding in order to give valid consent, i.e. considered to be *Gillick competent* (*Gillick v West Norfolk and Wisbech AHA* 1985). Although Gillick competence was originally intended to decide whether a child under 16 years can receive contraception without parental knowledge it has, since 1986, had wider applications in health provision and is also referred to as *Fraser competence* (DH 2009a). It is also advisable that the child's parents or other accompanying adults are kept informed of any clinical decisions that are made. Where there is a conflict of opinion regarding consent between child and parent, the health professional should always act in the child's best interest which in some instances may involve the courts determining whether it is lawful to treat the child (DH 2009a).

It is good practice that the health professional who is to perform the procedure should be the one to obtain the woman's consent. Such details of the discussion and decision should be clearly documented in the woman's records for colleagues to see that consent has been duly obtained or declined.

Consent can be *implied*, *verbal* or *written*. It is a common misconception that written consent is more valid than verbal consent when in fact written consent merely serves as evidence of consent. If appropriate information has not been provided, the woman feels that she is under duress or undue influence or she does not have capacity, then a signature on a form will make the consent *invalid*. It is advised that written consent for significant interventions such as surgery should always be obtained (DH 2009a) but for many procedures such as vaginal examination or phlebotomy verbal consent is sufficient. In an absolute emergency, it may be more appropriate to take witnessed verbal consent for caesarean section rather than spending time on paperwork.

Although the law protects the rights of the woman, the fetus does not have any rights until it is born. A mentally competent woman cannot be legally forced to have a caesarean section because of risks to the fetus. However, whilst accepting the law and respecting the woman's right to refuse such an intervention that may further endanger the life of the fetus, such a situation will be very uncomfortable for any midwife or obstetrician to sit back and allow a fetus to die. Cases such as this can be referred to court for an emergency application to determine whether the intervention can proceed lawfully.

Negligence

It is recognized that the most significant claims in obstetrics arise from birth trauma resulting in cerebral palsy. These are usually based on the allegation that there was negligence on the part of the health professionals involved in the intrapartum care and management, resulting in fetal asphyxia and consequently neurological damage to the baby.

The Congenital Disabilities (Civil Liability) Act 1976 enables a child who is born disabled as a result of negligence prior to birth to claim compensation from the person(s) responsible for the negligent act. A mother can only be sued for negligence to her unborn baby if this occurred through dangerous driving. In such cases, the child would sue the mother's insurance company. There has been an amendment to the Act so that children who have suffered damage during in vitro fertilization (IVF) treatment may also obtain compensation. As with all medicolegal cases, for the claimant to be successful, the following need to be proved:

- the health professional owed the woman a duty of care
- there was a *breach of duty of care* to the woman by the health professional such that the standard of care afforded to her was *below the standard that she could reasonably have expected*
- the harm/injury sustained was *caused by the breach of duty* and
- damages or other losses such as psychiatric injury (post-traumatic stress disorder/nervous shock, anxiety disorder or adjustment disorder), financial loss (loss of earnings) and future healthcare provision, recognized by the courts as being subject to compensation, have resulted from that harm.

In many cases where a baby suffers neurological damage and develops cerebral palsy, although it may be accepted that the care was substandard, proving *causation* is more difficult. i.e. whether the substandard care actually resulted in the disability. The situation is complicated by the fact that only a small percentage of babies born with significant neurological damage acquire their disability as a result of events that took place during labour and birth. However, parents will seek to assign the damage to issues of management during the intrapartum period when the health and wellbeing of some babies may have already been chronically compromised before this time.

Experts are therefore required to assess the case on behalf of the claimant (the woman or mother on behalf of the baby) and the defendant (usually the hospital Trust) to consider the issues of causation. This may mean that many medicolegal expert opinions are obtained from neonatologists, paediatric neurologists and obstetricians before finally reaching a conclusion.

The *burden of proof of negligence* is on the claimant to prove that on the *balance of probabilities* it is more likely than not that the defendant was negligent in order for them to be awarded any compensation by the courts. In cases of negligence, compensation is determined by agreeing the *liability* and the amount (*quantum*). However, if as a result of negligence the baby has died, then the parents can only recover bereavement costs. Where a fetus dies there is no bereavement costs as the unborn child does not have any legal rights.

Vicarious liability

In the event of an employed midwife being negligent, it would be usual for her employer to be sued. The doctrine of vicarious liability exists to ensure that any innocent victim obtains compensation for injuries caused by an employee. Under this doctrine the employer is responsible for compensation payable for the harm. For vicarious liability to be established the following elements must exist:

- there must be negligence: a duty of care has been breached and as a reasonably foreseeable consequence has caused harm/other failure by the employee
- the negligent act, omission or failure must have been by an employee
- the negligent employee must have been acting in the course of their employment.

It is worth noting that even where the employer is held to be vicariously liable, the midwife who is responsible for harm, such as death of a woman or baby, could be found guilty of manslaughter for their gross negligence which led to the death, could lose their job following disciplinary action and also be struck off the Register following a hearing by the NMC Conduct and Competence Committee.

The doctrine of vicarious liability does not necessarily deprive the employer of their rights against the negligent employee. If a midwife has been negligent then they are in breach of their contract of employment that requires them to take all reasonable care and skill. This breach gives the employer a right to be indemnified against the negligent midwife.

From 2013 the Health Care and Associated Professions (Indemnity Arrangements) Order 2013 (referred to as *The Indemnity Order*) specifies that all healthcare professionals, including midwives and nurses, are expected to have indemnity arrangements in place as *a condition of their registration*. The Clinical Negligence Scheme for Trusts (CNST) fulfils this requirement so each midwife should be covered via their employer's membership to CNST.

In the case of independent midwives who are self-employed, they have no vicarious liability or indemnity by an employer and are *personally liable* for the health and safety of themselves and others. However, from October 2013 all independent midwives in the UK are unable to practise without indemnity cover (The Indemnity Order 2013). It is therefore advisable they secure their own personal indemnity insurance cover as even though they have to have a supervisor of midwives, the supervisor is not liable; neither is supervisor's employer vicariously liable for the negligence of the independent midwife. However due to the increase in compensation paid out to maternity cases and subsequent rising costs of insurance premiums, many independent midwives are no longer able to function alone. They have either established social enterprise schemes where they commission care from maternity care providers with whom they negotiate professional indemnity insurance cover, or have returned to employment in the NHS.

ETHICAL ISSUES AND THE MIDWIFE

Although the area of ethics is complex and perceived as difficult and daunting, it is a major part of midwifery education and practice and should be seen as a daily tool to support a midwife's decision-making with childbearing women. Being ethically aware is a step towards being an autonomous practitioner: taking responsibility, empowering others and facilitating professional growth and development. The language and terminology, however, can be hard to comprehend and need greater explanation (see Box 2.4).

Ethics is often about exploring values and beliefs and clarifying what people understand, think and feel in a certain situation, often from what they say as much as what they do – such actions being underpinned by morality. Beliefs and values are very personal and dependent on many things, such as a person's background, the society they have been brought up in and the principles and concepts learned since early childhood, such as veracity (truth telling). It is important to reflect on these issues and be open and honest about dilemmas faced in practice. A potential area of conflict is that of law, as law and ethics are often seen as complementary to one another, yet they can also be placed at opposite ends of the spectrum, either creating overlap or creating conflict. Exploring ethics provides a framework to aid resolution of such dilemmas.

Ethical frameworks and theories

There are many ethical frameworks that could be adopted to use in clinical situations and Edwards (1996) advocates a four-level system of moral thinking based on the work

Box 2.4 **Terminology**	
Informed consent	Information regarding options for care/treatment
Rights	Justified claim to a demand
Duty	A requirement to act in a certain manner
Justice	Being treated fairly
Best interests	Deciding on best course for an individual
Utilitarian	Greatest good for greatest number
Deontological	Duty of care
Beneficence	Doing good
Non-maleficence	Avoiding harm

of Melia (1989) that can assist in formulating arguments and discussions and ultimately solving moral dilemmas (see Box 2.5).

Level one: Judgements

Judgements are usually readily made, based on information on individual gains. Such judgements may have no real foundation except the belief of the individual who made it. They may therefore be biased and not necessarily well thought through or based on all the available evidence. What informs a judgment is often linked to personal values and beliefs, societal influences as well as experiences of similar past events. It is important that midwives reflect on past judgements to consider if in retrospect they were well founded or based on personal bias or prejudice.

Level two: Rules

Rules govern our daily lives and are determined by the society or culture in which we live. In terms of ethics, rules are what guide the midwife's practice and control their actions. According to Beauchamp and Childress (2012) rules come in different forms:

- *Substantive rules:* cover issues such as privacy, confidentiality or truth telling
- *Authority rules:* are determined by those in power and enforced on a country or section of society
- *Procedural rules:* define a set course of action or line that should be followed.

The midwife should recognize that rules can be enabling in that they define clear limits or boundaries of practice, allowing freedom to act knowing the safe limits of those actions. The NMC (2012b) Midwives Rules and Standards are statutory rules bound by legal processes but can guide and enable practice when used appropriately and as a consequence ease any ethical dilemmas. The Code (NMC 2008) is less formal or obligatory than rules and is viewed as a set of guidelines to support safe practice among midwives as well as nurses.

Level three: Principles

There are four main principles which are usually applied specifically within health care and midwifery practice:

- *Respect for autonomy:* respecting another's right to self-determine a course of action: e.g. placing women at the centre of maternity care where their views and wishes are seen as key to the decision-making process in care delivery.
- *Non-maleficence: Primum non nocere* – above all, do no harm or cause no hurt.
- *Beneficence:* compassion, taking positive action to do good or balance the benefits or harm in a given situation. This principle can cause a particular dilemma when a woman chooses a course of action that may not be in her and her fetus/baby's best interests.
- *Justice:* to treat everyone fairly and as equals. This principle also encompasses fair access for all women to the same level and options of health and maternity services, including place of birth.

Level four: Ethical theories

There are a number of theories that could be explored and applied to healthcare and midwifery practice, e.g. liberalism, ethical relativism, feminism and casuistry are just some of them. The two main normative ethical theories that are at either end of the spectrum are *utilitarianism* (consequentialism) and *deontology.*

Utilitarianism

This theory considers actions in terms of their probable consequences and originates from the Greek *telos* meaning *end* or *purpose,* such that this theory is sometimes referred to as *teleological theory.* Although the original theory's aim was for all actions to create the greatest happiness for the greatest number of people, the word *happiness* has been criticized, as for some individuals actions may result in a degree of *unhappiness.* It is therefore more apt to consider this theory as substituting *happiness* for the word *good* or *benefit:* that is, *the greatest good/benefit for the greatest number.*

Many aspects of midwifery practice have been implemented on utilitarian principles: e.g. antenatal and neonatal screening tests are offered to all women irrespective of need or individual assessment to benefit society as a whole. However, midwives do need to be mindful that whilst the majority of women may opt for the testing to identify any potential health risks and consequential treatment, *unhappiness* may be evoked for some women as fear and anxiety is associated with the choice to accept or decline such a test.

There are two types of this theory: act utilitarianism and rule utilitarianism. *Act utilitarianism* was developed by Bentham, Mill and Sidgwick in the 18th and 19th centuries and is the purer form of the two types. The theory expects every potential action to be assessed according to its predicted outcomes in terms of benefit. In comparison, *rule utilitarianism* considers moral rules that are intended

- Self
- Colleagues
- Women (mothers)/patients
- Relatives
- Fetus/baby
- Employer
- Profession (NMC)

to ensure the greatest benefit, such that each act is assessed to how it conforms to the rules. Practically, utilitarianism theory is attractive in that it can aid decision making for the masses, such that an action is good if it provides benefits for the majority.

Deontology

This particular ethical theory derives from the Greek term *deon*, meaning *duty, rule* or *obligation*, and was formulated around the right thing to do *without regard to the consequences* by the German metaphysician, Immanuel Kant. All health professionals would appreciate they have a duty towards their patients/clients, but as shown in Box 2.6, they may have duties in other areas that they need to consider and balance in order to make appropriate decisions to take the best course of action. How duty is interpreted may vary according to the individual's personal situation, their values or beliefs with some individuals basing their duty on natural laws, religion and the Ten Commandments (*traditional deontology*).

The philosophy behind Kant's theory reflects that to act morally is concerned with truth-telling and out of respect for duty, *regardless* of the circumstances. Kant believed that the actions of an individual should always be rational and stem from good will, that is to say, duty for its own sake, namely the *categorical imperative*, which is expressed as follows:

- Act only according to that maxim by which you can also will that it would become a universal law.
- Act in such a way that you always treat humanity, whether in your own person or in the person of any other, never simply as a means, but always at the same time as an end.

This highlights that an action can only be moral if it can be applied to everyone universally: if everyone was to do it. Kant believed all individuals to be autonomous and rational and should be treated with respect rather merely as a means to an end. Beauchamp and Childress (2012) consider that if an action necessitates treating someone *without* respect then it is the *action that is wrong*. In maternity care, respecting women as individuals with their own personal experiences is fundamental to the role of the midwife.

Although the NHS and other healthcare providers are generally utilitarian, midwifery, nursing, medicine and other such disciplines adopt a more deontological approach. *The duty of care* which is the duty that health professionals are most familiar with, is in essence embedded in the text of The Code (NMC 2008).

Conflicting duties can cause dilemmas in deciding the best course of action. *Casuistry* is a system that can assist in prioritizing duties according to the circumstances. However, most people deal with conflicts and dilemmas in their lives without having an appreciation of these theories. Nevertheless, whether midwives opt to utilize formal or informal approaches to assist their ethical decision-making in practice, to have knowledge of each of them is important in order to understand how some decisions are made. Furthermore, having knowledge of ethical theories can help midwives to appreciate why certain approaches are taken by the employing organization/management when changes or implementation of innovations are proposed in practice.

THE STATUTORY SUPERVISION OF MIDWIVES

The purpose of supervision of midwives is to protect women and babies by actively promoting safe standards of midwifery practice. Supervision is a statutory responsibility that provides a mechanism for support and guidance to all midwives practising in the UK, empowering them to work within the full scope of their role (NMC 2013). The philosophy of midwifery supervision and the standards it develops reflect the key themes of clinical governance described in NHS First Class Service (DH 1998). These themes are:

- professional self-regulation
- clinical governance
- life-long learning.

Historical context

The concept of the supervision of midwives was established in the UK in Edwardian times with the passing of the 1902 Midwives Act (England and Wales), the Midwives (Scotland) Act in 1915 and the Midwives (Ireland) Act in 1918 that led to the setting up of a Central Midwives Board (CMB) in the respective countries. Under these Acts, the CMBs that initially had a medical majority had the power to frame the rules to govern midwifery practice and the authority to enforce their compliance. Midwives who disobeyed or ignored the rules or who were guilty of negligence, malpractice or personal or professional misconduct were consequently disciplined or suspended from practice. At this time, failure to submit an intention to practise

(ITP) form or submitting incomplete details would result in the midwife incurring a fine.

Although the CMBs had the responsibility for supervising the effective running of the profession, much of the responsibility for the supervision of midwives lay with Local Authorities (LA) that were under the control of county councils/county borough councils. As a consequence of the LAs acquiring extensive powers by the CMBs, they eventually became known as Local Supervising Authorities (LSA). The extent of the functioning powers of the LSA included:

- the supervision of midwives practising within their district in accordance with the CMB rules;
- investigating allegations of malpractice, negligence or misconduct;
- reporting the names of any practising midwife convicted of an offence;
- suspending a midwife from practice if they were likely to be a source of infection;
- reporting the death of any midwife;
- receiving the notification of intention to practise from each practising midwife within their district; and
- submitting a roll of midwives annually to the CMB.

The role of the LSA Officer was undertaken by the Medical Officer of Health (MOH) who passed on the bulk of their LSA work to non-medical inspectors. The first inspectors were often clergymen's daughters, members of the local gentry, or relatives of the MOH (Heagerty 1996). These individuals were used to supervising subordinates and had domestic standards much higher than those of the working-class midwives. As a result, they were extremely critical of the poor environments in which many of the midwives lived and practised at this time. The inspectors were at liberty to inspect the midwives in any way they felt appropriate. They could follow them on their rounds, visit their homes, question the women they had cared for and even investigate their personal lives in addition to inspecting their equipment (Kirkham 1996). Records could not be checked as they were rarely made due to the fact that many midwives were illiterate, notwithstanding their immense practical knowledge and independence.

The Midwives Act 1936 empowered the CMB to set rules requiring midwives to attend refresher courses and determined the qualifications of medical and non-medical inspectors: the latter being practising midwives. In 1937, further expansion of the 1936 Midwives Act stated that inspectors of midwives were to be known as 'supervisors of midwives' with their role being more of a *counsellor* and *friend*.

In 1974 the National Health Service (Reorganization) Act 1973 designated Regional Health Authorities in England and Area Health Authorities in Wales as LSAs. By 1977 the medical supervisor role had been abolished with all subsequent supervisors being practising midwives. The reorganization also led to supervision being introduced into the hospital environment as well as in the community.

The Midwives Act 1951 and Midwives (Scotland) Act 1951 required LSAs, through the supervisors of midwives, to ensure midwives attended statutory postgraduate courses (refresher courses). This statutory requirement continued until 2001 when Rule 37 (UKCC 1998) was superseded by the Post Registration Education and Practice (PREP) standards (UKCC 1997) and the subsequent developments in midwives' continuing professional development as a consequence of the Nursing and Midwifery Order 2001 and its amendments.

The responsibility for monitoring the statutory supervision of midwives is through the regulator, the NMC and detailed in the Midwives Rules and Standards (NMC 2012b). The Standards for the Preparation and Practice of Supervisors of Midwives (NMC 2006b) provides further detail and clarity about the statutory supervision of midwives.

Supervision of midwives in the 21st century

Many of the historic functions of the statutory supervision of midwives continue today, although they exist in a much more supportive fashion. The principal aim of statutory supervision of midwives is still the protection of the public, however the philosophy is centred on promoting best practice and excellence in care, preventing poor practice and intervening in unacceptable practice. Effective use of the supervisory framework leads to improvements in the standard of midwifery care and better outcomes for women. This endorses the need for midwives and supervisors of midwives to work towards a common aim of providing the best possible care for women and babies through a mutual responsibility for effective communication. Consequently, there is much more emphasis placed on discussion, support and continuing professional development needs with the supervisor of midwives providing a confidential framework for a supportive relationship with the midwife.

Midwives are still required to give notice to each LSA in whose area they intend to practise, before commencing to practise there. Subsequently midwives must give notice in respect of each 12 month period in which they intend to continue practising within a specific location (NMC 2012b: Rule 3). The intention to practise (ITP) documentation is now linked to the registrant's entry on the midwives part of the NMC register. This confirms the midwife's *eligibility to practise* to an employer and the public rather than the midwife merely having an effective registration.

Local Supervising Authorities

Local Supervising Authorities (LSA) are organizations within geographical areas, responsible for ensuring that statutory supervision of midwives is undertaken according to the standards set by the NMC under article 43 of the Nursing and Midwifery Order (The Order) 2001: details of which are set out in the Midwives Rules and Standards (NMC 2012b).

The Order states that each LSA shall:

1. exercise general supervision over all midwives practising in its area;
2. where it appears that the fitness to practise of a midwife in its area is impaired, report it to the Council; and
3. have power in accordance with the rules made under Article 42 [of The Order] to suspend a midwife from practice.

Local Supervising Authority arrangements differ across the UK. In England the LSA is NHS England, in Wales, it is Healthcare Inspectorate Wales, in Scotland it rests with the Health Boards and in Northern Ireland, the LSA is the Public Health Agency. Although the LSA role has no management responsibility to these organizations, it does act as a focus for issues relating to midwifery practice with its strength lying in its influence on quality in local maternity services.

Role of the LSA Midwifery Officer

Each LSA has an appointed LSA Midwifery Officer (LSAMO) employed to carry out the LSA function who is professionally accountable to the NMC. The LSAMO is a practising midwife with experience in statutory supervision and who provides an essential point of contact for supervisors of midwives to consult for advice on aspects of supervision. Members of the public who seek help or support concerning the provision of midwifery care can also contact the LSAMO directly.

The LSAMO provides leadership, support and guidance on a range of matters including professional development and also contributes to the wider NHS agenda by supporting public health and inter-professional activities at national level. It is a unique role in that it does not represent the interests of either the commissioners or providers of NHS maternity services. A list of the functions of the LSA, as discharged by the LSAMO, can be found in Box 2.7.

Box 2.7 Duties of the Local Supervising Authority Midwifery Officer (LSAMO)

Ensures that supervision is carried out to a satisfactory standard for all midwives within the geographical boundaries of the LSA

Provides impartial, expert advice on professional matters

Provides a framework for supporting supervision and midwifery practice

Operates a system that ensures each midwife meets the statutory requirements for practice

Selects and appoints supervisors of midwives and deselects if necessary

Ensures the supervisor of midwives to midwives ratio does not normally exceed 1:15

Provides a formal link between midwives, their supervisors and the statutory bodies

Implements the NMC's rules and standards for supervision of midwives

Provides advice and guidance to supervisors of midwives

Participates in the development and facilitation of programmes of preparation for prospective supervisors of midwives

Provides initial training and continuing education opportunities for supervisors of midwives

Provides advice on midwifery matters to maternity care providers

Works in partnership with other agencies and promotes partnership working with women and their families

Provides a point of contact for women to discuss any aspect of their midwifery care that they do not feel has been addressed through other channels

Manages communications within supervisory systems with a direct link between supervisors of midwives and the LSA

Conducts regular meetings with supervisors of midwives to develop key areas of practice

Investigates cases of alleged misconduct or lack of competence

Determines whether to suspend a midwife from practice, in accordance with Rule 14 of the Midwives Rules and Standards (NMC 2012b)

Conducts investigations and initiates legal action in cases of practice by persons not qualified to do so under the Nursing and Midwifery Order (2001)

Receives reports of maternal deaths

Leads the development of standards and audit of supervision

Maintains a list of current supervisors of midwives

Receives intention to practise data from every midwife practising in the LSA

Prepares an annual report of supervisory activities within the report year, including audit outcomes and emerging trends affecting maternity services for the NMC, DH and Trusts

Publishes details of how to contact supervisors of midwives

Publishes details of how the practice of midwives will be supervised

Publishes the local mechanism for confirming any midwife's eligibility to practise.

Having regular contact with supervisors of midwives and being part of the LSAMO Forum UK ensures that each LSA Midwifery Officer has detailed knowledge of contemporary issues to enable the development of midwifery practice in meeting the needs of women and their families (Bacon 2011). One of the many aims of the LSAMO Forum UK is to ensure that it contributes to maintaining a consistent and equitable approach to supervision through UK wide guidance.

Selection and preparation of supervisors of midwives

The statutory supervision of midwives is a valuable component of midwifery practice, however its success reflects the ability of those who are appointed as supervisors of midwives. It is therefore important to have robust high-quality preparation and ongoing assessment of performance. However, formal courses of instruction for supervisors of midwives did not exist until 1978, and it was not until the English National Board for Nursing, Midwifery and Health Visiting (ENB) developed an Open Learning Programme at Diploma level in 1992 (ENB 1992) that training to become a supervisor of midwives *prior to appointment* became a requirement.

The *standards for the preparation and practice of supervisors of midwives* (NMC 2006b) outline the standards of competence that underpin the principles of statutory supervision of midwives, in accordance with the Midwives Rules and Standards (NMC 2012b: Rule 9). Programmes of education are now delivered at first degree or masters level by Higher Education Institutions (HEI) and are approved and monitored annually by the NMC (NMC 2006b). Midwives must complete the course successfully *before* being eligible for appointment as a supervisor of midwife.

Role and responsibilities of the supervisor of midwives

Supervisors of midwives are independent of the employer and often work in a team. Their role is different from the midwifery manager, who is responsible to the employer to make sure that maternity services run effectively. Supervisors of midwives are accountable to the LSA and are supported in their role by the LSAMO. They provide leadership and guidance to midwives that include a 24-hour service provision for midwives and women (NMC 2007b; LSAMO Forum UK 2009).

Each supervisor has a *professional* and *practice* responsibility to ensure that the practice within their own clinical area is evidence-based, to challenge and monitor midwifery practice, set standards and carry out clinical audit. They must ensure that their personal supervisees have access to the NMC statutory rules and standards (NMC 2012b) and The Code (NMC 2008), and to local and national clinical guidelines. Among their many duties, a

---

Box 2.8 **Responsibilities of a supervisor of midwives include**

Being accountable to the Local Supervising Authority for all supervisory activities

Maintaining an awareness of local, regional and national health-related issues

Providing professional leadership

Being an effective change agent

Liaising with clinicians, managers and educationalists

Providing practical advice, guidance and support on all midwifery matters, including ethical issues

Supporting best practice and ensuring women-centred, evidence-based midwifery care

Offering guidance and support to women accessing maternity services

Being a confident advocate for midwives and childbearing women

Empowering women and midwives

Being a professional role model to midwives and student midwives

Facilitating a supportive partnership with midwives in clinical practice

Being approachable and accessible to midwives

Supporting midwives through dilemmas

Facilitating midwives' reflection on critical incidents

Assisting midwives with their personal and professional development plans

Undertaking annual supervisory reviews with personal supervisees

Supporting midwives undertaking LSA Practice Programmes [*The Programme*]

Being a mentor to midwives undertaking preparation of supervisor of midwives programmes

Maintaining records of all supervisory activities

---

supervisor is responsible to audit records, arrange regular meetings with their supervisees at least annually and work with them to identify any areas of practice requiring development. A list of the responsibilities of a supervisor of midwives is provided in Box 2.8.

Statutory supervision in action

Each supervisor of midwives is in an excellent position to identify good practice and also to learn of examples of good practice in other maternity units through the supervisory network that can be adopted within their own units. Where midwives have ideas for changing and improving practice, supervisors should be able to empower them to introduce such change and support them in their initiatives, acting as their advocate with senior staff.

Partnership between supervisor and midwife/supervisee

To benefit from supervision, mutual respect between the supervisor of midwives and their midwives/supervisees is essential. Midwives should work in partnership with their supervisors and make the most of supervision (LSAMO Forum UK 2009), so that it can be effective not only for themselves but also for the mothers and babies for whom they care.

The primary responsibilities of a midwife are to ensure the safe and efficient care of women and their babies, and to maintain personal fitness for practice to sustain their registration with the NMC. The supervisory relationship enables, supports and empowers midwives to fulfil these responsibilities. Figure 2.1 demonstrates how midwives can make the most of supervision and the benefits of a professional relationship with their named supervisor of midwives.

Supervisory reviews

Supervisory reviews provide midwives with an opportunity to take time out with their named supervisor of midwives to consider personal learning needs and professional development requirements. These review meetings can be used to consider mechanisms for gaining relevant experience in other areas and receiving the necessary professional knowledge and skills.

Midwives are responsible for meeting their own PREP requirements before re-registering with the NMC (2011) and these requirements can be discussed with the supervisor of midwives during the review. The supervisor will be able to guide the midwife if further academic study is being considered. The review also provides an opportunity to evaluate practice and share any practice issues causing concern. If it is felt necessary, the supervisor will investigate the matter and take appropriate action.

Although it is customary for only one supervisory review a year, midwives are able to access their supervisor as and when required. As many supervisors hold clinical posts, they often work alongside the midwives they supervise and have more regular contact on an informal basis. Being valued and supported by supervisors and having achievements recognized enhances midwives' professional confidence and practice. The supervisory decisions perceived as empowering are those made by a consensus between the supervisor and the midwife (Stapleton et al 1998). If this relationship is not recognized by either midwife or supervisor, then the opportunity to change supervisor should be taken by the midwife to enable the necessary rapport and confidence in the supervisory relationship for it to be successful. It benefits some midwives to change their supervisor every few years, while others feel the need for a longer-term relationship.

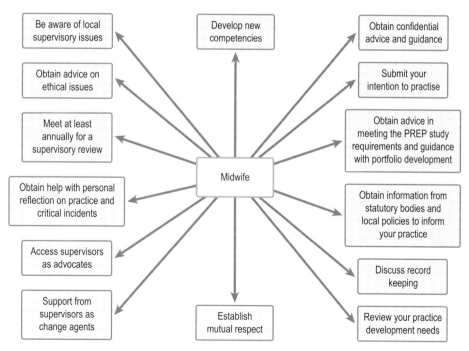

Fig. 2.1 Making the most of supervision.
(From Modern supervision in action, a practical guide for midwives, LSAMO Forum UK 2009, with permission from the Local Supervising Authority Midwifery Officers Forum UK.)

CLINICAL GOVERNANCE

Clinical governance was introduced in British health policy as a term to describe the accountability processes for the *safety*, *quality* and *effectiveness* of clinical care delivered to service users (DH 1997; Scottish Executive 1997; Welsh Office 1998; Department of Health, Social Services and Public Safety [DHSSPS] 2001). It was originally defined in First Class Service (DH 1998: 33) as

> *a framework through which NHS organizations are accountable for continuously improving the quality of their services and safeguarding high standards of care by creating an environment in which excellence in clinical care will flourish.*

According to Jaggs-Fowler (2011), clinical governance has developed beyond simply being a moral principle and is now a *statutory duty* for all NHS organizations to address, forming part of the overall drive to improve quality. It is just one component of the management tools variously known as *total quality management* and *continuous quality improvement*.

As part of implementing the concept of clinical governance, two government-appointed bodies, the National Institute for Health and Clinical Excellence [NICE] (known as the National Institute for Health and Care Excellence from 2013) and the National Commissioning Board (a peer and lay body), were initially introduced in England to standardize, improve and assess the quality of clinical practice on a national basis. However, with the extensive reorganization of the National Health Service (NHS) as a result of the Health and Social Care Act 2012, five key national bodies have been assigned to coordinate consistent governance of the NHS in England:

- The Department of Health
- The NHS Commissioning Board: NHS England
- The National Institute for Health and Care Excellence
- The Care Quality Commission
- The economic regulator Monitor.

Clinical Commissioning Groups (CCGs) now operate as statutory bodies replacing Primary Care Trusts (PCTs) and Strategic Health Authorities (SHAs) and consequently have taken over the responsibility for commissioning the vast majority of NHS services, including hospital care, community and mental health services. In addition, local CCGs are responsible for monitoring the quality of the care provided.

Within the context of local midwifery practice, the focus of clinical governance lies in the effective partnership between women and health professionals and the establishment of midwifery networks where the voice of service users assists in shaping local maternity services, policies,

protocols, guidelines and standards. In addition, professional bodies endorse the importance of health professionals working, learning and collaborating to provide safe and effective care to childbearing women, their babies and families (Royal College of Obstetricians and Gynaecologists [RCOG], RCM, Royal College of Anaesthetists [RCoA], Royal College of Paediatrics and Child Health [RCPCH] 2007; RCOG, RCM, RCoA 2008; RCOG 2009). Regular monitoring visits by the LSA Midwifery Officer, and by national bodies such as the Care Quality Commission (CQC) (England), Healthcare Improvement Scotland, Healthcare Inspectorate Wales, the Regulation and Quality Improvement Authority (Northern Ireland) and periodical assessments by the NMC means that, from a clinical governance perspective, there can be confidence in the standard of care provided in each maternity unit.

The key components of clinical governance

Clinical governance should be an integrated process in all aspects of health care delivery and the various processes underpinning it should in themselves be integrated with each other (Jaggs-Fowler 2011). With this in mind the key components of clinical governance can be grouped into three main categories: *clinical effectiveness, risk management* and *patient focus and public involvement,* all of which contribute to the delivery of high-quality care as summarized in Box 2.9. However, it may also be prudent to acknowledge that effective leadership and interpersonal skills are also vital components to the successful governance of an organization.

Policies, protocols, guidelines and standards

All healthcare providers are required to have policies, protocols, guidelines and standards in place to govern safe, effective and quality care to the public. It is important that midwives understand the differences between these definitions in order to utilize them appropriately in their clinical practice.

Policies are general principles or directions, usually without the mandatory approach for addressing an issue. They are a means of ensuring a consistent standard of care to avoid any confusion over practice and are often set at national level, for example *Midwifery 2020* (DH 2010) and *A Refreshed Framework for Maternity Services in Scotland* (Scottish Government 2011). Policies should make clear the procedures that will be followed by midwives, doctors and support staff. There are differing views about the benefits of policies, ranging from ensuring safe practice and providing consistency, to restricting midwives' autonomy. Indeed, if a midwife's clinical judgement on an individual woman's care is at odds with policy, she may be in breach

---

Box 2.9 Key components of clinical governance

Clinical effectiveness	• evidence-based practice
	• quality improvement tools (such as clinical audit and evaluation) to review and improve treatments and services based on:
	  – the views of patients, service users and staff
	  – evidence from incidents, near-misses, clinical risks and risk analysis
	  – outcomes from treatments or services
	  – measurement of performance to assess whether the team/department/organization is achieving the desired goals
	  – identifying areas of care that need further research
	• information systems to assess current practice and provide evidence of improvement
	• assessment of evidence as to whether services/treatments are cost effective
	• high-quality data and record keeping
	• workforce planning
	• promoting individual learning and learning across the organization
	  – professional development programmes
	  – dissemination of good practice, ideas and innovation
	  – supervision of midwives

Risk management	• clinical risk reduction • supervision of midwives • learning lessons from near misses • detection of adverse events • ensuring action is taken to prevent recurrence • addressing poor clinical performance
Patient focus and public involvement	• involving patients in decisions about their care • involving patients and carers in improving services • learning lessons from complaints

of her contract of employment unless she can justify her actions.

The term *protocol* is often used interchangeably with 'guideline'. A protocol is usually regarded as a local initiative that practitioners are expected to follow, but may also vary in meaning, e.g. a written agreement between parties, a multidisciplinary action plan for managing care, or an action plan for a clinical trial. Protocols therefore determine individual aspects of practice and should be based on the latest evidence. Most protocols are binding on employees as they usually relate to the management of individuals with urgent, life-threatening conditions, for example antepartum haemorrhage, such that if the practitioner does not work within the protocol they would be deemed to be in breach of their employment contract. However, it would not be expected to have protocols for the care of healthy women experiencing a physiological labour and birth.

Guidelines are usually less specific than protocols and may be described as suggestions for criteria or levels of performance that are provided to implement agreed *standards*. Both guidelines and standards should be based on contemporary, reliable research findings and include specific outcomes which act as performance indicators, upon which progress can be measured as evidence of achievement within an agreed timescale. The National Institute

for Health and Care Excellence (NICE) sets guidelines for clinical practice in all areas of health care, including maternity and neonatal care to provide good practice guidance for midwives and obstetricians. Supervisors of midwives play an important role in facilitating midwives to implement these guidelines within their own scope of practice. The interpretation and application of a guideline remains the responsibility of individual practitioners, as they should be aware of local circumstances and the needs and wishes of informed women. Guidelines are therefore tools to assist the midwife in making the most appropriate clinical decision in partnership with the woman, based on best available evidence.

It is acknowledged that there is a plethora of clinical guidelines not only produced by NICE but also organizations such as the Scottish Intercollegiate Guidelines Network (SIGN), RCOG and RCM. However, as variations in outcomes persist, it is essential that commissioners build into their contracts the requirements to deliver services to national standards and to manage performance against these. It is the responsibility of the Care Quality Commission in England, Healthcare Improvement Scotland, the Regulator and Quality Improvement Authority in Northern Ireland and Healthcare Inspectorate Wales to monitor health services against national standards in the respective UK countries.

Audit

Clinical audit is a process that is undertaken to review and evaluate the effectiveness of practice by measuring standards of health/midwifery care against national benchmarks. It is important to ensure that the auditing process is comprehensive, multidisciplinary and centred upon the women who receive the care and that the audit loop is closed completely. This means that should the data collected reveal any shortfall in meeting clinical standards, strategies to rectify such a deficit should always be implemented. Furthermore, when a change in practice is implemented, there should always be an evaluation to ensure the audit cycle develops into an audit spiral, leading to improved health care.

In midwifery, local surveys should take place regularly to monitor women's satisfaction with their maternity care to ensure these achieve the expected standards as well as identify areas for improvement. To address clinical governance, each maternity unit/service is expected to publish its local statistics and monitor generic indicators of the effectiveness and efficiency of health care. Such outcomes include healthcare-acquired infection (HCAI), infant mortality, neonatal mortality and stillbirths, women's experiences of childbirth and admission of full-term babies to neonatal care (DH 2012), as shown in Box 2.10.

Health care-associated infections (HCAIs) have become the subject of considerable public interest as a consequence in the rise in methicillin-resistant *Staphylococcus aureus* ('MRSA') and *Clostridium difficile* ('C. diff'). This is of particular concern to the maternity services as the latest Confidential Enquiries into maternal deaths reported that the leading cause of *direct* deaths during the triennium 2006–2008 was *sepsis*, accounting for 26 deaths (Harper 2011). Consequently, the prevention of infection was one of the top 10 recommendations from the report. However, with the introduction of a national strategy to reduce the rates of MRSA and C. diff, there is evidence that the rates of both types of infection have more than halved (National Patient Safety Agency [NPSA] 2007a, 2007b; National Audit Office 2009).

Box 2.10	**NHS outcomes framework relating to maternity care**	

Domain	Overarching indicators	Improvement areas

1. **Preventing people from dying prematurely**
 	
4. **Ensuring that people have a positive experience of care**
	1a. Potential Years of Life Lost (PYLL) from causes amenable to health care:
	   ii. *Children and young people*
	4a. Patient experience of primary care:
	   i. *GP services*
	   ii. *GP out of hours services*
	   iii. *NHS dental services*
	4b. Patient experience of hospital care
	4c. Friends and family test
		Reducing deaths in babies and young children:
		1.6.i. *infant mortality*
		   ii. *neonatal mortality and stillbirths*
		Improving people's experiences of outpatient care:
		4.1. *Patient experience of outpatient services*
		Improving hospitals' responsiveness to personal needs:
		4.2. *Responsiveness to in-patient personal needs*
		Improving access to primary care services:
		4.4. *Access to*
		   i. *GP services and*
		   ii. *NHS dental services*
		Improving women and their families' experience of maternity services:
		4.5. *Women's experiences of maternity services*

5. **Treating and caring for people in a safe environment and protect them from avoidable harm**	5a. Patient safety incidents reported
	5b. Safety incidents involving severe harm or death
	5c. Hospital deaths attributable to problems in care
		Reducing the incidence of avoidable harm:
		5.1. *Incidence of hospital-related venous thromboembolism (VTE)*
		5.2. *Incidence of healthcare associated infection (HCAI)*
		   i. *MRSA*
		   ii. *C. difficile*
		5.3. *Incidence of newly acquired category 2,3 and 4 pressure ulcers*
		5.4. *Incidences of medication errors causing serious harm*
		Improving the safety of maternity services:
		5.5. *Admission of full-term babies to neonatal care*

Source: NHS outcomes framework, 2013–2014 (DH 2012)

Risk management

Risk management is the systematic identification, analysis and control of any potential and actual risk and of any circumstances that put individuals at risk of harm. The concept was introduced in the mid-1990s with the principal aim of reducing litigation costs. Organizations such as the UK NHS are expected to adhere to the legislation pertaining to health and safety in the work place and other legal principles such as *the duty of care* to both the public and employees as part of their risk management strategy (CQC 2010; NHSLA 2013). Managing risk is therefore a fundamental component of clinical governance.

When a risk is evaluated it is not only important to consider the *probability* of something adverse happening but also the *consequences* if it should happen. In the context of health care, risk is usually associated with health risks, injury and death. More specifically within the context of maternity care, the *risk of harm* would include injury to a woman and/or her baby during childbirth or to a health professional engaged in providing maternity care. The *risk of detriment* is associated with some form of economic/social loss, which may not only include a valuation of harm to individuals but also damage on a much wider scale, such as adverse publicity for the local maternity services. All health service managers are expected to be conversant in risk management theory in order to identify and manage risk so that the probability of harm or detriment is lessened and the consequences of risk are reduced.

The introduction of the *Modified Early Obstetric Warning Scoring* (MEOWS) system (NICE 2007; DH 2009b; Centre for Maternal and Child Enquiries [CMACE] 2011) has contributed to the recognition of early warning signs in those women identified at risk of developing serious complications and life-threatening conditions to prompt earlier initiation of high-level care and more senior involvement in care planning and management.

Poor communication among health professionals is often criticized as being the commonest cause of preventable adverse outcomes in hospitals and a significant cause of written complaints (Health and Social Care Information Centre [HSCIC] 2012). An inquiry into the safety of birth in England found that when there are increased risks to the woman or baby, that render some births *less safe*, *functioning teams* are the key to improving the outcome for the woman and baby (Kings Fund 2008).

The use of the *Situation, Background, Assessment* and *Recommendation* (SBAR) tool (NHS Institute for Innovation and Improvement 2008) can assist in improving communication among members of the multiprofessional team. Its purpose is to enable health professionals to frame concise and focused information about the condition of a childbearing woman that requires immediate attention and action. Consequently, the SBAR tool assists in clarifying which information should be communicated between health professionals, enabling the development of efficient teamwork and the fostering of a culture of safety (RCOG 2009).

Clinical Negligence Scheme for Trusts (CNST)

The Clinical Negligence Scheme for Trusts (CNST) is a voluntary risk-pooling scheme for negligence claims arising out of incidents occurring after 1 April 1995. It is administered by the NHSLA, and all NHS Trusts, Foundation Trusts and Clinical Commissioning Groups (formerly PCTS) in England subscribe to CNST by paying an insurance premium based on their individual compliance to certain general standards. There are equivalent schemes in Scotland (Clinical Negligence and Other Risks Indemnity Scheme [CNORIS]), in Wales (the Welsh Risk Pool) and Northern Ireland. The NHSLA (2013) have produced a special standard for maternity services with a set of additional criteria and minimum requirements for specific situations. The basis of the standard relate to the following:

- organization
- clinical care
- high-risk conditions
- communication
- postnatal and neonatal care.

Consequently, risk management is an essential mission with significant funding implications for all healthcare providers striving for excellence.

It has been reported by the NHSLA (2012) that within the decade 2000–2010 over £3.1 billion was paid out in damages in a total of 5087 maternity claims to babies and mothers who were injured as a result of harm incurred during childbirth. In this period there were 5.5 million births, thus less than 1 in every 1000 births (0.1%) had become the subject of a claim, indicating that the vast majority of births do *not* result in a clinical negligence claim. Nevertheless, although obstetric and gynaecology claims accounted for 20% of the total number of claims the NHSLA received, it is significant to note that this area of practice was in fact responsible for 49% of the total value as compensation often involves 24-hour care for the claimant for the rest of their lives.

Clinical governance, risk management and statutory supervision of midwives

The statutory supervision of midwives is a vital element of leadership and clinical governance within the maternity services that also supports risk management by monitoring the development of maternity services and standards of midwifery practice such that women receive care that is both safe and of a high quality. An illustration of how the statutory supervision of midwives sits within clinical governance.

The nature of statutory supervision of midwives can limit the volume of *serious adverse incidents* within an organization by its supportive educative function to each individual midwife. In addition, the LSA Midwifery Officers regularly monitor standards of practice against documented evidence such as the Confidential Enquiries into Maternal Deaths, stillbirths and infant deaths reports as well as national standards and guidelines, through their supervisory audit visits to each maternity unit. Where there are unacceptable variations in clinical midwifery practice or care is inappropriate for women's needs, the LSA Midwifery Officer as an outside assessor is in a position to recommend remedial action (NMC 2012a). In addition, the LSA can contribute to the dissemination of national standards, such as safeguarding practices, to ensure the implementation of the most effective care at a local level.

Local Supervising Authorities (LSAs) must publish guidelines for investigating incidents including *near misses*, complaints or concerns relating to midwifery practice or allegations of impaired fitness to practice against a midwife

(NMC 2012b: Rule 10). The guidelines should include a time frame for the investigation and a communication strategy between the supervisor of midwives, the LSA and the employer (if the midwife is employed), a support mechanism for the midwife undergoing investigation and a procedure for obtaining an account of the woman and her family's experience. There should also be details of the action to be taken upon completion of the investigation, including disseminating the report and reporting to the midwife's employer or other healthcare regulators should the investigation find issues with systems or governance or other professions that may have contributed to unsafe practice. On occasion supervisory investigations are conducted by supervisors outside of the area where the practice concern arose. The benefits of externally led investigations as determined by Paeglis (2012: 25) include:

- no confusion for the midwives or employers that this is a LSA and not a management process;
- complete objectivity;
- a *fresh eyes* approach to practice issues that might previously have been accepted as custom and practice;

Box 2.11 **Outcomes arising from a Local Supervisory Authority investigation and subsequent actions taken**

No action	Local Action Plan with supervisor of midwives	LSA practice programme [*The Programme*]	NMC referral
It is advisable to share good practice arising from the investigation with stakeholders.	Minor mistakes. No risk of recurrence. Undertaken as soon as possible after event. Corrected through: • Reflection on the incident. • Continuing professional development relevant to the issue that caused concern. LSA informed of successful completion. Records kept of: • Discussions between the midwife and supervisor. • All actions taken. • Learning outcomes achieved.	Undertaken when development and assessment of a midwife's practice is required. LSA retains oversight of the programme which should be: • Planned jointly between investigating supervisor, the midwife, her named supervisor of midwives and a midwife educator. • Structured to include objectives and learning outcomes. • Based on competencies and essential skills clusters set in the Standards for pre-registration midwifery education (NMC 2009a). • Completed within a minimum of 150 hours and a maximum of 450 hours (extension of 150 hours permitted in some instances). LSA should allow protected time for the midwife to undertake *The Programme*.	Required if investigation or *The Programme* subsequently identifies the midwife's fitness to practise may be impaired. LSA may decide it is appropriate to *suspend a midwife from practice* in accordance with Rule 14 (NMC 2012b).

Source: Midwives Rules and Standards (NMC 2012b)

- sharing of good midwifery and supervisory practice and of lessons learned.

Should there be an appeal against a decision, the LSA Midwifery Officer is responsible for convening a local panel to review the handling of the investigation and the outcome in order to decide upon any further action.

Following an investigation, the LSA may recommend *no action, local action under the supervision of a named supervisor of midwives* or a *LSA practice programme/referral to the NMC*. Box 2.11 identifies the outcomes arising from a LSA investigation and the subsequent actions taken.

REFERENCES

Bacon L 2011 What does the future hold for the role of the local supervising authority? British Journal of Midwifery 19:439–42

Beauchamp T L, Childress J F 2012 Principles of biomedical ethics, 7th edn. Oxford University Press, Oxford

Bergman R 1981 Accountability: definition and dimensions. International Nursing Review 28(2):53–9

Bristol Royal Infirmary Inquiry (chair I Kennedy) 2001 Learning from Bristol: Report of the Public Inquiry into children's heart surgery at the Bristol Royal Infirmary 1984–1995. TSO, London

CQC (Care Quality Commission) 2010 Guidance about compliance: essential standards of quality and safety. CQC, London

CMACE (Centre for Maternal and Child Enquiries) 2011 Saving mothers' lives: reviewing maternal deaths to make motherhood safer: 2006–08. The Eighth Report on Confidential Enquiries into Maternal Deaths in the United Kingdom. BJOG: An International Journal of Obstetrics and Gynaecology 118(Suppl 1): 1–203

Clothier C, Macdonald C A, Shaw D A 1994 The Allitt Inquiry: Independent Inquiry relating to deaths and injuries on the children's ward at Grantham and Kesteven General Hospital during the period February to April 1991. HMSO, London

CHRE (Council for Healthcare Regulatory Excellence) 2008 Special report to the Minister of State for Health on the Nursing and Midwifery Council. CHRE, London

DH (Department of Health) 1997 The new NHS: modern, dependable. TSO, London

DH (Department of Health) 1998 First class service. HMSO, London

DH (Department of Health) 2007 Trust, assurance and safety: the regulation of health professions in the 21st century. CM7013. TSO, London

DH (Department of Health) 2009a Reference guide to consent for examination or treatment, 2nd edn. TSO, London

DH (Department of Health) 2009b Competencies for recognising and responding to acutely ill patients in hospital. TSO, London

DH (Department of Health) 2010 Midwifery 2020: delivering expectations. TSO, London

DH (Department of Health) 2011 Safeguarding adults: the role of health service practitioners. DH, London

DH (Department of Health) 2012 NHS outcomes framework, 2013–2014. TSO, London

DHSSPS (Department of Health, Social Services and Public Safety) 2001 Best practice – best care: a framework for setting standards, delivering services and improving monitoring and regulation in the HPSS. DHSSPS, Belfast

Edwards S D 1996 Nursing ethics: a principle-based approach. Macmillan, Basingstoke

ENB (English National Board for Nursing, Midwifery and Health Visiting) 1992 Preparation of supervisors of midwives: an open learning programme. ENB, London

Harper A 2011 Sepsis. In: Centre for Maternal and Child Enquiries (CMACE) Saving mothers' lives: reviewing maternal deaths to make motherhood safer: 2006–2008. The Eighth Report on Confidential

Enquiries into Maternal Deaths in the United Kingdom. BJOG: An International Journal of Obstetrics and Gynaecology 118(Suppl 1): 85–96

Heagerty B V 1996 Reassessing the guilty: the Midwives Act and the control of English midwives in the early 20th century. In: Kirkham M (ed) Supervision of midwives. Books for Midwives, Hale, Cheshire, p 13–27

HSCIC (Health and Social Care Information Centre) 2012 Data on written complaints in the NHS 2011–2012. NHS Office of Statistics, Leeds

HM Government 2007 Learning from tragedy: keeping patients safe. Overview of the government's action programme in response to the recommendations of the Shipman Inquiry. Cm 7014. TSO, London

HM Government 2013 Working together to safeguard children: a guide to inter-agency working to safeguard and promote the welfare of children. Available at: www.education.gov.uk/aboutdfe/statutory/g00213160/working-together-to-safeguard-children (accessed 28 August 2013).

ICM (International Confederation of Midwives) 2011 Definition of the midwife. Available at www.internationalmidwives.org (accessed 13 August 2013)

Jaggs-Fowler R M 2011 Clinical governance. InnovAiT 4:592–5

Kings Fund 2008 Safe births: everybody's business. An independent inquiry into the safety of maternity services in England. Kings Fund, London

Kirkham M (ed) 1996 Supervision of midwives. Books for Midwives, Hale, Cheshire

LSAMO (Local Supervising Authority Midwifery Officer) Forum UK 2009 Modern Supervision in action: a practical guide for midwives. Available at www.lsamoforumuk .scot.nhs.uk/midwives.aspx (accessed 30 July 2013)

Melia K 1989 Everyday nursing ethics. Macmillan, London

Mid Staffordshire NHS Foundation Trust Public Inquiry (chair R Francis) 2013 Report of the Mid Staffordshire NHS Foundation Trust Public Inquiry. Executive Summary. HC 947. TSO, London. Available at www.midstaffspublicinquiry.com (accessed 20 August 2013)

National Audit Office 2009 Reducing healthcare associated infections in hospitals in England. TSO, London

National Health Service Institute for Innovation and Improvement 2008 SBAR: Situation, Background, Assessment and Recommendation Tool. Available at www.institute .nhs.uk/quality_and_service _improvement_tools/quality (accessed 30 July 2013)

NHSLA (National Health Service Litigation Authority) 2012 Ten years of maternity claims: an analysis of the NHS litigation authority data. NHSLA, London

NHSLA (National Health Service Litigation Authority) 2013 Clinical negligence for trusts: maternity clinical risk management standards. NHSLA, London

NICE (National Institute for Health and Clinical Excellence) 2007 Acutely ill patients in hospital: recognition of and response to acute illness in adults in hospital. NICE, London

National Patient Safety Agency 2007a The national specifications for cleanliness in the NHS: a framework for setting and measuring performance outcomes. NPSA, London

National Patient Safety Agency 2007b Clean hands save lives: patient safety alert, 2nd edn. NPSA, London

NMC (Nursing and Midwifery Council) 2006a Standards of proficiency for nurse and midwife prescribers. NMC, London

NMC (Nursing and Midwifery Council) 2006b Standards for the preparation and practice of supervisors of midwives. NMC, London

NMC (Nursing and Midwifery Council) 2007a Standards for medicines management. NMC, London

NMC (Nursing and Midwifery Council) 2007b Statutory supervision of midwives: a resource for midwives and mothers. Quay Books, London

NMC (Nursing and Midwifery Council) 2008 The NMC Code: standards of conduct, performance and ethics for nurses and midwives. NMC, London

NMC (Nursing and Midwifery Council) 2009a Standards for pre-registration midwifery education. NMC, London

NMC (Nursing and Midwifery Council) 2009b Record keeping: guidance for nurses and midwives. NMC, London

NMC (Nursing and Midwifery Council) 2011 The PREP handbook. NMC, London

NMC (Nursing and Midwifery Council) 2012a Annual fitness to practise report 2011–2012: presented to Parliament pursuant to Article 50 (2) of the Nursing and Midwifery Order 2001, as amended by the Nursing and Midwifery (Amendment) Order 2008. TSO, London

NMC (Nursing and Midwifery Council) 2012b Midwives Rules and Standards. NMC, London

NMC (Nursing and Midwifery Council) 2012c Social networking sites. Available at www.nmc-uk.org .nurses-and-midwives/Advice-by -topic/A/Advice/Social-neworking -sites/ (accessed 13 August 2013)

NMC (Nursing and Midwifery Council) 2013 Midwifery regulation. Available at www.nmc-uk.org/Nurses-and -midwives/Midwifery-New/ (accessed 13 August 2013)

Paeglis C 2012 Supervision: a 'fresh eyes approach', The Practising Midwife 15(1):24–6

RCOG (Royal College of Obstetricians and Gynaecologists) 2009 Improving patient safety: risk management for maternity and gynaecology: Clinical Governance Advice 2. RCOG Press, London

RCOG, RCM, RCoA (Royal College of Obstetricians and Gynaecologists, Royal College of Midwives, Royal College of Anaesthetists) 2008 Standards for maternity care: report of a working party. RCOG Press, London

RCOG, RCM, RCoA, RCPCH (Royal College of Obstetricians and Gynaecologists, Royal College of Midwives, Royal College of Anaesthetists, Royal College of Paediatrics and Child Health) 2007 Safer childbirth: minimum standards for the organisation and delivery of care in labour. RCOG Press, London

Scottish Executive 1997 Designed to care: renewing the National Health Service in Scotland. Edinburgh: Scottish Executive Health Department

Scottish Government 2011 Framework for maternity care in Scotland. The Maternity Services Action Group. Scottish Government, Edinburgh. Available at www.scotland.gov.uk/ Resource/Doc/337644/0110854.pdf (accessed 2 August 2013)

Stapleton H, Duerden J, Kirkham M 1998 Evaluation of the impact of the supervision of midwives on professional practice and the quality of midwifery care. ENB, London

UKCC (United Kingdom Central Council for Nursing Midwifery and Health Visiting) 1997 Midwives refresher courses and PREP. UKCC, London

UKCC (United Kingdom Central Council for Nursing Midwifery and Health Visiting) 1998 Midwives rules and code of practice. UKCC, London

Welsh Office 1998 NHS Wales quality care and clinical excellence. Welsh Office, Cardiff

CASES

Bolam v Friern Hospital Management Committee [HMC] 1957 1 WLR 582

Gillick v West Norfolk and Wisbech AHA 1985 3 All ER 402

STATUTES, ORDERS AND DIRECTIVES

Charities Act 1993. HMSO, London

Congenital Disabilities (Civil Liability) Act 1976. HMSO, London

Data Protection Act 1998. HMSO, London

Directive 2005/36/EC of the European Parliament and of the Council of 7 September 2005 on the recognition of professional qualifications. Article 42 Pursuit of the professional activities of a midwife. http://eur-lex. europa.eu/LexUriServ/LexUriServ.do? uri=OJ:L:2005:255:0022:0142:en: PDF

European Convention for the Protection of Human Rights and Fundamental Freedoms 1951. HMSO, London

Health Act 1999. HMSO, London

Health Care and Associated Professions (Indemnity Arrangements) Order 2013 [The Indemnity Order]. TSO, London

Health and Safety at Work etc. Act 1974. HMSO, London

Health and Social Care Act 2007. TSO, London

Health and Social Care Act 2008. TSO, London

Health and Social Care Act 2012. TSO, London

Human Medicines Regulations 2012 Statutory Instrument 2012 No. 1916. TSO, London

Human Rights Act 1998. HMSO, London

Medicines Act 1968. HMSO, London

Mental Capacity Act 2005. TSO, London

Midwives Act 1902 (England and Wales). HMSO, London

Midwives (Scotland) Act 1915. HMSO, London

Midwives (Ireland) Act 1918. HMSO, London

Midwives Act 1936. HMSO, London

Midwives Act 1951. HMSO, London

Midwives (Scotland) 1951 Act. HMSO, London

National Health Service (Reorganisation) Act 1973. HMSO, London

Nursing and Midwifery Order 2001 Statutory Instrument 2002 No. 253 [The Order]. TSO, London

Nurses, Midwives and Health Visitors Act 1979. HMSO, London

Nurses, Midwives and Health Visitors Act 1992. HMSO, London

Nurses, Midwives and Health Visitors Act 1997. HMSO, London

Protection of Vulnerable Groups (Scotland) Act 2007. TSO, Edinburgh

Safeguarding Vulnerable Groups (Northern Ireland) Order 2007 Statutory Instrument No. 1351 (NI 11). TSO, Belfast

Safeguarding Vulnerable Groups Act 2006 (Controlled Activity and Miscellaneous Provisions) Regulations 2010 Statutory Instrument 2010 No. 1146. TSO, London

FURTHER READING

Beauchamp T L, Childress J F 2012 Principles of biomedical ethics, 7th edn. Oxford University Press, Oxford
This popular best-selling text provides a highly original, practical and insightful guide to morality in the health professions. Drawing from contemporary research and integrating detailed case studies and vivid real-life examples and scenarios, the authors demonstrate how ethical principles can be expanded to apply to various conflicts and dilemmas in clinical practice.

LSA Midwifery Officers Forum UK 2009 Modern supervision in action – a practical guide for midwives. NMC, London
This useful book helps midwives to get the most out of supervision. It is very user-friendly and explains the supervision of midwives very succinctly from the perspective of the midwife rather than the supervisor of midwives.

USEFUL WEBSITES

Care Quality Commission (CQC) (England): www.cqc.org.uk

Government departments (including Health): www.gov.uk

HealthCare Improvement (Scotland): www.healthcareimprovement scotland.org

Healthcare Inspectorate (Wales): www.hiw.org.uk

International Confederation of Midwives (ICM): www.internationalmidwives.org

Medicines and Healthcare Products Regulatory Agency (MHPRA): www.mhra.gov.uk

National Health Service Improving Quality (formerly NHS Institute for Innovation and Improvement): www.hsiq.nhs.uk

National Health Service Litigation Authority (NHSLA): www.nhsla.com

NHS England: www.england.nhs.uk

Nursing and Midwifery Council (NMC): www.nmc-uk.org

Professional Standards Authority (PSA): www.professionalstandards.org.uk

Regulation and Quality Improvement Authority (Northern Ireland): www.rqia.org.uk

Royal College of Anaesthetists: www.rcoa.ac.uk

Royal College of Midwives: www.rcm.org.uk

Royal College of Obstetricians and Gynaecologists: www.rcog.org.uk

Royal College of Paediatrics and Child Health: www.rcpch.ac.uk

Scottish Intercollegiate Guidelines Network: www.sign.ac.uk

The Scottish Government: www.scotland.gov.uk

Section | 2 |

Human anatomy and reproduction

Chapter | 3 |

The female pelvis and the reproductive organs

Ranee Thakar, Abdul H Sultan

It is important that midwives are well versed in the applied anatomy of the female pelvis and understand the processes of reproduction.

THE CHAPTER AIMS TO:

- cover the basic anatomy of the female and male reproductive system
- identify the main functions of the internal and external female and male genital organs.

FEMALE EXTERNAL GENITAL ORGANS

The female external genitalia (the vulva) include the mons pubis, labia majora, labia minora, clitoris, vestibule, the greater vestibular glands (Bartholin's glands) and bulbs of the vestibule (Fig. 3.1).

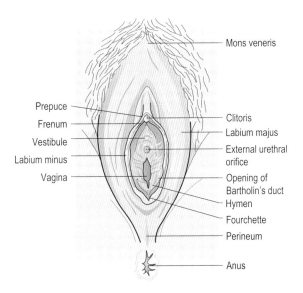

Fig. 3.1 Female external genital organs (vulva).

- The mons pubis is a rounded pad of fat lying anterior to the symphysis pubis. It is covered with pubic hair from the time of puberty.
- The labia majora ('greater lips') are two folds of fat and areolar tissue which are covered with skin and pubic hair on the outer surface and have a pink, smooth inner surface.
- The labia minora ('lesser lips') are two small subcutaneous folds, devoid of fat, that lie between the labia majora. Anteriorly, each labium minus divides into two parts: the upper layer passes above the clitoris to form along with its fellow a fold, the prepuce, which overhangs the clitoris. The prepuce is a retractable piece of skin which surrounds and protects the clitoris. The lower layer passes below the clitoris to form with its fellow the frenulum of the clitoris.
- The clitoris is a small rudimentary sexual organ corresponding to the male penis. The visible knob-like portion is located near the anterior junction of the labia minora, above the opening of the urethra and vagina. Unlike the penis, the clitoris does not contain the distal portion of the urethra and functions solely to induce the orgasm during sexual intercourse.
- The vestibule is the area enclosed by the labia minora in which the openings of the urethra and the vagina are situated.
- The urethral orifice lies 2.5 cm posterior to the clitoris and immediately in front of the vaginal orifice. On either side lie the openings of the Skene's ducts, two small blind-ended tubules 0.5 cm long running within the urethral wall.

- The vaginal orifice, also known as the introitus of the vagina, occupies the posterior two-thirds of the vestibule. The orifice is partially closed by the hymen, a thin membrane that tears during sexual intercourse. The remaining tags of hymen are known as the 'carunculae myrtiformes' because they are thought to resemble myrtle berries.
- The greater vestibular glands (Bartholin's glands) are two small glands that open on either side of the vaginal orifice and lie in the posterior part of the labia majora. They secrete mucus, which lubricates the vaginal opening. The duct may occasionally become blocked, which can cause the secretions from the gland to accommodate within it and form a cyst.
- The bulbs of the vestibule are two elongated erectile masses flanking the vaginal orifice.

Blood supply

The blood supply comes from the internal and the external pudendal arteries. The blood drains through corresponding veins.

Lymphatic drainage

Lymphatic drainage is mainly via the inguinal glands.

Innervation

The nerve supply is derived from branches of the pudendal nerve.

THE PERINEUM

The perineum corresponds to the outlet of the pelvis and is somewhat lozenge-shaped. Anteriorly, it is bound by the pubic arch, posteriorly by the coccyx, and laterally by the ischiopubic rami, ischial tuberosities and sacrotuberous ligaments. The perineum can be divided into two triangular parts by drawing an arbitrary line transversely between the ischial tuberosities. The anterior triangle, which contains the external urogenital organs, is known as the *urogenital triangle* and the posterior triangle, which contains the termination of the anal canal, is known as the *anal triangle*.

The urogenital triangle

The urogenital triangle (Fig. 3.2a) is bound anteriorly and laterally by the pubic symphysis and the ischiopubic rami. The urogenital triangle has been divided into two compartments: the superficial and deep perineal spaces, separated by the perineal membrane which spans the space between the ischiopubic rami. The levator ani muscles are attached to the cranial surface of the perineal membrane. The vestibular bulb and clitoral crus lie on the caudal surface of the membrane and are fused with it. These erectile tissues are covered by the bulbospongiosus and the ischiocavernosus muscles.

Superficial muscles of the perineum

Superficial transverse perineal muscle

The superficial transverse muscle is a narrow slip of a muscle that arises from the inner and forepart of the ischial tuberosity and is inserted into the central tendinous part of the perineal body (Fig. 3.2a). The muscle from the opposite side, the external anal sphincter (EAS) from behind, and the bulbospongiosus in the front, all attach to the central tendon of the perineal body.

Bulbospongiosus muscle

The bulbospongiosus (previously known as bulbocavernosus) muscle runs on either side of the vaginal orifice, covering the lateral aspects of the vestibular bulb anteriorly and the Bartholin's gland posteriorly (Fig. 3.2b). Some fibres merge posteriorly with the superficial transverse perineal muscle and the EAS in the central fibromuscular perineal body. Anteriorly, its fibres pass forward on either side of the vagina and insert into the corpora cavernosa clitoridis, a fasciculus crossing over the body of the organ so as to compress the deep dorsal vein. This muscle diminishes the orifice of the vagina and contributes to the erection of the clitoris.

Ischiocavernosus muscle

The ischiocavernosus muscle is elongated, broader at the middle than at either end and is situated on the side of the lateral boundary of the perineum (Fig. 3.2a). It arises by tendinous and fleshy fibres from the inner surface of the ischial tuberosity, behind the crus clitoridis, from the surface of the crus and from the adjacent portions of the ischial ramus.

Innervation

The nerve supply is derived from branches of the pudendal nerve.

The anal triangle

This area includes the anal canal, the anal sphincters and the ischioanal fossae.

Anal canal

The rectum terminates in the anal canal (Fig. 3.3). The anal canal is attached posteriorly to the coccyx by the anococcygeal ligament, a midline fibromuscular structure that runs between the posterior aspect of the EAS and the coccyx. The anus is surrounded laterally and posteriorly by loose adipose tissue within the ischioanal fossae, which is a potential pathway for spread of perianal sepsis from one side to the other. The pudendal nerves pass over the ischial spines at this point and can be accessed for injection of local anaesthetic into the pudendal nerve at this site. Anteriorly, the perineal body separates the anal canal from the vagina.

The anal canal is surrounded by an inner epithelial lining, a vascular subepithelium, the internal anal sphincter (IAS), the EAS and fibromuscular supporting tissue. The lining of the anal canal varies along its length due to its embryologic derivation. The proximal anal canal is lined with rectal mucosa (columnar epithelium) and is arranged in vertical mucosal folds called the columns of Morgagni (Fig. 3.3). Each column contains a terminal radical of the superior rectal artery and vein. The vessels are largest in the left-lateral, right-posterior and right-anterior quadrants of the wall of the anal canal where the subepithelial tissues expand into three *anal cushions*. These cushions seal the anal canal and help maintain continence of flatus and liquid stools. The columns are joined together at their inferior margin by crescentic folds called anal valves. About 2 cm from the anal verge, the anal valves create a demarcation called the dentate line. Anoderm covers the last 1–1.5 cm of the distal canal below the dentate line and consists of modified squamous epithelium that lack skin adnexal tissues such as hair follicles and glands, but contains numerous somatic nerve endings. Since the epithelium in the lower canal is well supplied with sensory nerve endings, acute distension or invasive treatment of haemorrhoids in this area causes profuse discomfort, whereas treatment can be carried out with relatively few symptoms in the upper canal lined by insensate columnar epithelium. As a result of tonic circumferential contraction of the sphincter, the skin is arranged in radiating folds around the anus and is called the anal margin. These folds appear to be flat or ironed out when there is underlying sphincter damage. The junction between the columnar and squamous epithelia is referred to as the anal transitional zone, which is variable in height and position and often contains islands of squamous epithelium extending into columnar epithelium. This zone probably has a role to play in continence by providing a highly specialized sampling mechanism.

Anal sphincter complex

The anal sphincter complex consists of the EAS and IAS separated by the conjoint longitudinal coat (Fig. 3.3). Although they form a single unit, they are distinct in structure and function.

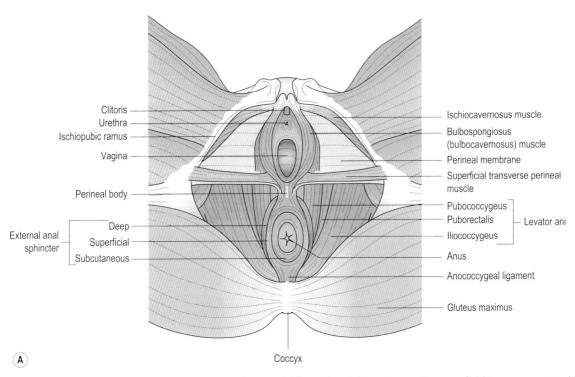

Clitoris
Urethra
Ischiopubic ramus
Vagina

Perineal body

Deep
External anal
sphincter
Superficial
Subcutaneous

Ischiocavernosus muscle
Bulbospongiosus
(bulbocavernosus) muscle
Perineal membrane
Superficial transverse perineal
muscle
Pubococcygeus
Puborectalis ⎤ Levator ani
Iliococcygeus ⎦
Anus
Anococcygeal ligament

Gluteus maximus

Coccyx

(A)

Fig. 3.2a Diagram of the perineum demonstrating the superficial muscles of the perineum. The superficial transverse perineal muscle, the bulbospongiosus and the ischiocavernosus form a triangle on either side of the perineum with a floor formed by the perineal membrane.

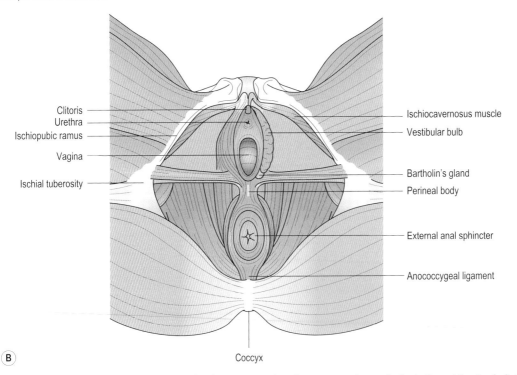

Clitoris
Urethra
Ischiopubic ramus
Vagina
Ischial tuberosity

Ischiocavernosus muscle
Vestibular bulb

Bartholin's gland
Perineal body

External anal sphincter

Anococcygeal ligament

Coccyx

(B)

Fig. 3.2b The left bulbospongiosus muscle has been removed to demonstrate the vestibular bulb and the Bartholin's gland.

58

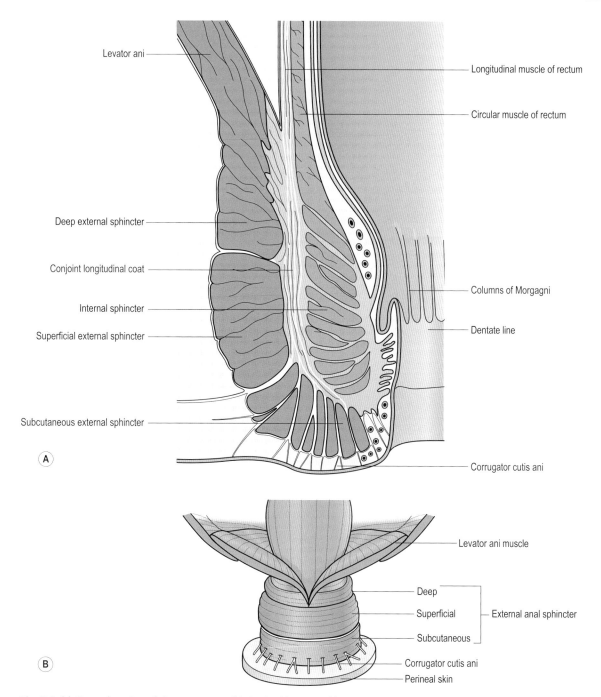

Fig. 3.3 (a) Coronal section of the anorectum. (b) Anal sphincter and levator ani.

External anal sphincter

The EAS comprises of striated muscle and appears red in colour (similar to raw red meat) (Fig. 3.4). As the EAS is normally under tonic contraction, it tends to retract when completely torn. A defect of the EAS can lead to urge faecal incontinence.

Internal anal sphincter

The IAS is a thickened continuation of the circular smooth muscle of the bowel and ends with a well-defined rounded edge 6–8 mm above the anal margin at the junction of the superficial and subcutaneous part of the EAS. In contrast to the EAS, the IAS has a pale appearance to the naked eye (Fig. 3.5). Defect of the IAS can lead to passive soiling of stools and flatus incontinence.

The longitudinal layer and the conjoint longitudinal coat

The longitudinal layer is situated between the EAS and IAS and consists of a fibromuscular layer, the conjoint longitudinal coat and the intersphincteric space with its connective tissue components (see Fig. 3.3).

Innervation of the anal sphincter complex

The nerve supply is derived from branches of the pudendal nerve.

Vascular supply

The anorectum receives its major blood supply from the superior haemorrhoidal (terminal branch of the inferior mesenteric artery) and inferior haemorrhoidal (branch of the pudendal artery) arteries, and to a lesser degree, from the middle haemorrhoidal artery (branch of the internal iliac), forming a wide intramural network of collaterals. The venous drainage of the upper anal canal mucosa, IAS and conjoint longitudinal coat passes via the terminal branches of the superior rectal vein into the inferior mesenteric vein. The lower anal canal and the EAS drain via the inferior rectal branch of the pudendal vein into the internal iliac vein.

Lymphatic drainage

The anorectum has a rich network of lymphatic plexuses. The dentate line represents the interface between the two different systems of lymphatic drainage. Above the dentate line (the upper anal canal), the IAS and the conjoint longitudinal coat drain into the inferior mesenteric and internal iliac nodes. Lymphatic drainage below the dentate line, which consists of the lower anal canal epithelium and the EAS, proceeds to the external inguinal lymph nodes.

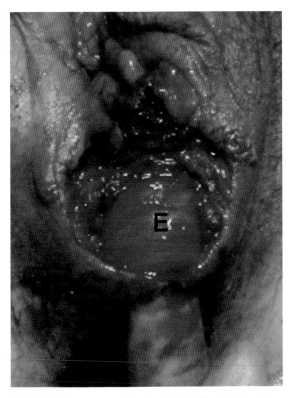

Fig. 3.4 An intact external anal sphincter (E) which is red in colour and appears like raw red meat.

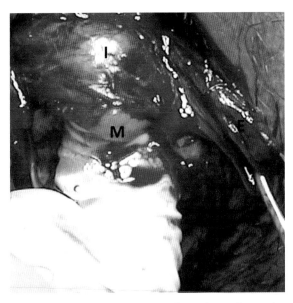

Fig. 3.5 The internal anal sphincter (I) is pale in colour and appears like raw white meat: E = external anal sphincter, M = mucosa.

The ischioanal fossa

The ischioanal fossa (previously known as the 'ischiorectal fossa') extends around the anal canal and is bound anteriorly by the perineal membrane, superiorly by the fascia of the levator ani muscle and medially by the EAS complex at the level of the anal canal. The ischioanal fossa contains fat and neurovascular structures, including the pudendal nerve and the internal pudendal vessels.

The perineal body

The perineal body is the central point between the urogenital and the anal triangles of the perineum (see Fig. 3.2a). Within the perineal body there are interlacing muscle fibres from the bulbospongiosus, superficial transverse perineal and EAS muscles. Above this level there is a contribution from the conjoint longitudinal coat and the medial fibres of the puborectalis muscle. Therefore, the support of the pelvic structures, and to some extent the hiatus urogenitalis between the levator ani muscles, depends upon the integrity of the perineal body.

THE PELVIC FLOOR

The pelvic floor is a musculotendinous sheet that spans the pelvic outlet and consists mainly of the symmetrically paired levator ani muscle (LAM) (Fig. 3.6), which is a broad muscular sheet of variable thickness attached to the internal surface of the true pelvis. Although there is controversy regarding the subdivisions of the muscle, it is broadly accepted that it is subdivided into parts according to their attachments, namely the pubovisceral (also known as pubococcygeus), puborectal and iliococcygeus. The pubovisceral part is further subdivided according to its relationship to the viscera, i.e. puboperinealis, pubovaginalis and puboanalis. The puborectalis muscle is located lateral to the pubovisceral muscle, cephalad to the deep component of the EAS, from which it is inseparable posteriorly.

The muscles of the levator ani differ from most other skeletal muscles in that they:

- maintain constant tone, except during voiding, defaecation and the Valsalva manoeuvre;

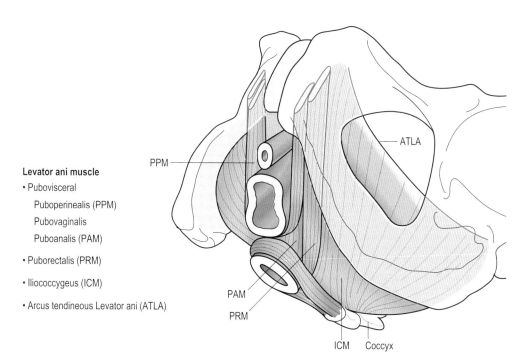

Levator ani muscle
- Pubovisceral
    Puboperinealis (PPM)
    Pubovaginalis
    Puboanalis (PAM)
- Puborectalis (PRM)
- Iliococcygeus (ICM)
- Arcus tendineous Levator ani (ATLA)

Fig. 3.6 The levator muscle (reproduced courtesy of Professor John DeLancey).
Schematic view of the levator ani muscles from below after the vulvar structures and perineal membrane have been removed showing the arcus tendineus levator ani (ATLA); external anal sphincter (EAS); puboanal muscle (PAM); perineal body (PB) uniting the two ends of the puboperineal muscle (PPM); iliococcygeal muscle (ICM); puborectal muscle (PRM). Note that the urethra and vagina have been transected just above the hymenal ring.

- have the ability to contract quickly at the time of acute stress (such as a cough or sneeze) to maintain continence;
- distend considerably during parturition to allow the passage of the term infant and then contract after birth to resume normal functioning.

Until recently, the concept of pelvic floor trauma was attributed largely to perineal, vaginal and anal sphincter injuries. However, in recent years, with advances in magnetic resonance imaging and three-dimensional ultrasound, it has become evident that LAM injuries form an important component of pelvic floor trauma. LAM injuries occur in 13–36% of women who have a vaginal birth. Injury to the LAM is attributed to vaginal birth resulting in reduced pelvic floor muscle strength, enlargement of the vaginal hiatus and pelvic organ prolapse. There is inconclusive evidence to support an association between LAM injuries and stress urinary incontinence and there seems to be a trend towards the development of faecal incontinence.

Innervation of the levator ani

The levator ani is supplied on its superior surface by the sacral nerve roots (S2–S4) and on its inferior surface by the perineal branch of the pudendal nerve.

Vascular supply

The levator ani is supplied by branches of the inferior gluteal artery, the inferior vesical artery and the pudendal artery.

THE PUDENDAL NERVE

The pudendal nerve is a mixed motor and sensory nerve and derives its fibres from the ventral branches of the second, third and fourth sacral nerves and leaves the pelvis through the lower part of the greater sciatic foramen. It then crosses the ischial spine and re-enters the pelvis through the lesser sciatic foramen. It accompanies the internal pudendal vessels upward and forward along the lateral wall of the ischioanal fossa, contained in a sheath of the obturator fascia termed Alcock's canal (Fig. 3.7). It is presumed that during a prolonged second stage of labour, the pudendal nerve is vulnerable to stretch injury due to its relative immobility at this site.

The inferior haemorrhoidal (rectal) nerve then branches off posteriorly from the pudendal nerve to innervate the EAS. The pudendal nerve then divides into two terminal branches: the perineal nerve and the dorsal nerve of the clitoris. The perineal nerve divides into posterior labial and muscular branches. The posterior labial branches supply the labium majora. The muscular branches are distributed to the superficial transverse perineal, bulbospongiosus, ischiocavernosus and constrictor urethræ muscles. The dorsal nerve of the clitoris, which innervates the clitoris, is the deepest division of the pudendal nerve (Fig. 3.8).

THE PELVIS

Knowledge of anatomy of a normal female pelvis is key to midwifery and obstetrics practice, as one of the ways to estimate a woman's progress in labour is by assessing the relationship of the fetus to certain bony landmarks of the pelvis. Understanding the normal pelvic anatomy helps to detect deviations from normal and facilitate appropriate care.

The pelvic girdle

The pelvic girdle is a basin-shaped cavity and consists of two innominate bones (hip bones), the sacrum and the coccyx. It is virtually incapable of independent movement except during childbirth as it provides the skeletal framework of the birth canal. It contains and protects the bladder, rectum and internal reproductive organs. In addition it provides an attachment for trunk and limb muscles. Some women experience pelvic girdle pain in pregnancy and need referral to a physiotherapist (see Chapter 12).

Innominate bones

Each innominate bone or hip bone is made up of three bones that have fused together: the ilium, the ischium and the pubis (Fig. 3.9). On its lateral aspect is a large, cup shaped acetabulum articulating with the femoral head, which is composed of the three fused bones in the following proportions: two-fifths ilium, two-fifths ischium and one-fifth pubis (Fig. 3.9). Anteroinferior to this is the large oval or triangular obturator foramen. The bone is articulated with its fellow to form the pelvic girdle.

The ilium has an upper and lower part. The smaller lower part forms part of the acetabulum and the upper part is the large flared-out part. When the hand is placed on the hip, it rests on the iliac crest, which is the upper border. A bony prominence felt in front of the iliac crest is known as the anterior superior iliac spine. A short distance below it is the anterior inferior iliac spine. There are two similar points at the other end of the iliac crest, namely the posterior superior and the posterior inferior iliac spines. The internal concave anterior surface of the ilium is known as the iliac fossa.

The ischium is the inferoposterior part of the innominate bone and consists of a body and a ramus. Above it forms part of the acetabulum. Below its ramus ascends anteromedially at an acute angle to meet the descending

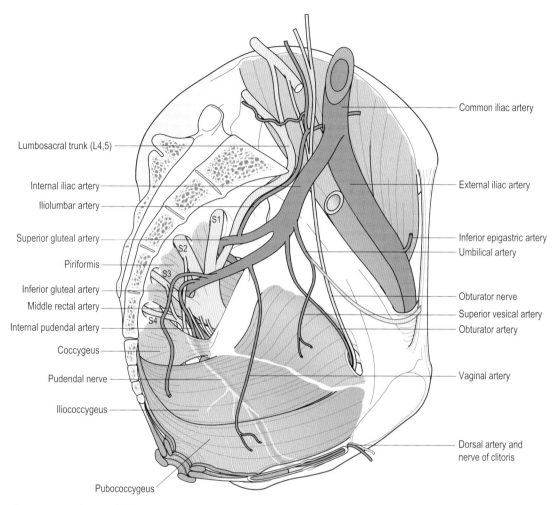

Fig. 3.7 Sagittal view of the pelvis demonstrating the pathway of the pudendal nerve and blood supply.

Labels on figure:
Common iliac artery
Lumbosacral trunk (L4,5)
Internal iliac artery
Iliolumbar artery
External iliac artery
Superior gluteal artery
Inferior epigastric artery
Umbilical artery
Piriformis
Inferior gluteal artery
Middle rectal artery
Obturator nerve
Superior vesical artery
Internal pudendal artery
Obturator artery
Coccygeus
Pudendal nerve
Vaginal artery
Iliococcygeus
Dorsal artery and nerve of clitoris
Pubococcygeus
S1 S2 S3 S4

pubic ramus and complete the obturator foramen. It has a large prominence known as the ischial tuberosity, on which the body rests when sitting. Behind and a little above the tuberosity is an inward projection, the ischial spine. This is an important landmark in midwifery and obstetric practice, as in labour, the station of the fetal head is estimated in relation to the ischial spines allowing assessment of progress of labour.

The pubis forms the anterior part. It has a body and two oar-like projections, the superior ramus and the inferior ramus. The two pubic bones meet at the symphysis pubis and the two inferior rami form the pubic arch, merging into a similar ramus on the ischium. The space enclosed by the body of the pubic bone, the rami and the ischium is called the obturator foramen.

The sacrum

The sacrum is a wedge-shaped bone consisting of five fused vertebrae, and forms the posterior wall of the pelvic cavity as it is wedged between the innominate bones. The caudal apex articulates with the coccyx and the upper border of the first sacral vertebra (sacral promontory) articulates with the first lumbar vertebra. The anterior surface of the sacrum is concave and is referred to as the hollow of the sacrum. Laterally the sacrum extends into a wing or ala. Four pairs of holes or foramina pierce the sacrum and, through these, nerves from the cauda equina emerge to innervate the pelvic organs. The posterior surface is roughened to receive attachments of muscles.

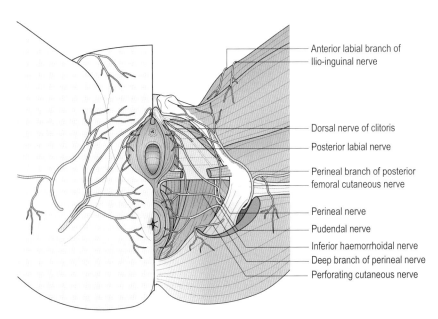

Anterior labial branch of
Ilio-inguinal nerve

Dorsal nerve of clitoris

Posterior labial nerve

Perineal branch of posterior
femoral cutaneous nerve

Perineal nerve

Pudendal nerve

Inferior haemorrhoidal nerve

Deep branch of perineal nerve

Perforating cutaneous nerve

Fig. 3.8 Branches of the pudendal nerve.

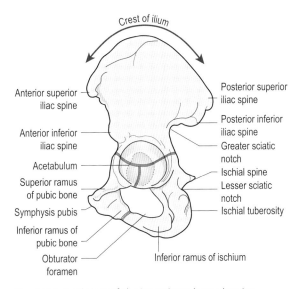

Crest of ilium

Anterior superior
iliac spine

Anterior inferior
iliac spine

Acetabulum

Superior ramus
of pubic bone

Symphysis pubis

Inferior ramus of
pubic bone

Obturator
foramen

Posterior superior
iliac spine

Posterior inferior
iliac spine

Greater sciatic
notch

Ischial spine

Lesser sciatic
notch

Ischial tuberosity

Inferior ramus of ischium

Fig. 3.9 Lateral view of the innominate bone showing important landmarks.

The coccyx

The coccyx is a vestigial tail. It consists of four fused vertebrae, forming a small triangular bone, which articulates with the fifth sacral segment.

Pelvic joints

There are four pelvic joints: one symphysis pubis, two sacroiliac joints and one sacrococcygeal joint.

The symphysis pubis is the midline cartilaginous joint uniting the rami of the left and right pubic bones.

The sacroiliac joints are strong, weight-bearing synovial joints with irregular elevations and depressions that produce interlocking of the bones. They join the sacrum to the ilium and as a result connect the spine to the pelvis. The joints allow a limited backward and forward movement of the tip and promontory of the sacrum, sometimes known as 'nodding' of the sacrum.

The sacrococcygeal joint is formed where the base of the coccyx articulates with the tip of the sacrum. It permits the coccyx to be deflected backwards during the birth of the fetal head.

Pelvic ligaments

The pelvic joints are held together by very strong ligaments that are designed not to allow movement. However, during pregnancy the hormone relaxin gradually loosens all the pelvic ligaments allowing slight pelvic movement providing more room for the fetal head as it passes through the pelvis. A widening of 2–3 mm at the symphysis pubis during pregnancy above the normal gap of 4–5 mm is normal but if it widens significantly, the degree of movement permitted may give rise to pain on walking.

The ligaments connecting the bones of the pelvis with each other can be divided into four groups:

* those connecting the sacrum and ilium – the sacroiliac ligaments;
* those passing between the sacrum and ischium – the sacrotuberous ligaments and the sacrospinous ligaments (Fig. 3.10);

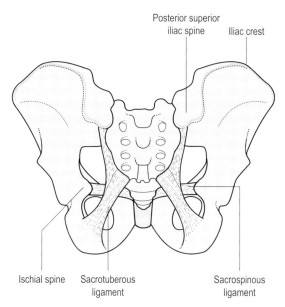

Fig. 3.10 Posterior view of the pelvis showing the ligaments.

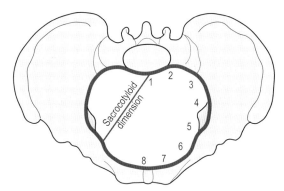

Fig. 3.11 Brim of female pelvis (for detail, see text).

Midwives need to be familiar with the fixed points on the pelvic brim that are known as its landmarks. Commencing posteriorly, these are (Fig. 3.11):

- sacral promontory (1)
- sacral ala or wing (2)
- sacroiliac joint (3)
- iliopectineal line, which is the edge formed at the inward aspect of the ilium (4)
- iliopectineal eminence, which is a roughened area formed where the superior ramus of the pubic bone meets the ilium (5)
- superior ramus of the pubic bone (6)
- upper inner border of the body of the pubic bone (7)
- upper inner border of the symphysis pubis (8).

- those uniting the sacrum and coccyx – the sacrococcygeal ligaments;
- those between the two pubic bones – the inter-pubic ligaments.

The pelvis in relation to pregnancy and childbirth

The term pelvis is applied to the skeletal ring formed by the innominate bones and the sacrum, the cavity within and even the entire region where the trunk and the lower limbs meet. The pelvis is divided by an oblique plane which passes through the prominence of the sacrum, the arcuate line (the smooth rounded border on the internal surface of the ilium), the pectineal line (a ridge on the superior ramus of the pubic bone) and the upper margin of the symphysis pubis, into the true and the false pelves.

The true pelvis

The true pelvis is the bony canal through which the fetus must pass during birth. It is divided into a brim, a cavity and an outlet.

The pelvic brim

The superior circumference forms the brim of the true pelvis, the included space being called the inlet. The brim is round except where the sacral promontory projects into it.

The pelvic cavity

The cavity of the true pelvis extends from the brim superiorly to the outlet inferiorly. The anterior wall is formed by the pubic bones and symphysis pubis and its depth is 4 cm. The posterior wall is formed by the curve of the sacrum, which is 12 cm in length. Because there is such a difference in these measurements, the cavity forms a curved canal. With the woman upright, the upper portion of the pelvic canal is directed downward and backward, and its lower course curves and becomes directed downward and forward. Its lateral walls are the sides of the pelvis, which are mainly covered by the obturator internus muscle.

The cavity contains the pelvic colon, rectum, bladder and some of the reproductive organs. The rectum is placed posteriorly, in the curve of the sacrum and coccyx; the bladder is anterior behind the symphysis pubis.

The pelvic outlet

The lower circumference of the true pelvis is very irregular; the space enclosed by it is called the outlet. Two outlets are described: the anatomical and the obstetrical.

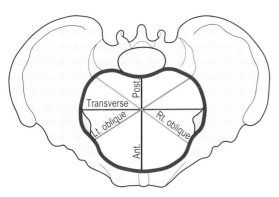

Fig. 3.12 View of pelvic brim showing diameters.

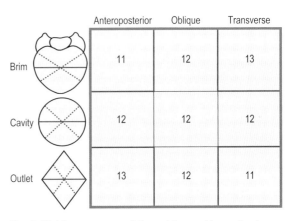

	Anteroposterior	Oblique	Transverse
Brim	11	12	13
Cavity	12	12	12
Outlet	13	12	11

Fig. 3.13 Measurements of the pelvic canal in centimetres.

The anatomical outlet is formed by the lower borders of each of the bones together with the sacrotuberous ligament. The obstetrical outlet is of greater practical significance because it includes the narrow pelvic strait through which the fetus must pass. The narrow pelvic strait lies between the sacrococcygeal joint, the two ischial spines and the lower border of the symphysis pubis. The obstetrical outlet is the space between the narrow pelvic strait and the anatomical outlet. This outlet is diamond-shaped.

The false pelvis

It is bounded posteriorly by the lumbar vertebrae and laterally by the iliac fossae, and in front by the lower portion of the anterior abdominal wall. The false pelvis varies considerably in size according to the flare of the iliac bones. However, the false pelvis has no significance in midwifery.

Pelvic diameters

Knowledge of the diameters of the normal female pelvis is essential in the practice of midwifery because contraction of any of them can result in malposition or malpresentation of the presenting part of the fetus.

Diameters of the pelvic inlet

The brim has four principal diameters: the anteroposterior diameter, the transverse diameter and the two oblique diameters (Figs 3.12, 3.13).

The anteroposterior or conjugate diameter extends from the midpoint of the sacral promontory to the upper border of the symphysis pubis. Three conjugate diameters can be measured: the anatomical (true) conjugate, the obstetrical conjugate and the internal or diagonal conjugate (Fig. 3.14).

The anatomical conjugate, which averages 12 cm, is measured from the sacral promontory to the uppermost point of the symphysis pubis. The obstetrical conjugate,

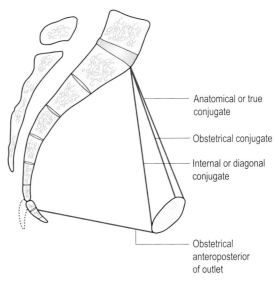

Fig. 3.14 Median section of the pelvis showing anteroposterior diameters.

which averages 11 cm, is measured from the sacral promontory to the posterior border of the upper surface of the symphysis pubis. This represents the shortest anteroposterior diameter through which the fetus must pass and is hence of clinical significance to midwives (Fig. 3.15). The obstetrical conjugate cannot be measured with the examining fingers or any other technique.

The diagonal conjugate is measured anteroposteriorly from the lower border of the symphysis to the sacral promontory.

The transverse diameter is constructed at right-angles to the obstetric conjugate and extends across the greatest width of the brim; its average measurement is about 13 cm.

Each oblique diameter extends from the iliopectineal eminence of one side to the sacroiliac articulation of the

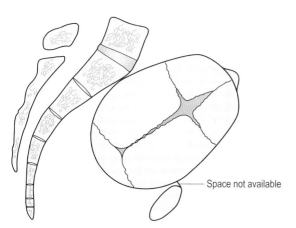

Fig. 3.15 Fetal head negotiating the narrow obstetrical conjugate.

— Space not available

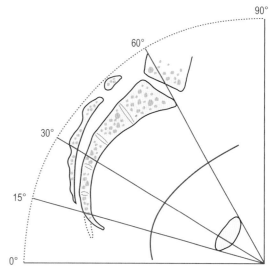

Fig. 3.16 Median section of the pelvis showing the inclination of the planes and the axis of the pelvic canal.

opposite side; its average measurement is about 12 cm. Each takes its name from the sacroiliac joint from which it arises, so the left oblique diameter arises from the left sacroiliac joint and the right oblique from the right sacroiliac joint.

Another dimension, the sacrocotyloid (see Fig. 3.11), passes from the sacral promontory to the iliopectineal eminence on each side and measures 9–9.5 cm. Its importance is concerned with posterior positions of the occiput when the parietal eminences of the fetal head may become caught (see Chapter 20).

Diameters of the cavity

The cavity is circular in shape and although it is not possible to measure its diameters exactly, they are all considered to be 12 cm (see Fig. 3.13).

Diameters of the outlet

The outlet, which is diamond-shaped, has three diameters: the anteroposterior diameter, the oblique diameter and the transverse diameter (see Fig. 3.13).

The anteroposterior diameter extends from the lower border of the symphysis pubis to the sacrococcygeal joint. It measures 13 cm; as the coccyx may be deflected backwards during labour, this diameter indicates the space available during birth.

The oblique diameter, although there are no fixed points, is said to be between the obturator foramen and the sacrospinous ligament. The measurement is taken as being 12 cm.

The transverse diameter extends between the two ischial spines and measures 10–11 cm. It is the narrowest diameter in the pelvis. The plane of least pelvic dimensions is said to be at the level of the ischial spines.

Orientation of the pelvis

In the standing position, the pelvis is placed such that the anterior superior iliac spine and the front edge of the symphysis pubis are in the same vertical plane, perpendicular to the floor. If the line joining the sacral promontory and the top of the symphysis pubis were to be extended, it would form an angle of 60° with the horizontal floor. Similarly, if a line joining the centre of the sacrum and the centre of the symphysis pubis were to be extended, the resultant angle with the floor would be 30°. The angle of inclination of the outlet is 15° (Fig. 3.16). When in the recumbent position, the same angles are made as in the vertical position; this fact should be kept in mind when carrying out an abdominal examination.

Pelvic planes

Pelvic planes are imaginary flat surfaces at the brim, cavity and outlet of the pelvic canal at the levels of the lines described above (Fig. 3.17).

Axis of the pelvic canal

A line drawn exactly half-way between the anterior wall and the posterior wall of the pelvic canal would trace a curve known as the curve of Carus. The midwife needs to become familiar with this concept in order to make accurate observations on vaginal examination and to facilitate the birth of the baby.

The four types of pelvis

The size of the pelvis varies not only in the two sexes, but also in different members of the same sex. The height of the individual does not appear to influence the size of the pelvis in any way, as women of short stature, in general, have a broad pelvis. Nevertheless, the pelvis is occasionally equally contracted in all its dimensions, so much so that all its diameters can measure 1.25 cm less than the average. This type of pelvis, known as a justo minor pelvis, can result in normal labour and birth if the fetal size is consistent with the size of the maternal pelvis. However, if the fetus is large, a degree of cephalopelvic disproportion will result. The same is true when a malpresentation or malposition of the fetus exists.

The principal divergences, however, are found at the brim (Fig. 3.18) and affect the relation of the antero-posterior to the transverse diameter. If one of the measurements is reduced by 1 cm or more from the normal, the pelvis is said to be contracted and may give rise to difficulty in labour or necessitate caesarean section.

Classically, pelves have been described as falling into four categories: the gynaecoid pelvis, the android pelvis, the anthropoid pelvis and the platypelloid pelvis (Table 3.1).

The gynaecoid pelvis (Fig. 3.19)

This is the best type for childbearing as it has a rounded brim, generous forepelvis, straight side walls, a shallow cavity with a well-curved sacrum and a sub-pubic arch of 90°.

The android pelvis

The android pelvis is so called because it resembles the male pelvis. Its brim is heart-shaped, it has a narrow forepelvis and its transverse diameter is situated towards the back. The side walls converge, making it funnel-shaped,

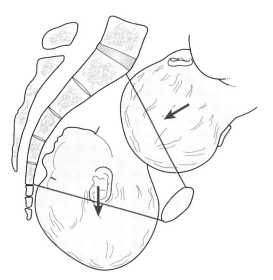

Fig. 3.17 Fetal head entering plane of pelvic brim and leaving plane of pelvic outlet.

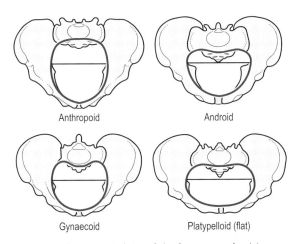

Anthropoid Android

Gynaecoid Platypelloid (flat)

Fig. 3.18 Characteristic brim of the four types of pelvis.

Table 3.1 Features of the four types of pelvis

Features	Gynaecoid	Android	Anthropoid	Platypelloid
Brim	Rounded	Heart-shaped	Long oval	Kidney-shaped
Forepelvis	Generous	Narrow	Narrowed	Wide
Side walls	Straight	Convergent	Divergent	Divergent
Ischial spines	Blunt	Prominent	Blunt	Blunt
Sciatic notch	Rounded	Narrow	Wide	Wide
Sub-pubic angle	90°	<90°	>90°	>90°
Incidence	50%	20%	25% (50% in non-Caucasian)	5%

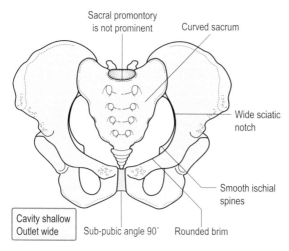

Sacral promontory
is not prominent
Curved sacrum

Wide sciatic
notch

Smooth ischial
spines

| Cavity shallow
Outlet wide |

Sub-pubic angle 90° Rounded brim

Fig. 3.19 Normal female pelvis (gynaecoid).

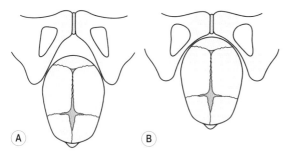

Fig. 3.20 (A) Outlet of android pelvis. The fetal head, which does not fit into the acute pubic arch, is forced backwards onto the perineum. (B) Outlet of the gynaecoid pelvis. The head fits snugly into the pubic arch.

and it has a deep cavity and a straight sacrum. The ischial spines are prominent and the sciatic notch is narrow. The sub-pubic angle is less than 90°. It is found in short and heavily built women, who have a tendency to be hirsute.

Because of the narrow forepelvis and the fact that the greater space lies in the hindpelvis the heart-shaped brim favours an occipitoposterior position. Furthermore, funnelling in the cavity may hinder progress in labour. At the pelvic outlet, the prominent ischial spines sometimes prevent complete internal rotation of the head and the anteroposterior diameter becomes caught on them, causing a deep transverse arrest. The narrowed sub-pubic angle cannot easily accommodate the biparietal diameter (Fig. 3.20) and this displaces the head backwards. Because of these factors, this type of pelvis is the least suited to childbearing.

The anthropoid pelvis

The anthropoid pelvis has a long, oval brim in which the anteroposterior diameter is longer than the transverse

diameter. The side walls diverge and the sacrum is long and deeply concave. The ischial spines are not prominent and the sciatic notch and the sub-pubic angle are very wide. Women with this type of pelvis tend to be tall, with narrow shoulders. Labour does not usually present any difficulties, but a direct occipitoanterior or direct occipitoposterior position is often a feature and the position adopted for engagement may persist to birth.

The platypelloid pelvis

The platypelloid (flat) pelvis has a kidney-shaped brim in which the anteroposterior diameter is reduced and the transverse diameter increased. The sacrum is flat and the cavity shallow. The ischial spines are blunt, and the sciatic notch and the sub-pubic angle are both wide. The head must engage with the sagittal suture in the transverse diameter, but usually descends through the cavity without difficulty. Engagement may necessitate lateral tilting of the head, known as asynclitism, in order to allow the biparietal diameter to pass the narrowest anteroposterior diameter of the brim (Box 3.1).

Other pelvic variations

High assimilation pelvis occurs when the 5th lumbar vertebra is fused to the sacrum and the angle of inclination of the pelvic brim is increased. Engagement of the head is difficult but, once achieved, labour progresses normally.

Deformed pelvis may result from a developmental anomaly, dietary deficiency, injury or disease (Box 3.2).

Box 3.2 **Deformed pelves**

Developmental anomalies

The Naegele's and Robert's pelves are rare malformations caused by a failure in development. In the Naegele's pelvis, one sacral ala is missing and the sacrum is fused to the ilium causing a grossly asymmetric brim. The Robert's pelvis has similar malformations which are bilateral. In both instances, the abnormal brim prevents engagement of the fetal head.

Dietary deficiency

Deficiency of vitamins and minerals necessary for the formation of healthy bones is less frequently seen today than in the past but might still complicate pregnancy and labour to some extent.

A *rachitic pelvis* is a pelvis deformed by rickets in early childhood, as a consequence of malnutrition. The weight of the upper body presses downwards on to the softened pelvic bones, the sacral promontory is pushed downwards and forwards and the ilium and ischium are drawn outwards resulting in a flat pelvic brim similar to that of the platypelloid pelvis (Fig. 3.21). The sacrum tends to be straight, with the coccyx bending acutely forward. Because the tuberosities are wide apart, the pubic arch is wide. The clinical signs of rickets are bow legs and spinal deformity.

If severe contraction is present, caesarean section is required to deliver the baby. The fetal head will attempt to enter the pelvis by asynclitism.

Osteomalacic pelvis. The disease osteomalacia is rarely encountered in the United Kingdom. It is due to an acquired deficiency of calcium and occurs in adults. All bones of the skeleton soften because of gross calcium deficiency. The pelvic canal is squashed together until the brim becomes a Y-shaped slit. Labour is impossible. In early pregnancy, incarceration of the gravid uterus may occur because of the gross deformity.

Injury and disease

Trauma. A pelvis that has been fractured will develop callus formation or may fail to unite correctly. This may lead to reduced measurements and therefore to some degree of contraction. Conditions sustained in childhood such as fractures of the pelvis or lower limbs, congenital dislocation of the hip and poliomyelitis may lead to unequal weight-bearing, which will also cause deformity.

Spinal deformity. If kyphosis (forward angulation) or scoliosis (lateral curvature) is evident, or is suggested by a limp or deformity, the midwife must refer the woman to a doctor. Pelvic contraction is likely in these cases.

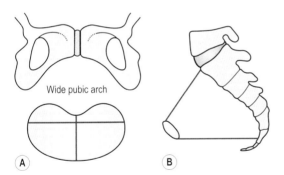

Fig. 3.21 Rachitic flat pelvis. (A) Note wide pubic arch and kidney-shaped brim. (B) The lateral view shows the diminished anteroposterior diameter of the brim and the increased anteroposterior diameter of the outlet.

THE FEMALE REPRODUCTIVE SYSTEM

The female reproductive system consists of the external genitalia, known collectively as the vulva, and the internal reproductive organs: the vagina, the uterus, two uterine tubes and two ovaries. In the non-pregnant state, the internal reproductive organs are situated within the true pelvis.

The vagina

The vagina is a hollow, distensible fibromuscular tube that extends from the vestibule to the cervix. It is approximately 10 cm in length and 2.5 cm in diameter (although there is wide anatomical variation). During sexual intercourse and when a woman gives birth, the vagina temporarily widens and lengthens.

The vaginal canal passes upwards and backwards into the pelvis with the anterior and posterior walls in close contact along a line approximately parallel to the plane of the pelvic brim. When the woman stands upright, the vaginal canal points in an upward-backward direction and forms an angle of slightly more than 45° with the uterus.

Function

The vagina allows the escape of the menstrual fluids, receives the penis and the ejected sperm during sexual intercourse, and provides an exit for the fetus during birth.

Relations

Knowledge of the relations of the vagina to other pelvic organs is essential for the accurate examination of

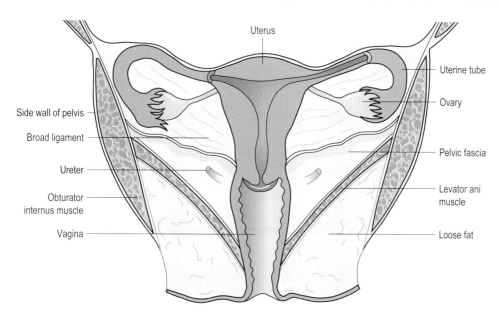

Fig. 3.22 Coronal section through the pelvis.

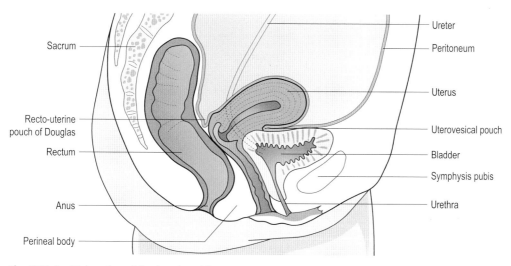

Fig. 3.23 Sagittal section of the female pelvis.

the pregnant woman and the safe birth of the baby (Figs 3.22, 3.23).

- **Anterior** to the vagina lie the bladder and the urethra, which are closely connected to the anterior vaginal wall.
- **Posterior** to the vagina lie the pouch of Douglas, the rectum and the perineal body, which separates the vagina from the anal canal.
- **Laterally** on the upper two-thirds are the pelvic fascia and the ureters, which pass beside the cervix;

on either side of the lower third are the muscles of the pelvic floor.
- **Superior** to the vagina lies the uterus.
- **Inferior** to the vagina lies the external genitalia.

Structure

The posterior wall of the vagina is 10 cm long whereas the anterior wall is only 7.5 cm in length; this is because the cervix projects into its upper part at a right-angle.

The upper end of the vagina is known as the vault. Where the cervix projects into it, the vault forms a circular recess that is described as four arches or fornices. The posterior fornix is the largest of these because the vagina is attached to the uterus at a higher level behind than in front. The anterior fornix lies in front of the cervix and the lateral fornices lie on either side.

Layers

The vaginal wall is composed of three layers: mucosa, muscle and fascia. The mucosa is the most superficial layer and consists of stratified, squamous non-keratinized epithelium, thrown in transverse folds called rugae. These allow the vaginal walls to stretch during intercourse and childbirth. Beneath the epithelium lies a layer of vascular connective tissue. The muscle layer is divided into a weak inner coat of circular fibres and a stronger outer coat of longitudinal fibres. Pelvic fascia surrounds the vagina and adjacent pelvic organs and allows for their independent expansion and contraction.

There are no glands in the vagina; however, it is moistened by mucus from the cervix and a transudate that seeps out from the blood vessels of the vaginal wall.

In spite of the alkaline mucus, the vaginal fluid is strongly acid (pH 4.5) owing to the presence of lactic acid formed by the action of Doderlein's bacilli on glycogen found in the squamous epithelium of the lining. These lactobacilli are normal inhabitants of the vagina. The acid deters the growth of pathogenic bacteria.

Blood supply

The blood supply comes from branches of the internal iliac artery and includes the vaginal artery and a descending branch of the uterine artery. The blood drains through corresponding veins.

Lymphatic drainage

Lymphatic drainage is via the inguinal, the internal iliac and the sacral glands.

Nerve supply

The nerve supply is derived from the pelvic plexus. The vaginal nerves follow the vaginal arteries to supply the vaginal walls and the erectile tissue of the vulva.

The uterus

The uterus is a hollow, pear-shaped muscular organ located in the true pelvis between the bladder and the rectum. The position of the uterus within the true pelvis is one of anteversion and anteflexion. Anteversion means that the uterus leans forward and anteflexion means that

it bends forwards upon itself. When the woman is standing, the uterus is in an almost horizontal position with the fundus resting on the bladder if the uterus is anteverted (see Fig. 3.23).

Function

The main function of the uterus is to nourish the developing fetus prior to birth. It prepares for pregnancy each month and following pregnancy expels the products of conception.

Relations

Knowledge of the relations of the uterus to other pelvic organs (Figs 3.24, 3.25) is desirable, particularly when giving women advice about bladder and bowel care during pregnancy and childbirth.

- **Anterior** to the uterus lie the uterovesical pouch and the bladder.
- **Posterior** to the uterus are the recto-uterine pouch of Douglas and the rectum.
- **Lateral** to the uterus are the broad ligaments, the uterine tubes and the ovaries.
- **Superior** to the uterus lie the intestines.
- **Inferior** to the uterus is the vagina.

Supports

The uterus is supported by the pelvic floor and maintained in position by several ligaments, of which those at the level of the cervix (Fig. 3.24) are the most important.

- The transverse cervical ligaments fan out from the sides of the cervix to the side walls of the pelvis. They are sometimes known as the 'cardinal ligaments' or 'Mackenrodt's ligaments'.

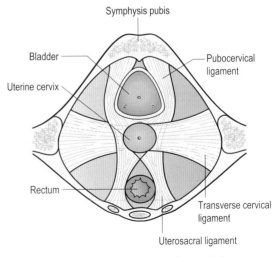

Fig. 3.24 Supports of the uterus, at the level of the cervix.

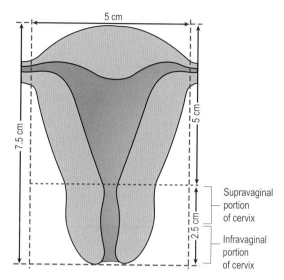

Fig. 3.25 Measurements of the uterus.

- The cornua are the upper outer angles of the uterus where the uterine tubes join.
- The fundus is the domed upper wall between the insertions of the uterine tubes.
- The body or corpus makes up the upper two-thirds of the uterus and is the greater part.
- The cavity is a potential space between the anterior and posterior walls. It is triangular in shape, the base of the triangle being uppermost.
- The isthmus is a narrow area between the cavity and the cervix, which is 7 mm long. It enlarges during pregnancy to form the lower uterine segment.
- The cervix or neck protrudes into the vagina. The upper half, being above the vagina, is known as the supravaginal portion while the lower half is the infravaginal portion.
- The internal os (mouth) is the narrow opening between the isthmus and the cervix.
- The external os is a small round opening at the lower end of the cervix. After childbirth, it becomes a transverse slit.
- The cervical canal lies between these two ostia and is a continuation of the uterine cavity. This canal is shaped like a spindle, narrow at each end and wider in the middle.

- The uterosacral ligaments pass backwards from the cervix to the sacrum.
- The pubocervical ligaments pass forwards from the cervix, under the bladder, to the pubic bones.
- The broad ligaments are formed from the folds of peritoneum, which are draped over the uterine tubes. They hang down like a curtain and spread from the sides of the uterus to the side walls of the pelvis.
- The round ligaments have little value as a support but tend to maintain the anteverted position of the uterus; they arise from the cornua of the uterus, in front of and below the insertion of each uterine tube, and pass between the folds of the broad ligament, through the inguinal canal, to be inserted into each labium majus.
- The ovarian ligaments also begin at the cornua of the uterus but behind the uterine tubes and pass down between the folds of the broad ligament to the ovaries.

It is helpful to note that the round ligament, the uterine tube and the ovarian ligament are very similar in appearance and arise from the same area of the uterus. This makes careful identification important when tubal surgery is undertaken.

Structure

The non-pregnant uterus is 7.5 cm long, 5 cm wide and 2.5 cm in depth, each wall being 1.25 cm thick (see Fig. 3.25). The cervix forms the lower third of the uterus and measures 2.5 cm in each direction. The uterus consists of the following parts:

Layers

The uterus has three layers: the endometrium, the myometrium and the perimetrium, of which the myometrium, the middle muscle layer, is by far the thickest.

The endometrium forms a lining of ciliated epithelium (mucous membrane) on a base of connective tissue or stroma. In the uterine cavity, this endometrium is constantly changing in thickness throughout the menstrual cycle (see Chapter 5). The basal layer does not alter, but provides the foundation from which the upper layers regenerate. The epithelial cells are cubical in shape and dip down to form glands that secrete an alkaline mucus.

The cervical endometrium does not respond to the hormonal stimuli of the menstrual cycle to the same extent. Here the epithelial cells are tall and columnar in shape and the mucus-secreting glands are branching racemose glands. The cervical endometrium is thinner than that of the body and is folded into a pattern known as the 'arbor vitae' (tree of life). This is thought to assist the passage of the sperm. The portion of the cervix that protrudes into the vagina is covered with squamous epithelium similar to that lining the vagina. The point where the epithelium changes, at the external os, is termed the squamo-columnar junction.

The myometrium is thick in the upper part of the uterus and is sparser in the isthmus and cervix. Its fibres run in all directions and interlace to surround the blood vessels and lymphatics that pass to and from the endometrium. The outer layer is formed of longitudinal fibres that are continuous with those of the uterine tube, the uterine ligaments and the vagina.

In the cervix, the muscle fibres are embedded in collagen fibres, which enable it to stretch in labour.

The perimetrium is a double serous membrane, an extension of the peritoneum, which is draped over the fundus and the anterior surface of the uterus to the level of the internal os. It is then reflected onto the bladder forming a small pouch between the uterus and the bladder called the uterovesical pouch. The posterior surface is covered to where the cervix protrudes into the vagina and is then reflected onto the rectum forming the recto-uterine pouch. Laterally the perimetrium extends over the uterine tubes forming a double fold, the broad ligament, leaving the lateral borders of the body uncovered.

Blood supply

The uterine artery arrives at the level of the cervix and is a branch of the internal iliac artery. It sends a small branch to the upper vagina, and then runs upwards in a twisted fashion to meet the ovarian artery and form an anastomosis with it near the cornu. The ovarian artery is a branch of the abdominal aorta, leaving near the renal artery. It supplies the ovary and uterine tube before joining the uterine artery. The blood drains through corresponding veins (Fig. 3.26).

Lymphatic drainage

Lymph is drained from the uterine body to the internal iliac glands and from the cervical area to many other pelvic lymph glands. This provides an effective defence against uterine infection.

Nerve supply

The nerve supply is mainly from the autonomic nervous system, sympathetic and parasympathetic, via the inferior hypogastric or pelvic plexus.

Uterine malformations

The prevalence of uterine malformation is estimated to be 6.7% in the general population. The female genital tract is formed in early embryonic life when a pair of ducts develops. These paramesonephric or Müllerian ducts come together in the midline and fuse into a Y-shaped canal. The open upper ends of this structure lead into the peritoneal cavity and the unfused portions become the uterine tubes. The fused lower portion forms the uterovaginal area, which further develops into the uterus and vagina. Abnormal development of the Müllerian duct(s) during embryogenesis can lead to uterine abnormalities (Box 3.3) (Fig. 3.27).

Structural abnormality of the uterus can lead to various problems during pregnancy and childbirth. The outcome depends on the ability of the uterus to accommodate the growing fetus. A problem exists only if the tissue is insufficient to allow the uterus to enlarge for a full-term fetus lying longitudinally. If there is insufficient hypertrophy, the possible difficulties are miscarriage, premature labour and abnormal lie of the fetus. In labour, poor uterine

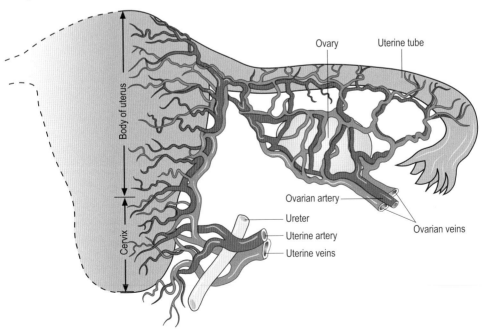

Fig. 3.26 Blood supply of the uterus, uterine tubes and ovaries.

Types of uterine malformation

Various types of structural abnormality can result from failure of fusion of the Müllerian ducts. Three of these abnormalities can be seen in Fig. 3.27. A double uterus with an associated double vagina will develop where there has been complete failure of fusion. Partial fusion results in various degrees of duplication. A single vagina with a double uterus is the result of fusion at the lower end of the ducts only. A bicornuate uterus (one with two horns) is the result of incomplete fusion at the upper portion of the uterovaginal area. In rare cases, one Müllerian duct regresses and the result is a uterus with one horn – termed a unicornuate uterus.

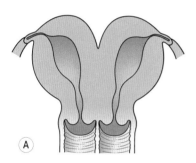

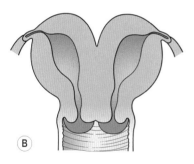

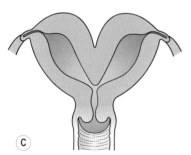

Fig. 3.27 Uterine malformations. (A) Double uterus with duplication of body of uterus, cervix and vagina.
(B) Duplication of uterus and cervix with single vagina.
(C) Duplication of uterus with single cervix and vagina.

function may be experienced. Minor defects of structure cause little problem and might pass unnoticed, with the woman having a normal outcome to her pregnancy. Occasionally problems arise when a fetus is accommodated in one horn of a double uterus and the empty horn has filled the pelvic cavity. In this situation, the empty horn has grown owing to the hormonal influences of the pregnancy, and its size and position will cause obstruction during labour. Caesarean section would be the method of delivery.

The fallopian tubes

The uterine tubes, also known as fallopian tubes, oviducts and salpinges, are two very fine tubes leading from the ovaries into the uterus.

Function

The uterine tube propels the ovum towards the uterus, receives the spermatozoa as they travel upwards and provides a site for fertilization. It supplies the fertilized ovum with nutrition during its continued journey to the uterus.

Position

The uterine tubes extend laterally from the cornua of the uterus towards the side walls of the pelvis. They arch over the ovaries, the fringed ends hovering near the ovaries in order to receive the ovum.

Relations

- **Anterior,** posterior and superior to the uterine tubes are the peritoneal cavity and the intestines.
- **Lateral** to the uterine tubes are the side walls of the pelvis.
- **Inferior** to the uterine tubes lie the broad ligaments and the ovaries.
- **Medial** to the two uterine tubes lies the uterus.

Supports

The uterine tubes are held in place by their attachment to the uterus. The peritoneum folds over them, draping down below as the broad ligaments and extending at the sides to form the infundibulopelvic ligaments.

Structure

Each tube is 10 cm long. The lumen of the tube provides an open pathway from the outside to the peritoneal cavity. The uterine tube has four portions (Fig. 3.28):

- **The interstitial portion** is 1.25 cm long and lies within the wall of the uterus. Its lumen is 1 mm wide.

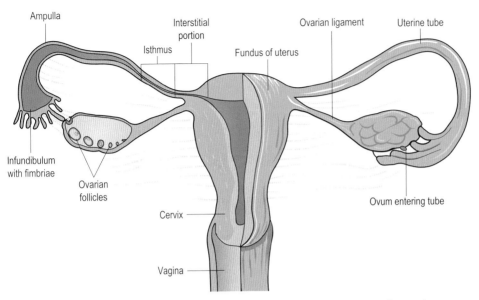

Fig. 3.28 The uterine tubes in section. Note the ovum entering the fimbriated end of one tube.

- **The isthmus** is another narrow part that extends for 2.5 cm from the uterus.
- **The ampulla** is the wider portion, where fertilization usually occurs. It is 5 cm long.
- **The infundibulum** is the funnel-shaped fringed end that is composed of many processes known as fimbriae. One fimbria is elongated to form the ovarian fimbria, which is attached to the ovary.

Layers (Fig. 3.29)

The lining of the uterine tubes is a mucous membrane of ciliated cubical epithelium that is thrown into complicated folds known as plicae. These folds slow the ovum down on its way to the uterus. In this lining are goblet cells that produce a secretion containing glycogen to nourish the oocyte.

Beneath the lining is a layer of vascular connective tissue.

The muscle coat consists of two layers: an inner circular layer and an outer longitudinal layer, both of smooth muscle. The peristaltic movement of the uterine tube is due to the action of these muscles.

The tube is covered with peritoneum but the infundibulum passes through it to open into the peritoneal cavity.

Blood supply

The blood supply is via the uterine and ovarian arteries, returning by the corresponding veins.

Lymphatic drainage

Lymph is drained to the lumbar glands.

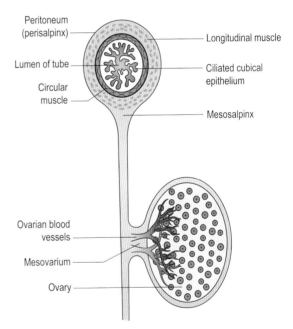

Fig. 3.29 Cross-section of a uterine tube and ovary.

Nerve supply

The nerve supply is from the ovarian plexus.

The ovaries

The ovaries are components of the female reproductive system and the endocrine system.

Function

The ovaries produce oocytes and the hormones, oestrogen and progesterone.

Position

The ovaries are attached to the back of the broad ligaments within the peritoneal cavity.

Relations

- **Anterior** to the ovaries are the broad ligaments.
- **Posterior** to the ovaries are the intestines.
- **Lateral** to the ovaries are the infundibulopelvic ligaments and the side walls of the pelvis.
- **Superior** to the ovaries lie the uterine tubes.
- **Medial** to the ovaries lie the ovarian ligaments and the uterus.

Supports

The ovary is attached to the broad ligament but is supported from above by the ovarian ligament medially and the infundibulopelvic ligament laterally.

Structure

The ovary is composed of a medulla and cortex, covered with germinal epithelium.

The medulla is the supporting framework, which is made of fibrous tissue; the ovarian blood vessels, lymphatics and nerves travel through it. The hilum where these vessels enter lies just where the ovary is attached to the broad ligament and this area is called the mesovarium (see Fig. 3.29).

The cortex is the functioning part of the ovary. It contains the ovarian follicles in different stages of development, surrounded by stroma. The outer layer is formed of fibrous tissue known as the tunica albuginea. Over this lies the germinal epithelium, which is a modification of the peritoneum.

The cycle of the ovary is described in Chapter 5.

Blood supply

Blood is supplied to the ovaries from the ovarian arteries and drains via the ovarian veins. The right ovarian vein joins the inferior vena cava, but the left returns its blood to the left renal vein.

Lymphatic drainage

Lymphatic drainage is to the lumbar glands.

Nerve supply

The nerve supply is from the ovarian plexus.

THE MALE REPRODUCTIVE SYSTEM

The male reproductive system (Fig. 3.30) consists of a set of organs that are partly visible and partly hidden within the body. The visible parts are the scrotum and the penis.

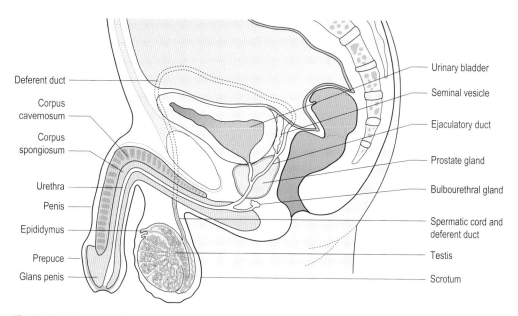

Deferent duct
Corpus cavernosum
Corpus spongiosum
Urethra
Penis
Epididymus
Prepuce
Glans penis

Urinary bladder
Seminal vesicle
Ejaculatory duct
Prostate gland
Bulbourethral gland
Spermatic cord and deferent duct
Testis
Scrotum

Fig. 3.30 Male reproductive system.

Inside the body are the prostate gland and tubes that link the system together. The male organs produce and transfer sperm to the female for fertilization. The organs are the scrotum, testis, rete and epididymis, ductus deferens, seminal vesicles prostate gland, bulbourethral glands and penis with the urethra.

The scrotum

The scrotum is part of the external genitalia. Also called the scrotal sac, the scrotum is a thin-walled, soft, muscular pouch located below the symphysis pubis, between the upper parts of the thighs behind the penis.

Function

The scrotum forms a pouch in which the testes are suspended outside the body, keeping them at a temperature slightly lower than that of the rest of the body. A temperature around 34.4 °C enables the production of viable sperm, whereas a temperature of or above 36.7 °C can be damaging to sperm count.

Structure

The scrotum is formed of pigmented skin and has two compartments, one for each testis.

The testes

Like the ovaries, to which they are homologous, the testes (also known as testicles) are components of both the reproductive system and the endocrine system. Each testis weighs about 25 g.

Function

The testes produce and store spermatozoa, and are the body's main source of the male hormone testosterone. Testosterone is responsible for the development of secondary sex characteristics.

Position

In the embryo, the testes develop high up in the lumbar region of the abdominal cavity. In the last few months of fetal life they descend through the abdomen, over the pelvic brim and down the inguinal canal into the scrotum outside the body. The testes are contained within the scrotum.

Structure

Each testis is an oval structure about 5 cm long and 3 cm in diameter.

Layers

There are three layers to the testis:

The **tunica vasculosa** is an inner layer of connective tissue containing a fine network of capillaries.

The **tunica albuginea** is a fibrous covering, ingrowths of which divide the testis into 200–300 lobules.

The **tunica vaginalis** is the outer layer, which is made of peritoneum brought down with the descending testis when it migrated from the lumbar region in fetal life.

The duct system within the testes is highly intricate:

The **seminiferous** ('seed-carrying') tubules are where spermatogenesis, or production of sperm, takes place. There are up to three of them in each lobule. Between the tubules are interstitial cells that secrete testosterone. The tubules join to form a system of channels that lead to the epididymis.

The **epididymis** is a comma-shaped, coiled tube that lies on the superior surface and travels down the posterior aspect to the lower pole of the testis, where it leads into the deferent duct or vas deferens.

The spermatic cord

The spermatic cord is the name given to the cord-like structure consisting of the vas deferens and its accompanying arteries, veins, nerves and lymphatic vessels.

Function

The function of the deferent duct is to carry the sperm to the ejaculatory duct.

Position

The cord passes upwards through the inguinal canal, where the different structures diverge. The deferent duct then continues upwards over the symphysis pubis and arches backwards beside the bladder. Behind the bladder, it merges with the duct from the seminal vesicle and passes through the prostate gland as the ejaculatory duct to join the urethra.

Blood supply

The testicular artery, a branch of the abdominal aorta, supplies the testes, scrotum and attachments. The testicular veins drain in the same manner as the ovarian veins.

Lymphatic drainage

Lymphatic drainage is to the lymph nodes round the aorta.

Nerve supply

The nerve supply to the spermatic cord is from the 10th and 11th thoracic nerves.

The seminal vesicles

The seminal vesicles are a pair of simple tubular glands.

Function

The function of the seminal vesicles is production of a viscous secretion to keep the sperm alive and motile. This secretion ultimately becomes semen.

Position

The seminal vesicles are situated posterior to the bladder and superior to the prostate gland.

Structure

The seminal vesicles are 5 cm long and pyramid-shaped. They are composed of columnar epithelium, muscle tissue and fibrous tissue.

The ejaculatory ducts

These small muscular ducts carry the spermatozoa and the seminal fluid to the urethra.

The prostate gland

The prostate is an exocrine gland of the male reproductive system.

Function

The prostate gland produces a thin lubricating fluid that enters the urethra through ducts.

Position

The prostate gland surrounds the urethra at the base of the bladder, lying between the rectum and the symphysis pubis.

Structure

The prostate gland measures $4 \times 3 \times 2$ cm. It is composed of columnar epithelium, a muscle layer and an outer fibrous layer.

The bulbourethral glands

The bulbourethral glands are two very small glands, which produce yet another lubricating fluid that passes into the urethra just below the prostate gland.

The penis

The penis is the male reproductive organ and additionally serves as the external male organ of urination.

Functions

The penis carries the urethra, which is a passage for both urine and semen. During sexual excitement it stiffens (an erection) in order to be able to penetrate the vagina and deposit the semen near the woman's cervix.

Position

The root of the penis lies in the perineum, from where it passes forward below the symphysis pubis. The lower two-thirds are outside the body in front of the scrotum.

Structure

The penis has three columns of erectile tissue:

The corpora cavernosa are two lateral columns that lie one on either side in front of the urethra.

The corpus spongiosum is the posterior column that contains the urethra. The tip is expanded to form the glans penis.

The lower two-thirds of the penis are covered in skin. At the end, the skin is folded back on itself above the glans penis to form the prepuce or foreskin, which is a movable double fold. The penis is extremely vascular and during an erection the blood spaces fill and become distended.

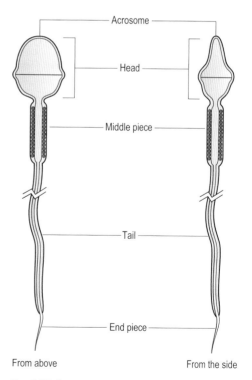

From above   From the side

Fig. 3.31 Spermatozoon.

The male hormones

The control of the male gonads is similar to that in the female, but it is not cyclical. The hypothalamus produces gonadotrophin-releasing factors. These stimulate the anterior pituitary gland to produce follicle stimulating hormone (FSH) and luteinizing hormone (LH). FSH acts on the seminiferous tubules to bring about the production of sperm, whereas LH acts on the interstitial cells that produce testosterone.

Testosterone is responsible for the secondary sex characteristics: deepening of the voice, growth of the genitalia and growth of hair on the chest, pubis, axilla and face.

Formation of the spermatozoa

Production of sperm begins at puberty and continues throughout adult life. Spermatogenesis takes place in the seminiferous tubules under the influence of FSH and testosterone. The process of maturation is a lengthy one and takes some weeks. The mature sperm are stored in the epididymis and the deferent duct until ejaculation. If this does not happen, they degenerate and are reabsorbed. At each ejaculation, 2–4 ml of semen is deposited in the vagina. The seminal fluid contains about 100 million sperm/ml, of which 20–25% are likely to be abnormal. The remainder move at a speed of 2–3 mm/min. The individual spermatozoon has a head, a body and a long, mobile tail that lashes to propel the sperm along (Fig. 3.31). The tip of the head is covered by an acrosome; this contains enzymes to dissolve the covering of the oocyte in order to penetrate it.

FURTHER READING

Kearney R, Sawhney R, DeLancey J O 2004. Levator ani muscle anatomy evaluated by origin-insertion pairs. Obstetrics and Gynecology 104: 168–73

A comprehensive and up-to-date description of levator ani muscle anatomy.

Schwertner-Tiepelmann N, Thakar R, Sultan A H et al 2012 Obstetric levator ani muscle injuries – current status. Ultrasound in Obstetrics and Gynecology 39: 372–83

This review article critically appraises the diagnosis of obstetric LAM injuries, to establish the relationship between LAM injuries and pelvic floor dysfunction and to identify risk factors and preventive strategies to minimize such injuries.

Stables D, Rankin J 2010 Physiology in childbearing: with anatomy and related biosciences, 3rd edn. Baillière Tindall, Edinburgh

This textbook presents a comprehensive and clear account of anatomy and physiology and related biosciences at all stages of pregnancy and childbirth.

Standring S (ed) 2008 Gray's anatomy: the anatomical basis of clinical practice, 40th edn. Elsevier Churchill Livingston, London

This large volume, with detailed information about the anatomy of every part of the human body, provides the reader with much more insight into the structure and function of the reproductive organs. This edition includes specialist revision of topics such as the anatomy of the pelvic floor.

Sultan A H, Thakar R, Fenner D E 2007 Perineal and anal sphincter trauma: diagnosis and clinical management. Springer-Verlag, London

This is a comprehensive text that focuses on the maternal morbidity associated with childbirth. It is essential reading for anyone involved in obstetric care such as obstetricians, midwives and family practitioners but will also be of interest to colorectal surgeons, gastroenterologists, physiotherapists, continence advisors and lawyers.

Chapter | 4 |

The female urinary tract

Jean Rankin

The midwife must have a sound knowledge of the anatomy of the structures of the urinary tract and the basics of normal renal physiology to then understand the changes that take place during pregnancy and how they may impact on the health and wellbeing of the childbearing woman.

THE CHAPTER AIMS TO:

- provide an overview of the anatomy and functions of the various structures of the urinary system
- describe the processes of *excretion*, *elimination* and *homeostatic regulation* of the volume and solute concentration of blood plasma
- explain how urine is produced and eliminated through the process of micturition
- provide an overview of how the physiological effects of pregnancy and its hormonal influences may impact on the functioning of the urinary tract.

THE KIDNEYS

The kidneys are excretory glands with both endocrine and exocrine functions. They perform the excretory functions of the urinary system by removing metabolic waste products from the circulation to produce urine. In addition to removing waste products the urinary system has a broad range of other essential homeostatic functions (see Box 4.1).

A typical adult kidney is a bean-shaped reddish-brown organ. Each kidney is about 10 cm long, 6.5 cm wide, 3 cm thick and weighs about 100 g (Coad and Dunstall 2011). Although similar in shape, the left kidney is a longer and more slender organ than the right kidney. Congenital absence of one or both kidneys, known as unilateral or bilateral renal agenesis, can occur (Jones 2012). Bilateral renal agenesis is uncommon but is a serious failure in the development of both kidneys in the fetus. It is one causative agent of the Potter sequence (also known as *Potter's syndrome*). This absence of fetal kidneys causes *oligohydramnios*, a deficiency of amniotic fluid in a pregnant woman which can place extra pressure on the developing fetus and can cause further malformations. Non-pregnant adults with unilateral renal agenesis have a considerably higher risk of developing hypertension, which will become even more pronounced during pregnancy.

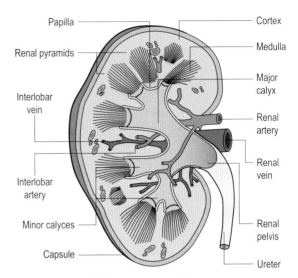

Fig. 4.1 Longitudinal section of the kidney.

Box 4.1 **Functions of the kidney**

- Regulation of water balance
- Regulation of blood pressure (renin–angiotensin system)
- Regulation of pH (acid–base balance) and inorganic ion balance (potassium, sodium and calcium)
- Control of formation of red blood cells (via erythropoietin)
- Secretion of hormones – renin, erythropoietin, 1.25-dihydroxyvitamin D3 (1,25-dihydroxycholecatciferol (also called calcitriol) and prostaglandins
- Vitamin D activation and calcium balance
- Gluconeogenesis (formation of glucose from amino acids and other precursors)
- Excretion of metabolic and nitrogenous waste products (urea from protein, uric acid from nucleic acids, creatinine from muscle creatine and haemoglobin breakdown products)
- Removal of toxic chemicals (drugs, pesticides and food additives)

Position and relations

The kidneys are situated in the posterior part of the abdominal cavity, one on either side of the vertebral column between the eleventh thoracic vertebra (T11) and the third lumbar vertebra (L3) (Jones 2012). The right kidney is slightly lower than the left kidney owing to its relationship to the liver (Coad and Dunstall 2011). The anterior and posterior surfaces of the kidneys are related to numerous structures, some of which come into direct contact with the kidneys whereas others are separated by a layer of peritoneum:

Posteriorly, the kidneys are related to rib 12 and the diaphragm, psoas major, quadratus lumborum and transversus abdominis muscles.

Anteriorly, the right kidney is related to the liver, duodenum, ascending colon and small intestine. The left kidney is related to the spleen, stomach, pancreas, descending colon and small intestine.

The triangular-shaped adrenal (suprarenal) glands are situated in the upper pole of the kidneys (Coad and Dunstall 2011).

Supports

The kidneys are maintained in position within the abdominal cavity by the overlying peritoneum, contact with adjacent visceral organs, such as the gastrointestinal tract, and by supporting connective tissue (Martini et al 2011).

Structure

Each kidney has a smooth surface covered by a tough fibrous capsule. There is a concave side facing medially. On this medial aspect is an opening called the *hilum*. The hilum is the point of entry for the renal artery and renal nerves, and the point of exit for the renal vein and the ureter (Fig. 4.1). Internally the hilum is continuous with the renal sinus.

Each kidney is enclosed by a thick fibrous capsule and has two distinct layers: the reddish-brown renal *cortex*, which has a rich blood supply, and the inner renal *medulla* where the structural and functional units of the kidney are located (Coad and Dunstall 2011). The renal medulla lies below the renal cortex and consists of between 8 and 18 distinct cone-shaped structures called *medullary* or *renal pyramids*. Each renal pyramid (which is striped in appearance) together with the associated overlying renal cortex forms a *renal lobe*. The base of each pyramid is broad and faces the cortex, while the pointed apex (*papilla*) projects into a minor *calyx*. Several minor calyces open into each of two or three major calyces, which then open into the *renal pelvis*. The renal pelvis is a flat funnel-shaped tube that is continuous with the *ureter*. Urine produced by the kidney flows continuously from the renal pelvis into the ureter and then into the bladder for storage (Stables and Rankin 2010).

The nephron

Each kidney has over 1 million nephrons, which are the functional units of the kidney. The nephron is approximately 3 cm long and is a tubule that is closed at one end and opens into the collecting duct at the other (Coad and

Dunstall 2011). The nephron has five distinct regions, each of which is adapted to a specific function:

- *Bowman's capsule* containing the glomerulus (renal corpuscle)
- the *proximal convoluted tubule*
- the *loop of Henle*
- the distal convoluted tubule and
- the collecting duct (Jones 2012).

There are two types of nephrons: *cortical nephrons* and *juxtomedullary nephrons*. The majority are cortical nephrons (85–90%) and these have short loops of Henle. Their main function is to control plasma volume during normal conditions. The juxtamedullary nephrons have longer loops of Henle extending into the medulla. These nephrons facilitate increased water retention when there is restricted water available (Coad and Dunstall 2011).

Each nephron begins at the renal corpuscle, which comprises the Bowman's capsule, which is a blind-ended cup-shaped chamber, and the glomerulus, a coiled arranged capillary network incorporated within the capsule (Fig. 4.2).

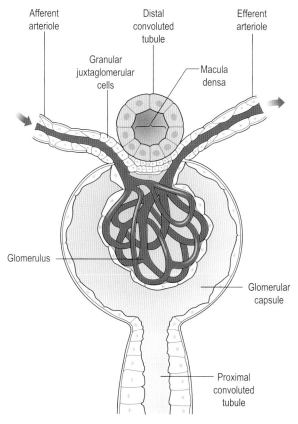

Afferent arteriole

Distal convoluted tubule

Efferent arteriole

Granular juxtaglomerular cells

Macula densa

Glomerulus

Glomerular capsule

Proximal convoluted tubule

Fig. 4.2 A glomerular body.
Reproduced from Coad J, Dunstall M 2011 Anatomy and physiology for midwives, 3rd edn. Edinburgh, Churchill Livingstone Elsevier, figure 2.2, p 30, after Brooker 1998.

Blood enters the renal corpuscle by way of the afferent arteriole which delivers blood to the glomerulus, with blood leaving by way of the efferent arteriole. This is the only place in the body where an artery collects blood from capillaries. The pressure within the glomerulus is increased because the afferent arteriole has a wider bore than the efferent arteriole and this factor forces the filtrate out of the capillaries into the capsule. At this stage any substance with a small molecular size will be filtered out.

The cup of the capsule is attached to the tubule of the nephron (Fig. 4.3). The proximal convoluted tubule initially winds and twists through the cortex, then forms a straight loop of Henle that dips into the medulla (descending arm), rising up into the cortex again (ascending arm) to wind and turn as the distal convoluted tubule before joining the straight collecting tubule. The straight collecting tubule runs from the cortex to a *medullary pyramid* where it forms a *medullary ray* and receives urine from many nephrons along its length (Martini et al 2011).

The distal convoluted tubule returns to pass alongside granular cells (also known as *juxtaglomerular cells*) of the afferent arteriole and this part of the tubule is called the *macula densa* (see Fig. 4.2). The granular cells and *macula densa* are known as the juxtaglomerular apparatus. The granular cells secrete renin whereas the *macula densa* cells monitor the sodium chloride concentration of fluid passing through.

Blood supply

The kidneys receive about 20–25% of the total cardiac output (Jones 2012). In healthy individuals, about 1200 ml of blood flows through the kidneys each minute. This is a phenomenal amount of blood for organs that have a combined weight of less than 300 g to experience (Martini et al 2011).

Each kidney receives blood through the renal artery, which originates from the lateral surface of the descending abdominal aorta near the level of the superior mesenteric artery. The artery enters at the renal hilum, transmitting numerous branches into the cortex to form the glomerulus for each nephron. Blood is collected up and returned via the renal vein.

Lymphatic drainage

A rich supply of lymph vessels lies under the cortex and around the urine-bearing tubules. Lymph drains into large lymphatic ducts that emerge from the hilum and lead to the aortic lymph glands.

Nerve supply

The kidneys are innervated by renal nerves. A renal nerve enters each kidney at the hilum and follows tributaries of renal arteries to reach individual nephrons. The

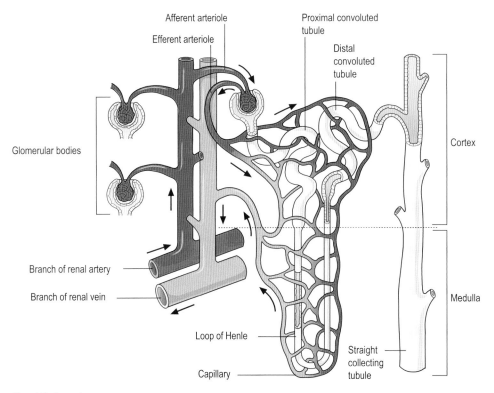

Afferent arteriole

Efferent arteriole

Proximal convoluted tubule

Distal convoluted tubule

Glomerular bodies

Cortex

Branch of renal artery

Branch of renal vein

Medulla

Loop of Henle

Straight collecting tubule

Capillary

Fig. 4.3 A nephron.

sympathetic innervation adjusts rates of urine formation by changing blood flow and blood pressure at the nephron and mobilizes the release of renin, which ultimately restricts losses of water and salt in urine by stimulating re-absorption at the nephron (Martini et al 2011).

Endocrine activity

The kidney secretes two hormones: *renin* and *erythropoietin*. Renin is produced in the afferent arteriole and is secreted when the blood supply to the kidneys is reduced and in response to lowered sodium levels. It acts on *angiotensinogen*, which is present in the blood, to form angiotensin, which raises blood pressure and encourages sodium re-absorption. The kidneys produce the hormone erythropoietin, in response to low oxygen levels that stimulate an increase in the production of red blood cells from the bone marrow (Coad and Dunstall 2011).

Table 4.1 Characteristics of urine	
Characteristics	**Normal range**
pH	4.5–8.0 (average 6.0)
Specific gravity	1.010–1.030
Osmotic concentration (osmolarity)	855–1335 mOsmol/l
Water content	93–97%
Volume	Varies depending on intake but usually 1000–1500 ml/day
Colour	Clear pale straw (dilute) Dark brown (very concentrated) Clear (in babies)
Odour	Varies with composition
Bacterial content	None (sterile)

URINE

Urine is usually acid and contains no glucose or ketones, nor should it carry blood cells or bacteria. The amber colour is due to the bile pigment *urobilin* and the colour varies depending on the concentration (see Table 4.1). In the newborn baby, it is almost clear. The volume and final concentration of urea and solutes depend on fluid intake. An adult can void between 1000 ml and 2000 ml of urine daily. Urine has a characteristic smell, which is not unpleasant when fresh. Strong odour or cloudiness generally indicates a bacterial infection.

Women are susceptible to urinary tract infection, usually due to ascending infection acquired via the urethra. A colony bacterial count of more than 100 000/ml is considered to be pathologically significant and is often referred to as bacteraemia (Coad and Dunstall 2011).

The production of urine

The production of urine takes place in three stages: *filtration*, *selective reabsorption* and *secretion*.

Filtration

Filtration is a largely passive, non-selective process that occurs through the semipermeable walls of the glomerulus and glomerular capsule. Fluids and solutes are forced through the membrane by hydrostatic pressure. The passage of water and solutes across the filtration membrane of the glomerulus is similar to that in other capillary beds: moving down a pressure gradient. However, the glomerular filtration membrane is thousands of times more permeable to water and solutes, and glomerular pressure is much higher than normal capillary blood pressure (Stables and Rankin 2010). Water and small molecules such as glucose, amino acids and vitamins escape through the filter as the *filtrate* and enter the nephron, whereas blood cells, plasma proteins and other large molecules are usually retained in the blood (Fig. 4.4). The content of the Bowman's capsule is referred to as the *glomerular filtrate* (GF) and the rate at which this is formed is referred to as the *glomerular filtration rate* (GFR). The kidneys form about 180 l of dilute filtrate each day (125 ml/min). Most of this is selectively reabsorbed so that the final volume of urine produced daily is about 1000–1500 ml/day (Coad and Dunstall 2011).

Selective reabsorption

Substances from the glomerular filtrate are reabsorbed from the rest of the nephron into the surrounding capillaries. Some substances, such as amino acids and glucose, are completely reabsorbed and are not normally present in urine. The reabsorption of other substances is under the regulation of several hormones. Water balance is mainly regulated by the *antidiuretic hormone* (ADH) produced by the posterior pituitary gland. This is regulated through a negative feedback loop (Fig. 4.5).

The secretion of ADH is initiated by an increase in plasma osmolality, by a decrease in circulating blood volume and by lowered blood pressure (e.g. through reduced fluid intake or sweating). The action of ADH is to increase permeability of the renal tubular cells. More water is reabsorbed, resulting in reduced volume of more concentrated urine. When the body has sufficient fluid intake and physiological paramenters are within normal range then the production of ADH is inhibited and urine

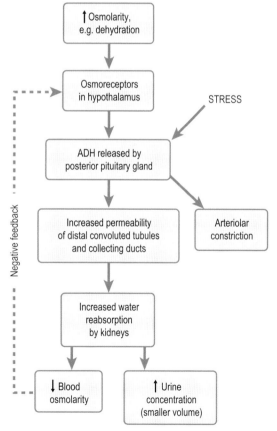

Fig. 4.5 The action of ADH.
Reproduced from Coad J, Dunstall M 2011 Anatomy and physiology for midwives, 3rd edn. Edinburgh, Churchill Livingstone Elsevier, figure 2.5, p 33.

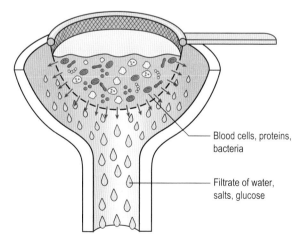

Blood cells, proteins, bacteria

Filtrate of water, salts, glucose

Fig. 4.4 Filtration: larger molecules stay in the sieve (glomerulus) and smaller molecules filter out (into the glomerular capsule).

increases in volume and is more dilute. One exception to note relates to the consumption of alcohol, which inhibits the effect of ADH on the kidneys, thereby inducing diuresis that is out of proportion to the volume of fluid ingested (Weise et al 2000). Newborn babies have poor ability to concentrate and dilute their urine and this is even more so for preterm infants. For this reason they are unable to tolerate wide variations in their fluid intake.

Minerals are selected according to the body's needs. Calcitonin increases calcium excretion and parathyroid hormone enhances reabsorption of calcium from the renal tubules (Coad and Dunstall 2011). The reabsorption of sodium is controlled by aldosterone, which is produced in the cortex of the suprarenal gland. The interaction of aldosterone and ADH maintains water and sodium balance. It is vital that the pH of the blood is controlled in the body and if it is tending towards acidity then acids will be excreted in urine. However, if the opposite situation arises then alkaline urine will be produced. Often this is the result of an intake of an alkaline substance. A diet high in meat and cranberry juice will keep the urine acidic whilst a diet rich in citrus fruit, most vegetables and legumes will keep the urine alkaline. Bacteria causing a urinary tract infection or bacterial contamination will also produce alkaline urine.

Secretion

Tubular secretion is an important mechanism in clearing the blood of unwanted substances. Secreted substances into the urine include hydrogen ions, ammonia, creatinine, drugs and toxins.

THE URETERS

The ureters are hollow muscular tubes. The upper end is funnel-shaped and merges into the renal pelvis, where urine is received from the renal tubules.

Function

The ureters transport urine from the kidneys to the bladder by waves of peristalsis. About every 30 seconds a peristaltic contraction begins at the renal pelvis and sweeps along the ureter, forcing urine towards the urinary bladder (Martini et al 2011).

Structure

Each ureter is about 0.3 cm in diameter and 25–30 cm long, running from the renal hilum to the posterior wall of the bladder (Fig. 4.6).

The ureters extend inferiorly and medially, passing over the anterior surfaces of the *psoas major muscle* and are

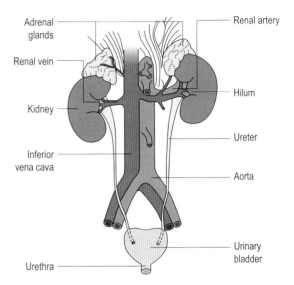

Fig. 4.6 The ureters.
Reproduced from Coad J, Dunstall M 2011 Anatomy and physiology for midwives, 3rd edn. Edinburgh, Churchill Livingstone Elsevier, figure 2.1, p 30, after Brooker 1998.

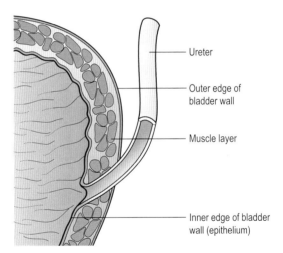

Fig. 4.7 Diagram to show the entry of the ureter into the posterior wall of the bladder.

firmly attached to the posterior abdominal wall. At the pelvic brim the ureters descend along the side walls of the pelvis to the level of the ischial spines and then turn forwards to pass beside the uterine cervix and enter the bladder from behind (Fig. 4.7). The ureters penetrate the posterior wall of the urinary bladder without entering the peritoneal cavity. They pass through the bladder wall at an oblique angle, and the ureteral openings are slit-like rather than rounded. This shape helps prevent the backflow of urine toward the ureter and kidneys when the urinary bladder contracts (Martini et al 2011).

Layers

The ureters are composed of three layers: an *inner lining*, a *middle muscular layer* and an *outer coat* (Martini et al 2011). The *inner lining* comprises of transitional epithelium arranged in longitudinal folds. This type of epithelium consists of several layers of pear-shaped cells and makes an elastic and waterproof inner coat.

The *middle muscular layer* is made up of longitudinal and circular bands of smooth muscle.

The *outer coat* comprises of fibrous connective tissue that is continuous with the fibrous capsule of the kidney.

Blood supply

The blood supply to the upper part of the ureter is similar to that of the kidney. In its pelvic portion, it derives blood from the common iliac and internal iliac arteries and from the uterine and vesical arteries, according to its proximity to the different organs. Venous return is along corresponding veins.

Lymphatic drainage

Lymph drains into the internal, external and common iliac nodes.

Nerve supply

The nerve supply is from the renal, aortic, superior and inferior hypogastric plexuses.

THE BLADDER

The bladder is a distensible, hollow, muscular, pelvic organ that functions as a temporary reservoir for the storage of urine until it is convenient for it to be voided. Pregnancy and childbirth can affect bladder control and thus midwives need to be familiar with the anatomy and physiology of the bladder.

Position, shape and size

The empty bladder lies in the pelvic cavity and is described as being *pyramidal* with its triangular base resting on the upper half of the vagina and its apex directed towards the symphysis pubis. However, as it fills with urine it rises up out of the pelvic cavity becoming an abdominal organ and more globular in shape as its walls are distended. It can be palpated above the symphysis pubis when full. During labour the bladder is an abdominal organ, as it is displaced by the fetus as it descends into the pelvic cavity.

The empty bladder is of similar size to the uterus, but when full of urine it becomes much larger. The normal capacity of the bladder is approximately 600 ml although the capacity in individuals does vary between 500 ml (Stables and Rankin 2010) and 1000 ml (Martini et al 2011).

Relations (see Fig. 4.8)

- *Anterior* to the bladder is the symphysis pubis, which is separated from it by a space filled with fatty tissue called the *Cave of Retzius*.

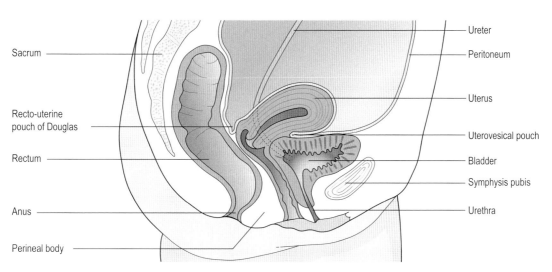

Fig. 4.8 Sagittal section of the pelvis showing the relations of the bladder.

- *Posterior* to the bladder is the cervix and ureters.
- *Laterally* are the lateral ligaments of the bladder and the side walls of the pelvis.
- *Superiorly* lie the intestines and peritoneal cavity. In the non-pregnant female the anteverted, ante-flexed uterus lies partially over the bladder.
- Inferior to the bladder is the urethra and the muscular diaphragm of the pelvic floor, which forms its main support, and on which its function partly depends.

Supports

There are five ligaments attached to the bladder (Stables and Rankin 2010). A fibrous band called the *urachus* extends from the apex of the bladder to the umbilicus. Two lateral ligaments extend from the bladder to the side walls of the pelvis. Two *pubovesical ligaments* attach from the bladder neck anteriorly to the symphysis pubis and they also form part of the pubocervical ligaments of the uterus.

Structure

The base of the bladder is termed the *trigone.* It is situated at the back of the bladder, resting against the vagina. Its three angles are the exit of the urethra below and the two slit-like openings of the ureters above. The apex of the trigone is thus at its lowest point, which is also termed *the* neck (Fig. 4.9).

The anterior part of the bladder lies close to the symphysis pubis and is termed the *apex of the bladder.* From the apex of the bladder, the urachus runs up the anterior abdominal wall to the umbilicus. In fetal life, the urachus is the remains of the yolk sac but in the adult is simply a fibrous band.

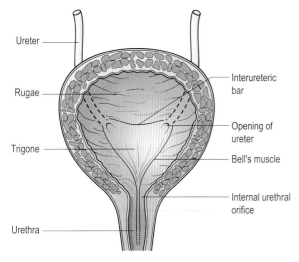

Ureter

Rugae

Trigone

Urethra

Interureteric bar

Opening of ureter

Bell's muscle

Internal urethral orifice

Fig. 4.9 Section through the bladder.

Layers

The lining of the bladder, like that of the ureter, is formed of transitional epithelium, which helps to allow the distension of the bladder without losing its water-holding effect. The lining, except over the trigone, is thrown into *rugae*, which flatten out as the bladder expands and fills. The mucous membrane lining lies on a submucous layer of areolar tissue that carries blood vessels, lymph vessels and nerves.

The epithelium over the trigone is smooth and firmly attached to the underlying muscle. The musculature of the bladder consists chiefly of the large *detrusor muscle* whose function is to expel urine. This muscle has three coats of smooth muscle: an *inner longitudinal, a middle circular* and an *outer longitudinal* layer. Around the neck of the bladder, the circular muscle is thickened to form the internal urethral sphincter (Stables and Rankin 2010). The general elasticity of the numerous muscle fibres around the bladder neck tends to keep the urethra closed (Standring 2009). In the trigone, the muscles are somewhat differently arranged. A band of muscle between the ureteric openings forms the *interureteric bar.* The *urethral dilator muscle* lies in the ventral part of the bladder neck and the walls of the urethra and it is thought to be of significance in overcoming urethral resistance to micturition (Standring 2009).

The outer layer of the bladder is formed of visceral pelvic fascia, except on its superior surface, which is covered with peritoneum (see Fig. 4.8).

Blood supply

Blood supply is from the superior and inferior vesical arteries and drainage is by the corresponding veins.

Lymphatic drainage

Lymph drains into the internal iliac and the obturator nodes.

Nerve supply

The nerve supply is parasympathetic and sympathetic and comes via the *Lee–Frankenhauser pelvic plexus* in the pouch of Douglas. The stimulation of sympathetic nerves causes the internal urethral sphincter to contract and the detrusor muscle to relax, whereas the parasympathetic nerve fibres cause the sphincter to relax and the bladder to empty.

THE URETHRA

In the female the urethra is a narrow tube, about 4 cm long, that is embedded in the lower half of the anterior vaginal wall. It passes from the internal meatus of the bladder to the vestibule of the vulva, where it opens externally as the urethral meatus. The internal sphincter surrounds the urethra as it leaves the bladder. As the urethra passes between the levator ani muscles it is enclosed by bands of striated muscle known as the membranous sphincter of the urethra, which is under voluntary control (Stables and Rankin 2010). During labour, the urethra becomes elongated as the bladder is drawn up into the abdomen, extending several centimetres.

Structure

The urethra forms the junction between the urinary tract and the external genitalia. The epithelium of its lining reflects this. The upper half is lined with transitional epithelium whereas the lower half is lined with squamous epithelium. The lumen is normally closed unless urine is passing down it or a catheter is in situ. When closed, it has small longitudinal folds. Small blind ducts called urethral crypts (of which the two largest are the *paraurethral glands* or *Skene's ducts*) open into the urethra near the urethral meatus (Martini et al 2011).

The submucous coat of the urethra is composed of epithelium, which lies on a bed of vascular connective tissue.

The musculature of the urethra is arranged as an inner longitudinal layer, continuous with the inner muscle fibres of the bladder, and an external circular layer. The *inner muscle fibres* help to open the internal urethral sphincter during micturition.

The *outer layer* of the urethra is continuous with the outer layer of the vagina and is formed of connective tissue.

At the lower end of the urethra, voluntary, striated muscle fibres form the so-called membranous sphincter of the urethra. This is not a true sphincter but it gives some voluntary control to the woman when she desires to resist the urge to void urine. The powerful levator ani muscles, which pass on either side of the uterus, also assist in controlling continence of urine.

Blood supply

The blood to the urethra is circulated by the inferior vesical and pudendal arteries and veins.

Lymphatic drainage

Lymph drains through the internal iliac glands.

Nerve supply

The internal urethral sphincter is supplied by sympathetic and parasympathetic nerves but the membranous sphincter is supplied by the pudendal nerve and is under voluntary control.

MICTURITION

The process of micturition (urination) is a coordinated response that is due to the contraction of the muscular wall of the bladder, reflex relaxation of the internal sphincter of the urethra and voluntary relaxation of the external sphincter (Coad and Dunstall 2011). As the bladder fills with urine, stretch receptors in the wall of the urinary bladder are stimulated which then relay parasympathetic sensory nerve impulses to the brain generating awareness of fluid pressure in the bladder. This usually occurs when the bladder contains approximately 200–300 ml of urine (with increasing discomfort as the volume increases). The urge to micturate can be voluntarily resisted and postponed until a suitable time. This is due to the conscious descending inhibition of the reflex bladder contraction and relaxation of the external sphincter. If the urge to micturate is not voluntarily resisted then the bladder will empty of urine by the muscle wall contracting, the internal sphincter opening by the action of Bell's muscles (see Fig. 4.9) and voluntary relaxation of the external sphincter. This is assisted by the increased pressure in the pelvic cavity as the diaphragm is lowered and the abdominal muscles contract. The tone of the external sphincter is also affected by psychological stimuli (such as waking or leaving home) and external stimuli (such as the sound of running water). Any factor that raises the intra-abdominal and intra-vesicular pressures (such as laughter or coughing) in excess of the urethral closing pressure can result in incontinence (Coad and Dunstall 2011).

Infants lack voluntary control over micturition because the necessary corticospinal connections have yet to be established (Martini et al 2011). Cortical control of micturition occurs from learned behaviour and is usually achieved by about 2 years of age.

CHANGES TO THE URINARY TRACT IN PREGNANCY AND CHILDBIRTH

The urinary system can be markedly stressed by pregnancy, mostly because of its close proximity to the reproductive organs and the major changes in fluid balance resulting in fluid retention during pregnancy (Coad and Dunstall 2011). In pregnancy the enlarging uterus affects all the parts of the urinary tract (see Chapter 9) at various times. In early pregnancy, bladder capacity is compromised by the growing uterus within the pelvic cavity which is relieved once the uterus becomes an abdominal organ. Once the presenting part engages through the pelvic brim in late pregnancy this again restricts space available for bladder capacity. The hormones of pregnancy also have an

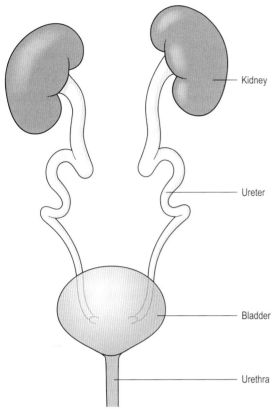

Kidney

Ureter

Bladder

Urethra

Fig. 4.10 Dilated, kinked ureters in pregnancy.

influence on the urinary tract. Under the influence of progesterone, bladder capacity increases to about 1000 ml by late pregnancy and the walls of the ureters relax, which allows them to dilate, bend or 'kink' (Fig. 4.10). If this occurs in the ureters, then it tends to result in a slowing down or stasis of urinary flow, causing women to be more at risk from infection.

During pregnancy large amounts of urine are produced due to an increase in glomerular filtration as this helps to eliminate the additional wastes created by maternal and fetal metabolism. In labour, the urethra becomes elongated as the bladder is drawn up into the abdomen.

During the postnatal period there is a rapid and sustained loss of sodium and a major diuresis occurs, especially on the 2nd to 5th postnatal day. A normal urine output for a woman during this time may be up to 3000 ml/day with voiding of 500–1000 ml at any one micturition (Stables and Rankin 2010).

CONCLUSION

The kidneys are excretory glands with both endocrine and exocrine functions. Urine produced by the kidney flows continuously from the renal pelvis into the ureter and then into the bladder for storage. The three major functions are: excretion, elimination and homeostatic regulation of the volume and solute concentration of blood plasma. Water balance is mainly regulated by the antidiuretic hormone (ADH) through a negative feedback loop.

During pregnancy the urinary system can be markedly stressed, mostly because of its close proximity to the reproductive organs, the major changes in fluid balance and the hormones of pregnancy. It is therefore important that the midwife recognizes what effects these can have on childbearing women to offer them appropriate advice and support in relieving any discomfort.

REFERENCES

Coad J, Dunstall M 2011 Anatomy and physiology for midwives, 3rd edn. Churchill Livingstone Elsevier, Edinburgh

Jones T L 2012 Crash course: renal and urinary system, 4th edn. Mosby Elsevier, London

Martini F H, Nath J L, Bartholomew E F 2011 Fundamentals of anatomy and physiology, 9th edn. Pearson International, London

Stables D, Rankin J 2010 Physiology in childbearing with anatomy and related biosciences, 3rd edn. Elsevier, Edinburgh

Standring S 2009 Gray's anatomy: the anatomical basis of clinical practice, 40th edn. Churchill Livingstone, New York

Weise J G, Shlipak M G, Browner W S 2000 The alcohol hangover. Annals of Internal Medicine 132(11):897–902

FURTHER READING

Coad J, Dunstall M 2011 Anatomy and physiology for midwives, 3rd edn. Churchill Livingstone, Elsevier, Edinburgh

Chapter 2 of this book includes several stylized diagrams related to urine production. The diagrams are detailed and

well explained and may help the individual who learns best from visual representation.

Stables D, Rankin J 2010 Physiology in childbearing with anatomy and related biosciences, 3rd edn. Elsevier, Edinburgh

Chapter 19 offers a fuller and more in-depth account of the physiology related to the renal and urinary system, including changes in pregnancy and a short account of the postnatal period.

Chapter | 5 |

Hormonal cycles: fertilization and early development

Jenny Bailey

Monthly physiological changes take place in the ovaries and the uterus, regulated by hormones produced by the hypothalamus, anterior pituitary gland and ovaries. These monthly cycles commence at puberty and occur simultaneously and together are known as the female reproductive cycle.

THE CHAPTER AIMS TO:

- explore in detail the events that occur during the ovarian and menstrual cycles
- describe in detail the process of fertilization followed by the subsequent development of the conceptus into the pre-embryonic period.

INTRODUCTION

The functions of the female reproductive cycle are to prepare the *egg*, often referred to as the *gamete* or *oocyte*, for fertilization by the *spermatozoon* (sperm), and to prepare the uterus to receive and nourish the fertilized oocyte. If fertilization has not taken place the inner lining of the uterus or endometrium and the oocyte are shed and bleeding occurs per vagina, and the cyclic events begin again.

Before the onset of puberty, luteinizing hormone (LH) and follicle stimulating hormone (FSH) levels are low. Pulsatile increases in gonadotrophin releasing hormone (GnRH), particularly at night, cause increase in LH secretion. This increasing surge of LH is established prior to menarche (Wennink et al 1990). It is also thought that the interaction of leptin with GnRH may have a role in the initiation of puberty. The first-ever occurrence of cyclic events is termed *menarche*, meaning the first menstrual bleeding. The average age of menarche is 12 years, although between the ages 8 and 16 is considered normal. The onset of menstrual bleeding ('periods' or menses) is a major stage in a girl's life, representing the maturation of the reproductive system and physical transition into womanhood. For many women this monthly phenomenon signals and embodies the quintessence of being a 'woman'. Similarly, for other women it is regarded as an inconvenience, causing pain, shame and embarrassment (Chrisler 2011). Cultural and religious traditions affect how women and their communities feel about menstruation. The advent of hormonal contraception (Chapter 27) affords women, especially those in Western society, an element of control over their periods. Factors such as heredity, diet, obesity and overall health can accelerate or delay menarche.

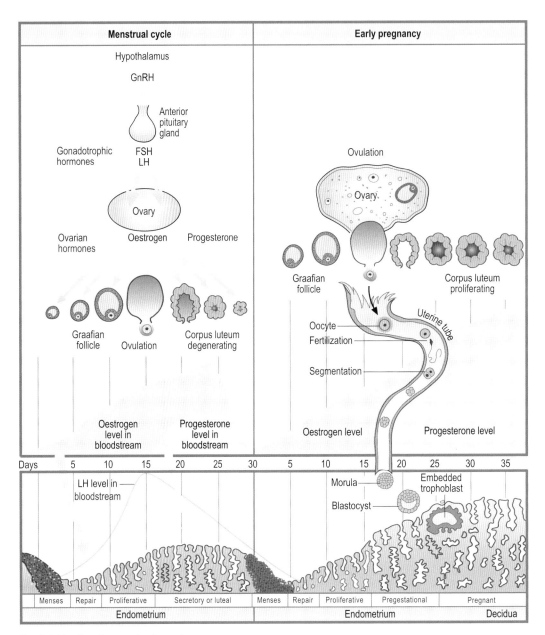

Fig. 5.1 The female reproductive cycle.

Interference with the hormonal–organ relationship prior to and during the reproductive years is likely to cause menstrual cycle dysfunction which may result in failure to ovulate. The cessation of cyclic events is referred to as the *menopause*, and signifies the end of reproductive life. Each woman has an individual reproductive cycle that varies in length, although the average cycle is normally 28 days long, and recurs regularly from puberty to the menopause except when pregnancy intervenes (Fig. 5.1).

THE OVARIAN CYCLE

The ovarian cycle (Fig. 5.2) is the name given to the physiological changes that occur in the ovaries essential for the preparation and release of an oocyte. The ovarian cycle consists of three phases, all of which are under the control of hormones.

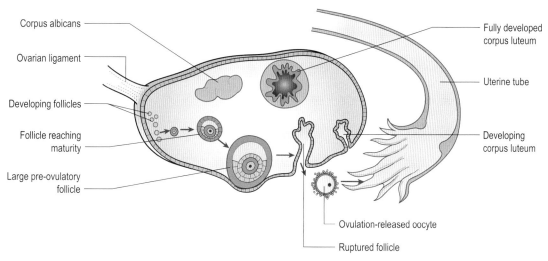

Fig. 5.2 The cycle of a Graafian follicle in the ovary.

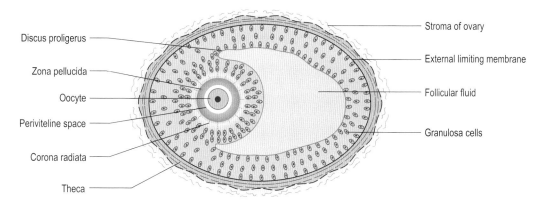

Fig. 5.3 A ripe Graafian follicle.

The follicular phase

The formation of oogonia in the germinal epithelium of the ovaries is known as *oogenesis*. Primordial germ cells differentiate into oogonia in the ovaries during fetal life. These diploid stem cells divide mitotically and proliferate into millions of germ cells. Most of the germ cells degenerate (by atresia), however some develop further into *primary oocytes*, and enter the prophase of meiosis I cell division. Meiotic arrest occurs and the process does not continue until after puberty (further meiotic division takes place at ovulation of the secondary oocyte and the process is only completed if fertilization occurs).Whilst in this arrested prophase stage of meiosis I the primary oocyte is surrounded by follicular cells and is hence known as the *primordial follicle*. There are up to 2 million primary oocytes in each ovary at birth and due to atresia the number is reduced to approximately 40 000 at puberty; 400 of these

will mature and ovulate during the woman's lifetime (Tortora and Derrickson 2011). Following puberty FSH and LH further stimulate the development of primordial follicles into *primary* and *secondary follicles* and subsequently into large *preovulatory or Graafian follicles* (Fig. 5.3) by a process known as folliculogenesis.

Low levels of oestrogen and progesterone stimulate the hypothalamus to produce GnRH. This releasing hormone causes the production of FSH and LH by the anterior pituitary gland. FSH controls the growth and maturity of the Graafian follicles. The Graafian follicles begin to secrete oestrogen, which comprises oestradiol, oestrone and oestriol. Rising levels of oestradiol cause a surge in LH. When oestradiol reaches a certain peak, the secretion of FSH is inhibited. The reduced FSH secretion causes a slowing in follicle growth and eventually leads to follicle death, known as *atresia*. The largest and dominant follicle secretes *inhibin*, which further suppresses FSH. This dominant follicle prevails and forms a bulge near the surface of the ovary, and soon becomes competent to ovulate. The time from the growth and maturity of the Graafian follicles to ovulation is normally around 1 week. Occasionally the follicular phase may take longer if the dominant follicle does not ovulate, and the phase will begin again. The differing lengths of menstrual cycle reported between individual women are as a result in the varying timespans in this pre-ovulatory phase. It can last 6–13 days in a 28-day cycle (Tortora and Derrickson 2011).

Ovulation

High oestrogen levels cause a sudden surge in LH around day 12–13 of a 28 day cycle, which lasts for approximately 48 hours. This matures the oocyte and weakens the wall of the follicle and causes *ovulation* to occur on day 14.

Ovulation is the process whereby the dominant Graafian follicle ruptures and discharges the secondary oocyte into the pelvic cavity. Fimbrae guide it into the uterine tube where it awaits fertilization. During the time of ovulation, meiotic cell division resumes and the diploid oocyte becomes haploid (with a first polar body). During ovulation some women experience varying degrees of abdominal pain known as *mittelschmerz*, which can last several hours. There may be some light bleeding caused by the hormonal changes taking place. Stringy clear mucus appears in the cervix, ready to accept the sperm from intercourse. Following ovulation the fertilized or unfertilized oocyte travels to the uterus.

The luteal phase

The *luteal phase* is the process whereby the cells of the residual ruptured follicle proliferate and form a yellow irregular structure known as the *corpus luteum*. The corpus luteum produces oestrogen, relaxin, inhibin and progesterone for approximately 2 weeks, to develop the endometrium of the uterus, which awaits the fertilized oocyte. Small amounts of relaxin cause uterine quiescence, which is an ideal environment for the fertilized oocyte to implant. The corpus luteum continues its role until the placenta is adequately developed to take over. During the luteal phase the cervical mucus becomes sticky and thick. In the absence of fertilization the corpus luteum degenerates and becomes the corpus albicans (white body), and progesterone, oestrogen, relaxin and inhibin levels decrease. In response to low levels of oestrogen and progesterone the hypothalamus produces GnRH. The rising levels of GnRH stimulate the anterior pituitary gland to produce FSH and the ovarian cycle commences again (Stables and Rankin 2010). The luteal phase is the most constant part of the ovarian cycle, lasting 14 days out of a 28 day cycle (Tortora and Derrickson 2011).

THE MENSTRUAL OR ENDOMETRIAL CYCLE

The *menstrual cycle* is the name given to the physiological changes that occur in the endometrial layer of the uterus, and which are essential to receive the fertilized oocyte. The menstrual cycle consists of three phases.

The menstrual phase

This phase is often referred to as *menstruation, bleeding, menses,* or a *period*. Physiologically this is the terminal phase of the reproductive cycle of events and is simultaneous with the beginning of the follicular phase of the ovarian cycle. Reducing levels of oestrogen and progesterone stimulate prostaglandin release that causes the spiral arteries of the endometrium to go into spasm, withdrawing the blood supply to it, and the endometrium dies, referred to as *necrosis*. The endometrium is shed down to the basal layer along with blood from the capillaries, the unfertilized oocyte tissue fluid, mucus and epithelial cells. Failure to menstruate *(amenorrhoea)* is an indication that a woman may have become pregnant. The term *eumenorrhoea* denotes normal, regular menstruation that lasts for typically 3–5 days, although 2–7 days is considered normal. The average blood loss during menstruation is 50–150 ml. The blood is inhibited from clotting due to the enzyme plasmin contained in the endometrium. The menstrual flow passes from the uterus through the cervix and the vagina to the exterior. The term *menorrhagia* denotes heavy bleeding. Some women experience uterine cramps caused by muscular contractions to expel the tissue. Severe uterine cramps are known as *dysmenorrhoea*.

The proliferative phase

This phase follows menstruation, is simultaneous with the follicular phase of the ovary and lasts until ovulation. There is the formation of a new layer of endometrium in the uterus, referred to as the proliferative endometrium. This phase is under the control of oestradiol and other oestrogens secreted by the Graafian follicle and consist of the re-growth and thickening of the endometrium in the uterus. During the first few days of this phase the endometrium is re-forming, described as the *regenerative phase*. At the completion of this phase the endometrium consists of three layers. The *basal layer* lies immediately above the myometrium and is approximately 1 mm thick. It contains all the necessary rudimentary structures for building new endometrium. The *functional layer*, which contains tubular glands, is approximately 2.5 mm thick, and lies on top of the basal layer. It changes constantly according to the hormonal influences of the ovary. The *layer of cuboidal ciliated epithelium* covers the functional layer. It dips down to line the tubular glands of the functional layer. If fertilization occurs, the fertilized oocyte implants itself within the endometrium.

The secretory phase

This phase follows the proliferative phase and is simultaneous with ovulation. It is under the influence of progesterone and oestrogen secreted by the corpus luteum. The functional layer of the endometrium thickens to approximately 3.5 mm and becomes spongy in appearance because the glands are more tortuous. The blood supply to the area is increased and the glands produce nutritive secretions such as glycogen. These conditions last for approximately 7 days, awaiting the fertilized oocyte.

FERTILIZATION

Human fertilization, known as conception, is the fusion of genetic material from the haploid sperm cell and the secondary oocyte (now haploid), to form the zygote (Fig. 5.4). The process takes approximately 12–24 hours and normally occurs in the ampulla of the uterine tube. Following ovulation, the oocyte, which is about 0.15 mm in diameter, passes into the uterine tube. The oocyte, having no power of locomotion, is wafted along by the cilia and by the peristaltic muscular contraction of the uterine tube. At the same time the cervix, which is under the influence of oestrogen, secretes a flow of alkaline mucus that attracts the spermatozoa. In the fertile male at intercourse approximately 300 million sperm are deposited in the posterior fornix of the vagina. Approximately 2 million reach the loose cervical mucus, survive and propel themselves towards the uterine tubes while the rest are destroyed by the acid medium of the vagina. Approximately 200 sperm will ultimately reach the oocyte (Tortora and Derrickson 2011). Sperm swim from the vagina and through the cervical canal using their whip-like tails (flagella). Prostaglandins from semen and uterine contractions as a result of intercourse facilitate the passage of the sperm into the uterus and beyond. Once inside the uterine tubes (within minutes of intercourse), the sperm undergo a process known as *capacitation*. This process takes up to 7 hours. Influenced by secretions from the uterine tube the sperm undergo changes to the plasma membrane, resulting in the removal of the glycoprotein coat and increased flagellation. The zona pellucida of the oocyte produces chemicals that attract capacitated sperm only. The acrosomal layer of the capacitated sperm becomes reactive and releases the enzyme hyaluronidase known as the *acrosome reaction*, which disperses the corona radiata (the outermost layer of the oocyte) allowing access to the zona pellucida (see Fig. 5.4C). Many sperm are involved in this process. Other enzymes, such as acrosin, produce an opening in the zona

pellucida. The first sperm that reaches the zona pellucida penetrates it (see Fig. 5.4D).

Upon penetration the oocyte releases corticol granules; this is known as the *cortical reaction*. The cortical reaction and depolarization of the the oocyte cell membrane makes it impermeable to other sperm. This is important as there are many sperm surrounding the oocyte at this time. The plasma membranes of the sperm and oocyte fuse. The oocyte at this stage completes its second meiotic division, and becomes mature. The pronucleus now has 23 chromosomes, referred to as *haploid*. The tail and mitochondria of the sperm degenerate as the sperm penetrates the oocyte, and there is the formation of the male pronucleus. The male and female pronuclei fuse to form a new nucleus that is a combination of the genetic material from both the sperm and oocyte, referred to as a *diploid* cell. The male and the female gametes each contribute half the complement of chromosomes to make a total of 46 (Box 5.1). This new cell is called a *zygote*.

Dizygotic twins (fraternal twins) are produced from two oocytes released independently but in the same time frame fusing with two different sperm; they are genetically different from each other. Monozygotic twins develop

---

Box 5.1 **Chromosomes**

Each human cell has a complement of 46 chromosomes arranged in 23 pairs, of which one pair are sex chromosomes. The remaining pairs are known as autosomes. During the process of maturation, both gametes shed half their chromosomes, one of each pair, during a reduction division called *meiosis*. Genetic material is exchanged between the chromosomes before they split up. In the male, meiosis starts at puberty and both halves redivide to form four sperm in all. In the female, meiosis commences during fetal life but the first division is not completed until many years later at ovulation. The division is unequal; the larger part will eventually go on to form the oocyte while the remainder forms the first polar body. At fertilization the second division takes place and results in one large cell, which is now mature, and a much smaller one, the second polar body. At the same time, division of the first polar body creates a third polar body.

When the gametes combine at fertilization to form the zygote, the full complement of chromosomes is restored. Subsequent division occurs by mitosis where the chromosomes divide to give each new cell a full set.

Sex determination

Females carry two similar sex chromosomes, XX; males carry two dissimilar sex chromosomes, XY. Each sperm will carry either an X or a Y chromosome, whereas the oocyte always carries an X chromosome. If the oocyte is fertilized by an X-carrying sperm a female is conceived, if by a Y-carrying one, a male.

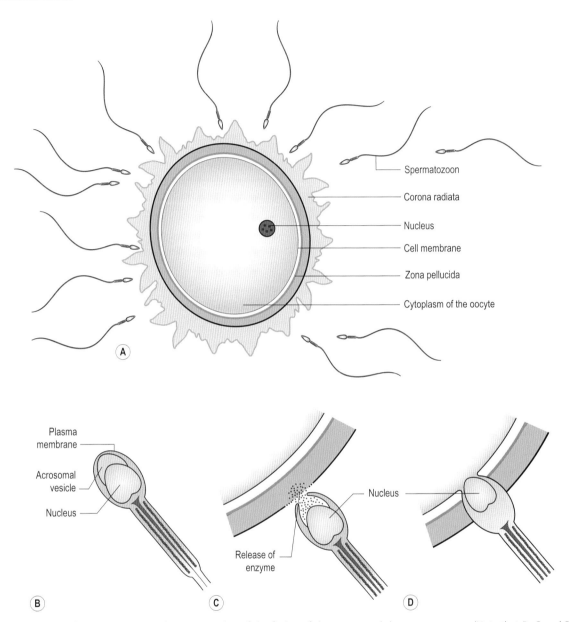

Fig. 5.4 Fertilization. Diagrammatic representation of the fusion of the oocyte and the spermatozoon. (Note that B, C and D are more greatly magnified than A.)

from a single zygote for a variety of reasons, where cells separate into two embryos, usually before 8 days following fertilization. These twins are genetically identical.

DEVELOPMENT OF THE ZYGOTE

The development of the zygote can be divided into three periods. The first 2 weeks after fertilization, referred to as the *pre-embryonic period*, includes the implantation of the zygote into the endometrium; weeks 2–8 are known as the *embryonic period*; and weeks 8 to birth are known as the *fetal period*.

The pre-embryonic period

During the first week the zygote travels along the uterine tube towards the uterus. At this stage a strong membrane of glycoproteins called the zona pellucida surrounds the zygote. The zygote receives nourishment, mainly glycogen, from the goblet cells of the uterine tubes and later the secretory cells of the uterus. During the travel the zygote undergoes mitotic cellular replication and division referred to as *cleavage*, resulting in the formation of smaller cells known as *blastomeres*. The zygote divides into two cells at 1 day, then four at 2 days, eight by 2.5 days, 16 by 3 days, now known as the *morula*. The cells bind tightly together in a process known as *compactation*. Next *cavitation* occurs whereby the outermost cells secrete fluid into the morula and a fluid-filled cavity or *blastocele* appears in the morula. This results in the formation of the blastula or *blastocyst*, comprising 58 cells. The process from the development of the morula to the development of the blastocyst is referred to as *blastulation* and has occurred by around day 4 (Fig. 5.5).

The zona pellucida remains during the process of cleavage, so that despite an increase in number of cells the overall size remains that of the zygote and constant at this stage. The zona pellucida prevents the developing blastocyst from increasing in size and therefore getting stuck in the uterine tube; it also prevents embedding occurring in the tube rather than the uterus, which could result in an ectopic pregnancy. Around day 4 the blastocyst enters the uterus. Endometrial glands secrete glycogen-rich fluid into the uterus which penetrates the zona pellucida. This and nutrients in the cytoplasm of the blastomeres provides nourishment for the developing cells. The blastocyst digests its way out of the zona pellucida once it enters the uterine cavity. The blastocyst possesses an *inner cell mass* or *embryoblast*, and an *outer cell mass* or *trophoblast*. The trophoblast becomes the placenta and chorion, while the embryoblast becomes the embryo, amnion and umbilical cord (Carlson 2004; Tortora and Derrickson 2011).

During week 2, the trophoblast proliferates and differentiates into two layers: the outer *syncytio-trophoblast* or *syncytium* and the inner *cytotrophoblast* (cuboidal dividing cells) (Fig. 5.6). Implantation of the trophoblast layer into the endometrium, now known as the *decidua*, begins. Implantation is usually to the upper posterior wall. At the implantation stage the zona pellucida will have totally disappeared. The syncytiotrophoblast layer invades the decidua by forming finger-like projections called *villi* that make their way into the decidua and spaces called *lacunae* that fill up with the mother's blood. The villi begin to branch, and contain blood vessels of the developing embryo, thus allowing gaseous exchange between the mother and embryo. Implantation is assisted by proteolytic enzymes secreted by the syncytiotrophoblast cells that erode the decidua and assist with the nutrition of the embryo. The syncytiotrophoblast cells also produce human chorionic gonadotrophin (hCG), a hormone that prevents menstruation and maintains pregnancy by sustaining the function of the corpus luteum.

Simultaneous to implantation, the embryo continues developing. The cells of the embryoblast differentiate into two types of cells: the *epiblast* (closest to the trophoblasts) and the *hypo-blast* (closest to the blastocyst cavity). These two layers of cells form a flat disc known as the *bilaminar embryonic disc*. A process of *gastrulation* turns the bilaminar disc into a tri-laminar embryonic disc (three layers). During gastrulation, cells rearrange themselves and migrate due to predetermined genetic coding. Three primary germ layers are the main embryonic tissues from which various structures and organs will develop. The first appearance of these layers, collectively known as the primitive streak, is around day 15.

- The **ectoderm** is the start of tissue that covers most surfaces of the body: the epidermis layer of the skin, hair and nails. Additionally it forms the nervous system.
- The **mesoderm** forms the muscle, skeleton, dermis of skin, connective tissue, the urogenital glands, blood vessels, and blood and lymph cells.
- The **endoderm** forms the epithelial lining of the digestive, respiratory and urinary systems, and glandular cells of organs such as the liver and pancreas.

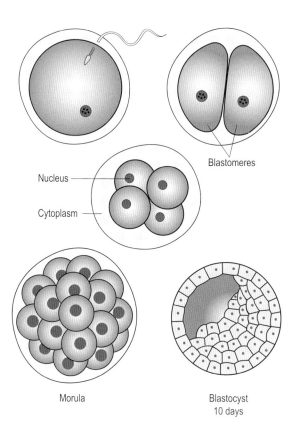

Fig. 5.5 Diagrammatic representation of the development of the zygote.

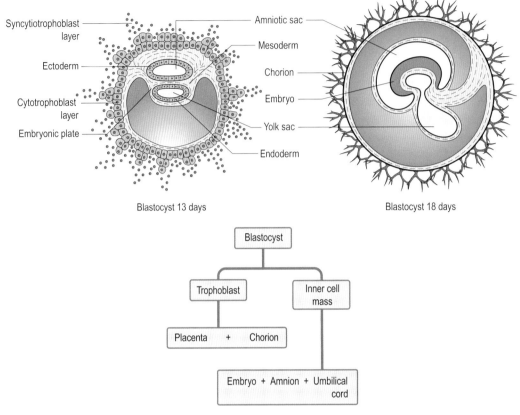

Fig. 5.6 The development of the blastocyst.

The epiblast separates from the trophoblast and forms the floor of a cavity, known as the *amniotic cavity*. The amnion forms from the cells lining the cavity. The cavity is filled with fluid, and gradually enlarges and folds around the bilaminar disc to enclose it. This amniotic cavity fills with fluid (amniotic fluid) derived initially from maternal filtrate; later the fetus contributes by excreting urine. Fetal cells can be found in the amniotic fluid and can be used in diagnostic testing for genetic conditions via a procedure known as amniocentesis (Chapter 11).

At about 16 days mesodermal cells form a hollow tube in the midline called the *notochordal process*; this becomes a more solid structure, the *notochord*, about a week later. Specialized inducing cells and responding tissues cause development of the vertebral bodies and intervertebral discs to occur. The neural tube is developed from further cell migration, differentiation and folding of embryonic tissue. This occurs in the middle of the embryo and develops towards each end. The whole process is known as *neurulation*. Teratogens, diabetes or folic acid deficiency may lead to neural tube defects.

The hypoblast layer of the embryoblast gives rise to extra-embryonic structures only, such as the yolk sac. Hypoblast cells migrate along the inner cytotrophoblast lining of the blastocele-secreting extracellular tissue which becomes the yolk sac. The yolk sac is lined with extraembryonic endoderm, which in turn is lined with extraembryonic mesoderm. The yolk sac serves as a primary nutritive function, carrying nutrients and oxygen to the embryo until the placenta fully takes over this role. The endoderm and mesoderm cells contribute to the formation of some organs, such as the primitive gut arising out of the endoderm cells. An outpouching of endodermic tissue forms the *allantois*, this extends to the connecting stalk around which the umbilical cord later forms. Growth of blood vessels is induced, connecting separately to vessels of the embryo and placenta (Kay et al 2011). Blood islands that later go on to develop blood cells arise from the mesodermal layer; the remainder resembles a balloon floating in front of the embryo until it atrophies by the end of the 6th week when blood-forming activity transfers to embryonic sites. After birth, all that remains of the yolk

---

Box 5.2 **Stem cells**

- Stem cells are unspecialized and give rise to specialized cells.
- The zygote can give rise to a whole organism, known as a **totipotent** stem cell.
- Stem cells such as those in the inner cell mass can give rise to many different types of cells and are consequently known as **pluripotent**.
- Further specialization of pluripotent stem cells gives rise to cells with more specific functions, known as **multipotent** stem cells.

Stem cells in adult organs (also known as adult stem cells, somatic or tissue-specific cells) have the potential to become *any* type of cell in a specific organ – **multipotent**. These cells facilitate repair of a damaged or diseased organ. Adult stem cells may have some 'plasticity' and may have the potential to be used in other organs of the body.

In the United Kingdom, cell cleavage up to 14 days after fertilization can be used for research. This tends to be undertaken at 5–6 days. As research occurs on the cells at this stage the embryo does not exist as a 3-D entity and its properties are changed – in essence it is no longer an 'embryo'.

Stem cell harvesting

Stem cells from an embryo, if transferred into another individual where there is no genetic match, will cause rejection issues similar to tissue transplantation.

Stem cells found in the umbilical cord, which can be collected, have originated in the fetal liver; most stem cells found in cord are progenitor cells and have differentiated further – usually into haematopoetic stem cells.

These cells may cause transplant issues if used in other people unless there is a very close genetic match, such as a sibling. The cells could then be used to treat acute lymphoblastic leukaemia.

In the United Kingdom, the Human Tissue Authority (HTA 2010), the Royal College of Obstetricians and Gynaecologists (RCOG)/Royal College of Midwives (RCM) (2011) and Trotter (2008) have produced useful guidance papers to help inform midwifery practice around the issue of stem cell harvesting and routine commercial umbilical cord blood collection.

---

sac is a vestigial structure in the base of the umbilical cord, known as the *vitelline duct*.

The pre-embryonic period is crucial in terms of initiation and maintenance of the pregnancy and early embryonic development. Inability to implant properly can results in ectopic pregnancy or miscarriage. Additionally chromosomal defects and abnormalities in structure and organs can occur during this time (Moore and Persaud 2003).

During embryological development stem cells under predetermined genetic control become specialized giving rise to further differentiation with a varying functionality according to their predefined role (Box 5.2).

REFERENCES

Carlson B M 2004 Human embryology and developmental biology, 3rd edn. Mosby, Philadelphia

Chrisler J C 2011 Leaks, lumps, and lines: stigma and women's bodies. Psychology of Women Quarterly 35(2):202–14

Human Tissue Authority (HTA) 2010 guidance for licensed establishments involved in cord blood collection. Accessed online at www.hta.gov.uk (11 April 2013)

Kay H H, Nelson D M, Wang Y 2011 The placenta. From development to disease. Oxford, Wiley–Blackwell

Moore K L, Persaud T V N 2003 Before we are born: essentials of embryology and birth defects, 8th edn. Saunders, London

Royal College of Obstetricians and Gynaecologists (RCOG)/Royal College of Midwives (RCM) 2011 Statement on umbilical cord blood collection and banking. Available at www.rcog.org.uk (accessed 11 April 2013)

Stables D, Rankin J 2010 Physiology in childbearing: with anatomy and related biosciences, 3rd edn. Baillière Tindall, Edinburgh

Tortora G J, Derrickson B 2011 Principles of anatomy and physiology. Maintenance and continuity of the human body, 13th edn. John Wiley & Sons, Hoboken, NJ

Trotter S 2008 Cord blood banking and its implications for midwifery practice: time to review the evidence? MIDIRS Midwifery Digest 18(2):159–64

Wennink J M B, Delemarre-van de Waal H A, Schoemaker R et al 1990 Luteinizing hormone and follicle stimulating hormone secretion patterns in girls throughout puberty measured using highly sensitive immunoradiometric assays. Clinical Endocrinology 33(3):333–44

FURTHER READING

Coad J, with Dunstall M 2011 Anatomy and physiology for midwives, 3rd edn. Churchill Livingstone, Edinburgh
A very full and clear explanation of endocrine activity is given in Chapter 3. Chapter 4 addresses the reproductive cycles in similar detail with clear diagrams to assist the reader.

Johnson M H, Everitt B J 2000 Essential reproduction, 5th edn. Blackwell Science, Oxford
This authoritative volume provides the interested reader with a much greater depth of information than is possible in the present book and is recommended for those who wish to study the hormonal patterns of reproduction in detail.

Schoenwolf G C, Bleyl S B, Brauer P R, Francis-West P H 2009 Larsen's human embryology, 9th edn. Churchill Livingstone, Philadelphia
Detailed embryology for those students wanting greater depth.

The placenta

Jenny Bailey

CHAPTER CONTENTS

This chapter discusses the development of the placenta – a complex organ, deriving from two separate individuals, the mother and the fetus (Tortora and Derrickson 2011). It is formed from the merging of the chorion and the allantois (see Chapter 5) in early pregnancy (Rampersad et al 2011). The process of forming a placenta (known as *placentation*) involves prevention of immune rejection, transfer of nutrients and waste products and the secretion of hormones to maintain the pregnancy. In addition, the chapter includes details of anatomical variations of the placenta and umbilical cord, highlighting their significance to midwifery practice.

THE CHAPTER AIMS TO:

- outline the development of the placenta
- explore variations of the placenta and umbilical cord and highlight their significance to midwifery practice.

EARLY DEVELOPMENT

Within a few days of fertilization, the trophoblasts (see Chapter 5) begin to produce human chorionic gonadotrophin (hCG), ensuring that the endometrium will be receptive to the implanting embryo. The endometrium increases in vascularity and undergoes a series of structural changes in a process known as *decidualization* in preparation for implantation; hence the endometrium is referred to as the *decidua* in pregnancy. Interconnecting arteriovenous shunts form between the maternal spiral arteries and veins which persist into the immediate postpartum period. A reduction of the number of shunts leading to narrower uterine arteries is involved with complications of pregnancy such as pre-eclampsia (Burton et al 2009).

The decidua has regions named according to its relationship to the implantation site:

- The *decidua basalis* lies between the developing embryo and the stratum basalis of the uterus at the implantation site.
- The *decidua capsularis* covers the developing embryo separating it from the uterine cavity.
- The *decidua vera* (otherwise known as the *decidua parietalis*) lines the remainder of the uterine cavity.

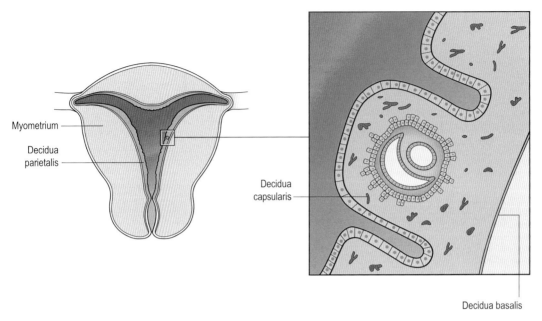

Myometrium

Decidua
parietalis

Decidua
capsularis

Decidua basalis

Fig. 6.1 Early implantation of the blastocyst.

Uterine glands secrete nutrients such as glycogen, to maintain the developing conceptus until the intraplacental blood flow is fully developed, some 10–12 weeks later (Burton et al 2002).

In pregnancy a sophisticated immune adaptation occurs to prevent rejection of the fetus. The decidua is invaded by macrophages, which become immunosuppressive. Adapted T-regulator cells, known as Tregs, become less effective as part of the specific hormonal response to antigens and the effect of natural killer (NK) cells is reduced such that their cytotoxicity becomes impaired and they are less likely to destroy any foreign cells.

Microchimerism is the term for the presence of a small number of cells in one individual that originated in a different individual. Some fetal cells actively move into the mother's circulation, tissues and organs in the first trimester of pregnancy without triggering an immune response. The role of these cells in maternal systems is unclear. They could have an immunosuppressant effect to protect the fetus and they also can facilitate growth and repair in maternal systems.

Implantation

Implantation involves two stages: prelacunar and lacunar.

Prelacunar stage

Seven days post conception the blastocyst makes contact with the decidua (*apposition*) and the process of

placentation begins (Fig. 6.1). The process of implantation is extremely aggressive: chemical mediators, prostaglandins and proteolytic enzymes are released by both the decidua and the trophoblasts and maternal connective tissue is invaded. Nearby maternal blood vessels ensure there is optimum blood flow to the placenta. At this stage the cytotrophoblasts form a double layer and further differentiate into various types of syncytiotrophoblasts. The supply of syncytiotrophoblasts is as a result of continued mitotic proliferation of the cytotrophoblastic layer below.

Lacunar stage

Increasing numbers of syncytiotrophoblasts surround the blastocyst and small lakes form within these cells known as *lacunae*, which will become the *intervillous spaces* between the villi (Fig. 6.2) and will be bathed in blood as maternal spiral arteries are eroded some 10–12 weeks following conception. Prior to this the embryo is nourished from uterine glands (see Chapter 5).

The trophoblasts have a potent invasive capacity, which if left unchecked would spread throughout the uterus. This potential is moderated by the decidua, which secretes cytokines and protease inhibitors that modulate trophoblastic invasion. The *layer of Nitabusch* is a collaginous layer between the endometrium and myometrium which assists in preventing invasion further than the decidua. Trophoblastic invasion into the myometrium can give rise to a morbidly adhered placenta, known as *placenta accreta* (see Chapter 18).

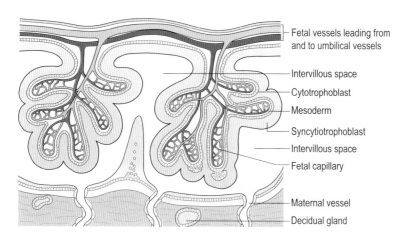

Fig. 6.2 Chorionic villi.

Fetal vessels leading from and to umbilical vessels

Intervillous space

Cytotrophoblast

Mesoderm

Syncytiotrophoblast

Intervillous space

Fetal capillary

Maternal vessel

Decidual gland

The chorionic villous tree

Chorionic villi are finger-like projections of chorion surrounded by cytotrophoblastic and syncytiotrophoblastic layers. Initially new blood vessels develop from progenitor cells within the chorionic villi of the placenta (known as vasculogenesis). A relatively low level of oxygen promotes this. Further growth of these vessels (angiogenesis) produces a vascular network that ultimately connects with those blood vessels developed independently in the embryo via the umbilical arteries and vein through the connecting stalk.

The villi proliferate and branch out approximately three weeks after fertilization. Over time the villi can differentiate and specialize, resulting in different functions. Villi become most profuse in the area where the blood supply is richest, the *decidua basalis*. This part of the trophoblastic layer, which is known as the *chorion frondosum*, eventually develops into the placenta. The villi under the decidua capsularis gradually degenerate due to lack of nutrition, forming the *chorion laeve*, which is the origin of the chorionic membrane (Fig. 6.3). As the fetus enlarges and grows, the decidua capsularis is pushed towards the decidua vera on the opposite wall of the uterus until, at about 27 weeks of gestation, the decidua capsularis subsequently disappears.

The syncytiotrophoblasts surrounding the villi erode the walls of maternal vessels as they penetrate the lower myometrium, opening them up into a funnel shape, forming a lake of maternal blood in which the villi float. This opening up reduces the velocity at which maternal blood enters the central cavity of the cotyledon (lobule) and villous tree (Burton et al 2009). The maternal blood circulates, enabling the villi to absorb nutrients and oxygen and to excrete waste. These are known as the *nutritive villi*. A few villi are more deeply attached to the decidua and are called *anchoring villi*.

Each chorionic villus is a branching structure like a tree arising from one stem. Its centre consists of mesoderm and

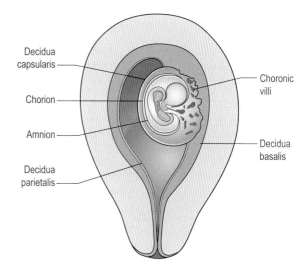

Decidua capsularis

Chorion

Amnion

Decidua parietalis

Choronic villi

Decidua basalis

Fig. 6.3 Implantation site at 3 weeks.

fetal blood vessels, as well as branches of the umbilical artery and vein. These are covered by a single layer of *cytotrophoblast* cells and the external layer of the villus is the *syncytiotrophoblast* (see Fig. 6.2). This means that four layers of tissue separate the maternal blood from the fetal blood making it impossible for the two circulations to mix unless any villi are damaged.

THE PLACENTA AT TERM

At term the placenta is discoid in shape, about 20 cm in diameter and 2.5 cm thick at its centre and weighing approximately 470 g, which is directly proportional to the weight of the fetus. Rampersad et al (2011) state that, by term, the ratio of fetal size to that of the placenta is about 7 to 1. Placental pathology and maternal disease can affect

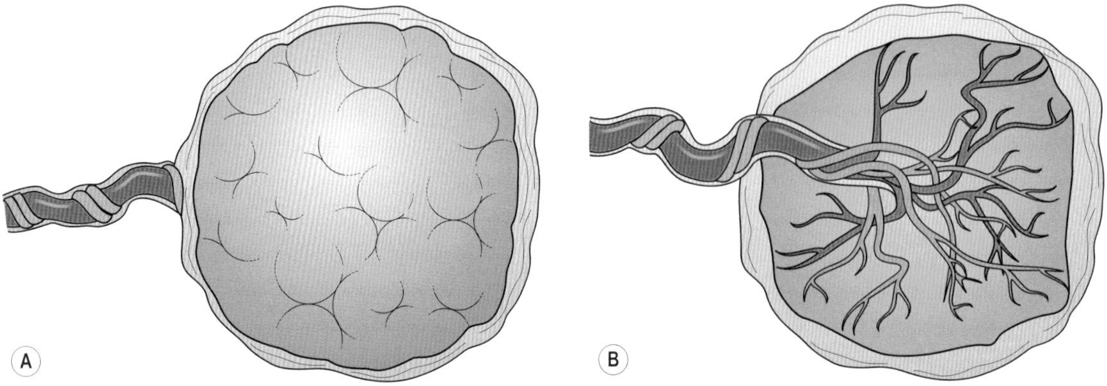

Fig. 6.4 The placenta at term. (A) Maternal surface. (B) Fetal surface.

this ratio: such sequelae being diabetes, pre-eclampsia, pregnancy-induced hypertension or intrauterine growth restriction (IUGR) (see Chapter 13). The weight of the placenta may be affected by physiological or active management of the third stage of labour owing to the varying amounts of fetal blood retained in the vessels. The placenta is no longer routinely weighed in clinical practice; however some maternity units may do so as part of clinical trials and research activities.

The maternal surface of the placenta (i.e. the *basal plate*) is dark red in colour due to maternal blood and partial separation of the basal decidua (Fig. 6.4A). The surface is arranged in up to 40 cotyledons (lobes), which are separated by *sulci* (furrows), into which the decidua dips down to form *septa* (walls). The cotyledons are made up of lobules, each of which contains a single villus with its branches. Sometimes deposits of lime salts may be present on the surface, making it slightly gritty. This has no clinical significance.

The fetal surface of the placenta (i.e. the *chorionic plate*) has a shiny appearance due to the amnion covering it (Fig. 6.4B). Branches of the umbilical vein and arteries are visible, spreading out from the insertion of the umbilical cord, which is normally in the centre. The amnion can be peeled off the surface of the chorion as far back as the umbilical cord, whereas the chorion, being derived from the same trophoblastic layer as the placenta, cannot be separated from it.

Functions

The placenta performs a variety of functions for the developing fetus which can be determined by the pneumonic SERPENT (Fig. 6.5).

Storage

The placenta metabolizes glucose, stores it in the form of glycogen and reconverts it to glucose as required. It can also store iron and the fat-soluble vitamins.

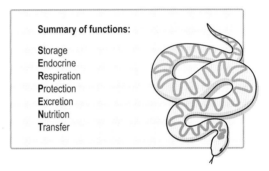

Summary of functions:

Storage
Endocrine
Respiration
Protection
Excretion
Nutrition
Transfer

Fig. 6.5 Summary of the functions of the placenta (SERPENT).

Endocrine

The many and varied endocrine functions of the placenta are complex, requiring maternal and fetal input. Both types of trophoblasts produce steroidal hormones (oestrogens and progesterone) in addition to many placental protein hormones necessary for pregnancy (Kay et al 2011).

Steroid hormones

There are three important *oestrogens: oestrone, oestradiol* and *oestriol.* Both maternal and fetal adrenal production provide precursors for oestrogen production by the placenta. *Pregnalone sulphate* is converted to oestriol by the feto-placental unit from 6 to 12 weeks onwards, rising steadily until term. Oestrogens influence uterine blood flow, enhance ribonucleic acid (RNA) and protein synthesis and aid growth of uterine muscle. They also increase the size and mobility of the maternal nipple and cause alveolar and duct development of the breast tissue. Serial serum (mmol/l) oestriol measurements can indicate the level of feto-placental wellbeing.

Progesterone production is maintained by the corpus luteum for approximately 8 weeks until the placenta takes over this function and is dependent on maternal cholesterol stores. Progesterone is thought to play an important part in immunosuppression to maintain the pregnancy (Kay et al 2011). Progesterone is produced in the syncytial layer of the placenta in increasing quantities until immediately before the onset of labour when its level falls. It maintains the myometrium in a quiescent state, during pregnancy. It is involved in preparing breast tissue during pregnancy and when levels reduce after birth of the placenta, prolactin stimulates lactation.

Protein hormones

Human chorionic gonadotrophin (hCG) is produced under the influence of placental gonadotrophic releasing hormone (GnRH) by the trophoblasts. Initially it is present in very large quantities, with peak levels being achieved between the 7th and 10th week, but these gradually reduce as the pregnancy advances. The function of hCG is to stimulate the corpus luteum to produce mainly progesterone. It also increases *fetal leydig cells* to affect male sexual development prior to fetal luteinizing hormone (LH) production (Kay et al 2011). Human chorionic gonadotrophin forms the basis of the many pregnancy tests available, as it is excreted in the mother's urine.

Human placental lactogen (hPL) is sometimes known as *human chorionic somatomammotropin hormone* (hCS) as it not only stimulates somatic growth but also stimulates proliferation of breast tissue in preparation for lactation. In early pregnancy, HPL stimulates food intake and weight gain, mobilizing free fatty acids, and functions with prolactin to increase circulating insulin levels (Barbour et al 2007; Kay et al 2011). Human placental lactogen is no longer considered the primary agent of insulin resistance as other growth hormones, such as human placental growth hormone (hPGH), appear to be the main determinants for this. Levels of hPL have been used as a screening tool in pregnancy to assess placental function.

Human placental growth hormone (hPGH) levels rise throughout pregnancy. This hormone is involved with hPL as a determinant of insulin resistance in late pregnancy. It mobilizes maternal glucose for transfer to the fetus and contributes to lipolysis, lactogenesis and fetal growth.

There are also many other factors, such as *insulin growth factor* (IGF) and *vascular endothelial growth factor* (VEGF), playing a variety of roles in metabolism, growth, vasculogenesis and regulation of utero-placental blood flow.

Respiration

Gaseous exchange to and from the fetus occurs as a result of diffusion. Transfer of gases is assisted by a slight maternal respiratory alkalosis in pregnancy. The fetal haemoglobin level is high *in utero* to facilitate transport of gases. The fetal haemoglobin also has a high affinity for oxygen.

Protection

The placenta provides a limited barrier to infection. Few bacteria can penetrate with the exception of the treponema of syphilis and the tubercle bacillus. However, many types of virus can penetrate the placental barrier, such as human immunodeficiency virus (HIV), hepatitis strains, Parvo virus B19, human cytomegalovirus (CMV) and rubella. In addition to this, some parasitic and protozoal diseases, such as malaria and toxoplasmosis, will cross the placenta.

The placenta filters substances of a high molecular weight therefore some drugs and medicines may transfer to the fetus. Although such drugs will cross the placental barrier to the fetus, many will be harmless, and others, such as antibiotics administered to a pregnant woman with syphilis, are positively beneficial (see Chapter 13). Substances including alcohol and some chemicals associated with smoking cigarettes and recreational drug use are not filtered out. These substances can cross the placental barrier freely and may cause congenital malformations and subsequent problems for the baby.

Immunoglobulins will be passed from mother to fetus transplacentally in late pregnancy, providing about 6–12 weeks' naturally acquired passive immunity to the baby.

In the case of Rhesus disease, if sensitization occurs and fetal blood cells enter the maternal circulation, responding antibodies produced by the mother may cross the placenta and destroy fetal surface antigens and consequently fetal cells, causing haemolysis, hydrops fetalis and potential fetal demise.

Excretion

The main substance excreted from the fetus is carbon dioxide. Bilirubin will also be excreted as red blood cells are replaced relatively frequently. There is very little tissue breakdown apart from this and the amounts of urea and uric acid excreted are very small.

Nutrition

The fetus requires nutrients for its ongoing development, such as amino acids and glucose which are required for growth and energy, calcium and phosphorus for bones and teeth, and iron and other minerals for blood formation. These nutrients are actively transferred from the maternal to the fetal blood through the walls of the villi. The placenta is able to select those substances required by the fetus, even depleting the mother's own supply in some instances. Water, vitamins and minerals also pass to the fetus. Fats and fat-soluble vitamins (A, D and E) cross the placenta only with difficulty and mainly in the later stages of pregnancy. Some substances, including amino acids, are found at higher levels in the fetal blood than in the maternal blood.

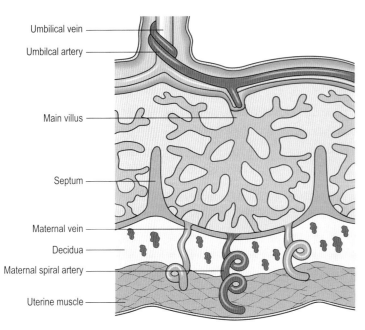

Fig. 6.6 Blood flow around chorionic villi.

Umbilical vein

Umbilcal artery

Main villus

Septum

Maternal vein

Decidua

Maternal spiral artery

Uterine muscle

Transfer of substances

Substances transfer to and from the fetus by a variety of transport mechanisms, as stated below:

- Simple diffusion of gases and lipid soluble substances.
- Water pores transfer water-soluble substances as a result of osmotic and potentially hydrostatic forces.
- Facilitated diffusion of glucose using carrier proteins.
- Active transport against concentration gradients of ions, calcium (Ca) and phosphorus (P).
- Endocytosis (pinocytosis) of macromolecules.

Placental circulation

Invading trophoblasts modify maternal spiral arterioles to accommodate a 10-fold increase in blood flow where there is open circulation around the chorionic villi. Maternal blood is discharged in a pulsatile fashion into the intervillous space by 80–100 spiral arteries in the decidua basalis after 10–12 weeks of gestation. The blood flows slowly around the villi, eventually returning to the endometrial veins and the maternal circulation. There are about 150 ml of maternal blood in the intervillous spaces, which is exchanged three or four times per minute.

Fetal blood, which is low in oxygen, is pumped by the fetal heart towards the placenta along the umbilical arteries and transported along their branches to the capillaries of the chorionic villi where exchange of nutrients takes place between the mother and fetus. Having yielded carbon dioxide and waste products and absorbed oxygen

and nutrients, the blood is returned to the fetus via the umbilical vein (Fig. 6.6).

The membranes

The basal and chorionic plates come together and meet at the edges to form the chorioamnion membrane where the amniotic fluid is contained. The chorioamnion membrane is composed of two membranes: the *amnion* and the *chorion*.

The *amnion* is the inner membrane derived from the inner cell mass and consists of a single layer of epithelium with a connective tissue base. It is a tough, smooth and translucent membrane, continuous with the outer surface of the umbilical cord which moves over the chorion aided by mucous. The amnion contains amniotic fluid, which it produces in small quantities as well as prostaglandin E2 (PGE2) which plays a role in the initiation of labour. In rare instances, the amnion can rupture, causing amniotic bands that can affect the growth of fetal limbs.

The *chorion*, which is the outer membrane that is continuous with the edge of the placenta, is composed of mesenchyme, cytotrophoblasts and vessels from the extended spiral arteries of the decidua basalis. It is a rough, thick, fibrous, opaque membrane which lines the decidua vera during pregnancy, although loosely attached. It produces enzymes that can reduce progesterone levels and also produces prostaglandins, oxytocin and platelet-activating factor which stimulate uterine activity. This membrane is friable and can rupture easily, so it can be retained in the uterus following birth.

Amniotic fluid

Amniotic fluid is a clear alkaline and slightly yellowish liquid contained within the amniotic sac. It is derived essentially from the maternal circulation across the placental membranes and exuded from the fetal surface. The fetus contributes to the amniotic fluid through metabolism in small quantities of urine and fluid from its lungs. This fluid is returned to the fetus by intramembranous flow across the amnion into the fetal vessels and through the mechanism of the fetus swallowing.

Functions of the amniotic fluid

Amniotic fluid distends the amniotic sac allowing for the growth and free movement of the fetus and permitting symmetrical musculoskeletal development. It equalizes pressure and protects the fetus from jarring and injury. The fluid maintains a constant intrauterine temperature, protecting the fetus from heat loss and providing it with small quantities of nutrients. In labour, as long as the membranes remain intact the amniotic fluid protects the placenta and umbilical cord from the pressure of uterine contractions. It also aids effacement of the cervix and dilatation of the uterine os, particularly where the presenting part is poorly applied.

Constituents of the amniotic fluid

Amniotic fluid consists of 99% water with the remaining 1% being dissolved solid matter including food substances and waste products. In addition, the fetus sheds skin cells, *vernix caseosa* and *lanugo* into the fluid. Abnormal constituents of the liquor, such as *meconium* in the case of fetal compromise, may give valuable diagnostic information about the condition of the fetus. Aspiration of amniotic fluid for diagnostic examination is termed *amniocentesis.*

Research has found that amniotic fluid is a plentiful source of non-embryonic stem cells (De Coppi et al 2007). These cells have demonstrated the ability to differentiate into a number of different cell-types, including brain, liver and bone.

Volume of amniotic fluid

During pregnancy, amniotic fluid increases in volume as the fetus grows: from 20 ml at 10 weeks to approximately 500 ml at term.

The umbilical cord (funis)

The umbilical cord, which extends from the fetal surface of the placenta to the umbilical area of the fetus, is formed by the 5th week of pregnancy. It originates from the duct that forms between the amniotic sac and the yolk sac, which transmits the umbilical blood vessels (see Chapter 5).

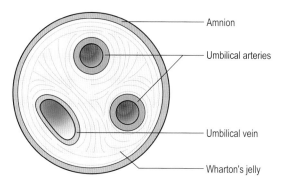

Fig. 6.7 Cross-section through the umbilical cord.

Functions

The umbilical cord transports oxygen and nutrients to the developing fetus, and removes waste products.

Structure

The umbilical cord contains two arteries and one vein (Fig. 6.7), which are continuous with the blood vessels in the chorionic villi of the placenta. The blood vessels are enclosed and protected by *Wharton's jelly*, a gelatinous substance formed from primary mesoderm. The whole cord is covered in a layer of amnion that is continuous with that covering the placenta. There are no nerves in the umbilical cord, so cutting it following the birth of the baby is not painful.

The presence of only two vessels in the cord may indicate renal malformations in the fetus; however, in some instances this has little significance to the subsequent health of the baby.

Measurements

The cord is approximately 1–2 cm in diameter and 50 cm in length. This length is sufficient to allow for the birth of the baby without applying any traction to the placenta.

A cord is considered *short* when it measures <40 cm. There is no specific agreed length for describing a cord as *too long*, but the disadvantages of a very long cord are that it may become wrapped round the neck or body of the fetus or become knotted. Either event could result in occlusion of the blood vessels, especially during labour.

Compromise of the fetal blood flow through the umbilical cord vessels can have serious detrimental effects on the health of the fetus and baby. *True knots* should always be noted on examination of the cord, but they must be distinguished from *false knots*, which are lumps of Wharton's jelly on the side of the cord and do not have any physiological significance.

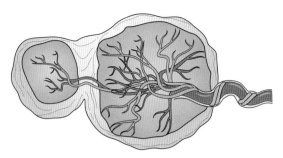

Fig. 6.8 Succenturiate lobe of placenta.

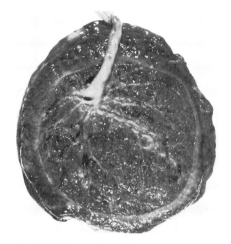

Fig. 6.9 Circumvallate placenta.

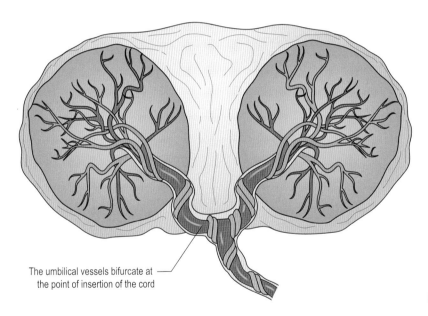

The umbilical vessels bifurcate at
the point of insertion of the cord

Fig. 6.10 Bipartite placenta.

Anatomical variations of the placenta and cord

A *succenturiate lobe* of placenta is the most significant of the variations in conformation of the placenta. A small extra lobe is present that is separate from the main placenta, and joined to it by blood vessels that run through the membranes to connect it (Fig. 6.8). The danger is that this small lobe may be retained *in utero* after the placenta is expelled, and if it is not removed, it may lead to haemorrhage and infection. Every placenta must be examined for evidence of a retained succenturiate lobe, which can be

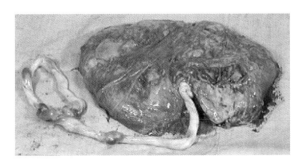

Fig. 6.11 Battledore insertion of the cord.

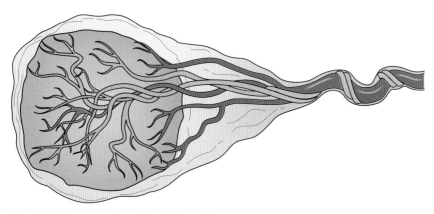

Fig. 6.12 Velamentous insertion of the cord.

identified by a hole in the membranes with vessels running to it.

In a *circumvallate* placenta, an opaque ring is seen on the fetal surface of the placenta. It is formed by a doubling back of the fetal membrane onto the fetal surface of the placenta and may result in the membranes leaving the placenta nearer the centre instead of at the edge as usual (Fig. 6.9). This placental variation is associated with *placental abruptio* and intrauterine growth restriction (IUGR).

In a *bipartite placenta*, there are two complete and separate lobes where the main cord bifurcates to supply both parts (Fig. 6.10). A *tripartite placenta* is similar to a bipartite placenta but it has three distinct parts.

In a *battledore* insertion of the cord, the cord is attached at the very edge of the placenta, and where the attachment is fragile it may cause significant problems with active management of the third stage of labour (Fig. 6.11).

A *velamentous* insertion of the cord, occurs when the cord is inserted into the membranes some distance from the edge of the placenta. The umbilical vessels run through the membranes from the cord to the placenta (Fig. 6.12). If the placenta is normally situated, no harm will result to the fetus, but the cord is likely to become detached upon applying traction during active management of the third stage of labour. However, if the placenta is low-lying, the vessels may pass across the uterine os (*vasa praevia*). In this case, there is great danger to the fetus when the membranes rupture and even more so during artificial rupture of the membranes, as the vessels may be torn, leading to rapid exsanguination of the fetus. If the onset of haemorrhage coincides with rupture of the membranes, fetal haemorrhage should be assumed and the birth expedited. It is possible to distinguish fetal blood from maternal blood by Singer's alkali-denaturation test, although, in practice, time is so short that it may not be possible to save the life of the baby. If the baby survives, haemoglobin levels should be estimated after birth and blood transfusion considered.

CONCLUSION

Development of the placenta requires complex processes involving enzymes, hormones and growth factors which remodel maternal tissue in addition to constructing new tissue specifically for the sustenance of the fetus. The placenta acts as a life support system for the developing embryo and fetus until birth.

REFERENCES

Barbour L A, McCurdy C E, Hernandez T L et al 2007 Cellular mechanisms for insulin resistance in normal pregnancy and gestational diabetes. Diabetes Care 30(Suppl 2): 112–19

Burton G J, Woods A W, Jauniaux E et al 2009 Rheological and physiological consequences of conversion of maternal spiral arteries for unteroplacental blood flow during human pregnancy. Placenta 30(6):473–82

Burton G J, Watson A L, Hempstock J et al 2002 Uterine glands provide histiotrophic nutrition for the human fetus during the first trimester of pregnancy. Journal of Clinical Endocrinology and Metabolism 87(6):2954–9

De Coppi P, Bartsch G Jr, Siddiqui M M et al 2007 Isolation of amniotic stem cell lines with potential for therapy. Nature Biotechnology 25(1):100–5

Kay H H, Nelson D M, Wang Y 2011 The placenta: from development to disease. Blackwell, Oxford

Rampersad R, Cerva-Zivkovic M, Nelson D M 2011 Development and anatomy of the human placenta. In: Kay H H, Nelson DM, Wang Y (eds)

The placenta: from development to disease. Blackwell, Oxford

Tortora G J, Derrickson B 2011 Principles of anatomy and physiology:

maintenance and continuity of the human body, 13th edn. John Wiley & Sons, Hoboken, NJ

FURTHER READING

Coad J, with Dunstall M 2011 Anatomy and physiology for midwives, 3rd edn. Churchill Livingstone/Elsevier, London

Chapter 8 of this comprehensive text provides a detailed account of the placenta.

Kay H H, Nelson D M, Wang Y 2011 The placenta: from development to disease. Blackwell, Oxford

Chapters 3 and 4 provide details regarding placental development for students who wish a more in-depth knowledge.

Oats J K, Abraham S (2010) Llewellyn-Jones fundamentals of obstetrics and gynaecology, 9th edn. Mosby/Elsevier, London

This book has a section on the placenta (Chapter 3) that the reader may find useful.

Stables D, Rankin J (2010) Physiology in childbearing with anatomy and related biosciences, 3rd edn. Elsevier, Edinburgh

Section 2A in Chapter 12 considers the placenta, membranes and amniotic fluid

Chapter | 7 |

The fetus

Jenny Bailey

This chapter provides a system-by-system approach for the reader to appreciate the complexities surrounding embryonic and fetal development and the subsequent changes that occur in the baby at the time of birth. In addition, discussion of the fetal skull and the significance of its diameters in late pregnancy and during labour in influencing an optimum birth outcome is provided.

An understanding of the detail is of value to the midwife when providing parents with information about the effects of maternal lifestyle, such as diet, smoking, alcohol intake, drug use and exercise, on fetal growth and development (see Chapter 8) and when a baby is born before term (see Chapter 30).

THE CHAPTER AIMS TO:

- outline the early development of the embryo and subsequent development of the fetus
- discuss the fetal circulation and the changes that occur at birth
- discuss the significance of the fetal skull and the significance of its diameters in determining a successful birth outcome.

TIME SCALE OF DEVELOPMENT

Embryological development is complex and occurs from the 2nd to the 8th week of pregnancy and includes the development of the *zygote* in the first 2–3 weeks following fertilization. *Fetal* development occurs from the 8th week until birth. The interval from the beginning of the last menstrual period (LMP) until fertilization is not part of pregnancy, however this period is important for the calculation of the expected date of birth. Figure 7.1 illustrates the comparative lengths of these prenatal events.

A summary of embryological and fetal development categorized into 4-week periods is provided in Box 7.1. This should be used to complement the text below.

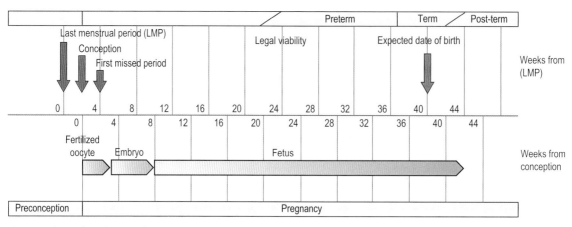

Fig. 7.1 Timescales of prenatal events.

FETAL GROWTH AND MATURATION

From the 9th week of pregnancy, fetal growth is rapid. Tissues grow by cell proliferation, cell enlargement and accretion of extracellular material. An adequate supply of nutrients and oxygen from the placenta to the fetus is crucial for growth. In developed countries the average birth weight is around 3400 g of which 50% is acquired by 30 weeks' gestation. The fetus gains approximately 25 g/day between weeks 32 and 40. A visual representation of growth in terms of height is provided in Fig. 7.2.

As fetal growth is an indicator of fetal health and wellbeing, monitoring of growth is crucial. This is done by visual observation of the uterus for size, symphysis fundal height measurements and ultrasonography.

The cardiovascular system

The early development of the cardiovascular system in the 3rd week of pregnancy coincides with the lack of the yolk sac, and the urgent need to supply the growing embryo with oxygen and nutrients from the maternal blood through the placenta.

The cardiovascular system is the first system to function in the embryo. The heart and vascular system commences development in the 3rd week, and by the 4th week a primitive heart is visible and is beginning to function, beating at around 22 days (Schoenwolf et al 2009). Vascular endothelial growth factor is a protein that causes vasculogenesis and subsequent angiogenesis to occur. Initially a vascular plexus is formed in the embryo, which is continually remodeled into a system of arteries and veins to accommodate the growing and developing embryo.

The first signs of the heart are the appearance of paired endothelial strands in the cardiogenic mesoderm, which canalize to become heart tubes and then fuse to become a tubular-shaped heart. The development continues to include remodeling and septation while the heart continues to beat. Blood is pumped around the vessels from the 4th week, by which time three major vascular systems have developed.

Arteries

Vitelline arteries link the aorta with the yolk sac which subsequently supplies the gut and other arteries in the neck and thorax. Mid gestation they are remodelled to form three main arteries which supply the gastrointestinal tract.

Two *umbilical* arteries deliver deoxygenated blood to the placenta.

Veins

The embryo has three major venous systems draining into the tubular-shaped heart: vitelline, umbilical and cardinal (Schoenwolf et al 2009).

The *vitelline* veins return poorly oxygenated blood from the gut and yolk sac. The hepatic veins and the portal vein develop from the vitelline veins and their networks. A temporary shunt, the *ductus venosus*, also develops from these veins.

Umbilical veins form in the body stalk. The right umbilical vein anastomoses with the ductus venosus shunting oxygenated placental blood into the inferior vena cava leaving the left umbilical vein to continue carrying oxygenated blood from the placenta to the embryo. Between 5–7 weeks of pregnancy, the foramen ovale is formed. From here on there is shunting of highly oxygenated blood from the right to left atrium, bypassing the right ventricle and pulmonary system, allowing the higher oxygenated blood to be pumped immediately to the brain and upper body.

The *cardinal* veins drain the head, neck and body wall into the heart.

Development over time ensures that the three systems develop into the adult pattern whilst maintaining some

Box 7.1 **Summary of embryological and fetal development**

Embryo
0–4 weeks
- Blastocyst implants
- Primitive streak appears
- Conversion of bilaminar disc into trilaminar disc
- Some body systems laid down in primitive form
- Primitive central nervous system forms (*neurulation*)
- Primitive heart develops and begins to beat
- Covered with a layer of skin
- Limb buds form
  - Optic vessels develop
  - Gender determined

4–8 weeks
- Very rapid cell division
- More body systems laid down in primitive form and continue to develop
- Spinal nerves begin to develop
- Blood is pumped around the vessels
- Lower respiratory system begins to develop
- Kidneys begin to develop
- Skeletal ossification begins developing
- Head and facial features develop
- Early movements
- Embryo visible on ultrasound from 6 weeks

Fetus
8–12 weeks
- Rapid weight gain
- Eyelids meet and fuse
- Urine passed
- Swallowing begins
- Distinguishing features of external genitalia appear
- Fingernails develop
- Some primitive reflexes present

12–16 weeks
- Rapid skeletal development – visible on X-ray
- Lanugo appears
- Meconium present in gut
- Nasal septum and palate fuse
- Eternal genitalia fully differentiate into male or female by week 12
- Fetus capable of sucking thumb

16–20 weeks
- Constant weight gain
- 'Quickening' – mother feels fetal movements
- Fetal heart heard on auscultation
- Vernix caseosa appears
- Skin cells begin to be renewed
- Brown adipose tissue (BAT) forms

20–24 weeks
- Most organs functioning well
- Eyes complete
- Periods of sleep and activity
- Ear apparatus developing
- Responds to sound
- Skin red and wrinkled
- Surfactant secreted in the lungs from week 20

24–28 weeks
- Legally viable and survival may be expected if born
- Eyelids open
- Respiratory movements

28–32 weeks
- Begins to store fat and iron
- Testes descend into scrotum
- Lanugo disappears from face
- Skin becomes paler and less wrinkled

32–36 weeks
- Weight gain 25 g/day
- Increased fat makes the body more rounded
- Lanugo disappears from body
- Hair on fetal head lengthens
- Nails reach tips of fingers and toes
- Ear cartilage soft
- Plantar creases visible.

36 weeks to birth
- Birth is expected
- Body round and plump
- Skull formed but soft and pliable

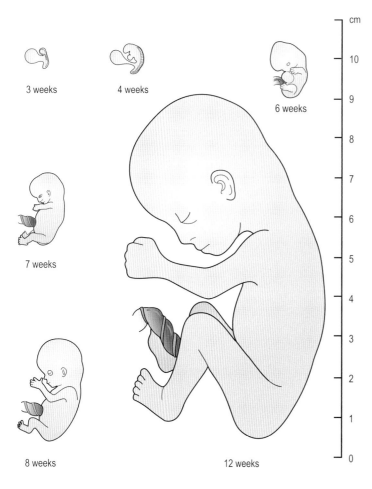

cm

Fig. 7.2 Sizes of embryos and fetus between 3 and 12 weeks' gestation.

3 weeks 4 weeks

6 weeks

7 weeks

8 weeks 12 weeks

temporary structures in the fetus which resolve at, or soon after, birth.

There are three phases of red blood cell formation:

- the *yolk sac* period, between weeks 3 and 13;
- the *hepatic/liver* period, between weeks 5 and 36 (Stables and Rankin 2010); and
- the *bone marrow* period, from the 10th week throughout life (Schoenwolf et al 2009).

Red blood cells, known as *erythrocytes*, which are produced from 'blood islands' in the extra embryonic mesoderm lining the yolk sac and liver, contain fetal haemoglobin. Fetal haemoglobin (HbF) has a much greater affinity for oxygen and is found in greater concentrations (18–20 g/dl at term) in the blood than adult haemoglobin (HbA), thus enhancing the transfer of oxygen across the placental site. Fetal erythrocytes have a life span of 90 days, shorter than adult erythrocytes, which is around 120 days. The short life span of fetal erythrocytes contributes to neonatal physiological jaundice (see Chapter 33). Genes passed

from both parents determine the fetal blood group and Rhesus factor.

The respiratory system

The development of the respiratory system begins in the 3rd week. The lower respiratory tract and lungs develop simultaneously. The lungs originate from a 'lung bud' growing out of the foregut, which repeatedly subdivides to form the branching structure of the bronchial tree. By 36 weeks of pregnancy, respiratory bronchioles have a capillary network and culminate in terminal sacs (*alveoli*). Lung development occurs on several levels and continues after birth until about 8 years of age when the full number of bronchioles and alveoli will have developed. The development of type II alveolar cells commences around 20 weeks of fetal life. These cells are necessary for the production of *surfactant*, a lipoprotein that reduces the surface tension in the alveoli and assists gaseous exchange. The amount of surfactant increases until the alveoli mature between 36 weeks and birth.

There is some movement of the thorax from the 12th week of fetal life and more definite diaphragmatic movements from the 24th week. This does not constitute breathing as gaseous exchange is via the placenta.

At term, the lungs contain about 100 ml of lung fluid. About one-third of this is expelled during birth and the rest is absorbed and transported by the lymphatics and blood vessels as air takes its place.

Babies born before 24 weeks of pregnancy have a reduced chance of survival owing to the immaturity of the capillary system in the lungs and the lack of surfactant (see Chapter 33).

The urogenital system

The urogenital system is divided functionally into the *urinary/renal* system and the *genital/reproductive* system. Both systems develop from the intermediate mesoderm. The kidneys develop from the 4th week of fetal life and produce small amounts of urine between the 6th and 10th week. They become more functional around the 15th week when more urine is produced. The urine does not constitute a route for excretion as elimination of waste products is via the placenta. The urine forms much of the amniotic fluid and production increases with fetal maturity.

The superior vesical arteries arise from the first few centimetres of the hypogastric arteries, which lead to the umbilical arteries. A single umbilical artery at birth is suggestive of malformations of the renal tract (see Chapter 32).

The sex of the embryo is determined at fertilization: either two X chromosomes (in the female) or one X and one Y chromosome (in the male) are inherited. The gonads develop from the 5th week from the intermediate mesoderm. In the two sexes, genital development is similar and is referred to as the *indifferent state of sexual development*. A single sex determining protein on the gene of the Y chromosome (SRY) controls the subsequent male development pattern (Schoenwolf et al 2009). Differentiation occurs from the 7th week, but female gonad development occurs slowly under the influence of *pro-ovarian* genes and the ovaries may not be identifiable until the 10th week. The external genitalia in both sexes develop in the 9th week, but males and females are not distinguishable until about the 12th week.

The endocrine system

The adrenal glands develop from mesoderm and neural crest cells from the 6th week of fetal life, and grow to 10–20 times larger than the adult adrenals. Their size regresses during the first year of life. They produce the precursors for placental formation of oestriols and influence maturation of the lungs, liver and epithelium of the digestive tract. It is also thought that the adrenal glands play a part in the initiation of labour, but the exact mechanism is not fully understood (Johnson and Everitt 2000).

The pituitary gland develops and takes on its characteristic shape from between the 9th and 17th week of fetal life. The fetal pituitary produces gonadotrophins, i.e. luteinizing hormone (LH) and follicle stimulating hormone (FSH) from weeks 13–14, and human growth hormone (hGH) is present by weeks 19–20.

The digestive system

The primitive gut develops from the endodermal layer of the yolk sac in the 4th week of fetal life. It begins as a straight tube, and proceeds on several levels: foregut, midgut and hindgut.

By the 5th week, the *foregut* (oesophagus, stomach and duodenum) is visible. The liver, gallbladder and pancreas bud form the gut tube around the 4th to 5th week of fetal life. The liver grows rapidly from the 5th week and by the 10th week occupies much of the abdominal cavity, constituting about 10% of the fetal weight by the 9th week. Towards the end of pregnancy, iron stores are laid down in the liver and the liver cells produce bile from the 12th week.

The *midgut* (small intestine, caecum and vermiform appendix, ascending colon and transverse colon) undertakes much of its development in the 6th week, while *the hindgut* (rectum and anal canal) completes its development in the 7th week of fetal life.

Around 12 weeks, the digestive tract is well formed and the lumen is patent. Most digestive juices are present before birth and act on the swallowed substances to form *meconium*. Bile enters the duodenum from the bile duct during the 13th week, giving the intestinal contents a dark green colour. Meconium is *normally* retained in the gut until after birth when it is passed as the first stool of the baby.

Insulin is secreted from 10 weeks of fetal life and glucagon from 15 weeks, both of which rise steadily with increasing fetal age.

The nervous system

The brain begins to develop from around day 19 and three structures are visible: *forebrain*, *midbrain* and *hindbrain*. By the 5th week, there is differentiation between the major regions, namely the thalamus and the hypothalamus.

The neural tube is derived from the *ectoderm* which folds inwards by a complicated process to form the neural tube, which is then covered over by skin. Closure of the neural tube is essential and takes place by 26 days. This process is occasionally incomplete, leading to open neural tube defects (see Chapter 32).

The development of the sense organs, including the transmission of sensory input to the brain and output from the brain, occurs under complex processes. The eyes and ears are associated with the development of the head and neck, which begin early and continue until the cessation of growth in the late teens. Although the eyes develop from around 22 days, for normal vision to occur many complex structures within the eye must properly relate to neighbouring structures. The eye is completely formed by 20 weeks but the eyelids are fused until around 24 weeks. The developing eyes are sensitive to light.

The development of the inner ear, which contains the structures for hearing and balance, commences early in embryological life but is not complete until around 25 weeks.

Motor output controlled by the basal ganglia in the form of movement, begins around 8 weeks, however these movements are not usually felt by the mother until around 16 weeks, and are referred to as *quickening*. As the nervous system matures fetal behaviour becomes more complex and more defined. The fetus develops behavioural patterns: sleep with no eye or body movements; sleep with periodic eye and body movements, known as *REM sleep*; wakefulness with subtle eye and limb movements; active phase with vigorous eye and limb movements.

Integumentary, skeletal and muscular systems

The epidermis develops from a single layer of ectoderm to which other layers are added. By the end of 4 weeks, a thin outer layer of flattened cells covers the embryo. Further development continues until 24 weeks. Brown adipose tissue (BAT) develops from 18 weeks' gestation; this plays an important part in thermoregulation after birth. From 18 weeks, the fetus is covered with a white, creamy substance called *vernix caseosa*, which protects the skin from the amniotic fluid and from any friction against itself. Hair begins to develop between the 9th and 12th week. By 20 weeks the fetus is covered with a fine downy hair called *lanugo*; at the same time the hair on the head and eyebrows begin to form. Lanugo is shed from 36 weeks and by term, there is little left. Fingernails develop from about 10 weeks but the toenails do not form until about 18 weeks. By term the nails usually extend beyond the fingertips and so it is not unusual to see scratches on the baby's face.

Most skeletal tissue arises from the mesodermal and neural crest cells but skeletal tissue in different parts of the body are diverse in morphology and tissue architecture. The skull develops during the 4th week from the mesenchyme surrounding the developing brain. It consists of two major parts: the *neurocranium*, which forms the bones of the skull, and the *viscerocranium*, which forms the bones of the face (Tortora and Derrickson 2011). The neurocranium forms flat bones at the roof and sides of the skull. Ossification here is intramembranous and the membranous separations between the flat bones are known as

sutures and *fontanelles*. The functions of these will be discussed later in the chapter.

THE FETAL CIRCULATION

The placenta is the source of oxygenation, nutrition and elimination of waste for the fetus. There are several temporary structures in addition to the placenta and the umbilical cord that enable the fetal circulation to occur (Fig. 7.3). These include:

- The *ductus venosus*, which connects the umbilical vein to the inferior vena cava.
- The *foramen ovale*, which is an opening between the right and left atria.
- The *ductus arteriosus*, which leads from the bifurcation of the pulmonary artery to the descending aorta.
- The *hypogastric arteries*, which branch off from the internal iliac arteries and become the umbilical arteries when they enter the umbilical cord.

The fetal circulation takes the following course:

Oxygenated blood from the placenta travels to the fetus in the umbilical vein. The umbilical vein divides into two branches – one that supplies the portal vein in the liver, the other anastomosing with the ductus venosus and joining the inferior vena cava. Most of the oxygenated blood that enters the right atrium passes across the foramen ovale to the left atrium, which mixes with a very small amount of blood returning from the lungs from where it passes into the left ventricle via the bicuspid valve, and then the aorta. The head and upper extremities receive approximately 50% of this blood via the coronary and carotid arteries, and the subclavian arteries respectively. The rest of the blood travels down the descending aorta, mixing with deoxygenated blood from the right ventricle via the ductus arteriosus.

Deoxygenated blood collected from the head and upper parts of the body returns to the right atrium via the superior vena cava. Blood that has entered the right atrium from the superior vena cava enters at a different angle to the blood that enters from the inferior vena cava and heads towards the foramen ovale. Hence there are two distinct blood flows entering the right atrium. Most of the lesser oxygenated blood entering the right atrium from the superior vena cava passes behind the flow of highly oxygenated blood going to the left atrium and enters the right ventricle via the tricuspid valve. There is a small amount of blood mixing where the two blood flows meet in the atrium. From the right ventricle a little blood travels to the lungs in the pulmonary artery, for their development. Most blood, however, passes from the pulmonary artery through the ductus arteriosus into the descending aorta. This blood, although low in oxygen and nutrients, is

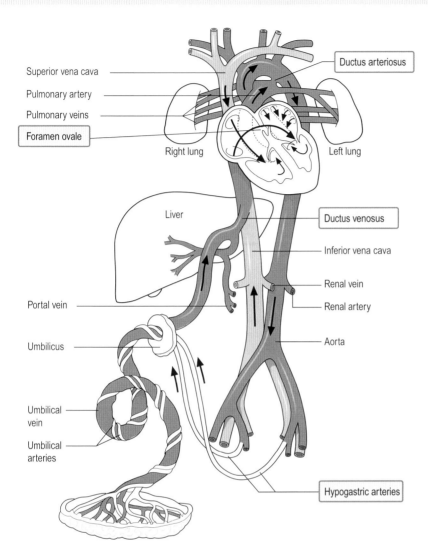

Fig. 7.3 A diagram of the fetal circulation. The arrows show the course taken by the blood. The temporary structures are labelled in colour.

Superior vena cava

Pulmonary artery

Pulmonary veins

Foramen ovale

Ductus arteriosus

Right lung

Left lung

Liver

Ductus venosus

Inferior vena cava

Renal vein

Renal artery

Portal vein

Umbilicus

Aorta

Umbilical vein

Umbilical arteries

Hypogastric arteries

sufficient to supply the lower body of the fetus. It is also by this means that deoxygenated blood travels back to the placenta via the internal iliac arteries, which lead into the hypogastric arteries, and ultimately into the umbilical arteries. This circulation means that the fetus has a well-oxygenated and perfused head, brain and upper body compared to its lower extremities.

ADAPTATION TO EXTRAUTERINE LIFE

At birth, there is a dramatic alteration to the fetal circulation and an almost immediate change occurs. The cessation of umbilical blood flow causes a cessation of flow in the ductus venosus and a fall in pressure in the right atrium. As the baby takes its first breath, blood is drawn along the pulmonary system via the pulmonary artery and

as a consequence, pressure increases in the left atrium due to the increased blood supply returning to it via the pulmonary veins. The alteration of pressures between the two atria causes a mechanical closure of the foramen ovale. In addition, as the baby takes its first breath, the lungs inflate, and there is a rapid fall in pulmonary vascular resistance of approximately 80%, a slight reverse flow of oxygenated aortic blood along the ductus arteriosus and a rise in the oxygen tension. This causes the smooth muscle in the walls of the ductus arteriosus to contract and constrict, usually within 24 hours following birth, though it can remain patent for a few days.

As these structural changes become permanent, the following fetal structures arise:

- The umbilical vein becomes the *ligamentum teres.*
- The ductus venosus becomes the *ligamentum venosum.*

117

- The ductus arteriosus becomes the *ligamentum arteriosum*.
- The foramen ovale becomes the *fossa ovalis*.
- The hypogastric arteries become the *obliterated hypogastric arteries* except for the first few centimetres, which remain open and are known as the *superior vesical arteries*.

Adaptation to extrauterine life also involves:

- Maintenance of a nutritional state through the establishment of breastfeeding.
- Elimination of waste via the kidneys and gastrointestinal system.
- Establishment of the portal and liver circulation.
- Temperature control.
- Communication developed through parent–baby interactions (Stables and Rankin 2010).

THE FETAL SKULL

The fetal head is large in relation to the fetal body compared with the adult (Fig. 7.4). Additionally, it is large in comparison with the maternal pelvis and is the largest part of the fetal body to be born.

Adaptation between the skull and the pelvis is necessary to allow the head to pass through the pelvis during labour without complications. The bones of the vault are thin and

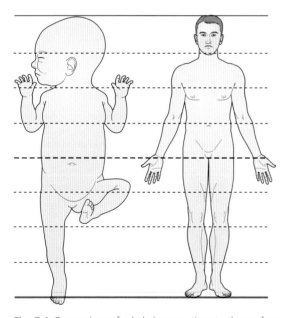

Fig. 7.4 Comparison of a baby's proportions to those of an adult. The baby's head is wider than the shoulders and one-quarter of the total length.

pliable, and if subjected to great pressure damage to the underlying delicate brain may occur. Important intracranial membranes, venous sinuses and structures can be seen in Figs 7.5, 7.6.

Divisions of the fetal skull

The skull is divided into the *vault*, the *base* and the *face* (Fig. 7.7).

The *vault* is the large, dome-shaped part above an imaginary line drawn between the orbital ridges and the nape of the neck.

The *base* comprises bones that are firmly united to protect the vital centres in the medulla oblongata.

The face is composed of 14 small bones that are also firmly united and non-compressible.

The bones of the vault

The bones of the vault (Fig. 7.8) are laid down in membrane. They harden from the centre outwards in a process known as *ossification*. Ossification is incomplete at birth, leaving small gaps between the bones, known as the *sutures* and *fontanelles*. The ossification centre on each bone appears as a *protuberance*. Ossification of the skull is not complete until early adulthood.

The bones of the vault consist of:

- The *occipital bone*, which lies at the back of the head. Part of it contributes to the base of the skull as it contains the *foramen magnum*, which protects the spinal cord as it leaves the skull. The ossification centre is the *occipital protuberance*.
- The two *parietal bones*, which lie on either side of the skull. The ossification centre of each of these bones is called the *parietal eminence*.
- The two *frontal bones*, which form the forehead or *sinciput*. The ossification centre of each bone is the *frontal eminence*. The frontal bones fuse into a single bone by eight years of age.
- The upper part of the *temporal bone* on both sides of the head forms part of the vault.

Sutures and fontanelles

The *sutures* are the cranial joints formed where two bones meet. Where two or more sutures meet, a *fontanelle* is formed (see Fig. 7.8). The sutures and fontanelles described below permit a degree of overlapping of the skull bones during labour, which is known as *moulding*.

- The *lambdoidal suture* separates the occipital bone from the two parietal bones.
- The *sagittal suture* lies between the two parietal bones.
- The *coronal suture* separates the frontal bones from the parietal bones, passing from one temple to the other.

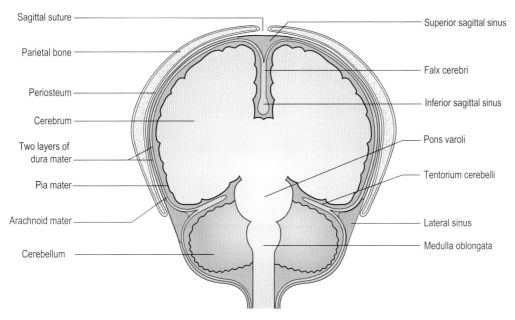

Fig. 7.5 Coronal section through the fetal head to show intracranial membranes and venous sinuses.

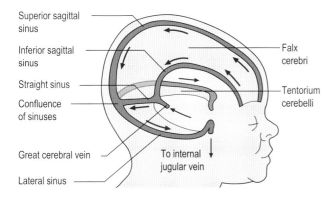

Fig. 7.6 Diagram showing intracranial membranes and venous sinuses. Arrows show direction of blood flow.

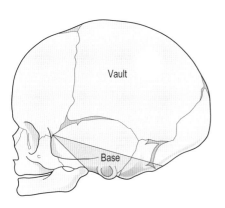

Fig. 7.7 Divisions of the skull showing the large, compressible vault and the non-compressible face and base.

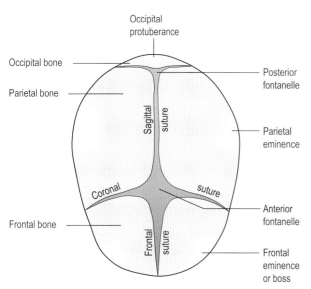

Fig. 7.8 View of fetal head from above (head partly flexed), showing bones, sutures and fontanelles.

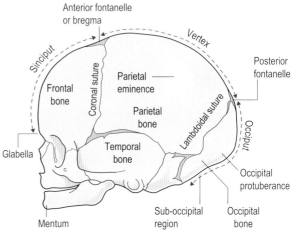

Fig. 7.9 Fetal skull showing regions and landmarks of clinical importance.

- The *frontal suture* runs between the two halves of the frontal bone. Whereas the frontal suture becomes obliterated in time, the other sutures eventually become fixed joints.
- The *posterior fontanelle* or *lambda* (shaped like the Greek letter lambda λ) is situated at the junction of the lambdoidal and sagittal sutures. It is small, triangular in shape and can be recognized vaginally because a suture leaves from each of the three angles. It normally closes by 6 weeks of age.
- The *anterior fontanelle* or *bregma* is found at the junction of the sagittal, coronal and frontal sutures. It is broad, kite-shaped ◆ and recognizable vaginally because a suture leaves from each of the four corners. It measures 3–4 cm long and 1.5–2 cm wide and normally closes by 18 months of age. Pulsations of cerebral vessels can be felt through this fontanelle.

Regions and landmarks of the fetal skull

The skull is further separated into regions, and within these there are important landmarks as shown in Fig. 7.9. These landmarks are useful to the midwife when undertaking a vaginal examination as they help ascertain the position of the fetal head.

- The *occiput region* lies between the foramen magnum and the posterior fontanelle. The part below the *occipital protuberance* (landmark) is known as the *sub-occipital region*.
- The *vertex region* is bounded by the posterior fontanelle, the two parietal eminences and the anterior fontanelle.

- The *forehead/sinciput region* extends from the anterior fontanelle and the coronal suture to the orbital ridges.
- The face extends from the orbital ridges and the root of the nose to the junction of the *chin* or *mentum* (landmark) and the neck. The point between the eyebrows is known as the *glabella*.

Diameters of the fetal skull

Knowledge of the diameters of the skull alongside the diameters of the pelvis allows the midwife to determine the relationship between the fetal head and the mother's pelvis.

There are six longitudinal diameters (Fig. 7.10).

The longitudinal diameters are:

- The *sub-occipitobregmatic* (SOB) diameter (9.5 cm) measured from below the occipital protuberance to the centre of the anterior fontanelle or bregma.
- The *sub-occipitofrontal* (SOF) diameter (10 cm) measured from below the occipital protuberance to the centre of the frontal suture.
- The *occipitofrontal* (OF) diameter (11.5 cm) measured from the occipital protuberance to the glabella.
- The *mentovertical* (MV) diameter (13.5 cm) measured from the point of the chin to the highest point on the vertex.
- The *sub-mentovertical* (SMV) diameter (11.5 cm) measured from the point where the chin joins the neck to the highest point on the vertex
- The *sub-mentobregmatic* (SMB) diameter (9.5 cm) measured from the point where the chin joins the neck to the centre of the bregma (anterior fontanelle).

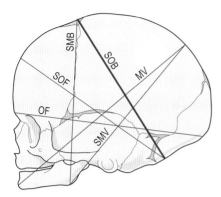

Fig. 7.10 Diagram showing the longitudinal diameters of the fetal skull.

Diameter	Length (cm)
SOB, sub-occipitobregmatic	9.5
SOF, sub-occipitofrontal	10.0
OF, occipitofrontal	11.5
MV, mentovertical	13.5
SMV, sub-mentovertical	11.5
SMB, sub-mentobregmatic	9.5

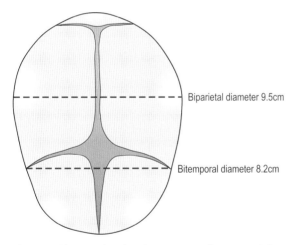

Biparietal diameter 9.5cm

Bitemporal diameter 8.2cm

Fig. 7.11 Diagram showing the transverse diameters of the fetal skull.

There are also two transverse diameters, as shown in Fig. 7.11.

- The *biparietal diameter* (9.5 cm) – the diameter between the two parietal eminences.
- The *bitemporal diameter* (8.2 cm) – the diameter between the two furthest points of the coronal suture at the temples.

Knowledge of the diameters of the trunk is also important for the birth of the shoulders and breech (as detailed in Box 7.2).

> ### Box 7.2 **Diameters of the fetal trunk**
>
> #### Bisacromial diameter 12 cm
>
> This is the distance between the acromion processes on the two shoulder blades and is the dimension that needs to pass through the maternal pelvis for the shoulders to be born. The articulation of the clavicles on the sternum allows forward movement of the shoulders, which may reduce the diameter slightly.
>
> #### Bitrochanteric diameter 10 cm
>
> This is measured between the greater trochanters of the femurs and is the presenting diameter in breech presentation.

Presenting diameters

Some presenting diameters are more favourable than others for easy passage through the maternal pelvis and this will depend on the attitude of the fetal head. This term *attitude* is used to describe the degree of flexion or extension of the fetal head on the neck. The attitude of the head determines which diameters will present in labour and therefore influences the outcome.

The presenting diameters of the head are those that are at right-angles to the *curve of Carus* of the maternal pelvis. There are always two: a *longitudinal* diameter and a *transverse* diameter. The presenting diameters determine the *presentation* of the fetal head, for which there are three:

1. *Vertex presentation.* When the head is well flexed the sub-occipitobregmatic diameter (9.5 cm) and the biparietal diameter (9.5 cm) present (Fig. 7.12). As these two diameters are the same length the presenting area is circular, which is the most favourable shape for dilating the cervix and birth of the head. The diameter that distends the vaginal orifice is the sub-occipitofrontal diameter (10 cm). When the head is deflexed, the presenting diameters are the occipitofrontal (11.5 cm) and the biparietal (9.5 cm). This situation often arises when the occiput is in a posterior position. If it remains so, the diameter distending the vaginal orifice will be the occipitofrontal (11.5 cm).

2. *Face presentation.* When the head is completely extended the presenting diameters are the sub-mentobregmatic (9.5 cm) and the bitemporal (8.2 cm). The sub-mentovertical diameter (11.5 cm) will distend the vaginal orifice.

3. *Brow presentation.* When the head is partially extended, the mentovertical diameter (13.5 cm) and the bitemporal diameter (8.2 cm) present. If this presentation persists, vaginal birth is unlikely.

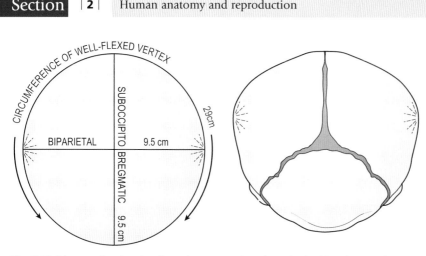

Fig. 7.12 Diagram showing the dimensions presenting when the fetal head is well flexed in a vertex presentation.

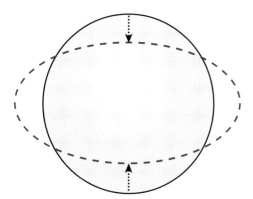

Fig. 7.13 Demonstration of the principle of moulding. The diameter compressed is diminished; the diameter at right-angles to it is elongated.

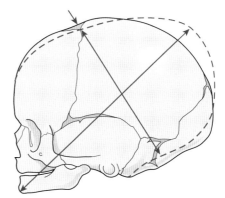

Fig. 7.14 Moulding in a normal vertex presentation with the head well flexed. The sub-occipitobregmatic diameter is reduced and the mentovertical elongated.

Moulding

The term *moulding* is used to describe the change in shape of the fetal head that takes place during its passage through the birth canal. Alteration in shape is possible because the bones of the vault allow a slight degree of bending and the skull bones are able to override at the sutures. This overriding allows a considerable reduction in the size of the presenting diameters, while the diameter at right-angles to them is able to lengthen owing to the give of the skull bones (Fig. 7.13). The shortening of the fetal head diameters may be by as much as 1.25 cm. The dotted lines in Figs 7.14–7.19 illustrate moulding in the various presentations.

Additionally, moulding is a protective mechanism and prevents the fetal brain from being compressed as long as it is not excessive, too rapid or in an unfavourable direction. The skull of the pre-term infant is softer and has wider sutures than that of the term baby, and hence may mould excessively should labour occur prior to term.

Venous sinuses are closely associated with the intracranial membranes, as shown in Fig. 7.6, and if membranes are torn due to excessive moulding or precipitate labour there is danger of bleeding. A tear of the tentorium cerebelli may result in bleeding from the great cerebral vein.

CONCLUSION

Embryonic and fetal development occurs alongside placental development. There is constant growth and remodelling of cells, tissues, organs and systems prior to birth. Several temporary structures in the fetus support systems *in utero*; these consequently become redundant at birth and they either disappear or become ligaments. At birth all organs are functioning but some may be immature and continue to develop as part of extra-uterine life.

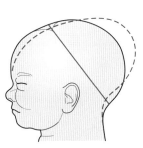

Fig. 7.15 Vertex presentation, head well flexed.

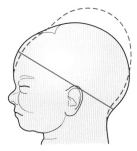

Fig. 7.16 Vertex presentation, head partially flexed.

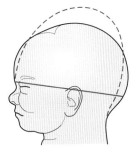

Fig. 7.17 Vertex presentation, head deflexed.

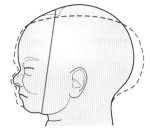

Fig. 7.18 Face presentation.

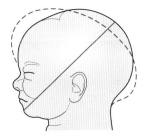

Fig. 7.19 Brow presentation.

Figs 7.15–7.19 Series of diagrams showing moulding when the head presents. Moulding is shown by the dotted line.

REFERENCES

Johnson M H, Everitt B J 2000 Essential reproduction, 5th edn. Blackwell, Oxford

Schoenwolf G, Bleyl S, Brauer P, Francis-West P (2009) Larsens human embryology, 4th edn.

Churchill Livingstone, Philadelphia

Stables D, Rankin J 2010 Physiology in childbearing with anatomy and related biosciences, 3rd edn. Elsevier, Edinburgh

Tortora G J, Derrickson B 2011 Principles of anatomy and physiology: maintenance and continuity of the human body, 13th edn. John Wiley & Sons, Hoboken, NJ

FURTHER READING

Coad J, Dunstall M 2011 Anatomy and physiology for midwives, 3rd edn. Churchill Livingstone/Elsevier, London
A detailed discussion of embryonic and fetal development appears in Chapter 9. The fetal circulation and transition to neonatal life are addressed in Chapter 15.

England M A 1996 Life before birth, 2nd edn. Mosby–Wolfe, London

This text serves to illustrate embryological and fetal development in photographic form. For the student who requires a detailed understanding of prenatal events and in particular the hormonal influences, this book is unsurpassed.

Schoenwolf G C, Bleyl S B, Brauer P R et al (eds) 2009 Larson's human embryology, 4th edn. Churchill Livingstone, Philadelphia

Originating in a series of Christmas lectures at the Royal Institution, this text explores the unifying principles that may account for the way embryos develop. Written for the non-specialist, it invites the reader to think broadly and aims to inspire as well as instruct.

Section | 3 |

Pregnancy

Chapter | 8 |

Antenatal education for birth and parenting*

Mary Louise Nolan

*Please note that although the Nursing and Midwifery Council replaced the term 'Health Visitor' with the title of 'Specialist Community Public Health Nurse' in 2002, the former continues to be widely used in practice and for the purposes of this chapter will be used throughout.

This chapter discusses the special opportunities that antenatal sessions provide for midwives to help mothers and fathers make a happy and successful transition to parenthood. It explores new thinking about the content of antenatal education provided to groups, and describes skills and activities which midwives can use to enable parents to acquire information, problem-solving skills and support relevant to their individual circumstances.

THE CHAPTER AIMS TO:

- justify the allocation of time and resources to providing antenatal education in groups
- place new thinking about antenatal education in the context of research and health policy
- build midwives' confidence and skills to facilitate antenatal sessions that effectively meet the needs of women and men making the transition to parenthood.

PARENT EDUCATION: THE RESEARCH AND POLICY BACKGROUND

In 2007, a survey of 3682 women (Nolan 2008) from all parts of the United Kingdom (UK) revealed that a large number had been offered no or very few antenatal classes during their most recent pregnancy. Many of those who had attended classes were dissatisfied with their quality, criticizing in particular the unrealistic portrayal of labour, birth and early parenting, lack of practical skills work to help them use their own resources for coping with the pain of labour, and being given no opportunity to discuss how to cope with being a mother.

These comments are in line with research carried out over the past 20 years. The study by Spiby and coworkers (1999) found that women were dissatisfied with the time given to practising self-help skills for labour during antenatal classes and cited this as a reason for not being able to put such skills into practice when they were actually in labour. The study by Ho and Holroyd (2002) of Hong Kong women's experience of classes highlighted the lack of engagement of midwives with women's individual worries. Women felt that the sessions were not organized around their life situations rather than according to subject matter. Too much information was given in the short time available and there was too little emphasis on discussion to enable women to hear each other's viewpoints and move towards deciding what was best for them in their particular circumstances. The women especially highlighted that they had not been able to make friends. The importance of antenatal classes as an opportunity for developing a peer support network has featured repeatedly in the literature over many years; for example, the study by Stamler (1998) found that the seven women interviewed wanted 'more socialization' and considered classes unsatisfactory that did not encourage this by facilitating discussion. More recently, Nolan et al (2012) explored the nature of friendships made at antenatal classes and identified their role in securing women's mental health in the early months of new motherhood by allowing them to share information about babycare, normalizing their experiences and increasing their confidence to manage their own and their babies' welfare.

In the year of publication of the survey carried out by Nolan during 2007 which highlighted the steady decrease in the availability of antenatal education (Nolan 2008), the Child Health Promotion Programme (Department of Health [DH] 2008) described the government's commitment to a new emphasis on parenting support, especially for first-time mothers and fathers. This document spoke of the need for stable positive relationships within families in order to provide the best possible home environment for babies to develop robust physical and emotional health. It advocated approaches to educating and supporting parents that focused on their strengths rather than on their deficits. Fathers were brought to the fore and services were reminded that men must be included in all perinatal and childcare services, to ensure that they were equally as well informed as mothers and able to make a strong, positive contribution to the upbringing of their children.

This focus on supporting families with babies stemmed from the increasingly public profile of new evidence from neuroscience showing that the development of the unborn baby was affected not only by genetic heritage, the efficiency of the placenta, the quality of the mother's diet, whether she smoked, her use of alcohol, prescribed and street drugs, *but also by her mental and emotional wellbeing.*

Wadhwa et al (1993: 858) concluded that 'independent of biomedical risk, maternal prenatal stress factors are significantly associated with infant birth weight and with gestational age at birth'. At the beginning of the 21st century, Glover and O'Connor (2002) produced evidence from 7448 women participating in the Avon Longitudinal Study of Parents and Children that the pregnant woman's mood could have a direct effect not just on newborn babies' weight, but also on their brain development, with later consequences for behavioural development throughout childhood. A meta-analysis (Talge et al 2007) of studies looking at the relationship between maternal mental health, babies' development *in utero* and their progress during the first years of life, concluded that maternal stress in pregnancy makes it substantially more likely that children will have emotional, cognitive and physical problems. Neuroscience also explained how the architecture of the brain is shaped by new babies' earliest experiences, that is, by their relationship with their primary caregiver(s). While antenatal education had traditionally focused on helping mothers (and sometimes fathers) acquire practical babycare skills such as changing nappies, feeding and bathing babies, neuroscience suggested that equal emphasis should be placed on helping parents understand how their newborn babies are primed to enter into a relationship with them, and how they invite interaction through a variety of cues.

A generation of childcare gurus had battled for supremacy over the hearts and minds of new parents, from those advocating 'attachment parenting' (Liedloff 1986; Jackson 2003) to those requiring that both parents and baby adhere to a strict routine as soon as the baby is born (Ford 2006). Parents had also been persuaded that 'early education' in the form of playing Mozart through headphones placed on the pregnant woman's abdomen, or teaching infants to 'sign' would give them a head start. Now the evidence was supporting parents' basic instinct to respond to their children when they cried, to enjoy playing with them and to 'watch, wait and wonder' (Cohen et al 1999). The importance of 'mutual gaze' (simply looking at the baby), talking and singing to the baby (with nursery rhymes very much back in fashion) and baby massage to promote the release of the 'social hormone', oxytocin, were all established on a solid evidence base that was also in tune with most parents' instinctive understanding of how to meet their babies' needs.

This evidence, coupled with uncomfortable reports stating that Britain's children and young people were amongst the unhappiest in Europe (Children's Society 2012), impelled government to reconsider the value of pregnancy as an educational opportunity. Pregnancy is an ideal opportunity for helping women acquire understanding, skills and support networks to make the transition to motherhood less stressful and more fulfilling, both for them and for their infants. Midwives, health visitors and childbirth educators had long known that pregnancy was 'a teachable moment', a period of crisis that renders women and men unusually open to reflecting on their self concept, lifestyle, values and ideas about parenthood. The Department of Health (DH 2009) set up an Expert Reference Group to devise a programme of high-quality antenatal education which would 'help prepare parents for parenthood from early pregnancy onwards' (section 3.36).

ANTENATAL EDUCATION: THE EVIDENCE

The Expert Reference Group (DH 2009) commissioned a systematic review of antenatal education to inform its work. This review (McMillan et al 2009) found that the quality of research into antenatal group-based education was generally poor. The Review's conclusions were, therefore, tentatively presented. Some evidence was found for a positive effect on maternal psychological wellbeing when antenatal programmes focused on:

- the emotional changes that men and women experience across the transition to parenthood
- the couple relationship
- parenting skills and early childcare
- bonding and attachment
- problem-solving skills.

The review by McMillan et al (2009) also found evidence that programmes focusing on strengthening the couple's relationship in preparation for parenting improved parental confidence and satisfaction with the couple and parent–infant relationship in the postnatal period. No evidence was found of a link between attending antenatal classes and improved birth outcomes in terms of reduced caesarean section or instrumental delivery rates.

Effective facilitation of antenatal programmes was found to be dependent on their being sensitive to people's cultures, responsive to both parents, participative and focused on building social support. This was in agreement with a powerful study of 'maternal health literacy' carried out by Renkert and Nutbeam (2001) which noted that 'teaching methods (in antenatal classes) were heavily weighted towards the transfer of factual information, as distinct from the development of decision making skills, and practical skills for childbirth and parenting'. The study concluded that, 'if the purpose of antenatal classes is to improve maternal health literacy, then women need to leave a class with the skills and confidence to take a range of actions that contribute to a successful pregnancy, childbirth and early parenting' (Renkert and Nutbeam 2001: 381). Women need to know where they can find more information, how to access support and what resources are available to them in the community.

LEADING ANTENATAL SESSIONS: AIMS AND SKILLS

There is a popular myth, much detested by teachers, that 'those who can, do, and those who can't, teach'. Leading a group of adults may not primarily be about teaching, although in the case of antenatal sessions, there is likely to be an element of instruction. However, ensuring that participants find the experience of attending classes as relevant and useful as possible, demands sophisticated skills on the part of the group leader. It is unfortunate that while the potential of antenatal and postnatal groups has been recognized anew, there is an increasing tendency to use unqualified maternity support workers and parent link workers to lead them rather than midwives. The quality of health and social care services has regularly been linked to the level of training of those who deliver them. Recently, nursery provision has come under scrutiny and a clear link established between how well carers understand the needs of very small children, and the optimal development of those children (Department for Children, Schools and Families [DCSF] 2012). The same is true of antenatal sessions. If the aim is to run a peer support group where mothers and fathers can get to know each other, then little more is required than an accessible venue, a pleasant room, comfortable seating, refreshments and someone to introduce people to each other. However, the presence of an educated, confident, competent and empathic group leader is essential if antenatal sessions are to help participants identify and acquire information relevant to their life circumstances and practise new skills. Trained facilitators can help parents challenge each other's beliefs and change or renew them in the light of ideas they might not have considered before.

While ideally, antenatal group courses would be led by the same person throughout, this is not always possible 'in the real world', just as it is not always possible for a woman to have the same midwife throughout childbirth. If several people are taking responsibility for antenatal sessions, it is vital that they have spent time together, talking about and agreeing what it is they want to achieve. These aims then underpin every session, whoever is the group leader, and ensure that the mothers and fathers attending have an integrated learning experience. The aims for one Community Healthcare Trust's antenatal programme are given in Box 8.1.

Sharing information

Any antenatal group session is likely to involve information-sharing, discussion and practical skills work. Of these, the first is probably the area in which many group leaders who are health professionals feel most competent, and the one

Box 8.1 **Aims of antenatal education**

- To provide a high-quality pregnancy programme that reflects the most recent evidence regarding what is effective in group-based antenatal education.
- To help mothers and fathers recognize and build on their strengths as parents-to-be.
- To enhance the physical and mental wellbeing of participants so that they can provide a secure environment for their new baby.
- To equip participants with knowledge of a range of resources to enable them to acquire the information and support they need during pregnancy and new parenthood.
- To maximize the potential of group antenatal education to build positive social capital on which mothers and fathers can draw after the birth of their babies.

Box 8.2 **Sharing group knowledge and experience**

It is often the case that group members know far more about a topic than might be expected. Finding out what the group knows, and building on that knowledge is an important skill for the group leader. The example below is taken from a recent antenatal session.

When asked to talk about friends' experiences of having a caesarean section, group members' pooled knowledge proved extensive:
- some friends had had planned caesareans and some emergency
- emergency caesareans were more traumatic for both mother and father (and probably the baby)
- the surgery proceeded quickly until the birth of the baby; once the baby was born, the mother remained in theatre for quite a long time
- some fathers found being present during surgery daunting
- often the father held the baby first because the mother had drips in both arms
- there was an unexpected amount of pain afterwards and it could be difficult for the mother to hold the baby for feeding
- some mothers recovered quickly and were back to normal in a few weeks; some took months
- some mothers felt fine about their caesarean and some felt as if they had 'failed'.

In this session, the group leader had little to do beyond answering a few questions raised by the group and stressing the importance of asking for help with the baby on the postnatal ward, keeping the wound clean, recognizing signs of infection, and not expecting to do too much once home.

in which they are often, in fact, least. There are two pitfalls: first, to believe that the more information given, the better; and the second, that giving information will change people's behaviour.

The fact that many group leaders know from personal experience that most information is forgotten as soon as individuals leave a lecture, does not deter them from overloading mothers and fathers with information. In order for people to retain information:

- it must be the information that they want at that moment in their lives;
- it must be linked either to first-hand or to vicarious experiences;
- it must be presented succinctly in as many different forms as possible.

Many topics that might be covered in antenatal sessions are huge, for example, 'Labour and Birth'. Yet mothers and fathers do not need to know the anatomy and physiology or the clinical management of labour and birth in the depth that a midwife needs to know these things. What group participants need to know is 'what will it be like for me?'

A fascinating experiment was conducted in an old-fashioned 'Nightingale Ward' in the 1950s (Janis 1958) with patients undergoing prostate surgery. The patients on one side of the ward were given detailed, technical information about the surgical procedures they would undergo, including the names of the instruments and drugs employed. The patients on the other side of the ward were given descriptions of the sensations involved in having an anaesthetic, waking up after surgery and recovering from an abdominal wound. The patients who had received this kind of information made far speedier recoveries than those given 'textbook' information.

Mothers and fathers attending antenatal sessions already know a great deal – they will be the repositories of both correct and incorrect information. The task of the group leader is to elicit what they know so that she can reinforce what is correct and restructure what is not. Asking participants to share their own experiences of a particular aspect of labour, for example having an induction, or what they have heard about it from friends and other informants, enables her to judge the level of knowledge in the group and to find out what parents want to know. By exploring the details of the experience as described by members of the group, acknowledging accurate information, asking group members themselves to correct misinformation (which they are often able to do), answering questions raised by people on a need to know basis, a rich learning experience is provided (as seen in Box 8.2). Embedding new information in a web made up of what people already

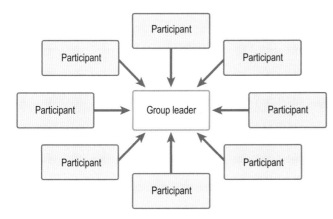

Fig. 8.1 Leader–participant interaction without group discussion.

know and their shared ideas of what an experience might be like, provides the most effective means of transmitting information that may influence their decision-making.

A study by Stapleton et al (2002) of the effectiveness of the MIDwives Information Resource Service (MIDIRS) information leaflets came to the conclusion that women did not value or use information that was presented to them 'cold', in this case, in leaflet form. They *did* value having the opportunity to discuss the information in the leaflets with a midwife or well-informed person who could answer their questions. This research constitutes a warning to group leaders who believe that information-giving is satisfactory without interaction with the recipient and discussion as to its relevance to the woman's circumstances.

The more varied the means by which information is transmitted, the more locations in the brain will be used to store it. This increases the likelihood that information will be retained. The repertoire of creative ideas for facilitating learning that is demonstrated by any primary school teacher is just as relevant for the person leading an antenatal group session with adults. The adult brain is assisted to retain information in the same way as the child's. Pictures that present information visually aid memory and enhance enjoyment of learning, which in itself makes learning more effective. Today, there is a huge range of video material available which can be used to present facts in an exciting way, or provide material to trigger discussion. A quick foray into YouTube will produced a multitude of video clips ideal for antenatal sessions.

Three-dimensional models that parents can handle to enable learning to take place through the hands and eyes, such as plastic pelves, dolls, different kinds of nappies and pieces of clinical equipment, help in the journey from simply knowing facts to understanding them and ultimately to applying them. Role-play is also a form of three-dimensional modelling that is enormously effective in enriching mothers' and fathers' concept of 'what it will be like'.

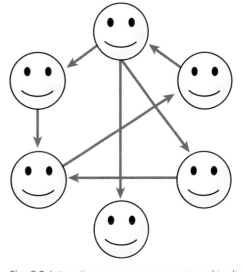

Fig. 8.2 Interactions among a group engaged in discussion.

Promoting discussion

It is often mistakenly assumed that an educational group in which the leader gives information and the group members are free to ask questions is having a discussion. However, a group whose interactions can be charted as in Fig. 8.1 is not having a discussion but rather, a question and answer session.

A group whose interactions can be charted as in Fig. 8.2 depicts a more engaging discussion.

In order to have a discussion, group members need to know a little about each other and therefore to feel at ease. A group consisting of more than six will deter many people from contributing and the group leader therefore has to break a big group into smaller units so that making a contribution becomes less daunting. Ice-breakers are important to help people start to learn each other's names and something of each other's history, as well as because they make a statement that this group is going to be as much about participants talking as about the group leader talking.

The first 10 minutes of a group session are an excellent learning opportunity. People are usually excited about joining the group, perhaps slightly anxious. As long as they are not paralysed with nerves, a little adrenalin in the system primes them for learning. Ice-breakers can incorporate both a 'getting to know you' element and an exchange of ideas on topics integral to the antenatal course. Having invited group members to form small groups or three or four people, they might talk about:

- What they already know about their unborn babies. *Aim*: to develop the relationship between parents and their babies.
- Where they are planning on giving birth and why they have chosen this location. *Aim*: to establish parents as the individuals who make decisions for themselves and their babies.
- What they see as the most enjoyable aspects of parenting, and what the most challenging. *Aim*: to encourage reflection on parenting, and project beyond the birth of the baby.

Sharing thoughts and feelings, even if cautiously in the beginning, enables group members to appreciate that there is much they have in common as 'becoming parents', and to have their fears and worries 'normalized'. Establishing the commonalities that mark everyone's journey into parenthood provides a secure basis from which group members can develop friendships and engage in future, perhaps more profound discussions.

Research by Nolan et al 2012 has shown that friendship formation may proceed at a faster pace when happening in pregnancy, and bypass much of the 'social chit-chat' that generally characterizes the early stages of relationships. An emerging appreciation of the responsibilities that parenting entails and of the extent to which current lifestyles will change following the birth of a baby motivates people, in the interests of survival, to reach out to others for support and companionship. Perhaps the overriding duty of antenatal group sessions is to facilitate the forming of friendships and this is dependent on providing multiple opportunities for people to get to know each other.

The use of open-ended questions such as 'How do you feel about that?', 'Could you say a little more?', and of reflecting questions raised by group members back to the group 'Would anyone like to answer that from their point of view?', are key tools in promoting discussion. Discussion may also be facilitated by prompts such as pictures and video clips, by inviting new parents to visit the group to talk about their experiences and by engaging the group in activities that require them to do more than simply write down facts. Finding the right trigger for discussion can transform a group that appears disinterested in the

Box 8.3 **Promoting valuable discussion**

A fairly reserved group of young mothers quickly began to function as a group in which quality learning was taking place when asked to discuss how to manage with a new baby with only £67 a week. During the vigorous exchanges that took place, the teenagers learned from each other which shops offered the best prices for nappies and an array of household items; how to prepare a variety of easy-to-make, inexpensive (and often nutritious) meals; how to avoid bank charges; where to go to find out about benefit entitlements; and what each thought about the amount of help boyfriends and partners should give with the new baby.

session into one where everyone is contributing and learning (see Box 8.3).

Practical skills work

The survey by Nolan (2008) of antenatal education noted that many women wanted more time in their antenatal sessions to be devoted to practising self-help skills for labour such as breathing and other relaxation techniques, different positions and massage. While fathers may not ask to learn babycare skills, group leaders should make it a priority to help men learn how to change nappies, bathe, soothe and settle babies. If men feel confident and competent to care for their babies, they are able to offer practical support to the mother in the early postnatal period. High levels of father involvement are strongly linked with both mothers' and fathers' satisfaction with their relationship and with family life (Craig and Sawriker 2006).

Many antenatal group leaders are daunted at the prospect of leading practical sessions. This discomfort may be attributed to lack of ease with their own bodies, lack of belief that teaching such skills makes a difference in labour, a perception that group members might be reluctant to participate, and poor quality venues where there is insufficient space for people to move around freely. Leaders whose only preparation for antenatal group sessions was a couple of lectures during their pre-registration training, and whose apprenticeship as group leaders has been spent observing other group leaders equally diffident about introducing practical work, are understandably nervous. Yet labour, birth and caring for babies are intensely physical activities (as is midwifery) and people need practice to be well prepared for their role either as parent (or as midwife).

The best way to gain in confidence to teach physical skills is to observe and speak to as many skilled practitioners as possible. Active Birth teachers, Hypnobirthing

Box 8.4 **Practical skills: a significant impact**

A group that included a very young father who was clearly attending antenatal sessions under a certain amount of duress was taught some simple baby massage skills. While everyone was practising, the group leader put on a CD of nursery rhymes and talked about how massaging a baby and singing or reciting nursery rhymes would make the baby feel secure, help him or her develop language, and be a source of enjoyment for both parent and child. At the end of the session, the young father asked the leader where he could get a copy of the CD she had used and where he could attend baby massage sessions with his baby.

therapists, Birth Dance teachers, antenatal teachers trained by the National Childbirth Trust (NCT) – all of these are able to demonstrate and analyse the facilitation of practical skills work.

These are some of the ways of making practical work easier for both group leaders and mothers and fathers:

- Ensure that you know why you are teaching these skills, and that group participants have a strong rationale for why they should practise them.
- Ask everyone to try the same exercises at the same time.
- Demonstrate what you want people to do – with confidence.
- Support people constantly while they are practising, giving positive feedback and making suggestions to each woman or couple individually.
- Have a laugh with the group.
- Relate the skills being practised to the stage of labour for which they are relevant.
- If practising babycare skills, separate the fathers from the mothers because women tend to mock men's efforts while men will strongly support each other. So the men can practise bathing and dressing a doll at one end of the room, and the women at the other.

Group members may seem reluctant to participate in practical work, but provided that the group leader is sufficiently confident, she will be able to help people overcome their anxiety. The learning that is achieved through practical work can be dramatic (see Box 8.4).

CONTENT OF ANTENATAL EDUCATION IN GROUPS

The Expert Reference Group convened by the Department of Health in 2007 devised an antenatal programme based

on six themes which they felt best captured what the literature said was important to people making the journey into parenthood. These six themes – *Getting to Know Your Unborn Baby; Changes for Me and Us; Giving Birth and Meeting Our Baby; Our Health and Wellbeing; Caring for Our Baby;* and *Who is There for Us? People and Resources* – were not necessarily meant to be delivered in six sessions, with one session for each theme. Instead, the themes were intended to permeate every session.

Getting to Know Our Unborn Baby

Given recent research indicating that the development of the baby's brain is affected by maternal physical and emotional wellbeing, topics such as healthy diet and lifestyle and coping with stress are very important. The difficulty is that the best time to discuss these topics is prior to pregnancy. Even early pregnancy classes happen too late since they are difficult to arrange before the end of the first trimester (and many women are reluctant to acknowledge their pregnancy publicly before they are safely past the first three months). By the second trimester, making changes in lifestyle will have less impact, although by no means, none. A strong case should therefore be made by the midwifery profession for midwives to be active in schools, leading the curriculum on pregnancy, birth and parenting.

There is scope, however, for antenatal group sessions to increase participants' understanding of how the unborn baby is affected by the mother's state of mind. This is not so as to induce guilt in mothers who are experiencing stress over which they have no control (living with domestic abuse; unable to speak English; isolated from family and friends; burdened with financial worries etc.) but to emphasize that every mother and baby are uniquely in harmony with each other, and respond to each other's moods. The closeness of the relationship is designed to ensure the survival of the baby. Topics that might, therefore, be covered under the heading of Getting to Know Our Unborn Baby (see Box 8.5) are how the baby's brain develops during pregnancy; what the baby can see, hear, taste, touch and smell and at what stage of pregnancy; what part the baby plays in the initiation of labour, and how recreating the experience of the uterus can comfort newborn babies (being held close, hearing their mothers' heartbeat and voice, being kept warm through contact with their mothers' skin, being fed on demand). Relaxation can be taught as a skill to reduce adrenalin levels and optimize the uterine environment for the baby as well as conferring health benefits on the mother.

Changes for Me and Us

The Expert Reference Group acknowledged the difficulties inherent in covering lifestyle issues specifically in relation

---

Box 8.5 **Getting to Know Our Unborn Baby: Activity**

Ask mothers and fathers to consider what life is like for their unborn baby in the womb.

- What do they know about their baby; what are the baby's patterns or waking and sleeping?
- Does the baby have particular likes or dislikes?
- Does the baby have his own idiosyncrasies?
- How will the baby feel when she leaves the womb and is born?
- How can that change from womb to world be made as easy as possible for the baby?

Box 8.6 **Changes for Me and Us: Activity**

Invite participants to complete a 24-hour clock representing the activities of their current life. Then ask them to complete another showing their life after their baby is born with time allocated to feeding, changing, comforting and playing with the baby.

The discussion that follows focuses on how their lives are going to change, who is there to support them, what kind of support they want and how they can access it. Also how life will change for other family members, such as grandparents, and the baby's siblings.

What kind of mother or father do they want to be? Do they have parental role models? Do they know what they definitely want to do and not do as parents?

Box 8.7 **Giving Birth and Meeting Our Baby: Activity**

While playing some relaxing background music, ask group members to make themselves comfortable and to try to imagine what might be happening to them at different points in labour:

'Think about the start of labour, when you're not quite sure what's happening.

Where are you? Where do you feel safe to labour? There's a contraction now – what position are you in?

If you're the woman's birth companion, how do you see yourself helping her with this contraction?

It's eight hours later in the labour now, and you're both in hospital. What is the room like? How are you feeling? When you have a strong contraction, how are you coping with it and what are you, as the person supporting her, doing at this point?

Can you imagine the moment when your baby is born? How do you feel? Ecstatic? Exhausted? Very emotional? Confused?

Your baby needs to be close to you both. How are you getting to know him or her now?'

---

to pregnancy, and preferred to set these issues in the broader context of family life. Making decisions about reducing smoking and alcohol intake as well as improving diet may help parents provide a better environment for their new baby to grow up in as well as improving the quality of their own lives. Pregnancy also provides a 9-month period of reflection for mothers and fathers to consider how this baby will affect their network of relationships, personal interests, social obligations and work commitments. Babies enter their parents' complex world, and planning ahead may ensure that adding one more element does not cause the whole world to fall apart (see Box 8.6).

Giving Birth and Meeting Our Baby

The theme of Giving Birth and Meeting Our Baby focuses on normal labour and birth, drawing on group members' knowledge of how labour starts , how long it lasts, what helps and what does not. Since people often attack their antenatal classes postnatally on the grounds of lack of realism, it is important to use as many different teaching and learning strategies as possible to convey what labour 'is really like'. A picture of a woman in labour can be a trigger for discussion of upright positions and birth companions' role; pictures of the hospital environment are very helpful in contextualizing information (How might being in this room affect your labour? Who are the staff you will meet and what is their role?). Labour and birth stories are invaluable in telling it from the woman's (or man's) point of view and there are also YouTube videos that recount parents' birth stories in their own words. In addition, mental rehearsal is a useful technique for helping mothers and fathers create an experience in their own minds and imagine their own roles (see Box 8.7).

Our Health and Wellbeing

The birth of the first child has been shown to precipitate a sudden deterioration in couples' relationship functioning (Doss et al 2009). As the baby is completely dependent on the mother to stay alive physically and to develop emotionally and cognitively, it is vital that the mother should feel supported. For most women, the person most likely to offer that support is her partner. However, tiredness, an overwhelming sense of new responsibility, worries about diminished income, lack of couple time without the baby – all these factors contribute to minor tensions

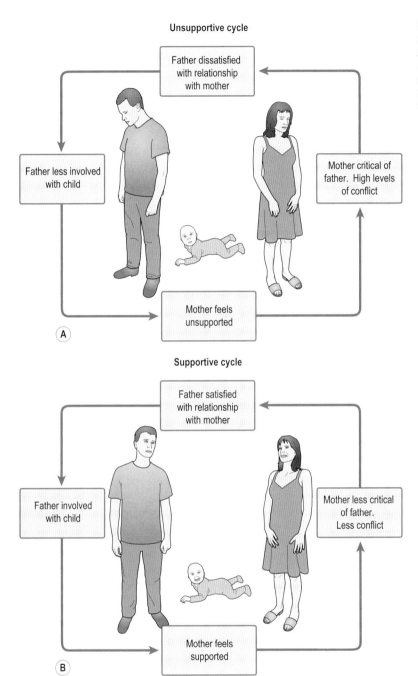

Unsupportive cycle

Father dissatisfied with relationship with mother

Father less involved with child

Mother critical of father. High levels of conflict

Mother feels unsupported

(A)

Supportive cycle

Father satisfied with relationship with mother

Father involved with child

Mother less critical of father. Less conflict

Mother feels supported

(B)

Fig. 8.3 (A) Unsupportive cycle. (B) Supportive cycle.
Adapted from OneplusOne e-learning modules, Transition to Parenthood Information Sheet (2005) and Supporting Couple Relationships (2008), reproduced with permission OneplusOne.

between couples escalating into major arguments. Understanding how to change vicious circles into virtuous ones gives parents a model to which they can refer in the critical early months of their baby's life. Figure 8.3 illustrates how fathers' involvement with their baby, or lack of involvement, can make mothers feel supported and content with their relationship with their partner, or unsupported and discontented. Helping fathers learn basic babycare skills in antenatal sessions is a very useful strategy for enabling them to play a full part in the early weeks of their new babies' lives when mothers are most in need of help.

Depending on how many sessions the antenatal course involves and how strong a relationship the group leader is able to build up with the people attending, there may be scope for more in-depth work on relationships, such as exploring how individuals typically respond when unhappy with their partner's behaviour – criticism, contempt, defensiveness, stonewalling (Gottman 1994) and strategies for tackling conflict.

The theme of Our Health and Wellbeing also involves looking at mental illness starting in the postnatal period, antenatal depression that gets worse after the birth of a baby (rather than talking about 'postnatal depression', which is not recognized in The Diagnostic and Statistical Manual of Mental Disorders IV [DSM IV] (American Psychiatric Association 1994) as a separate diagnosis) *and* looking at how mothers and fathers can keep themselves mentally healthy. It is very important to have an emphasis on mental health as everyone has to work at that, but only a few people will experience clinical depression. This topic provides another opportunity to look at lifestyles and the contribution a good diet, taking some exercise and a moderate intake of alcohol and other stimulants make to feeling mentally strong and able to cope.

Caring for Our Baby

Caring for Our Baby covers both the physical care of the baby and the emotional. The importance of helping parents acquire skills to be able to meet the daily physical needs of their baby has already been mentioned. Feeding is a huge area to cover and the risk of information overload is a very real one. As always with topics that are potentially information-heavy, the group leader needs to be clear in her own mind as to what are the most important things to get across, and then provide additional information in response to the questions uppermost in parents' mind at the time. In terms of breastfeeding, it may be that the group leader feels the need to give very little information, but to address some common fears (it's going to hurt; I won't have enough milk; how do I know my baby's getting sufficient milk?) and focus on ensuring that everyone in the group knows where she or he would get help if problems arise. While brief antenatal information giving sessions on breastfeeding have been found to greatly increase fathers' understanding of how breastfeeding works and their support of mothers (Wolfberg et al 2004), it is the couples' confidence to ask for help and their knowledge of where to find it that may be key in helping the woman to have a successful and enjoyable experience of feeding her baby.

The majority of parents are capable of meeting their baby's emotional and learning needs if left to their own devices and not sidetracked by manuals which they erroneously believe know more about how to look after their baby than they do. Some parents will have very little of

---

> ### Box 8.8 **Caring for Our Baby: Activity**
>
> Ask group participants to split into smaller groups and set up a competition (adult learners enjoy competitions every bit as much as children do!) How many nursery rhymes can they write down in a minute. (The average is around eight.)
>
> Congratulate everyone. Ask each group to choose one nursery rhyme they all know and sing it to the other groups. Discuss how the rhythms of nursery rhymes exaggerate the rhythms of normal speech and fire the baby's brain to make 'language connections'.

---

this innate understanding however, having been the recipients of very poor parenting or none at all. All parents like learning about how babies communicate and what they enjoy, about how babies comfort themselves and what is happening when babies 'look away' from their parents' faces. Helping parents rediscover nursery rhymes (as illustrated in Box 8.8), poems for children and singing will give them ideas, or reinforce innate ideas, about what babies need to develop trust in human relationships and to start to learn their own language. Baby massage is a wonderful way of ensuring that mothers, fathers and babies have 'conversations'.

Who Is There for Us? People and Resources

Very little time is devoted by maternity care professionals to antenatal education and even though more is likely to be required as government takes up the challenge of supporting new parents better, there is never likely to be enough time to discuss everything that might be relevant to parents. With this in mind, the group leader has to take responsibility for knowing where to signpost parents who want more information or help now, or in the future. Signposting will probably be a part of every topic covered in the antenatal course and what kind of signposting will depend on the needs and interests of the particular group of parents participating in the course. Some examples of signposting are given in Box 8.9.

DEFINING LEARNING OUTCOMES

There is never enough time for antenatal sessions. This being the case, it is very important that group leaders are clear about what it is they want to achieve (their aims) and what they want participants to learn. Aims have already

> **Box 8.9 Who Is There for Us?**
> **Signposting people and resources**
>
> - To health and social care professionals
> - To benefits agencies
> - To groups for parents with particular needs
> - To Children's Centres
> - To buggy push/baby swim groups
> - To parent and baby groups
> - To Internet chat rooms
> - To high-quality Internet sites
> - To books
> - To NICE (National Institute of Health and Care Excellence) guidelines
> - To research

been discussed in this chapter. Learning outcomes are vital for ensuring that the group leader and the group remain on task and all leave the session feeling they have gained something in terms of enhanced adulthood (Knowles 1984). They are not all about head knowledge. There is also learning that takes place in the heart and learning that is physical. Therefore, a list of learning outcomes for an individual session will include learning in various 'domains'. In order to ensure that leaders define the learning that will have taken place, rather than the process by which it will be achieved, every learning outcome needs to begin with the stem: *'by the end of this session, participants will be able to …'* (rather than, 'by the end of this session, participants will have …').

Learning outcomes for a session covering the relationship between unborn babies and their mother, start of labour, comfort positions for labour, healthy eating during and after pregnancy, and looking after myself and my partner might be expressed as follows:

By the end of this session, participants will be able to …

- describe the importance of relaxation during pregnancy (and after)
- state five signs that labour is about to start or has started
- demonstrate three positions that might make contractions easier to manage
- suggest two easy-to-make, inexpensive and nutritious meals for the first months after the baby is born
- agree with their partners how to divide household chores and babycare between them
- list Internet sites where they can find more information about healthy eating, and list sessions that provide more opportunities to practise self-help skills for labour.

MAXIMIZING ATTENDANCE AT ANTENATAL SESSIONS

If antenatal education is to be universally available to all pregnant women and their partners, the way in which it is provided needs to be tailored to the needs of local communities. Time and again, when accounts are given of successful groups, it is evident that their success lies in group leaders having identified where and when to run sessions, and topics specifically relevant to the people attending.

Women and men who are highly motivated to attend antenatal sessions, perhaps because their experiences of education have led them to value it, and, more pragmatically, because they are not dependent on public transport for access, tend to go to all the sessions that are on offer. They will go to sessions led by midwives at the hospital or clinic, and also to the NCT. They may also attend yoga for pregnancy and aquanatal classes. Other parents-to-be, a very significant minority, have no antenatal education.

The reasons for nonattendance have been explored, notably by Cliff and Deery (1997) in an article entitled 'Too like school'. These researchers identified the following barriers to attendance:

- young age
- less privileged socioeconomic background
- perception that the content of sessions was not relevant.

A Swedish study (Fabian et al 2004) of nonattendance at antenatal sessions found, against a background of 93% attendance of first-time mothers, that primigravid nonattenders were:

- more likely not to speak Swedish as their first language
- to be smokers
- to have considered abortion
- to have missed several antenatal checks.

Multigravid women who did not attend were:

- poorly educated
- pregnant with an unplanned baby
- abnormally frightened of childbirth.

These studies are helpful in terms of identifying the population of women less likely to attend antenatal sessions and some of the reasons why. Perhaps the most important reason would seem to be the fear of being judged – for smoking, for having considered a termination, for failing to attend antenatal clinic appointments, for not having planned the pregnancy and for not having done well at school. It is difficult to persuade women that they will not be judged until they have had at least one non-judgemental, respectful and person-centred experience of adult education. This requires them to come to a session. Planning to ensure sessions are as welcoming as

137

possible to local women is therefore vital if the considerable psychological, as well as physical, barriers that many face are to be overcome.

Availability of the intended participants is the first thing to take into account:

- When are women, and the people whom they want with them at the birth and who will be helping them care for the baby, free to attend sessions?
- Can women drive to sessions or do they take public transport?
- Which community centres are the best used, and safest (for both participants and group leaders)? Children's Centres may be ideal in terms of their location and facilities, but not all are open in the evening when sessions may be best suited to working mothers and fathers.

Planners also need to find out what is already available in the community for pregnant women. If successful hypnobirthing sessions are running, or women regularly attend aquanatal classes at the local leisure centre, or meet at a school where basic maths and English are being taught to women who missed out on education in childhood, or socialize at Asian Women's groups, it may be possible to link antenatal sessions to these activities.

While the Expert Reference Group carried out a stakeholders' review (summarized in DH 2011) of what people wanted to talk about and learn in their antenatal sessions and reflected the findings in the *Preparation for Birth and Beyond* programme's themes, some women will have very specific needs that may be best addressed in groups run just for them. Women asylum seekers will need help in understanding the UK maternity care system. In areas where smoking rates are very high and there is a significant problem with drug abuse, antenatal education may need to focus on helping women manage these problems as well as prepare for labour, birth and early parenting. There may be areas where facilitating women-only antenatal sessions is appropriate, and areas where large numbers of women belong to faith communities that preclude their attending sessions on certain days of the week.

If women are unlikely to attend sessions for cultural reasons, antenatal education can be provided through home-based learning materials. There is a vast range of information sheets, video clips and online activities that can be brought together in a 'pack' and offered to pregnant women. A small group of dedicated midwives, using their in-depth knowledge of the communities they serve, could, with a little time, compile such a pack. Consulting with local childbirth and parenting educators, social workers, faith leaders and youth workers may help ensure that both the content of the pack and the way in which it is presented maximize its use and usefulness.

Young mothers may prefer to attend sessions with peers of their own age. There is evidence that they may feel inhibited at antenatal group sessions with older mothers who are in stable relationships. The most vulnerable young women may be offered the Family–Nurse Partnership (FNP) programme, which is often delivered through Sure Start Children's Centres. This is an evidence-based intervention providing education and support from pregnancy through to the baby's second year of life. FNP nurses, who work closely with midwives and health visitors, aim to build a strong, trusting relationship with young mothers to help them achieve a healthy pregnancy and provide a physically and emotionally safe environment for their babies. The insights gained from many years of running and evaluating the FNP in the UK informed the work of the Expert Reference Group in devising the *Preparation for Birth and Beyond* antenatal education package.

Personal invitation seems to be the most effective means of encouraging attendance at antenatal group sessions. The invitation is likely to be delivered by the midwife, and she should be very clear that it is an invitation both to the mother and to the person the mother would most like to bring with her. If this is the father, and the midwife knows him, using his name when issuing the invitation is both polite and an excellent way of gaining his goodwill. Texting women with the time and venue for each antenatal session is very useful, especially when reaching out to pregnant teenagers. Letters addressed to both parents can be sent out, but must start with their names, rather than 'Dear parents'.

Including fathers

Research into the impact on fathers of attending antenatal sessions where their needs are identified and responded to, and the focus is on their transition to parenthood equally with the mothers', is very positive. Studies have reported better couple relationships (Diemer 1997), mothers reporting greater satisfaction with the division of labour in relation to home and babycare tasks (Matthey et al 2004), and greater parental sensitivity (Pfannenstiel and Honig 1995).

There are various key strategies for attracting fathers to antenatal group sessions and to retaining their attendance. First, it is important to ensure that the invitation to attend is addressed both to the mothers and the fathers. Fathers Direct (now The Fatherhood Institute) (2007) recommends avoiding the term '*parent*' as this is commonly interpreted by both men and women as meaning mothers. The Institute also recommends not using the words '*classes*', '*groups*' or '*education*' in the name of the programme, but instead to use a title that indicates a practical focus, such as '*How to Have a Baby and Look After It*'. It is essential to provide sessions at times that make it possible for the fathers in the area that is being targeted to attend. Fathers who work away from home, or undertake long daily commutes, will need weekend sessions. There may be a possibility to run fathers' sessions at the workplace, given a sympathetic employer.

Sessions need to provide opportunity for fathers to talk to each other. This means at least occasionally splitting the group by gender to allow for male bonding. When men are in a single-sex group, they interrupt each other with supportive comments, but supportive comments decrease as the number of female members in the group increases (Smith-Lovin and Brody 1989). When sessions have included single-sex small group work, group members are more likely to discuss issues with their partners after the class has ended (Symon and Lee 2003). Whole-group sessions need to include the men's perspective on every topic. For example, 'start of labour' needs to consider both how the mothers may feel *and* the fathers. 'Keeping mentally healthy' needs to be about more than what the fathers can do to support the mothers, but also about what they can do to look after themselves, as shown in Box 8.10.

It is very important to make sure that visual aids depict fathers as often as mothers, and that there are handouts and literature available that are pitched specifically at them.

Box 8.10 Fathers' perspectives

The Fatherhood Institute (formerly Fathers Direct) suggests that expectant fathers commonly have the following issues uppermost in their minds:
- What happens if something is wrong with the baby?
- What can I do to help my partner through the pregnancy?
- What happens if something goes wrong at the birth?
- What if I am not ready to be a father?
- What will happen to our relationship?
- How can we still earn enough money?

Source: Fathers Direct, 2007. Including new fathers: a guide for maternity professionals. Fathers Direct, London.

Young fathers have been shown to want:
- reassurance and to grow in self-confidence
- help with decision-making
- greater self-awareness
- childcare knowledge, skills and awareness
- social contact and new friends
- practical information and advice
- 'political' recognition

Source: Key issues raised by the Trust for the Study of Adolescence (2005). The Young Fathers Project: A project to develop and evaluate a model of working with young vulnerable fathers. TSA, Brighton.

How many mothers and fathers in the group?

Traditionally, antenatal classes provided in hospitals have been open to all who wish to attend, resulting in extremely large groups. This almost certainly proves to be an unfavourable learning environment. The sessions in Ho and Holroyd's study (2002) were attended by between 48 and 95 women. The women identified that it was impossible to engage in questioning and discussion, impossible to have their personal problems addressed, impossible to make friends and impossible for the educators to seek appropriate feedback from them.

Groups function best when they are composed of about 8 to 16 people. This ensures that the more shy members can contribute if they want to, and gives everyone an opportunity to be heard and have his or her personal needs addressed. It may be acceptable to offer information to larger groups but the expense of bringing people together has to be questioned if what is going to be achieved could equally well have been achieved by giving a handout at the antenatal clinic.

How many sessions and how long?

A 2007 survey of antenatal education (Nolan 2008) found that women wanted to attend more than one antenatal session. They felt that meeting over a number of weeks gave them the opportunity to get to know other women, and made it more likely that friendships would continue into the postnatal period. In addition, a single session was considered simply inadequate to cover the many topics on which they wanted information and which they wanted to discuss.

Information is retained according to its perceived relevance to learners. Antenatally, mothers and fathers will be interested especially in issues relating to pregnancy, labour, birth and the first weeks of their new baby's life. Following the birth, as they begin to experience all the dimensions of their new role, the need for more information on some topics, and for support from other new parents and health professionals becomes apparent. For this reason, antenatal groups that continue into the postnatal period offer midwives a wonderful opportunity to help mothers and fathers cope with problems that could only be dimly anticipated antenatally. Information about infant feeding, sleeping, weaning and emotional development becomes immediately relevant in the postnatal period. Listening to the stories of people whom parents have already met in their antenatal group provides a wonderful way of normalizing experiences. The ideal therefore is to move away from *antenatal* education to one of *transition to parenthood* education, with sessions starting from mid-pregnancy and continuing into the first 3–6 months of the babies' lives. While this may sound utopian, it would be reasonable to argue that this level of support might well reduce demands on community midwives, specialist community public health nurses (health visitors) and General Practitioners (GPs), and lead to a reduction in the incidence of mental ill health and relationship breakdown following childbirth. One study (Nolan et al 2012) has noted that women can manage anxiety about their baby's development if they can 'compare notes' with other women and gain a broad concept of what is 'normal'.

The length of individual sessions may well be determined by the availability of the venue. Shorter sessions may be more tolerable for heavily pregnant women and tired fathers, but whatever the length of the session, it is important to recognize certain key features of adult learning. The average attention span of an adult is about 10 minutes. This means that activities, discussions and information-giving that continue for longer than this may result in a diminishing return as far as learning is concerned. In order to retain people's interest, every session needs a variety of learning opportunities and the leader needs to set a pace that is acceptable to both activists and reflectors (Honey and Mumford 1982).

The brain needs water, glucose and protein in order to be able to function. A break half way through the session allows time for parents to socialize and to have a drink and something to eat – thus enhancing attention and learning power when they return to the group.

The aim of the group leader is to achieve a number of balances in each session:

- between her doing the talking and the mothers and fathers doing the talking
- between people sitting in their seats and moving around
- between work done with the whole group and work done in small groups
- between single-sex small group work and mixed small group work
- between focusing on themes to do with pregnancy and birth and those to do with living with a new baby
- between group participants determining the agenda and how long to give to each topic, and the group leader leading the session.

Effective evaluation of any session could be carried out using the bullet-point list above. However, in order to see herself as group members are seeing her, it is important for the group leader to have a skilled outsider present at her sessions occasionally, someone who can give detailed feedback on which she can build so as to provide ever-more effective learning opportunities.

CONCLUSION

It is anticipated that antenatal education will once again become widespread throughout the UK, be properly funded, valued by midwives and valuable to mothers and fathers. While there are many questions for midwives to answer in terms of how best to provide sessions that will be relevant and useful to mothers and fathers from the communities they serve, what potential group participants want is very clear.

- They want sessions that cover a variety of topics from pregnancy to birth to feeding and caring for their babies and looking after themselves.
- They do not want just one class that is rushed and does not answer their questions.
- They want to be part of a small group where they can make friends.
- They do not want huge numbers at classes because they do not feel able to ask questions and cannot interact with other people.
- They want group leaders to use up-to-date videos and teaching aids that help them prepare for labour, birth and parenting in the 21st century.

Mothers and fathers are very quick to spot poor facilitation skills and biased teaching. This places a requirement upon midwife lecturers to ensure that their students acquire group skills during their pre-registration or post-registration programmes.

The best classes, in the view of mothers and fathers:

- are where the facilitator respects their right to make up their own minds about what they want in labour and how they will care for their babies;
- welcome questions;
- provide lots of opportunities for talking;
- provide information in a way that empowers them rather than frightening them; and
- are structured, responsive to their individual needs, relaxed and fun (based on Nolan 2008).

REFERENCES

American Psychiatric Association 1994 Diagnostic and Statistical Manual of Mental Disorders, 4th edn (DSM-IV). American Psychiatric Association, Arlington, VA

Children's Society 2012 The Good Childhood Report 2012. The Children's Society, London

Cliff D, Deery R 1997 Too much like school: social class, age, marital status and attendance/ non-attendance at antenatal classes. Midwifery 13(3):139–45

Cohen N, Muir E, Lojkasek M et al 1999 Watch, wait, and wonder: testing the effectiveness of a new approach to mother–infant psychotherapy. Infant Mental Health Journal 20(4):429–51

Craig L, Sawrikar P 2006 Work and family balance: transitions to high school. Unpublished Draft Final Report. Social Policy Research Centre, University of New South Wales

DCSF (Department for Children, Schools and Families) 2012 The Early Years: foundations for life, health and learning. DCSF, London

DH (Department of Health) 2008 The Child Health Promotion Programme: pregnancy and the first five years of life. DH/DCSF, London

DH (Department of Health) 2009 Healthy lives, brighter futures: the strategy for children and young people's health. DH/DCSF, London

DH (Department of Health) 2011 Preparation for birth and beyond. available at: www.dh.gov.uk/en/Publicationsandstatistics/Publications/PublicationsPolicyAndGuidance/DH_130565 (accessed 3 May 2013)

Diemer G 1997 Expectant fathers: influence of perinatal education on coping, stress and spousal relations. Research in Nursing and Health 20:281–93

Doss B D, Rhoades G K, Stanley S M et al 2009 The effect of the transition to parenthood on relationship quality: an 8-year prospective study. Journal of Personality and Social Psychology 96(3):601–19

Fabian H M, Rådestad I J, Waldenström U 2004 Characteristics of Swedish women who do not attend childbirth and parenthood education classes during pregnancy. Midwifery 20(3):226–35

Fathers Direct 2007 Including new fathers: a guide for maternity professionals. Fathers Direct, London

Ford G 2006 The complete sleep guide for contented babies and toddlers. Vermilion, London

Glover V, O'Connor T G 2002 Effects of antenatal stress and anxiety:

implications for development and psychiatry. British Journal of Psychiatry 180:389–91

Gottman J 1994 Why marriages succeed or fail. Bloomsbury, London

Ho I, Holroyd E 2002 Chinese women's perceptions of the effectiveness of antenatal education in the preparation for motherhood. Journal of Advanced Nursing 38(1):74–85

Honey P, Mumford A 1982 Manual of learning styles. P Honey, London

Jackson D 2003 Three in a bed: the benefits of sleeping with your baby. Bloomsbury, London

Janis I L 1958 Psychological stress: psychoanalytic and behavioral studies of surgical patients. Academic Press, New York

Knowles M 1984 Andragogy in action. Jossey–Bass, London

Liedloff J 1986 The continuum concept: in search of happiness lost. Da Capo Press, Cambridge, MA

Matthey S, Kavanagh D J, Howie P et al 2004 Prevention of postnatal distress or depression: an evaluation of an intervention at preparation for parenthood classes. Journal of Affective Disorders 79(1-3): 113–26

McMillan A S, Barlow J, Redshaw M 2009 Birth and beyond: a review of the evidence about antenatal education. University of Warwick, Warwick. Available at: www.dh.gov.uk/en/Healthcare/Children/Maternity/index.htm (accessed 3 May 2013)

Nolan M 2008 Antenatal survey (1). What do women want? The Practising Midwife 11(1):26–8

Nolan M, Mason V, Snow S et al 2012 Making friends at antenatal classes: a qualitative exploration of friendship across the transition to motherhood. Journal of Perinatal Education 21(3):178–85

Pfannenstiel A E, Honig A S 1995 Effects of a prenatal 'Information and insights about infants' program on the knowledge base of first-time low-education fathers one month postnatally. Early Childhood Development and Care 111: 87–105

Renkert S, Nutbeam D 2001 Opportunities to improve maternal health literacy through antenatal education: an exploratory study. Health Promotion International 16(4):381–8

Smith-Lovin L, Brody C 1989 Interruptions in group discussions: the effects of gender and group composition. American Sociological Review 54(3):424–35

Spiby H, Henderson B, Slade P et al 1999 Strategies for coping with labour: does antenatal education translate into practice? Journal of Advanced Nursing 29(2):388–94

Stamler L L 1998 The participants' views of childbirth education: is there congruency with an enablement framework for patient education? Journal of Advanced Nursing 28:939–47

Stapleton H, Kirkham M, Thomas G 2002 Qualitative study of evidence based leaflets in maternity care. British Medical Journal 324:639

Symon A, Lee J 2003 Including men in antenatal education: evaluating innovative practice Evidence Based Midwifery 1(1):12–19

Talge N M, Neal C, Glover V 2007 Antenatal maternal stress and long-term effects on child neurodevelopment: how and why? Journal of Child Psychology and Psychiatry 48(3/4):245–61

Trust for the Study of Adolescence (TSA) 2005 The Young Fathers Project: a project to develop and evaluate a model of working with young vulnerable fathers. TSA, Brighton

Wadhwa P D, Sandman C A, Porto M et al 1993 The association between prenatal stress and infant birth weight and gestational age at birth: a prospective investigation. American Journal of Obstetrics and Gynecology 169(4):858–65

Wolfberg A J, Michels K B, Shields W et al 2004 Dads as breastfeeding advocates: results from a randomized controlled trial of an educational intervention. American Journal of Obstetrics and Gynecology 191(3):708–12

FURTHER READING

Department of Health 2011 Preparation for birth and beyond: a resource pack for leaders of community groups and activities. DH, London. Available at: www.dh.gov.uk/en/Publicationsandstatistics/Publications/PublicationsPolicyAndGuidance/DH_130565

This package encapsulates a fresh approach to antenatal education and considers relationships and emotions across the transition to parenthood as well as preparation for labour and birth. Lots of practical activities for use with diverse groups of parents are described and copyright free worksheets can be downloaded.

Gerhardt S 2004 Why love matters: how affection shapes a baby's brain. Routledge, London

This inspiring book explains how newborn babies' brains are moulded in response to their earliest experiences with their mothers and other primary caregivers. It explains why positive interaction is essential for babies' healthy social and emotional development.

Sunderland M 2007 What every parent needs to know: the incredible effects of love, nurture and play on your child's development. Dorling Kindersley, London

This well-referenced book provides an accessible account of the latest findings from neurobiology regarding how the baby's brain develops in utero and during the first years of life.

Chapter 9

Change and adaptation in pregnancy

Irene Murray, Jenny Hassall

Anatomical and physiological adaptations occurring throughout pregnancy affect virtually every body system. The timing and intensity of the changes vary between systems but all are designed to support fetal growth and development, and prepare the woman for birth and motherhood. The midwife's appreciation of the physiological adaptations to pregnancy and recognition of abnormal findings is fundamental in the management of all pregnancies, enabling her to provide appropriate midwifery care to each woman, including those affected by pre-existing illness. A common feature of these changes is the dynamic and symbiotic partnership between the uteroplacental unit and the woman influenced by physical, mechanical, genetic and hormonal factors. Many aspects of the physiology of pregnancy remain poorly understood and controversies continue to be researched. (Changes in the woman's emotional state due to hormonal factors are discussed in Chapter 25 and changes in the breast are detailed in Chapter 34.)

THE CHAPTER AIMS TO:

- provide an overview of the adaptation of each body system during pregnancy and the underlying hormonal changes
- identify the physiological changes that mimic or mask disease in pregnancy
- provide the rationale for common disorders in pregnancy in order for the midwife to facilitate appropriate advice
- review the diagnosis of pregnancy.

PHYSIOLOGICAL CHANGES IN THE REPRODUCTIVE SYSTEM

The uterus

The uterus plays a remarkable role in pregnancy by stretching and expanding to accommodate and nurture the growing fetus (Hudson et al 2012). This expansion and activation takes place in the middle muscle layer of the uterine wall, the *myometrium*, which is partly covered and protected by an outer layer of peritoneum, the *perimetrium*. An internal layer, the *endometrium*, lines the uterine wall (Abbas et al 2010).

Perimetrium

The perimetrium is a thin layer of peritoneum composed of connective tissue that comprises collagen and elastin fibres, which is draped over the uterus and uterine tubes and is continuous laterally with the broad ligaments (Impey and Child 2012) (see Chapter 3). During pregnancy, the peritoneal sac is greatly distorted as the uterus enlarges and rises out of the pelvis, drawing up the two folds of broad ligament on either side. Stretching of the peritoneum makes it difficult to localize pain late in pregnancy which may delay diagnosis of disease (Casciani et al 2012).

By the third trimester the ligaments and uterine tubes appear lower on the sides of the uterus. The tubes run downwards, with the fimbriae spread out on its surface and bound to the sides of the uterus by the narrowed broad ligaments. The ovaries have become abdominal structures lying laterally to the gravid uterus (Standring et al 2008). As the uterus expands there is increasing stress and tension on the round ligaments which run almost perpendicularly downwards from the fundus. Spasm of the round ligaments may cause painful cramps which are usually more pronounced on the right side due to the dextrorotation of the uterus (see below) and are relieved by more gradual movement (Beckman et al 2010).

Myometrium

The myometrium is the muscular wall of the uterus that undergoes dramatic remodelling during pregnancy to provide support for the growing fetus and ultimately to expel it during labour (Ciarmela et al 2011). It is composed mainly of bundles of smooth myometrial cells (myocytes) embedded in a supporting extracellular matrix (ECM). The myocytes are elongated, spindle-shaped cells which are functionally different between upper and lower uterine segments having a contractile phenotype in the upper segment and a more relaxed phenotype in the lower segment (Mosher et al 2013). Smooth muscle cells increase in length from 50 μm in the non-pregnant uterus to about

500 μm or longer in the pregnant uterus (Abbas et al 2010). Each bundle of myocytes is approximately 300 μm in diameter and is further organized into fasciculi each of which measures 1–2 mm in diameter (Blanks et al 2007). The ECM is composed of tension-bearing proteins such as collagen, fibronectin and elastin, all of which increase significantly in mass and composition under the influence of progesterone and oestrogen, providing a scaffold for the smooth muscle cells, mast cells, blood and lymphatic vessels (Åkerud 2009). The increase in elastin in particular assists in accommodating the physical strain within the uterine muscle during pregnancy. Both myocytes and the ECM play an important role in contractility and are synchronously regulated to enable the uterus to change from the relative quiescence of pregnancy to maximal contractility during labor.

Phases of myometrial development

Myometrial development in pregnancy begins with an early *proliferative phase* activated by oestrogen and other hormones (Shynlova et al 2010), resulting in a rapid increase in myocytes (*hyperplasia*) by at least 10-fold. This is followed by a *synthetic phase* when myocytes increase in size (*hypertrophy*) and further remodelling of the ECM (Shynlova et al 2009). Myometrial hypertrophy and hyperplasia is initiated and finalized early in gestation. Subsequent enlargement in length and volume is mainly through mechanical stretch, which transforms the uterus into a relatively thin-walled muscular organ capable of accommodating fetal growth and movement. In the *contractile phase* hypertrophy stabilizes and the muscle prepares for the *labour phase* of intense coordinated contractions (Shynlova et al 2009).

Myometrial layers

The classic description of three layers of myometrium (*stratum supravasculare, stratum vasculare* and *stratum subvasculare*) found in most major texts was observed during research in other species such as the mouse. In spite of extensive investigation since the end of the 19th century, the debate continues concerning the organization of human myometrial muscle fibres. Young and Hession (1999) described the bulk of the myometrium (*stratum vasculare*) to be composed of a thick layer of myocytes organized into cylindrical, sheet-like and *fibre* bundles or *fasciculata* with communicating bridges that merge and intertwine to form an interlacing network and a contiguous pathway allowing coordinated contraction. The myocytes within each bundle all contract and relax in a longitudinal direction only (as with a spring). These fasciculi are well ordered, running transversely across the fundus of the uterus, obliquely down the anterior and posterior walls of the uterus and transversely across the lower uterine segment (Fig. 9.1). Other investigators describe a homogenous structure of one continuous layer

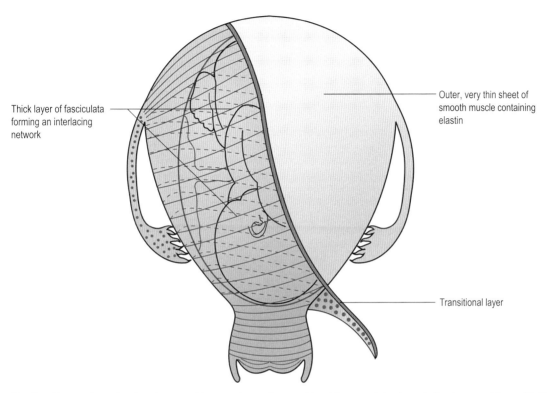

Fig. 9.1 Myometrium showing the very thin outer layer, the transitional layer and the inner bulk of myometrium with the arrangement of the fasciculata running transversely across the fundus between the fallopian tubes, obliquely down anterior and posterior walls and transversely around the lower uterine segment.

of smooth muscle cells organized in large interwoven bundles where longitudinal and circumferential muscle fibres are mixed with fasciculi running at right angles within them (Miftahof and Nam 2011).

The inner third of the myometrium (*stratum subvascu-lare*) and its underlying endometrium is known as the *endo–myometrial junctional zone* (Aguilar and Mitchell 2010). In the non-pregnant state it measures less than 5 mm thick but during pregnancy it becomes indistinct. The peristaltic waves of the junctional zone change direction depending on the stage of parturition thus playing an integral part in both sperm transport and implantation (Aguilar and Mitchell 2010). Failure in the remodelling of the junctional zone segment of the spiral arteries during placentation can result in impaired placental perfusion which may lead to pregnancy complications (Brosens et al 2010).

There is little change in the myometrial thickness of the uterine body across pregnancy in spite of the increased volume. The mean thickness is 0.6 cm at 15 weeks and 0.7 cm at 36 weeks with only a very slight decline in later weeks. At term the pregnant uterus is described as a thin, soft biological shell or *bioshell* with readily indentable walls through which the fetus can easily be palpated

Table 9.1 Increases in weight and size of the uterus during pregnancy			
	Nulliparous	**Parous**	**At term**
Weight of uterus (g)	44	80–110	1100
Size of uterus (cm)	6–8 × 5 × 2.5	9–10	40 × 22.5 × 20
Sources: Cunningham et al 2010; Abduljalil et al 2012			

(Cunningham et al 2010). It is pear-shaped and measures about 40 cm in height although the dimensions vary considerably depending on maternal height, weight, parity and ethnic origin (Gardosi 2012) (Table 9.1). During normal pregnancy the weight of the uterus increases 10- to 20-fold from about 44 g in the primigravida to 1100 g at term. It increases with successive pregnancies and may weigh more than 110 g in a non-pregnant woman who is para 5 or more (Abduljalil et al 2012).

There is a dynamic balance in pregnancy between forces promoting uterine quiescence with a cervix that remains closed or contractility with a cervix that softens and dilates (Petraglia et al 2010). The quiescent phase is controlled by prostacyclin, corticotropin-releasing hormone (CRH), relaxin, parathyroid hormone, nitric oxide and a complex interplay of signals between fetus and mother (Mesiano et al 2011). Progesterone's relaxing effect blocks the myometrial response to oxytocin. The changing oestrogen and progesterone concentration within the uterus causes an increase in the expression of calcium and potassium channels which dampens electrical activity (Soloff et al 2011). Cell-to-cell gap junctions are present in very low density, indicating poor coupling and limited electrical conduction between the cells. The fragmented bursts of irregular, poorly coordinated, low electrical activity that takes place over several minutes are known as *Braxton Hicks contractions*, initially described by Braxton Hicks in 1872. They are painless, non-rhythmic uterine contractions that are easily palpated from about 12 weeks' gestation and are unpredictable, sporadic and of variable intensity. During the last few weeks of pregnancy they may become more rhythmic, increase in frequency and may occur every 10–20 minutes. The woman is usually unaware of Braxton Hicks contractions unless the uterus is particularly sensitive, which may cause some degree of pain. Some women may find them very uncomfortable such that they may confuse them with *false labour* (Cunningham et al 2010).

In contrast to many other species, progesterone levels remain relatively high throughout pregnancy decreasing only after the birth of the placenta. Awakening of the quiescent uterus is due therefore not to withdrawal of progesterone but rather to resistance of the tissues to its action (Mesiano et al 2011). As term approaches, progesterone resistance increases, gap junction density rises and excitation of myocytes causes the forceful, synchronous contractions of labour.

Endometrium (decidua)

Remodelling of the endometrium begins spontaneously in stromal cells adjacent to spiral arterioles during the mid-secretory phase of the menstrual cycle. If implantation occurs the endometrial cells undergo a transformation known as the *decidual reaction* which extends into the junctional zone and forms the *decidua of pregnancy*. The primary function of *decidualization* is to provide nutrition and an immunologically privileged site for the early embryo. Triggered by maternal immune cells the *decidual cells* swell due to the accumulation of glycogen and lipid (Moore et al 2013). Their secretions dampen the local immune response to the invading trophoblast enhancing its invasiveness (Gellersen et al 2013) (see Chapter 5). Implantation of the trophoblast usually occurs on the anterior or posterior wall of the body of the uterus where the decidua is better developed than in the cervix or isthmus.

Profound changes take place in cellular function during decidualization. Spindle-shaped endometrial stromal cells become round and produce hormones, growth factors and cytokines. Uterine glands and arteries become coiled and the recognizable pattern of three distinct layers can be identified: a superficial compact layer, an intermediate spongy layer and a thin basal layer (see Chapter 5). Under the influence of progesterone, the decidua achieves maximum thickness at 6 weeks' gestation then gradually becomes less distinct until it is not identifiable by 10 weeks (Wong et al 2009). Effective decidualization is essential for the formation of a functional placenta.

Blood flow to the body of the uterus and placenta from a convoluted network of uterine and ovarian arteries and veins is fully established by the end of the first trimester. Remodelling of spiral arteries into large low-resistance uteroplacental vessels begins after implantation and by 7 weeks' gestation the diameter of the vessels almost doubles in size to accommodate the massive increase in uterine perfusion from 45 ml to 750 ml per minute at term. By mid-pregnancy 90% of uterine blood supply is flowing into the intervillous spaces of the placenta (Brosens et al 2012).

In early pregnancy the tips of the spiral arteries are plugged by the invading trophoblast cells so there is little blood flow into the placenta. With increasing trophoblast invasion the tips of the spiral arteries are enormously dilated, particularly beneath the implantation site, often reaching a four-fold increase of 2–3 mm in diameter. Loss of smooth muscle in their walls and their elastic lamina results in their dilatation and conversion into *flaccid conduits* (Burton et al 2009). About 120 spiral arteries enter the intervillous space and extend from the decidua to the myometrium (Pijnenborg et al 2011). They also become longer as the uterus enlarges circumferentially due either to longitudinal growth or progressive straightening of the coiled vessel. Transformation of these spiral arteries has a profound effect on the rate and constancy of delivery of maternal blood to the placenta at an optimal pressure and velocity.

The passage of blood through the dilated uterine arteries of the pregnant uterus produces a soft blowing sound like the continuous murmur of the sea, known as the *uterine souffle*. It can be detected from 15 weeks' gestation, is synchronous with the maternal pulse and heard most distinctly near the lower portion of the uterus and in both inguinal regions. In contrast, the *placental souffle* can be heard over the placenta and is produced by the blood flowing through it. This should not be confused with the *funic souffle*, a muffled swooshing sound produced by the pulsation of blood as it is propelled through the arteries in the umbilical cord. Although synchronous with the fetal heart rate and found in the immediate vicinity of the placenta, it is quite different to the very distinct sound of the fetal heart.

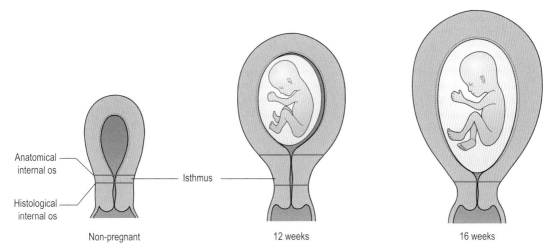

Fig. 9.2 Changes in the uterus from non-pregnant to 16 weeks' gestation.
From Hanretty K 2010 Obstetrics illustrated, 7th edn. Churchill Livingstone, Edinburgh, p 34, with permission of Churchill Livingstone, Elsevier.

Changes in uterine shape and size

Making comparisons between the uterus and fruit is a fairly reliable mental benchmark for uterine sizing in early pregnancy. At 5 weeks' gestation the uterus feels like a small unripe *pear*. By 8 weeks it feels like a large *navel orange*. By 10 weeks it is about the size of a *grapefruit* and by 12 weeks it is the size of a *cantaloupe melon* (Sage-Femme Collective 2008). Traditionally, gestational age was assessed by comparing uterine height with abdominal landmarks (Hargreaves et al 2011). Although the current standard practice of symphysis-fundal height measurement is flawed, its continued use is advised until proven alternatives are found (Neilson 2009).

12th week of pregnancy

For the first few weeks of pregnancy the uterus maintains its original pear shape but as pregnancy advances the corpus and fundus become globular and by 12 weeks it is almost spherical. Thereafter it increases in length more rapidly than in width and becomes ovoid in shape. By the end of the 12th week it can usually be palpated just above the symphysis pubis (Cunningham et al 2010). Changes in uterine position are normal during pregnancy. The fundus of the uterus is able to move relatively freely in all planes and is frequently retroverted in the first trimester (Fig. 9.2).

16th week of pregnancy

Between 12 and 16 weeks' gestation, the fundus becomes dome-shaped. When the uterus enlarges it comes into contact with the anterior abdominal wall and the bladder is displaced superiorly (Theodorou and Larentzakis 2012). As it rises it rotates to the right (*dextrorotation*) due to the rectosigmoid on the left side of the pelvis, and tension is exerted on the broad and round ligaments (Cunningham et al 2010).

20th week of pregnancy

By the 20th week of pregnancy the uterine fundus is at the level of the umbilicus. The uterus is an ovoid shape and the round ligaments appear to be inserted slightly above the middle of the uterus and the uterine tubes elongate.

30th week of pregnancy

The enlarging uterus displaces the intestines laterally and superiorly. The caecum and appendix, which have been progressively rising upwards from 12 weeks, now reach the iliac crest. The abdominal wall supports the uterus and maintains the relation between the long axis of the uterus and the axis of the pelvic inlet. In the supine position the uterus falls back to rest on the vertebral column, the inferior vena cava and aorta (Cunningham et al 2010).

36th week of pregnancy

By the end of the 36th week the enlarged uterus almost fills the abdominal cavity. The fundus is at the tip of the xiphoid cartilage which is pushed forward and continues to rise almost to the liver (Cunningham et al 2010). The diaphragm is raised by about 4 cm and the anteroposterior diameter of the thoracic cavity increases (Theodorou and Larentzakis 2012). With the gradual upward displacement of the abdominal organs there is stretching of the abdominal and peritoneal cavity. The liver is no longer palpable having been forced upwards, backwards and to the right by the expanding uterus. The transverse colon, stomach and spleen are crowded into the vault of the abdominal cavity and the small intestines lie above, behind and to the sides of the uterus.

38th week of pregnancy

Between 38 and 40 weeks the increase in myometrial tone leads to smoothing and shortening of the lower uterine segment. The uterus becomes more rounded with a decrease in fundal height although this is influenced by the lie of the fetus. Tension on the uterine tubes and broad ligaments increase (Cunningham et al 2010).

Uterine divisions

The development of the uterine divisions in pregnancy is asymmetric (Hamdi et al 2010). The muscular upper uterine segment of the uterus grows faster in the first seven months of pregnancy while the lower uterine segment grows more rapidly towards the end of pregnancy. During the first trimester the isthmus hypertrophies and triples in length to about 3 cm (Standring et al 2008). In the second trimester the walls of the isthmus are of a similar thickness to the walls of the body. By term the walls of the lower uterine segment may be as little as 0.4 cm thick.

In the primigravida, during the last two weeks of pregnancy, the low-intensity Braxton Hicks contractions cause shortening of the passive lower segment in preparation for cervical dilatation. The contractile upper segment of the corpus pulls the isthmus open over the presenting part converting it into a thinned out cone of circular fibres to develop into the lower uterine segment. This is detected clinically when the previously *floating* presenting part becomes fixed in the pelvic inlet. In the multigravida, the lower uterine segment usually develops in the early part of labour. In all cases, the isthmus changes from a sphincter into a thinned out tendon-like structure that pulls the cervix open. With the development of the lower uterine segment a transverse depression or ridge forms at its junction with the thickened upper uterine segment. This ridge becomes the *physiological retraction ring* during the second stage of physiological labour. It is a landmark that is used to ensure that the incision at caesarean section is in the less vascular lower uterine segment where there is less risk of dehiscence in subsequent pregnancies compared to the classical caesarean section scar (Standring et al 2008).

Descent of the fetal head into the pelvic brim (*engagement*) at 38 weeks' gestation in the primigravida has traditionally been considered a reassuring sign that labour will proceed normally without risk of dystocia. The primigravida with an unengaged head at term or onset of labour is more likely to need intervention (Iqbal and Sumaira 2009). In African women, engagement often does not occur until labour is well established, perhaps because of their shape of pelvis or stronger pelvic support structures, but this should not preclude a normal birth. Descent of the fetal head into the pelvic inlet causes a change in shape of the abdomen and is accompanied by the feeling of the

baby dropping known as *lightening* (Cunningham et al 2010). The woman may feel a sense of relief as the rib cage expands more easily, enabling her to breathe more deeply and to tolerate more substantial meals. Although heartburn may reduce, there may be an increase in other symptoms. Sharp pains may occur in the rectum and cervix, and constipation is common. Increased pressure of the fetal head on the bladder may lead to urinary frequency and an increased risk of urinary incontinence (Gabbe et al 2012).

The cervix

The cervix has been described as the *gatekeeper of pregnancy* as it is transformed from a closed, rigid, collagen-dense structure with a closed os in early pregnancy to one that is soft, distensible and effaced at the time of birth (Larsen and Hwang 2011). It is less contractile than the lower uterine segment as it contains less smooth muscle. The initial *softening phase* of the cervix, which is dependent on progesterone, begins at conception and continues until approximately 32 weeks. This softening in early pregnancy was first described by Hegar in 1895 and became known as *Hegar's sign*. There are changes in the structural organization of cervical tissue leading to a decline in tensile strength and an increase in compliance. *Crvical ripening* is a more accelerated phase occurring in the final weeks of pregnancy. Collagen is reduced or disorganized leading to degradation of the ECM. The cervix becomes thin, more elastic and pliable (Hassan et al 2011). Increased blood flow to the cervix results in a bluish-purple coloration known as *Goodell's sign* (Geraghty and Pomeranz 2011). These changes are intricately timed to coincide with uterine contractions and the initiation of cervical dilatation (Larsen and Hwang 2011). Pro-inflammatory agents, anti-inflammatory cytokines, prostaglandins, stromal factors and nitric oxide all contribute to the inflammatory process of cervical ripening. The gradual remodelling of the cervix enables progressive softening to take place while at the same time ensuring the cervix remains closed (Timmons et al 2010). The glands of the cervix undergo such marked hypertrophy and hyperplasia that by the end of pregnancy they occupy half of the entire cervical mass. They become everted so that the tissue tends to become red and velvety and bleeds even with minor trauma such as taking *Papanicolaou smears* (Pap test). The basal cells near the squamocolumnar junction are more prominent in shape and size due to oestrogen which renders the Pap smear less efficient (Cunningham et al 2010).

The endocervical mucosal cells produce copious amounts of a tenacious mucus which creates an antibacterial plug in the cervix. The consistency of the mucus changes during pregnancy under the influence of progesterone. When cervical mucus is spread and dried on a glass slide it is characterized by crystallization or *beading*. If there is leakage of amniotic fluid *ferning* may be visualized due to *arborization* (a branching, treelike arrangement) of the crystals (Cunningham et al 2010).

Taking up or *effacement* of the cervix is the shortening of the cervical canal from about 2 cm in length to a circular orifice with paper-thin edges. Muscle fibres at the level of the internal os are pulled upwards to become part of the lower uterine segment. This *funneling* process takes place from above downwards because there is less resistance in the lower uterine segment and cervix. The centrifugal pull on the cervix can be visualized on transvaginal sonography whereby the relationship of the cervical canal to the lower uterine segment changes from a T shape to the notched Y shape. With further effacement the uterine segment then becomes a V shape and ultimately a U shape (Iams 2010). In the primigravida effacement usually takes place prior to the commencement of labour but in the multigravida effacement may take place simultaneous with cervical dilatation (Cunningham et al 2010).

There is still no agreement about what constitutes a normal length of cervix, however a cervical length of less than 2.5 cm is strongly predictive of preterm birth regardless of gestational age. Differences in cervical length may be associated with race, maternal age, parity and past obstetric history (Slager and Lynne 2012).

The vagina

Increased blood flow to the vagina results in a bluish-purple coloration of the vagina known as *Chadwick's sign* (Geraghty and Pomeranz 2011). In preparation for the distension that occurs in labour, the vaginal walls undergo striking changes: the mucosa thickens, the connective tissue loosens and the smooth muscle cells hypertrophy. The increased volume of vaginal secretions due to high levels of oestrogen results in a thick, white discharge known as *leucorrhoea* (Cunningham et al 2010). The dominant vaginal flora is the *Lactobacillus acidophilus* (Doderlein's bacillus). During pregnancy the higher levels of oestrogen favour an increase in the activity and proliferation of the lactobacilli, a byproduct of which is lactic acid which leads to the increased vaginal acidity of pregnancy (pH varying from 3.5 to 6). This is particularly important in protecting women from genital tract infection in pregnancy which may lead to perinatal complications (Donati et al 2010).

CHANGES IN THE CARDIOVASCULAR SYSTEM

During pregnancy profound but predominantly reversible changes occur in maternal haemodynamics and cardiac function. These complex adaptations are necessary to:

- meet evolving maternal changes in physiological function

- promote the growth and development of the uteroplacental–fetal unit
- compensate for blood loss at the end of labour.

These physiological adaptations are extensive, with all components undergoing a degree of modification in pregnancy (Table 9.2). It is critical to achieve a balance between fetal requirements and maternal tolerance. In most women, these demands are effectively accommodated by physiological adaptations without compromising the mother.

Table 9.2 A summary of the key components of the cardiovascular system and adaptations in pregnancy

Component	Key change in pregnancy
The heart	Increases in size Shifted upwards and to left
Arteries	Dramatic systemic and pulmonary vasodilatation to increase blood flow
Capillaries	Increased permeability
Veins	Vasodilatation and impeded venous return in lower extremities
Blood	Haemodilution Increased capacity for clot formation

Adapted from Torgersen and Curran 2006

Anatomical changes in the heart and blood vessels

The heart is enlarged by chamber dilatation and a degree of myocardial hypertrophy in early pregnancy leading to a 10–15% increase in ventricular wall muscle (Monga 2009). The progressive blood volume expansion throughout pregnancy results in increased diastolic filling (particularly in the left ventricle) and progressive distension of the heart chambers. Despite cardiac enlargement, efficiency is maintained by lengthening of myocardial fibres and reduction in after load facilitated by peripheral vasodilatation. These structural changes in the heart mimic *exercise-induced cardiac remodelling* (Baggish and Wood 2011), which occurs in response to physical training, and, similarly, they are reversible after pregnancy.

The enlarging uterus raises the diaphragm, and the heart is correspondingly displaced upward and to the left to produce a slight anterior rotation of the heart on its long axis. This partially accounts for pregnancy variations in key parameters used for cardiac assessment, including electrocardiography (ECG) and radiographic assessments and can give an exaggerated impression of cardiac enlargement (Gordon 2012). Atrial or ventricular extrasystoles are relatively common in pregnancy along with increased

Table 9.3 Key physiological changes in the cardiovascular system in pregnancy

Parameter	Adaptation	Magnitude	Non-pregnant (average value)	Timing of peak/ average peak value
Oxygen consumption	Increase	20–30%	180 ml/min	Term
Total body water	Increase	6–8 l		Term
Plasma volume	Increase	45–50%	2600 ml	32–34 weeks; 3850 ml
Red cell mass	Increase	20–30%	1400 ml	Term 1650 ml
Total blood volume	Increase	30–50%	4000 ml	32 weeks; 5500 ml
Cardiac output	Increase	30–50%	4.9 l/min	28 weeks; 7 l/min
Stroke volume	Increase			20 weeks
Heart rate	Increase	10–20 bpm	75 bpm	Trimester 1; 90 bpm
Systemic vascular resistance	Decrease	21%	–	Trimester 2
Pulmonary vascular resistance	Decrease	35%	–	34 weeks
Diastolic blood pressure	Decrease, returning to normal by term	10–15 mmHg	–	24 weeks
Systolic blood pressure	Minimal, no decrease	5–10 mmHg	–	24 weeks
Serum colloid osmotic pressure	Decrease	10–15%	–	14 weeks

Sources: Nelson-Piercy 2009; Blackburn 2012

susceptibility to supraventricular tachycardia, however it is imperative that signs of severe disease such as angina or resting dyspnoea are not overlooked (Adamson et al 2011).

Within 5 weeks of conception changes in maternal blood vessels are evident, including an increase in aortic size and venous blood volume. Compliance of the entire vasculature is increased, partially due to the softening of the collagen and smooth muscle hypertrophy (Blackburn 2012). While influenced by progesterone, relaxin and endothelial-derived relaxant factors such as nitric oxide and prostacyclin, the exact mechanism underlying these changes is not yet fully understood.

Alongside these anatomical changes are complex physiological changes which are summarized in Table 9.3. They are accompanied by widespread peripheral vasodilatation resulting in the high flow, low resistance haemodynamic state with marked haemodilution characteristic of a healthy pregnancy.

Blood volume

The increase in total blood volume (TBV) is essential to:
- meet the demands of the enlarged uterus with a significantly hypertrophied vascular system and provide extra blood flow for placental perfusion
- supply extra metabolic needs of the fetus

- protect the woman (and fetus) against the harmful effects of impaired venous return
- provide extra perfusion of maternal organs
- counterbalance the effects of increased arterial and venous capacity
- safeguard against adverse effects of excessive maternal blood loss at birth.

The first step is extreme vasodilatation for which several possible explanations are suggested; the dramatically vasodilated, uteroplacental vasculature contributes to this change supported by evidence that fetal weight correlates directly with the rise in blood volume (Blackburn 2012). This only partially explains the reduced systemic vascular resistance, since a significant proportion of the decrease occurs outside the uteroplacental circulation. Increased vasodilatation is probably facilitated by a systemic and renal vasodilator unique to pregnancy. Current studies suggest that relaxin is also a key factor (Conrad 2011). Vasodilatation is partly mediated by rising pregnancy hormone levels, particularly progesterone and oestrogen. These hormones are associated with the stimulation of nitric oxide production and enhancement of endothelial function which induce the renin–angiotensin–aldosterone system (RAAS) and stimulates sodium and water retention (Monga 2009). The RAAS is important in fluid and electrolyte homeostasis and maintaining arterial blood pressure (Fig. 9.3). It has also been postulated that

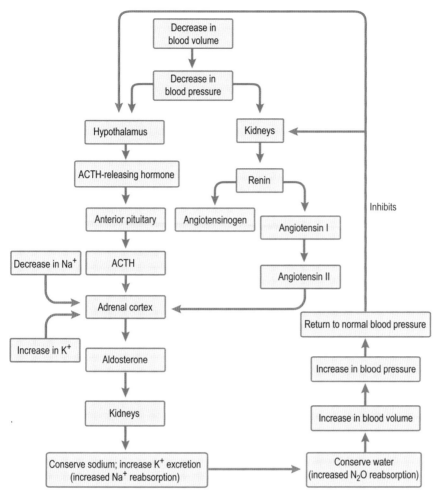

Fig. 9.3 The renin–angiotensin–aldosterone system (RAAS).
From Wallace W 2005 Endocrine function. In: Montague S, Watson R, Hubert R (eds) Physiology for nursing practice, 3rd edn. Elsevier, p 232, with permission of Elsevier.

hormonal factors and expansion of blood volume associated with pregnancy may affect sympathetic nervous activity, inhibiting both its vasoconstrictor effect and baroreflex control of heart rate (Fu and Levine 2009).

Vasodilatation causes an *underfilling* of the maternal circulation which subsequently initiates fluid and electrolyte retention, expansion of the plasma and extracellular fluid volumes and a concurrent increase in cardiac output. This occurs prior to full placentation and is accompanied by a parallel increase in renal blood flow and glomerular filtration rate. Fluid balance and osmoregulation are regulated through the modification of homeostatic mechanisms to accommodate and maintain these changes. There is a marked increase in all components of the RAAS leading to increased fluid and electrolyte retention. Oestrogen reduces the transcapillary escape rate of albumin, which promotes intravascular protein retention and shifts

extracellular fluid volume distribution while lowering the osmotic threshold for antidiuretic hormone (ADH) release. Levels of ADH appear to remain relatively stable despite heightened production, owing to a three- to four-fold increase in metabolic clearance as a consequence of the placental enzyme vasopressinase, which inactivates ADH and oxytocin.

Atrial natriuretic peptide (ANP) and brain natriuretic peptide (BNP) secreted in response to heart dilatation, raised end diastolic pressure and volume, have similar physiologic actions, both acting as antagonists to the RAAS. Gestational modifications of ANP and BNP are controversial and research has been unable to confirm when plasma levels are modified. Reported increases do not reach pathological levels associated with heart failure. Inconsistencies in study findings may be due to postural effects, namely aortocaval compression by the enlarged uterus on maternal haemodynamics (Gordon 2012) (see Box 9.1).

Cardiac output

The profound increase in cardiac output (30–50%) ensures blood flow to the brain and coronary arteries is maintained, while distribution to other organs is modified as pregnancy advances. Increased cardiac output is due to increases in stroke volume and heart rate. The relative contributions of these factors vary with gestational age. The increase in heart rate mainly occurs during the first trimester, thus contributing to early changes in cardiac output. Increases in stroke volume facilitate second trimester increases in cardiac output, augmented by plasma volume expansion. The stroke volume increases by 10% during the first half of pregnancy, reaching a peak at 20 weeks that is maintained until term (Nelson-Piercy 2009) (Fig. 9.4).

Cardiac output in pregnancy is extremely sensitive to changes in body position. This increases with advancing pregnancy, as the gravid uterus impinges on the inferior vena cava, thereby decreasing blood return to the heart (see Box 9.1). Large variations in cardiac output, pulse rate, blood pressure and regional blood flow may follow slight changes of posture, activity or anxiety.

Blood pressure and vascular resistance

While cardiac output is raised, arterial blood pressure is reduced by 10% in pregnancy. The decrease in systemic vascular resistance accounts for this, particularly in the peripheral vessels. The decrease begins at 5 weeks'

Box 9.1 **Supine hypotensive syndrome**

In later pregnancy (from 24 weeks) the gravid uterus occludes the inferior vena cava and laterally displaces the subrenal aorta, this is particularly so when the mother lies supine. This *aortocaval* compression has a profound effect on venous return to the heart.

Turning from a lateral to a supine position can reduce maternal cardiac output by 10–30% (Gordon 2012). The event is often concealed, because only 10% of pregnant women will exhibit supine hypotension syndrome (Bamber and Dresner 2003). The majority of women are able to compensate by raising systemic vascular resistance and heart rate. Blood from the lower limbs may also return through the development of paravertebral collateral circulation, however if these are not well developed or adequately perfused, the pregnant woman may experience *supine hypotensive syndrome*. This occurs in around 10% of the childbearing population and consists of *hypotension*, *bradycardia*, *dizziness*, *light-headedness* and *nausea*, if the woman remains in the supine position too long. The fall in blood pressure may be severe enough for the woman to lose consciousness due to reduced cerebral blood flow.

Pregnant women usually avoid lying supine, however they are often subjected to such a position during maternity care with technicians reporting unawareness of this condition (McMahon et al 2009).

The consequent aortocaval compression can be relieved by placing a wedge under the woman's hip or by tilting the operating table to displace the uterus. Compression of the aorta may lead to reduced uteroplacental and renal blood flow and fetal compromise.

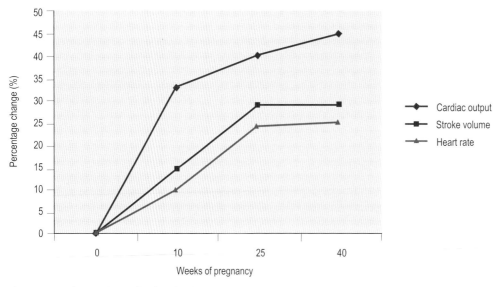

Fig. 9.4 Key changes in cardiac function in pregnancy.
Data from Cunningham et al 2010.

gestation, reaches a nadir in the second trimester (a 21% reduction) and then gradually rises as term approaches (Blackburn 2012). Numerous modifications occur in the mechanisms controlling vascular activity. Agents responsible for peripheral vasodilatation include prostacyclin, nitric oxide and progesterone and vasoactive prostaglandins. The changes are not limited to the uteroplacental circulation but are apparent throughout the body in a healthy pregnancy. Increased heat production further contributes to the reduced resistance, stimulating vasodilatation in heat loss areas particularly.

Early pregnancy is associated with a marked decrease in diastolic blood pressure but minimal reduction in systolic pressure. With reduced peripheral vascular resistance the systolic blood pressure decreases an average of 5–10 mmHg below baseline levels and the diastolic pressure reduces 10–15 mmHg by 24 weeks' gestation. Thereafter blood pressure gradually rises, returning to the pre-pregnant levels at term. Despite increased blood volume systemic venous pressures do not rise significantly. The exception to this is in the legs due to the gravid uterus impeding venous return.

Regional blood flow

As blood volume increases with gestation, a substantial proportion (10–20%) is distributed to the uteroplacental unit. Renal vasodilatation early in pregnancy initiated prior to implantation in the luteal phase (Gordon 2012) results in a dramatic increase in renal blood flow and glomerular filtration rate which facilitates efficient excretion.

As a percentage of total cardiac output blood flow to the brain, coronary arteries and liver is reduced, the overall increase in cardiac output compensates for this and the blood flow to these regions is not significantly changed. Pulmonary blood flow increases secondary to the increase in cardiac output, further facilitated by reduced pulmonary vascular resistance. Blood flow in the lower limbs decelerates in late pregnancy by compression of the iliac veins and inferior vena cava by the enlarging uterus and the hydrodynamic effects of increased venous return from the uterus. Reduced venous return and increased venous pressure in the legs contributes to the increased distensibility and pressure in the veins of the legs, vulva, rectum and pelvis, leading to dependent oedema, varicose veins of the legs, vulva and anus (see Box 9.2). These changes are more pronounced in the left leg due to compression of the left iliac vein by the overlying right iliac artery and the ovarian artery, accounting for 85% of venous thrombosis in pregnancy occurring in the left leg (Nelson-Piercy 2009).

A rise in temperature by 0.2–0.4 °C occurs as a result of the effects of progesterone and the increased basal metabolic rate (BMR). To eliminate the excess heat produced there is an increased blood flow to the capillaries of the

---

Box 9.2 **Varicosities**

Varicosities develop in approximately 40% of women, and are usually seen in the veins of the legs, but may also occur in the vulva and as haemorrhoids in the anal area.

The effects of progesterone and relaxin on the smooth muscles of the vein walls and the increased weight of the growing uterus all contribute to the increased risk of valvular incompetence. A family tendency is also a factor (Blackburn 2012).

Some suggestions for alleviating them include: spraying the legs with hot and cold water, resting with the legs elevated and wearing supportive stockings.

---

mucous membranes and skin, particularly in the hands and feet. This peripheral vasodilatation explains why pregnant women are often heat-intolerant: more prone to perspire, to nasal congestion and to nosebleeds.

Haematological changes

In parallel with the 30–45% increase in maternal blood volume, plasma volume increases by 50% (1250–1600 ml) over the course of the pregnancy (Monga 2009), followed by a relatively smaller increase in red blood cell volume (Table 9.4). These changes are responsible for the *hypervolaemia of pregnancy* leading to numerous modifications to parameters commonly assessed in blood tests (Table 9.5). Changes are detectable at 6–8 weeks. In pregnancy, plasma volume, placental mass and fetal birth weight positively correlate with these changes (Rasmussen and Yaktine 2009). Excessive increases in plasma volume have been associated with multiple pregnancy, prolonged pregnancy, maternal obesity and large for gestational age babies, while inadequate increases have been associated with pre-eclampsia.

Red cell mass (the total volume of red cells in circulation) increases during pregnancy by approximately 18% in response to increased levels of erythropoietin stimulated by maternal hormones (prolactin, progesterone, human placental lactogen and oestrogen) and oxygen requirements of maternal and placental tissue (Cunningham et al 2010). This homeostatic mechanism is discrete from that which controls fluid balance and increased plasma volume. Therefore, in spite of the increased production of red blood cells, the marked increase in plasma volume causes dilution of many circulating factors. As a result the red cell count, haematocrit and haemoglobin concentration all decrease, resulting in *apparent anaemia*, characteristic of a healthy pregnancy (Fig. 9.5). This trend reverses towards term as red cell mass continues to increase after 30 weeks when the plasma volume expansion has

Table 9.4 Key haematological changes in pregnancy

	Non-pregnant	Weeks of pregnancy		
		20	30	40
Plasma volume (ml)	2600	3150	3750	3850
Red cell mass (ml)	1400	1450	1550	1650
Total blood volume (ml)	4000	4600	5300	5500
Haematocrit (PCV) (%)	35–47	32.0	29.0	30.0
Haemoglobin (g/l)	115–165	110	105	110

Source: Llewellyn-Jones 2010

plateaued. The disproportionate increase in plasma volume is advantageous: i.e. by reducing blood viscosity, resistance to blood flow is reduced leading to improved placental perfusion and reduced maternal cardiac effort (Cunningham et al 2010).

Red blood cells become more spherical with increased diameter due to the fall in plasma colloid pressure encouraging more water to cross the erythrocyte cell membrane. Mean cell volume (MCV) also increases due to the higher proportion of young larger red blood cells (reticulocytes). The exact increase in red cell mass remains inconclusive, partly because assessments have been influenced by routine iron medication.

While total haemoglobin increases from 85 to 150 g the mean haemoglobin decreases. In healthy women with adequate iron stores this reduces by about 20 g/l from an average of 133 g/l in the non-pregnant state to 110 g/l in early pregnancy. It is at its lowest at around 32 weeks' gestation when plasma volume expansion is maximal, and after this time rises by approximately 5 g/l, returning to 110 g/l around the 36th week of pregnancy. A haemoglobin level below 105 g/l at 28 weeks should be investigated (National Institute for Health and Clinical Excellence [NICE] 2008) (see Chapter 13).

Iron metabolism

Iron requirements increase significantly in pregnancy, with estimates for the total iron requirements of pregnancy ranging from 500 to 1150 mg (Cao and O'Brien 2013). While there is an initial net saving from amenorrhoea, in late pregnancy iron requirements increase dramatically to 3–8 mg iron/day. About 500 mg are required to increase the maternal red blood cell mass, 300 mg are transported to the fetus, while the remaining 200 mg are utilized in compensating for insensible loss in skin, stool and urine. In spite of the moderate increase in iron absorption from the gut, woman require an iron-rich diet and have approximately 500 mg of stored iron prior to conception to accommodate the requirements of pregnancy. Since this amount is not available from body stores in most women, the red cell volume and haemoglobin level decrease with the rising plasma volume.

Many women conceive with insufficient iron reserves, but research to date has not fully established the benefits and drawbacks of iron supplementation or the optimal biomarkers for interpreting circulating iron status. In spite of this apparent imbalance, even with severe maternal iron deficiency anaemia, the placenta is able to provide sufficient iron from maternal serum for fetal production of haemoglobin. *Hepcidin* has recently been identified as a key hormone in the homeostasis of maternal, placental and fetal iron levels and studies have identified the differential metabolism of *haem* and *non-haem* sources in pregnancy (Young et al 2012). Furthermore the impact of neonatal iron status on long-term health is only recently being fully appreciated and warrants further study (Cao and O'Brien 2013).

Plasma protein

Haemodilution leads to a decrease in total serum protein content within the first trimester which remains reduced throughout pregnancy. Despite oestrogen reducing the transcapillary escape rate of albumin, concentration declines abruptly in early pregnancy and then more gradually (see Table 9.5). Albumin is important as a carrier protein for hormones, drugs, free fatty acids and unconjugated bilirubin, and its influence in decreasing colloid osmotic pressure. A 10–15% fall in colloid osmotic pressure allows water to move from the plasma into the cells or out of vessels, and plays a part in the increased fragility of red blood cells and oedema of the lower limbs (Nelson-Piercy 2009). It is now accepted that peripheral oedema in the lower limbs in late pregnancy is a feature of physiological, uncomplicated pregnancy.

Table 9.5 Normal values in pregnant/non-pregnant women

Test	Non-pregnant (typical range)	Pregnant (typical range)	Comments
Biochemistry			
Alanine transaminase (ALT) (U/L)	6–40	No change	Raised levels indicate liver damage
Alkaline phosphatase (IU/L)	40–120	Doubled by late pregnancy	Usually elevated in third trimester due to placental production of enzyme
Bile acids (total) (µmol/l)	<9		Values of total bile acids ≥14 µmol/l are viewed as abnormal, indicating cholestasis
Bilirubin (µmol/l)	<17		Little change in non-pregnant range
Creatinine (µmol/l)	50–100	75 approximately is upper limit of normal	Lower in mid-pregnancy but rises towards term
Potassium (mmol/l)	3.5–5.3	Unchanged	Unchanged in pregnancy
Albumin (g/l)	30–48	25–35	Total protein and albumin are both lower in pregnancy
Urea (mmol/l)	2–6.5	Usually ≤4.5	Lower in pregnancy
Uric acid (µmol/l)	150–350	Lowest values in second trimester, 10 × gestational age in weeks is approximately upper limit of normal	Increases with gestation, although lower levels than non-pregnant
Haematology			
Clotting time (min)	12	8	Observe for clotting or oozing from venepuncture sites in women of higher risk
Fibrin degradation products (µg/ml)	Mean 1.04	High values in third trimester and especially around time of birth	
Fibrinogen (g/l)	1.7–4.1	By term 2.9–6.2	Marked increase in pregnancy especially in third trimester and around time of birth
Haemotocrit (%)	35–47	31–35	Lower in pregnancy
Haemoglobin (g/l)	115–165	100–120 should be >100 in third trimester	Good iron stores needed to maintain pregnancy levels. Fall in first trimester whether or not iron and folate taken
Platelets (× 10^9/l)	150–400	Slight decrease in pregnancy lower limit of *normal* = 120	No functional significance
White cell count (× 10^9/l)	4.0–11.0	9.0–15.0; higher values up to 25.0 around time of birth	Normal increase in pregnancy Rise in infections

Source: Ramsay 2000

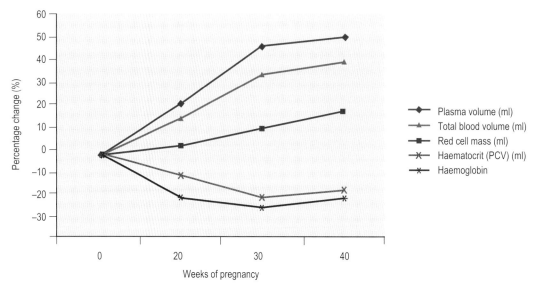

Fig. 9.5 Key haematological changes in pregnancy.
Data from Cunningham et al 2010.

Clotting factors

In pregnancy, adaptations occur in the coagulation system to protect the woman from peripartum haemorrhage while also maintaining the uteroplacental interface. The cumulative effect of these is commonly described as *the characteristic hypercoagulable state* of pregnancy. The increased tendency to clot is caused by increases in clotting factors and fibrinogen accompanied by reduced plasma fibrinolytic activity and an increase in circulating fibrin degradation products in the plasma. Due to these changes pregnant women have a five-to six-fold increased risk for thromboembolic disease (Gordon 2012).

From 12 weeks' gestation there is a 50% increase in synthesis of plasma fibrinogen concentration (Factor I) rising to 200% pre-pregnancy levels at term (Thornton and Douglas 2010). This is critical for the prevention of haemorrhage at the time of placental separation. The development of a fibrin mesh to cover the placental site to control the bleeding requires 5–10% of all the circulating fibrinogen. When this process is impaired, for example by inadequate uterine action or incomplete placental separation, compounded by placental blood flow of up to 700 ml/min at term, there is rapid depletion of fibrinogen reserves, putting the woman at risk of haemorrhage.

Coagulation factors VII, VIII and X increase in pregnancy, while factors II (*prothrombin*) and V remain constant or show a slight fall. Both the prothrombin time (normal 10–14 secs) and the partial thromboplastin time (normal 35–45 secs) are slightly shortened as pregnancy advances. The clotting times of whole blood, however, are not significantly different in pregnancy to non-pregnant values. The platelet count declines slightly as pregnancy advances, which is explained by haemodilution and increased consumption in the uteroplacental circulation. The increased production of platelets results in a slight increase in mean platelet volume (MPV), which is due to immature platelets being larger than old ones resulting in an overall increase in average size. Substantial increases in MCV could indicate excessive platelet consumption and is often used as a marker for hypertensive disease.

A decrease in some endogenous anticoagulants (antithrombin, protein S and activated protein C resistance) occur in pregnancy along with the physiological vasodilatation of pregnancy, this contributes to a six-fold increase in the risk of thromboembolism in pregnancy (Nelson-Piercy 2009).

White blood cells (leucocytes) and immune function

Pregnancy presents a paradox for the woman's immune system as the mechanisms that are essential to protect her from infection have the potential to destroy the genetically disparate conceptus. It is clear that the immunological relationship between the mother and the fetus involves a two-way communication involving fetal antigen presentation and maternal recognition of and reaction to these antigens by the immune system (Chen et al 2012). There is evidence that progesterone plays a major role in the immunological tolerance seen in pregnancy.

The total white cell count rises from 8 weeks' gestation and reaches a peak at 30 weeks. This is mainly because of the increase in numbers of neutrophil polymorphonuclear leucocytes, monocytes and granulocytes, the latter two producing a far more active and efficient phagocytosis function. This enhances the blood's phagocytic and bactericidal properties. Numbers of eosinophils, basophils, monocytes, lymphocytes and circulating T cells and B cells remain relatively constant. Lymphocyte function is depressed, and natural killer cytokine activity is reduced regulated by progesterone, particularly in the latter stages of pregnancy. Chemotaxis is suppressed resulting in a delayed response to some infections. There is decreased resistance to viral infections such as herpes, influenza, rubella, hepatitis, poliomyelitis and malaria. The metabolic activity of granulocytes increases during pregnancy, possibly resulting from the stimulation of rising oestrogen and cortisol levels (Gordon 2012).

The maternal immune response is biased toward an enhancement of innate (*humoral*) immunity and away from cell-mediated response that could be harmful to the fetus. The stimulus for these changes is predominantly hormonal involving progesterone, human placental lactogen (hPL), prostaglandins, corticosteroids, human chorionic gonadotrophin (hCG), prolactin and serum proteins.

CHANGES IN THE RESPIRATORY SYSTEM

To accommodate increased oxygen requirements and the physical impact of the enlarging uterus intricate changes occur in respiratory physiology. These are mediated by an interaction of hormonal, biochemical and mechanical factors and are summarized in Table 9.6. Progressive increases in maternal and fetal metabolic demands are reflected in a marked increase in resting oxygen consumption reaching a 20–30% peak from non-pregnant values at term.

The driving force for change is the respiratory stimulatory effect of progesterone initiating hyperventilation by increasing sensitivity to carbon dioxide through lowering the threshold at which the respiratory centre is stimulated (Jensen et al 2009). Overcompensation to respiratory demand causes arterial oxygen tension to increase and arterial carbon dioxide tension to decrease, accompanied by a compensatory decline in serum bicarbonate; mild

Table 9.6 Summary of changes in respiratory function				
Parameter	Adaptation	Magnitude (%)	Non-pregnant (average value)	Timing of peak/ average peak value
Oxygen consumption	Increase	18	250 ml/min	300 ml/min
Metabolic rate	Increase	15		Peaks at term with increases up to eight-fold reported (Blackburn 2012)
Minute volume: amount of air/minute moved into and out of the lungs	Increase	40	7.5 l/min	Peaks at term; 10.5 l/min
Tidal volume: amount of air inspired and expired with normal breath	Increase	40	500 ml	700 ml
Vital capacity: maximum amount of air that can be forcibly expired after maximum inspiration	No change	–	3200 ml	3200 ml
Functional residual capacity: amount of air in lungs at resting expiratory level	Decrease	20	1700 ml	1350 ml
Blood gas analysis:				
Arterial oxygen tension (PaO_2).	Increase		95–100 mmHg	Peak end trimester 1; 106–8 mmHg
Arterial carbon dioxide tension ($PaCO_2$)	Decrease		35–40 mmHg	27–32 mmHg
Serum bicarbonate	Decrease			18–22 mmol/l
Arterial Ph	Small increase			7.44 (a mild respiratory alkalosis)
Source: Nelson-Piercy 2009				

Box 9.3 Breathlessness

The respiratory changes can be extremely uncomfortable and may lead to dyspnoea, dizziness and altered exercise tolerance. Up to 75% of pregnant women with no underlying pre-existing respiratory disease experience some dyspnoea, possibly due to an increased awareness of the physiological hyperventilation (Nelson-Piercy 2009). This physiological dyspnoea often occurs early in pregnancy and does not interfere with daily activities and usually diminishes as term approaches.

Although mechanical impediment by the uterus is often blamed, hyperventilation is due to altered sensitivity to CO_2. Although it is not usually associated with pathological processes, care must be taken not to dismiss this lightly and miss a warning sign of cardiac or pulmonary disease (Hegewald and Crapo 2011).

Breathlessness can be alleviated by maintaining an upright posture and holding hands above the head while taking deep breaths. Women may need to modify their physical activity levels to accommodate these symptoms, however studies have shown that exercising in pregnancy can help to alleviate them (Lewis et al 2010).

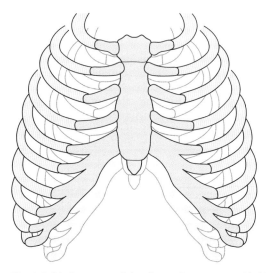

Fig. 9.6 Displacement of the ribcage in pregnancy (dark) and the non-pregnancy state (light) showing elevated diaphragm, the increased transverse diameter and circumference, flaring out of ribs and the increased subcostal angle.
From de Swiet M 1998 The respiratory system. In: Chamberlain G, Broughton Pipkin F (eds) Clinical physiology in obstetrics, 3rd edn. Blackwell Science, Oxford, p 115, with permission from Wiley Publishing Ltd.

respiratory alkalosis is consequently physiologically normal in pregnancy (Bobrowski 2010) (see Box 9.3).

From early pregnancy, the overall shape of the chest alters as the anteroposterior and transverse diameters increase by about 2 cm resulting in a 5–7 cm expansion of the chest circumference. The lower ribs flare outwards prior to any mechanical pressure from the growing uterus. This progressively increases the subcostal angle, from 68° in early pregnancy to 103° at term (Fig. 9.6). Although the expanding uterus causes the diaphragm to rise by up to 4 cm above its usual resting position, diaphragmatic movement during respiration is not impaired as chest wall mobility increases and lower ribs flare, increasing the thoracic space. Changes are mediated by progesterone and relaxin which increase ribcage elasticity by relaxing ligaments in a similar mechanism to that occurring in the pelvis. Inspiratory and expiratory maximum pressures appear to remain stable throughout pregnancy. Lemos et al (2010) have suggested that the stretching of the muscles involved in ventilating the lungs is accompanied by the significant addition of *sarcomeres* (the basic unit of a muscle), thereby maintaining muscle strength. Progesterone also facilitates bronchial and tracheal smooth muscle relaxation, thereby reducing airway resistance. This improves air flow and explains why the health of women with existing respiratory problems rarely deteriorates in pregnancy.

Expansion of the rib cage causes the *tidal volume* to increase by 30–40% gradually rising from approximately 8 weeks' gestation to term (Jensen et al 2009). Studies report that the normal respiratory rate of 14–15 breaths/

min may demonstrate minimal increase in pregnancy, though pregnant women do breathe more deeply, even at rest. The *minute volume* that facilitates gas exchange is increased by 30–40%, from 7.5–10.5 l/min, and minute oxygen uptake increases appreciably as pregnancy advances (Cunningham et al 2010). The enhanced tidal volume contributes to an increase in inspiratory capacity while *vital capacity* is unchanged. As a result, the *functional residual capacity* is decreased by 20%. This reduces the amount of used gas mixing with each new inspiration thereby enhancing alveolar gas exchange by 50–70%. While making ventilation more efficient this may result in rapid falls in arterial oxygen tension even with short periods of apnoea which is further compounded by the reduced buffering capacity. Whether from obstruction of the airway or inhalation of a hypoxic mixture of gas the consequence of these adaptations is that pregnant women have less reserve if they become hypoxic.

Blood volume expansion and vasodilatation of pregnancy result in hyperaemia and oedema of the upper respiratory mucosa, which predispose the pregnant woman to nasal congestion, epistaxis and even changes in voice. The changes to the upper respiratory tract may lead to upper airway obstruction and bleeding making both mask anaesthesia and tracheal intubation more difficult. These can be further exacerbated by fluid overload or oedema associated with pregnancy-induced hypertension or pre-eclampsia.

Blood gases

Changes in respiratory function result in a state of compensated respiratory alkalosis. Arterial oxygen partial pressure (PaO_2) is slightly increased from non-pregnant values (98–100 mmHg) to pregnant values of (101–104 mmHg). In addition, the *hyperventilation of pregnancy* causes a 15–20% decrease in maternal arterial carbon dioxide partial pressure ($PaCO_2$) from an average of 35–40 mmHg in the non-pregnant woman to 30 mmHg or lower in late pregnancy. Because fetal $PaCO_2$ is 44 mmHg these changes not only safeguard adequate oxygenation but also maintain an exaggerated carbon dioxide gradient from fetus to mother. This facilitates the transfer of CO_2 from the fetus to the mother and the subsequent expiration of CO_2 from the maternal lungs. It is important that clinicians consider these changes when undertaking assessment of maternal blood gases. A $PaCO_2$ of 35–40 mmHg which might ordinarily be considered borderline low is markedly abnormal in a pregnant woman and can even represent impending respiratory failure (Nelson-Piercy 2009).

The body has a considerable capacity for storing carbon dioxide in blood, largely as bicarbonate. To compensate, renal excretion of bicarbonate is significantly increased which may limit the buffering capacity in pregnancy. The fall in $PaCO_2$ is matched by an equivalent fall in plasma bicarbonate concentration. Although maternal arterial pH changes very little, the resulting mild *alkalaemia* (arterial pH 7.40–7.45) further facilitates oxygen release to the fetus.

CHANGES IN THE CENTRAL NERVOUS SYSTEM

Adaptations of the central nervous system (CNS) are probably the least well understood compared to other body systems. The adaptive changes encompass diverse scientific disciplines, including neuroendocrinology, neuroscience, physiology and psychology such that failure of adaptation can lead to disorders that have profound and long lasting consequences for the woman. Russell et al (2001) affirm that the hormonal fluctuations occurring throughout pregnancy may remodel the female brain, increasing the size of neurones in some regions and producing structural changes in others. These manifest in various ways, e.g. the substantial increase in size and activity of the pituitary gland by 30–50%.

Adaptations in neural circuitry in the maternal brain are initiated by pregnancy hormones. Oestrogen and progesterone readily enter the brain to act on nerve cells changing the balance between inhibition and stimulation. Other pregnancy hormones, such as relaxin, prolactin and lactogen, also have an impact. Progression of pregnancy is signalled to the brain by the pattern of secretion of these

Box 9.4 **Sleep disturbances**

Various hormonal and mechanical influences promote insomnia leading to disturbed sleep during pregnancy, i.e. sleep fragmentation with greater amounts of light sleep and fewer periods of deep sleep. These disturbances tend to worsen as pregnancy advances, with up to 90% of women reporting frequent night awakenings (Wilson et al 2011) that for some continue postpartum. As a consequence, sleep disturbance has been associated with increased labour length and caesarean section rates and may also contribute to the tendency for some women becoming depressed postpartum compared to other periods in their life (Goyal et al 2007).

Interventions include establishing sleep–wake habits, avoiding caffeine, relaxation techniques, massage, heat and support for lower back pain, modifying sleep environment, limiting fluids in the evening and avoiding passive smoking. Sleep medications should be avoided, although psycho-educational interventions are being explored as a potentially affective alternative (Kempler Sharp et al 2012).

hormones culminating in a complex interplay of communications between the mother and fetoplacental unit.

Up to 80% of pregnant women report symptoms of 'baby brain'. There is growing evidence that fetal microchimeric cells participate in the maternal response to injury. Although it is known that hormonal changes during pregnancy can affect neurogenesis, there is no substantive evidence that pregnancy itself influences certain areas in the brain into being more receptive for fetal cells. Consequently, Tan et al (2011) suggest that further studies are required to determine whether there is any biological significance to this.

A pregnant woman's sleep pattern can be affected by both mechanical and hormonal influences. These include nocturia, dyspnoea, nasal congestion, stress and anxiety as well as muscular aches and pains, leg cramps and fetal activity (see Box 9.4).

CHANGES IN THE URINARY SYSTEM

The striking anatomical and physiological changes occurring in the urinary system are critical for an optimal pregnancy outcome. Systemic vasodilatation in the first trimester and an increase in blood volume and cardiac output results in a massive vasodilatation of the renal circulation that increases the renal plasma flow (RPF) (Baidya et al 2012). According to Pipkin (2012), there is an 85% increase in RPF above non-pregnant values after

6 weeks' gestation; this falls in the second trimester to about 65%.

In a healthy pregnancy the kidneys lengthen by up to 1.5 cm and kidney volume increases by as much as 30% (Abduljalil et al 2012). Growth is less in the right kidney due to its proximity to the liver and greater in the left kidney due to increased blood supply via the shorter left renal artery (Ugboma et al 2012). Dilatation of the renal pelvis and ureters (*hydronephrosis of pregnancy*) with reduced peristalsis starts as early as 7 weeks' gestation, peaks at between 22 and 26 weeks and by the third trimester is marked in approximately 90% of women. It is due to relaxation of the smooth muscle of the urinary collecting system under the influence of progesterone (Pepe and Pepe 2013). Hydronephrosis is usually only present above the pelvic brim due to compression and lateral displacement of the ureters after the uterus rises out of the pelvis. Dilatation is asymmetric, being greater on the right side due to dextrorotation of the uterus and dilatation of the right ovarian vein complex, and less on the left side due to the cushioning effect of the sigmoid colon. The ureters also become longer and are thrown into single or double curves of various sizes (Cunningham et al 2010).

Dilated ureters with reduced peristalsis and mechanical obstruction by the enlarged uterus all contribute to urinary stasis leading to the increased risk of urinary tract infection in pregnancy. More than 200 ml of urine can collect in the ureters serving as an excellent reservoir for pathogenic bacteria (Ansari and Rajkumari 2011) (Fig. 9.7) (see Chapter 13). Other factors that increase the potential for colonization and susceptibility for ascending infection are alkaline urine, increased bladder volume, reduced detrusor tone, vesico-ureteric reflux and dysfunctional ureteric valves. Glucose excretion in the urine which increases in pregnancy 100-fold due to the increased glomerular filtration rate (GFR) also provides an excellent medium for bacterial proliferation (see Box 9.5).

Significant anatomical changes also occur in the bladder. The blood vessels in the mucosa increase in size and become more tortuous. After 12 weeks' gestation the bladder trigone is elevated causing thickening of the posterior margin due to the increased uterine size, hyperaemia of all pelvic organs and hyperplasia of the bladder muscle and connective tissues. The trigone becomes deeper and wider as pregnancy progresses leading to reduced bladder capacity. To compensate for this the urethra lengthens by about 0.5 cm and the bladder tone increases to help maintain continence (Cunningham et al 2010). In spite of this, urinary incontinence can be troublesome in pregnancy (see Box 9.6).

As the uterus enlarges the bladder becomes distorted and is drawn upwards anteriorly, becoming an abdominal

---

Box 9.5 **Asymptomatic bacteriuria**

Asymptomatic bacteriuria is defined as the presence of more than 100 000 organisms per ml in two consecutive urine samples in the absence of declared symptoms. It occurs in 2–10% of the pregnant population.

If not treated, up to 20% of women will develop a lower urinary tract infection (UTI) and the condition will develop into pyelonephritis in 30% of pregnant women if not properly treated (Asali et al 2012; Law and Fiadjoe 2012).

It is usually caused by *Escherichia coli* (*E. coli*) and has been associated with adverse pregnancy outcomes such as preterm birth, miscarriage and pregnancy-induced hypertension.

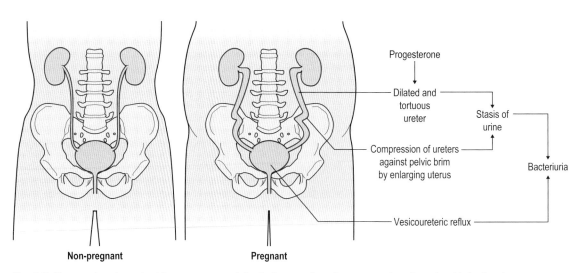

Fig. 9.7 Changes in urinary tract in pregnancy and the factors predisposing women to urinary tract infection in pregnancy.

organ by the third trimester (Fiadjoe et al 2010). When engagement of the head takes place in the primigravida the base of the bladder is pushed forward and upward converting the normal convex surface into a concavity that complicates diagnostic tests. The pressure of the presenting part impairs drainage of blood and lymph from the bladder base causing oedema and greater susceptibility to trauma and infection (Cunningham et al 2010).

As a result of renal vasodilatation and increased RPF, the GFR increases by 25% by the second week after conception and by 45% by the 9th week, only rising thereafter by another 5–10%, from which it remains elevated until term. The filtered load of metabolites increases markedly and tubular reabsorption is unable to compensate. This has a profound effect on the concentration of certain plasma metabolites (Pipkin 2012).

Creatinine clearance, which measures glomerular filtration, is one of the main physiological parameters of renal function (Abduljalil et al 2012). It increases significantly by 4 weeks, peaks at 9–11 weeks and then is sustained until the 36th week of gestation after which it reduces by 15–20%. As renal clearance of creatinine and urea increases plasma levels decrease from 70 µmol/l and 5 µmol/l respectively in the non-pregnant woman to mean values of 50 µmol/l and 3 µmol/l before rising again near term. Due to the increased GFR there is also increased uric acid clearance. As tubular reabsorption of uric acid is decreased, serum uric acid concentration falls by about 25% in early pregnancy but during the second half of pregnancy it rises again as the kidney excretes a progressively smaller proportion of filtered uric acid. Thus *normal* laboratory reference ranges may reflect renal impairment in a pregnancy (Pipkin 2012).

Due to the changes in glomerular permeability and altered tubular reabsorption proteinuria is common in pregnancy, with increases of 300 mg per day being considered normal (Baidya et al 2012). Urinary calcium excretion is also two to three times higher in pregnancy even though tubular reabsorption is enhanced. To counter this, intestinal absorption doubles by week 24, after which it stabilizes. Although there is an increased filtration of potassium in pregnancy, Pipkin (2012) purports that it is reabsorbed effectively in the renal tubules.

The increased GFR also causes an increased filtration of glucose. Tubular capacity to reabsorb glucose is decreased, resulting in a 10-fold increase in glucose excretion (Baidya et al 2012). As a consequence, glycosuria can be detected in around 50% of pregnant women. Clinicians should be aware that although glycosuria may be common in pregnancy, it should not be overlooked as some women may have diabetes mellitus (Cunningham et al 2010).

By day an increased urinary output leads to frequency and urgency of micturition affecting 81% of women by the third trimester. The accumulation of oedema in the lower extremities by day is reabsorbed more quickly at night, particularly in the lateral recumbent position, resulting in increased diuresis at night with more dilute urine by the third trimester in up to 66% of pregnant women.

CHANGES IN THE GASTROINTESTINAL SYSTEM

Anatomical and physiological changes take place in each organ of the gastrointestinal system. Influenced by oestrogen and progesterone the gums become highly vascularized, oedematous, have less resistance to infection and are more easily irritated. Bleeding and tender gums are commonly reported by women in pregnancy and can be a sign of periodontal disease. Minor trauma or inflammation occurring in the presence of bacterial plaque can lead to gingivitis. This can develop into a localized hyperplasia known as *pyogenic granuloma* or *pregnancy epulis*, a benign vascular lesion of the skin and mucosa occurring in up to 10% of pregnant women (Saravanan et al 2012). Such a lesion is purplish-red to pink in colour and is a reactive inflammatory mass of loose granulation tissue rich in capillary vessels, endothelial and inflammatory cells situated between the upper maxillary teeth. It is usually painless but may ulcerate due to trauma and become painful. Although the lesion normally regresses postpartum, it may recur in the same place in subsequent pregnancies. In a minority of cases, surgical excision may be required.

Peridontal infections occur more frequently in women who smoke or who have diabetes. Whether suppurative and painful or silent they will lead to loss of bone support for the teeth (Saravanan et al 2012). Although there is little evidence that dental caries increases more rapidly during pregnancy, good oral and dental hygiene consisting of brushing and flossing during pregnancy is essential for the overall health of mother and baby (Kloetzel et al 2011; Kumar et al 2013). The fetus draws the calcium required from the maternal skeleton rather than the

Box 9.7 **Ptyalism**

Ptyalism is the excessive production of saliva throughout pregnancy. Its cause is unknown but progesterone and/or hCG may be responsible for the increased viscosity which reduces with advancing gestation. Gastric acid is also thought to affect the volume of saliva.

Ptyalism causes a bad taste in the mouth and women complain that swallowing the excessive or thickened saliva perpetuates a sense of nausea and that they need to spit it out. Ptyalism may either diminish during sleep or cause the woman to waken more frequently at night. If associated with *hyperemesis gravidarum* it may continue until term.

Central nervous system depressants (e.g. barbiturates), anticholinergics (e.g. belladonna alkaloid), or phosphorylated carbohydrate have been recommended to improve the woman's distress. Using gum or ice are temporary coping strategies the woman can use. Although ptyalism has not previously been considered a serious condition, it has recently been postulated that it may lead to adverse perinatal outcomes (Suzuki and Fuse 2013).

Box 9.8 **Nausea and vomiting**

Nausea and vomiting (*morning sickness*) has varying levels of severity and has far-reaching effects for some women in terms of ability to carry out day-to-day tasks, care for children and take part in full-time employment.

Symptoms usually begin in the 4th week of pregnancy with a marked increase between 5 and 10 weeks when hCG levels are at their highest, followed by a steady decline until 20 weeks (Jarvis and Nelson-Piercy 2011).

Nausea and vomiting is associated with enlarged placental size with increased amounts of hCG that occurs in the female fetus, multiple pregnancy or hydatidiform mole. It is more prevalent in younger women, multigravida, multiple pregnancies, alcohol use during pregnancy (Naumann et al 2012) or those with eating disorders. However, it has been suggested that nausea and vomiting is a protective mechanism against the ingestion of harmful substances.

The possible causes are varied and include: genetic, cultural, endocrine, environmental and psychosocial factors as well as reduced gastric oesophageal pressure and delayed gastric emptying due to the effects of progesterone (Jarvis and Nelson-Piercy 2011).

Pregnancies complicated by nausea and vomiting are less likely to result in miscarriage (Jarvis and Nelson-Piercy 2011). It does not appear to adversely affect the fetus and no significant difference has been found in birthweight, gestational age, or premature birth (Naumann et al 2012). There is currently limited evidence in the form of RCTs to demonstrate the effectiveness of various treatments which makes it difficult for professionals to offer clear guidance (Matthews et al 2010). Women should, however, be advised of the lower level evidence demonstrating considerable relief of nausea and vomiting with vitamin B6 (Koren et al 2011).

systemic circulation. It is the increased acidity of the saliva in pregnancy which predisposes temporarily to dental caries and erosion (see Box 9.7). A more acidic oral environment develops as a result of dietary changes, the urge to snack frequently, increased consumption of carbohydrates, substance misuse, poor oral hygiene and an increase in the frequency of vomiting. The higher incidence of untreated decay and teeth extraction in the grand multigravida may relate more to socio-behavioural causes rather than biological (Russell et al 2010). It is recommended by Detman et al (2010) that improved oral health education is required to remove persisting misconceptions about dental care in pregnancy.

Upper gastrointestinal symptoms complicate the majority of pregnancies, with most women complaining of either heartburn, nausea and vomiting of pregnancy or both. Nausea and vomiting of pregnancy is experienced by 70–85% of pregnant women and many feel that their distressing symptoms are trivialized (Naumann et al 2012) (see Box 9.8).

A cascade of complex interacting factors, including hormones, is thought to influence the hypothalamic control of food and the pregnancy-induced increase in appetite. However, women often eat significantly more than is required. Riley (2011) affirms that excessive weight gain is associated with higher fetal birthweights and postpartum weight retention.

Oral and olfactory cravings and aversions in pregnancy are well documented but much of the data is conflicting, making conclusions about their cause difficult. Cravings and aversions vary between high- and low-income countries. Common cravings are fruit, strongly flavoured or savoury food, liquorice, potato crisps, cheese and milk. Common aversions are tea and coffee, fried foods, eggs and sweet foods later in pregnancy (Patil and Young 2012). Investigation into cravings and aversions is required since there is increasing evidence that some micronutrients in early pregnancy can influence postnatal development of obesity and chronic diseases (Weigel et al 2011). *Pica*, which describes persistent eating of non-food substances such as earth, chalk or soap, occurs frequently in pregnancy but should not be diagnosed unless it is of unusual extent or causes health concerns (see Box 9.9).

The increased abdominal pressure due to the enlarging uterus causes a shift in pressure gradient between the abdomen and the thorax (Bredenoord et al 2013). The angle of the gastro-oesophageal junction is altered and the lower oesophageal sphincter is displaced into the negative

Box 9.9 **Pica**

Pica is the persistent craving and compulsive consumption of substances such as ice, clay, soap, coal or starch. It has been reported to be as high as 74% in Kenya but as low as 0.02% in Denmark.

The consequences for mother and baby remain unknown (López et al 2012). However, if lead enters the bloodstream due to pica in pregnancy following previous exposure, the elevated maternal lead levels are associated with significant risks for mother and baby. Immigrant women are at particular risk of this and they should therefore be screened antenatally for potential prior exposure to lead in their country of origin (Alba et al 2012).

Box 9.10 **Heartburn**

Up to 85% of pregnant women experience heartburn in pregnancy. Troublesome symptoms of retrosternal and epigastric pain, regurgitation and acid taste in the mouth can all affect the woman's quality of life. Increasing gestational age, heartburn before pregnancy and multiparity may also predispose women to gastro-oesophageal reflux in pregnancy which usually resolves after the birth of the baby (Katz et al 2013).

In most pregnant women reflux symptoms can be managed by lifestyle modifications such as small frequent meals, not eating or drinking late at night, sleeping semi-recumbent or on the left side, avoiding food and medication causing reflux, chewing gum and abstinence from alcohol and tobacco.

Intermittent use of *antacids* such as Gaviscon® (Reckitt Benckiser), metoclopramide, sucralfate and H_2 *receptor blockers* (ranitidine) are all safe to use in pregnancy (Cuckson and Germain 2011). For women with severe symptoms, a *proton pump inhibitor (PPI)* such as omeprazole should be the treatment of choice as it is the most effective, with no safety concerns for the fetus.

pressure of the intrathoracic cavity. These mechanical changes, along with the relaxing effects of progesterone which reduces gastrointestinal transit, all contribute to the reflux of gastric contents into the lower oesophagus leading to *heartburn* (Naumann et al 2012) (see Box 9.10).

Gastric acid production is reduced in pregnancy secondary to increased levels of progesterone. The gastric pH and volume in pregnant and non-pregnant women show no differences in the proportion of women meeting *at risk* criteria (pH <2.5, volume >25 ml) for pulmonary aspiration of gastric contents. In addition, studies using serial gastric ultrasound examinations have demonstrated no change in gastric emptying in healthy pregnant women throughout *all trimesters* compared with non-pregnant women (Abduljalil et al 2012). The risk of aspiration in pregnant women, however, is still increased because of the reduced pressure at the lower oesophageal sphincter (Reitman and Flood 2011).

Progesterone combined with the pressure of the gravid uterus on the rectosigmoid colon decreases motility of the small intestine and colon and increases transit time in the second and third trimesters. This leads to frequent complaints of bloating and abdominal distension (see Box 9.11), constipation and haemorrhoids (see Box 9.12).

Identifying the position of the appendix in the later stages of pregnancy can be challenging due to anatomical alterations. The enlarging uterus displaces the appendix and caecum superiorly to the level of the liver and laterally to the right upper quadrant of the abdomen. The tip of the appendix may be close to the right flank in late second trimester and consequently localizing the pain of appendicitis can be difficult. As Wild et al (2013) conclude, clinicians should be mindful that the gravid uterus often leads to atypical presentations of appendicitis in pregnancy.

The gall bladder enlarges in pregnancy and emptying is slower due to reduced motility. This promotes bile stasis and increased concentrated bile content which can predispose to physiological cholestasis and pruritis (Abduljalil

Box 9.11 **Abdominal distension**

Abdominal distension and a bloated feeling occur when nutrients and fluids remain in the intestinal tract for longer, particularly in the third trimester due to prolonged transit time. Increased flatulence may also occur due to decreased motility and pressure of the uterus on the bowel (Blackburn 2012). The increased sodium and water absorption secondary to the increased aldosterone levels during pregnancy leads to reduced stool volume and further prolonged colonic transit time. The functional changes that occur with the enlarging uterus may mechanically limit colonic emptying, which is probably the main reason for constipation in late pregnancy.

et al 2012; Pipkin 2012). The large residual volume of bile is more saturated with cholesterol resulting in the retention of cholesterol crystals and increased risk of gallstone formation, particularly in the multigravida (Cuckson and Germain 2011).

Liver size is unchanged but by the third trimester it is forced into a more superior posterior position to the right (Joshi et al 2010). Increased hepatic perfusion after 26 weeks' gestation is due to the increase in portal venous return (Abduljalil et al 2012). Reference ranges for many liver function tests are altered and would be considered abnormal in the non-pregnant woman. Serum albumin

Constipation affects up to 40% of pregnant women, further exacerbated by factors such as dehydration, poor dietary intake, opiate analgesia and iron supplements. Treatment consists of non-pharmacological measures such as increased fluid intake and dietary fibre and temporary cessation of oral iron (Cuckson and Germain 2011).

There are no definitive guidelines on laxative prescribing in pregnancy, but the British National Formulary (2013) suggests that if dietary and lifestyle measures fail, bulk-forming laxatives should be prescribed first, then an osmotic laxative such as lactulose or macrogols (polyethylene glycols), followed by a stimulant such as senna if required.

Constipation indirectly predisposes to the development of haemorrhoids, which occur in up to 85% of women in late pregnancy. Haemorrhoids are varicosities of the anal and perianal venous plexus. They are caused by the rise in intra-abdominal pressure and restriction of venous return in the lower extremities and pelvis due to the enlarging uterus and the resulting venous stasis, stagnation of blood and arteriovenous shunting in the compressed rectal veins.

Pregnancy may be the first time that haemorrhoids become symptomatic, presenting with pain, bleeding and irritation. For many women symptoms will resolve soon after the birth but for others it may become worse. Treatment consists of the correction of constipation and the application of topically applied local anaesthetic, anti-inflammatory or emollient creams and suppositories. In more severe cases oral flavonoids or phlebotonics may be beneficial for strengthening and improving the tone of blood vessel walls. Occasionally surgery may be required (Avsar and Keskin 2010; Perera et al 2012).

concentration falls due to plasma volume expansion. Gestation-specific alkaline phosphatase rises due to increased placental secretion, while aminotransferase and gamma-glutamyl transaminase are reduced (Cuckson and Germain 2011) (see Table 9.5).

CHANGES IN METABOLISM

A well-integrated metabolic shift is required by the woman to provide for the increased physiological demands of pregnancy, labour and lactation, increased BMR, increased cost of physical activity, and to ensure provision of adequate nutrients critical for maintaining a healthy, viable and optimally growing fetus (Hadden and McLaughlin 2009). These adaptations are orchestrated within a few weeks of conception by oestrogen and progesterone originating from the fetoplacental unit and by prolactin and hPL from the maternal pituitary gland (Freemark 2010) (see Chapter 6). Energy metabolism changes during the course of pregnancy, differs considerably between women and is influenced by body mass index (BMI), maternal age, stage of gestation, BMR and level of physical activity (Blumfield et al 2012). In order to give appropriate advice on diet and nutrition, clinicians should be aware of the religious teachings and eating habits of immigrant women, particularly those from the Indian subcontinent where pregnant Muslim women are expected to observe total fasting during Ramadam. Estimates of energy costs range from 80 000 kcal to an actual saving of 10 000 kcal in different parts of the world (Hadden and McLaughlin 2009). With less physical activity occurring in pregnancy, women should not *eat for two*. The Scientific Advisory Committee on Nutrition (SACN) (2012) recommends that a daily increase of 191 kcal should be sufficient for most women during the last trimester of pregnancy.

The BMR increases during pregnancy because of the increased mass of metabolically active tissues as well as new tissue synthesis which leads to increased oxygen consumption, increased cardiac output and expansion of blood volume. Average increases in BMR have been observed to be around 5% in the first trimester, 10% in the second trimester and 25% in the third trimester (SACN 2012). The increased maternal BMR plus energy released by the developing fetus and uteroplacental unit lead to changes in temperature regulation with increased heat production particularly in the first trimester.

The changes in carbohydrate metabolism are the most dramatic of all. The production of glucose from carbohydrate in the maternal diet increases while glucose intolerance restricts its uptake to guarantee sufficient availability of glucose for the fetus as its primary source of energy for cellular metabolism (McGowan and McAuliffe 2010). Normally the maternal blood glucose is 10–20% higher than fetal blood glucose. This gradient, along with resistance to the glucose-lowering effects of insulin, favours transfer of a continuous, uninterrupted supply of glucose to the fetus through the placenta by diffusion. Insulin resistance is a normal physiological adaptation of pregnancy manifest by a fasting plasma insulin that triples as pregnancy progresses due to placental hormones (*cortisol, growth hormone, hPL*).

During early pregnancy increased levels of oestrogen and progesterone promote pancreatic beta cell hyperplasia causing a rapid increase in insulin production. This lowers plasma glucose by moving it into cells and by inhibiting hepatic glucose release, but also reduces plasma amino acids and free fatty acids. These adjustments result in a sparing of glucose for the fetus (Hadden and McLaughlin 2009). Hyperinsulinaemia leads to a decline in fasting plasma glucose levels by 10–15%, higher postprandial glucose values and increased uptake of glucose by muscles for storage as glycogen, increased storage of fats and decreased lipolysis. Following a meal containing glucose, pregnant women demonstrate prolonged hyperglycaemia, hyperinsulinaemia and a greater suppression of glucagon, the purpose of which is to ensure a sustained postprandial supply of glucose to the fetus (Hauth et al 2011). This is followed by a progressive reduction in glucose resulting in relative fasting hypoglycaemia known as *accelerated starvation*. Omitting meals or prolonged periods between food intake can provoke this condition, resulting in deleterious effects for both woman and fetus, such that pregnancy is described as a *diabetogenic state* (Pipkin 2012).

Normal glucose ranges during pregnancy are 3.4–5.5 mmol/l except immediately after meals, when levels can rise to 6.5 mmol/l (McGowan and McAuliffe 2010). In response to a 75 g glucose load the recommendation by the International Association of Diabetes and Pregnancy Study Groups Consensus Panel for cut-off points in the diagnosis of *gestational diabetes* is a fasting glucose of 5.1 mmol/l, at 1 hour post prandial a value of 10.0 mmol/l, and 8.5 mmol/l at 2 hours post prandial (Metzger et al 2010). In late pregnancy when the rate of weight gain reduces, maternal energy metabolism shifts from carbohydrate to lipid oxidation, thus further sparing glucose for the fetus to ensure a continuous supply of fuel when its needs are greatest (Herring et al 2012).

Complex changes take place in lipid metabolism during pregnancy influenced by oestrogen, progesterone, hPL and insulin resistance. Increased lipid synthesis and appetite in the first two trimesters of pregnancy lead to hyperlipidaemia, hypertrophy of adipocytes and the accumulation of fat in maternal depots. Adipose tissue becomes more responsive to insulin, which facilitates increased fat storage (Hadden and McLaughlin 2009). It is usual for women to build up an increased store of 2–5 kg fat mainly in the second trimester (Abduljalil et al 2012).

Maternal tissue lipid is used as an energy source in order to spare glucose and amino acids for the fetus. By 36 weeks fasting plasma triglycerides are two to four times the pre-pregnancy level. Maternal hypertriglyceridaemia contributes to fetal growth and development and serves as an energy depot for maternal dietary fatty acids (Hadden and McLaughlin 2009). Cholesterol is also available for fetal use to build cell membranes and as a precursor of bile acids and steroid hormones. Plasma cholesterol levels decline slightly in early pregnancy and then rise steadily, as do other lipids. Elevated free fatty acid levels have been associated with excess fetal adiposity and childhood obesity (Hadden and McLaughlin 2009).

The protein intake of a pregnant woman is particularly important. Amino acids are required by both woman and fetus for energy and growth (Hadden and McLaughlin 2009). About half the protein gained is deposited in the fetus and the remainder accumulates in the placenta, uterine muscle, breast and other maternal tissues in late pregnancy. In most cases total serum protein content

reduces within the first trimester due to increased placental uptake, increased insulin levels, diversion of amino acids for gluconeogenesis and transfer of amino acids to the fetus for use in glucose formation. By 20 weeks the mean serum albumin in healthy pregnant women decreases from 46 to 38 g/l. This reduces the plasma oncotic pressure and predisposes to oedema. Following a meal the amino acid levels rise briefly. These changes in amino acids occurring after fasting further reflect *accelerated starvation* (Hadden and McLaughlin 2009).

When women consume adequate amounts of *calcium* in the diet, parathyroid hormone (PTH) levels decrease in the first trimester. By 36 weeks calcium absorption doubles to support maternal and fetal bone mineralization with the fetus accumulating 250–350 mg of calcium per day. This increase in maternal calcium absorption leads to a physiological hypercalciuria after meals which can increase the risk of renal calculi (Hacker et al 2012). Guidance on calcium intake in pregnancy varies between countries. While the UK does not recommend supplementation (Olausson et al 2012), other countries advise calcium supplementation to reduce the risk of excessive bone loss, pre-eclampsia and preterm birth (Hacker et al 2012). *Vitamin D* supplementation is advised due to the re-emergence of rickets and the low vitamin D status of many women, particularly women of South Asian, African, Caribbean or Middle Eastern family origin. Global recommendations advise supplementation with 10–50 µg of vitamin D per day (NICE 2008; Olausson et al 2012).

MATERNAL WEIGHT

A healthy pre-conception body weight should be attained as maternal diet and nutritional status at the time of conception influence fetal outcome and the risk of later chronic disease (Riley 2011) (see Chapter 13). A variety of components contribute to weight gain during pregnancy (Table 9.7). The fetus accounts for approximately 27% of the increase in weight, the placenta, amniotic fluid and uterus 20%, the breasts 3%, blood volume and extravascular fluid 23%, and maternal fat stores 27% (Herring et al 2012). Most weight is gained in the second and third trimesters at rates of 0.45 kg and 0.40 kg per week respectively compared with 1.6 kg throughout the first trimester (SACN 2012). In early to mid-pregnancy, underweight and normal weight women deposit fat on their hips, back and upper thighs, which are important as a calorie reserve for late pregnancy and lactation (Herring et al 2012).

Although there are guidelines for clinicians to advise women about weight management during childbirth (NICE 2010), there remains an absence of official recommendations in the UK for specific weight gain parameters. Consequently the United States (US) Institute of Medicine (IOM) 2009 guidelines (Rasmussen and Yaktine 2009)

Table 9.7 Distribution of average increase in weight

	Weight gain (kg)	Percentage of total weight
Maternal		
Uterus	0.9	
Breasts	0.4	
Fat	4.0	64
Blood	1.2	
Extracellular fluid	1.2	
Total	7.7	
Fetal		
Fetus	3.3	25
Placenta	0.7	11
Amniotic fluid	0.8	
Total	4.8	
Grand total	12.5	

Table 9.8 Breast changes in chronological order

Time of occurrence	Changes
3–4 weeks	Prickling, tingling sensation due to increased blood supply particularly around the nipple
6–8 weeks	Increase in size, painful, tense and nodular due to hypertrophy of the alveoli. Delicate, bluish surface veins become visible just beneath the skin
8–12 weeks	Montgomery's tubercles become more prominent on the areola. These hypertrophic sebaceous glands secrete sebum, which keeps the nipple soft and supple. The pigmented area around the nipple (*the primary areola*) darkens, may enlarge and become more erectile
16 weeks	Colostrum can be expressed. The secondary areola develops with further extension of the pigmented area that is often mottled in appearance
Late pregnancy	Colostrum may leak from the breasts and progesterone causes the nipple to become more prominent and mobile

are often used by UK health professionals as a guide based on World Health Organization (WHO) cut-off points. Different levels of weight gain are recommended depending on the women's pre-pregnancy BMI (Riley 2011). Women with a BMI of *less than 18.5* should gain 12.5–18 kg; healthy women who have a BMI *between 18.5 and 24.9* should gain 11.5–16 kg during pregnancy; those with a BMI *between 25.9 and 29.9* should gain 7–11.5 kg and women with a BMI *over 30* should gain only 5–9 kg (Rasmussen and Yaktine 2009).

Total body water increases gradually with gestational age from 6 to 8 l due to retention of extracellular water and sodium which helps to maintain normal blood pressure. This leads to oedema and increased hydration and swelling of connective tissue (Pipkin 2012). The most marked expansion occurs in extracellular fluid volume and accounts for 8–10 kg of the average maternal weight gain during pregnancy (O'Donoghue 2011). This increase is important in expanding the plasma volume to fill the increased vascular bed in normal pregnancy. It activates the RAAS which stimulates increased reabsorption of sodium and water in the renal tubules thus maintaining normal blood pressure.

Fluid balance is maintained in pregnancy by a decrease in both plasma osmolality and *thirst threshold* so that pregnant women feel the urge to drink at a lower level of plasma osmolality than non-pregnant women. *Plasma oncotic pressure* is also reduced and, along with compression of pelvic and femoral vessels by the gravid uterus and prostaglandin-induced vascular relaxation, may contribute to the development of peripheral oedema (O'Donoghue 2011).

Physiological oedema of the lower leg is found in about 80% of all women in late pregnancy which causes discomfort, a feeling of heaviness, night cramps and painful paraesthesia. Regular foot massage is suggested to provide effective relief (Çoban and Şirin 2010). Fluid retention and accumulation of fat may result in larger shoes being required in the last trimester of pregnancy (Ponnapula and Boberg 2010).

The placenta and fetus follow different growth patterns during gestation. While fetal growth is very slow in the first trimester during organogenesis, placental growth is more rapid, reaching peak growth at 28–30 weeks' gestation. With the onset of fetal insulin secretion at 24–26 weeks' gestation fetal growth then increases more rapidly, with the highest growth achieved close to term (Abduljalil et al 2012; Kumar et al 2012). A birth weight between 3 kg and 4 kg is associated with optimal maternal and fetal outcomes (Herring et al 2012). Amniotic fluid volume during pregnancy is a dynamic process, accounting for 6% of gestational weight.

The weight of the breasts increases during pregnancy, with considerable variability between women (Riley 2011). Changes in the breasts are summarized in Table 9.8.

MUSCULOSKELETAL CHANGES

Relaxation of pelvic joints commences at 10–12 weeks gestation. An increased concentration of relaxin increases pelvic laxity and may be responsible for loosening pelvic ligaments and increasing instability, causing some degree of discomfort for the woman (Aldabe et al 2012). The increase in weight and the anterior shift in the centre of gravity lead to biomechanical changes and the characteristic *waddling* gait of pregnancy. Progesterone and oestrogen change the structure of connective tissue and increase mobility of joint capsules and spinal segment as well as pelvic joint structure in preparation for birth (Yousef et al 2011). There is decreased neuromuscular control and coordination, decreased abdominal strength, increased spinal lordosis and changes in mechanical loading and joint kinetics. All of these influence postural control and may be related to the increased risk of falling (McCrory et al 2010). There is a significant increase in the angles of thoracic kyphosis, lumbar lordosis and pelvic inclination (Yousef et al 2011).

Because of the many changes in load and body mechanics many women experience low back pain (see Box 9.13). Hormonal and biomechanical imbalances in addition to an increased functional demand on the ankle plantar flexors during pregnancy exacerbate *leg cramp syndrome*. This is caused by the sudden involuntary spasm of the gastrocnemius muscle. Treatment for leg cramps is not usually required, however a balanced diet and calcium gluconate supplements may help to relieve symptoms (Ponnapula and Boberg 2010).

SKIN CHANGES

Pregnancy causes a variety of common changes in skin, hair and nails, which in the majority of cases is a normal physiological response modulated by hormonal, immunologic and metabolic factors (see Box 9.14). Those attributed to hormonal changes are often seen in women on the combined oral contraceptive pill (Farage et al 2009). Certain changes have been shown to have a genetic predisposition, particularly *striae gravidarum* (stretch marks) and pigmentation changes.

Almost all women note some degree of skin darkening as one of the earliest signs of pregnancy. While the exact physiology remains unclear, it is generally attributed to an increase in melanocyte stimulating hormone, progesterone and oestrogen serum levels. Hyperpigmentation is more marked in dark-skinned women, being pronounced in areas that are normally pigmented, e.g. areola, genitalia and umbilicus. This also occurs in areas prone to friction, such as the axillae and inner thighs, and in recent scars.

Box 9.13 **Back pain**

As a result of the many changes in load and body mechanics, many women experience low back pain. The stretched abdominal muscles lose their ability to maintain posture so that the lower back has to support the majority of the weight.

Women who exercise prior to and during pregnancy can strengthen abdominal, back and pelvic muscles to improve posture and increased weight-bearing ability. Exercise in the second half of pregnancy focusing on abdominal strength, pelvic tilts and water aerobics are particularly effective in reducing low back pain. Pelvic girdle support belts and corsets are also useful in supporting the back. Simple home remedies such as heat pads and over-the-counter medication may ease the pain before muscle relaxants or opioids are prescribed. However, many women experience low back pain and inflammation in the first trimester before mechanical changes have occurred, suggesting that some pain may be due to the effects of relaxin rather than mechanical load.

Box 9.14 **Hair growth**

Hair growth has been shown to follow a common pattern in pregnancy. Women commonly report a thickening and increased volume of scalp hair. Stimulated by oestrogen, the growing period for hairs is increased in pregnancy so the woman reaches the end of pregnancy with many over-aged hairs. This ratio is reversed after birth, so that sometimes alarming amounts of hair are shed during brushing or washing. Normal hair growth is usually restored by 6–12 months. Mild hirsutism is common during pregnancy, particularly on the face (Muallem and Rubeiz 2006). Actions that may help include reducing damage to the hair by not combing when it is wet, and avoiding hairstyles that pull and stress hair, using shampoos and conditioners that contain biotin and silica. Diet that is high in fruit and vegetables containing flavonoids and antioxidants may provide protection for the hair follicles and encourage growth.

The *linea alba* is a line that lies over the midline of the rectus muscles from the umbilicus to the symphysis pubis. Hyperpigmentation causes it to darken resulting in the *linea nigra*. Pigmentation of the face affects up to 50–70% of pregnant women (Bolanca et al 2008) and is known as *chloasma* or *melasma*, or *mask of pregnancy*. It is caused by melanin deposition into epidermal or dermal macrophages, further exacerbated by sun exposure. The chloasma usually regresses postpartum but may persist in approx 10% of women and may be aggravated by oral contraceptives, which should thus should be avoided in susceptible women (Bolanca et al 2008). If chloasma persists post-partum, Katsambas and Stratigos (2001) suggest that it can be treated with a variety of topical agents, including *hydroquinone, tretinoin, kojic acid* and *vitamin C*.

As maternal size increases in pregnancy, stretching occurs in the collagen layer of the skin, particularly over the breasts, abdomen and thighs. In some women, this results in *striae gravidarum* caused by thin tears occurring in the dermal collagen. These appear as red stripes changing to glistening, silvery white lines approximately 6 months postpartum. The aetiology of striae has yet to be defined but may be compounded by adrenocorticoids, oestrogens and relaxin which modify collagen and possibly elastic tissue. Longstanding attempts to identify an effective treatment remain inconclusive. Recent studies using olive oil and cocoa butter have been unable to demonstrate any significant reduction in the incidence or severity of striae gravidarum (Osman et al 2008; Soltanipoor et al 2012).

Pruritus in pregnancy is characterized by intense itching either with or without a rash. It occurs in up to 20% of pregnancies (Nelson-Piercy 2009) with numerous potential differential diagnoses, including infection, eczema, or related to drug therapy. Although it usually clears spontaneously after pregnancy, pruritus should be investigated to exclude *obstetric cholestasis* which can have serious fetal and maternal consequences if untreated (see Chapter 13).

Angiomas or vascular spiders (minute red elevations on the skin of the face, neck, arms and chest) and *palmar erythema* (reddening of the palms) frequently occur, possibly as a result of high oestrogen levels. They are rarely of clinical significance and usually resolve spontaneously within a few months postpartum. Nevertheless changes may mask more serious conditions such as *malignant neoplasms* or *herpes gestationis*. It is therefore imperative to assess for specific dermatoses of pregnancy which may be associated with maternal disease and fetal mortality and morbidity if severe and left untreated.

CHANGES IN THE ENDOCRINE SYSTEM

The changes in all compartments of the endocrine system and their timing are critical for the initiation and maintenance of pregnancy, for fetal growth and development and for parturition (Feldt-Rasmussen and Mathiesen 2011) (see Chapter 5). Hormone levels are influenced by and vary according to parity, BMI, age, gestation, ethnicity and smoking.

Placental hormones

Human chorionic gonadotrophin (hCG) produced by the placental syncytiotrophoblast and cytotrophoblast cells and

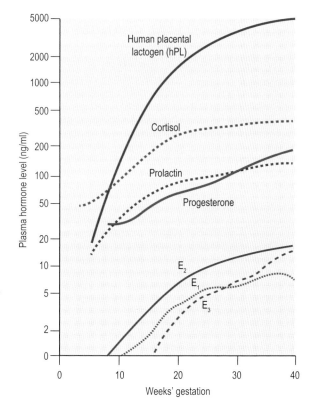

Fig. 9.8 Variations in plasma hormone concentrations during a normal pregnancy.
From Heffner L, Schust D 2010 The reproductive system at a glance. Wiley–Blackwell, Oxford, ch 20, with permission of Wiley–Blackwell.

by the pituitary gland is a hormone with multiple functions during pregnancy (Cole 2012). It can be detected in maternal serum from the 8th day after ovulation so is useful as a diagnostic marker for pregnancy. The unique role of this hormone is to rescue the corpus luteum from involution so that it can continue to produce progesterone which in turn maintains the decidua (Feldt-Rasmussen and Mathiesen 2011). Secretion of hCG commences at implantation, peaks at concentrations of 100–200 IU/ml at 8–10 weeks then declines to 20 IU/ml by 20 weeks' gestation, remaining stable until labour (Fig. 9.8).

Human chorionic gonadotrophin drives hemochorial placentation and nutrient transfer to the fetus and promotes the development and growth of uterine spiral arteries, the formation of the umbilical circulation in villous tissue and the formation of the umbilical cord. It is also important in preventing rejection of fetoplacental tissue during pregnancy (Cole 2012).

Relaxin is produced by the corpus luteum and contributes to the process of decidualization and to the vasodilatation of healthy pregnancy (Conrad 2011).

Human placental lactogen (hPL) is secreted into the maternal circulation by the syncytiotrophoblast and can be detected in the maternal circulation as early as 6 weeks' gestation with concentrations increasing up to 30-fold throughout pregnancy. This hormone regulates maternal carbohydrate, lipid and protein metabolism and fetal growth. Maternal glucose uptake and glycogen synthesis are increased along with glucose oxidation and insulin secretion as a result of hPL function: producing maternal diabetogenic effects. It also acts to promote the growth of breast tissue in preparation for lactation (Braun et al 2013).

The placenta secretes over 20 different *oestrogens* into the maternal circulation but the major ones are *oestradiol*, *oestrone* and *oestriol*, the latter being the most predominant in pregnancy. Whilst oestrogens are produced primarily by the developing follicles and corpus luteum, they are also produced by the placenta, liver, adrenal glands, fat and breast cells. Oestrogen concentrations greatly increase during pregnancy, reaching levels 3–8 times higher than those observed in the non-pregnant woman. Oestradiol concentrations peak at around 6–7 weeks' gestation when the production and secretion shifts from the corpus luteum to the placenta. It then rises steadily throughout pregnancy, particularly in the second and third trimesters.

Oestrogen increases uterine blood flow and facilitates placental oxygenation and nutrition to the fetus. It also prepares the breasts for lactation, affects the RAAS and stimulates the production of hormone-binding globulins in the liver (Myatt and Powell 2010). It is also responsible for changes in the nasal, gingival and laryngeal mucosa when it peaks during the third trimester.

Progesterone is a pro-gestational hormone. It is the key hormone in the initial stages of pregnancy and is essential for creating a suitable endometrial environment for implantation and maintenance of the pregnancy (Mesiano et al 2011). Progesterone is produced predominantly by the corpus luteum in the first 9 weeks, after which production shifts to the placenta. Concentrations plateau around 8–10 weeks and remain relatively stable until around 16 weeks, when they begin to rise again. At 32 weeks there is a second rise in levels due to placental use of fetal precursors. At term the placenta produces about 250 mg progesterone per day.

Progesterone promotes decidualization, inhibits smooth muscle contractility, maintains myometrial quiescence and prevents the onset of uterine contractions (Feldt-Rasmussen and Mathiesen 2011). A decrease or disruption of its production or activity promotes cervical re-modelling and initiates labour (Mesiano et al 2011). It is the precursor of some fetal hormones and plays an important role in suppressing the maternal immunological response to fetal antigens thereby preventing rejection of the trophoblast.

The pituitary gland and its hormones

The maternal pituitary gland enlarges two- to three-fold during pregnancy due to hypertrophy and hyperplasia of the lactotrophs (*prolactin-secreting cells*) under the influence of oestrogen. As a result, prolactin levels increase. Insulin-like growth factor levels increase in the second half of pregnancy contributing to the acromegaloid features of some pregnant women. Corticotrophin-releasing hormones rise several hundred-fold by term. Adrenocorticotrophic hormone (ACTH) and cortisol levels rise progressively throughout pregnancy, with a further increase in labour. Free cortisol rises three-fold with a two- to three-fold increase in urinary free cortisol which makes diagnosis and treatment challenging in the event of pituitary or adrenal pathology (Feldt-Rasmussen and Mathiesen 2011).

Maternal serum *follicle stimulating hormone* (FSH) levels during pregnancy are stable and almost undetectable, possibly due to the excessive production of oestrogen by the placenta. Maternal serum levels of *leuteinizing hormone* (LH) increase rapidly in the first trimester to a maximum of 3 IU/l and then decline slowly until birth.

Prolactin is produced by the anterior lobe of the pituitary gland and by amniotic fluid. It stimulates mammary growth and development and lactation (Feldt-Rasmussen and Mathiesen 2011) (see Chapter 34). Prolactin levels increase progressively throughout pregnancy and by term serum levels are about 10 times the non-pregnant level.

The posterior pituitary gland produces two hormones: *vasopressin* and *oxytocin*. However, *vasopressin* does not play a significant role in pregnancy. *Oxytocin* levels are low during pregnancy but increase in labour (Feldt-Rasmussen and Mathiesen 2011), its function being to act on the myometrium to increase the length, strength and frequency of contractions. It is responsible for the milk-ejecting action of the posterior lobe of the pituitary gland and is thought to play a role in regulating milk production through control of prolactin (Chapter 34) and in the establishment of complex social and bonding behaviours related to birth and care of the baby (Petraglia et al 2010).

Thyroid function

The thyroid gland is moderately enlarged during pregnancy due to hormone-induced glandular hyperplasia and increased vascularity (Baba and Azar 2012). Thyroid size is influenced by different factors, including iodine supply, genetics, gender, age, parity and smoking. There is a positive correlation in pregnancy between thyroid volume and BMI (Gaberšček and Zalatel 2011). The function of the thyroid gland is to produce sufficient thyroid hormones necessary to meet the demands of peripheral tissues. Maintaining euthyroidism during pregnancy is essential for the growth and development of the fetus. In the first trimester the fetus depends solely on thyroid hormones and iodine

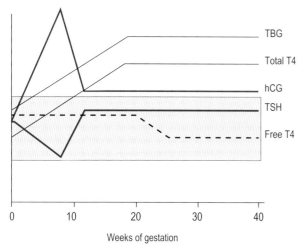

TBG

Total T4

hCG

TSH

Free T4

0   10   20   30   40

Weeks of gestation

Fig. 9.9 Change in thyroid function indices throughout getstation. The shaded area represents the normal range of thyroid-binding globulin (TBG), total T4 thyroxine, thyroid stimulating hormone (TSH) and free T4. hCG = human chorionic gonadotrophin.

Reproduced with permission from Casey B M, Leveno K J 2006 Thyroid disease in pregnancy. Obstetrics and Gynaecology 108:1283–9.

from the mother, such that subtle changes in thyroid function can have detrimental effects on the fetus.

Maternal thyroid function alters dramatically during pregnancy due to the physiological changes of pregnancy and fetal requirements. Since the fetal thyroid does not function until mid-pregnancy the fetus is dependent on maternal thyroid function for its normal brain development. Increased *thyroxine* production is required for metabolic changes as well as transfer of thyroxine to the fetal brain cells (Rebagliato et al 2010; Lazarus 2011). Healthy pregnant women are usually able to adjust their thyroid function in pregnancy if an adequate store of iodine exists prior to conception (Rebagliato et al 2010). However, maternal thyroid failure during the first half of pregnancy has been associated with several pregnancy complications as well as intellectual impairment in the child (Baba and Azar 2012).

The steep rise in hCG levels during the first trimester may result in an increased production of thyroid hormones and thus decreased *thyroid stimulating hormone* (TSH) levels (Fig. 9.9). Higher levels of oestrogen lead to a two- and three-fold increase in the levels *of thyroxine-binding globulin* (TBG) which causes a 50% increase in total thyroxine. Total *thyroxine* (T4) and total *triiodothyronine* (T3) concentrations increase sharply in early pregnancy and plateau early in the second trimester at concentrations 30–100% greater than pre-pregnancy values (Lazarus 2011; Baba and Azar 2012). In the second and third trimesters when stimulation by hCG declines, T3 and T4 levels remain above the non-pregnant levels and TSH levels

remain low, however this does not result in hyperthyroidism due to the parallel increase in TBG.

The increased GFR and renal blood flow improves the clearance of *renal iodide*. This reflects the additional demand for iodine in pregnancy to protect the woman and provide for the needs of the fetus. Iodide levels increase a few weeks after conception and reach a plateau during mid-pregnancy. Iodine requirements intensify in pregnancy because of the increase in synthesis of thyroid hormone, urinary iodine excretion, placental transfer and metabolism of thyroid hormones. Total body iodine stores decrease by 40% during pregnancy ranging from 15 mg to 50 mg of which two-thirds is stored hormone in the thyroid gland (Rebagliato et al 2010). Excretion of iodine in the urine rises and iodine deficiency is common in pregnancy even in areas where there is generally sufficient iodine (Kennedy et al 2010), consequently there is an association with maternal goitre and reduced maternal thyroxine (T4) level (Lazarus 2011). Severe iodine deficiency leads to *cretinism* in the newborn therefore an adequate intake of iodine is essential during pregnancy to maximize fetal outcome, particularly appropriate maturation of the fetal brain to improve early neurological development (Rebagliato et al 2010).

Routine iodine supplementation is advised in parts of the world where the risk of iodine deficiency is endemic and should commence before conception (Kennedy et al 2010). It is generally recommended that all pregnant women should increase their intake of iodine to 250 µg per day before and during pregnancy but should not exceed 500 µg per day as a higher intake may cause thyroid dysfunction.

Due to the many changes in thyroid function there is a real risk of misinterpretation of thyroid function tests in pregnancy and it is recommended that pregnancy reference ranges are used as markers (Feldt-Rasmussen and Mathiesen 2011). As T4 and T3 levels define thyroid status in early pregnancy while TSH concentrations provide indication of thyroid status in later pregnancy, Kennedy et al (2010) advises that laboratories should establish their own trimester-specific reference ranges for thyroid hormones and TSH.

Adrenal glands

Adrenal metabolism changes significantly, with adrenal steroid levels increasing throughout pregnancy. Adrenocorticotrophic hormone (ACTH) levels escalate dramatically, with the initial peak at 11 weeks, a significant rise after 16–20 weeks and a final surge during labour. Despite these increases in plasma and urinary free cortisol levels, pregnant women do not show any features of hypercortisolism. *Renin* and *angiotensin* levels rise leading to elevated levels of angiotensin II and aldosterone (Feldt-Rasmussen and Mathiesen 2011) and plasma *aldosterone* levels increase 5- to 20-fold during pregnancy, with a plateau at 38 weeks.

Aldosterone secretion continues to respond to physiological stimuli such as posture and varies according to salt intake. The increase in aldosterone promotes sodium retention in the distal renal tubules.

Cortisol produced by the decidua acts in combination with hCG and progesterone secreted by the conceptus to suppress maternal immune response (Feldt-Rasmussen and Mathiesen 2011). There is a steady rise in serum cortisol as pregnancy advances, which decreases the inflammatory response resulting in improvement in dermatological and rheumatoid conditions. This rise in serum cortisol also causes relative gestational immunosuppression which leads to reactivation of latent viral infections, suggesting that endocrine and immune systems are closely related.

DIAGNOSIS OF PREGNANCY

Women who are aware of their bodies might begin to suspect that they are pregnant within the first few days of pregnancy but for most, the first sign is missing a period (Table 9.9). Other symptoms include nausea and vomiting, breast tenderness and fullness, urinary frequency and fatigue. Most women use a home pregnancy test (HPT) to determine their pregnancy status before seeking professional health care.

Traditionally diagnosis has been based on history and physical examination. Issues that may confuse the diagnosis of early pregnancy are an atypical last menstrual period, contraceptive use and a history of irregular periods. Spotting or light bleeding is common in early pregnancy between weeks 6 and 7 (Hasan et al 2010), which may further complicate the assessment. The signs of pregnancy described below are mainly of historic significance. Although they may still be of value in some parts of the world, they have generally been rendered obsolete in the developed world by more modern and sophisticated methods.

Hegar's (or Goodell's) sign

Softening of the lower parts of the isthmus is felt in contrast to a firm cervix at about 6–8 weeks' gestation on bimanual pelvic examination (Davis Jones 2011).

Chadwick's sign

The cervix, vagina, vulva and vaginal mucous membranes become darker or blue in colour at 8 weeks' gestation (Geraghty and Pomeranz 2011). It is caused by the greatly increased blood supply to the pelvic organs. It is also known as *Jacquemier's sign*. While this sign indicates pregnancy, it does not necessarily indicate viability.

Osiander's sign

Stronger pulsations can be felt in the lateral vaginal fornix due to increased blood supply from the enlarged uterine artery (Davis Jones 2011). This may also occur in the non-pregnant woman due to fibroids and pelvic inflammation.

Quickening

It is a pivotal moment in pregnancy when the first fluttering movements of the growing fetus are felt. Quickening occurs at 18–20 weeks although many women experience it at an earlier gestation. Fetal movements can begin to be palpated around 20 weeks (see Table 9.9).

Measurement of hyperglycosylated hCG (hCG-H) produced by trophoblast cells is the principal form of total hCG made in early pregnancy and forms the basis for pregnancy testing, using either maternal urine or serum. Urine pregnancy tests and one-step point-of-care (POC) tests are widely used both at home and in laboratories. However, some serum hCG, POC and HPTs poorly detect hCG-H, which limits their use in early pregnancy testing; consequently, manufacturers have attempted to produce a specific hCG-H assay, but without success (Brezina et al 2011). Reliability of the HPT depends on the correct adherence to both instructions and timing of the test. Tests routinely claim to have an accuracy of 99% in the detection of hCG concentrations. The most accurate tests are First Response™ Early Result Pregnancy Test (Church & Dwight Co., Inc.) and Clear Choice™ At Home Pregnancy Test (Pharmatech Inc.) (Cole 2010).

Early pregnancy detection is critical as it allows prenatal care to begin during the most vulnerable stages of fetal development. Research has shown that women who access prenatal care early in their pregnancy have improved outcomes than women who delay or have inadequate prenatal care (Quelopana et al 2009).

COMMON DISORDERS ARISING FROM ADAPTATIONS TO PREGNANCY

Throughout this chapter reference has been made to the multitude of symptoms produced by the physiological changes occurring in pregnancy. While deemed physiological, women may experience these as unpleasant, and even distressing or debilitating. Due to their common, natural and non-pathological nature and the fact that they generally resolve spontaneously, caregivers are often guilty of a dismissive or trivializing approach towards them.

Table 9.9 Signs of pregnancy

Sign	Time of occurrence	Differential diagnosis
Possible (presumptive) signs		
Early breast changes (*unreliable in multigravida*)	3–4 weeks +	Contraceptive pill
Amenorrhoea	4 weeks +	Hormonal imbalance Emotional stress Illness
Nausea and vomiting	4–14 weeks	Gastrointestinal disorders Pyrexial illness Cerebral irritation, etc.
Bladder irritability	6–12 weeks	Urinary tract infection Pelvic tumour
Quickening	16–20 weeks +	Intestinal movement, wind
Probable signs		
Presence of human chorionic gonadotrophin (*hCG*) in: Blood Urine	9–10 days 14 days	Hydatidiform mole Choriocarcinoma
Softened isthmus (Hegar's sign)	6–12 weeks	
Blueing of vagina (Chadwick's sign)	8 weeks +	
Pulsation of fornices (Osiander's sign)	8 weeks +	Pelvic congestion Tumours
Changes in skin pigmentation	8 weeks +	
Uterine souffle	12–16 weeks	Increased blood flow to uterus as in large uterine myomas or ovarian tumours
Braxton Hicks contractions	16 weeks	
Ballottement of fetus	16–28 weeks	
Positive signs		
Visualization of gestational sac by: Transvaginal ultrasound Transabdominal ultrasound	4.5 weeks 5.5 weeks	
Visualization of heart pulsation by: Transvaginal ultrasound Transabdominal ultrasound	5 weeks 6 weeks	
Fetal heart sounds by: Doppler Fetal stethoscope	11–12 weeks 20 weeks +	No alternative diagnosis
Fetal movements Palpable Visible	22 weeks + Late pregnancy	
Fetal parts palpated	24 weeks +	
Visualization of fetus by X-ray (*superseded by ultrasound*)	16 weeks +	

The two key issues for midwives to build into their practice are:

1. Ensure assessment of a woman's symptoms is accurate, differentiating clearly between physiological and potentially pathological symptoms.

2. Develop a sympathetic approach to women experiencing these discomforts and ensure appropriate advice is offered to ameliorate or better tolerate the symptoms of pregnancy.

REFERENCES

Abbas K, Monaghan S, Campbell I 2010 Uterine physiology. Anaesthesia and Intensive Care Medicine 12(3): 108–10

Abduljalil K, Furness P, Johnson T et al. 2012 Anatomical, physiological and metabolic changes with gestational age during normal pregnancy. Clinical Pharmacokinetics 51(6):365–6

Adamson D, Dhanjal M, Nelson-Piercy C 2011 Heart disease in pregnancy. Oxford, Oxford University Press

Aguilar H, Mitchell B 2010 Physiological pathways and molecular mechanisms regulating uterine contractility. Human Reproduction Update 16(6):725–44

Åkerud A 2009 Uterine remodelling during pregnancy. Lund University, Lund, Sweden, p 21–2

Alba A, Carleton L, Dinkel L et al 2012 Increased lead levels in pregnancy among immigrant women. Journal of Midwifery and Women's Health 57:509–14

Aldabe D, Ribeiro D, Milosavljevic S et al 2012 Pregnancy-related pelvic girdle pain and its relationship with relaxin levels during pregnancy: a systematic review. European Spine Jourrnal 21:1769–76

Ansari H, Rajkumari A 2011 Prevalence of asymptomatic bacteriuria and associated risk factors among antenatal women attending a tertiary care hospital. Journal of Medical and Allied Sciences 1(2):74–8

Asali F, Mahfouz I, Phillips C 2012 The management of urogynaecological problems in pregnancy and the early postpartum period. The Obstetrician and Gynaecologist 14:153–8

Avsar A, Keskin H 2010 Haemorrhoids during pregnancy. Journal of Obstetrics and Gynaecology, 30(3):231–7

Baba K, Azar S 2012 Thyroid dysfunction in pregnancy. International Journal of General Medicine 5:227–30

Baggish A, Wood M 2011 Athlete's heart and cardiovascular care of the athlete. Circulation 123:2723–35

Baidya D, Maitra S, Chhabra A et al 2012 Pregnancy with renal disease: pathophysiology and anaesthetic management. Trends in Anaesthesia and Critical Care 2:281–6

Bamber J, Dresner M 2003 Aortocaval compression in pregnancy: the effect of changing the degree and direction of lateral tilt on maternal cardiac output. Anesthesia and Analgesia 97:256–8

Beckman C, Ling F, Barzanski B et al 2010 Obstetrics and gynaecology, 6th edn. Lippincott Williams and Wilkins, Baltimore, p 74

Blackburn S 2012 Maternal, fetal and neonatal physiology, 4th edn. Philadelphia, WB Saunders

Blanks A, Shmygol A, Thornton S 2007 Myometrial function in prematurity. Best Practice and Research: Clinical Obstetrics and Gynaecology 21(5):807–19

Blumfield M, Hure A, Macdonald-Wicks L 2012 Systematic review and meta-analysis of energy and macronutrient intakes during pregnancy in developed countries. Nutrition Reviews 70(6):322–36

Bobrowski R A 2010 Pulmonary physiology in pregnancy. Clinical Obstetrics and Gynecology 53(2):285–300

Bolanca I, Bolanca Z, Kuna K et al 2008 Chloasma: the mask of pregnancy. Collegium Antropologicum 32(Suppl 2):139–41

Braun T, Husar A, Challis R et al 2013 Growth restricting effects of a single course of antenatal betamethasone treatment and the role of human

placental lactogen. Placenta 34(5):407–15

Bredenoord A, Pandolfi J, Smout A 2013 Gastro-oesophageal reflux disease. The Lancet 381(9881):1933–42

Brezina P, Haberl E, Wallach E 2011 At home testing: optimizing management for the infertility physician. Fertility and Sterility 95(6):1867–78

British National Formulary 2013 Edition 63. Pharmaceutical Press, London, 1.6. www.medicinescomplete.com/mc/bnf/current/PHP546-laxatives.htm

Brosens I, Derwig I, Brosens J et al 2010 The enigmatic uterine junctional zone: the missing link between reproductive disorders and major obstetrical disorders? Human Reproduction 25(3): 569–74

Brosens I, Ghaem-Maghami S, Pijnenborg R 2012 Uterus transplantation in the human: a complex surgical, medical and ethical challenge. Human Reproduction 28(2):292–3

Burton G, Woods A, Jauniaux E et al 2009 Rheological and physiological consequences of conversion of the maternal spiral arteries for uteroplacental blood flow during human pregnancy. Placenta 30:473–82

Cao C, O'Brien O 2013 Pregnancy and iron homeostasis: an update. Nutrition Reviews 71(1): 35–51

Casciani E, Masselli G, Luciani M et al 2012 Errors in imaging of emergencies in pregnancy. Seminars in Ultrasound, CT and MRI 33(4):347–70

Chen S J, Liu Y L, Sytwu H K 2012 Immunologic regulation in pregnancy:from mechanism to therapeutic strategy. Clinical and

Developmental Immunobiology 258391 (accessed online at www .hindawi.com/journals/ cdi/2012/258391/ 3 March 2013)

Ciarmela P, Islam S, Reis F et al 2011 Growth factors and myometrium: biological effects in uterine fibroid and possible clinical implications. Human Reproduction Update 17(6):772–90

Çoban A, Şirin A 2010 Effect of foot massage to decrease physiological lower leg oedema in late pregnancy: a randomized controlled trial in Turkey. International Journal of Nursing Practice 16:454–60

Cole L 2010 Hyperglycosylated hCG: a review. Placenta 31: 653–64

Cole L 2012 hCG: the wonder of today's science. Reproductive Biology and Endocrinology 10:24

Conrad K P 2011 Emerging role of relaxin in the maternal adaptations to normal pregnancy: implications for pre-eclampsia. Seminars in Nephrology 31(1):15–32

Cuckson C, Germain S 2011 Hyperemesis, gastro-intestinal and liver disorders in pregnancy. Obstetrics, Gynaecology and Reproductive Medicine 21:3

Cunningham F, Leveno K, Bloom S et al 2010 William's obstetrics, 23rd edn. New York, McGraw-Hill

Davis Jones B 2011 Comprehensive medical terminology, 4th edn. New York, Delmar Cengage Learning

Detman L, Cottrell B, Denis-Luque M 2010 Exploring dental care: misconceptions and barriers in pregnancy. Birth 37:4

Donati L, Augusto Di Vico A, Nucci M et al 2010 Vaginal microbial flora and outcome of pregnancy. Archives of Gynecology and Obstetrics 281:589–600

Farage M A, MacLean A B, Neill S 2009 Physiological changes associated with the menstrual cycle: a review. Obstetrical Gynecological Survey 64(1):58–72

Feldt-Rasmussen U, Mathiesen E 2011 Endocrine disorders in pregnancy: physiological and hormonal aspects of pregnancy. Best Practice and Research Clinical Endocrinology and Metabolism 25:875–84

Fiadjoe P, Kannan K, Rane A 2010 Maternal urological problems in pregnancy. European Journal of Obstetrics & Gynecology and Reproductive Biology 152:13–17

Freemark M 2010 Placental hormones and the control of fetal growth. Journal of Clinical Endocrinology and Metabolism 95(5):2054–7

Fu Q, Levine B 2009 Autonomic circulatory control during pregnancy in humans. Seminars in Reproductive Medicine 27(4):330–7

Gabbe S, Galan H, Niebyl J et al (eds) 2012 Obstetrics: normal and problem pregnancies, 6th edn. Philadelphia, Elsevier Saunders

Gaberšćek S, Zalatel K 2011 Thyroid physiology and autoimmunity in pregnancy and after delivery. Expert Reviews on Clinical Immunology 7(5):697–707

Gardosi J 2012 Customised assessment of fetal growth potential: implications for perinatal care. Archives of Diseases in Childhood Fetal and Neonatal Edition 97(5):F314–17

Gellersen B, Wolf A, Kruse M et al 2013 Human endometrial stromal cell–trophoblast interactions: mutual stimulation of chemotactic migration and pro-migratory roles of cell surface molecules CD82 and CEACAM1. Biology of Reproduction 88(3):1–13

Geraghty L, Pomeranz M 2011 Physiologic changes and dermatoses of pregnancy. International Journal of Dermatology 50:771–82

Gordon M 2012 Maternal physiology. In: Gabbe S, Galan H, Niebyl J et al (eds), Obstetrics: normal and problem pregnancies, 6th edn. Philadelphia, Elsevier Saunders, p 55–84

Goyal D, Gay C L, Lee K A 2007 Patterns of sleep disruption and depressive symptoms in new mothers. Journal of Perinatal and Neonatal Nursing 21(2):123–9

Hacker A, Fung E, King J 2012 Role of calcium during pregnancy: maternal and fetal needs. Nutrition Reviews 70(7):397–409

Hadden D, McLaughlin C 2009 Normal and abnormal maternal metabolism during pregnancy. Seminars in Fetal and Neonatal Medicine 14:66–71

Hamdi K, Bastani P, Saheb-Madarek E et al 2010 Prediction of latency interval in preterm premature rupture of membranes using sonographic myometrial thickness. Pakistan Journal of Biological Sciences 13(17):841–6

Hanretty K 2010 Obstetrics illustrated. Churchill Livingstone, Elsevier, p 34

Hargreaves K, Cameron M, Edwards H et al 2011 Is the use of symphysis–fundal height measurement and ultrasound examination effective in detecting small or large fetuses? Journal of Obstetrics and Gynaecology 31(5):380–3

Hasan R, Baird D, Herring A et al 2010 Patterns and predictors of vaginal bleeding in the first trimester of pregnancy. Annals of Epidemiology 20:524–31

Hassan S, Romero R, Gotsch F et al 2011 Cervical insufficiency. In: Winn HN, Chervenak FA, Romero R (eds), Clinical Maternal-Fetal Medicine Online, 2nd edn, ch 3, p 6. Available at: http://informahealthcare.com/ doi/book/ 10.3109/9780203347263

Hauth J, Clifton R, Roberts J et al 2011 Maternal insulin resistance and preeclampsia. American Journal of Obstetrics and Gynecology 204:327, e1–6

Heffner L, Schust D 2010 The reproductive system at a glance. Wiley–Blackwell, Oxford, ch 20

Hegewald M, Crapo R 2011 Respiratory physiology in pregnancy. Clinical Chest Medicine 32:1–13

Herring S J, Rose M Z, Skouteris H et al 2012 Optimizing weight gain in pregnancy to prevent obesity in women and children. Diabetes Obesity & Metabolism 14(3):195–203

Hudson C, Heesom K, Bernal A 2012 Phasic contractions of isolated human myometrium are associated with Rhokinase (ROCK)-dependent phosphorylation of myosin phosphatase-targeting subunit (MYPT1). Molecular Human Reproduction 18(5):265–79

Iams J 2010 Cervical remodelling in pregnancy. In: Creasy R, Resnik R, Iams J et al (eds), Creasy and Resnik's maternal fetal medicine: principles and practice, 6th edn. Philadelphia, Saunders, ch 30

Impey L, Child T 2012 Obstetrics and gynaecology, 4th edn. Chichester, Wiley–Blackwell

Iqbal S, Sumaira S 2009 Outcome of primigravida with unengaged versus engaged fetal head at term or onset of labour. Biomedica 25:159–62

Jarvis S, Nelson-Piercy C 2011 Management of nausea and vomiting in pregnancy. British Medical Journal 342:1407–12

Jensen D, Webb K A, Davies G A et al. 2009 Mechanisms of activity-related breathlessness in healthy human pregnancy. European Journal of Applied Physiology 106(2): 253–65

Joshi D, James A, Quaglia A et al 2010 Liver disease in pregnancy. The Lancet 375:594–605

Katsambas A D, Stratigos A J 2001 Depigmenting and bleaching agents: coping with hyperpigmentation. Clinical Dermatology 19:483–8

Katz P, Gerson L, Vela M 2013 Guidelines for the diagnosis and management of gastroesophageal reflux disease. Americal Journal of Gastroenterology 108:308–28

Kempler Sharp L, Bartlett D 2012 Sleep education during pregnancy for new mothers. Biomedical Central Pregnancy and Childbirth 12:155 (available online at www .biomedcentral.com/1471-2393/12/155 accessed 3 March 2013)

Kennedy R, Malabu U, Jarrod G et al 2010 Thyroid function and pregnancy: before, during and beyond. Journal of Obstetrics and Gynaecology 30(8):774–83

Kloetzel M, Hueber C, Milgrom P 2011 Referrals fof dental care during pregnancy. Journal of Midwifery and Women's Health 65(2):110–17

Koren G, Maltepe C, Gow R 2011 Therapeutic choices for nausea and vomiting of pregnancy: a critical review of a systematic review. Journal of Obstetrics and Gynaecology 33(7):733–5

Kumar A, Basra M, Begum N et al 2013 Association of maternal periodontal health with adverse pregnancy outcome. Journal of Obstetrics and Gynaecological Research 39(1): 40–5

Kumar N, Leverence J, Bick D et al 2012 Ontogeny of growth-regulating genes in the placenta. Placenta 33:94–9

Larsen B, Hwang J 2011 Progesterone interactions with the cervix: translational implications for term and preterm birth. Infectious Diseases in Obstetrics and Gynecology. Open access article ID 353297

Law H, Fiadjoe P 2012 Urogynaecological problems in pregnancy. Journal of Obstetrics and Gynaecology 32:109–12

Lazarus J H 2011 Thyroid function in pregnancy. British Medical Bulletin 97:137–48

Lemos A, Figueiroa J N, de Souza A I et al 2010 Respiratory muscle strength in pregnancy. Respiratory Medicine 104(11):1638–44

Lewis B, Avery M, Jennings E et al 2010 The effect of exercise during pregnancy on maternal outcomes: practical implications for practice. American Journal of Lifestyle Medicine 2(5):441–55

Llewellyn-Jones D 2010 Fundamentals of obstetrics and gynaecology, 9th edn. London, Mosby

López L, Marigual M, Martín N et al 2012 Characteristics of pica practice during pregnancy in a sample of Argentine women. Journal of Obstetrics and Gynaecology 32:150–3

Matthews A, Dowswell T, Haas D et al 2010 Interventions for nausea and vomiting in early pregnancy. Cochrane Database of Systematic Reviews 2010, Issue 9. Art. No. CD007575. doi: 10.1002/14651858. CD007575.pub2

McCrory J, Chambers A, Daftary A et al 2010 Dynamic postural stability during advancing pregnancy. Journal of Biomechanics 43:2434–9

McGowan C, McAuliffe F 2010 The influence of maternal glycaemia and dietary glycaemic index on pregnancy outcome in healthy mothers. British Journal of Nutrition 104:153–9

McMahon M A, Banks A, Fenwick A et al 2009 Prevention of supine hypotensive syndrome in pregnant women undergoing computed tomography: a national survey of current practice. Radiography 15(2):97–100

Mesiano S, Wang Y, Norwitz E 2011 Progesterone receptors in the human pregnancy uterus: do they hold the key to birth timing? Reproductive Sciences 18(1):6–19

Metzger B, Gabbe S, Persson B et al (International Association of Diabetes and Pregnancy Study Groups Consensus Panel) 2010 International Association of Diabetes and Pregnancy Study Groups recommendations on the diagnosis and classification of hyperglycemia in pregnancy. Diabetes Care 33(3):676–82

Miftahof R, Nam H 2011 Biomechanics of the gravid human uterus. Springer-Verlag, Berlin

Monga M 2009 Maternal cardiovascular and renal adaptation to pregnancy. In: Creasy R, Resnik R, Iams J et al (eds), Creasy and Resnik's maternal fetal medicine: principles and practice, 6th edn. Philadelphia, Saunders, p 101–10

Moore K, Persaud T, Torchia M et al 2013 The developing human: clinically orientated embryology, 9th edn. Elsevier Saunders

Mosher A, Rainey K, Bolstad S et al 2013 Development and validation of primary human myometrial cell culture models to study pregnancy and labour. Biomedical Central Pregnancy and Childbirth 13 (Suppl 1):S7

Muallem M, Rubeiz N 2006 Physiological and biological skin changes in pregnancy. Clinics in Dermatology 24(2):80–3

Myatt L, Powell T 2010 Maternal adaptations to pregnancy and the role of the placenta. In: Symonds M, Ramsay M (eds) Maternal–fetal nutrition during pregnancy and lactation. Cambridge, Cambridge University Press, p 1–10

NICE (National Institute for Health and Clinical Excellence) 2008 Antenatal care: routine care for the healthy pregnant woman. CG 62. NICE, London

NICE (National Institute for Health and Clinical Excellence) 2010 Weight management before, during and after pregnancy. PHG 27. NICE, London

Naumann C, Zelig C, Napolitano P et al 2012 Nausea, vomiting, and heartburn in pregnancy: a prospective look at risk, treatment, and outcome. Journal of Maternal–Fetal and Neonatal Medicine 25(8):1488–93

Neilson J P 2009 Symphysis–fundal height measurement in pregnancy.

Cochrane Database of Systematic Reviews 1998, Issue 1. Art. No. CD000944. doi: 10.1002/14651858

Nelson-Piercy C 2009 Handbook of obstetric medicine, 4th edn. Oxford, Taylor and Francis

O'Donoghue K 2011 Physiological changes in pregnancy. In: Baker P, Kenny L (eds) Obstetrics by ten teachers, 19th edn. London, Hodder and Stoughton, p 20–37

Olausson H, Goldberg G, Laskey M et al 2012 Calcium economy in human pregnancy and lactation. Nutrition Research Reviews 25:40–67

Osman H, Usta I, Rubeiz N et al. 2008 Cocoa butter lotion for prevention of striae gravidarum: a double-blind, randomized and placebo-controlled trial. BJOG: An International Journal of Obstetrics and Gynaecology 115(9):1138–42

Patil C, Young S 2012 Biocultural considerations of food cravings and aversions: an introduction. Ecology of Food and Nutrition 51(5):365–73

Pepe F, Pepe P 2013 Color Doppler ultrasound (CDU) in the diagnosis of obstructive hydronephrosis in pregnant women. Archives in Gynecology and Obstetrics 288(3):489–93

Perera N, Liolitsa D, Iype S et al 2012 Phlebotonics for haemorrhoids (Review). Cochrane Database of Systematic Reviews, Issue 8 Art. No. CD004322. doi: 10.1002/14651858.CD004322.pub3

Petraglia F, Imperatore A, Challis J 2010 Neuroendocrine mechanisms in pregnancy and parturition. Endocrine Reviews 31:6783–816

Pijnenborg R, Vercruysse L, Brosens I 2011 Deep placentation. Best Practice and Research Clinical Obstetrics and Gynaecology 25:273–85

Pipkin F 2012 Maternal physiology. In: Edmonds K (eds), Dewhurst's textbook of obstetrics and gynaecology, 8th edn. Wiley–Blackwell, Oxford, p 5–15

Ponnapula P, Boberg J 2010 Lower extremity changes experienced during pregnancy. Journal of Foot and Ankle Surgery 49:452–8

Quelopana M, Champion J, Salazar B 2009 Factors predicting the initiation of prenatal care in Mexican women. Midwifery 25:277–85

Ramsay M, James D, Steer P et al 2000 Normal values in pregnancy, 2nd edn. Bailliere Tindall, Oxford

Rasmussen K M, Yaktine A L (eds) 2009 Weight gain during pregnancy: re-examining the Guidelines. Institute of Medicine (IOM) US and National Research Council (US) Committee to Reexamine IOM Pregnancy Weight Guidelines. National Academies Press, Washington, DC

Rebagliato M, Murcia M, Espada M et al 2010 Iodine intake and maternal thyroid function during pregnancy. Epidemiology 21:1

Reitman E, Flood P 2011 Anaesthetic considerations for non-obstetric surgery during pregnancy. British Journal of Anaesthesia 107:S1, i72–i78

Riley H 2011 Weight management before, during and after pregnancy: what are the 'rules'? British Nutrition Foundation Nutrition Bulletin 36:212–15

Russell J, Douglas A, Windle R 2001 The maternal brain: neurobiological and neuroendocrine adaptation and disorders in pregnancy and postpartum. Elsevier Science, Edinburgh

Russell S, Ickovics J, Yaffee R 2010 Parity and untreated dental caries in US women. Journal of Dental Research 89:1091–6

Sage-Femme Collective 2008 Every woman's guide: natural liberty. Sage-Femme Collective, Las Vegas

Saravanan T, Shakila K R, Shanthini K 2012 Pregnancy epulis. Multidisciplinary Dentistry 2(3): 514

Scientific Advisory Committee on Nutrition (SACN) 2012 Dietary reference values for energy 2011. TSO, London

Shynlova O, Kwong R, Lye S 2010 Mechanical stretch regulates hypertrophic phenotype of the myometrium during pregnancy. Reproduction 139:247–53

Shynlova O, Tsui P, Jaffer S et al 2009 Integration of endocrine and mechanical signals in the regulation of myometrial functions during pregnancy and labour. European Journal of Obstetrics, Gynecology and Reproductive Biology 144S:S2–S10

Slager J, Lynne S 2012 Assessment of cervical length and the relationship between short cervix and preterm birth. Journal of Midwifery and Women's Health 57(1):S4–11

Soloff M, Jeng Y, Izban M et al 2011 Effects of progesterone treatment on expression of genes involved in uterine quiescence. Reproductive Sciences 18(8):781–97

Soltanipoor F, Delaram M, Taavoni S et al 2012 The effect of olive oil on prevention of striae gravidarum: a randomized controlled clinical trial. Complementary Therapies in Medicine 20:263–6

Standring S, Borley N, Collins P et al 2008 Gray's anatomy of the human body. The anatomical basis of clinical practice, 40th edn. Churchill Livingstone, London

Suzuki S, Fuse Y 2013 Clinical significance of ptyalism gravidarum. Archives of Gynecology and Obstetrics 287:629–31

Tan K, Zeng X, Sasajala P et al 2011 Fetomaternal microchimerism. Chimerism 2(1):16–18.

Theodorou D, Larentzakis A 2012 The pregnant patient. In: Velmahos G, Degianis E, Doll D (eds), Penetrating trauma. A practical guide on operative technique and peri-operative management. Springer-Verlag, Berlin, p 529–36

Thornton P, Douglas J 2010 Coagulation in pregnancy. Best Practice and Research in Clinical Obstetrics and Gynaecology 24(3):339–52

Timmons B, Akins M, Mahend M 2010 Cervical remodeling during pregnancy and parturition. Trends in Endocrinology and Metabolism 21:353–61

Torgersen K L, Curran C A 2006 A systematic approach to the physiologic adaptations of pregnancy. Critical Care Nursing Quarterly 29:2–19

Ugboma E, Ugboma H, Nwankwo N et al 2012 Sonographic evaluation of the renal volume in normal pregnancy. Journal of Clinical and Diagnostic Research 6(2): 234–8

Weigel M, Coe K, Castro N et al 2011 Food aversions and cravings during early pregnancy: association with nausea and vomiting. Ecology of Food and Nutrition 50(3):197–214

Wild J, Abdul N, Ritchie J et al 2013 Ultrasonography for diagnosis of acute appendicitis (Protocol). Cochrane Database of Systematic Reviews 2013, Issue 2. Art. No. CD010402. doi: 10.1002/14651858. CD010402

Wilson D L, Barnes M, Ellett L et al 2011 Decreased sleep efficiency, increased wake after sleep onset and increased cortical arousals in late pregnancy. Australian and New Zealand Journal of Obstetrics Gynaecology 51(1):38–46

Wong H, Cheung Y, Tait J 2009 Sonographic study of the deciduas basalis in the first trimester of pregnancy. Ultrasound Obstetrics and Gynecology 33:634–7

Young M F, Griffin I, Pressman E et al 2012 Maternal hepcidin is associated with placental transfer of iron derived from dietary heme and nonheme sources. Journal of Nutrition 142(1):33–9

Young R, Hession R 1999 Three-dimensional structure of the smooth muscle in the term-pregnant human uterus. Obstetrics and Gynecology 93(1):94–9

Yousef A, Hanfy H, Elshamy F et al 2011 Postural changes during normal pregnancy. Journal of American Science 7(6):1013–18

Chapter |10|

Antenatal care

Helen Baston

Antenatal care is the care given to a pregnant woman from the time conception is confirmed until the beginning of labour. The midwife facilitates woman-centred care by providing her with accessible and relevant information to help her make informed choices throughout pregnancy. The foundation of this process is the development of a trusting relationship in which the midwife engages with the woman and listens to her story.

THE CHAPTER AIMS TO:

- describe current models of antenatal care
- explore the role of the midwife in providing woman-centred care, identifying the woman's physical, psychological and sociological needs
- discuss the initial assessment visit, define its objectives and consider the significance of the woman's health and social history
- describe the physical examination and psychological support of the woman provided throughout pregnancy.

THE AIM OF ANTENATAL CARE

The aim of antenatal care is to monitor the progress of pregnancy to optimize maternal and fetal health. To achieve this, the midwife critically evaluates the physical, psychological and sociological effects of pregnancy on the woman and her family. This process requires engagement by the midwife, as outlined in Box 10.1.

Historical background

Antenatal care has been provided in the United Kingdom (UK) for almost a century and was first offered in the late 1920s (Ministry of Health 1929). The model of antenatal

---

Box 10.1 **Key principles of antenatal care by the midwife**

- Developing a trusting relationship with the woman.
- Providing a holistic approach to the woman's care that meets her individual need.
- Making a comprehensive assessment of the woman's health and social status, accessing all relevant sources of information.
- Promoting an awareness of the public health issues for the woman and her family.
- Exchanging information with the woman and her family, enabling them to make informed choices about pregnancy and birth.
- Being an advocate for the woman and her family during her pregnancy, supporting her right to choose care appropriate for her own needs and those of her family.
- Identifying potential risk factors and taking the appropriate measures to minimize them.
- Timely sharing of information with relevant agencies and professionals.
- Accurate, contemporaneous documentation of assessments, plans, care and evaluation.
- Recognizing complications of pregnancy and appropriately referring women to the obstetric team or relevant health professionals or other organizations (see Chapters 11–14).
- Preparing the woman and her family to meet the challenges of labour and birth, and facilitating the development of a birth plan.
- Facilitating the woman to make an informed choice about methods of infant feeding and giving appropriate and sensitive advice to support her decision (Chapter 34).
- Offering parenthood education within a planned programme or on an individual basis (Chapter 8).

---

care followed a regime of monthly visits until 28 weeks' gestation, then fortnightly visits until 36 weeks, then weekly visits until the birth of the baby. This model continued for decades but was eventually challenged in the 1980s by Hall et al (1980), whose retrospective analysis demonstrated that conditions requiring hospitalization, including pre-eclampsia, were neither prevented nor detected by antenatal care; and intrauterine growth restriction was over-diagnosed. It was felt that reducing visits for those who did not need them would mean that more support could be given to vulnerable women to improve their outcomes.

To evaluate the impact of reduced antenatal visiting, Sikorski et al (1996) conducted a randomized controlled trial, with low-risk pregnant women, to compare the acceptability and effectiveness of a reduced antenatal visit schedule of six to seven routine visits with the traditional 13 routine visits. No differences in clinical outcome between the two groups were found, but twice as many women in the reduced-visit group were dissatisfied with the frequency of attendance, compared with women who received the full range of visits. The World Health Organization trialled a system of four routine antenatal visits for women assessed as being low risk (Villar et al 2001). They found no statistically significant differences between the outcomes of pre-eclampsia, severe anaemia, urinary tract infection and low birth-weight infants between the intervention group and standard care, in the 24, 678 women enrolled in the study.

Patterns of visiting continue to be investigated and Dowswell et al (2010) compared standard care with reduced visiting schedules investigated in seven randomized controlled trials. They concluded that for high income countries there was no difference between the groups but for low to medium income countries, perinatal mortality was increased in those receiving reduced visits and the authors conclude that visits should not be reduced without close monitoring of the impact on neonatal outcome. As previous research had demonstrated (Clement et al 1996; Villar et al 2001), women prefer more scheduled visits, but as outlined in National Institute for Health and Clinical Excellence (NICE) (2008) guidance, women who had a midwife willing to spend time with them and encourage them to ask questions were more likely to be satisfied with reduced visits than those whose midwife did not offer this.

NICE (2003, 2008) has endorsed a schedule of seven visits for parous women and 10 for primigravid women and this pattern is often reflected in the service specification commissioned (see Box 10.2 for the NICE 2008 recommended visiting pattern). The midwife must continue to use her knowledge and judgement when providing care, as there will be situations where deviation from the pathway will be necessary to ensure safety for either the woman or her unborn baby. In such situations, the midwife should clearly document her rationale and ensure

Box 10.2 **Antenatal visiting pattern as advocated by NICE**

- Booking appointment(s) with midwife by 10 weeks if possible
- 10–14 weeks: ultrasound scan for gestational age
- 16 weeks: midwife
- 18–20 weeks: ultrasound scan for fetal anomalies
- 25 weeks: midwife (nulliparous women)
- 28 weeks: midwife
- 31 weeks: midwife (nulliparous women)
- 34 weeks: midwife
- 36, 38 weeks: midwife
- 40 weeks: midwife (nulliparous women)
- 41 weeks: midwife (discuss options)

Source: NICE 2008

Box 10.3 **Antenatal Quality Standard: quality statements**

Statement 1: Pregnant women are supported to access antenatal care, ideally by 10 weeks 0 days.

Statement 2: Pregnant women are cared for by a named midwife throughout their pregnancy.

Statement 3: Pregnant women have a complete record of the minimum set of antenatal test results in their hand-held maternity notes.

Statement 4: Pregnant women with a body mass index of 30 kg/m^2 or more at the booking appointment are offered personalized advice from an appropriately trained person on healthy eating and physical activity.

Statement 5: Pregnant women who smoke are referred to an evidence-based stop smoking service at the booking appointment.

Statement 6: Pregnant women are offered testing for gestational diabetes if they are identified as at risk of gestational diabetes at the booking appointment.

Statement 7: Pregnant women at high risk of pre-eclampsia at the booking appointment are offered a prescription of 75 mg of aspirin to take daily from 12 weeks until at least 36 weeks.

Statement 8: Pregnant women at intermediate risk of venous thromboembolism at the booking appointment have specialist advice provided about their care.

Statement 9: Pregnant women at high risk of venous thromboembolism at the booking appointment are referred to a specialist service.

Statement 10: Pregnant women are offered fetal anomaly screening in accordance with current UK National Screening Committee programmes.

Statement 11: Pregnant women with an uncomplicated singleton breech presentation at 36 weeks or later (until labour begins) are offered external cephalic version.

Statement 12: Nulliparous pregnant women are offered a vaginal examination for membrane sweeping at their 40- and 41-week antenatal appointments, and parous pregnant women are offered this at their 41-week appointment.

Source: NICE 2012 http://publications.nice.org.uk/quality-standard-for-antenatal-care-qs22/list-of-quality-statements

that she continues to evaluate the care she provides or has requested from other members of the team. If the deviation falls outside the midwife's current remit, she is obliged to 'call such health or social care professionals as may reasonably be expected to have the necessary skills and experience to assist you in the provision of care' (Nursing and Midwifery Council [NMC] 2012: 15).

Current practice

National evidence-based guidelines, in relation to antenatal care have been developed and circulated in the UK since 2003. They were updated in 2008 and reviewed again in 2011 when it was decided that there was insufficient new evidence to warrant a change. They are next due for review in 2014.

In addition to full national clinical guidance, NICE also produce 'Quality Standards' that are 'a concise set of statements designed to drive and measure priority quality improvements within a particular area of care' (NICE 2012). The Antenatal Quality Standard comprises 12 statements and these are detailed in Box 10.3. They are a useful framework for examining maternity services and provide benchmarks for audit and commissioning purposes, although most of them relate to women with risk factors.

Public health role of the midwife

Midwives have always held a privileged position in relation to their ability to influence the health and wellbeing of women and their families. With access to women at a time in their life when they may be open to change their behaviour to achieve a healthy baby, midwives can offer support, information and referral. The public health remit of the midwives was strengthened when their unique position to address inequality was formally recognized in the government White Paper *Saving Lives: Our Healthier Nation* (Department of Health [DH] 1999). It has since been recognized as a significant part of the midwife's role and deeply embedded in the Midwifery 2020 strategy (McNeill et al 2010) and future government policy (DH & National Health Service [NHS] Commissioning Board 2012).

There are a range of health behaviours that impact on life chances and these follow a social gradient. By addressing these public health issues and working together with other agencies, midwives can influence the future health of the population. Extending the boundaries of midwifery care to offer social support can result in positive outcomes in terms of lifestyle, employment and the growth and development of children (Leamon and Viccars 2007). The Marmot Review (2010) examined strategies that could be implemented in order to reduce inequalities in health. It focused on the challenges people face throughout the life course and highlighted the importance of children getting 'the best start in life' (2010: 173). It identified the need to give priority to maternal health interventions and evidence-based parenting support programmes, children's centres, advice and assistance.

Access to care

Early contact with the maternity services, ideally by 10 weeks' gestation, is important so that appropriate and valuable advice relating to screening, nutrition and optimum care of the developing fetus can be given. Medical conditions, infections and lifestyle behaviours may all have a profound and detrimental effect on the fetus during this time.

Women are encouraged to access their midwife through their local health or children's centre on confirmation or suspicion of a positive pregnancy test and should be facilitated to do this. They do not require a formal referral from a General Practitioner (GP). It has been a longstanding conundrum that the people who are most likely to need or benefit from health services are least likely to access them. Often referred to as 'hard to reach' groups, it might be more accurate to describe some *services* as 'hard to reach' and particularly useful to do this when considering how access to services can be increased.

Late booking for antenatal care has been recognized as a feature of many maternal deaths (Lewis 2007; CMACE [Centre for Maternal and Child Enquiries] 2011a). The recent Confidential Enquiry into Maternal Deaths (CMACE 2011a) noted improvement and applauded the fact that recommendations from previous Confidential Enquiries into Maternal Deaths reports are being acted on. However, late booking and poor attendance remains a feature of many maternal deaths. Indeed, 87% of the population at the time of the report had booked by 13 weeks' gestation (DH 2010a) compared with 58% of the women who died from Direct and Indirect causes.

For some women, late booking cannot be avoided if they have arrived only recently in the country. However, these women are particularly vulnerable as they may be naive about how maternity services work, not knowing where they are located, be unable to negotiate public transport and not speak English. Services can be made more accessible if community-based outreach workers and bilingual link/advocacy workers recruited from the target population are employed to provide care (Hollowell et al 2012).

Maternity services can also be difficult to access for indigenous women. They may not recognize the importance of attending early for care to enable valuable health and social care screening to be undertaken. They may be juggling childcare demands with work and financial pressures. Centralization of services may mean that the consultant maternity unit is located in towns or cities, many miles from home. Whilst low-risk women receive the majority of their care in the community, closer to home, for those where there is a complication or a medical condition that requires close monitoring, regular attendance at the consultant unit can be a real challenge.

A flexible approach to the timing of visits and the place of consultation has been incorporated into many maternity services to address issues of access, choice and maternal satisfaction (DH 2007). However, it is equally important that women perceive antenatal care as a valuable resource and an opportunity to receive effective, relevant care from staff who treat them with respect and kindness.

Models of midwifery care

Women can choose from a variety of midwifery care options depending on local availability and their level of risk. The majority of low-risk women receive antenatal care in the community, either at a Children's Centre, GP surgery, or in their own home. Hospital- or community-based clinics are available for women who receive care from an obstetrician or physician in addition to their midwife. Midwifery teams, case loading and independent midwifery (IM) are all examples of how antenatal care can be provided flexibly to meet the needs of individual women. In the UK from early in 2014 IMs will be required to have professional indemnity insurance (PII) for all aspects of midwifery care. The NMC Midwifery Order 2001 will be amended, giving the NMC the power to refuse the right to registration or remove from the register any IM who does not have PII cover (DH 2013).

Options for place of birth include the home, a birth centre (stand-alone or alongside) or a consultant-led unit. National maternity policy promotes birth at home as an option for all women with low-risk pregnancies (DH 2007), but fundamental to this is women's choice and local configuration of services. Women who have identified risk factors or develop complications during pregnancy will usually plan for a hospital birth. However, some women with potentially complex needs may request midwifery-led care, for a range of reason. They should have the opportunity to discuss their hopes and expectations so that a mutually acceptable plan can be agreed, and supported by appropriately skilled midwives.

THE INITIAL ASSESSMENT (BOOKING VISIT)

The purpose of this visit is to initiate the development of a trusting relationship that facilitates the positive engagement of the woman with the maternity service; this is the most important element of antenatal care. Whilst it is crucial that risk assessment and identification of clinical relevant information is obtained, none of these can be undertaken if the woman does not feel able to communicate with the midwife.

Meeting the midwife

The woman's first introduction to midwifery care is crucial in forming her initial impressions of the maternity service. A friendly, professional approach will enable the development of a positive partnership between the woman and the midwife. The initial visit focuses on the exchange of information (Box 10.4) and identification of factors that may require referral to another member of the multi-professional team (Box 10.5). It is a key opportunity for the midwife and the woman to get to know each other. The midwife may meet other members of the family and in this way gain a more informed view of the woman's circumstances. However, the midwife will also recognize that there are occasions when the woman may need to spend time alone with her to facilitate discussion, which she may not feel able to have in the presence of family members.

Box 10.4 Objectives for the initial assessment (booking visit)

- To build the foundation for a trusting relationship in which the woman and midwife are partners in care.
- To assess health by taking a detailed history and offering appropriate screening tests.
- To ascertain baseline recordings of blood pressure, urinalysis, blood values, uterine growth and fetal development to be used as a standard for comparison as the pregnancy progresses.
- To identify risk factors by taking accurate details of past and present midwifery, obstetric, medical, family and personal history.
- To provide an opportunity for the woman and her family to express and discuss any concerns they might have about the current pregnancy and previous pregnancy loss, labour, birth or puerperium.
- To give public health advice pertaining to pregnancy in order to maintain the health of the mother and fetus.
- Make appropriate referral where additional healthcare or support needs have been identified.

Communication

The midwife requires many skills to provide optimal antenatal care: fundamentally, the ability to communicate effectively and sensitively. Listening skills involve focusing on what the woman is saying and how she is saying it, considering the content and tone. In addition, non-verbal

---

Box 10.5 Factors that may require additional antenatal support or referral to an obstetrician/physician/other health professional

Initial assessment
- Age less than 18 years or 40 years and over
- Grande multiparity
- Vaginal bleeding at any time during pregnancy
- Unknown or uncertain expected date of birth
- Late booking

Past obstetric history
- Stillbirth or neonatal death
- Baby small or large for gestational age
- Congenital abnormality
- Rhesus isoimmunization
- Pregnancy-induced hypertension
- Two or more terminations of pregnancy
- Three or more spontaneous miscarriages
- Previous pre-term labour
- Cervical cerclage in past or present pregnancy
- Previous caesarean section or uterine surgery
- Ante- or postpartum haemorrhage
- Precipitate labour
- Multiple pregnancy

Maternal health
- Previous history of deep vein thrombosis or pulmonary embolism
- Chronic illness, e.g. epilepsy, severe asthma, hepatic or renal disease, cystic fibrosis
- Hypertension, cardiac disease
- History of infertility
- Uterine anomalies
- Family history of diabetes or genetic disorders
- Type I or Type II diabetes
- Substance abuse (drugs, alcohol or smoking)
- Psychological or psychiatric disorders

Examination at the initial assessment
- Blood pressure 140/90 mmHg or above
- Maternal obesity or underweight according to BMI
- Blood disorders

Source: NICE 2008

---

responses, including facial expression, body position and eye contact, will influence the quality of the interaction and have the potential to enhance or detract from the development of a positive relationship between woman and midwife (Allison 2012).

The midwife can promote communication with the woman during discussion by gentle questioning, open-ended statements and reflecting back keywords from what is said, to encourage and facilitate exploration of what is meant (Rungapadiachy 1999). Midwives also need to be aware of the language they use, avoiding unnecessary jargon and technical language (Lucas 2006). Communication encompasses writing accurate, comprehensive and contemporaneous records of information given and received and the plan of care that has been agreed (NMC 2009). The midwife must also communicate relevant information with the multiprofessional team (NMC 2008) and with the GP and health visitor in particular (CMACE 2011a).

Taking an antenatal booking history involves a lot of questioning and data collection. However, in completion of the documentation the midwife must be mindful that she needs to have eye contact with the woman in order to facilitate discussion and observe her responses to particular questions. General conversation about the woman's experiences can be a more useful way of sharing information between woman and midwife compared with asking a list of questions or filling in computer data in a mechanistic manner (McCourt 2006).

Personal information

As part of getting to know each other the midwife will introduce herself as the woman's named midwife. She will then clarify the woman's name and the relationship to her of anyone accompanying her. Important details such as date of birth, address and current occupation are written down and provide a useful means of breaking the ice. The woman's age should be considered in relation to local guidelines. For example, it may be a recommendation that women who are 40 years of age or more are offered induction of labour at term (Royal College of Obstetricians and Gynaecologist [RCOG] 2013a). If this is the case, the woman will need to know what her care pathway will be so that she can be fully involved in all decisions. The midwife will explain that she will be asking lots of questions and encourage the woman to ask if anything is unclear.

Social circumstances

It is useful to explore the woman's response to the pregnancy. Some women may be overwhelmed by having to care for a new baby along with other children, they may be isolated or living in poverty. The woman may be a teenager, and experiencing conflict with her parents, social stigma and accommodation concerns. The midwife will need to have a contemporary knowledge of local services and initiatives, such as the Family–Nurse Partnership for pregnant teenagers (DH 2010b), social services and voluntary agencies to make appropriate referrals, in partnership with the woman.

Many women live in complex circumstances and the midwife will sometimes need to ask a range of questions to untangle the details. For example, what are their living arrangements, are there any children from previous relationships and who has custody, to identify if there are any child protection concerns that may need further follow up.

If the woman appears to have difficulty understanding information that is being given, she may have a learning disability or difficulty. It is important to liaise closely with her GP to establish if any diagnosis has been made. Further referral and engagement with social care services may be necessary to ensure that appropriate advocacy and assessment is put in place. There are also many useful visual aids that can support communication where written word is inappropriate.

Domestic abuse is also a possible concern, with a prevalence of 5% to 21% in pregnancy (Leneghan et al 2012). It is important for the midwife to explore this issue sensitively and be aware of the signs or symptoms of domestic abuse. The woman may only disclose information if she is alone hence the midwife should endeavour to provide such opportunities and do so in a secure environment (NICE 2008). Support can then be offered in collaboration with the multi-agency team.

It may become clear that the woman and her unborn baby are potentially vulnerable, for a range of reasons. It is important that the midwife does not display a negative attitude to vulnerable women as this can be a barrier for future access to care (NICE 2010a). There are a range of agencies that can be engaged to provide additional support, including link workers, social workers, health visitors and doulas, depending on local provision. The midwife may need to consider implementation of the Common Assessment Framework (CAF) process in order to make the most appropriate request for additional services (Department for Education [DfE] 2012). This should be undertaken after the booking appointment in line with local policy and with the mother's consent. Any immediate cause for concern should be escalated in line with national guidelines and local policy.

Menstrual history and expected date of birth

The next topic of conversation is the reason that has brought the woman to this appointment. An accurate menstrual history helps determine the expected date of birth (EDB), enables the midwife to predict a birth date and subsequently calculate gestational age at any point in the pregnancy. This is particularly important for the timing of fetal anomaly screening and measuring fetal growth.

The EDB is calculated by adding 9 calendar months and 7 days to the date of the first day of the woman's last menstrual period (known as Naegele's Rule). This method assumes that:

- the woman takes regular note of regularity and length of time between periods;
- conception occurred 14 days after the first day of the last period; this is true only if the woman has a regular 28-day cycle;
- the last period of bleeding was true menstruation; implantation of the ovum may cause slight bleeding;
- breakthrough bleeding and anovulation can be affected by the contraceptive pill thus impacting on the accuracy of a last menstrual period (LMP).

The duration of pregnancy based on Naegele's rule is 280 days. However, if the woman has a 35-day cycle then 7 days should be added; if her cycle is less than 28 days then the appropriate number of days is subtracted. A definitive EDB will be given when the woman attends for her 'dating' ultrasound scan at around 12 weeks of pregnancy.

Obstetric history

Previous childbearing history is important in considering the possible outcome of the current pregnancy and also in relation to how the woman feels about the future. In order to give a summary of a woman's childbearing history, the descriptive terms gravida and para are used. 'Gravid' means 'pregnant', gravida means 'a pregnant woman', and a subsequent number indicates the number of times she has been pregnant regardless of outcome. 'Para' means 'having given birth'; a woman's parity refers to the number of times that she has given birth to a child, live or stillborn, excluding termination of pregnancy. A grande multigravida is a woman who has been pregnant five times or more, irrespective of outcome. A grande multipara is a woman who has given birth five times or more.

Previous childbearing experiences

A sympathetic non-judgemental approach is required to elicit information and encourage the woman to talk freely about her experiences of previous births, miscarriages or terminations. Confidential information may be recorded in a clinic-held summary of the pregnancy and not in the woman's handheld record if she requests this. Where a woman has had a previous traumatic birth experience, subsequent pregnancy may evoke panic and fear (Nilsson et al 2010). This impending birth has the potential to heal or harm and the woman may benefit from being able to talk through what happened and/or engage with a psychological intervention to enable her to achieve closure (Beck and Watson 2010). Where a woman or her partner has lost

a child due to Sudden Infant Death Syndrome (SIDS) or has a close relative who has had this experience, she is likely to be very anxious about the prospect of this happening again. Care of the Next Infant (CONI) is a programme of support facilitated by The Lullaby Trust (previously Foundation for the Study of Infant Deaths FSID) and provided by health visitors (Lullaby Trust 2013). Eligible parents are offered training in resuscitation, monitoring equipment and extra visits and it is paramount that they are referred to the scheme in the antenatal period to ensure that this care can be facilitated in a timely way to allay anxiety.

Repeated spontaneous fetal loss may indicate such conditions as genetic abnormality, hormonal imbalance or incompetent cervix (see Chapter 12). The woman and her partner are likely to be worried about the pregnancy and continuity of carer in these circumstances will be particularly valuable. If there is a history of unexplained stillbirth, the woman should be referred for obstetric antenatal care (RCOG 2010). Some maternity units have special clinics for women who have experienced late fetal loss and most have some means of alerting staff that a woman has previously lost a baby, often with tear-drop sticker in the hospital case notes (SANDS [Stillbirth and Neonatal Death Society] 2012). Staff do need to be mindful of painful anniversaries and be prepared for parents to express a range of emotions, depending on their own particular circumstances (Chapter 26).

Medical and surgical history

During pregnancy both the mother and the fetus may be affected by a medical condition, or a medical condition may be altered by the pregnancy; if untreated there may be serious consequences for the woman's health (CMACE 2011a). For example:

- Women with a history of thrombosis are at greater risk of recurrence during pregnancy, more when over 30 years; have a Body Mass Index (BMI) over 25; have prolonged bed rest; a family history of venous thromboembolism (VTE); have a caesarean birth or travel by air (Farquharson and Greaves 2006). Thromboembolism is the second highest cause of direct maternal death in the UK (CMACE 2011a). All women should have a documented risk assessment for VTE at booking, using a structured tool, and repeated if hospitalized (RCOG 2009). Appropriate thromboprophylaxis and expert referral can be initiated depending on the level of risk identified (Chapter 13).
- Hypertensive disorders encompass gestational hypertension (pre-eclampsia and eclampsia) and chronic/essential hypertension. Essential hypertension is the underlying factor in 90% of chronic cases (Walfish and Hallak 2006). NICE

(2010b) have produced evidence-based guidelines to support monitoring, referral and care (Chapter 13).

- Other conditions, including asthma, epilepsy, infections and psychiatric disorders may require medication, which may adversely affect fetal development. Suicide is a leading cause of maternal death (Lewis 2007; CMACE 2011a), therefore any psychiatric illness prior to the pregnancy must be fully explored so that the most appropriate multidisciplinary care can be offered (NICE 2007) (see Chapter 25). Major medical complications such as diabetes and cardiac conditions require the involvement and support of a medical specialist (Chapter 13).

- Previous surgery should be documented as it may highlight previous problems with anaesthesia or other conditions or complications of relevance. Any surgery of the spine should be noted as this may have an impact on the woman's ability to have an epidural or spinal in labour. Breast surgery may impact on her ability to breastfeed depending on the technique involved. Previous pelvic or abdominal surgery may have consequences requiring specialist advice.

- The woman should be asked if she is taking any medication, either prescribed or over the counter. She should be advised not to take supplements that contain vitamin A and seek advice from the pharmacist before taking any medication throughout pregnancy and when breastfeeding.

Family history

Birth outcomes are multifactorial and may relate to familial or ethnic predisposition as well as economic and social deprivation. The risk of black and Asian mothers having a stillbirth is 2.1 and 1.6 respectively when compared to white mothers (CMACE 2011b). Black African and black Caribbean women have a significantly higher maternal mortality rate than white women, although the trend is declining. Overall, 42% of direct deaths were from minority ethnic or black groups and 1 in 10 maternal deaths were to non-English speaking woman (CMACE 2011a).

Genetic disease in the baby is more likely to occur if the biological parents are close relatives such as first cousins. In a large prospective study (Bundey and Aslam 1993), it is reported that the prevalence of recessive disorders in European babies was 0.28%, compared with 3% in the British Pakistanis in the study. Hence, while there is an increased risk of recessive genetic disorders in babies born to married cousins, most babies are healthy. However, there is a lack of information for parents at risk and they face the additional barriers of fear, stigma and language barriers (Khan et al 2010). Where it has been identified that a couple are first cousins, genetic counselling should be offered.

Diabetes, although not inherited, leads to a predisposition in other family members, particularly if they become pregnant or obese. Screening for gestational diabetes is now recommended for women with a BMI of 30 or more; previous baby weighing 4.5 kg or more; previous gestational diabetes and/or first-degree relative with diabetes (NICE 2008). Hypertension also has a familial component and multiple pregnancy has a higher incidence in certain families. Some conditions such as sickle cell anaemia and thalassaemia are more common in those of black Caribbean, African-Caribbean, African, Pakistani, Cypriot, Bangladeshi and Chinese ethnicity (NICE 2008); and the Family Origin Questionnaire (FOQ) is used at the booking visit to screen couples at risk (Chapter 11).

Lifestyle

Healthy eating

General health should be discussed and good habits reinforced, giving further advice when required. All women should be provided with information about healthy eating, and vitamin D supplementation (10 micrograms per day) is suggested for all women during pregnancy and breastfeeding to maintain bone and teeth health (NICE 2008). Particular recommendation should be given to women at risk of deficiency (NICE 2008). Women should take 400 micrograms of folic acid each day prior to pregnancy and until 12 weeks' gestation to reduce the risk of a neural tube defect. Some women, such as those on anticonvulsant medication, especially sodium valproate, are at increased risk of having a fetus affected by a neural tube defect. In such cases it is recommended that the woman consults her GP and takes a higher dose of 5 milligrams (5 mg) of folic acid.

The midwife should advise the woman about eating a balanced diet during pregnancy and not 'eating for two' (NICE 2010c). It is currently not recommended that women attempt to lose weight during pregnancy. Women should also be informed about which foods they should avoid, e.g. pate, liver products and soft cheeses; food to limit, e.g. tuna, caffeine; and foods where precaution is needed, e.g. sushi and eggs. Full details can be found on the Food Standards Agency (2013) website.

Exercise

NICE (2010c) require health professionals to discuss how physically active a woman is at her first antenatal visit, providing her with tailored information and advice. Usual aerobic or strength conditioning exercise should be continued (RCOG 2006). Not only will this enhance general wellbeing, but also reduce stress and anxiety and prepare the body for the challenge of labour. Any activity that can cause trauma or physical injury to the woman or fetus should be avoided (RCOG 2006). In addition, NICE

(2010c) also recommend at least 30 minutes of moderate activity each day, keeping sedentary activities to a minimum. Sexual intercourse during pregnancy may continue and has been found to reduce the likelihood of preterm labour between 29 and 36 weeks (Sayle et al 2001).

Smoking

Approximately 13.3% of women are smokers at the time they give birth (DH 2011), however the rate varies between cities and between wards within cities. Some women may be ready to cut down or give up smoking, while others may not want to change their smoking behaviour (Prochaska 1992). The midwife can be influential in motivating the woman to quit smoking by complying with NICE guidelines (2010d). She should offer carbon monoxide (CO) screening to all women at each antenatal contact and refer women to a stop smoking service if they smoke or their CO level is 7 parts per million (ppm) or more. This provides an opportunity to provide non-judgemental advice and support (Grice and Baston 2011). Smoking in pregnancy is associated with birth defects (Huckshaw et al 2011) and a range of conditions that compromise the infant's health and wellbeing including: low birth weight, intellectual impairment, respiratory dysfunction, Sudden Infant Death Syndrome and premature birth (Godfrey et al 2010).

Nicotine replacement therapy should be discussed with women having difficulty quitting smoking (NICE 2010d) but only used if she is abstaining from smoking. The woman, her partner and other family members should be informed about the direct and passive effects of smoking on the baby and aim to have a smoke-free home. Family members should be directed to Stop Smoking Services as living with a smoker makes it very difficult for pregnant women to quit (Koshy et al 2010).

Alcohol and drug misuse

The effects of excessive maternal alcohol on the fetus are marked, particularly in the 1st trimester when fetal alcohol syndrome can develop. This syndrome consists of restricted growth, facial abnormalities, central nervous system problems, behavioural and learning difficulties and is entirely preventable (Thackray and Tifft 2001). It is recommended that pregnant women abstain from alcohol during the first trimester and drink no more than one to two UK units once or twice a week thereafter (NICE 2008). The midwife also needs to ask prospective parents if they take illicit drugs, regardless of their social status. Many maternity units have a substance misuse team that can support the care of women who abuse alcohol/drugs. Such care should be provided by a named midwife or doctor who has specialized knowledge and experience in this field (NICE 2010a).

Risk assessment

The booking assessment shapes the direction of a woman's antenatal pathway. It is where her 'risk status' (CMACE 2011a) is determined and appropriate referral made. The information gathered regarding the woman's obstetric, medical and social history and current pregnancy enables the midwife to assess her risk status. The midwife must also seek additional information from the GP (CMACE 2011a) and access previous case notes to elicit all the relevant information. If a risk factor is identified (see Box 10.4) the woman should be referred to a consultant obstetrician, who will discuss a plan for care for her based on the need to access additional expertise and resources. Place of birth may also be influenced by the risk assessment but in all cases the ultimate decision is taken by the woman. Where a woman choses a path of care that could cause significant harm to her or her baby, the midwife should discuss the evidence with her, document these discussions and inform someone in authority of her concerns (NMC 2008: 5). The midwife should listen to a woman's rationale for requesting a particular path of care and respect her right to decline treatment (NMC 2008:3). Advice can always be sought from a supervisor of midwives, 24 hours a day (NMC 2012).

PHYSICAL EXAMINATION

Prior to conducting the physical examination of a pregnant woman, her consent and comfort are primary considerations. Observation of physical characteristics is important. Poor posture and gait can indicate back problems or previous trauma to the pelvis. The woman may be lethargic, which could be an indication of extreme tiredness, anaemia, malnutrition or depression. It is therefore important to look holistically at the woman and her family and assess fetal growth and development by recognized markers in conjunction with this knowledge.

Weight

Obesity is literally a growing problem, with approximately 16% of women starting pregnancy with a BMI of 30 kg/m² (Heslehurst et al 2010). There are no evidence-based UK guidelines regarding what constitutes normal weight gain in pregnancy (NICE 2010c). However, in the United States (US) it is recommended that women of normal BMI should gain between 11.5 and 16 kg (Rasmussen and Yaktine 2009). Referral to an obstetrician should be made if the woman's BMI is <18 kg/m² or ≥30 kg/m² (NICE 2008). Women with a BMI in the obese range are more at risk of complications of pregnancy. These may include gestational diabetes, pregnancy-induced hypertension (PIH) and shoulder dystocia. There may also be difficulty in palpating the fetal parts and defining presentation, position or engagement of the fetus. Overweight or underweight women should be carefully monitored, have additional care from an obstetrician, and be offered appropriate support, including nutritional counselling within the multiprofessional team (see Chapter 13). Women with a BMI of 30 or more should be offered a glucose tolerance test. There is emerging evidence (Thangaratinam et al 2012) that maternal and neonatal outcomes can be improved by lifestyle and dietary interventions that reduce maternal weight gain, but is currently not advised to lose weight during pregnancy.

Blood pressure

Blood pressure is taken in order to ascertain normality and provide a baseline reading for comparison throughout pregnancy. Systolic blood pressure does not alter significantly in pregnancy, but diastolic falls in mid-pregnancy and rises to near non-pregnant levels at term. The systolic recording may be falsely elevated if a woman is nervous or anxious, if a small cuff is used on a large arm, the arm is unsupported or if the bladder is full. The woman should be comfortably seated or resting in a lateral position on the couch for the measurement. Brachial artery pressure is highest when the subject is sitting and lower when in the recumbent position. Current opinion is that Korotkoff V should be used (Walfish and Hallak 2006).

Urinalysis

At the first visit the woman should be offered screening to exclude asymptomatic bacteriuria (NICE 2008; NSC [National Screening Committee] 2012a). Because the condition is asymptomatic the woman is unaware of disease; treatment could reduce the risk of pyelonephritis and preterm labour (Williams 2006) (see Chapter 11).

Urinalysis is performed at every visit to exclude proteinuria which may be a symptom of pre-eclampsia (NICE 2008) (see Chapter 13). NICE (2008) does not currently recommend routine testing for glycosuria.

Blood tests

The midwife should explain why blood tests are carried out at the booking visit to facilitate informed decision making about the tests that are available. There are many views as to the ethical issues involved in screening. It is important to gain informed consent for any blood tests undertaken (NMC 2008) and offer appropriate counselling before and after the screening is carried out.

The midwife should be fully aware of the difference between screening and diagnostic tests, and their accuracy, and discuss these options with women. Blood tests offered at the initial assessment include the following.

ABO blood group and Rhesus (Rh) factor

It is important to identify the blood group, RhD status and red cell antibodies in pregnant women, so haemolytic disease of the newborn (HDN) can be prevented and preparations made for blood transfusion if it becomes necessary. Blood will be taken at booking and again at 28 weeks to determine if antibodies are present (NICE 2008). All Rh-negative women will be offered two doses of prophylactic anti-D 500 International Units (IU) at 28 and 34 weeks' gestation or a single dose of 1500 IU at 28–30 weeks' gestation (NICE 2008). Threatened miscarriage, amniocentesis, chorionic villus sampling, external cephalic version or any other uterine trauma are indications for the administration of anti-D gammaglobulin within a 72 hours of the event in pregnancy in addition to that given at 28 and 34 weeks (RCOG 2011a). A Kleihauer test should be undertaken to assess how much anti-D is required (RCOG 2011a). If the titration demonstrates a rising antibody response then more frequent assessment will be made in order to plan management by a specialist in Rhesus disease (see Chapter 11).

Full blood count

This is taken to observe the woman's general blood condition, and includes haemoglobin (Hb) estimations. If the mean cell volume (MCV) is found to be low on the full blood count result, serum ferritin levels are also taken in order to assess the adequacy of iron stores. Iron supplementation is not considered necessary in women who are taking adequate dietary iron and who have a normal Hb and MCV at the initial assessment.

There is evidence that supplementing non-anaemic women with iron can increase the risk of hypertension and the small for gestational age birth rate (Ziaei et al 2007). The decision to use supplements should be made on an individual woman's circumstances and include clear information about dietary iron sources. Maximum absorption of iron in meat or green leafy vegetables will be achieved by consuming vitamin C at the same time and avoiding caffeine. The intestinal mucosa has a limited ability to absorb iron and when this is exceeded extra iron is excreted in the stools.

Other screening tests

Venereal disease research laboratory (VDRL) test

This is performed for syphilis. Not all positive results indicate active syphilis; early testing will allow a woman to be treated in order to prevent infection of the fetus (see Chapter 11).

HIV antibodies

Routine screening to detect HIV infection should be offered in pregnancy (NSC 2013) as treatment in pregnancy is beneficial in reducing vertical transmission to the fetus (Chapter 11). Specialist teams should be involved in the subsequent care and management of women with a positive diagnosis.

Rubella immune status

This is determined by measuring the rubella antibody titre (Chapter 11). Women who are not immune must be advised to avoid contact with anyone with the disease. The live vaccination is offered postnatally, and subsequent pregnancy must be avoided for at least 3 months.

Haemoglobinopathies

All women should be offered screening for sickle cell disease or thalassaemias early in pregnancy. Some ethnic groups have a higher incidence than others and the type of screening will depend on the prevalence (NICE 2008). If a woman either has or is a carrier of one of these diseases her partner's blood should also be tested. The couple will be offered genetic counselling and management during pregnancy will be explained (Chapter 11).

Hepatitis B

Screening is offered in pregnancy so that infected women can be offered postnatal intervention to reduce the risk of mother-to-baby transmission (NICE 2008). Chapter 11 explores this issue in more detail.

Screening for fetal anomaly

The midwife will also explain to the woman the current options regarding fetal anomaly screening and provide her with written information to enable her to make an informed choice. She will inform her about the routine dating and anomaly scans which are part of the screening programme. See Chapter 11 for further details.

Infections NOT routinely screened for in pregnancy

Hepatitis C

This is currently not recommended as a routine screening test in pregnancy because there is insufficient evidence regarding the prevalence and effectiveness of treatments to reduce transmission to the baby (NSC 2013).

Chlamydia

It is not recommended that all women are routinely screened (NSC 2011), however women under 25 years of age are offered this as part of the National Chlamydia Screening Programme (Public Health England 2013).

Cytomegalovirus and toxoplasmosis

These are not routinely tested in pregnancy because tests do not currently determine which pregnancies may result in an infected fetus (NICE 2008). Toxoplasmosis screening is not recommended because the risks of screening may outweigh the benefits; however, women need to be informed of how to avoid contracting the infection (NICE 2008).

Group B streptococcus

The NSC (2012b) reviewed this guidance and conclude that screening should not be offered currently but might be a consideration in the future (see Chapter 11).

THE MIDWIFE'S EXAMINATION

The midwife's general examination of the woman should be holistic and encompass the woman's physical, social and psychological wellbeing. This antenatal contact gives the midwife an opportunity to look at the woman's face and assess her health and general wellbeing, including demeanour and signs of fatigue. If at any time the midwife notices any sign of ill health she should discuss this with the woman, and advocate referral to the most appropriate health professional (NMC 2012).

The midwife should facilitate discussion about infant feeding throughout pregnancy (UNICEF [United Nations Children's Fund] 2012). Where breastfeeding peer support is available, introductions should be made so that postnatal support can be more easily accessed. Breastfeeding should be promoted in a sensitive manner, and information given about the benefits to both mother and baby (Chapter 34). Most women will not require an examination of their breasts. Current evidence does not support the benefits of nipple preparation (see Chapter 34). The midwife may also discuss the woman's experiences of breast changes so far in her pregnancy, and expected changes as pregnancy progresses.

Some women will appreciate information about the body changes taking place during pregnancy. Increasing abdominal size may be an acceptable body change but breast changes may not have been anticipated. For most women, breast size and appearance are an important part of their body image. Partners may also be affected by the changes and the midwife can encourage open and honest discussion between the woman and her partner to help to resolve anxieties.

Bladder and bowel function may be discussed; dietary advice may be necessary at this visit or later in the pregnancy with reference to how hormonal changes may alter normal bowel and kidney function. Early referral within the multidisciplinary team will be necessary if treatment is required or problems identified. Vaginal discharge (leucorrhoea) increases in pregnancy; the woman may discuss any increase or changes with the midwife. If the discharge is itchy, causes soreness, is any colour other than creamy-white or has an offensive odour then infection is likely, and should be investigated further. Later in pregnancy the woman may report a change from leucorrhoea to a heavier mucous discharge.

Early bleeding is not uncommon, however if this is reported the woman can be referred to an Early Pregnancy Assessment Unit for confirmation of pregnancy and advice and appropriate care and follow-up. Ultrasound will usually confirm a diagnosis. The woman may require anti-D immunoglobulin if she is Rhesus-negative within 72 hours (see Chapter 22 for management of antepartum haemorrhage).

In the past midwives have palpated the uterus once it has entered the abdomen, from about 12 weeks' gestation; however, current guidelines suggest that because of sophisticated scanning techniques there is no benefit in palpating the uterus prior to 24 weeks' gestation, at which time uterine growth can be measured (NICE 2008).

Oedema

This should not be evident during the initial assessment but may occur as the pregnancy progresses. Physiological oedema occurs after rising in the morning and worsens during the day; it is often associated with daily activities or hot weather. At visits later in pregnancy the midwife should observe for oedema and ask the woman about symptoms. Often the woman may notice that her rings feel tighter and her ankles are swollen. Pitting oedema in the lower limbs can be identified by applying gentle fingertip pressure over the tibial bone: a depression will remain when the finger is removed. If oedema reaches the knees, affects the face or is increasing in the fingers it may be indicative of hypertension of pregnancy if other markers are also present.

Varicosities

These are more likely to occur during pregnancy and are a predisposing cause of deep vein thrombosis. The woman should be asked if she has any pain in her legs. Reddened areas on the calf may be due to varicosities, phlebitis or deep vein thrombosis. Areas that appear white as if deprived of blood could be caused by deep vein thrombosis. The woman should be asked to report any tenderness that she feels either during the examination or at any time during the pregnancy. Referral should be made to medical colleagues as appropriate (NMC 2012). Support stockings will help alleviate symptoms although not prevent varicose veins occurring (NICE 2008).

Abdominal examination

Abdominal examination is carried out from 24 weeks' gestation to establish and affirm that fetal growth is consistent with gestational age during the pregnancy. The specific aims are to:

- observe the signs of pregnancy
- assess fetal size and growth
- auscultate the fetal heart when indicated
- locate fetal parts
- detect any deviation from normal.

Preparation

The woman should be asked to empty her bladder before making herself comfortable on the couch. A full bladder will make the examination uncomfortable; this can also make the measurement of fundal height less accurate. The midwife washes her hands and exposes only that area of the abdomen she needs to palpate, and covers the remainder of the woman to promote privacy and protect her dignity. The woman should be lying comfortably with her arms by her sides to relax the abdominal muscles. The midwife should discuss her findings throughout the abdominal examination with the woman.

Inspection

The uterus is first assessed by observation. A full bladder, distended colon or obesity may give a false impression of fetal size. The shape of the uterus is longer than it is broad when the lie of the fetus is longitudinal, as occurs in the majority of cases. If the lie of the fetus is transverse, the uterus is low and broad.

The multiparous uterus may lack the snug ovoid shape of the primigravid uterus. Often it is possible to see the shape of the fetal back or limbs. If the fetus is in an occipitoposterior position a saucer-like depression may be seen at or below the umbilicus. The midwife may observe fetal movements, or the mother may feel them; this can help the midwife determine the position of the fetus. The woman's umbilicus becomes less dimpled as pregnancy advances and may protrude slightly in later weeks.

Lax abdominal muscles in the parous woman may cause the uterus to sag forwards; this is known as pendulous abdomen or anterior obliquity of the uterus. In the primigravida it is a significant sign as it may be due to pelvic contraction.

Skin changes

Stretch marks from previous pregnancies appear silvery and recent ones appear pink. A linea nigra may be seen; this is a normal dark line of pigmentation running longitudinally in the centre of the abdomen below and sometimes above the umbilicus. Scars may indicate previous obstetric or abdominal surgery or self-harm.

Palpation

The midwife's hands should be clean and warm; cold hands do not have the necessary acute sense of touch, they tend to induce contraction of the abdominal and uterine muscles and the woman may find palpation uncomfortable. Arms and hands should be relaxed and the pads, not the tips, of the fingers used with delicate precision. The hands are moved smoothly over the abdomen to avoid causing contractions.

Measuring fundal height

In order to determine the height of the fundus the midwife places her hand just below the xiphisternum. Pressing gently, she moves her hand down the abdomen until she feels the curved upper border of the fundus (Fig. 10.1).

Clinically assessing the uterine size to compare it with gestation does not always produce an accurate result, although there are landmarks that can be used as an approximate guide (see Fig. 10.2). From 25 weeks of pregnancy, the midwife should commence serial symphysis fundal height (SFH) measurements (Fig. 10.3). She uses a tape measure (with the centimetres facing the mother's abdomen) held at the fundus and extended down to the symphysis pubis, to take a single measurement. This should be recorded in the pregnancy record and plotted on a customized chart rather than a population-based chart (RCOG 2013b).

Further investigation is warranted and an ultrasound scan will usually be required alongside appropriate medical referral, if:

- a single measurement plots below the 10th centile; *or*
- serial measurements show slow growth by crossing centiles (RCOG 2013b).

If the uterus is unduly big the fetus maybe large or it may indicate multiple pregnancy or polyhydramnios. When the uterus is smaller than expected the LMP date may be incorrect, or the fetus may be small for gestational age (SGA). Fetal growth restriction (FGR) is associated with stillbirth and expert opinion suggests that early detection and management can reduce the incidence by 20% (Imdad et al 2011).

Fundal palpation

This determines the presence of the breech or the head in the fundus. This information will help to diagnose the lie and presentation of the fetus. Talking through the palpation with the woman, making eye contact with her during the procedure, the midwife lays both hands on the sides of the fundus, fingers held close together and curving round the upper border of the uterus. Gentle yet deliberate pressure is applied using the palmar surfaces of the fingers to determine the soft consistency and indefinite outline that denotes the breech. Sometimes the buttocks feel rather firm but they are not as hard, smooth or well defined as the head. With a gliding movement the fingertips are separated slightly in order to grasp the fetal mass, which may be in the centre or deflected to one side, to assess its size and mobility. The breech cannot be moved independently of the body but the head can (Fig. 10.4). The head is much more distinctive in outline than the breech, being hard and round; it can be balloted (moved from one hand to the other) between the fingertips of the two hands because of the free movement of the neck.

Lateral palpation

This is used to locate the fetal back in order to determine position. The hands are placed on either side of the uterus

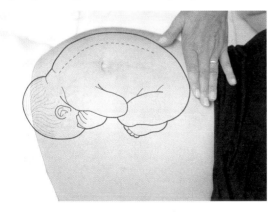

Fig. 10.1 Assessing the fundal height in finger-breadths below the xiphisternum.

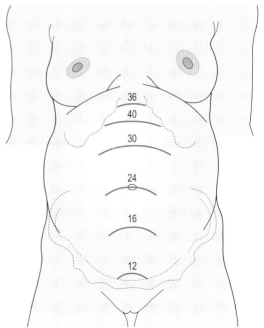

Fig. 10.2 Growth of the uterus, showing the fundal heights at various weeks of pregnancy.

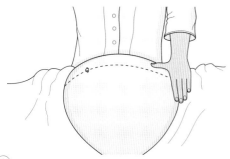

(A)   Palpate to determine fundus with two hands

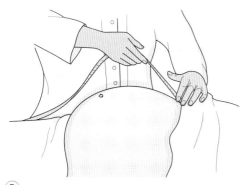

(B)   Secure tape with hand at top of fundus

Fig. 10.3 Measuring fundal height.
(From Morse K, Williams A, Gardosi J 2009 Fetal growth screening by fundal height measurement. Best Practice & Research Clinical Obstetrics and Gynaecology 23:809–18. www.perinatal.org.uk/ FetalGrowth/FundalHeight.aspx. Reproduced with permission.)

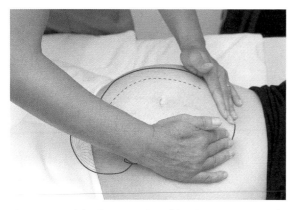

Fig. 10.4 Fundal palpation. Palms of hands on either side of the fundus, fingers held close together palpate the upper pole of the uterus.

at the level of the umbilicus (Fig. 10.5). Gentle pressure is applied with alternate hands in order to detect which side of the uterus offers the greater resistance. More detailed information is obtained by feeling along the length of each side with the fingers. This can be done by sliding the hands down the abdomen while feeling the sides of the uterus alternately. Some midwives prefer to steady the uterus with one hand, and using a rotary movement of the opposite hand, to map out the back as a continuous smooth resistant mass from the breech down to the neck; on the other side the same movement reveals the limbs as small parts that slip about under the examining fingers.

'Walking' the fingertips of both hands over the abdomen from one side to the other is another method of locating the fetal back (Fig. 10.6).

Pelvic palpation

Pelvic palpation will identify the pole of the fetus in the pelvis; it should not cause discomfort to the woman. NICE

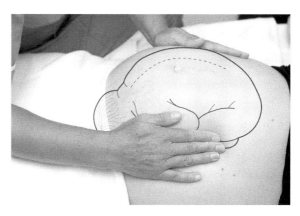

Fig. 10.5 Lateral palpation. Hands placed at umbilical level on either side of the uterus. Pressure is applied alternately with each hand.

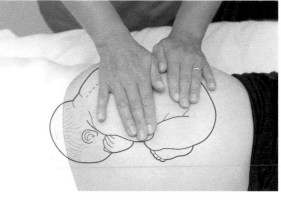

Fig. 10.6 'Walking' the fingertips across the abdomen to locate the position of the fetal back.

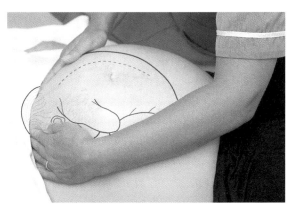

Fig. 10.7 Pelvic palpation. The fingers are directed inwards and downwards.

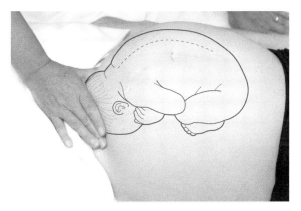

Fig. 10.8 Pawlik's manoeuvre. The lower pole of the uterus is grasped with the right hand, the midwife facing the woman's head.

(2008) recommend this is done only from 36 weeks onwards.

The midwife should ask the woman to bend her knees slightly in order to relax the abdominal muscles and also suggest that she breathe steadily; relaxation may be helped if she sighs out slowly. The sides of the uterus just below umbilical level are grasped snugly between the palms of the hands with the fingers held close together, and pointing downwards and inwards (Fig. 10.7).

If the head is presenting (towards the lower part of the uterus), a hard mass with a distinctive round smooth surface will be felt. The midwife should also estimate how much of the fetal head is palpable above the pelvic brim to determine engagement. This two-handed technique appears to be the most comfortable for the woman and gives the most information.

Pawlik's manoeuvre, where the practitioner grasps the lower pole of the uterus between her fingers and thumb, which should be spread wide enough apart to accommodate the fetal head (Fig. 10.8), is sometimes used to judge

the size, flexion and mobility of the head, but undue pressure must not be applied. It should be used only if absolutely necessary as it can be very uncomfortable for the woman: There is no research evidence to support one method over the other.

Engagement

Engagement is said to have occurred when the widest presenting transverse diameter of the fetal head has passed through the brim of the pelvis. In cephalic presentations this is the biparietal diameter and in breech presentations the bitrochanteric diameter. In a primigravid woman, the head normally engages at any time from about 36 weeks of pregnancy, but in a multipara this may not occur until after the onset of labour. Engagement of the fetal head is usually measured in fifths palpable above the pelvic brim. When the vertex presents and the head is engaged the following will be evident on clinical examination:

- only two- to three-fifths of the fetal head is palpable above the pelvic brim (Fig. 10.9);
- the head will not be mobile.

On rare occasions, the head is not palpable abdominally because it has descended deeply into the pelvis. If the head is not engaged, the findings are as follows:

- more than half of the head is palpable above the brim
- the head may be high and freely movable (ballotable) or partly settled in the pelvic brim and consequently immobile.

In a primigravid woman, it is usual for the head to engage by 37 weeks' gestation; however this is not always the case. When labour starts, the force of labour contractions encourages flexion and moulding of the fetal head and the relaxed ligaments of the pelvis allow the joints to give. This is usually sufficient to allow engagement and descent. Other causes of a non-engaged head at term include:

- occipitoposterior position
- full bladder
- wrongly calculated gestational age
- polyhydramnios
- placenta praevia or other space-occupying lesion
- multiple pregnancy
- pelvic abnormalities
- fetal abnormality.

Presentation

Presentation refers to the part of the fetus that lies at the pelvic brim or in the lower pole of the uterus. Presentations can be vertex, breech, shoulder, face or brow (Fig. 10.10). Vertex, face and brow are all head or cephalic presentations.

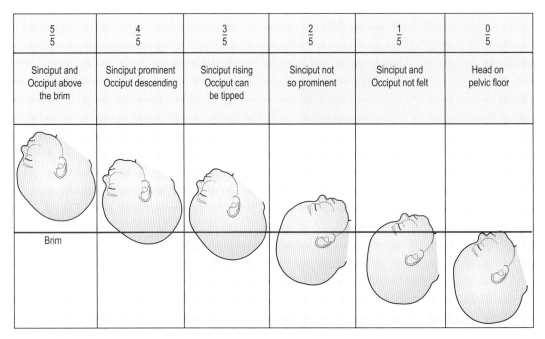

$\frac{5}{5}$	$\frac{4}{5}$	$\frac{3}{5}$	$\frac{2}{5}$	$\frac{1}{5}$	$\frac{0}{5}$
Sinciput and Occiput above the brim	Sinciput prominent Occiput descending	Sinciput rising Occiput can be tipped	Sinciput not so prominent	Sinciput and Occiput not felt	Head on pelvic floor

Fig. 10.9 Descent of the fetal head estimated in fifths palpable above the pelvic brim.

When the head is flexed the vertex presents; when it is fully extended the face presents; and when it is partially extended the brow presents (Fig. 10.11). It is more common for the head to present because the bulky breech finds more space in the fundus, which is the widest diameter of the uterus, and the head lies in the narrower lower pole. The muscle tone of the fetus also plays a part in maintaining its flexion and consequently its vertex presentation.

Auscultation

Listening to the fetal heart has historically been an important part of the process. However, NICE (2008) does not recommend routine listening other than at maternal request because there is no clinical benefit. A Pinard's fetal stethoscope will enable the midwife to hear the fetal heart directly and determine that it is fetal and not maternal. The stethoscope is placed on the mother's abdomen, at right-angles to it over the fetal back (Fig. 10.12). The ear must be in close, firm contact with the stethoscope but the hand should not touch it while listening because then extraneous sounds are produced. The stethoscope should be moved about until the point of maximum intensity is located where the fetal heart is heard most clearly. The midwife should count the beats per minute, which should be in the range of 110–160. The midwife should take the woman's pulse at the same time as listening to the fetal heart to enable her to distinguish between the two. In addition, ultrasound equipment (e.g. a sonicaid or

Doppler) can be used for this purpose so that the woman and her partner/children may also hear the fetal heartbeat.

Lie

The lie of the fetus is the relationship between the long axis of the fetus and the long axis of the uterus (Figs 10.13–10.15). In the majority of cases the lie is longitudinal due to the ovoid shape of the uterus; the remainder are oblique or transverse. Oblique lie, when the fetus lies diagonally across the long axis of the uterus, must be distinguished from obliquity of the uterus, when the whole uterus is tilted to one side (usually the right) and the fetus lies longitudinally within it. When the lie is transverse the fetus lies at right angles across the long axis of the uterus. This is often visible on inspection of the abdomen.

Attitude

Attitude is the relationship of the fetal head and limbs to its trunk. The attitude should be one of flexion. The fetus is curled up with chin on chest, arms and legs flexed, forming a snug, compact mass, which utilizes the space in the uterine cavity most effectively. If the fetal head is flexed the smallest diameters will present and, with efficient uterine action, labour will be most effective.

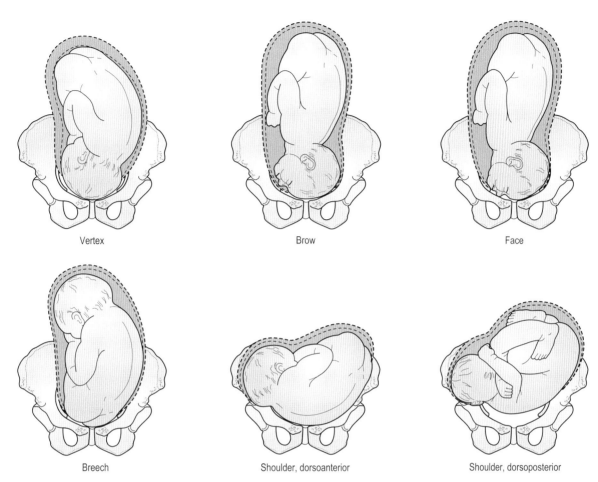

Fig. 10.10 **The five presentations.**

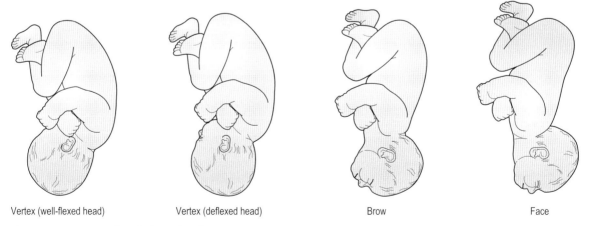

Fig. 10.11 **Varieties of cephalic or head presentation.**

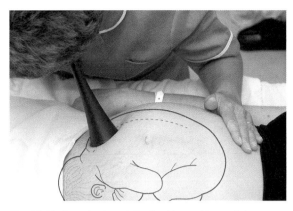

Fig. 10.12 Auscultation of the fetal heart. Vertex right occipitoanterior.

Denominator

'Denominate' means 'to give a name to'; the denominator is the name of the part of the presentation, which is used when referring to fetal position. Each presentation has a different denominator and these are as follows:

- in the vertex presentation it is the occiput
- in the breech presentation it is the sacrum
- in the face presentation it is the mentum.

Although the shoulder presentation is said to have the acromion process as its denominator, in practice the dorsum is used to describe the position. In the brow presentation no denominator is used.

Position

The position is the relationship between the denominator of the presentation and six points on the pelvic brim (Fig. 10.16). In addition, the denominator may be found in the midline either anteriorly or posteriorly, especially late in labour. This position is often transient and is described as direct anterior or direct posterior.

Anterior positions are more favourable than posterior positions because when the fetal back is at the front of the uterus it conforms to the concavity of the mother's abdominal wall and the fetus can flex more easily. When the back is flexed the head also tends to flex and a smaller diameter presents to the pelvic brim. There is also more room in the anterior part of the pelvic brim for the broad biparietal diameter of the head. The positions in a vertex presentation are summarized in Box 10.6 and shown in Fig. 10.17.

Findings

The findings from the abdominal palpation should be considered part of the holistic assessment of the pregnant woman's health and fetal wellbeing. The midwife collates all the information she has gathered from inspection, palpation and auscultation and relays this to the woman. Deviation from the expected growth and development should be discussed with the woman and referral to an obstetrician or appropriate professional arranged and documented as appropriate (NMC 2012).

ONGOING ANTENATAL CARE

The information gathered during the antenatal visits will enable the midwife and pregnant woman to determine the appropriate pattern of antenatal care (NICE 2008). The timing and number of visits will vary according to individual need and changes should be made as circumstances dictate (e.g. as demonstrated in Box 10.7).

Indicators of maternal wellbeing

The woman's general health and wellbeing is observed throughout and the midwife must remain vigilant for signs of domestic abuse, emotional fragility and social instability. Endeavouring to maintain continuity of carer will be a key process for identifying impending problems and for encouraging free exchange of information between the woman and her midwife. There should be clear referral pathways for the midwife to follow when she has cause for concern regarding a woman's obstetric, social or emotional wellbeing.

Surveillance for symptoms of pre-eclampsia is ongoing throughout pregnancy. It has been recommended by NICE (2008: para 1.9.2.5) that if there is a 'single diastolic blood pressure of 110 mmHg or two consecutive readings of 90 mmHg at least 4 hours apart and/or significant proteinuria (1+)', there should be an increase in surveillance (see Chapter 13).

Indicators of fetal wellbeing

These include:

- increasing uterine size compatible with the gestational age of the fetus;
- fetal movements that follow a regular pattern from the time when they are first felt;
- fetal heart rate that is regular and variable with a rate between 110 and 160 beats/minute.

Eliciting information about recent fetal movements reminds the woman of the importance of noticing this feedback from her baby. Women should be reminded that there should be no reduction in fetal movements in the last trimester (RCOG 2011b) and to contact their midwife if they notice a reduction. Recurrent reduction in fetal movements is associated with a poor fetal outcome (O'Sullivan et al 2009). However, NICE (2008), and

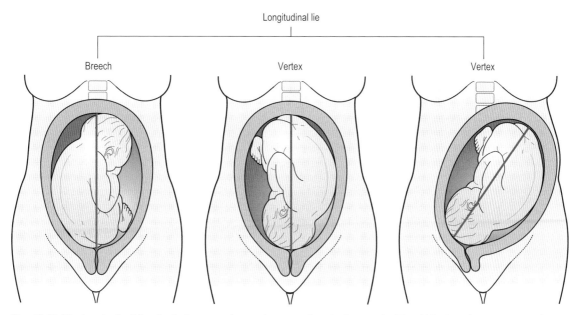

Longitudinal lie

Breech   Vertex   Vertex

Fig. 10.13 The longitudinal lie. Confusion sometimes exists regarding the lie seen in (C), which gives the impression of an oblique lie, but the fetus is longitudinal in relation to the uterus and merely moving the uterus abdominally rectifies the presumed obliquity.

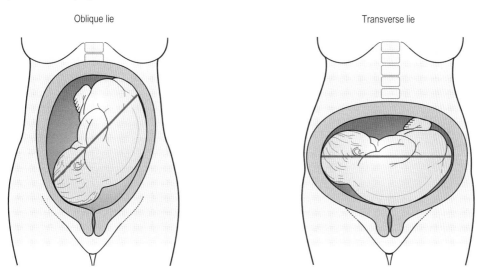

Oblique lie   Transverse lie

Fig. 10.14 Shows an oblique lie because the long axis of the fetus is oblique in relation to the uterus.

Fig. 10.15 Shows a transverse lie with shoulder presentation.

Figs 10.13–10.15 **The lie of the fetus.**

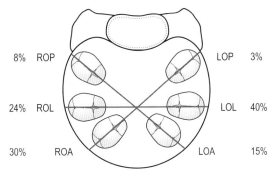

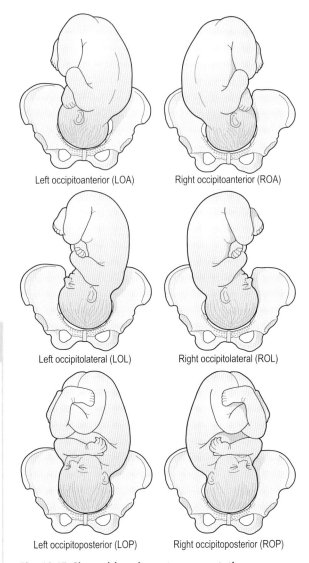

8%	ROP		LOP	3%
24%	ROL		LOL	40%
30%	ROA		LOA	15%

Fig. 10.16 Diagrammatic representation of the six vertex positions and their relative frequency. LOA, left occipitoanterior; LOL, left occipitolateral; LOP, left occipitoposterior; ROA, right occipitoanterior; ROL, right occipitolateral; ROP, right occipitoposterior.

Left occipitoanterior (LOA) Right occipitoanterior (ROA)

Left occipitolateral (LOL) Right occipitolateral (ROL)

Left occipitoposterior (LOP) Right occipitoposterior (ROP)

Fig. 10.17 Six positions in vertex presentation.

Box 10.6 **Positions in a vertex presentation**
(Fig. 10.16)

- **Left occipitoanterior (LOA)** The occiput points to the left iliopectineal eminence; the sagittal suture is in the right oblique diameter of the pelvis.
- **Right occipitoanterior (ROA)** The occiput points to the right iliopectineal eminence; the sagittal suture is in the left oblique diameter of the pelvis.
- **Left occipitolateral (LOL)** The occiput points to the left iliopectineal line midway between the iliopectineal eminence and the sacroiliac joint; the sagittal suture is in the transverse diameter of the pelvis.
- **Right occipitolateral (ROL)** The occiput points to the right iliopectineal line midway between the iliopectineal eminence and the sacroiliac joint; the sagittal suture is in the transverse diameter of the pelvis.
- **Left occipitoposterior (LOP)** The occiput points to the left sacroiliac joint; the sagittal suture is in the left oblique diameter of the pelvis.
- **Right occipitoposterior (ROP)** The occiput points to the right sacroiliac joint; the sagittal suture is in the right oblique diameter of the pelvis.
- **Direct occipitoanterior (DOA)** The occiput points to the symphysis pubis; the sagittal suture is in the anteroposterior diameter of the pelvis.
- **Direct occipitoposterior (DOP)** The occiput points to the sacrum; the sagittal suture is in the anteroposterior diameter of the pelvis.

In breech and face presentations the positions are described in a similar way using the appropriate denominator.

---

subsequently supported by Imdad et al (2011), does not recommend routine fetal movement counting as there is insufficient evidence that it improves fetal wellbeing.

Preparation for labour

Perineal massage

Women should be informed that there is evidence that perineal massage from 35 weeks of pregnancy is effective in reducing the likelihood of perineal damage during the birth (Beckmann and Garrett 2006) (and see Chapter 15). This can be undertaken by the woman or her partner just once or twice a week with a significant positive impact on her perineal integrity and postnatal pain (Chapter 23).

Box 10.7 **Risk factors that may arise during pregnancy**

- Any chronic or acute illness or disease in the woman Hb lower than 10.5 g/dl
- Proteinuria
- BP: single diastolic of 110 mgHg or two of 90 mmHg at least 4 hours apart; two systolic of above 160 mmHg at least 4 hours apart
- Uterus large or small for gestational age
- Excess or decreased liquor
- Malpresentation
- Fetal movement pattern significantly reduced or changed
- Any vaginal, cervical or uterine bleeding
- Premature labour
- Infection
- Sociological or psychological factors

Stretch and sweep

NICE guidelines (2008) recommend that the midwife offers a membrane sweep to women who have not given birth by 41 weeks. More recently, the Antenatal Quality Standard (NICE 2012) recommends at 40 and 41 weeks for a primigravida (see Box 10.2). This procedure has been shown to reduce the number of women who require induction of labour, and although this can be uncomfortable it is a safe and simple technique (Boulvain et al 2005) (see Chapter 19).

Birth plans

During the latter weeks of pregnancy, expectations and plans for labour and birth will be a focus of discussion. Women should know when they should contact a midwife

and how to do so. If the woman has planned a home birth, she will be visited by her midwife to make final preparations. Most maternity units provide a list of items that women will need to bring with them if they are planning to birth away from home. In all situations it is important to ensure that women know how to get advice if they have any concerns.

A birth plan can be instrumental in assisting the woman towards having the birth experience of her choice and to consider what she might like to do during labour and what is important to her. Lundgren et al (2003) suggest that birth plans do not enhance the childbirth experience for all but some women felt that aspects of pain, fear and concern for their baby were alleviated by having a birth plan. Birth plans are likely to be most effective if they are written with the midwife sharing information to enable the woman to make plans that are informed by what is available locally and what is considered current best practice and care.

Flexibility and adaptability should be built into the labour and birth plans to ensure an individual approach is adopted and the woman's wishes are carefully considered. Parents' wishes should be revisited when labour commences and discussions recorded in the labour notes. Each woman should be aware that it may be necessary to adapt her plans depending on the circumstances at the time, but be reassured that she will be fully involved in all decisions made.

Home visit and safe sleeping advice

It is practice in many units to undertake one of the antenatal visits at the woman's home, in order to discuss arrangements for caring for the baby when it is born. This may include seeing where the baby will sleep and advising on safe sleeping principles (see Chapter 34). It provides another opportunity to discuss keeping a smoke-free home and ensuring that the woman knows how and when to make contact when labour starts.

REFERENCES

Allison R 2012. Language matters. The Practising Midwife 15(1):14–16

Beck C T, Watson S 2010 Subsequent childbirth after a previous traumatic birth. Nursing Research 59(4): 241–9

Beckmann M, Garrett A 2006 Antenatal perineal massage for reducing perineal trauma. Cochrane Database of Systematic Reviews, Issue 1. Art. No.: CD005123. doi: 10.1002/ 14651858.CD005123.pub2

Boulvain M, Stan C, Irion O 2005 Membrane sweeping for induction of

labour. Cochrane Database of Systematic Reviews, Issue 1. Art. No. CD000451. doi: 10.1002/14651858. CD000451.pub2

Bundey S, Aslam H 1993 A five-year prospective study of the health of children in different ethnic groups, with particular reference to the effect of inbreeding. European Journal of Human Genetics 1: 206–9

CMACE (Centre for Maternal and Child Enquiries) 2011a Saving mothers' lives: reviewing maternal deaths to

make motherhood safer: 2006–08. The Eighth Report on Confidential Enquiries into Maternal Deaths in the United Kingdom. BJOG: An International Journal of Obstetrics and Gynaecology 118(Suppl 1): 1–203

CMACE (Centre for Maternal and Child Enquiries) 2011b Perinatal mortality 2009: United Kingdom. CMACE, London. Available at www.hqip.org .uk/assets/NCAPOP-Library/ CMACE-Reports/35.-March-2011

-Perinatal-Mortality-2009.pdf (accessed 12 May 2013)

Clement S, Candy B, Sikorski J et al 1996 Does reducing the frequency of routine antenatal visits have long term effects? Follow up of participants in a randomised controlled trial. British Journal of Obstetrics and Gynaecology 106 (4):367–70

Department for Education (DfE) 2012 The CAF process. Available at www.education.gov.uk/ childrenandyoungpeople/strategy/ integratedworking/caf/a0068957/ the-caf-process (accessed 11 May 2013)

DH (Department of Health) 1999 Our healthier nation: reducing health inequalities: an action report. DH, London

DH (Department of Health) 2007 Maternity matters: choice, access and continuity of care in a safe service. DH, London

DH (Department of Health) 2010a Statistical press notice: Vital Signs Monitoring Return – quarterly update return – May. DH, London

DH (Department of Health) 2010b Healthy lives, healthy people. www .gov.uk/government/uploads/system/ uploads/attachment_data/ file/151764/dh_127424.pdf.pdf

DH (Department of Health) 2011. Statistical release: smoking at delivery – Quarter 2. 2011/12. www.dh.gov.uk/en/ Publicationsandstatistics/ Publications/PublicationsStatistics/ DH_130858

DH (Department of Health) 2013 Health Care and Associated Professions (Indemnity Arrangements) Order 2013 A paper for consultation. www.gov.uk/ government/uploads/system/ uploads/attachment_data/ file/143273/Indemnity -Consultation1.pdf (accessed 18 May 2013)

DH and NHS Commissioning Board 2012 Compassion in practice. www.commissioningboard.nhs.uk/ files/2012/12/compassion-in-practice .pdf (accessed 31 December 2012)

Dowswell T, Carroli G, Duley L et al 2010 Alternative versus standard packages of antenatal care for low-risk pregnancy. Cochrane

Database of Systematic Reviews, Issue 10. Art. No.: CD000934. doi:10.1002/14651858.CD000934. pub2

Farquharson R, Greaves M 2006 Thromboembolic disease. In: James, D, Steer P, Weiner C et al (eds), High risk pregnancy, 3rd edn. Saunders, London, p 938–48

Food Standards Agency 2013 What foods should I eat and stay away from in pregnancy? www.food.gov .uk/about-us/about-the-fsa/ faqsconsumer/pregnancy#.UY_wdL -LG-I (accessed 12 May 2013)

Godfrey C, Pickett K, Parrott S et al 2010 Estimating the costs to the NHS of smoking in pregnancy for pregnant women and infants. Public Health Research Consortium, University of York

Grice J, Baston H 2011 Carbon monoxide screening in pregnancy. The Practising Midwife 14(10):36, 38–41

Hall M H, Cheng P K, MacGillivray I 1980 Is routine antenatal care worth while? Lancet ii: 78–80

Heslehurst N, Rankin J, Wilkinson J R et al 2010. A nationally representative study of maternal obesity in England, UK: trends in incidence and demographic inequalities in 619 323 births, 1989–2007. International Journal of Obesity 34(3): 420–8

Hollowell J, Oakley L, Vigurs C et al 2012 Increasing the early initiation of antenatal care by Black and Minority Ethnic women in the United Kingdom: a systematic review and mixed methods synthesis of women's views and the literature on intervention effectiveness. Final Report. Perinatal Epidemiology Unit, University of Oxford Available at www.npeu.ox.ac.uk/files/downloads/ infant-mortality/Infant-Mortality— DIVA-final-report-Oct-2012.pdf (accessed 12 May 2013)

Huckshaw A, Rodeck C, Boniface S 2011 Maternal smoking in pregnancy and birth defects: a systematic review based on 173 687 malformed cases and 11.7 million controls. Human Reproduction Update 17(5):589–604

Imdad A, Yakoob M, Siddiqui S et al 2011 Screening and triage of intrauterine growth restriction (IUGR) in general population and

high risk pregnancies: a systematic review with a focus on reduction of IUGR related stillbirths. BMC Public Health 11(Suppl 3):S1

Khan N, Benson J, MacLeod, R et al 2010 Developing and evaluating a culturally appropriate genetic service for consanguineous. South Asian families Journal of Community Genetics 1(2):73–81

Koshy P, Mackenzie M, Tappin D et al 2010 Smoking cessation during pregnancy: the influence of partners, family and friends on quitters and non-quitters. Health and Social Care in the Community 18 (5):500–10

Leamon J, Viccars A 2007 West Howe midwifery evaluation: the with me study. Bournemouth University, Bournemouth

Leneghan S, Gillen P, Sinclair M 2012. Interventions to reduce domestic abuse in pregnancy: a qualitative systematic review. Evidence Based Midwifery 10(4):137–42

Lewis G (ed) 2007 The Confidential Enquiry into Maternal and Child Health (CEMACH) Saving mothers' lives: reviewing maternal deaths to make motherhood safer – 2003–2005. The Seventh Report on Confidential Enquiries into Maternal Deaths in the United Kingdom. CEMACH, London

Lucas M (2006) Think before you speak. The Practising Midwife 9(4):46

Lullaby Trust (2013) Care of the next infant. Available at www.lullabytrust .org.uk/new-design/support/coni (accessed 11 May 2013)

Lundgren I, Berg M, Lindmark G 2003 Is the childbirth experience improved by a birth plan? Journal of Midwifery and Women's Health 48(5):322–8

Marmot Review 2010 Fair society, healthy lives. A strategic review of health inequalities in England post-2010. Available at www .instituteofhealthequity.org/projects/ fair-society-healthy-lives-the-marmot -review (accessed 12 May 2013)

McCourt C 2006 Supporting choice and control? Communication and interaction between midwives and women at the antenatal booking visit. Social Science and Medicine 62(6):1307–18

McNeill J, Lynn F, Alderdice F 2010 Systematic review of reviews: The

Public Health Role of the Midwife. School of Nursing & Midwifery, Queen's University Belfast

Ministry of Health 1929 Maternal mortality in childbirth. Antenatal clinics: their conduct and scope. HMSO, London

NICE (National Institute for Clinical Excellence) 2003 Antenatal care: routine care for the pregnant woman. NICE, London

NICE (National Institute for Health and Clinical Excellence) 2007 Antenatal and postnatal mental health. CG45. NICE, London

NICE (National Institute for Health and Clinical Excellence) 2008 Antenatal care: routine care for the healthy pregnant woman. CG62. NICE, London

NICE (National Institute for Health and Clinical Excellence) 2010a Pregnancy and complex social factors. NICE Clinical guideline 110 http://guidance.nice.org.uk/CG110/NICEGuidance/pdf/English (accessed 10 February 2013)

NICE (National Institute for Health and Clinical Excellence) 2010b Hypertension in pregnancy. NICE Clinical Guideline 107. www.nice.org.uk/nicemedia/live/13098/50418/50418.pdf (accessed 12 May 2013)

NICE (National Institute for Health and Clinical Excellence) 2010c Dietary interventions and physical activity interventions for weight management before, during and after pregnancy. Public Health Guidance 27. www.nice.org.uk/nicemedia/live/13056/49926/49926.pdf (accessed 31 December 2012)

NICE (National Institute for Health and Clinical Excellence) 2010d Quitting smoking in pregnancy and following childbirth. Public health guidance 26. http://guidance.nice.org.uk/PH26/Guidance/pdf/English (accessed 10 February 2013)

NICE (National Institute for Health and Clinical Excellence) 2012 Antenatal quality standard: quality statements. Available at http://www.nice.org.uk/aboutnice/qualitystandards/qualitystandards.jsp (accessed 27 December 2012)

NSC (National Screening Committee) 2011 Screening for chlamydia infection in pregnancy www.screening.nhs.uk/chlamydia-pregnancy (accessed 12 May 2013)

NSC (National Screening Committee) 2012a Asymptomatic bacteriuria screening in pregnancy policy position statement 25 April. Available at www.screening.nhs.uk/asymptomaticbacteriuria (accessed 23 April 2013)

NSC (National Screening Committee) 2012b Group B streptococcus. Available at www.screening.nhs.uk/groupbstreptococcus (accessed 23 April 2013)

NSC (National Screening Committee) 2013 Policy Review. Screening in the UK 2011–2012. Available at www.screening.nhs.uk (accessed 18 May 2013)

Nilsson C, Bondas T, Lundgren I. 2010 Previous birth experience in women with intense fear of childbirth. Journal of Obstetric, Gynecological and Neonatal Nursing 39(3): 298–309

NMC (Nursing and Midwifery Council) 2008 The code. Standards of conduct, performance and ethics for nurses and midwives. NMC, London

NMC (Nursing and Midwifery Council) 2009 Record keeping for nurses and midwives. NMC, London

NMC (Nursing and Midwifery Council) 2012 The midwives rules and standards. NMC, London

O'Sullivan O, Stephen G, Martindale E et al 2009 Predicting poor perinatal outcome in women who present with decreased fetal movements. J Obstet Gynaecol 29(8):705–10

Prochaska J 1992 What causes people to change from unhealthy to health enhancing behaviour? In: Heller T, Bailey L, Patison S (eds) Preventing cancers. Open University Press, Buckingham, p 147–53

Public Health England 2013. National Chlamydia Screening Programme. Available at www.chlamydiascreening.nhs.uk (accessed 23 April 2013)

Rasmussen K, Yaktine A, eds 2009 Committee to Reexamine Institute of Medicine Pregnancy Weight Guidelines (Weight gain during pregnancy: re-examining the guidelines [online]). Available from http://books.nap.edu/openbook.php?record_id=12584 (accessed 31 December 2012)

RCOG (Royal College of Obstetricians and Gynaecologists) 2006 Exercise in pregnancy. www.rcog.org.uk/files/rcog-corp/Statement4-14022011.pdf (accessed 31 December 2012)

RCOG (Royal College of Obstetricians and Gynaecologists) 2009 Green top guideline No. 37. Reducing the risk of thrombosis and embolism during pregnancy and the puerperium. Available at www.rcog.org.uk/files/rcog-corp/GTG37aReducingRiskThrombosis.pdf (accessed 12 May 2013)

RCOG (Royal of Obstetricians and Gynaecologists) 2010. Green top guideline No. 55. Late intrauterine fetal death and stillbirth. www.rcog.org.uk/files/rcog-corp/GTG%2055%20Late%20Intrauterine%20fetal%20death%20and%20stillbirth%2010%2011%2010.pdf (accessed 31 December 2012)

RCOG (Royal College of Obstetricians and Gynaecologists) 2011a Green top guideline No. 22. The use of anti-D immunoglobulin for Rhesus D prophylaxis. www.rcog.org.uk/files/rcog-corp/GTG22AntiD.pdf (accessed 31 December 2012)

RCOG (Royal College of Obstetricians and Gynaecologists) 2011b Green top guideline No. 57. Reduced fetal movements www.rcog.org.uk/files/rcog-corp/GTG57RFM25022011.pdf (accessed 31 December 2012)

RCOG (Royal College of Obstetricians and Gynaecologists) 2013a Scientific Impact Paper No. 34. Induction of labour at term in older mothers. Available at www.rcog.org.uk/files/rcog-corp/1.2.13%20SIP34%20IOL.pdf (accessed 12 May 2013)

RCOG (Royal College of Obstetricians and Gynaecologists) 2013b Green top guideline No. 31. The investigation and management of the small for gestational age fetus. www.rcog.org.uk/files/rcog-corp/22.3.13GTG31SGA.pdf (accessed 20 April 2013)

Rungapadiachy D 1999 Interpersonal Communication and Psychology. Butterworth Heinemann, Oxford

Sayle A, Savitz D, Thorp J et al 2001 Sexual activity during late pregnancy and risk of pre-term delivery. Obstetrics and Gynecology 97:283–9

Sikorski J, Wilson J, Clement S et al 1996 A randomised controlled trial comparing two schedules of antenatal visits: the antenatal care project. British Medical Journal 312(7030):546–53

SANDS (Stillbirth and Neonatal Death Society) 2012 Antenatal care. www .uk-sands.org/Support/Another-pregnancy/Antenatal-care.html (accessed 31 December 2012)

Thackray H, Tifft C 2001 Fetal alcohol syndrome. Pediatrics in Review 22(2): 47–55

Thangaratinam S, Jolly K, Rogozinska S et al 2012 Effects of interventions in pregnancy on maternal weight and obstetric outcomes: meta-analysis of randomised evidence. British

Medical Journal 344:e2088. Available at www.bmj.com/content/344/bmj .e2088 (accessed 31 December 2012)

UNICEF (United Nations Children's Fund) 2012 UK Baby Friendly Initiative 2012 Guide to the Baby Friendly Initiative standards. Available at www.unicef.org.uk/ Documents/Baby_Friendly/ Guidance/Baby_Friendly_ guidance_2012.pdf (accessed 12 May 2013)

Villar J, Hassan B, Piaggio G et al 2001a WHO antenatal care randomized trial for the evaluation of a new model of routine antenatal care. The Lancet 357(9268):1551–64

Walfish A, Hallak M 2006 Hypertension. In: James P, Steer C, Weiner B et al (eds) High risk pregnancy, 3rd edn. Elsevier, Philadelphia, p 772–97

Williams D 2006 Renal disorders. In: James D, Steer P, Weiner B et al (eds) High risk pregnancy, 3rd edn. Elsevier, Philadelphia, p 1098–124

Ziaei S, Norozzi M, Faghihzadeh S et al 2007 A randomised placebo-controlled trial to determine the effect of iron supplementation on pregnancy outcome in pregnant women with haemogloblin ≥13.2 g/ dl. BJOG: An International Journal of Obstetrics and Gynaecology 114(6): 684–8

FURTHER READING

Downe S, Finlayson K, Walsh D, et al 2009 'Weighing up and balancing out': a meta-synthesis of barriers to antenatal care for marginalised women in high-income countries. BJOG: An International Journal of Obstetrics and Gynaecology 116 (4): 519–529

This article examines how care can be improved for disadvantaged pregnant women.

Raine R, Cartwright M, Richens Y et al 2010 A qualitative study of women's experiences of communication in antenatal care: identifying areas for action. Maternal and Child Health Journal 14: 590–599

An interesting paper highlighting the importance of effective communication as a hallmark of high quality antenatal care.

Thomson G, Dykes F, Singh et al 2013 A public health perspective of women's experiences of antenatal care: an exploration of insights from community consultation. Midwifery 29 (30): 211–216

A useful read that identifies why inequalities in antenatal care persist for the most vulnerable in society.

USEFUL WEBSITES

Child and Maternal Health Intelligence Network: www.chimat.org.uk

Cochrane Library – database of systematic reviews: www.thecochranelibrary.com

National Institute for Health and Care [formerly Clinical] Excellence: www.nice.org.uk

Royal College of Obstetricians and Gynaecologists – guidance: www.rcog.org.uk/womens-health

Chapter |11|

Antenatal screening of the mother and fetus

Lucy Kean, Angie Godfrey, Amanda Sullivan

Screening has now become such a routine part of antenatal care that many women accept this, often with little thought. There is no aspect of the screening programme that does not, however, have the potential to raise huge social, emotional and health issues for pregnant women. The role of the midwife is to guide women through the wealth of tests available, with the best advice possible. This can only be achieved by excellent training and regular updates for all midwives and doctors. Screening develops and moves forward every few months and so vigilance on behalf of us all is needed to ensure we provide the best care.

THE CHAPTER AIMS TO:

- discuss the principles of screening, good counseling techniques and the potential impact of positive results on women
- describe the currently available screening tests, their aims, and the efficiency of each test
- define what consent is and how the consent process should be undertaken
- provide information regarding how to deal with positive tests and what negative results mean.

SCREENING PRINCIPLES

Screening of a mother and baby is now a major part of care for all pregnancies. The underlying principles of screening are that the condition being screened for must be important and well understood (i.e. something that makes a difference to health and wellbeing and does more good than harm). Treatment should be available and at a stage where the outcome can be changed. There should be an appropriate and acceptable test that is available to a defined group, making the screening cost effective in reducing poorer health outcomes.

The National Screening Committee of the United Kingdom (NSC 2013) defines screening as:

> *a process of identifying apparently healthy people who may be at an increased risk of a disease or condition, they can then be offered information, further tests and appropriate treatment to reduce their risk and/or any complications arising from the disease or condition.*

Broadly speaking, the conditions that form the national programme for screening in the United Kingdom (UK) meet these criteria. When screening for currently unscreened conditions is considered (e.g. Group B streptococcus), it is weighed against these important criteria.

Screening in pregnancy can be divided into looking for conditions in the mother that, if untreated or undetected, could affect her health or the health of the baby or both, and screening for conditions in the fetus that could impact significantly on the health of the baby.

Limitations of screening

Screening has important ethical differences from clinical practice as the health service is targeting apparently healthy people, offering to help individuals to make better informed choices about their health. There are risks involved, however, and it is important that people have realistic expectations of what a screening programme can deliver.

While screening has the potential to save lives or improve life through early diagnosis of serious conditions, it is not a foolproof process. Equally, some screening is directed at detecting conditions in the fetus that may lead to significant handicap, and to provide prospective parents with choices regarding continuation or otherwise of the pregnancy.

Screening can reduce the risk of developing a condition or its complications but it cannot offer a guarantee of protection. In any screening programme there is a minimum of false-positive results (wrongly reported as having the condition) and false-negative results (wrongly reported as not having the condition). The UK NSC is increasingly presenting screening as *risk reduction* to emphasize this point.

Screening can be an emotive issue. While screening for fetal problems is often considered the most emotionally charged area, it is important to realize that maternal screening can also raise issues and challenges that all health professionals involved in the service need to be equipped to help with. Imagine the emotional journey a mother embarks on when faced with a new diagnosis of Human Immunodeficiency Virus (HIV) in early pregnancy.

Social and psychological impact of screening investigations

Pregnancy is a profound and life-changing event. During this time the mother has to adapt physically, socially and psychologically to the forthcoming birth of her child. Many women feel more emotional than usual (Raphael-Leff 2005) and may have heightened levels of anxiety (Kleinveld et al 2006; Raynor and England 2010). As Green et al (2004) state, the increasing availability of fetal investigations has been shown to cause women even greater anxiety and stress. Any feelings of excitement and anticipation can quickly change when the mother is introduced to the idea that she is 'at risk' of having a baby with a particular problem (Fisher 2006).

There is evidence that mothers nearing the end of their reproductive years (with a higher risk of chromosomal abnormality) experience pregnancy in a way that is different to younger women. Older mothers are often more anxious and have fewer feelings of attachment to the fetus at 20 weeks of pregnancy (Berryman and Windridge 1999). Psychologists, sociologists and health professionals now generally accept the finding that high-risk women delay attachment to the fetus until they receive reassuring test results. Rothman (1986) classically termed this the *'tentative pregnancy'*, in a study of women undergoing amniocentesis.

Anxiety caused by consideration of possible fetal abnormality may be accompanied by moral or religious dilemmas. Tests that can diagnose chromosomal or genetic abnormalities also carry a risk of procedure-induced miscarriage. Many parents agonize about whether to subject a potentially normal fetus to this risk in order to obtain this information. Parents may then need to consider whether they wish to terminate or continue with an affected pregnancy. Some religious authorities only support prenatal testing so long as the integrity of the mother and fetus are maintained. There are also opposing views about the legitimacy of terminating a pregnancy, even when a serious disorder has been diagnosed. Such dilemmas are an unfortunate but inevitable cost of the choices associated with some fetal investigations.

Despite this, there are important advantages to the acquisition of knowledge about the fetus before birth. First, society greatly values the freedom of individuals to choose. People are encouraged to accept some responsibility when making decisions about treatment options, in partnership with healthcare professionals. A second advantage is that reproductive autonomy may be increased. Women can choose for themselves whether they wish to embark upon the lifelong care of a child with special needs. This may be viewed as empowering and as a means of preventing later suffering and hardship for child and family alike.

In summary, prenatal testing is a two-edged sword. It enables midwives and doctors to give people choices that were unheard of in previous generations and that may prevent much suffering. However, in some circumstances they actually increase the amount of anxiety and psychological trauma experienced in pregnancy. The long-term effects of such trauma on family dynamics are not currently understood.

HOW SCREENING IS SET UP AND THE MIDWIFE'S ROLE AND RESPONSIBILITIES

All midwives need to have a broad understanding of screening investigations because they are responsible for offering, interpreting and communicating the results. In the UK, the Midwives Rules and Standards (NMC 2012) state that midwives should work in partnership with women to provide safe, responsive and compassionate care. This implies that the midwife as a key public health agent should enable women to make decisions about their care based on individual needs. Some midwives specialize in discussing complex testing issues with parents and become antenatal screening coordinators.

In England from 1 April 2013, 27 Screening and Immunisation Teams will have the responsibility for commissioning and oversight of the UK National Screening Committee (NSC) Antenatal and Newborn Screening programmes. The UK NSC has the overall responsibility for determining these programmes and will ensure the Quality Assurance aspect via Regional Quality Assurance Teams.

The UK NSC (2011a) recommends that dedicated screening coordinators oversee the running of screening programmes in every Trust. Screening coordinators also provide specialist advice and ensure that there is a line of referral for women whose needs are not met by routine services. Screening for pregnant women and newborn babies is now such a complex process that the role of screening coordinator has become a full-time role in most services.

The UK NSC publishes an extremely helpful timeline for antenatal and newborn screening that will help

individuals to see what is required and by when (http://cpd.screening.nhs.uk/timeline).

Each of the individual screening programmes has a number of key performance indicators (KPI) on which the performance of individual National Health Service (NHS) Trusts is measured. The most recent KPI document runs to 45 pages. Overseeing the delivery of the KPIs is the remit of the screening coordinator in each Trust, but it is the hard work of the professionals on the ground that ensures targets are met. As an example, the KPI for screening for hepatitis B states that at least 70% of pregnant women who are hepatitis B positive should be referred and seen by an appropriate specialist within an effective timeframe (6 weeks from identification).

The KPI for screening for Down syndrome at between 10 weeks + 0 days and 20 weeks + 0 days states that in 97% of women there must be sufficient information for the woman to be uniquely identified, and the woman's correct date of birth, maternal weight, family origin, smoking status and ultrasound dating assessment in millimetres, with associated gestational date and sonographer ID, must be included on the request form.

Failsafe procedures are a necessary part of the screening process. In the UK these have been implemented to ensure all screening processes are complete. There are back-up mechanisms in addition to usual care, which ensures if something goes wrong in the screening pathway, processes are in place firstly to identify what is going wrong and secondly to determine what action should follow to ensure a safe outcome.

All professionals undertaking screening must be appropriately trained and confident in discussing the risks and benefits of all screening programmes, and in the UK they must adhere to the NSC recommendations and standards.

Documentation

In whatever system is practised, good documentation is vital. The midwife should discuss and offer screening tests, record that the discussion has taken place, that the offer has been made, that the offer has been either accepted or declined. It is very helpful for the whole team engaged in antenatal care to understand from the documentation why screening is declined, if this is the case. Women find being persistently re-offered a screening test that they have declined frustrating and annoying, and simply documenting the discussion properly, rather than ticking a box to indicate that screening was declined, is helpful. This can sometimes also lead on to discussion that can reveal that a woman has not understood the test, the purpose or the benefits, which can help to improve understanding.

In the event of decline for infectious diseases screening at the antenatal 'booking' appointment, a routine re-offer should be made at about 28 weeks. From a litigation perspective, it is not uncommon for women who have declined screening but experienced a poor outcome to suggest that they were not offered screening or did not understand the purpose of the test on offer. Good documentation and being able to show that written information was given can help in the comprehension of such cases.

Discussion of options

When offering tests, it is necessary for the midwife to present and discuss the options, so that women can make an informed choice that best suits their circumstances and preferences. Midwives are required to discuss options for testing in a manner that enables shared decision-making (Sullivan 2005). This means providing the opportunity to discuss choices with a trained professional who is impartial and supportive as the women make decisions along the screening and diagnostic pathway.

There may be mixed feelings about the final decision. Sometimes it is helpful to consider what the mother's worst-case scenario would be, as that can help to decide the best way forward. The principles for consent for shared decision-making are shown in Box 11.1.

Midwives commonly recommend antenatal tests such as infectious disease screening, full blood count or cardiotocograph for reduced fetal movements. However, tests for fetal anomaly require a non-directive approach that enables the mother to make an informed choice (Clarke 1994). Consent must be obtained prior to all tests and this must be documented. Standardized processes allow systems to serve women uniformly and allow good quality of care to be offered to all. In the UK, the NSC (2011a) has published Consent Standards and Guidance for the fetal anomaly screening process which can be used as a model in any healthcare system.

- Standard 1: All hospital trusts must have a care pathway to provide evidence that the UK National Screening Committee (UK NSC) and NHS Fetal Anomaly Screening Programme (FASP) information booklet and leaflets are being used.

Box 11.1 **Principles for obtaining informed consent**

- Purpose of the procedure/test
- All risks and benefits to be reasonably expected
- Details of all possible future treatments that could arise as a consequence of testing
- Disclosure of all available options (this may include tests that are offered by private providers where relevant)
- The option of refusing any tests
- The offer to answer any queries

- Standard 2: All pregnant women must be offered, at least 24 hours before decisions are made, up-to-date information on fetal anomaly screening based on the current available evidence. The NHS FASP recommends the use of the UK NSC (2012) leaflet entitled *Screening tests for you and your baby*, available on the NHS FASP website: www.fetalanomaly.screening.nhs.uk. This is available in many different languages and, where needed, resources are available as audio and easy reading.
- Standard 3: All eligible pregnant women must be offered 'testing' and this offer must be recorded in the woman's notes and/or hospital electronic records at the antenatal 'booking' appointment.
- Standard 4: All decisions about the test itself must be recorded in the woman's hand-held notes and/or in the hospital records.

It is important all documentation is dated and signed by the health professional involved.

The UK NSC (2011a) guidance is very complete and it is a useful document for all midwives to read. Key aspects are shown in Box 11.2.

Assumptions must never be made regarding knowledge about the conditions being screened for. Common misunderstandings are that Down syndrome cannot occur if it has not previously occurred in a family or that a woman is too young to have an affected baby. Many women (and their partners) do not understand that syphilis is a sexually transmitted infection, but that the initial result can show positive if there have been similar non-sexually transmitted infections (such as Yaws).

Women who decline first trimester screening should know that they can take up second trimester screening for Down's syndrome if they change their mind and that they can undergo second trimester screening for fetal anomaly at $18+^0$ to $20+^6$ weeks.

Women who decline initial screening for infections can and should be offered screening later in the pregnancy.

Importantly, only the woman has the right to consent to or decline the screening tests. A partner or family member has no right to consent or decline on her behalf. Women can withdraw consent for testing at any time. This decision should be recorded.

The process of consent

Consent is a complex process not a single entity, and requires adequate time. It is important to ensure that the woman has had the time she needs to consider the information and come to a decision. That there has been enough time to ask questions, that she feels comfortable and has involved those she would wish to in reaching a decision. The extent to which women want to involve others is very variable.

- The pregnant woman must understand the condition being screened for.
- The midwife should explain about the nature, purpose, risks, benefits, timing, limitations and potential consequences of screening.
- The woman should understand that screening is optional, and understand the risks and benefits of not undergoing screening.
- In the UK there is the choice of continuing or terminating a pregnancy for serious fetal abnormalities.

Local knowledge should be shared: how, where and when the test is done:

- What the test results mean and potential significant clinical and emotional consequences.
- The decisions that might need to be made at each point along the pathway and their consequences.
- How and when the results will be given.
- How women progress through the pathway, including those who opt out of screening.
- The possibility that screening can provide information about other conditions.
- The fact that screening may not provide a definitive diagnosis.
- What further tests might be needed, e.g. chorionic villus sampling (CVS) and amniocentesis.
- That confirmatory/repeat testing may occasionally be required.
- Balanced and accurate information about the various conditions being screened should be provided.

The amount of information needed will vary between women. Women who do not understand English will require interpreting services and other services might be needed for some women. Not all women will have the capacity to consent. Where capacity is in doubt there are usually local guidelines as to how this should progress forward that are beyond the scope of this chapter.

Issues to consider when presenting information

When discussing tests, it is important to understand the motivations and thought processes of pregnant women. The motivation for testing is often different for mother and practitioner. For the fetal anomaly screening programme, the UK NSC rationale for testing is to identify fetal anomalies; however mothers commonly accept these tests in order to gain reassurance that their fetus is normal

(Hunt et al 2005). Mothers often think that fetal anomaly tests such as ultrasound scans are an integral or mandatory part of their antenatal care. They may also be unaware of the reasons for performing the test and this can compound the shock of finding problems or abnormalities (Health Technology Assessment 2000).

When women are anxious or under stress, they are less able to remember the information provided (Ingram and Malcarne 1995). Parents may feel vulnerable and less able to ask questions. This may lead to dissatisfaction with the quality of communications with health carers. Since an unborn fetus is something of an enigma to parents, this may increase anxiety and sensitivity to real or imaginary cues. For example, professionals practising non-directive counselling may be perceived as evasive and as concealing bad news. One particular aspect of counselling that has been criticized by parents is the portrayal of risk estimates (Al-Jader et al 2000).

There is much evidence that people do not make consistent decisions about undertaking tests in pregnancy on the basis of the risk information received. For instance, a mother with a risk of Down syndrome of 1:150 may perceive herself to be at a very high risk and may request amniocentesis. However, others may view that same risk as very low. The phenomenon of how parents interpret risk information is not fully understood, although it is clear that personal circumstances, preferences and beliefs are an integral part of this process. For this reason, it is vital that, with any screening, the midwife begins a consultation by investigating how much the mother knows about the condition being tested for, and what she already knows about the test risks, benefits and the consequences of results.

There are also common biases in the way people interpret risk information. The midwife should be aware of these in order to help parents choose the most appropriate course of action. For example, people tend to view an event as more likely if they can easily imagine or recall instances of it. This means that a mother whose friend or neighbour has a baby with Down syndrome may be sensitized to this possibility and overestimate the chances of it happening to her. Mothers who work with infirm people, or those with a disability, are most likely to seek prenatal diagnosis (Sjögren 1996). Perhaps these mothers are easily able to imagine the lifelong commitment of caring for a child with special needs. This common bias in risk perception is important because it means that some mothers may not easily be reassured by reiteration of the fact that the risk of a problem may be comparatively rare.

Explaining risk

The way in which the midwife tells a mother about risk will also greatly influence how that risk is perceived. For example, a mother who is told that her risk of a particular condition is 1 in 10 may be more alarmed than if she had been informed that there was a 90% chance of normality, or 9 out of 10 babies will not be affected by the condition. This is known as the *'framing'* effect (Kessler and Levine 1987).

People vary considerably in the ways that they consider and understand risk, so it is important that this information is presented in a variety of ways using appropriate language. The UK NSC (2011a) recommend the use of the word 'chance' rather than 'risk' and that the chance of the outcome (which for antenatal screening now mainly relates to screening for Down syndrome) be given as a percentage as well as a ratio 1 in *x*. As such, a midwife discussing a 1 in 100 chance of a disorder should also point out the fact that 99% or 99 out of 100 similar people will not experience that disorder. This may help people cope when considering tests or when anxiously awaiting results.

There are other general considerations to take into account when providing information (Hunter 1994), as delineated in Box 11.3.

If a test is undertaken in pregnancy, it is good practice to ensure that the woman is clear about how, when and from whom she will be able to obtain the result. If possible, there should be some options available.

The UK NSC (2011a) is clear that the person ordering the test has the responsibility to ensure that the test is properly completed and that the woman is informed of the result. The National Institute for Health and Clinical Excellence (NICE 2008) antenatal care guidelines state that every woman should have the results of all of their screening tests recorded in their hand-held notes within 14 days or at the 16 week antenatal appointment. It therefore requires each midwifery team to have a process for the management of tracking tests performed and the results, a means to inform women, a process of fail-safe so that when, as will inevitably happen, a test is not performed or sample not processed because in some way the process failed, this is recognized in a timely enough fashion for the test to be repeated, and that the results are recorded in the woman's hand-held notes.

On a logistical front, this is no mean task. Failings in the screening system are identified as serious incidents and there is a formal process in the UK that must be undertaken when failings are identified. In practice, the majority of women who fall between stools are those whose pregnancies do not follow the routine process, for instance those who move or whose pregnancy does not continue. These women, as much as anyone else, still should be informed of results that are important to them, such as the results of infection screening.

INDIVIDUAL SCREENING TEST CONSIDERATIONS

Antenatal screening tests are broadly divided into those that are looking for a problem in the mother that could affect the fetus, such as an infection, the presence of a red-cell antibody, or a particular haemoglobin variant, which if passed on by both parents could cause an issue, or those looking directly for a problem in the fetus.

FETAL SCREENING TESTS

Population screening of the fetus (i.e. that offered to everyone) is now directed at two areas: defining the risk of a baby having Down syndrome (trisomy 21), and the detection of specific abnormalities.

Screening for Down syndrome

Down syndrome is the most common cause of severe learning difficulty in children. In the absence of antenatal screening, around 1 in 700 births would be affected (Kennard et al 1995). While some children with Down syndrome learn literacy skills and lead semi-independent lives, others remain completely dependent. Around one in three of these babies are born with a serious heart defect. The average life expectancy is about 60 years, although most people develop pathological changes in the brain

---

Box 11.3 General principles when providing information

1. Be clear: explain everything in terms that are not medical jargon or complex terminology.
2. Be aware that people can remember only a limited amount of information at one time – be simple, concise and to the point.
3. Give important information first. This will then be remembered best.
4. Group pieces of information into logical categories, such as treatment, prognosis and ways to cope.
5. Information may be recalled more easily if it has been presented in several forms. For example, leaflets can be helpful.
6. Offer to answer any queries. Give contact numbers, in case people think of questions at a later date.
7. Do not make assumptions about information requirements on the basis of social class, profession, age or ethnic group.
8. Summarize, check understanding and repeat the information. Ask whether there is anything that remains unclear.

Source: Hunter 1994

(associated with Alzheimer's disease) after the age of 40 (Kingston 2002).

Screening for Down syndrome has been driven by both health economics and maternal choice. That is not to say, however, that all mothers wish to be screened, or would act to end a pregnancy if they knew they were carrying an affected fetus. Uptake rates for screening vary depending on the population being screened. Some mothers will chose screening despite knowing that they would not act on a result that gave them a high chance. Interestingly, the single largest factor in deciding whether to take further tests after a high chance result is the degree of magnitude of the change in risk. In other words, a mother who has a pre-test chance (based on age alone) of 1 in 100 (1%), who has a screening result of 1 in 120 (0.83%) will be less likely to wish to proceed to further testing than a woman who has a pre-test chance of 1 in 1000, who then receives a result of 1 in 120 chance, even though both are at equal risk of giving birth to a baby with Down syndrome.

The national screening programme for Down syndrome in the UK comprises the offer of one of two tests. The gestational age window for a combined test starts from $10+^0$ weeks to $14+^1$ weeks in pregnancy.

The combined test comprises measurement of the crown–rump length (CRL) (Fig. 11.1) to estimate fetal gestational age (dating scan), measurement of the nuchal translucency (NT) space at the back of the fetal neck (Fig. 11.2) and maternal blood to measure the serum markers of pregnancy-associated plasma protein A (PAPP-A) and human chorionic gonadotrophin hormone (hCG).

Using this test, 90% of fetuses affected with Down syndrome would be expected to fall into the high-chance category (a chance of 1 in 150 or more) (the detection rate) with 2% of women carrying unaffected babies having a chance of 1 in 150 or higher (a screen positive rate of 2%).

The quadruple test window starts from $14+^2$ weeks to $20+^0$ weeks. A maternal blood sample is required for the analysis of hCG, alpha-fetoprotein (aFP), unconjugated oestriol (uE3) and inhibin-A.

As stated in the UK NSC (2011b), Model of Best Practice 2011–2014, this test has a lesser detection rate of 75% and a screen positive rate of less than 3%, but has been retained because there will always be women who book too late in pregnancy for combined testing (about 15% of the pregnant population) and wish to have screening. Women presenting after 20 weeks are offered ultrasound for abnormality screening, which will occasionally detect an abnormality that increases the chance that the baby has Down syndrome, but there is no population screening available at this gestation.

Women need to decide as early in their pregnancy as possible if they wish to undertake screening for Down syndrome as earlier testing is superior, and ease of access is important in facilitating testing.

In counselling, women need to be clear that neither screening test gives a guarantee of normality. With combined screening 10% of affected babies will be missed and with quadruple testing 25% of Down babies will be missed. This is termed the *false-negative rate*.

Diagnostic testing for Down syndrome

In the UK, women who receive a result of 1 in 150 or higher from either first or second trimester screening or those women who have previously had a chromosomal abnormality or who carry a genetic disorder will be offered diagnostic testing, i.e. CVS or amniocentesis. The NHS no longer provides diagnostic testing for maternal age alone or following a low chance screening test result, although privately available services are usually easy to access.

CVS can be performed from 11 weeks of pregnancy. Usually the procedure is carried out transabdominally (Fig. 11.3), though occasionally a transcervical (TC) route is needed. The miscarriage rate is often quoted as 2–3% but in most fetal medicine units the procedure-related

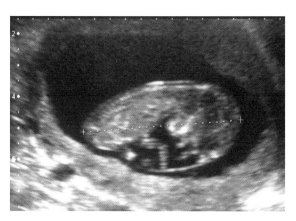

Fig. 11.1 Crown–rump length.

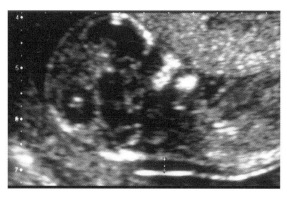

Fig. 11.2 Translucency measurement.

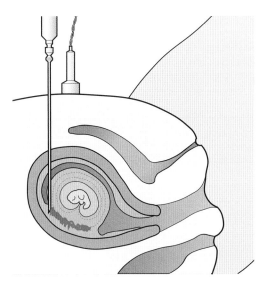

Fig. 11.3 Transabdominal CVS.

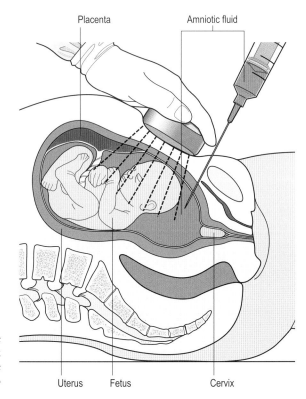

Fig. 11.4 Amniocentesis.

loss rate is closer to 1% (though TC sampling risks are higher). A provisional result is usually issued on a direct preparation at 1–2 days. If this result shows no evidence of an extra chromosome 21 it can be taken as 99.9% certain that the fetus does not have trisomy 21. However, as confined placental mosaicism can rarely occur, which gives a false-negative result, at this stage definite confirmation cannot be made until the culture result is available at 14–21 days.

Amniocentesis can be performed after 15 weeks (Fig. 11.4). The procedure-related loss rate is usually no higher than 1% and in many units is closer to 0.5%. Rapid testing using polymerase chain reaction or fluorescent in situ hybridization can usually mean that a result for trisomy 21 (and usually 13 and 18) is available in 2–3 working days.

A diagnosis of Down syndrome can be accurately made using CVS or amniocentesis, but it cannot give certainty as to the severity of the disorder or the quality of life of a particular individual. Responses to a diagnosis will vary, according to cultural, social, moral and religious beliefs.

Screening for haemoglobinopathies

The NHS NSC antenatal and newborn screening programmes include antenatal screening for fetal haemoglobinopathies. This should be linked with the newborn bloodspot screening programme, which tests for sickle cell disease. Linking results of parents and babies increases health professionals access to families with genetic disorders, allowing the results to be available throughout the individual's life, reducing repeat screening. Haemoglobinopathies are inherited disorders of haemoglobin and are more prevalent in certain racial groups. Antenatal screening identifies about 22,000 carriers of sickle cell disease and thalassaemia in the UK every year (NHS Sickle Cell and Thalassaemia Programme 2011).

Currently, in the UK, antenatal screening for haemoglobinopathy is based on population prevalence. High prevalence areas have universal screening (offer all pregnant women electrophoresis screening for haemoglobin variants and thalassaemia trait). Low prevalence areas use the national Family Origin Questionnaire (FOQ) to determine genetic ancestry for the last two generations (or more if possible). All areas collect information on the FOQ in their maternity population. This information is needed by laboratories to help interpret screening results.

In low-prevalence areas, women with genetic ancestry that includes high-risk racial groups are offered electrophoresis testing. If the mother is found to be a haemoglobinopathy carrier, partner testing is then recommended and should be offered soon after the result is available. Genetic ancestry is also important when interpreting screening results. It is important to establish maternal iron levels when carrier status for thalassaemia is suspected, since iron deficiency can give rise to similar red cell appearances.(e.g. alpha thalassaemia). Most haemoglobinopathies are recessively inherited, so the fetus would have a 1 in 4 chance of inheriting the disorder and a 1 in 2 chance of being a carrier.

Pre-test information for antenatal haemoglobinopathy screening

- In early pregnancy, information should be supplied. In the UK this means that all women should receive the NSC (2012) information booklet *Screening tests for you and your baby* as early in pregnancy as possible.
- The information should be provided in an appropriate language or format.
- Testing should be performed as early in pregnancy as possible, ideally at 8–10 weeks' gestation, as screening decisions are often gestation-dependent.
- Women who book late in pregnancy should be offered haemoglobinopathy screening in the same way at the first point of contact. Options for ending an affected pregnancy may be limited.

Where both parents are identified as carriers, they need urgent counselling. In the UK parents are referred urgently to the PEGASUS (Professional Education for Genetic Assessment and Screening) trained midwife for specialist counselling or to the combined obstetric/haematology clinic at the booking hospital. Diagnostic testing by CVS or amniocentesis should be offered.

Where paternity is unknown, the father of the baby is unavailable or declines testing, the woman should be offered a counselling appointment to calculate the possibility of the baby having an inherited haemoglobin disorder and an offer of diagnostic testing made if the risks warrant this. All women will be offered neonatal blood spot screening at 5 days, which will detect sickle cell disease (but not other haemoglobinopathies).

Ultrasonography for fetal screening

In the UK, the NSC (2011a) standards are that all pregnant women should be offered two routine ultrasound scans. These include an early pregnancy scan (usually timed to be able to perform the NT measurement if requested) and an 18–20 week fetal anomaly screening scan. Ultrasound works by transmitting sound at a very high frequency, via a probe, in a narrow beam. When the sound waves enter the body and encounter a structure, some of that sound is reflected back. The amount of sound reflected varies according to the type of tissue encountered; for example, fluid does not reflect sound and appears as a black image. Conversely, bone reflects a considerable amount of sound and appears as white or echogenic. Many structures appear as different shades of grey. Generally, pictures are transmitted in 'real time', which enables fetal movements to be seen.

Safety aspects of ultrasound

Ultrasound has been used as a diagnostic imaging tool since the 1950s, so we are now into the third generation of scanned babies. It seems reasonable to assume that any major adverse effects of this technology would have become apparent before now. However, modern machines have higher resolutions and indications for ultrasound scanning have greatly increased. This means that levels of exposure to ultrasound have increased in pregnancy. Although the technology is considered safe, it should be used with respect and only when there is good indication, and care should be taken to limit exposure time and the thermal indices should be controlled (European Committee of Medical Ultrasound Safety 2008). Ultrasound is a diagnostic tool, but diagnosis can only be as reliable as the expertise of the operator and the quality of the machine. As Wood (2000) states, abnormalities may be missed or incorrectly diagnosed if the operator is inexperienced or inadequately trained.

Women's experiences of ultrasound

In general, women experience ultrasound as a pleasurable opportunity to have visual access to their unborn baby (Sandelowski 1994). Indeed, ultrasound scans have been shown to increase psychological attachment to the fetus (Sedgman et al 2006). Parents have a profound curiosity about their baby and a scan can turn something nebulous into something that seems much more real as a living individual (Furness 1990). This can be particularly important for a woman's partner and family, who do not have the immediate physical experience of the pregnancy. Women tend to regard their scan as providing a general view of fetal well-being: the fact that the fetus is alive, growing and developing. However, this reassurance is temporary and begins to wear off after a few weeks (Clement et al 1998). Mothers may then seek other forms of reassurance (e.g. monitoring fetal movements, auscultation of the fetal heartbeat). This initial reassurance may also create an enthusiasm for scans when there is no clinical indication.

Scans may also cause considerable anxiety, however, particularly if there is a suspected or actual problem with the fetus. There is evidence to suggest that women who miscarry after visualization of the fetus on scan may feel a heightened sense of anguish because the fetus seemed more real. This may also be the case for parents considering termination of pregnancy on the grounds of fetal abnormality. However, others may view their scan as a treasured memory of the baby they lost (Black 1992).

The identification of fetal abnormality in the antenatal period has differing psychological effects for parents when the pregnancy is to continue. Some parents have reported feeling grateful that they were able to prepare for the birth of a child with a disability (Chitty et al 1996). However, others have reported feelings of wishing they had not known about their child's problems before birth because this created a powerful image of the fetus as a 'monster'. Some parents reported this to be far worse than the reality of caring for the baby after birth (Turner 1994). It is necessary for midwives to be mindful of the powerful psychological effects ultrasound scans have on pregnant women and their families, if sensitive and appropriate care is to be given at this potentially distressing time.

The midwife's role concerning ultrasound scans

As for all procedures, mothers should be fully informed about the purpose of the scan. Information should be given about which conditions are being checked for and which problems the scan would be unable to detect. Because of the pleasurable aspect of seeing the fetus, ultrasound scans have traditionally been tests that mothers undertake willingly, without prior discussion and consideration of potential consequences. Ultrasound screening for fetal abnormality is a screening test and as such women should be counselled as to the purpose, choices and pitfalls of screening so that they can decide whether or not they wish to undergo a procedure that may bring unwelcome news. Women should be aware that ultrasound scans are optional and not an inevitable part of their care.

Women should also understand that a normal 'scan' does not guarantee normality in the baby. Box 11.4 shows the detection rates for the commonly assessed abnormalities, which should be shared with women.

There is evidence that, although some mothers may find this information disturbing, most feel that this is outweighed by the positive aspects of seeing the baby and gaining reassurance (Oliver et al 1996). Indeed, extra

---

Box 11.4 **Detection rates for commonly assessed fetal abnormalities**	
Anencephaly	98%
Open spina bifida	90%
Cleft lip	75%
Diaphragmatic hernia	60%
Gastroschisis	98%
Exomphalos	80%
Serious cardiac abnormalities	50%
Bilateral renal agenesis	84%
Lethal skeletal dysplasia	60%
Edwards' syndrome (trisomy 18)	95%
Patau's syndrome (trisomy 13)	95%

Source: UK NSC 2010 NHS Fetal Anomaly Screening Programme: 18+^{0} to 20+^{6} Weeks Fetal Anomaly Scan National Standards and Guidance for England: Appendix 9

---

information about the purpose of the scan has been shown to increase women's understanding and satisfaction with the amount of information received, while the proportion of women accepting a scan (99%) appears to remain unchanged (Thornton et al 1995).

The Royal College of Obstetricians and Gynaecologists (RCOG 2000) recommends that, wherever scans are performed, a midwife or counsellor with a particular interest or expertise in the area should be available to discuss difficult news. All women with a suspected or confirmed fetal anomaly should be seen by an obstetric ultrasound specialist within three working days of the referral being made or seen by a fetal medicine unit within five working days of the referral being made (NSC 2011a: Standard 4). Effective multidisciplinary team working and communication are therefore essential. It is also good practice for the midwife to liaise with the primary healthcare team, who would normally carry out the majority of antenatal care. With the increasing use of client-held records, mothers may have more opportunity to scrutinize the written results of their scan. Midwives may increasingly be called upon to explain and discuss these findings, both in hospital and in the community setting.

First trimester pregnancy scans

All women should be offered a first trimester scan. The purpose of this is to establish:

- that the pregnancy is viable and intrauterine (not ectopic);
- to measure the NT if the gestation is appropriate and screening for Down syndrome is accepted;
- to accurately define the gestational age;
- to determine fetal number (and chorionicity or amnionicity in multiple pregnancies);
- to detect gross fetal abnormalities, such as anencephaly (absence of the cranial vault).

Early ultrasound scanning is beneficial, in reducing the need to induce labour for post-maturity (Whitworth et al 2010). A gestation sac can usually be visualized from 5 weeks' gestation and a small embryo from 6 weeks. Until 13 weeks, gestational age can be accurately assessed by CRL measurement (the length of the fetus from the top of the head to the end of the sacrum). Care must be taken to ensure that the fetus is not flexed at the time of measurement. Mothers are asked to attend with a full bladder, since this aids visualization of the uterus at an early gestation.

Dealing with increased nuchal translucency

A nuchal translucency of >3.5 mm occurs in about 1% of pregnancies (see Fig. 11.2). It is considered to be the threshold definition of an increased NT above which the risk of other (non-chromosomal) abnormalities increases. Increased NT is associated with a risk of chromosomal abnormalities and also with other structural (mainly cardiac) abnormalities (>10% risk), genetic syndromes and an increased fetal loss rate. Where an increased NT is seen regardless of whether screening for Down syndrome was declined, the potential for problems to be present must be discussed and ideally referral to specialist scanning and counselling arranged. In the presence of a normal karyotype, if no structural abnormalities are found the UK NSC (2011a) states that the incidence of adverse outcome is not increased, but also acknowledges that the chance of developmental delay is 2–4%.

Where diagnostic testing and 18–20 weeks ultrasound is normal it is reasonable to be optimistic regarding outcome, but it is worth recognizing that parents will carry the anxiety of uncertainty with them through and even beyond the end of the pregnancy and will often require a lot of support.

Second trimester ultrasound scans

After $13+^6$ weeks of pregnancy, gestational age is primarily assessed using the head circumference (HC).

The detailed fetal anomaly screening scan

This scan is usually performed at $18–20+^6$ weeks of pregnancy. The purpose of this scan is to reassure the mother that the fetus has no obvious structural anomalies that fall into the following categories:

- anomalies that are incompatible with life;
- anomalies that are associated with significant morbidity and long-term disability;
- anomalies that may benefit from intrauterine therapy;
- anomalies that may require postnatal treatment or investigation.

Detection rates should be in line with those outlined earlier. Technical difficulties, such as fetal position, multiple pregnancy, fibroids or maternal obesity may mean that a second scan before 23 weeks is offered. Some structural problems do not have sonographic signs that would be visible at this gestation or even at all. Anal atresia does not have a clear appearance on ultrasound; hydrocephalus and other bowel obstructions may not appear until later in pregnancy. Diagnosis may therefore not be possible. The UK NSC has defined which structures should be examined (Box 11.5) and which images should be stored as part of the woman's record.

Some features on ultrasound may be seen that increase the risk of another problem such as Down syndrome. An increased skin fold measurement of >6 mm at the level of the nuchal fold (a different entity to the nuchal translucency) should be noted as there is an associated increase in the risk for Down syndrome of at least 10-fold. Mild cerebral ventriculomegaly should be noted as there is

> ### Box 11.5 $18+^0$ to $20+^6$ weeks fetal anomaly ultrasound scan base menu
>
> - Spine, vertebrae and skin covering in transverse and longitudinal sections.
> - Head and neck: Head shape and internal structures (cavum pellucidum, cerebellum, ventricular size at atrium). Nuchal fold. Face and lips.
> - Thorax: Four-chamber view of heart, cardiac outflow tracts, lungs.
> - Abdominal shape and content – at level of the stomach with small portion of intrahepatic vein, abdominal wall, renal pelves, bladder.
> - Limbs: Arms – three bones and hand (metacarpals). Legs – three bones and foot (metatarsals).
> - Placental location and amniotic fluid.
>
> Source: UK NSC 2010 NHS Fetal Anomaly Screening Programme: $18+^0$ to $20+^6$ Weeks Fetal Anomaly Scan National Standards and Guidance for England: Appendix 1

again an increased risk of chromosomal abnormalities of about 10%. Echogenic bowel can be seen in cases of cystic fibrosis, fetal infection, and if associated with growth restriction and mild renal pelvis dilatation (>7 mm) can progress to significant hydronephrosis.

What used to be termed 'soft markers' are no longer considered to have any significant impact on the risk of chromosomal abnormality in isolation or combination, and are termed 'normal variants' and are therefore not usually reported (choroid plexus cysts, two-vessel cord, dilated cisterna magna, echogenic cardiac focus).

Advantages and disadvantages of fetal anomaly scans

Provided the sonographer has sufficient expertise, many lethal or severely disabling conditions can be detected during the 18–20 week scan. There is also an increase in first trimester diagnosis. Although this means that parents may be faced with difficult and unexpected decisions, it allows parents the choices that would be denied without this knowledge. Furthermore, many parents are offered reassurance that no obvious abnormalities were seen. For neonates requiring early surgical or paediatric interventions, prior knowledge of the abnormality allows a plan of care to be evolved in advance of the birth. The mother can then give birth in a unit with appropriate facilities. This has been shown to reduce morbidity in cases of gastroschisis (an abdominal wall defect, adjacent to the umbilicus, allowing the intestines and other abdominal organs to protrude outside the body), cardiac abnormalities and intestinal obstruction (Romero et al 1989). For parents who choose to continue the pregnancy knowing that the baby has a life-limiting condition, careful planning regarding place of birth, care of the baby after birth and multidisciplinary support can be provided.

In summary, the 18–20 week scan appears to confer psychological and health improvement benefits in some cases, but also has the capacity to cause great anxiety and distress. Care must be taken to ensure that parents are fully informed of the purpose, benefits and limitations of ultrasound scans before they consent to this procedure.

New and emerging technologies

Fetal imaging techniques

Ultrasound scans in pregnancy have been discussed at length in this chapter, since they are important fetal investigations. Women generally see two-dimensional (2-D) images of their unborn baby. However, there is a growing market for three-dimensional ultrasound imaging (3-D). As such, multiple images are stored digitally and then shaded to produce life-like pictures. This technique can assist the diagnosis of surface structural anomalies, such as cleft lip and spina bifida, and improvements are being seen in cardiac and neurological scanning (Sandelowski 1994; Sedgman et al 2006).

Magnetic resonance imaging (MRI) has also been applied in the examination of the fetus over the last two decades. This technique has not been widely applied because ultrasound can give similar diagnostic information at a lower cost. However, MRI has a contribution to make, particularly when examining the brain. There is evidence that this may provide additional information and change the counselling and management for a significant number of pregnancies where brain abnormalities are suspected (Glenn and Barkovich 2006). A further application is that MRI offers an alternative to postmortem following termination or perinatal death. This can offer information to parents who decline postmortem because of its invasive nature (Brookes and Hall-Craggs 1997). MRI imaging has been used to refine the diagnosis of many other conditions including diaphragmatic hernias and sacrococcygeal teratomas (Kumar and O'Brien 2004).

Free fetal DNA

Much work is now being done on the technology that identifies free fetal DNA in the maternal circulation. Already it is possible to identify with great (though not 100%) accuracy, fetal sex, blood group and some genetic disorders. Before long RAPID (Reliable Accurate Prenatal non-Invasive Diagnosis) study will report the results of the research into testing for Down syndrome using this technology. Already a test is available privately in the United States. This will undoubtedly increase the true-positive rate and decrease the false-negative rate for screening for

Down syndrome, which will become available as a blood test. Confirmatory testing will still be required, but fewer tests will be needed. Free fetal DNA is now routinely used to determine fetal blood group (see below).

SCREENING FOR MATERNAL CONDITIONS

The rationale for screening a mother is to detect conditions that are amenable to treatment and will have potential health benefits for her and her baby. In the main, in pregnancy, screening is focused on those that carry improved outcomes for the baby.

Infectious diseases

In the UK the NSC programme for screening of infectious diseases in pregnancy recommends that all pregnant women are screened for:

- HIV
- syphilis
- hepatitis B (HBV)
- rubella.

The infectious diseases screened for meet the screening criteria in that they are important and intervention can reduce harm. Rubella screening cannot reduce the risk if a mother develops the illness but allows immunization in the future to reduce risk.

Human immune deficiency virus (HIV)

Knowledge and adequate management of women with HIV can reduce mother to child transfer to less than 1% and improve maternal health. Screening should be offered at booking and again later in pregnancy in women at high risk (e.g. women who are paid for sex, women who have an untested partner from an area of high prevalence, intravenous drug users). Women who decline screening should also be re-offered testing later in pregnancy.

Hepatitis B (HB)

Adequate immunization programmes for infants at risk of vertical transmission of HBV can reduce infant infection rates by 90% and improvements in maternal health can be made.

Referral to a specialist is required for women who are found to be hepatitis B positive. Establishing the neonatal and maternal risk will be determined by testing of antibody and antigen status and viral DNA levels. Occasionally hepatitis B can reactivate in pregnancy and knowledge of status can aid management of the pregnant mother.

Syphilis

Syphilis used to be a rare infection in the UK, but the incidence is now inexorably rising. Treatment of syphilis can prevent pregnancy loss plus congenital syphilis, and prevent long-term problems for the mother. A positive screening result does not distinguish between syphilis and other treponemal infections, so specialist input is required if the initial screening test is positive.

In all three of the above infections, knowledge of infection can prevent unwitting infection of sexual partners.

Rubella

Screening for susceptibility to rubella aims to identify the 3% of women who are susceptible, to counsel about avoidance of potentially infected individuals during pregnancy and to offer postnatal vaccination.

For the above infections, testing in early pregnancy is recommended. Written information should be provided at least 24 hours prior to decisions being made. In order for the woman to make an informed choice, the midwife should discuss the following points:

- The infections that are screened for, their routes of transmission and the implications of a positive test.
- The benefits, to both mother and baby, to be gained from the identification and management of those with positive results.
- The results procedure, including the feedback of results and the possibility of a false- negative or false-positive result.
- All pregnant women should be advised that if they develop, or are exposed to, a rash during the pregnancy they should seek professional advice.

That the offer was made and the response to the offer should be documented with the date. Women who initially decline should be re-offered testing at a later date; usually it is best to do this before 28 weeks. If testing is declined it is good practice to enquire why and to explore and document the reasons. Women who book late or who arrive untested in labour can be urgently screened.

Women with a positive result for syphilis, HIV or HBV should be seen and counselled as soon as possible and within 10 days in the UK. Appropriate referrals should then be made to ensure that the correct care pathway is inducted.

Screening for infectious diseases in pregnancy can be enormously challenging for the mother and for the midwife. The cultural and social stigma that is still attached to a diagnosis of HIV means that some women will be reluctant to consider testing or may be devastated when a positive test is confirmed. Issues such as partner testing need sensitive exploration and should be undertaken by the wider multidisciplinary team that will care for these women. The midwife needs to have enough knowledge to understand the disease, the process following a positive test and the ability to answer questions or direct women to the answers.

New screening

In the UK screening does not exist on a population basis yet for Group B Streptococcus (GBS). GBS is carried in the genital tract and gut of many healthy people (between 10 and 40%). It is estimated that about 25% of pregnant women in the UK carry GBS. In the UK GBS is either detected opportunistically or by screening for high-risk situations, such as after premature or prolonged rupture of the membranes. Using this strategy 0.5/1000 babies are affected by early onset GBS disease, a disease that can cause severe problems for these babies, including meningitis and death. New work on why only some babies are affected has focused on the ability of the mother to pass on GBS antibodies, but this has not been able to identify a very high-risk group that could be effectively targeted.

In the United States screening is offered by vaginal swabs at 35–37 weeks. However, the risk of GBS in the United States is considerably higher, again for reasons that are not entirely understood.

The NSC (UK) is consulting on whether to include GBS screening within the programme for the future. Important considerations are the effect of antibiotics on as many as 25% of the pregnant population, weighed against the harm to about 340 babies per year.

Mid-stream urine testing

Screening for asymptomatic bacteriuria is recommended as in pregnancy progression to pyelonephritis can occur in up to 25% of women. Pyelonephritis can be life-threatening and can lead to miscarriage and premature labour. Treatment is simple and effective with appropriately targeted antibiotics.

Screening for anaemia

Anaemia is one of the commonest complications of pregnancy. The most common reason for iron deficiency anaemia in pregnancy is the increased demands of the fetus for iron. Risk factors for the development of iron deficiency in pregnancy include iron deficiency prior to pregnancy, hyperemesis, vegetarian or vegan diet, multiple pregnancies, pregnancy recurring after a short interval and blood loss.

Pregnant women should be offered screening for anaemia in early in pregnancy and at 28 weeks. This allows enough time for treatment if anaemia is detected.

Haemoglobin levels outside the normal UK range for pregnancy (that is, 11 g/dl at first contact and 10.5 g/dl at 28 weeks) should be investigated. Provided there are no unusual features to suggest another cause for the anaemia, treatment with iron can be started and a blood test for serum ferritin sent at the same time to confirm iron stores are low. The woman should be asked if she is known to have a haemoglobinopathy. These women should be directly referred to an Obstetric Haematology clinic for assessment.

Screening for red cell antibodies

All pregnant women should be offered antenatal testing to assess ABO and rhesus status and to look for red cell antibodies. There will usually be relevant national guidelines, which will specify the intervals at which this should take place. This will vary depending on the woman's Rhesus (Rh) type and whether any red cell antibodies are detected.

Red cell antibodies are antibodies against red cell antigens, and the relevance to pregnancy will vary depending on the type and level of the circulating antibody. Some antibodies occur naturally, without any sensitising event, but most of the important ones require a sensitising event such as a previous pregnancy or transfusion. Antibodies to the ABO system tend to be naturally occurring, as does anti-E.

Once an antibody has been identified it will be relevant to understand the issues for both the mother and baby.

For the mother with any red-cell antibody the major issue is related to increased difficulty in crossmatching blood. Women with antibodies will not be able to undergo rapid electronic crossmatching and therefore for women at any increased risk in labour of haemorrhage, crossmatching in the early stages or before planned birth may be prudent.

For the fetus, red-cell antibodies are of significance as IgG antibodies can cross the placenta. If the fetal red blood cells carry the antigen the antibody is directed against they will be destroyed. This can lead to fetal anaemia and in severe cases cause fetal hydrops. Jaundice and kernicterus (brain damage caused by very high unconjugated bilirubin levels) in the neonatal period are the major neonatal risks.

Routine antibody testing in pregnancy aims to:

- identify Rhesus-negative women who will be eligible for anti-D immunoglobulin prophylaxis
- identify women who are difficult to crossmatch so that steps can be taken to minimize risk
- identify women with antibodies that put the fetus at risk of haemolytic disease of the newborn (HDN).

The UK recommends that all women should be tested at booking and again at 28 weeks' gestation (NICE 2008).

There are many red cell antibodies and it is useful to understand which ones are important causes of HDN.

- Antibodies to the Rhesus antigens are the most common to cause problems.
- Rhesus D antibodies are the principle cause of severe HDN.

- Rhesus c can cause HDN, especially if antibodies to Rhesus E are also present
- Rarely antibodies to Rhesus E, e, C and CW can cause HDN.

Antibodies to non-Rhesus antigens can also cause HND. Anti-K (Kell) antibodies are an important cause of severe HDN. These antibodies not only destroy the fetal red cells, but inhibit production in the bone marrow, exacerbating any developing anaemia.

Other antibodies known to cause HDN less commonly include anti Fya (Duffy), anti Jka (Kidd) and anti S.

Antibodies to the ABO system may be detected on routine testing. In general these occur in Group O women and are naturally occurring anti-A and anti-B antibodies. Because these antibodies are IgM antibodies they do not cross the placenta and do not harm the fetus. Occasionally some group O women produce IgG antibodies when carrying group A or B infants. These IgG antibodies can cross the placenta and cause HDN, but this tends to be mild.

How the results are presented

Antibody levels are either given as the actual measured amount or as the dilution achieved before there is insufficient antibody to cause red cell clumping.

Rh-D and Rh-c are always measured and the result will be given in iu/ml; hence the higher the result the worse the effects are likely to be.

Other antibody levels are expressed as titres. A titre of 1:2 means that after a single dilution there was no clumping of the red cells. This would be a low level of antibody. A titre of 1:16 states that there were four dilutions before the antibody was too weak to clump cells, implying a much higher level of antibody. It is useful to understand that a jump from 1:2 to 1:4 is a single dilution, as is a jump from 1:16 to 1:32.

What parents need to know

Parents need to understand the purpose of blood group and red cell antibody screening, what is being tested for and what the test involves. This will involve discussion about the nature and effects of red cell antibodies, how and when test results will be available and the meaning of the results.

Management when an antibody is detected

When an antibody is detected it is important that the relevance of this is discussed with the mother. The discussion should cover the potential for difficulties in crossmatching blood and the potential for fetal or neonatal problems. If significant antibody titres are found management needs to be discussed, including the need for surveillance for fetal anaemia and the possibility of intrauterine transfusion – this would usually be done by the obstetrician managing the pregnancy.

Surveillance will depend on the type of antibody found; for some antibodies, the titre (level) of the antibody; and the gestation of pregnancy at which it is discovered.

Discussion with the consultant team is usually needed to define the steps that need to be taken.

When an antibody is detected that may cause HDN the next steps will usually be:

1. Referral for discussion with an appropriate consultant/haematology team.
2. Partner testing. This is to determine the potential for fetal risk. Only a fetus that is antigen positive for the antibody found can be at risk. This means that, for instance, if a woman has anti-D antibodies and a Rh-D-positive partner there will be a 50–100% risk of producing a baby who is Rh-D-positive, depending on whether the partner carries one or two Rh-D-positive genes. It is imperative that the woman understands the importance of partner testing, the need to be honest if there can be any doubt regarding paternity (and for this to be asked about sensitively, without the partner being present). Beware with IVF pregnancies also. Remember to ask whether there has been egg donation, as in these cases it may be the maternal genetic complement that differs and cases of HDN have occurred where this vital fact has not been ascertained.
3. Free fetal DNA testing. Where the fetus is potentially at risk because the partner is positive for the antigen to the detected antibody or where partner testing cannot be undertaken, typing of the fetal red cell status can be performed on a blood test from the woman. The test is usually carried out between 12–18 weeks. The results are accurate in 99% of cases but in some cases a result cannot be given.
4. Confirmatory testing. Invasive testing using CVS or amniocentesis is usually undertaken only where there is a need to establish fetal karyotype for other reasons. In cases where ultrasound suggests developing anaemia a fetal blood sample prior to

intrauterine transfusion will be tested for fetal blood typing.

On-going surveillance

Once the risk of a pregnancy being affected has been established the timing and frequency of repeat testing of antibody titres can be determined. The need for assessment of the fetus at risk can also be established.

Surveillance for fetal anaemia is now undertaken primarily using ultrasound measurement of the blood flow velocity within the fetal brain. Measurement of the maximum velocity in the fetal middle cerebral artery has been found to be as accurate as the old-fashioned measurement of bilirubin in amniotic fluid, but is without the attendant risks of serial amniocentesis.

The frequency of surveillance will be determined by the risk of anaemia, which is dependent on the type and level of antibody and the risk of the fetus being antigen-positive.

CONCLUSION

Fetal investigations are an integral aspect of antenatal care. Scientists and clinicians have developed a range of new diagnostic and imaging technologies. Some of these have been incorporated into national screening programmes and standards of care. The midwife must therefore ensure that women are informed about the benefits and risks associated with these technologies, so that they can make choices to suit their requirements. Undoubtedly, testing technologies profoundly influence women's experiences of pregnancy and their early attachment to their unborn child. Midwives therefore have a duty to prepare women for tests through sensitive and accurate communications and then to support parents in their assimilation of information and decision-making once the results are known.

Maternal investigations also require careful counselling and thought as a constellation of unintended consequences can arise if women do not think through their screening choices, or are inadequately counselled.

REFERENCES

Al-Jader L N, Parry Langdon N, Smith R J 2000 Survey of attitudes of pregnant women towards Down syndrome screening. Prenatal Diagnosis 20(1):23–9

Berryman J C, Windridge K C 1999 Women's experiences of giving birth after 35. Birth 26(1): 16–23

Black R B 1992 Seeing the baby: the impact of ultrasound technology. Journal of Genetic Counselling 1(1):45–54

Brookes J S, Hall-Craggs M A 1997 Postmortem perinatal examination: the role of magnetic resonance imaging. Ultrasound in Obstetrics and Gynaecology 9(3):45–7

Chitty L, Barnes C A, Berry C 1996 Continuing with the pregnancy after a diagnosis of lethal abnormality. British Medical Journal 313:478–80

Clarke A 1994 Genetic counselling: Practice and principles. Routledge, London

Clement S, Wilson J, Sikorski J 1998 Women's experiences of antenatal ultrasound scans. In: Clement S (ed.) Psychological perspectives on pregnancy and childbirth. Churchill Livingstone, Edinburgh, p 117–32

European Committee of Medical Ultrasound Safety (ECMUS) 2008 Clinical safety statement for diagnostic ultrasound. Available at www.efsumb.org/guidelines/2008safstat.pdf (accessed June 2013).

Fisher J 2006 Pregnancy loss, breaking bad news and supporting parents. In: Sullivan A, Kean L, Cryer A (eds) Midwife's guide to antenatal investigations. Elsevier, London, p 31–42

Furness M E 1990 Fetal ultrasound for entertainment? Medical Journal of Australia 153(7):371

Glenn O A, Barkovich A J 2006 Magnetic resonance imaging of the fetal brain and spine: an increasingly important tool in prenatal diagnosis, Part 1. American Journal of Neuroradiology 27:1604–11.

Green J M, Hewison J, Bekker H L et al 2004 Psychosocial aspects of genetic screening of pregnant women and newborns: a systematic review. Health Technology Assessment 8(33) (Executive summary)

Health Technology Assessment 2000 Ultrasound screening in pregnancy: a systematic review of the clinical effectiveness, cost-effectiveness and women's views. The National Coordinating Centre for HTA, Southampton

Hunt L M, de Voogd B, Castaneda H 2005 The routine and the traumatic in prenatal genetic diagnosis: does clinical information inform patient decision-making? Patient Education and Counselling 56(3):302–12

Hunter M 1994 Counselling in obstetrics and gynaecology. British Psychological Society Books, Leicester

Ingram R, Malcarne V 1995 Cognition in depression and anxiety. Same, different or a little of both. In: Craig K, Dobson K (eds) Anxiety and depression in adults and children. Sage, London, p 37–56

Kennard A, Goodburn S, Golightly S et al 1995 Serum screening for Down syndrome. Royal College of Midwives Journal 108:207–10

Kessler S, Levine E 1987 Psychological aspects of genetic counselling IV. The subjective assessment of probability. American Journal of Medical Genetics 28:361–70

Kingston H M 2002 ABC of clinical genetics, 3rd edn. BMJ Publishing, London

Kleinveld J H, Timmermans D R M, de Smit D J et al 2006 Does prenatal screening influence anxiety levels of pregnant women? A longitudinal randomised controlled trial. Prenatal Diagnosis 26(4):354–61

Kumar S, O'Brien A 2004 Recent developments in fetal medicine. British Medical Journal 328:1002–6

NICE (National Institute for Health and Clinical Excellence) 2008 Antenatal care. Routine care for the healthy pregnant woman, CG 62. NICE, London

NSC (National Screening Committee) 2011a NHS fetal anomaly screening programme. Consent standards and guidance. Developed by the National Health Service Fetal Anomaly Screening Programme (NHS FASP) Consent Standards Review Group. Available at www.screening.nhs.uk (accessed 11 April 2013).

NSC (National Screening Committee) 2011b Screening for Down's syndrome: UK NSC policy recommendations 2011–2014 model of best practice. Available at www.screening.nhs.uk (accessed 11 April 2013)

NSC (National Screening Committee) 2012 Screening tests for you and your baby: version 2. Available at www.screening.nhs.uk (accessed 11 April 2013)

NSC (National Screening Committee) 2013 What is screening? Available at www.screening.nhs.uk (accessed 11 April 2013)

NHS Sickle Cell and Thalassaemia Screening Programme Standards for the Linked Antenatal and Newborn Screening Programme 2011, 2nd edn. Available at http://sct.screening.nhs.uk

NMC (Nursing and Midwifery Council) 2012 Midwives rules and standards. NMC, London

Oliver S, Rajan L, Turner H et al 1996 A pilot study of informed choice' leaflets on positions in labour and routine ultrasound. NHS Centre for Reviews and Dissemination, York

Raphael-Leff J 2005 Psychological processes of childbearing. Anna Freud Centre, London

Raynor M D, England E 2010 Psychology for midwives: pregnancy, childbirth and puerperium. Open University Press/McGraw-Hill, Maidenhead

Romero R, Ghidini A, Costigan K et al 1989 Prenatal diagnosis of duodenal atresia: does it make any difference? Obstetrics and Gynaecology 71:739–41

Rothman B 1986 The tentative pregnancy. How amniocentesis changes the experience of motherhood. Norton Paperbacks, New York

RCOG (Royal College of Obstetricians and Gynaecologists) 2000 Routine ultrasound screening in pregnancy. Protocol, standards and training. Supplement to ultrasound screening for fetal abnormalities report of the RCOG working party. RCOG, London. Available at www.rcog.org.uk

Sandelowski M 1994 Channel of desire: fetal ultrasonography in two-use contexts. Qualitative Health Research 4:262–80

Sedgman B, McMahon C, Cairns D et al 2006 The impact of two-dimensional versus three-dimensional ultrasound exposure on maternal–fetal attachment and maternal health behavior in pregnancy. Ultrasound in Obstetrics and Gynecology 27:245–51

Sjögren B 1996 Psychological indications for prenatal diagnosis. Prenatal Diagnosis 16:449–54

Sullivan A. 2005 Skilled decision making: the blood supply of midwifery practice. In: Raynor M, Marshall J, Sullivan A (eds) Decision making in midwifery practice. Elsevier, London

Thornton J G, Hewison J, Lilford R J et al 1995 A randomised trial of three methods of giving information about prenatal testing. British Medical Journal 311: 1127–30

Turner L 1994 Problems surrounding late prenatal diagnosis. In: Abramsky L, Chapple J (eds) Prenatal

diagnosis: The human side. Chapman & Hall, London

Whitworth M, Bricker L, Neilson J P, et al 2010 Ultrasound for fetal assessment in early pregnancy. Cochrane Database of Systematic Reviews 2010, Issue 4. Art. No.

CD007058. doi: 10.1002/14651858. CD007058.pub2

Wood P 2000 Safe and (ultra) sound – some aspects of ultrasound safety. Royal College of Midwives Journal 3(2):48–50

FURTHER READING

Sullivan A, Kean L, Cryer A (eds) 2006 Midwife's guide to antenatal investigations. Elsevier, London

A practical guide for midwives to use when discussing and interpreting antenatal test results. Covers maternal and fetal investigations.

USEFUL WEBSITES

UK National Screening Committee: www.screening.nhs.uk

DIPEx – Patient experiences website: www.dipex.org

Includes a range of pregnancy and screening experiences from the woman's perspective. Includes video clips of interviews with women who talk about their experiences.

Chapter |12|

Common problems associated with early and advanced pregnancy

Helen Crafter, Jenny Brewster

Problems of pregnancy range from the mildly irritating to life-threatening conditions. Fortunately in the developed world, the life-threatening ones are rare because of improvements in the general health of the population, improved social circumstances and lower parity. However, as women delay childbearing, they become more at risk of disorders associated with increasing age, such as miscarriage and placenta praevia.

Regular antenatal examinations beginning early in pregnancy are undoubtedly valuable. They help to prevent many complications and their ensuing problems, contribute to timely diagnosis and treatment, and enable women to form relationships with midwives, obstetricians and other health professionals who become involved with them in striving to achieve the best possible pregnancy outcomes.

- provide an overview of problems of pregnancy
- describe the role of the midwife in relation to the identification, assessment and management of the more common disorders of pregnancy
- consider the needs of both parents for continuing support when a disorder has been diagnosed.

THE MIDWIFE'S ROLE

The midwife's role in relation to the problems associated with pregnancy is clear. At initial and subsequent encounters with the pregnant woman, it is essential that an accurate health history is obtained. General and specific physical examinations must be carried out and the results meticulously recorded. The examination and recordings enable effective referral and management. Where the midwife detects a deviation from the norm which is outside her sphere of practice, she must refer the woman to a suitable qualified health professional to assist her (NMC [Nursing and Midwifery Council] 2012a). The midwife will continue to offer the woman care and support throughout her pregnancy and beyond. The woman who develops problems during her pregnancy is no less in need of the midwife's skilled attention; indeed, her condition and psychological state may be considerably improved by the midwife's continued presence and support. It is also the midwife's role in such a situation to ensure that the woman and her family understand the situation; are enabled to take part in decision-making; and are protected from unnecessary fear. As the primary care manager, the midwife must ensure that all the attention the woman receives from different health professionals is balanced and integrated – in short, the woman's needs remain paramount throughout.

ABDOMINAL PAIN IN PREGNANCY

Abdominal pain is a common complaint in pregnancy. It is probably suffered by all women at some stage, and therefore presents a problem for the midwife of how to distinguish between the physiologically normal (e.g. mild indigestion or muscle stretching), the pathological but not dangerous (e.g. degeneration of a fibroid) and the dangerously pathological requiring immediate referral to the appropriate medical practitioner for urgent treatment (e.g. ectopic pregnancy or appendicitis).

The midwife should take a detailed history and perform a physical examination in order to reach a decision about whether to refer the woman. Treatment will depend on the cause (see Box 12.1) and the maternal and fetal conditions.

Many of the pregnancy-specific causes of abdominal pain in pregnancy listed in Box 12.1 are dealt with in this and other chapters. For most of these conditions, abdominal pain is one of many symptoms and not necessarily the overriding one. However, an observant midwife's skills may be crucial in procuring a safe pregnancy outcome for a woman presenting with abdominal pain.

BLEEDING BEFORE THE 24TH WEEK OF PREGNANCY

Any vaginal bleeding in early pregnancy is abnormal and of concern to the woman and her partner, especially if there is a history of previous pregnancy loss. The midwife can come into contact with women at this time either through the booking clinic or through phone contact. If bleeding in early pregnancy occurs a woman may contact the midwife, the birthing unit or a triage line for advice and support. The midwife should be aware of the local policies pertaining to her employment and how to guide the woman. In some areas of the United Kingdom (UK) women are reviewed within the maternity department from early pregnancy, whereas in others, they will be seen by the gynaecology team until 20 weeks' gestation, possibly in an early pregnancy clinic. However, women are often advised to contact their General Practitioner (GP) in the first instance, and many will visit an accident and emergency department.

In all cases, a history should be obtained to establish the amount and colour of the bleeding, when it occurred and whether there was any associated pain. Fetal well-being may be assessed either by ultrasound scan or, in the second trimester, using a hand-held Doppler device to hear the fetal heart sounds. Maternal reporting of fetal movements may also be useful in determining the viability of a pregnancy.

There are many causes of vaginal bleeding in early pregnancy, some of which can occasionally lead to life-threatening situations and others of less consequence for the continuance of pregnancy. The midwife should be aware of the different causes of vaginal bleeding in order to advise and support the woman and her family accordingly.

Implantation bleed

A small vaginal bleed can occur when the blastocyst embeds in the endometrium. This usually occurs 5–7 days after fertilization, and if the timing coincides with the

---

Box 12.1 **Causes of abdominal pain in pregnancy**

Pregnancy-specific causes

Physiological

Heartburn, soreness from vomiting, constipation

Braxton Hicks contractions

Pressure effects from growing/vigorous/malpresenting fetus

Round ligament pain

Severe uterine torsion (can become pathological)

Pathological

Spontaneous miscarriage

Uterine leiomyoma

Ectopic pregnancy

Hyperemesis gravidarum (vomiting with straining)

Preterm labour

Chorioamnionitis

Ovarian pathology

Placental abruption

Spontaneous uterine rupture

Abdominal pregnancy

Trauma to abdomen (consider undisclosed domestic abuse)

Severe pre-eclampsia

Acute fatty liver of pregnancy

Incidental causes

More common pathology

Appendicitis

Acute cholestasis/cholelithiasis

Gastro-oesophageal reflux/peptic ulcer disease

Acute pancreatitis

Urinary tract pathology/pyelonephritis

Inflammatory bowel disease

Intestinal obstruction

Miscellaneous

Rectus haematoma

Sickle cell crisis

Porphyria

Malaria

Arteriovenous haematoma

Tuberculosis

Malignant disease

Psychological causes

Source: Adapted from Cahill et al 2011; Mahomed 2011a

---

expected menstruation this may cause confusion over the dating of the pregnancy if the menstrual cycle is used to estimate the date of birth.

Cervical ectropion

More commonly known as *cervical erosion*. The changes seen in cases of cervical ectropion are as a physical response to hormonal changes that occur in pregnancy. The number of columnar epithelial cells in the cervical canal increase significantly under the influence of oestrogen during pregnancy to such an extent that they extend beyond to the vaginal surface of the cervical os, giving it a dark red appearance. As this area is vascular, and the cells form only a single layer, bleeding may occur either spontaneously or following sexual intercourse. Normally, no treatment is required, and the ectropion reverts back to normal cervical cells during the puerperium.

Cervical polyps

These are small, vascular, pedunculated growths on the cervix, which consist of squamous or columnar epithelial cells over a core of connective tissue rich with blood vessels. During pregnancy, the polyps may be a cause of

bleeding, but require no treatment unless the bleeding is severe or a smear test indicates malignancy.

Carcinoma of the cervix

Carcinoma of the cervix is the most common gynaecological malignant disease occurring in pregnancy with an estimated incidence of 1 in 2200 pregnancies (Copeland and Landon 2011). The condition presents with vaginal bleeding and increased vaginal discharge. On speculum examination the appearance of the cervix may lead to a suspicion of carcinoma, which is diagnosed following colposcopy or a cervical biopsy.

The precursor to cervical cancer is cervical intraepithelial neoplasia (CIN), which can be diagnosed from an abnormal Papanicolaou (Pap) smear. Where this is diagnosed at an early stage, treatment can usually be postponed for the duration of the pregnancy. The Pap smear is not routinely carried out during pregnancy, but the midwife should ensure that pregnant women know about the National Health Service Cervical Screening Programme (2013), recommending a smear 6 weeks postnatally if one has not been carried out in the previous 3 years.

Treatment for cervical carcinoma in pregnancy will depend on the gestation of the pregnancy and the stage of the disease, and full explanations of treatments and their possible outcomes should be given to the woman and her family. For carcinoma in the early stages, treatment may be delayed until the end of the pregnancy, or a cone biopsy may be performed under general anaesthetic to remove the affected tissue. However, there is a risk of haemorrhage due to the increased vascularity of the cervix in pregnancy, as well as a risk of miscarriage. Where the disease is more advanced, and the diagnosis made in early pregnancy, the woman may be offered a termination of pregnancy in order to receive treatment, as the effects of chemotherapy and radiotherapy on the fetus cannot be accurately predicted at the present time. During the late second and third trimester the obstetric and oncology teams will consider the optimal time for birth in order to achieve the best outcomes for both mother and baby.

Spontaneous miscarriage

The term *miscarriage* is used to describe a spontaneous pregnancy loss in preference to the term of *abortion* which is associated with the deliberate ending of a pregnancy. A miscarriage is seen as the loss of the products of conception prior to the completion of 24 weeks of gestation, with an early pregnancy loss being one that occurs before the 12th completed week of pregnancy (RCOG [Royal College of Obstetricians and Gynaecologists] 2006).

It is estimated that 10–20% of clinically recognized pregnancies will end in a miscarriage, resulting in 50 000 hospital admissions annually. Approximately 1–2% of second trimester pregnancies will result in a miscarriage (RCOG 2011a). Methods of managing pregnancy loss are currently evolving, with more emphasis being placed on medical intervention and/or management.

In all cases of miscarriage, the woman and her family will need guidance and support from those caring for her. In all areas of communication, the language used should be appropriate, avoiding medical terms, and be respectful of the pregnancy loss. Following the miscarriage, the parents may wish to see and hold their baby, and will need to be supported in doing this by those caring for them. Even where there is no recognizable baby, some parents are comforted by being given this opportunity (SANDS [Stillbirth and Neonatal Death Society 2007]). It is also important to create memories for the parents in the form of photographs, and, for pregnancy losses in the second and third trimesters, footprints and handprints may be taken (see Chapter 26).

For a pregnancy loss prior to 24 weeks' gestation, there is no legal requirement for a baby's birth to be registered or for a burial or cremation to take place. However, many National Health Service (NHS) facilities now make provision for a service for these babies, or parents may choose to make their own arrangements. In the case of cremation, the parents should be advised that there are very few or no ashes.

Following a miscarriage, blood tests may be carried out on the woman, and depending on gestational age, the parents may be offered a post mortem examination of the fetal remains in an effort to try to establish a reason for the pregnancy loss. However, in many cases there is no identifiable cause. Should this be the case, the outlook for future pregnancies is generally good. Many early pregnancy losses are due to chromosomal malformations, resulting in a fetus that does not develop. Should a reason for the miscarriage be identified, it may be of some comfort to the woman allowing for medical management to be put in place to enable a subsequent pregnancy to be more successful.

A spontaneous miscarriage may present in a number of ways, all associated with a history of bleeding and/or lower abdominal pain.

A *threatened miscarriage* occurs where there is vaginal bleeding in early pregnancy, which may or may not be accompanied by abdominal pain. The cervical os remains closed, and in about 80% of women presenting with these symptoms a viable pregnancy will continue.

Where the abdominal pain persists and the bleeding increases, the cervix opens and the products of conception will pass into the vagina in an *inevitable miscarriage*. Should some of the products be retained, this is termed an *incomplete miscarriage*. Infection is a risk with incomplete miscarriage and therapeutic termination of pregnancy. The signs and symptoms of miscarriage are present, accompanied by uterine tenderness, offensive vaginal discharge and pyrexia. In some cases this may progress to overwhelming sepsis, with the accompanying symptoms of hypotension, renal failure and disseminated intravascular coagulation (DIC). The remaining products may be passed spontaneously to become a *complete miscarriage*.

Where there is a *missed* or *silent miscarriage* a pregnancy sac with identifiable fetal parts is seen on ultrasound examination, but there is no fetal heart beat. There may be some abdominal pain and bleeding but the products of the pregnancy are not always passed spontaneously.

The first priority with any woman presenting with vaginal bleeding is to ensure that she is haemodynamically stable. Profuse bleeding may occur where the products of conception are partially expelled through the cervix.

Human chorionic gonadotrophic hormone (hCG) is present in the maternal blood from 9–10 days following conception, and assessing hCG levels may be used as an indication of the pregnancy's viability. Where a woman has persistent bleeding serial readings can be taken to assess the progress of a pregnancy or distinguish an ectopic pregnancy from a complete miscarriage where the uterus is empty on an ultrasound scan. The levels of hCG double every 48 hours in a normal intrauterine pregnancy from 4 to 6 weeks of gestation.

As a pregnancy progresses, transvaginal ultrasound and/or abdominal ultrasound may be used to confirm the presence or absence of a viable pregnancy sac (RCOG 2006). A gentle vaginal or speculum examination may also be performed to ascertain if the cervical os is open, and to observe for the presence of any products of conception within the vagina.

In the case of threatened miscarriage where viability of the pregnancy has been confirmed, there is no specific treatment as the likelihood of the pregnancy progressing is usually good. The practice of bed rest to preserve pregnancy is not supported by evidence so women should be neither encouraged nor discouraged from doing this.

For a complete miscarriage, there also is no required treatment if the woman's condition is stable, apart from the support and guidance she and her family will require to deal with their loss.

If there are retained products of conception, an incomplete or missed miscarriage, the options for treatment will often depend on gestational age and the condition of the woman. Miscarriages may be managed surgically, medically or expectantly. In many cases the appropriate management is to wait for the products of the conception to be passed spontaneously. However women should be aware that this can take several weeks (RCOG 2006). Women adopting this option should be given full information regarding the probable sequence of events and be provided with contact details for further advice, with the option of admission to hospital if required. It is important that women are educated to actively observe for signs of infection and know what to do if they suspect this.

The surgical method, where the uterine cavity is evacuated of the retained products of conception (ERPC) prior to 14 weeks' gestation is suitable for women who do not want to be managed expectantly and who are not suitable for medical management. Under either a general or local anaesthetic the cervix is dilated and a suction curettage is used to empty the uterus. The use of prostaglandins prior to surgery makes the cervix easier to dilate, thus reducing the risk of cervical damage. Between 1 and 2% of surgical evacuations result in serious morbidity for the woman with the main complications being perforation of the uterus, tears to the cervix and haemorrhage.

Medical management of miscarriages includes a variety of regimes involving the use of prostaglandins, such as misoprostol, and may include the use of an antiprogesterone such as mifepristone for a missed miscarriage, or progesterone alone for an incomplete miscarriage. The success rates for medically managed miscarriages vary from 13 to 96% (RCOG 2006) depending on the gestation and size of the gestational sac. Often women will spend time at home between the administration of the first drug and subsequent treatment, so it should be ensured that they have full knowledge of what might happen and a contact number to use at any time. Although the complications include abdominal pain and bleeding, overall the medical management of miscarriage reduces both the number of hospital admissions and the time women spend in hospital.

Recurrent miscarriage

Tests may be carried out on the woman and fetus following a miscarriage to try to establish any underlying cause. This is especially important where there is a history of recurrent miscarriage. Following a history of three or more miscarriages a referral is usually made to a specialist recurrent miscarriage clinic (RCOG 2011a), where appropriate and accurate information and support can be given.

Genetic reasons for the miscarriage may be identified through karyotyping of the fetal tissue, as well as both parents. This can cause difficult dilemmas to deal with but more recent genetic engineering is offering hope to some couples. Women should also be tested for *lupus anticoagulant* and *anticardiolipin antibodies*, with treatment of low dose aspirin and heparin being initiated if either of these is present. Other treatments depend on the cause, or causes, of the miscarriages being identified.

Ectopic pregnancy

An ectopic pregnancy occurs when a fertilized ovum implants outside the uterine cavity, often within the fallopian tube. However, implantation can also occur within the abdominal cavity (for instance on the large intestine or in the Pouch of Douglas), the ovary or in the cervical canal. The incidence is 11.1 per 1000 pregnancies (RCOG 2010a), with 6 deaths attributed to ectopic pregnancy in the 2006–2008 Saving Mother's Lives report (CEMACE [Centre for Maternal and Child Enquiries] 2011).

The conceptus produces hCG in the same way as for a uterine pregnancy, maintaining the corpus luteum, which leads to the production of oestrogen and progesterone and the preparation of the uterus to receive the fertilized ovum. However, following implantation in an abnormal site the conceptus continues to grow and in the more common case of an ectopic pregnancy in the fallopian tube, until the tube ruptures, often accompanied by catastrophic bleeding in the woman, or until the embryo dies.

Many ectopic pregnancies occur with no identifiable risk factors. However, it is recognized that damage to the fallopian tube through a previous ectopic pregnancy or previous tubular surgery increases the risk, as do previous ascending genital tract infections. Further risk factors include a pregnancy that commences with an intrauterine contraceptive device (IUCD) in situ or the woman conceives while taking the progestogen-only pill.

Ectopic (tubal) pregnancies present with vaginal bleeding and a sudden onset of lower abdominal pain, which is initially one sided, but spreads as blood enters the peritoneal cavity. There is referred shoulder tip pain caused by the blood irritating the diaphragm.

In 25% of cases, the presentation will be acute, with hypotension and tachycardia. On abdominal palpation there is abdominal distension, guarding and tenderness, which assists in confirming the diagnosis. However, in the majority of cases the presentation is less acute, so there should be a suspicion of ectopic pregnancy in any woman who presents with amenorrhea and lower abdominal pain. In these cases the presentation may be confused with that of a threatened or incomplete miscarriage, thus delaying appropriate treatment.

A transvaginal ultrasound of the lower abdomen is a useful diagnostic tool in confirming the site of the pregnancy. A single blood test for hCG level may be either positive (where the corpus luteum remains active) or negative, so is of limited diagnostic value. Serial testing is of greater value.

The basis of treatment in the acute, advanced presentation is surgical removal of the conceptus and ruptured fallopian tube as these threaten the life of the woman if she is not stabilized and treated rapidly. In the majority of cases, surgery is currently by laparoscopy as opposed to a laparotomy, as this reduces blood loss, as well as postoperative pain. The ectopic pregnancy may either be removed through an incision in the tube itself, a salpingotomy, or by removing part of the fallopian tube, i.e. a salpingectomy. Although a salpingotomy will enable a higher chance of a uterine pregnancy in the future, it is associated with a higher incidence of subsequent tubal pregnancies (RCOG 2010a).

Where the fetus has died, hCG levels will fall and the ectopic pregnancy may resolve itself, with the products either being reabsorbed or miscarried. Medical management is also a choice where the diagnosis of an ectopic pregnancy is made and the woman is haemodynamically stable. Methotrexate is given in a single dose according to the woman's body weight (RCOG 2010a), and works by interfering with DNA (deoxyribonucleic acid) synthesis, thus preventing the continued growth of the fetus (NHS Choices 2012). Should this be the treatment choice, the woman should be informed that further treatment may be needed as well as how to access support at any time should it be required (RCOG 2010a).

Women who are Rhesus-negative should be given anti-D immunoglobulin as recommended by national and local guidelines following any form of pregnancy loss (RCOG 2011b). (See Box 12.2 for further information.)

OTHER PROBLEMS IN EARLY PREGNANCY

Inelastic cervix

Formally known as *incompetent cervix*, an *inelastic cervix* will lead to silent, painless dilatation of the cervix and loss

---

> **Box 12.2 Note on anti-D immunoglobulin**
>
> For all women who are Rhesus-negative, there is an increased risk of sensitization occurring during any form of pregnancy loss, and threatened miscarriage (NICE 2011). Anti-D immunoglobulin prophylaxis should be considered for non-sensitized women presenting with a history of bleeding after 12 weeks' gestation. Where the bleeding persists throughout the pregnancy, anti-D should be repeated at 6-weekly intervals. Anti-D immunoglobulin should also be administered to all non-sensitized Rhesus-negative women following miscarriage, ectopic pregnancy or therapeutic termination of pregnancy (RCOG 2011b).

---

of the products of conception, either as a miscarriage, or a preterm birth. The incidence is 1 : 100–1 : 2000 pregnancies, the large variation being due to differences in populations (Ludmir and Owen 2007).

The cervix consists mainly of connective tissue, collagen, elastin, smooth muscle and blood vessels, and undergoes complex changes during pregnancy. The exact mechanism for inelastic cervix is unknown, but the risk is increased where there has been trauma to the cervix during surgical procedures such as a dilatation and curettage or cone biopsy, or the weakness may be of congenital origin.

The diagnosis of an inelastic cervix is usually made retrospectively on review of gynaecological and obstetric history. There will have been a painless dilatation of the cervix typically at around 18–20 weeks of gestation, or on digital vaginal or ultrasound examination, the length of the cervical canal may be noted to have shortened without any accompanying pain.

A cervical cerclage may be inserted. However the evidence to support this procedure is weak, and both the procedure and the implications should be fully discussed with the woman (NICE [National Institute for Health and Clinical Excellence] 2007). A suture is inserted from 14 weeks' gestation at the level of the internal os, and remains in situ until 38 weeks' gestation, unless there are earlier signs of labour. The associated risks are that the cervix may dilate with the suture in situ, leading to lacerations of the cervix, and infection. In 3% of cases, the cervix fails to dilate during labour, resulting in a caesarean section (Ludmir and Owen 2007).

Gestational trophoblastic disease (GTD)

In this condition there is abnormal placental development, resulting in either a complete *hydatidiform mole* or a *partial mole* and there is no viable fetus. The grape-like appearance of the mole is due to the over-proliferation of chorionic villi. Usually this is a benign condition which becomes apparent in the second trimester, characterized by vaginal bleeding, a larger than expected uterus, hyperemesis gravidarum and often symptoms of pre-eclampsia. However if a molar pregnancy does not spontaneously miscarry, two associated disorders can occur; *gestational trophoblastic neoplasia* (GTN) where the mole remains in situ and is diagnosed by continuing raised hCG levels and ultrasound scanning, and *choriocarcinoma*, which can arise as a malignant variation of the disease. It is thought that 3% of complete hydatidiform moles will progress to choriocarcinoma.

In the UK, GTD is a rare event, but women of Asian origin are at higher risk. Age is also a risk factor for both teenagers and women over 45 years of age. However, 90% of molar pregnancies occur in women between the ages of 18 and 40 years (Copeland and Landon 2011). Other risk factors include a previous molar pregnancy and those with blood type Group A. Treatment is by evacuation of the uterus, followed by histology of the tissue to enable accurate diagnosis of molar pregnancy (RCOG 2010b).

Due to the risk of carcinoma developing following a molar pregnancy, all cases should be followed up at a trophoblastic screening centre, with serial blood or urine hCG levels being monitored. In the UK, this programme has resulted in 98–100% of cases being successfully treated and only 5–8% requiring chemotherapy (RCOG 2010b). Where the hCG levels are within normal limits within 56 days of the end of the pregnancy, follow-up continues for a further 6 months. However, if the hCG levels remain raised at this point, the woman will continue to be assessed until the levels are within normal limits. Following subsequent pregnancies, hCG levels should be monitored for 6–8 weeks to ensure that there is no recurrence of the disease (RCOG 2010b).

Following a hydatidiform mole, those women who are Rhesus-negative should be administered anti-D immunoglobulin as recommended by national and local guidelines. (See Box 12.2. for further information.)

Uterine fibroid degeneration

Fibroids (leiomyomas) can degenerate during pregnancy as a result of their diminishing blood supply, resulting in abdominal pain as the tissue becomes ischaemic and necrotic. Suitable analgesia and rest are indicated until the pain subsides, although it can be a recurring problem throughout a pregnancy. Not all fibroids degenerate during pregnancy as some may receive an increased blood supply, causing enlargement with the consequential impact of obstructing labour.

Induced abortion/termination of pregnancy

Under the terms of the Abortion Act 1967, amended by the Human Fertilisation and Embryology Act 1990,

---

Box 12.3 Statutory grounds for termination of pregnancy

(a) that the pregnancy has not exceeded its twenty-fourth week and that the continuance of the pregnancy would involve risk, greater than if the pregnancy were terminated, of injury to the physical or mental health of the pregnant woman or any existing children of her family; or

(b) that the termination is necessary to prevent grave permanent injury to the physical or mental health of the pregnant woman; or

(c) that the continuance of the pregnancy would involve risk to the life of the pregnant woman, greater than if the pregnancy were terminated; or

(d) that there is a substantial risk that if the child were born it would suffer from such physical or mental abnormalities as to be seriously handicapped.

Abortion Act 1967; amended by the Human Fertilisation and Embryology Act 1990

---

provision is made for a pregnancy to be terminated up to 24 weeks of pregnancy for a number of reasons and with the written agreement of two registered medical practitioners The medical practitioners must agree that, in their opinion, the termination is justified under the terms of the statutory Act (see Box 12.3) In the UK, in 2011, 189 931 terminations of pregnancy were undertaken: the majority of these occurring before 20 weeks' gestation (Department of Health 2012). It should be noted that the law in Ireland does not allow for pregnancies to be terminated unless it is to preserve the life of the woman (RCOG 2011c).

The majority of terminations in the UK are carried out under clause (a) of the Abortion Act, meaning that continuing the pregnancy would involve a greater mental or physical risk to the woman or her existing family than if the pregnancy were terminated. Prior to any termination of pregnancy, the woman should receive counselling to discuss the options available. Whatever the reason for the termination, support should be offered before, during and following the procedure. In many cases the care and support provided for women experiencing a spontaneous miscarriage will also apply to those undergoing an induced termination of pregnancy. The reasons for the termination may include malformations of the fetus that are incompatible with life, or a condition that adversely affects the health of the women such that terminating the pregnancy offers the best option to expedite appropriate and timely treatment.

Before the commencement of the termination, it must be ensured that the HSA1 form, which is a legal requirement of the Abortion Act 1967 has been completed and signed by the two medical personnel agreeing to the termination. In addition, it is also a legal requirement that the Chief Medical Officer is notified of all terminations of pregnancy that take place, within 14 days of their occurrence (RCOG 2011c), by the practitioners completing form HSA4. The data on this form is then used for statistical purposes and monitoring terminations of pregnancies that take place within the UK. Only a medical practitioner can terminate a pregnancy. However, in practice, drugs that are prescribed to induce the termination may be administered by registered nurses and midwives working in this area of clinical practice.

The methods used for terminating the pregnancy will depend on the gestational age. Prior to 14 weeks' gestation, the pregnancy is generally terminated surgically by gradually dilating the cervix with a series of dilators and evacuating the uterus via vacuum aspiration or suction curettes. This may be carried out under general or local anaesthesia.

Terminations in later pregnancy are carried out medically, using a regime of drugs to prepare and dilate the cervix. The actual regime used may vary across healthcare providers. The cervix is initially prepared using mifepristone, which is a progesterone antagonist. This is given orally, and is followed 36–48 hours later by vaginal and/ or oral prostaglandins, such as misoprostol. The woman may return home in between the administration of the two drugs and should be provided with clear information about what to expect, the contact details of a named healthcare professional and the reassurance that admission to hospital can be at any time. During the termination, analgesia appropriate to her needs should be available.

A termination of pregnancy should not result in the live birth of the fetus. To this effect, should the procedure take place after 21 weeks and 6 days gestation, feticide may be performed prior to the commencement of the termination process. This involves an injection of potassium chloride being injected into the fetal heart to prevent the fetus being born alive (RCOG 2011c).

Where nurses and midwives have a conscientious objection to termination of pregnancy, they have the right to refuse to be involved in such procedures. However, they cannot refuse to give life-saving care to a woman, and must always be non-judgemental in any care and contact that they provide (NMC 2012b).

As with other pregnancy losses, those women who undergo a termination of pregnancy and are Rhesus-negative will require anti-D immunoglobulin as recommended by national and local guidelines. (See Box 12.2 for further information.)

Pregnancy problems associated with assisted conception

There are a number of techniques available to attempt assisted conception for women and couples who have fertility problems. However, achieving a pregnancy is not always the end of the difficulties that may occur.

A serious condition that may occur is that of *ovarian hyperstimulation syndrome.* When fertility drugs have been taken to stimulate the production of follicles, massive enlargement of the ovaries and multiple cysts can develop (RCOG 2007). Many women taking fertility drugs will experience a mild form of this syndrome, but in a considerable percentage (0.5–5%) this develops to include oliguria, renal failure and hypovolaemic shock (Mahomed 2011b). This risk increases when pregnancy has been achieved. The condition itself subsides spontaneously, but medical support and treatment is required for those who are severely unwell.

In assisted conception, the risk of miscarriage is approximately 14.7%. This rate is probably associated with the quality and length of freezing of the oocytes or embryos that are used. However there are no differences in the number of chromosomal malformations when compared with spontaneous pregnancies (Mahomed 2011b).

The number of multiple pregnancies increases with assisted conception, with rates of 27% for twins and 3% for triplets (Mahomed 2011b). Assisted reproductive technology accounts for 1% of all births, but 18% of all multiple births; consequently multiple birth in itself is a risk factor for pregnancy (see Chapter 14). With all pregnancies resulting from assisted techniques, there is an increase in the rate of pre-term birth, small for gestational age babies, placenta praevia, pregnancy induced hypertension and gestational diabetes. The reasons for these rates are not known, but it is considered that they relate to the original factors leading to the infertility (Mahomed 2011b).

Nausea, vomiting and hyperemesis gravidarum

Nausea and vomiting are common symptoms of pregnancy, affecting approximately 70% of women (Gordon 2007), with the onset from 4–8 weeks' gestation and lasting until 16–20 weeks (NICE 2010). Very occasionally the symptoms persist for the whole of pregnancy. From the woman's point of view, nausea and vomiting is frequently dismissed by others as being a common symptom of physiological pregnancy so the impact that it may have on her life and that of her family may be ignored (Tiran 2004).

The cause of these symptoms is thought to be due to the presence of hCG, which is present during the time that the nausea and vomiting is most prevalent, although oestrogen and/or progesterone are also thought to have some influence (Tiran 2004; Gordon 2007). According to NICE (2010), ginger may be of help in reducing the symptoms, as is wrist acupuncture, a form of treatment for nausea in pregnancy often chosen by women as it is drug-free.

According to Betts (2006: 25), the wrist area is seen to 'harmonise the stomach', thus working to reduce nausea.

Hyperemesis gravidarum is the severest form of nausea and vomiting and occurs in 3.5 per 1000 pregnancies (Gordon 2007). The woman presents with a history of vomiting that has led to weight loss and dehydration that may also be associated with postural hypotension, tachycardia, ketosis and electrolyte imbalance (Williamson and Girling 2011). This requires treatment in hospital, where intravenous fluids are given to re-hydrate the woman and correct the electrolyte imbalance, with anti-emetics being administered to control the vomiting. Very often a combination of drugs will be needed in order to achieve this. It is important to exclude other conditions, such as a urinary tract infection, disorders of the gastrointestinal tract, or a molar pregnancy, where vomiting may also be excessive.

The aim of treatment is not only to stabilize the woman's condition, but also to prevent further complications. Continual vomiting during the pregnancy may lead to vitamin deficiencies, and/or hyponatraemia, which can present with confusion and seizures, leading ultimately to respiratory arrest if left untreated (Williamson and Girling 2011). For women who are immobilized through the severity of the vomiting, deep vein thrombosis is also a potential complication due to the combination of dehydration and immobility. In cases of hyperemesis gravidarum the fetus may be at risk of being small for gestational age due to a lack of nutrients.

Pelvic girdle pain (PGP)

During pregnancy the activity of the pregnancy hormones, especially relaxin, can cause the ligaments supporting the pelvic joints to relax, allowing for slight movement. As a consequence, pelvic girdle pain (PGP), or formerly known as *symphysis pubis dysfunction*, occurs when this relaxation is excessive, allowing the pelvic bones to move up and down when the woman is walking. This leads to pain in the pubic area as well as backache, usually occurring any time from the 28th week of pregnancy. Approximately, 1 in 5 pregnant women are affected by PGP (ACPWH [Association of Chartered Physiotherapists in Women's Health] 2011), with symptoms varying from mild pain and discomfort to severe mobility difficulties. Some women also experience pain and discomfort when lying down in certain positions and on standing (ACPWH 2011). Very often, PGP occurs without identifiable risk factors, but these may include a history of lower back or pelvic girdle pain, and/or a job that is physically active.

On suspecting that a woman has PGP, the midwife should explain the condition and the possible causes to the woman and organize a referral to an obstetric physiotherapist. The woman should be advised to rest as much as possible and undertake activities that do not cause her further pain. Very often it is movement that involves abducting the hips which increases the pain and discomfort. A physiotherapist can be helpful in advising on mobility and coping with daily tasks and in supplying aids such as pelvic girdle support belts and in extreme cases, crutches, so that the pain may be reduced.

A plan for both pregnancy and care in labour should be developed and recorded, so that the midwives caring for the woman during the birth are aware of the PGP and any positions that can be beneficial, such as being upright and kneeling as well as the woman's analgesia requirements. As there may be a reduction in hip abduction, the midwife should take care when performing vaginal examinations, and if the lithotomy position is required during the birth, not to cause the woman unnecessary discomfort (ACPWH 2011). Following the birth, the ligaments slowly return to their pre-pregnant condition, but this may take some time. Extra support may be required and physiotherapy may need to be continued beyond the postnatal period.

BLEEDING AFTER THE 24TH WEEK OF PREGNANCY

Antepartum haemorrhage (APH)

Antepartum haemorrhage is bleeding from the genital tract after the 24th week of pregnancy, and before the onset of labour. As shown in Table 12.1, it is caused by:

Table 12.1 Causes of bleeding in late pregnancy	
Cause	Incidence (%)
Placenta praevia	31.0
Placental abruption	22.0
'Unclassified bleeding'	47.0
of which:	
Marginal	60.0
Show	20.0
Cervicitis	8.0
Trauma	5.0
Vulvovaginal varicosities	2.0
Genital tumours	0.5
Genital infections	0.5
Haematuria	0.5
Vasa praevia	0.5
Other	0.5
Source: Adapted from Navti and Konje 2011	

- Bleeding from local lesions of the genital tract (*incidental causes*).
- Placental separation due to *placenta praevia* or *placental abruption*.

Effect on the mother

A small amount of bleeding will not physically affect the woman (unless she is already severely anaemic) but it is likely to cause her anxiety. In cases of heavier bleeding, this may be accompanied by medical shock and blood clotting disorders. The midwife will be aware that the woman can die or be left with permanent morbidity if bleeding in pregnancy is not dealt with promptly and effectively.

Effect on the fetus

Fetal mortality and morbidity are increased as a result of severe vaginal bleeding in pregnancy. Stillbirth or neonatal death may occur. Premature placental separation and consequent hypoxia may result in severe neurological damage in the baby.

Initial appraisal of a woman with APH

Antepartum haemorrhage is unpredictable and the woman's condition can deteriorate at any time. A rapid decision about the urgency of need for a medical or paramedic presence, or both, must be made, often at the same time as observing and talking to the woman and her partner.

Assessment of maternal condition

- Take a history from the woman.
- Assess basic observations of temperature, pulse rate, respiratory rate and blood pressure, including their documentation.
- Observe for any pallor or restlessness.
- Assess the blood loss (consider retaining soiled sheets and clothes in case a second opinion is required).
- Perform a *gentle* abdominal examination, while assessing for signs of labour.
- **On no account must any vaginal or rectal examination be undertaken, nor should an enema or suppositories be administered to a woman experiencing an APH as these could result in torrential haemorrhage.**

Sometimes bleeding that the woman had presumed to be from the vagina may be from haemorrhoids. The midwife should consider this differential diagnosis and confirm or exclude this as soon as possible by careful questioning and examination.

Assessment of fetal condition

- The woman is asked if the baby has been moving as much as normal
- An attempt should be made to listen to the fetal heart. An ultrasound apparatus may be used in order to obtain information. However if the woman is at home and the bleeding is severe this would not be a priority. The midwife will need to ensure the women is transferred to hospital as soon as her condition is stabilized in order to give the fetus the best chance of survival. Speed of action is vital.

Supportive treatment for moderate or severe blood loss and/or maternal collapse would consist of:

- providing ongoing emotional support for the woman and her partner/relatives
- administering rapid fluid replacement (warmed) with a plasma expander, with whole blood if necessary
- administering appropriate analgesia
- arranging transfer to hospital by the most appropriate means, if the woman is at home.

Management of antepartum haemorrhage depends on the definite diagnosis (see Table 12.2).

Placenta praevia

In this condition the placenta is partially or wholly implanted in the lower uterine segment. The lower uterine segment grows and stretches progressively after the 12th week of pregnancy. In later weeks this may cause the placenta to separate and severe bleeding can occur. The amount of bleeding is not usually associated with any particular type of activity and commonly occurs when the woman is resting. The low placental location allows all of the lost blood to escape unimpeded and a retroplacental clot is not formed. For this reason, pain is not a feature of placenta praevia. Some women with this condition have a history of a small repeated blood loss at intervals throughout pregnancy whereas others may have a sudden single episode of vaginal bleeding after the 20th week. However, severe haemorrhage occurs most frequently after the 34th week of pregnancy. The degree of placenta praevia does not necessarily correspond to the amount of bleeding. A type 4 placenta praevia may never bleed before the onset of spontaneous labour or elective caesarean section in late pregnancy or, conversely, some women with placenta praevia type 1 may experience relatively heavy bleeding from early in their pregnancy.

Degrees of placenta praevia

Type 1 placenta praevia

The majority of the placenta is in the upper uterine segment (see Figs 12.1, 12.5). Blood loss is usually mild and the mother and fetus remain in good condition. Vaginal birth is possible.

Table 12.2 Comparison of clinical issues in placental abruption and placenta praevia

Comparison	Placental abruption	Placenta praevia
Onset of bleeding	May follow trauma (road traffic accident, domestic violence) but usually unprovoked Amount variable May contain clots	Almost always unprovoked Usually heavy No clots present
Signs	Generalized abdominal pain *if* some blood is trapped behind the placenta (concealed) When acute bleeding ceases, altered (old, brown) blood will continue vaginally for a few hours	Always painless Bleeding is always fresh (bright red)
Initial symptoms for moderate and severe blood loss:	Temperature may be raised if there is infection in the uterus (sepsis) Pulse and respirations may be raised due to blood loss and shock Blood pressure low due to blood loss and shock	Temperature normal Pulse and respirations may be raised due to blood loss and shock Blood pressure low due to blood loss and shock
On palpation	Uterus tense and painful *if* there is concealed blood loss If palpation is possible (i.e. not too painful for the woman), fetal presentation and engagement not affected by abruption Fetal heart rate may be normal, erratic or absent	Non-tender uterus Likely fetal malpresentation, as the placenta occupies the pelvis Fetal heart rate may be normal, erratic or absent
On diagnostic ultrasound scan	Normally situated placenta Blood clots may be seen in the cavity of the uterus	Placenta is lying in the lower segment of the uterus

Type 2 placenta praevia

The placenta is partially located in the lower segment near the internal cervical os (marginal placenta praevia) (see Figs 12.2, 12.6). Blood loss is usually moderate, although the conditions of the mother and fetus can vary. Fetal hypoxia is more likely to be present than maternal shock. Vaginal birth is possible, particularly if the placenta is anterior.

Type 3 placenta praevia

The placenta is located over the internal cervical os but not centrally (see Figs 12.3, 12.7). Bleeding is likely to be severe, particularly when the lower segment stretches and the cervix begins to efface and dilate in late pregnancy. Vaginal birth is inappropriate because the placenta precedes the fetus.

Type 4 placenta praevia

The placenta is located centrally over the internal cervical os (see Figs 12.4, 12.8) and torrential haemorrhage is very likely. Caesarean section is essential to save the lives of the woman and fetus.

Incidence

Placenta praevia affects 2.8 per 1000 of singleton pregnancies and 3.9 per 1000 of twin pregnancies (Navti and Konje 2011). There is a higher incidence of placenta praevia among women with increasing age and parity, in women who smoke and those who have had a previous caesarean section. Furthermore, it is known that there is also an increased risk of recurrence where there has been a placenta praevia in a previous pregnancy.

Management

Immediate re-localization of the placenta using ultrasonic scanning is a definitive aid to diagnosis, and as well as confirming the existence of placenta praevia it will establish its degree. Relying on an early pregnancy scan at 20 weeks of pregnancy is not very useful when vaginal bleeding starts in later pregnancy, as the placenta tends to migrate up the uterine wall as the uterus grows in a developing pregnancy.

Further management decisions will depend on:

- the amount of bleeding
- the condition of the woman and fetus
- the location of the placenta
- the stage of the pregnancy.

Conservative management

This is appropriate if bleeding is slight and the woman and fetus are well. The woman will be kept in hospital at rest until bleeding has stopped. A speculum examination will have ruled out incidental causes. Further bleeding is

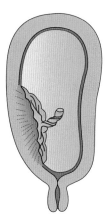

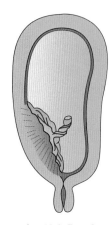

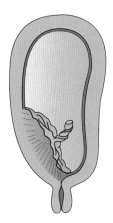

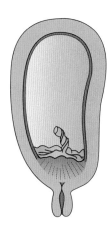

Fig. 12.1 Type 1.   Fig. 12.2 Type 2.   Fig. 12.3 Type 3.   Fig. 12.4 Type 4.

Figs 12.1–12.4 **Types and positions of placenta praevia.**

Fig. 12.5 Type 1.   Fig. 12.6 Type 2.   Fig. 12.7 Type 3.   Fig. 12.8 Type 4.

Figs 12.5–12.8 **Relation of placenta praevia to cervical os.**

almost inevitable if the placenta encroaches into the lower segment; therefore it is usual for the woman to remain in, or close to hospital for the rest of her pregnancy. A visit to the special care baby unit/neonatal intensive care unit and contact with the neonatal team may also help to prepare the woman and her family for the possibility of pre-term birth.

A decision will be made with the woman about how and when the birth will be managed. If there is no further severe bleeding, vaginal birth is highly likely if the placental location allows. The midwife should be aware that, even if vaginal birth is achieved, there remains a danger of postpartum haemorrhage because the placenta has been situated in the lower segment where there are fewer oblique muscle fibres and the action of the *living ligatures* is less effective.

Immediate management of life-threatening bleeding

Severe vaginal bleeding will necessitate immediate birth of the baby by caesarean section regardless of the location of the placenta. This should take place in a maternity unit with facilities for the appropriate care of the newborn, especially if the baby is preterm. During the assessment and preparation for theatre the woman will be extremely anxious and the midwife must comfort and encourage her,

sharing information with her as much as possible. The partner will also need to be supported, whether he is in the operating theatre or waits outside.

If the placenta is situated anteriorly in the uterus, this may complicate the surgical approach as it underlies the site of the normal incision. In major degrees of placenta praevia (types 3 and 4) caesarean section is required even if the fetus has died in utero. Such management aims to prevent torrential haemorrhage and possible maternal death.

Complications

Complication include:

- Maternal shock, resulting from blood loss and hypovolaemia.
- Anaesthetic and surgical complications, which are more common in women with major degrees of placenta praevia, and in those for whom preparation for surgery has been suboptimal.
- Placenta accreta, in up to 15% of women with placenta praevia.
- Air embolism, an occasional occurrence when the sinuses in the placental bed have been broken.
- Postpartum haemorrhage: occasionally uncontrolled haemorrhage will continue, despite the administration of uterotonic drugs at the birth, even

following the best efforts to control it, and a ligation of the internal iliac artery. A caesarean hysterectomy may be required to save the woman's life.

- Maternal death is rare in the developed world.
- Fetal hypoxia and its sequelae due to placental separation.
- Fetal death, depending on gestation and amount of blood loss.

Placental abruption

Premature separation of a normally situated placenta occurring after the 24th week of pregnancy is referred to as a placental abruption. The aetiology of this type of haemorrhage is not always clear, but it may be associated with:

- hypertension
- a sudden reduction in uterine size, for instance when the membranes rupture or after the birth of a first twin
- trauma, for instance external cephalic version of a fetus presenting by the breech, a road traffic accident or domestic violence, as these may partially dislodge the placenta
- high parity
- previous caesarean section
- cigarette smoking.

Incidence

Placental abruption occurs in 0.49–1.8% of all pregnancies with 30% of cases being classed as *concealed* and 70% being *revealed* (Navti and Konje 2011), although there is probably a combination of both in many situations (mixed haemorrhage). In any of these situations the blood loss may be mild, moderate or severe, ranging from a few spots to continually soaking clothes and bed linen.

In *revealed* haemorrhage, as blood escapes from the placental site it separates the membranes from the uterine wall and drains through the vagina. However in *concealed* haemorrhage blood is retained behind the placenta where it is forced back into the myometrium, infiltrating the space between the muscle fibres of the uterus. This extravasation (seepage outside the normal vascular channels) can cause marked damage and, if observed at operation, the uterus will appear bruised, oedematous and enlarged. This is termed *Couvelaire uterus* or *uterine apoplexy*. In a completely concealed abruption with no vaginal bleeding, the woman will have all the signs and symptoms of hypovolaemic shock and if the blood loss is moderate or severe she will experience extreme pain. In practice the midwife cannot rely on visible blood loss as a guide to the severity of the haemorrhage; on the contrary, the most severe haemorrhage is often that which is totally concealed.

As with placenta praevia, the maternal and fetal condition will dictate the management.

Mild separation of the placenta

Most commonly a woman self-admits to the maternity unit with slight vaginal bleeding. On examination the woman and fetus are in a stable condition and there is no indication of shock. The fetus is alive with normal heart sounds. The consistency of the uterus is normal and there is no tenderness on palpation. The management would include the following plan of care:

- An ultrasound scan can determine the placental localization and identify any degree of concealed bleeding
- The fetal condition should be assessed by frequent or continuous monitoring of the fetal heart rate while bleeding persists. Subsequently a cardiotocograph (CTG) should be undertaken once or twice daily
- If the woman is not in labour and the gestation is less than 37 weeks she may be cared for in the antenatal ward for a few days. She may return home if there is no further bleeding and the placenta has been found to be in the upper uterine segment. The woman should be encouraged to return to hospital if there is any further bleeding.
- Women who have passed the 37th week of pregnancy may be offered induction of labour, especially if there has been more than one episode of mild bleeding
- Further heavy bleeding or evidence of fetal compromise could indicate that a caesarean section is necessary.

The midwife should offer the woman comfort and encouragement by attending to her emotional needs, including her need for information. Physical domestic abuse should be considered by the midwife, which the woman may be frightened to reveal. It should also be noted that if the woman is already severely anaemic then even an apparently mild abruption may compromise her wellbeing and that of the fetus.

Moderate separation of the placenta

About a quarter of the placenta will have separated and a considerable amount of blood may be lost, although concealed haemorrhage must also be considered. The woman will be shocked and in pain, with uterine tenderness and abdominal guarding. The fetus may be alive, although hypoxic, however intrauterine death is also a possibility.

The priority is to reduce shock and to replace blood loss:

- Fluid replacement should be monitored with the aid of a central venous pressure (CVP) line. Meticulous fluid balance records must be maintained.
- The fetal condition should be continuously assessed by CTG if the fetus is alive, in which case immediate caesarean section would be indicated once the woman's condition is stabilized.

- If the fetus is in good condition or has died, vaginal birth may be considered as this enables the uterus to contract and control the bleeding. The spontaneous onset of labour frequently accompanies moderately severe placental abruption, but if it does not then amniotomy is usually sufficient to induce labour. Oxytocics may be used with great care, if necessary. The birth of the baby is often quite sudden after a short labour. The use of drugs to attempt to stop labour is usually inappropriate.

Severe separation of the placenta

This is an **acute obstetric emergency** where at least two-thirds of the placenta has detached and 2000 ml of blood or more are lost from the circulation. Most or all of the blood may be concealed behind the placenta. The woman will be severely shocked, perhaps far beyond the degree to which would be expected from the visible blood loss (see Chapter 22). The blood pressure will be lowered but if the haemorrhage accompanies pre-eclampsia the reading may lie within the normal range owing to a preceding hypertension. The fetus will almost certainly be dead. The woman will have very severe abdominal pain with excruciating tenderness and the uterus would have a board-like consistency.

Features associated with severe antepartum haemorrhage are:

- coagulation defects
- renal failure
- pituitary failure
- postpartum haemorrhage.

Treatment is the same as for moderate haemorrhage:

- Whole blood should be transfused rapidly and subsequent amounts calculated in accordance with the woman's CVP.
- Labour may begin spontaneously in advance of amniotomy and the midwife should be alert for signs of uterine contraction causing periodic intensifying of the abdominal pain.
- If bleeding continues or a compromised fetal heart rate is present, caesarean section will be required as soon as the woman's condition has been adequately stabilized.

Blood coagulation failure

Normal blood coagulation

Haemostasis refers to the arrest of bleeding, preventing loss of blood from the blood vessels. It depends on the mechanism of coagulation. This is counterbalanced by fibrinolysis which ensures that the blood vessels are reopened in order to maintain the patency of the circulation.

Blood clotting occurs in three main stages:

1. When tissues are damaged and platelets break down, *thromboplastin* is released.
2. Thromboplastin leads to the conversion of *prothrombin* into *thrombin*: a proteolytic (protein-splitting) enzyme.
3. Thrombin converts *fibrinogen* into *fibrin* to form a network of long, sticky strands that entrap blood cells to establish a *clot*. The coagulated material contracts and exudes *serum*, which is plasma depleted of its clotting factors. This is the final part of a complex cascade of coagulation involving a large number of different clotting factors (simply named Factor I, Factor II etc. in order of their discovery).

It is equally important for a healthy person to maintain the blood as a fluid in order that it can circulate freely. The coagulation mechanism is normally held at bay by the presence of *heparin*, which is produced in the liver.

Fibrinolysis is the breakdown of fibrin and occurs as a response to the presence of clotted blood. Unless fibrinolysis takes place, coagulation will continue. It is achieved by the activation of a series of enzymes culminating in the proteolytic enzyme *plasmin*. This breaks down the fibrin in the clots and produces *fibrin degradation products* (FDPs).

Disseminated intravascular coagulation (DIC)

The cause of disseminated intravascular coagulation (also known as disseminated intravascular coagulopathy) (DIC) is not fully understood. It is a complex pathological reaction to severe tissue trauma which rarely occurs when the fetus is alive and usually starts to resolve after birth. Inappropriate coagulation occurs within the blood vessels, which leads to the consumption of clotting factors. As a result, clotting fails to occur at the bleeding site. DIC is never a primary disease, as it always occurs as a response to another disease process.

Events that trigger DIC include:

- placental abruption
- intrauterine fetal death, including delayed miscarriage
- amniotic fluid embolism
- intrauterine infection, including septic miscarriage
- pre-eclampsia and eclampsia.

Management

The aims of the management of DIC are summarized in Box 12.4.

The midwife should be alert for conditions that affect DIC, as well as the signs that clotting is abnormal. The assessment of the nature of the clot should be part of the midwife's routine observation during the third stage of labour. Oozing from a venepuncture site or bleeding from

Box 12.4 **Aims of the management of DIC**

- To manage the underlying cause and remove the stimulus provoking DIC
- To ensure maintenance of the circulating blood volume
- To replace the used up clotting factors and destroyed red blood cells

Source: Lindow and Anthony 2011

Box 12.5 **Hepatic disorders of pregnancy**

Specific to pregnancy

Intrahepatic cholestasis of pregnancy
Acute fatty liver in pregnancy (see Chapter 13)
Pre-eclampsia and eclampsia (see Chapter 13)
Severe hyperemesis gravidarum.

Pre- or co-existing in pregnancy

Gall bladder disease
Hepatitis

Box 12.6 **Causes of jaundice in pregnancy**

Not specific to pregnancy

Viral hepatitis – A, B, C are the most prevalent
Hepatitis secondary to infection, usually cytomegalovirus, Epstein–Barr virus, toxoplasmosis or herpes simplex
Gall stones
Drug reactions
Alcohol/drug misuse
Budd–Chiari syndrome

Pregnancy-specific causes

Acute fatty liver
HELLP (haemolysis, elevated liver enzymes, low platelets) syndrome
Intrahepatic cholestasis of pregnancy
Hyperemesis gravidarum

Note: Jaundice is not an inevitable symptom of liver disease in pregnancy.

the mucous membrane of the woman's mouth and nose must be noted and reported. Blood tests should include assessing the full blood count and the blood grouping, clotting studies and the levels of platelets, fibrinogen and fibrin degradation products (FDPs).

Treatment involves the replacement of blood cells and clotting factors in order to restore equilibrium. This is usually done by the administration of fresh frozen plasma and platelet concentrates. Banked red cells will be transfused subsequently. Management is carried out by a team of obstetricians, anaesthetists, haematologists, midwives and other healthcare professionals who must strive to work together harmoniously and effectively to achieve the best possible clinical outcomes for the woman.

Care by the midwife

DIC causes a frightening situation that demands speed both of recognition and of action. The midwife has to maintain her own calmness and clarity of thinking as well as assisting the couple to deal with the situation in which they find themselves. Frequent and accurate observations must be maintained in order to monitor the woman's condition. Blood pressure, respirations, pulse rate and temperature are recorded. The general condition is noted. Fluid balance is monitored with vigilance for any sign of renal failure.

The partner in particular is likely to be confused by a sudden turn in events, when previously all seemed to be under control. The midwife must make sure that someone is giving him appropriate attention, keeping him informed of what is happening. All health professionals need to be aware that the partner may find it impossible to absorb all that he is told and may require repeated explanations. He may be the best person to help the woman to understand her condition. The death of the woman from organ failure as a result of DIC is a real possibility.

HEPATIC DISORDERS AND JAUNDICE

Some liver disorders are specific to pregnant women, and some pre-existing or co-existing disorders may complicate the pregnancy, as shown in Box 12.5.

Causes of jaundice in pregnancy are listed in Box 12.6.

Obstetric cholestasis (OC)

This is an idiopathic condition that usually begins in the third trimester of pregnancy, but can occasionally present as early as the first trimester. It affects 0.7% of pregnancies and resolves spontaneously following birth, but it has up to a 90% recurrence rate in subsequent pregnancies (Williamson and Girling 2011). Its cause is unknown, although genetic, geographical and environmental factors are considered to be contributory factors. It is not a life-threatening condition for the woman, but there is an increased risk of pre-term labour, fetal compromise and meconium staining, and the stillbirth risk is increased unless there is active management of the pregnancy.

Clinical presentation

The presentation may include:

- pruritus without a rash
- insomnia and fatigue as a result of the pruritus

- fever, abdominal discomfort, nausea and vomiting
- urine may be darker and stools paler than usual
- a few women develop mild jaundice.

Investigations

The following investigations should be done:

- Tests to eliminate differential diagnoses such as other liver disease or pemphigoid gestationalis (a rare autoimmune disease of late pregnancy that mimics OC) include hepatic viral studies, an ultrasound scan of the hepatobiliary tract and an autoantibody screen.
- Blood tests to assess the levels of bile acids, serum alkaline phosphatase, bilirubin and liver transaminases, which would be raised.

Management

Management consists of:

- Application of local antipruritic agents, such as antihistamines.
- Vitamin K supplements are administered to the woman, 10 mg orally daily, as her absorption will be poor, leading to prothombinaemia which predisposes her to obstetric haemorrhage if left untreated.
- Monitor fetal wellbeing possibly by Doppler of the umbilical artery blood flow.
- Consider elective birth when the fetus is mature, or earlier if the fetal condition appears to be compromised by the intrauterine environment, or the bile acids are significantly raised, as this is associated with impending intrauterine death.
- Provide sensitive psychological care to the woman.
- Advise the woman that her pruritus should disappear within 3–14 days of the birth.
- If the woman chooses to use oral contraception in the future, she should be advised that her liver function should be regularly monitored.

Gall bladder disease

Pregnancy appears to increase the likelihood of gallstone formation but not the risk of developing acute cholecystitis. Diagnosis is made by exploring the woman's previous history, with an ultrasound scan of the hepatobiliary tract. The treatment for gall bladder disease is based on providing symptomatic relief of biliary colic by analgesia, hydration, nasogastric suction and antibiotics. If at all possible, surgery in pregnancy should be avoided.

Viral hepatitis

Viral hepatitis is the most commonly diagnosed viral infection of pregnancy (Andrews 2011). See Table 12.3 for information about hepatitis A, B and C in pregnancy. Hepatitis D, E and G have more recently been described in medical literature but their relevance to pregnancy is not yet known.

SKIN DISORDERS

Many women suffer from physiological pruritus in pregnancy, particularly over the abdomen as it grows and stretches. The application of calamine lotion is often helpful. However pruritus can be a symptom of a disease process, such as OC and pemphigoid gestationalis, an auto-immune disease of pregnancy where blisters develop over the body as the pregnancy progresses.

Women with pre-existing skin conditions such as eczema and psoriasis should be advised about the use of steroid creams and applications containing nut oil derivatives, which may adversely affect the fetus.

ABNORMALITIES OF THE AMNIOTIC FLUID

The amount of liquor present in a pregnancy can be estimated by measuring 'pools' of liquor around the fetus with ultrasound scanning. The single deepest pool is measured to calculate the *amniotic fluid volume* (AFV). However, where possible a more accurate diagnosis may be gained by measuring the liquor in each of four quadrants around the fetus in order to establish an *amniotic fluid index* (AFI). There are two abnormalities of amniotic fluid: *hydramnios* (or polyhydramnios) and *oligohydramnios*.

Hydramnios

Hydramnios is present when there is an excess of amniotic fluid in the amniotic sac. Causes and predisposing factors include:

- twin to twin transfusion syndrome
- maternal diabetes
- fetal anaemia (maternal alloimmunization, syphilis/parvovirus infection)
- fetal malformation such as oesophageal atresia, open neural tube defect, anencephaly
- a fetal and placental tumour (rare).

However, in many cases the cause is unknown.

Types

Chronic hydramnios

This is gradual in onset, usually starting from about the 30th week of pregnancy. It is the most common type.

Table 12.3 Viral hepatitis in pregnancy

	Incidence	Clinical presentation	Mode of spread	Incubation period	Mother to baby (vertical) transmission	Diagnosis	Management	Complications	Other
Hepatitis A (HAV)	Endemic worldwide	Fatigue, malaise, fever, nausea, anorexia, weight loss, pruritus, jaundice, hepatosplenomegaly	Contaminated food and water (faecal matter), sexual contact	15–50 days	Possible at birth, but rare	HAV-specific IgM is a serological marker for acute infection Abnormal liver function tests	No specific antiviral treatment available May need to admit to hospital for fluid replacement (barrier nurse)	Usually complete recovery, but can last for 12 months	Vaccination is available for women who travel to high risk areas and is safe in pregnancy Immunoglobulin is available for babies born within 2 weeks of acute maternal infection Hepatitis A is a rare cause of acute hepatitis in pregnancy Breast feeding is safe
Hepatitis B (HBV)	2 billion infected worldwide In West 0.5–5% population are chronic carriers 600 000 deaths a year worldwide attributable to consequences	All of above plus arthralgia, rash and myalgia	Body fluids especially blood, semen and saliva	1–6 months	Possible in pregnancy, at birth making baby prone to liver damage in childhood	Woman's history and lifestyle Serological studies useful after antibodies for HBV have formed – serum markers	Caesarean birth not useful in preventing transmission Treat symptoms as they arise Infection control procedures while woman infective Nutrition and sexual advice Monitor long-term liver function if carrier, and baby is infected Vaccinate contacts Vaccinate baby postnatally	Longer-term liver damage can be fatal Danger of being mistaken for pre-eclampsia and HELLP syndrome because of liver pain and coagulopathy	8–10% of those infected become chronic carriers 25–30% of these will die from chronic liver failure years later if they do not receive a liver transplant In 90% of primary carriers symptoms resolve in 1–3 months Routine pregnancy screening enables neonatal prophylaxis Breastfeeding safe in acute disease if mother receives immunoprophylaxis
Hepatitis C (HCV)	In USA 2.3–4.5% in pregnant women No data from other countries	75% have no symptoms, but in 25% same as for Hepatitis A to a lesser extent	Shared needles, sexual contact (extent unknown) Blood transfusion since 1992 in USA Sharps injury	30–60 days	Thought to be 2–7% in preliminary studies	Woman's history and lifestyle HCV screening assays currently limited	None available No vaccine available yet	B cell lymphoma Chronic liver disease 75–85% acutely infected individuals will get chronic liver damage and require a liver transplant	Outcome for baby is not yet known Screening not recommended as there is no known treatment yet HCV infection is often accompanied by HIV infection Transmission rate in breastfeeding not yet known

Acute hydramnios

This is very rare. It usually occurs at about 20 weeks and develops very suddenly. The uterine size reaches the xiphisternum in about 3 or 4 days. Acute hydramnios is frequently associated with monozygotic twins or severe fetal malformation.

Diagnosis

The woman may complain of breathlessness and discomfort. If the hydramnios is acute in onset, she may experience severe abdominal pain. The condition may cause exacerbation of symptoms associated with pregnancy, such as indigestion, heartburn and constipation. Oedema and varicosities of the vulva and lower limbs may also be present.

Abdominal examination

On inspection, the uterus is larger than expected for the period of gestation and is globular in shape. The abdominal skin appears stretched and shiny, with marked striae gravidarum and superficial blood vessels.

On palpation, the uterus feels tense and it is difficult to feel the fetal parts, but the fetus may be balloted between the two hands. A *fluid thrill* may be elicited by placing a hand on one side of the abdomen and tapping the other side with the fingers.

Ultrasonic scanning is used to confirm the diagnosis of hydramnios and may also reveal a multiple pregnancy or fetal malformation.

Auscultation of the fetal hear may be difficult due to the hydramnios.

Complications

These include:

- maternal ureteric obstruction and urinary tract infection
- unstable lie and malpresentation
- cord presentation and prolapse
- prelabour (and often preterm) rupture of the membranes
- placental abruption when the membranes rupture
- preterm labour
- increased incidence of caesarean section
- postpartum haemorrhage
- increased perinatal mortality rate.

Management

Care will depend on the condition of the woman and fetus, the cause and degree of the hydramnios and the stage of pregnancy. The presence of fetal malformation will be taken into consideration in choosing the mode and timing of birth. If there is a gross malformation present, labour may be induced. Should the fetus have an operable condition, such as oesophageal atresia, transfer will be arranged to a neonatal surgical unit.

Mild hydramnios is managed expectantly. Regular ultrasound scans will reveal whether or not the hydramnios is progressive. Some cases of idiopathic hydramnios resolve spontaneously as pregnancy progresses.

For a woman with symptomatic hydramnios, an upright position will help to relieve any dyspnoea and antacids can be taken to relieve heartburn and nausea. If the discomfort from the swollen uterus is severe, then therapeutic *amniocentesis*, or *amnioreduction*, may be considered. However, this is not without risk, as infection may be introduced or the onset of labour provoked. No more than 500 ml of amniotic fluid should be withdrawn at any one time. It is at best a temporary relief as the fluid will rapidly accumulate again and the procedure may need to be repeated. Acute hydramnios managed by amnio-reduction has a poor prognosis for the fetus.

Labour may need to be induced in late pregnancy if the woman's symptoms become worse. The lie must be corrected if it is not longitudinal and the membranes ruptured cautiously, allowing the amniotic fluid to drain out slowly in order to avoid altering the lie and to prevent cord prolapse (see Chapter 22). In addition, placental abruption is also a risk if the uterus suddenly diminishes in size.

Labour usually progresses physiologically, but the midwife should be prepared for the possibility of postpartum haemorrhage. The baby should be carefully examined for malformations at birth and the patency of the oesophagus is ascertained by passing a nasogastric tube.

Oligohydramnios

Oligohydramnios is an abnormally small amount of amniotic fluid. It affects 3–5% of pregnancies (Beall et al 2011). At term there may be 300–500 ml but amounts vary and they can be even less. When diagnosed in the first half of pregnancy, oligohydramnios is often found to be associated with renal agenesis (absence of kidneys) or Potter's syndrome, in which the baby also has pulmonary hypoplasia. When diagnosed at any time in pregnancy before 37 weeks, oligohydramnios may be due to fetal malformation or to preterm prelabour rupture of the membranes where the amniotic fluid fails to re-accumulate. The lack of amniotic fluid reduces the intrauterine space and over time will cause compression malformations. The baby has a squashed-looking face, flattening of the nose, micrognathia (a malformation of the jaw) and talipes. The skin is dry and leathery in appearance.

Oligohydramnios can accompany maternal dehydration, and sometimes occurs in post-term pregnancies.

Diagnosis

On inspection, the uterus may appear smaller than expected for the period of gestation. The woman may have noticed a reduction in fetal movements if she is a multigravida and has experienced childbirth previously.

On palpation, the uterus is small and compact and fetal parts are easily felt.

Ultrasonic scanning will enable differentiation of oligo-hydramnios from intrauterine growth restriction (IUGR). Renal malformation may be visible on the scan.

Auscultation of the fetal heart should be heard without any undue difficulty.

Management

This will depend on the gestational age, the severity and the cause of the oligohydramnios. In the first trimester the pregnancy is likely to miscarry. The condition causes the greatest dilemmas in the second trimester but is often associated at this time with fetal death and congenital malformations. If the pregnancy remains viable the woman may wish to consider a termination of pregnancy. In the third trimester the condition is more likely associated with preterm prelabour rupture of the membranes (PPROM) and birth is usually indicated (Beall et al 2011).

Liquor volume will be estimated by ultrasound scan and the woman should be questioned about the possibility of pre-term rupture of the membranes. Doppler ultrasound of the uterine artery may be performed to assess placental function, although Neilson (2012), in a recent Cochrane review, suggests this is of limited clinical value. If the woman is dehydrated she should be encouraged to drink plenty of water, or offered intravenous hypotonic fluid.

Where fetal anomaly is not considered to be lethal, or the cause of the oligohydramnios is not known, prophylactic amnioinfusion may be performed in order to prevent compression malformations and hypoplastic lung disease, and prolong the pregnancy. Little evidence is available to determine the benefits and hazards of this intervention in mid-pregnancy. If the oligohydramnios is due to preterm prelabour rupture of the membranes and labour does not ensue, the woman should be observed for uterine infection (*chorioamnionitis*), and treated accordingly if it develops.

In cases of near-term and term pregnancy, induction of labour is likely to be advocated. Alternatively, fetal surveillance by cardiotocography, amniotic fluid measurement with ultrasound and Doppler assessment of fetal and uteroplacental arteries may be offered to the woman who prefers to await the onset of spontaneous labour. Regardless of whether labour commences spontaneously or is induced, epidural analgesia may be indicated because uterine contractions can be unusually painful due to the lack of amniotic fluid. Continuous fetal heart rate monitoring is desirable because of the potential for impairment of placental circulation and cord compression. Furthermore, if meconium is passed *in utero* it will be more concentrated and represent a greater danger to an asphyxiated fetus during birth.

Preterm prelabour rupture of the membranes (PPROM)

Preterm prelabour rupture of the membranes (PPROM) occurs before 37 completed weeks' gestation, where the fetal membranes rupture without the onset of spontaneous uterine activity and the consequential cervical dilatation.

It affects 2% of pregnancies and placental abruption is evident in 4–7% of women who present with PPROM. The condition has a 17–32% recurrence rate in subsequent pregnancies of affected women (Svigos et al 2011). There is a strong association between PPROM and maternal colonization (Bacterial vaginosis [BV]), with potentially pathogenic micro-organisms, with a 30% incidence of subclinical *chorioamnionitis* (Hay 2012). Infection may both precede (and cause) or follow PPROM. It is also more common in smokers and recreational drug users, for example cocaine users. Preterm prelabour rupture of the membranes is associated with 40% of preterm births (RCOG 2010c).

Risks of PPROM

Risks associated with PPROM include:

- imminent labour resulting in a preterm birth
- chorioamnionitis, which may be followed by fetal and maternal systemic infection if not treated promptly
- oligohydramnios if prolonged PPROM occurs
- cord prolapse
- malpresentation associated with prematurity
- antepartum haemorrhage
- neonatal sepsis
- psychosocial problems resulting from uncertain fetal and neonatal outcome and long-term hospitalization; increased incidence of impaired mother and baby bonding after birth

Management

If PPROM is suspected, the woman will be admitted to the maternity unit. A careful history is taken and rupture of the membranes confirmed by a sterile speculum examination of any pooling of liquor in the posterior fornix of the vagina. Saturated sanitary towels over a 6-hour period will also offer a reasonably conclusive diagnosis if urine leakage has been excluded. A Nitrazine test may be useful to confirm this. A fetal fibronectin immunoenzyme test is useful in confirming rupture of the membranes, and ultrasound scanning also has some value.

Digital vaginal examination should be avoided to reduce the risk of introducing infection. Observations are made of the fetal condition from the fetal heart rate, as an infected fetus may have a tachycardia, and also a maternal infection screen, temperature and pulse, uterine tenderness and any purulent or offensively smelling vaginal discharge. A decision on future management will then be made.

If the pregnancy is less than 32 weeks, the fetus appears to be uncompromised and APH and labour have been excluded, it will be managed expectantly.

- The woman is admitted to hospital.
- Frequent ultrasound scans are undertaken to assess the growth of the fetus and the extent and complications of any oligohydramnios.
- Corticosteroids are administered to mature the fetal lungs as soon as PPROM is confirmed, should the baby be born early.
- If labour intervenes the administration of a tocolytic drug (such as *atosiban acetate*) should be considered to prolong the pregnancy. In practice these are usually discontinued after the corticosteroids have had time to take effect.
- Known vaginal infections are treated with antibiotics. Prophylactic antibiotics may also be offered to women without symptoms of infection.
- If membranes rupture before 24 weeks of gestation the outlook is poor and the woman may be offered termination of the pregnancy.
- If the woman is more than 32 weeks pregnant, the fetus appears to be compromised and APH or intervening labour is suspected or confirmed, active management will ensue. The mode of birth will need to be decided and induction of labour or caesarean section performed.

Hindwater leakage of amniotic fluid, and resealing of the amniotic sac are currently poorly understood phenomena.

CONCLUSION

Midwives have an important role to play when women experience pathological problems in their pregnancy. The woman is likely to report symptoms firstly to a midwife, who will then make basic observations that confirm or exclude the likelihood of a deviation from normal. While explaining her findings to the woman and her partner, the midwife must make a decision about possible diagnoses, whether to transfer her to a high-risk obstetric unit and if this warrants transportation by ambulance. The midwife may be required to start managing the woman's condition prior to admission to hospital. In hospital the midwife is required to ensure the woman's care is coordinated with other healthcare professionals, who must be supplied with appropriate background information, that the woman and her partner receive psychological support and that contemporaneous records are kept (NMC 2012a). The midwife must report any deterioration in a woman's condition immediately to an appropriate healthcare professional. The midwife is responsible for maintaining continual updating of her professional knowledge and skills in all areas of practice to ensure that every woman receives optimal maternity care throughout her pregnancy.

REFERENCES

Abortion Act 1967. c. 87. London: HMSO. Accessed at www.legislation.gov.uk/ukpga/1967/87 (2 July 2013)

Andrews J I 2011 Hepatic viral infections. In: James D (ed) High risk pregnancy management options. Saunders Elsevier, Philadelphia, p 469–77

ACPWH (Association of Chartered Physiotherapists in Women's Health) 2011 Pregnancy-related pelvic girdle pain. www.csp.org.uk/sites/files/csp/secure/acpwh-pgppat_0.pdf (accessed 20 June 2013)

Beall M H, Beloosesky R, Ross M G 2011 Abnormalities of amniotic fluid volume. In: James D (ed) High risk pregnancy management options. Saunders Elsevier, Philadelphia, p 197–207

Betts D 2006 The essential guide to acupuncture in pregnancy and childbirth. Hove: The Journal of Chinese Medicine.

Cahill D J, Swingler R, Wardle P G 2011 Bleeding and pain in early pregnancy. In: James D (ed) High risk pregnancy management options. Saunders Elsevier, Philadelphia, p 57–74

CEMACE (Centre for Maternal and Child Enquiries) 2011 Saving mothers lives: reviewing maternal deaths to make motherhood safer: 2006–2008. The Eighth Report on Confidential Enquiries into Maternal Deaths in the United Kingdom. BJOG: An International Journal of Obstetrics and Gynaecology 118(Suppl 1):1–203

Copeland L J, Landon M B 2011 Malignant diseases and pregnancy. In: Gabbe S G, Niebyl J R, Simpson J L (eds) Obstetrics: normal and problem pregnancies. Churchill Livingstone, Philadelphia, p 1153–77

Department of Health 2012 Abortion Statistics, England and Wales: 2011

www.gov.uk/government/uploads/system/uploads/attachment_data/file/127785/Commentary1.pdf.pdf (accessed 20 June 2013)

Gordon M C 2007 Maternal physiology. In: Gabbe S G, Niebyl JR, Simpson J L (eds) Obstetrics: normal and problem pregnancies. Churchill Livingstone, Philadelphia, p 55–84

Hay P 2012 BASHH Guidelines, UK National Guideline for the management of Bacterial Vaginosis 2012. http://www.bashh.org/documents/4413.pdf (accessed 14 September 2014)

Human Fertilisation and Embryology Act 1990 c. 37. London: HMSO. Accessed at www.legislation.gov.uk/ukpga/1990/37/section/37 (2 July 2013)

Lindow S W, Anthony J 2011 Major obstetric haemorrhage and disseminated intravascular coagulation. In: James D (ed) High risk pregnancy management options. Saunders Elsevier, Philadelphia, p 1331–45

Ludmir J, Owen J 2007 Cervical incompetence. In: Gabbe S G, Niebyl J R, Simpson J L (eds) Obstetrics: normal and problem pregnancies. Churchill Livingstone, Philadelphia, p 650–67

Mahomed K 2011a Abdominal pain. In: James D (ed) High risk pregnancy management options. Saunders Elsevier, Philadelphia, p 1013–26

Mahomed K. 2011b Nonmalignant gynecology. In: James D (ed) High risk pregnancy management options. Saunders Elsevier, Philadelphia, p 1027–36

National Health Service Cervical Screening Programme 2013 www.screening.nhs.uk/cervicalcancer-england (accessed 2 July 2013)

Navti O B, Konje J C 2011 Bleeding in late pregnancy. In: James D (ed) High risk pregnancy management options. Saunders Elsevier, Philadelphia, p 1037–52

Neilson J P 2012 Biochemical tests of placental function for assessment in pregnancy. Cochrane Pregnancy and Childbirth Group. Available at http://onlinelibrary.wiley.com/doi/10.1002/14651858.CD000108.pub2/full (accessed 9 July 2012)

NHS (National Health Service) Choices 2012 Treating ectopic pregnancy. www.nhs.uk/Conditions/Ectopic-pregnancy/Pages/Treatment.aspx (accessed 20 June 2013)

NICE (National Institute for Health and Clinical Excellence) 2007 Laparoscopic cerclage for prevention of recurrent pregnancy loss due to cervical incompetence. NICE, London. Available at: www.nice.org.uk/nicemedia/live/11336/35859/35859.pdf (accessed 20 June 2013)

NICE (National Institute for Health and Clinical Excellence) 2010 Antenatal care. CG 62. NICE, London. Available at: www.nice.org.uk/nicemedia/live/11947/40115/40115.pdf (accessed 20 June 2013)

NICE (National Institute for Health and Clinical Excellence) 2011 Routine antenatal anti-D prophylaxis for women who are rhesus negative: review of NICE Technology Appraisal Guidance 41. NICE, London. Available at: www.nice.org.uk/nicemedia/pdf/TA156Guidance.pdf (accessed 20 June 2013)

NMC (Nursing and Midwifery Council) 2012a Midwives Rules and Standards. NMC, London. Available at www.nmc-uk.org/Documents/NMC-Publications/Midwives%20Rules%20and%20Standards%202012.pdf (accessed 20 June 2013)

NMC (Nursing and Midwifery Council) 2012b Conscientious objection by nurses and midwives. www.nmc-uk.org/Nurses-and-midwives/Regulation-in-practice/Regulation-in-Practice-Topics/Conscientious-objection-by-nurses-and-midwives-/ (accessed 20 June 2013)

RCOG (Royal College of Obstetricians and Gynaecologists) 2006 The management of early pregnancy loss. Green-top Guideline No. 25. RCOG, London. Available at www.rcog.org.uk/files/rcog-corp/uploaded-files/GT25ManagementofEarlyPregnancyLoss2006.pdf (accessed 20 June 2013)

RCOG (Royal College of Obstetricians and Gynaecologists) 2007 Ovarian hyperstimulation syndrome: what you need to know. RCOG, London. Available at www.rcog.org.uk/files/rcog-corp/Ovarian%20Hyperstimulation%20Syndrome.pdf (accessed 20 June 2013)

RCOG (Royal College of Obstetricians and Gynaecologists) 2010a The management of tubal pregnancy. Green-top Guideline No. 21. RCOG, London. Available at www.rcog.org.uk/files/rcog-corp/GTG21_230611.pdf (accessed 20 June 2013)

RCOG (Royal College of Obstetricians and Gynaecologists) 2010b The management of gestational trophoblastic disease. Green-top Guideline No. 38. RCOG, London. Available at www.rcog.org.uk/files/rcog-corp/GT38Management

Gestational0210.pdf (accessed 20 June 2013)

RCOG (Royal College of Obstetricians and Gynaecologists) 2010c Pre-term pre-labour rupture of the membranes. Green-top Guideline No. 44. RCOG, London. Available at www.rcog.org.uk/files/rcog-corp/GTG44PPROM28022011.pdf (accessed 20 June 2013)

RCOG (Royal College of Obstetricians and Gynaecologists) 2011a The investigation and treatment of couples with recurrent first-trimester and second-trimester miscarriage. Green-top Guideline No. 17. RCOG, London. Available at www.rcog.org.uk/files/rcog-corp/GTG17recurrentmiscarriage.pdf (accessed 20 June 2013)

RCOG (Royal College of Obstetricians and Gynaecologists) 2011b The use of anti-D immunoglobulin for rhesus D prophylaxis. Green-top Guideline No. 22. RCOG, London. Available at www.rcog.org.uk/files/rcog-corp/GTG22AntiD.pdf (accessed 22 June 2013)

RCOG (Royal College of Obstetricians and Gynaecologists) 2011c The care of women requesting induced abortion. Evidence-Based Clinical Guideline No. 7. RCOG, London. Available at www.rcog.org.uk/files/rcog-corp/Abortion%20guideline_web_1.pdf (accessed 20 June 2013)

SANDS (Stillbirth and Neonatal Death Society) 2007 Pregnancy loss and the death of a baby: guidelines for professionals. SANDS, London

Svigos J M, Dodd J M, Robinson J S 2011 Prelabour rupture of the membranes. In: James D (ed) High risk pregnancy management options. Saunders Elsevier, Philadelphia, p 1091–100

Tiran D 2004 Nausea and vomiting in pregnancy. Churchill Livingstone, Edinburgh

Williamson C, Girling J 2011 Hepatic and gastrointestinal disease. In: James D (ed) High risk pregnancy management options. Saunders Elsevier, Philadelphia, p 1032–60

FURTHER READING

Bothamley J, Boyle M 2009 Medical conditions affecting pregnancy and childbirth. Milton Keynes, Radcliffe

A midwifery textbook written for midwifery students with useful sections on hyperemesis gravidarum and obstetric cholestasis.

Boyle M (ed) 2011 Emergencies around childbirth. Milton Keynes, Radcliffe

This book has useful sections on antepartum haemorrhage and maternal collapse, written with student and newly qualified midwives in mind.

Monga A, Dobbs S 2011 Gynaecology by ten teachers. Hodder, London

A general gynaecology text book which will provide students and midwives with useful background information about early pregnancy and pregnancy-related gynaecology conditions.

Raynor M D, Marshall J E, Jackson K 2012 Midwifery practice: critical illness, complications and

emergencies casebook. McGraw–Hill/Open University Press, Maidenhead

Provides a useful case study approach with questions and answers for the reader to enhance their knowledge and understanding in recognizing the critically ill woman, and conditions such as APH, DIC and obstetric cholestasis.

World Health Organization (WHO) 2012 Facts on induced abortion worldwide. WHO, Geneva. Available at www.guttmacher.org/pubs/fb_IAW .html (accessed 2 July 2013)

Useful fact sheet looking at the incidence and trends of abortion worldwide.

World Health Organization 2012 Safe and unsafe induced abortion: global and regional levels in 2008, and trends during 1995–2008. Geneva, WHO. Available at http://apps.who. int/iris/bitstream/10665/75174/1/ WHO_RHR_12.02_eng.pdf (accessed 2 July 2013)

Useful information sheet examining global trends on both safe and unsafe abortion.

USEFUL WEBSITES

Antenatal Results and Choices: www.arc-uk.org

This charity website aims to offer information and support to parents and families following the diagnosis of a fetal abnormality, which may then lead to difficult decisions having to be made. Information, leaflets and training are also available for professionals.

Ectopic Pregnancy Trust: www.ectopic .org.uk

Website for professionals and women related to ectopic pregnancy.

ICP Support: www.icpsupport.org

Website offering support and information for women and professionals regarding intrahepatic cholestasis of pregnancy (obstetric cholestasis).

Miscarriage Association: www .miscarriageassociation.org.uk

Offers support and information to parents following the various forms of early pregnancy loss. Information also available for professionals.

NHS Cervical Screening Programme: www.cancerscreening.nhs.uk/ cervical/

Provides details of the cervical cancer screening programme offered in the UK, as well as information relevant for the public and professionals.

Pelvic Partnership: www.pelvic partnership.org.uk

This website is run by volunteers who all have personal experience of Pelvic Girdle Pain. The information provided is mainly provided for women, but provides additional knowledge and guidance for students and midwives alike.

Pregnancy Sickness Support: www .pregnancysicknesssupport.org.uk

A charity website that offers information and support to both women and professionals with regards to nausea and vomiting in pregnancy. There is also guidance regarding hyperemesis gravidarum.

Royal College of Obstetricians and Gynaecologists: www.rcog.org.uk

RCOG website that provides a wealth of information and guidance through the Green-top series on best practice relating to gynecological and obstetric-related situations.

SANDS (Stillbirth and Neonatal Death Society): www.uk-sands.org

This is a comprehensive website offering information and support for parents and families following the loss of a baby. SANDS also produces guidelines for professionals to help support those caring for bereaved families.

Chapter |13|

Medical conditions of significance to midwifery practice

S Elizabeth Robson, Jayne E Marshall, Rowena Doughty, Moira McLean

Medical disorders are of increasing significance in midwifery practice. A few years ago a student midwife would have learnt about a few of them during education and training, but this situation is changing. Increasing maternal age and advances in medical treatment have resulted in women who might have previously died, or been advised against pregnancy, now presenting for maternity care and bringing considerable challenges along with them (CMACE 2011). In addition to using this chapter as a resource, a midwife caring for such women may need to seek additional sources for advancing her knowledge as not every medical condition or infection could be fully explored within this chapter.

THE CHAPTER AIMS TO:

- provide an account of the most common medical conditions and their effect on childbearing women
- provide an overview of the less common medical conditions and their significance to the health and wellbeing of the woman and her family
- explain the importance of midwives having an in-depth knowledge of medical conditions in order to recognize women with such conditions and care for them effectively.

HYPERTENSIVE DISORDERS

Blood pressure – regulation and measurement

Blood pressure (BP) is the force exerted by blood volume on the blood vessel walls, known as peripheral resistance. This force is generated by contraction of the ventricles of the heart, and in the case of young, healthy adults blood enters the aorta at 120 mmHg at systole (contraction) and falls to 80 mmHg at diastole (relaxation) (Tortora and Derrickson 2010). As the blood is dispersed through the arterial system the pressure gradually lowers to 16 mmHg by the time it reaches the capillaries. Blood pressure is never zero unless there is a cardiac arrest (Webster et al 2013).

When cardiac output rises due to increased stroke volume or heart rate the BP rises, providing peripheral resistance remains constant, and BP lowers with a decrease in cardiac output. Haemorrhage lowers blood volume and cardiac output so the blood pressure will fall; conversely it will rise due to fluid retention increasing blood volume (Tortora and Derrickson 2010). Systolic pressure is relatively labile, and can be affected by emotional mood and body posture. BP rises with age as the arteries become thicker and harder and is exacerbated by conditions such as atherosclerosis.

Regulation of blood pressure

Blood pressure is regulated by neural, chemical and hormonal controls of which the midwife needs a basic knowledge because drugs to control BP often act on these pathways.

Baroreceptors are specialized nerve endings in the left ventricle, carotid sinus, aortic arch and pulmonary veins that act as stretch receptors. Increased pressure in these vessels stimulates the baroreceptors to relay this information to the cardiovascular centre of medulla oblongata in the brain. The cardiovascular centre responds by putting out parasympathetic impulses via the motor (*efferent*) fibres of the vagus nerve supplying the heart, causing fewer sympathetic impulses reaching the heart. This causes a lowered heart rate, lowered cardiac output and vasodilatation of arterioles giving rise to a fall in BP (Tortora and Derrickson 2010). Conversely, if pressure on the baroreceptors decreases, the feedback to the cardiovascular centre results in increased sympathetic impulses causing accelerated heart rate, increased force of contraction and vasodilatation. BP then rises.

Chemoreceptors monitor blood chemicals, in particular hydrogen ions, oxygen and carbon dioxide, and are situated close to the baroreceptors. They also relay information to the cardiovascular centre of the medulla oblongata (Tortora and Derrickson 2010). If there is a deficiency of oxygen (*hypoxia*) the carbon dioxide level rises and hydrogen ion concentration increases causing acidity, such that the chemoreceptors are stimulated and send responses to the medulla oblongata. In response the cardiovascular centre increases sympathetic nerve stimulation causing vasoconstriction of arterioles and veins, and BP rises.

Certain *hormones* influence blood pressure as follows (Tortora and Derrickson 2010):

- Epinephrine and norepinephrine from the adrenal medulla increase heart rate and raise BP.
- Antidiuretic hormone (ADH) released from the posterior pituitary gland causes vasoconstriction especially if there is hypovolaemia due to haemorrhage. Alcohol inhibits release of ADH leading to vasodilatation, which lowers BP.
- Angiotensin II causes vasoconstriction and stimulates secretion of aldosterone resulting in greater reabsorption of water by the kidneys, both resulting in raised BP.
- Atrial natriuretic peptide (ANP) from cells in the heart's atria causes vasodilatation, and lowers BP.
- Histamine released by mast cells in an inflammatory response is a vasodilator, decreasing BP.
- Progesterone of pregnancy causes vasodilatation and lowers BP (see below).

Blood pressure adaptation in pregnancy

In pregnancy blood plasma volume increases from approximately 2600 ml to 3800 ml by 32 weeks' gestation and red cell mass from 1400 to 1800 ml; consequently cardiac output increases by 40%, with the majority of the extra output directed to the uterus and kidneys (Greer et al 2007). This should result in raised BP, however the increasing release of progesterone throughout pregnancy causes vasodilatation, and systolic and diastolic pressures actually fall in the first and second trimesters by about 10 mmHg (Burrow et al 2004), which can predispose the pregnant woman to fainting due to hypotension (see Chapter 9). Systolic and diastolic measurements rise slowly to the pre-pregnancy levels in the third trimester (Redman et al 2010).

Measuring blood pressure

Accurate measurement of BP is essential in order to confirm wellness or to diagnose hypotension or hypertension at the earliest possibility. Traditionally blood pressure was measured using a mercury sphygmomanometer and stethoscope, but human errors in these readings resulted in greater use of manual (usually anaeroid) and digital devices (Waugh and Smith 2012), as well as health and safety concerns about mercury devices. Diastolic BP is now determined at Korotkoff Phase V (disappearance of sound) rather than Korotkoff Phase IV (muffling sound) when using manual devices. Box 13.1 outlines recommendations for measuring BP pressure.

The size of cuff is an important consideration as a cuff, and the bladder inside it, that are too small will *undercuff* the woman with risk of overestimating the blood pressure. About 25% of antenatal women could fall into this category, so both standard and large size cuffs should be available in all maternity clinics and wards (Waugh and Smith 2012).

A difference in systolic BP readings between left and right arms of >10 mmHg can be observed in general populations, including healthy women in the antenatal period, and is considered normal (Clarke et al 2012). If hypertension is suspected, the National Institute for Health and Clinical Excellence (NICE) (2011) recommends measuring BP in both arms and if the difference is ≥20 mmHg the measurements should be repeated. If the ≥20 mmHg difference remains, all subsequent readings should be measured in the arm with the higher reading and the midwife should bring this difference to the attention of a doctor (Nursing and Midwifery Council 2012).

Defining hypertension

Hypertension is systolic or diastolic BP that is raised from normal values. New guidelines recommend that a diagnosis of hypertension should be confirmed using 24-hour ambulatory blood pressure monitoring (ABPM) as gold

---

> ### Box 13.1 Blood pressure measurement
>
> - Patient/woman should be seated for at least 5 minutes, relaxed and not moving or speaking.
> - The arm must be supported at the level of the heart.
> - Ensure no tight clothing constricts the arm.
> - Place the cuff neatly, with the centre of its bladder over the brachial artery. This bladder should encircle at least 80% of the arm, but not more than 100%.
>
> #### Digital devices
> - Some monitors allow manual blood pressure setting selection, where you choose the appropriate setting.
> - Other monitors will automatically inflate and re-inflate to the next setting if required.
> - Repeat three times and record measurement as displayed.
> - Initially test blood pressure in both arms and use the arm with the highest reading for subsequent measurement.
>
> #### Manual devices
> - Estimate the systolic beforehand:
>   (a) Palpate the brachial artery
>   (b) Inflate cuff until pulsation disappears
>   (c) Deflate cuff
>   (d) Estimate systolic pressure.
> - Then inflate to 30 mmHg above the estimated systolic level needed to occlude the pulse.
> - Place the stethoscope diaphragm over the brachial artery and deflate at a rate of 2–3 mm/sec until you hear regular tapping sounds.
> - Measure systolic (*first sound*) and diastolic (*disappearance*) to nearest 2 mmHg.
>
> Source: NICE 2011

---

standard rather than be based solely on measurements of BP taken in clinical situations (NICE 2011). Definitions applied to the general, non-pregnant, population are outlined in Box 13.2.

Hypertension in pregnant women should be taken seriously; lower parameters of BP measurement apply and the definitions in Box 13.3 are used in midwifery and obstetric practice.

Hypertensive conditions of pregnancy

Over the years there have many classifications of hypertension in pregnancy and in particular the competing definitions of pregnancy-induced hypertension (PIH) have caused confusion. The midwife is therefore advised to use

---

Box 13.2 Definitions of hypertension in the general, non-pregnant population

Stage 1 hypertension

Blood pressure of 140/90 mmHg or higher *and* subsequent ambulatory blood pressure monitoring (ABPM) daytime average or home blood pressure monitoring (HBPM) average of 135/85 mmHg or higher

Stage 2 hypertension

Blood pressure of 160/100 mmHg or higher *and* subsequent ambulatory blood pressure monitoring (ABPM) daytime average or home blood pressure monitoring (HBPM) average of 150/95 mmHg or higher

Severe hypertension

Systolic blood pressure is 180 mmHg or higher, *or* clinical diastolic pressure is 110 mmHg or higher.

Source: NICE 2011

Box 13.3 Definitions of hypertension in pregnancy

Mild hypertension

Diastolic blood pressure 90–99 mmHg, systolic blood pressure 140–149 mmHg.

Moderate hypertension

Diastolic blood pressure 100–109 mmHg, systolic blood pressure 150–159 mmHg.

Severe hypertension

Diastolic blood pressure 110 mmHg or greater, systolic blood pressure 160 mmHg or greater.
   Note the lower measurements for this definition when compared with severe hypertension in the general population.

Chronic hypertension

This is hypertension that is present at the initial visit (booking) or before 20 weeks, or if the woman is already taking antihypertensive medication when referred to maternity services. It can be primary or secondary in aetiology.

Gestational hypertension

This is *new* hypertension presenting after 20 weeks without significant proteinuria.

Pre-eclampsia

This is *new* hypertension presenting after 20 weeks with significant proteinuria.

Severe pre-eclampsia

This is pre-eclampsia with severe hypertension and/or with symptoms, and/or biochemical and/or haematological impairment.

Source: NICE 2010a

---

the definitions in Box 13.3. The following will attempt to clarify how the conditions present and develop into the next stage, with inherent complications.

Chronic hypertension

Chronic hypertension encompasses hypertension >140/90 mmHg that existed before pregnancy (NICE 2010a). This was previously known as *benign* or *essential* hypertension. The earlier that hypertension is diagnosed in pregnancy the more likely it is to be pre-existing chronic hypertension (Webster et al 2013). Lack of *illness* symptoms implies the woman is unlikely to have had her BP measured pre-pregnancy and potentially it is diagnosed for the first time once she is pregnant.

Chronic hypertension has many associated factors, especially: obesity, black race, family history of hypertension and lifestyle factors such as lack of exercise, alcohol consumption and poor diet with high salt or fat intake. The risk of developing chronic hypertension increases with age and it can be primary or secondary in aetiology (NICE 2010a). If this condition is known pre-pregnancy, the women should be directed to pre-conception care. This is to ascertain the extent of the hypertension, treat the causes and assess co-morbidities such as renal impairment or diabetes mellitus where the BP may be lower than with hypertension alone, as the risk of cardiovascular disease is greater (Webster et al 2013). Current medication should be reviewed as angiotensin-converting enzyme (ACE) inhibitors, diuretics and angiotensin receptor blockers (ARB) increase the risk of congenital malformations (Waugh and Smith 2012) and safer alternatives might need to be prescribed (see Box 13.4).

Gestational hypertension

Gestational hypertension is hypertension >140/90 mmHg that presents after the 20th week of pregnancy and without significant proteinuria. The BP should return to normal values postnatally. It can be difficult to differentiate between the presentation of chronic hypertension and gestational hypertension, because the physiological fall in BP in the first trimester of pregnancy occurs with both normotensive and hypertensive women, and can mask the existence of chronic hypertension unless pre-pregnancy values are known (Webster et al 2013). The diagnosis of gestational versus chronic hypertension might be resolved only in retrospect when the six-week postnatal BP readings are performed.

Box 13.4 Antihypertensive drugs used in pregnancy

Beta-blockers

- Inhibit action of catecholamines on the adrenoreceptors
- Beta-1 affects heart rate and contractility
- Beta-2 affects vascular and smooth muscle
- Associated with neonatal hypoglycaemia and IUGR

Labetalol (first line treatment)

- Combined alpha- and beta-blocker that can be given orally or IV
- Licensed for use in pregnancy. Used IV for the acute treatment of severe hypertension
- Avoid use with asthmatic women as it causes bronchospasm
- Compatible with breastfeeding

Methyldopa

- Acts centrally to produce a decrease in vascular resistance
- Has a maximum effect 48 hours after commencement of treatment
- Small amounts are secreted into breastmilk, but it is classified as compatible with breastfeeding

Nifedipine

- Calcium channel-blocker that inhibits transport of calcium across cell membranes
- Causes vasodilatation, which reduces blood pressure

Source: NICE 2010a; Webster et al 2013

- Not licensed for pregnancy use before 20 weeks' gestation
- Probably compatible with breastfeeding

Hydralazine

- Direct-acting vasodilator
- No adverse fetal effects, but many maternal side effects, including acute hypotension, tachycardia and palpitations
- Initially 25 mg twice/day given orally in the third trimester only
- Compatible with breastfeeding

Diuretics

- Relieve oedema by inhibiting sodium re-absorption in the kidney and increasing urine production, thus lowering blood volume and in turn blood pressure
- Act within 1–2 hours of oral administration and last for 12–24 hours
- Usually administered in the morning so that diuresis does not interfere with sleep
- Loss of potassium (*hypokalaemia*) is a complication and potassium supplements may be given for long-term treatment of hypertension
- Use in pregnancy is restricted to treating complex disorders, e.g. heart disease or renal disease in combination with other drugs

Complications

According to Waugh and Smith (2012) and Webster et al (2013), the complications of gestational hypertension and chronic hypertension are the same:

- intrauterine fetal growth restriction (IUGR)
- placental abruption
- superimposed pre-eclampsia
- worsening hypertension leading to severe hypertension and risks of stroke (cerebral vascular accident [CVA] and organ damage).

Management

- The woman with known chronic hypertension should be booked at a consultant unit, and re-referred to any clinics treating her hypertension and co-existing conditions. If she is taking ACE inhibitors or ARB these are discontinued and alternative hypertensive therapy prescribed (see Box 13.4).

- The physiological fall of BP in early pregnancy might entail reducing or even ceasing antihypertensives in the first trimester, and then increasing doses gradually towards term based on BP readings.
- The woman who has a raised BP without proteinuria presenting during pregnancy is likely to have gestational hypertension and should be referred to a maternal medicine clinic and booked for labour and birth in a consultant-led unit.

Thereafter management of both chronic and gestational hypertension is the same and requires involvement of both doctor and midwife as follows:

- Schedule antenatal appointments, as for nulliparae, to see a doctor and midwife at 16, 25, 28, 31, 34, 36, 38 weeks (NICE 2010a).
- Additional appointments should be arranged for maternal medicine or hypertension clinics if indicated.
- At each appointment record BP, urinalysis with emphasis on proteinuria, and assess fetal growth by

symphysis–fundal height (SFH). Be alert for signs of pre-eclampsia.

- Review BP readings; adjust drug dosages accordingly, aiming to keep BP ≤150/100 mmHg in uncomplicated cases (NICE 2010a).
- The doctor should prescribe low-dose aspirin (75 mg once daily).
- Arrange ultrasound fetal growth and amniotic fluid volume assessment and umbilical artery Doppler velocimetry between 28 and 30 weeks and between 32 and 34 weeks. If results are normal, these are not repeated unless there is a clinical indication (NICE 2010a).
- Assess and manage co-existing conditions such as obesity or diabetes mellitus.
- Advise the woman to keep her dietary intake of sodium low (NICE 2010a).
- Hospital admission is unlikely with both chronic and gestational hypertension unless the hypertension becomes severe.
- Labour should be induced at 37 weeks or earlier if BP is uncontrolled, or fetal or antenatal complications develop.
- Labour will require hourly BP monitoring and administration of hypertensive drugs with dosages adjusted if BP fluctuates.
- An epidural may be advantageous in labour as this lowers BP.
- Continuous fetal monitoring is required in labour (NICE 2007).
- A normal birth by the midwife can be anticipated, and caesarean section should be performed for obstetric reasons only.
- The length of the second stage of labour should be shortened only if severe hypertension develops.
- Ergometrine and syntometrine should be avoided for the third stage of labour as these are acute vasoconstrictors. Use oxytocin in preference.
- Breastfeeding should be encouraged.
- The midwife should record BP daily in the postpartum period for the first 3 days and then on the 5th day.
- Postpartum BP should be maintained below 140/90 mmHg and, if necessary, medication adjusted (Waugh and Smith 2012).
- Prior to transfer home from hospital the woman should be seen by an obstetrician who is likely to stop methyldopa within two days of birth and restart the antihypertensive treatment the woman was taking before she planned the pregnancy.
- If BP falls below 130/80 mmHg the obstetrician should reduce the hypertensive treatment (NICE 2010a).
- The midwife should reinforce advice on lifestyle factors such as diet and exercise.

- The combined oral contraceptive pill might be contraindicated, so referral to a doctor or family planning clinic for specialist advice is essential.
- The midwife should not discharge the woman from her care if BP levels give concern and other members of the multidisciplinary team may need to be involved.
- A 2-week postnatal review with the general practitioner (GP) should be arranged where the continued use of antenatal hypertensive treatment should be reviewed.
- A medical review in combination with the 6-week postnatal review should also be arranged (NICE 2010a).

Superimposed pre-eclampsia

Women with chronic hypertension may develop pre-eclampsia as well, and the signs and symptoms are the same as for pre-eclampsia (see below). In these women the blood pressure profile may be more difficult to interpret as the baseline BP is likely to be higher and exacerbated by the effects of treatment with antihypertensives (Webster et al 2013). Development of significant proteinuria (see Box 13.3) is indicative of pre-eclampsia and often accompanied by fetal growth restriction (Webster et al 2013). Management and treatment are as for pre-eclampsia.

Secondary hypertension

Women may develop secondary hypertension as a complication of either underlying physiology or disease, most commonly caused by:

- *Renal disease*, which results in sodium retention by the kidney leading to water retention, an increased blood volume and thereafter hypertension. This may be classified as renal hypertension. Depending upon the nature of the renal disease the early birth of the baby may become necessary to prevent long-term kidney damage (Webster et al 2013).
- *Phaeochromocytoma*, an adrenal gland tumour secreting the hormones dopamine, adrenaline and noradrenaline (see section on regulation of blood pressure).
- *Congenital heart disease*, especially if there is constriction of the aorta.
- *Conn's syndrome:* an excess of aldosterone hormone causes sodium retention and associated hypokalaemia.
- *Cushing's syndrome:* an excess of glucocorticoid hormones.

Management

The management is to address the underlying cause. However, substantive treatment might have to wait until the woman has given birth and then treat the condition as for chronic hypertension.

Pre-eclampsia

Pre-eclampsia (formerly known as PET: pre-eclamptic tox-aemia) is an *idiopathic* (= cause unknown) condition of pregnancy characterized by proteinuria and hypertension presenting after 20 weeks of pregnancy in a woman who previously had normal blood pressure. The severity can be mild, moderate or severe, and may be pre-eclampsia or eclampsia (see below).

Pre-eclampsia occurs in 3% of all pregnancies (Hutcheon et al 2011) and >10% of women will develop this in their first pregnancy (Waugh and Smith 2012) (Box 13.5). Whilst most of these women will have a successful outcome to their pregnancy, some will proceed to multi-system complications. In the latest Centre for Maternal and Child Enquiries triennial report into maternal deaths (CMACE 2011), there were a total of 19 women in the United Kingdom (UK) who died as a result of pre-eclampsia or eclampsia (Neilson 2011), with an estimated 500–600 babies dying each year, mainly due to premature birth rather than the condition itself. The probability of a woman developing it in future pregnancies is 16%, rising to 25% in cases of severe pre-eclampsia and, where the woman's baby was born before 28 weeks, this probability rises to 55% (NICE 2011).

Pre-eclampsia is commonly known as a *disease of theories* and the pathophysiology is not fully understood. It is thought that the condition arises from the influence of placental tissue as it can arise in molar pregnancies (*gestational trophoblastic disease*) where there is placental tissue but no fetal tissue (Waugh and Smith 2012).

Management in pregnancy

Women at risk of pre-eclampsia should be investigated for underlying medical problems and will normally be commenced on aspirin from 12 weeks of pregnancy until the baby is born (see Table 13.1) (Webster et al 2013). Women at high risk have one of the following:

- hypertensive disease during a previous pregnancy
- chronic hypertension
- chronic kidney disease
- autoimmune disease, especially antiphospholipid syndrome (APS) or systemic lupus erythematosus (SLE) (NICE 2010a).

Early recognition of pre-eclampsia is paramount as the midwife is likely to be the first health professional to notice the clinical signs at an antenatal appointment, and prompt referral to an obstetrician is necessary for investigations, albeit the ultimate responsibility for the diagnosis lies with the doctor. Pre-eclampsia can be recognized by:

- blood pressure: systolic >140 mmHg or diastolic >90 mmHg (see Chronic hypertension)
- proteinuria (see Box 13.6 for principles of assessing proteinuria)
- oedema – may be detectable on examination. Ankle oedema is a common phenomenon in pregnancy and tends to diminish overnight. More generalized oedema that pits on pressure on the pre-tibial surface, face, hands, abdomen and sacrum, especially if sudden in onset, warrants further investigation. The severity of the oedema increases with the severity of the pre-eclampsia.

The midwife should appreciate that the woman may be feeling well and will need convincing that she requires a hospital referral. Referral should be to a consultant-led unit for investigations that, according to Williams and Craft (2012), are likely to include:

- Urine sample or 24 hour urine collection to quantify the proteinuria (>300 mg) and determine the ratio of protein to creatinine (>30 mg/mmol).

Box 13.5 **Associated factors for developing pre-eclampsia**

Maternal factors

- Primipaternity (first pregnancy with a new partner)
- Extremes of maternal age (<20 and >40 years)
- Family history of pre-eclampsia
- Pre-eclampsia in a previous pregnancy
- Pregnancy after assisted reproductive technology
- Obesity
- Pre-existing diabetes mellitus type 1
- Pre-existing hypertensive disease
- Pre-existing medical conditions, e.g. renal disease, systemic lupus erythematosus (SLE), rheumatoid arthritis

Pregnancy related factors

- First pregnancy
- Multiple pregnancy
- Developing a medical disorder during pregnancy, e.g. venous thromboembolic disease (VTE), such as antiphospholipid (Hughes) syndrome (APS), gestational diabetes, gestational hypertension
- Developing infection with inflammatory response
- Hydropic degeneration of the placenta

Source: NICE 2010a; James et al 2011

Table 13.1 Management of pregnancy with pre-eclampsia

Degree of hypertension	Mild	Moderate	Severe
	(140/90 to 149/99 mmHg)	**(150/100 to 159/109 mmHg)**	**(160/110 mmHg or higher)**
Admit to hospital	Yes	Yes	Yes
Treatment	Nil	Oral labetalol as first-line treatment to keep: diastolic blood pressure between 80–100 mmHg systolic blood pressure less than 150 mmHg Low-dose aspirin: 75 mg/day from 12 weeks	Oral labetalol as first-line treatment to keep: diastolic blood pressure between 80–100 mmHg systolic blood pressure less than 150 mmHg Low-dose aspirin: 75 mg/day from 12 weeks
Measure blood pressure	At least four times a day	At least four times a day	More than four times a day, depending upon clinical circumstances
Test for proteinuria	Do not repeat quantification of proteinuria	Do not repeat quantification of proteinuria	Do not repeat quantification of proteinuria
Blood tests	Monitor *twice* a week with the following tests: kidney function, electrolytes, full blood count, transaminases, bilirubin	Monitor *three* times a week with the following tests: kidney function, electrolytes, full blood count, transaminases, bilirubin	Monitor *three* times a week with the following tests: kidney function, electrolytes, full blood count, transaminases, bilirubin

---

Box 13.6 Determining proteinuria in pregnancy

- If using a dipstix to test the urine, ensure the reagent strips are in date and read according to the stipulated times along the exterior label.
- A mid-stream specimen of urine (MSSU) may be necessary to exclude urinary tract infection (UTI) as a cause of proteinuria.
- If an automated reagent-strip reading device is used to detect proteinuria and a result of 1+ or more is obtained, use a spot urinary protein : creatinine ratio or 24-hour urine collection to quantify proteinuria.
- Significant proteinuria is diagnosed when the urinary protein : creatinine ratio is >30 mg/mmol, or if a 24-hour urine collection result shows > 300 mg protein.
- Ensure 24 hour urine collections are complete before sending to the laboratory for analysis.

Source: NICE 2010a

- Full blood count to observe for platelet consumption and haemolysis. In pre-eclampsia the haemoglobin concentration may be raised (>120 g/l) due to haemoconcentration.
- Urea and electrolytes to assess renal dysfunction (raised serum creatinine >90 μmol/l).
- Liver enzymes to assess liver function and observe for transaminitis.
- Assessment of fetal wellbeing by ultrasound to monitor growth and volume of amniotic fluid and Doppler velocimetry of the umbilical arteries.

Once pre-eclampsia is diagnosed the woman should be offered hospital admission with an integrated package of care including investigations, assessment of fetal wellbeing and drug therapy, that will alter depending upon the severity of the pre-eclampsia as outlined in Table 13.1. Labetalol is the first-line treatment (unless the woman has asthma) and other antihypertensives such as methyldopa and nifedipine (see Box 13.4) might be offered after considering the side-effect profiles for woman and fetus (NICE 2010a). Popular theories about vitamins being *natural remedies* for pre-eclampsia have no sound research base (Talaulikar and Manyonda 2011) and a meta-analysis by

Basaran et al (2010) actually found vitamins C and E supplementation to be associated with an increased risk of gestational hypertension.

Whilst drugs will treat the hypertension, the solution for pre-eclampsia is to expedite the birth of the baby and placenta. Induction of labour will be determined by the obstetrician, and is likely to be at 37 weeks for mild pre-eclampsia 34–36 weeks for moderate pre-eclampsia and at 34 weeks for severe hypertension, following a course of corticosteroids to assist with fetal lung maturity (NICE 2010a; Vijgen et al 2010). Birth should be earlier in the event of uncontrolled blood pressure or fetal or antenatal complications, with caesarean section being undertaken for urgent clinical situations or if the fetus is very preterm (Webster et al 2013), ensuring close liaison with neonatal intensive care and anaesthetist teams (NICE 2010a).

Management in labour

Vigilant care by the midwife is paramount in labour, and whilst this is a high-risk labour the midwife may facilitate the birth of the baby in the absence of obstetric complications. Intrapartum care is similar to that provided to a woman with chronic hypertension and in particular there should be continuous fetal monitoring. An epidural anaesthetic is encouraged after review of the platelet count and continuation of antenatal antihypertensive drugs and blood tests according to previous results and the clinical picture are also warranted (Webster et al 2013). Oxytocin is used to control haemorrhage during the third stage of labour in preference to syntometrine or ergometrine. Blood pressure should be measured hourly, with the midwife being alert for signs of *fulminant eclampsia*.

Postnatal management

As with chronic hypertension, there should be regular measurement of blood pressure until hypertensive treatment has ceased. Blood pressure should be measured four times a day whilst in hospital, then recorded daily at home until the third day and once between days 3 to 5. On each occasion the midwife should ask the woman about severe headache and epigastric pain (NICE 2010a). Methyldopa is usually discontinued or replaced by another antihypertensive drug. If the BP is ≥150/100 mmHg the midwife should refer the woman for medical care, where the dosage of antihypertensives is likely to be increased.

The midwife should arrange for the woman to take drugs home before transfer from hospital as she is likely to continue with the antenatal drug regimen until her BP lowers to 130/80 mmHg when the dosage can be adjusted by the medical team. The woman should not be discharged from the midwife's care until the BP becomes stable and the maternal condition no longer gives any cause for concern. There should be a review of hypertensive treatment by the GP at 2 weeks and an obstetric with specialist review offered between 6 and 8 weeks to assess the hypertension (NICE 2010a).

Severe pre-eclampsia and eclampsia

Severe pre-eclampsia encompasses high blood pressure of systole ≥160 mmHg or diastole ≥110 mmHg on two occasions *and* significant proteinuria. Modern definitions also include women with moderate hypertension who have at least two of the features below:

- low blood platelet count <100 ×10⁶/l
- abnormal liver function
- liver tenderness
- Haemolysis Elevated Liver enzymes and Low Platelet count (HELLP) syndrome
- clonus (intermittent muscular contractions and relaxations)
- papilloedema
- epigastric pain
- vomiting
- severe headache
- visual disturbance (flashing light similar to migraine)

This condition, unless treated effectively, can lead to *eclampsia* with risk of mortality and morbidity. The woman **must** be admitted to a high-risk obstetric ward for medical treatment to bring her blood pressure under control, reduce the risk of fluid overload and prevent seizures. Oral labetalol or nifedipine may be used but if the BP is >170/110 mmHg, intravenous (IV) labetalol or hydrallazine are given in bolus doses to lower the BP and then as a continuous IV infusion (IVI). Intravenous magnesium sulphate may also be administered as this drug can reduce the chance of an eclamptic seizure by 50%. Fluid restriction and a low salt diet should be initiated and monitored with a fluid balance chart, including regular urinalysis to assess proteinuria. The midwife should also be aware that magnesium toxicity may present with a reduced urine output of <10 ml per hour. The effects on the fetus are as for pre-eclampsia, but there is an 80-fold increased risk of iatrogenic pre-term birth before 33 weeks, IUGR and consequent admission to neonatal intensive care (Hutcheon et al 2011).

Fulminant eclampsia

This is the acute worsening of symptoms, especially headache, epigastric pain and vomiting accompanied by high blood pressure, indicating that severe eclampsia is developing into eclampsia and that a **convulsion is imminent**. Consequently, emergency intervention is required.

Eclampsia

Eclampsia is a neurological condition associated with pre-eclampsia, manifesting with tonic-clonic convulsions in pregnancy that *cannot* be attributed to other conditions such as epilepsy (NICE 2010a; Hutcheon et al 2011). A national study undertaken throughout the UK through the United Kingdom (UK) Obstetric Surveillance System (UKOSS) between February 2005 and February 2006 identified 214 cases, indicating an estimated incidence of 27.5 cases per 100 000 births (Knight 2007) compared with a rate of 82 cases per 100 000 births in the United States of America (USA) (Hutcheon et al 2011). Rates of eclampsia have actually decreased in the developed world, due to improved antenatal care, timing of birth and use of magnesium sulphate (Knight 2007; Hutcheon et al 2011). However, as Neilson (2011) reports, when combining the UKOSS data and that of the latest CMACE triennial report into maternal deaths (CMACE 2011) the case fatality rate from eclampsia is estimated to be 3.1%.

Eclampsia can develop any time from 20 weeks' gestation up to 6 weeks postpartum and indeed 44% of cases occur postnatally (Shennan and Waugh 2003). The UKOSS data revealed that 63% of women in the UK who had eclampsia did *not* have established pre-eclampsia and over 20% of women had their first convulsion at home (Knight 2007) and were initially admitted to accident and emergency departments.

When a woman has an eclamptic seizure the midwife must summon medical aid immediately, initiate Airway, Breathing, Circulation (ABC) principles and then assist the doctor with treatment as outlined in Box 13.7.

The birth

If eclampsia arises during the antenatal or intrapartum period, the woman is likely to require an emergency caesarean section, so the midwife should prepare her for this type of birth and a potentially preterm baby. An epidural or spinal anaesthesia is preferred to reduce the consequences associated with general anaesthesia. If the woman gives birth vaginally, syntometrine and ergometrine should be avoided to manage the third stage of labour and oxytocin used instead.

Subsequent care

Once the woman's condition is stabilized she should have one-to-one care in either the Intensive Care Unit (ICU) or the High Dependency Care Unit (HDCU) attached to the labour ward. The aim of the care is to attain a BP of <150/80 mmHg. The woman will require an electrocardiogram (ECG) for one hour after the loading dose of magnesium sulphate, and this drug is continued by IVI for at least 24 hours. A blood sample to measure serum magnesium should be taken as this drug can reach a toxic level. If the urinary output reduces to <100 ml over 4 hours the magnesium sulphate may be reduced by 50% by the doctor, hence accurate fluid balance recording is essential.

Box 13.7 **Management of an eclamptic seizure**

- Do not leave the convulsing woman alone.
- Summon medical and senior midwifery aid to gather equipment to site an IVI, administer emergency drugs and set up bed rails.
- In the community, ambulance and paramedic team are required.
- Try to reassure the woman and her relatives.
- Prevent any subsequent injury to the mother with bed rails and by applying padding.

A: Airway. Protect from aspiration by placing woman in left lateral position, assisted by a wedge if still pregnant. Use suction for oral secretions.

B: Breathing. Anaesthetist should be called for possible intubation. Consider an oral airway. Administer supplementary oxygen by face mask.

C: Circulation. Observe the pulse, and if cardiac arrest occurs commence continuous chest compressions (cardiac massage).

- The doctor should site an IVI and take blood samples for: full blood count, group and save, clotting factors, uric acid, liver function tests, serum calcium, and urea and electrolytes.

- Accurate records of all fluid given should be maintained.
- A Foley's catheter should be inserted in the bladder to ensure accurate recording of the urinary output and regular urine testing for proteinuria.

D: Drugs. Administration of the anticonvulsant magnesium sulphate is given as 4 g by a slow IVI for 5 minutes. If recurrent seizures occur the IV rate is increased or a further bolus dose of 2–4 g is given. An electrocardiogram (ECG) should be conducted during the loading dose and for one hour afterwards. The maximum IV dose of magnesium sulphate is 9 g over the first hour. If the convulsions do not stop the medical team may consider administering 5 mg diazepam or 1 mg lorazepam.

D: Documents. All observations and treatment to be documented in the woman's case notes.

E: Environment. Ensure the woman keeps safe.

F: Fundus. If the woman is still pregnant, the uterus should be displaced by assisting her into the left lateral position, assisted by a wedge.

Source: Hull and Rucklidge 2009

Continuous monitoring of the woman's BP is warranted along with hourly monitoring of pulse, respiration, oxygen saturation, urine output and reflexes. Ongoing antihypertensive therapy should be continued and adjusted as determined by the woman's blood pressure readings (Hull and Rucklidge 2009). This monitoring usually continues for 24–48 hours, after which, providing the woman's condition improves, she can be transferred to the postnatal ward for a few more days until the medical team considers her condition is satisfactory for transfer home.

The baby is likely to be initially cared for on the neonatal unit and the woman should be taken to see her baby as soon as her condition permits. Breastfeeding is to be encouraged and psychological support given by the midwife and neonatal staff.

Haemolysis, Elevated Liver enzymes and Low Platelets (HELLP) syndrome

This is a multisystem disorder that can occur on its own or in association with pre-eclampsia. There is activation of the coagulation system causing increased deposits of protein fibrin throughout the body resulting in fragmentation of erythrocytes (Webster et al 2013). Fibrin deposits on blood vessel walls initiate clumping of platelets resulting in blood clots and lowering of the platelet count. These deposits decrease the diameter of the blood vessels, raising blood pressure and reducing the blood flow to organs (Webster et al 2013). The liver is especially affected, with destruction of liver cells leading to abnormal liver function and a distended liver with symptoms of epigastric discomfort.

HELLP syndrome presents antenatally in 70% of cases, most usually in the third trimester, and in the postnatal period it occurs in 30% of cases. If HELLP syndrome occurs before 26 weeks it is usually associated with antiphospholipid syndrome (APS) (Pawelec et al 2012). It also complicates 20% of severe pre-eclampsia cases resulting in high maternal and perinatal morbidity and mortality rates (Greer et al 2007). Of the 19 maternal deaths reported by Neilson (2011) in the latest CMACE triennial report, there was evidence of HELLP syndrome in eight of these women.

The woman will present with non-specific symptoms, often malaise, including nausea, vomiting and epigastric pain. In some cases there may be haematuria or jaundice. If there is pre-eclampsia there will be raised blood pressure and proteinuria. These symptoms are similar to acute fatty liver disease (AFLD) and the blood tests define the diagnosis. Complications can include:

- progressive disseminated intravascular coagulation (DIC)
- liver haematoma and rupture
- placental abruption
- pulmonary oedema and adult respiratory distress

- pleural effusions
- renal failure.

The main treatment is to expedite the birth of the baby with the management and midwifery care being similar to that for severe pre-eclampsia, with emphasis on the administration of magnesium sulphate to prevent convulsions. The condition usually resolves, however, 2 weeks after the baby's birth.

Acute fatty liver disease

Acute fatty liver disease of pregnancy is a rare and serious condition with uncertain aetiology, and current theory implies it is part of the pre-eclampsia spectrum (Doughty and Waugh 2013). Women with a raised body mass index (BMI), primigravidae and women with a multiple pregnancy appear to be at risk.

Five out of the following symptoms denote diagnosis, which usually present after 30 weeks of pregnancy: nausea, vomiting, polyuria, polydipsia, fever, headache, encephalopathy, pruritus, abdominal pain, tiredness, confusion, jaundice, anorexia, ascites, coagulopathy, hypertension, proteinuria, liver failure and hepatic encephalopathy (James et al 2011).

The condition of the woman can deteriorate rapidly, especially liver function, affecting both maternal and fetal morbidity and mortality. The woman must be referred to a specialist hepatologist for further investigation and to exclude alternative diagnoses such as HELLP. Management is to hasten the birth of the baby such that the midwife may need to prepare the woman for a preterm birth. Careful fluid balance is required in labour and vigilant observation, as DIC is a significant risk. Following the birth the woman is likely to be transferred to an ICU/HDCU where her condition should begin to improve after 48 hours (Doughty and Waugh 2013).

METABOLIC DISORDERS

Obesity

Obesity is considered to be one of the most significant health concerns affecting society, with significant impact on the maternity services (Modder and Fitzsimons 2010). Individual risk of serious morbidity or mortality is related to increasing weight through the development of disease pathways directly attributable to obesity, e.g. cardiovascular disease, certain cancers and type 2 diabetes mellitus. However, these pathways are unclear as individuals of normal body weight may also develop these conditions.

The increasing prevalence of obesity is commonly called an *epidemic* (World Health Organization [WHO] 2000), although obesity does not resemble an infectious disease; rather, it is used to describe a trend. Using BMI

Box 13.8 **WHO international body mass index (BMI) classifications (kg/m²)**

- Under-weight = <18.5
- Normal range = 18.5–24.9
- Pre-obese = 25.0–29.9
- Obese = ≥30.0
  - Obese Class I = 30.0–34.9
  - Obese Class II = 35.0–39.9
  - Obese Class III = ≥40.0

classification, statistics demonstrate 25% of adults over 16 years are obese (BMI ≥30 kg/m²) of which 18.5% are women of childbearing age (Modder and Fitzsimons 2010). These figures rise to almost 60% when those in the overweight category are included with a further 5% of the population having a BMI ≥40 kg/m² (Heslehurst et al 2010). In 2007, it was estimated that if this trend continues to rise, by 2050 more than 50% of women will be classed as obese (Foresight 2007). Currently only around 40% of women have a normal BMI.

Classifying size using body mass index (BMI)

Obesity is diagnosed using the BMI classification, implemented over 50 years ago as a *measure of fatness*, being considered a more robust way of assessing a person's level of body fat than measuring solely height and weight (Gard and Wright 2005). Obesity is defined as a BMI ≥30 kg/m² and can be subdivided into classes I, II and III (see Box 13.8). As a screening tool for fatness, the BMI is considered accurate in 75% of cases at best, failing to account for variations in body fat distributions, muscle and bone density, ethnic variations, gender specifics or age effect.

Distribution of body fat and disease

Distribution of body fat is considered a significant indicator of future ill-health, being suggestive of a disordered glucose tolerance (WHO 2000), which often contributes to medical complications such as type 2 diabetes mellitus. In such conditions, visceral fat (fat retained abdominally) is metabolically more active, contributing to *metabolic syndrome* which is directly associated with cardiovascular disease and type 2 diabetes (Gluckman and Hanson 2012).

Obesity as a concept

Being obese is not in itself a disease, although, as the level of obesity increases so does the individual risk of developing chronic disease (Gluckman and Hanson 2012). Social

scientists would agree that obesity is not a disease, but is a social construct defined as a disease, because it is considered abnormal in current Western culture (de Vries 2007). Obese individuals are consequently subject to significant stigma and discrimination directly attributed to their size and shape, even by healthcare professionals (Nyman et al 2010). This negative attitude probably reflects deeper cultural prejudices that exist towards obesity, reflected in the prevailing ideology of it being caused by the individual. However, the cause of obesity is multifactorial: it is considered a complex interplay of genetics, biology and behaviour on a background of cultural, environmental and social factors, where the individual plays a passive role within an *obesogenic* society (Foresight 2007).

Obesity demographics

A high incidence of obesity is associated with socioeconomic inequalities. Sellstrom et al (2009) identified increased rates of obesity in poorer societal groups, especially younger age groups. Children born into lower social class families are likely to become obese, although this trend is seen more in women than in men, probably because of the complexity of the role of women in society (Khlat et al 2009).

Pathophysiology of obesity

The main effect obesity has on an individual's health is increasing their risk of developing *metabolic syndrome*. Obesity, especially central obesity, causes metabolic dysfunction involving primarily lipids and glucose, which eventually results in organ dysfunction within many of the body systems, especially the cardiovascular system. Other risk factors for metabolic syndrome include family history, poor diet and a sedentary lifestyle.

Metabolic syndrome is thought to be caused by visceral adipose tissue causing the release of pro-inflammatory cytokines, known as *adipokines*, which promote insulin resistance. This causes a systemic inflammatory response, which over time results in microvascular and endothelial dysfunction in all of the body systems. The individual will have *atherogenic dyslipidaemia*, identified by low high density lipoprotein (HDL), raised triglycerides, hypertension and raised fasting blood glucose levels. As well as insulin resistance, such individuals develop a *prothrombotic state* with raised fibrinogen and plasminogen-activator-inhibitor levels (Miller and Mitchell 2006).

Nutritional needs in pregnancy

Weight gain is usual at certain times in a female's life, e.g. during infancy, between the ages of 5 and 7 years, adolescence, pregnancy and the menopause (Webb 2008). Maternal overnutrition has permanent effects on a fetus, that is, a higher birth weight tends to result in a higher BMI as an adult (Smith et al 2008). Physiological changes in pregnancy predispose to weight gain, essentially to provide energy for labour and lactation, and this storage is facilitated by the effect that increases in oestrogen, progesterone and human placental lactogen (HPL) have on glucose metabolism (Webb 2008). Women with a raised BMI should be advised and encouraged to lose weight pre-conceptually to optimize pregnancy outcomes (Modder and Fitzsimons 2010).

A woman's basal metabolic rate (BMR) increases during pregnancy due to the increased metabolic activity of the maternal and fetal tissues. The increased body weight and the increased maternal cardiovascular, renal and respiratory load also influence a rise in the basal metabolic rate (BMR), but in part this is counterbalanced by a general decrease in activity. The resulting increase in required calorie intake is therefore relatively small; an extra 200 kcal per day are required during the third trimester for most women (NICE 2010b). Weight gain in pregnancy is dependent on factors such as diet, activity and maternal wellbeing (Gardner et al 2011).

Antenatal care

The BMI is routinely calculated at the initial visit with the midwife (booking) and a discussion about the implications of a raised BMI should consequently take place between the midwife and the woman. Depending on local guidelines, women with a raised BMI are often referred to a multiprofessional antenatal clinic, which involves specialist midwives, obstetricians and dieticians (Modder and Fitzsimons 2010). Oteng-Ntim et al (2011) undertook a systematic review, consisting of 1228 women, and found that where lifestyle interventions were introduced for obese and overweight women during pregnancy, the gestational weight gain was reduced, along with a reduction in the prevalence of gestational diabetes. However, the quality of the published studies was mainly poor, so these results must be taken with caution.

Obesity is a significant risk factor for maternal mortality (CMACE 2011), with 16 of the women who died in the triennium 2006–2008 having a BMI ranging from $\geq$25 kg/m^2 to >40 kg/m^2. The subsequent risk of morbidity associated with childbearing of women who have a raised BMI is outlined in Box 13.9 (Smith et al 2008; Modder and Fitzsimons 2010). However, it is important to note that obesity alone is not associated with poor perinatal outcomes, but that it does increase the risk, which subsequently increases as the BMI increases (Scott-Pillai et al 2013). Women with obesity might find some *minor disorders of pregnancy*, such as back pain and fatigue, are exacerbated (see Chapter 9).

During pregnancy, women who are obese may report a range of psycho-social issues related to their increased BMI. For instance, they may feel disappointed at not being

---

Box 13.9 **Risks associated with obesity in pregnancy**

Maternal

- Miscarriage and stillbirth
- Gestational diabetes: offered a glucose tolerance test (GTT) at 24–28 weeks if BMI $\geq$30
- Hypertension: ensure correct size cuff and increase surveillance if BMI $\geq$35; increase antenatal appointments to screen for PET to every 3 weeks between 24 and 32 weeks and refer to specialist care if one or more additional risk factors are present, e.g. first baby, raised BP at booking
- Venous thromboembolism: assess risk at every visit; prophylaxis is recommended if two or more risk factors are present
- Prolonged pregnancy: risks associated with induction of labour
- Presence of pre-existing medical conditions, e.g. ischaemic heart disease
- Poorer mental health, e.g. depression

Fetal

- Neural tube defects (NTDs): all women should take 5 mg folic acid daily
- Macrosomia
- Preterm labour
- Lower Apgar scores
- Late stillbirth
- Neonatal mortality

Maternity services

- Increased hospital admissions
- Increased costs associated with managing complications
- Increased length of hospital stay
- Increased neonatal care requirements

Source: Smith et al 2008; Modder and Fitzsimons 2010

---

recognized as pregnant until later in pregnancy (Nash 2012a) and worry about their weight gain in pregnancy (Nash 2012b). They may also experience a variety of feelings towards their body image, but generally feel less stigma and discrimination, as weight gain is more socially acceptable while pregnant (Johnson et al 2004).

The maternity services need to ensure suitable equipment and staffing levels are available, e.g. suitable beds and chairs, large BP cuffs, sufficient operating department staff in respect of caring for women with obesity (Modder and Fitzsimons 2010). Risk assessments for labour should be undertaken antenatally for each woman, considering moving and handling issues in order to ensure suitable

Box 13.10 **Intrapartum risks associated with obesity**

- Prolonged pregnancy and induction of labour
- Prolonged labour: labour is slower and there is often a delay between 4–7 cm with syntocinon use being higher. There should be close observation of progress in labour with one-to-one care for women with a BMI ≥40
- Complications, e.g. shoulder dystocia
- Emergency caesarean birth: if a woman has a BMI >40 the incidence is almost 50%. There is an increased risk of malpresentation, e.g. occipito-posterior (OP) position and vaginal birth after caesarean (VBAC) is less successful
- Primary postpartum haemorrhage (PPH): venous access and active management of the third stage of labour is recommended for women with a BMI ≥40

Source: Kerrigan and Kingdon 2010; Modder and Fitzsimons 2010

Box 13.11 **Risks associated with obesity in the postnatal period**

Maternal
- Venous thromboembolism: early mobilization following birth encouraged. Prophylaxis considered even following vaginal birth
- Longer postoperative recovery
- Increased postoperative complications, e.g. wound dehiscence and infection
- Tendency to retain pregnancy weight gain
- Lowered rates of breastfeeding duration
- Reduced contraception choices: depending on presence of co-morbidities

Neonatal
- Increased risk of congenital abnormality, e.g. heart defects
- Macrosomia: increased risk of trauma from birth; practical difficulties associated with undertaking the neonatal examination
- Low birth weight: associated with the presence of antenatal maternal co-morbidity, with increased risk of possible long-term effects on health, e.g. increased rates of cardiovascular disease and diabetes mellitus in middle age

Source: Smith et al 2008; Modder and Fitzsimons 2010

aids are available to assist with movement (Modder and Fitzsimons 2010; Marshall and Brydon 2012). Furthermore, CMACE/Royal College of Obstetricians and Gynaecologists (Modder and Fitzsimons 2010) endorse that all maternity units should have documented environmental risk assessments regarding the availability of facilities for pregnant women presenting with a BMI of ≥30 kg/m² at the initial visit.

Intrapartum care

Obesity is a significant risk factor during labour, as detailed in Box 13.10. For women who have a BMI ≥35 kg/m² it is recommended that the birth should occur in a consultant-led environment (Kerrigan and Kingdon 2010). However, these women will benefit from good-quality midwifery-led care to promote optimal outcomes, e.g. encouraging mobility and an upright position. It could also be argued that these women might benefit from birthing in a midwife-led unit/birth centre alongside an obstetric unit. It is recommended by NICE (2007) that individual discussions with women whose BMI is between 30 and 34 kg/m² should take place regarding the local birth place options available.

It is worth noting that there may be difficulties in assessing maternal and fetal wellbeing during labour, e.g. ensuring a good quality cardiotocograph (CTG) recording, undertaking vaginal examinations and performing manoeuvres in an emergency such as shoulder dystocia (Doughty and Waugh 2013). In addition, there may be difficulties in managing intraoperative complications such as controlling haemorrhage.

Postnatal care

Obesity has a direct influence on short- and long-term health and wellbeing for the mother and the baby following birth, as indicated in Box 13.11.

Breastfeeding has been shown to reduce the weight a woman has gained in pregnancy more effectively than in those women who choose to artificially feed their babies (Baker et al 2008). Obese women are as likely to initiate breastfeeding as women of a normal weight, but tend to breastfeed for a shorter time (Amir and Donath 2007). It is known that obese women have delayed lactogenesis and a lowered response of prolactin to suckling, leading to reduced milk production and premature cessation of breastfeeding. However, the response to prolactin is reduced over time so extended support from midwives skilled at supporting the continuance of breastfeeding is especially important in this group of women (Jevitt et al 2007).

Weight gained in pregnancy is difficult to lose postnatally due to a number of factors such as the demands of caring for a new baby, eating irregular meals and an inability to exercise as frequently. This may result in higher rates of obesity in later life (Gardner et al 2011). Women who were obese during pregnancy also exhibit a tendency to retain fat centrally following the baby's birth, which may result in increased morbidity and mortality later in life (Villamor and Cnattingius 2006). However, interpregnancy weight reduction has been shown to improve outcomes in any subsequent pregnancy (Modder and Fitzsimons 2010). Discussions around weight, activity and healthy lifestyle modification behaviours by healthcare professionals during the 6–8 weeks postnatal examination are recommended by NICE (2010b) and the RCOG (2006). If co-morbidities such as gestational diabetes have been diagnosed during pregnancy a glucose tolerance test (GTT) should be undertaken at the postnatal examination and the woman should continue to have annual cardiometabolic screening (Modder and Fitzsimons 2010). The Royal College of Midwives (RCM) has collaborated with Slimming World® to develop strategies to positively influence and improve the health of childbearing women (Avery et al 2010; Pallister et al 2010).

Obstetric cholestasis

Obstetric cholestasis (OC) is also known as *intrahepatic cholestasis of pregnancy* and is a condition specific to pregnancy that denotes a disruption and reduction of bile products by the liver. It is diagnosed by the presence of raised serum bile acids and usually appears after the 28th week gestation, resolving a couple of weeks following the birth of the baby. Obstetric cholestasis manifests as intense itching (*pruritus*) that mainly affects the soles of the feet, hands and body, becoming worse at night, albeit there is no visible rash. The woman often complains of loss of sleep. Urinary tract infections (UTI) are common and jaundice may occur, with the woman stating that her faecal stools are pale.

Treatment is based on the use of topical creams, but medications such as ursodeoxycholic acid and chlorampheniramine may be prescribed. Obstetric cholestasis causes severe liver impairment and increases perinatal morbidity and mortality (Saleh and Abdo 2007). Timing of the birth depends on gestational age and fetal wellbeing, which is monitored through fetal growth and biophysical profiles, fetal movements and CTG. Birth before 38 weeks is usually advocated (RCOG 2011a). There is also an increased risk of postpartum haemorrhage (PPH) due to coagulation disruption. Oral vitamin K 10 mg is often prescribed to lessen the risk and active management of the third stage of labour is advised. Postnatal care is based on ensuring liver function tests (LFTs) return to normal. Recurrence in a subsequent pregnancy is high, at around 90%.

ENDOCRINE DISORDERS

Insulin is a polypeptide hormone produced in the pancreas by the beta cells of the islets of Langerhans. It has a pivotal role in the metabolism of carbohydrate, fat and protein and *lowers* the level of blood glucose. Conversely, the alpha cells produce the hormone *glucagon* which *increases* the blood glucose. In healthy individuals, the blood glucose level regulates the secretion of insulin and glucagon on a negative-feedback principal. Hence if the blood glucose level is high (*hyperglycaemia*) more insulin is released, whereas if the blood glucose level is low (*hypoglycaemia*) insulin is inhibited and glucagon is released (Tortora and Derrickson 2010). Excess glucose is stored in the liver where it can be released depending upon metabolic demands. In the longer term, excess glucose is stored as body fat and this is an important issue when considering obesity and also macrosomic babies of mothers with diabetes.

Diabetes mellitus

Diabetes mellitus is a metabolic disorder due to deficiency or diminished effectiveness of endogenous insulin affecting 5.5% of the adult population in the UK and is the most common pre-existing medical disorder complicating pregnancy in the UK (NICE 2008; James et al 2011). It is characterized by hyperglycaemia, deranged metabolism and complications mainly affecting blood vessels.

The classic presentation, especially in type 1 diabetes, is of weight loss and the occurrence of the three *polys: polydipsia* (excess thirst), *polyuria* (excessive, dilute urine production) and *polyphagia* (excessive hunger) (Tortora and Derrickson 2010). There may also be lethargy, prolonged infection, boils and pruritis vulvae. Conversely, with type 2 diabetes, individuals are often obese with few or no presenting symptoms.

A random blood glucose result ≥11.1 mmol/l is highly suggestive of diabetes and the diagnosis is confirmed by a fasting blood glucose test. A GTT entails taking a fasting blood sample, giving a 75 g glucose drink and a taking a further blood test 2 hours later to determine the plasma glucose levels. If the plasma level is ≥7.0 mmol/l following the fasting test, or ≥7.8 mmol/l following the 2-hour test, a diagnoses of diabetes is made by the physician.

There are several types of diabetes mellitus, as follows.

Type 1 diabetes (formally insulin-dependent or juvenile onset diabetes)

Type 1 diabetes develops as a result of progressive autoimmune destruction of the pancreatic beta cells, most probably initiated by infection, with the result that no, or an inadequate amount of, insulin is produced. Hyperglycaemia occurs leading to glycosuria, dehydration, lipolysis and proteolysis with the classic symptoms listed above. Metabolism of type 1 diabetes mimics starvation. In the absence of insulin the body cells use fatty acids to produce adenosine triphosphate (ATP). By-products of this process produce organic acids called *ketones*. As ketones accumulate they lower the pH of the blood making it acidic, known as *ketoacidosis* (Tortora and Derrickson 2010). This can be detected by the presence of ketones in the urine and the breath smelling of *pear drop* sweets. If untreated, the ketoacidosis will lead to coma and death.

In 85% of cases there is no first-degree family history of the condition; however, if one parent has type 1 diabetes, there is a 2–9% chance of an individual developing it, and if both parents have the condition the risk rises to 30%. Diagnosis is confirmed by raised blood glucose results. Complications include nephropathy, neuropathy, retinopathy and cataract formation. Microvascular complications arise if there is chronic hyperglycaemia, leading to secondary complications such as atherosclerosis and gangrene of the feet due to sensory neuropathy and ischaemia. For this reason individuals with diabetes are discouraged from walking barefooted and may need referral to a diabetic foot clinic.

Treatment is the lifelong administration of insulin, which has to be given by subcutaneous injections two to five times a day. This is usually self-administered. Traditionally animal-derived insulins from beef and pork were used, and from the 1980s *human* insulin was introduced prior to a genetically modified form known as *human analogue*. All of these can be short- and long-lasting, as shown in Table 13.2.

Treatment is based upon best practice guidelines and is determined for each individual person with diabetes and the specialist diabetes team (NICE 2008; Scottish Intercollegiate Guidelines Network [SIGN] 2010). The blood glucose levels aimed for are in the range of a person without diabetes, which are: *preprandial* (fasting/before a meal) between 3.5 and 5.9 mmol/l, and one hour *postprandial* <7.8.00 mmol/l. Insulin dosage is adjusted according to blood glucose levels and the individual needs to test their blood sugar at least twice a day using *finger*

prick tests and reagent strips read against a colour chart, or with a glucose meter (*glucometer*). In the home setting, urine is also tested for ketones using dipsticks.

Hypoglycaemia is a potential problem when insulin therapy is used, as insulin will decrease blood glucose levels. When the level is low, adrenergic symptoms of palpitations, perspiration, tremor and hunger alert the individual to take action and resolve this by eating a meal or taking glycogen sweets or gel (de Valk and Visser 2011). If the blood glucose decreases further the individual is likely to experience neuroglycogenic symptoms of altered behaviour and mood swings (de Valk and Visser 2011). If left untreated, convulsions and loss of consciousness can result, leading to coma and death.

Severe hypoglycaemia is associated with loss of consciousness and requires the assistance of another person to administer glucagon intramuscularly as there is a risk of asphyxiation with oral administration. Individuals who have diabetes should always carry glucagon *ready-to-use* devices with them for this purpose.

Where diabetes control cannot be achieved by a traditional basal/bolus regime, individuals with diabetes are increasingly being offered the choice of insulin pump therapy. Continuous subcutaneous insulin infusion pumps (CSII) are in common use in the USA and the midwife is increasingly likely to encounter them in the UK. The pump controls the constant administration of insulin as a basal dose, in *bursts* at 3-minute intervals with the individual self-administering a bolus dose via the pump when they consume carbohydrate, or if they need to reduce severely high blood glucose levels. This is not currently a *closed loop system*, as each individual has to have a good understanding of their own personal carbohydrate to insulin ratios in order to regulate the pump to administer an appropriate bolus dose whenever carbohydrate is consumed and set the pump up to follow their required

Table 13.2 Types of insulin according to origin and length of action

Insulin type	Rapid action	Short action	Intermediate action	Long action
Analogue	Apidra® Humalog® NovoRapid®			Lantus® Levemir®
Human		Actrapid® Humulin S® Insuman Rapid®	Humulin I® Insuman Basal Insulatard®	
Animal		Hypurin Bovine Neutral® Hypurin Porcine Neutral®	Hypurin Bovine Isophane® Hypurin Porcine Isophane®	Hypurin Bovine Lente® Hypurin Bovine Protamine Zinc®

NB: Pre-mixed insulin can be prescribed, but only when two injections a day are required.

basal dose profile. There are also some pumps that work in conjunction with a continuous glucose monitoring sensor which is injected into the skin, with a transmitter clipped to the surface. The transmitter sends readings to the pump once every 5 minutes. The pump can be set up to sound an alarm if the readings are outside limits defined by the individual and is particularly useful for diabetics who are susceptible to serious hypoglycaemic episodes while asleep. However, as the individual remains responsible for defining appropriate insulin doses based on the information provided by the sensor, they are still required to perform daily blood glucose and urinary ketones tests which necessitates the mental capacity to cope with the system and calculations.

A fully *closed loop system*, also known as the *artificial pancreas* which mimics normal pancreatic administration of insulin, has also been developed. As with the CSII there is a pump and a sensor, but there is an additional hand-held control device that contains an algorithm to calculate the insulin dose required. This information is transmitted to the pump and the insulin is administered automatically without any intervention from the individual. There is also a *suspend insulin* command to prevent hypoglycaemic episodes. Results from clinical trials are promising and this treatment may become mainstream in just a few years, with midwives encountering it soon in a research context with childbearing women. *Islet cell transplants* are now available in the UK for individuals who meet strict criteria, being intended for those unable to recognize severe hypoglycaemia or those who are otherwise healthy renal transplant recipients.

Regular attendance at outpatient clinics is necessary to monitor diabetic control. The glycated or glycosylated haemoglobin (HbA1c) test is performed every 2–6 months. This measures the average blood glucose level by analysing the molecule in the haemoglobin in the red blood cell where glucose binds. The higher the HbA1c the poorer is the diabetic control. Treatment aims to keep the HbA1c at <48 mmol/mol (6.5%). However, since 2011, HbA1c has been expressed in mmol/mol to comply with the International Federation of Clinical Chemistry (IFCC) Units.

Type 2 diabetes (formally non-insulin-dependent or maturity onset diabetes)

In type 2 diabetes there is a gradual resistance to the action of insulin in the liver and muscle. This can also be combined with impaired pancreatic beta cell function leading to a relative insulin deficiency. Type 2 diabetes accounts for 85% of cases of diabetes and tends to cluster in families. All racial groups are affected but it is six times more common in people of South Asian descent and three times more common among people of African and African-Caribbean origin. Traditionally it was associated with older people but it is increasingly diagnosed in children,

young adults and among those with a raised BMI and sedentary lifestyle (Gregory and Todd 2013).

The initial treatment is by strict diet to reduce weight and increased physical activity to improve glucose tolerance and control the diabetes. As the condition progresses oral diabetic agents such as *metformin* become necessary, and eventually insulin treatment might be required. Furthermore, ancillary medication such as ACE inhibitors and statins may be prescribed to prevent cardiovascular complications. Diabetic monitoring is the same as for type I diabetes.

Secondary diabetes

This is a type of diabetes that presents secondary to another medical condition such as pancreatic disease or cystic fibrosis (Dornhorst and Williamson 2012).

Maturity onset diabetes of the young (MODY)

In this type of diabetes, there is a genetic defect affecting pancreatic beta cell insulin secretion. Out of all cases presenting, 95% have a first-degree relative affected. However, maturity onset diabetes of the young (MODY) is not associated with obesity and it tends to be diagnosed in the second or third decade of life (Dornhorst and Williamson 2012).

Gestational diabetes mellitus (GDM)

This is a form of diabetes that arises in the second or third trimester of pregnancy, affecting up to 5% of all pregnancies, and resolves after the birth of the baby. There is intolerance to glucose which is attributed to increasing levels of placental hormones, in particular HPL and increasing maternal insulin resistance, especially after 20 weeks of gestation (Gregory and Todd 2013). Gestational diabetes is usually asymptomatic and according to Reece et al (2009) it is associated with:

- increasing maternal age
- family history of type 2 diabetes or GDM
- certain ethnic groups (Asian, African-Caribbean, Latin American, Middle Eastern)
- previous unexplained stillbirth
- previous macrosomia
- obesity (three-fold risk of GDM)
- smoking (two-fold risk of GDM: England et al 2004)
- change in weight between pregnancies: an inter-pregnancy gain of more than three BMI points doubles the risk of GDM (Villamor and Cnattingius 2006)

Gestational diabetes should resolve shortly after the birth of the baby. The finite diagnosis is therefore made in retrospect as it is not possible during pregnancy to differentiate between GDM and types 1 and 2 diabetes that present for the first time in pregnancy (the latter two of which do not resolve following the baby's birth). It is therefore important that observations and outpatient follow-up appointments are undertaken in the postnatal period. The lifetime risk of developing type 2 diabetes after gestational diabetes is seven-fold (Bellamy et al 2009). The treatment is referral to a dietician with adherence to a diet restricting sugar and fat, encouragement of 30 minutes exercise a day, self-monitoring of blood glucose and insulin therapy if necessary.

Pre-conception care

Pre-conception care is essential for any women with diabetes because of the potential pregnancy complications and four-fold increased risk overall of congenital malformations which are associated with hyperglycaemia. If the HbA1c is >58 mmol/mol (7.5%) at the initial visit to the midwife, this risk increases to nine-fold with a four-fold increase in spontaneous miscarriage (Temple 2011). Hughes et al (2010) therefore argue there is a requirement for formalized pre-conception clinics and midwifery involvement for women who have diabetes as approximately only a third of these women receive any such care from their GP or from a hospital clinic (Temple 2011). This should involve each woman taking a daily dose of 5 mg of folic acid prior to conception (NICE 2008) and having a thorough medical assessment, as existing complications such as retinopathy and nephropathy can deteriorate during pregnancy (Scanlon and Harcombe 2011; Gregory and Todd 2013). Any medication should be reviewed and ACE inhibitors discontinued.

Type 1 diabetes

Insulin might need to be changed and the regimen intensified to obtain optimal control. *NovoRapid®* is the only insulin licensed for use in pregnancy.

Type 2 diabetes

Pre-conception care is important as some anti-diabetic drugs may be teratogenic to early fetal development. Women with type 2 diabetes may also be on statins and ACE inhibitors, which should be discontinued. Consequently, insulin by subcutaneous injection should be commenced and contraception continued until the woman achieves optimal diabetic control. The BMI should be calculated and, if indicated, weight reduction should be encouraged prior to conception.

Pre-conception management

NICE (2008) advocates the following:

- Aim to maintain HbA1c <43 mmol/l (6.1%) to reduce the risk of congenital malformations.

- Strongly advise women with HbA1c >86 mmol/l (10%) to avoid pregnancy.
- Reinforce self-monitoring of blood glucose.
- Offer HbA1c testing monthly.
- Offer retinal assessment at the first pre-conception appointment and then annually if no retinopathy is found.
- Assess nephropathy risk including microalbuminuria estimation and serum creatinine/epidermal growth factor receptor (eGFR). If serum creatinine is ≥120 µmol/l, or the eGFR is <45 ml/min/1.73 m, a referral should be made to a nephrologist before contraception is discontinued.
- Discontinue statins before pregnancy or as soon as pregnancy is confirmed.

Antenatal management

The midwife will increasingly encounter women with pre-existing diabetes because of the increased prevalence of diabetes in young people. Furthermore, some multigravidae might silently develop type 2 diabetes, conceive their fourth or fifth child and present late for the initial appointment with the midwife due to being familiar with pregnancy, however they are at risk of developing complications associated with hyperglycaemia.

Existing medical complications can worsen during pregnancy, or be recognized for the first time. Furthermore, the midwife will care for women when diabetes presents during pregnancy: indeed the midwife is likely to be the first health professional to recognize the altered state of health. If diabetes is identified in the first trimester, then this is likely to be pre-existing diabetes diagnosed for the first time in pregnancy rather than GDM. Complications for the pregnancy encompass:

- pre-eclampsia
- macrosomic baby, due to hyperglycaemia, with risk of shoulder dystocia
- IUGR
- polyhydramnios
- exacerbation of diabetic complications in the woman, in particular retinopathy and nephropathy
- risk of iatrogenic preterm birth leading to the baby being admitted to the neonatal unit.

In addition, the risks to the fetus/baby born to a woman with diabetes are that they are:

- five times more likely to be stillborn
- three times more likely to die in the first few months of life
- four times more likely to have a major congenital malformation.

These risks, however, are substantially reduced if there is good blood glucose control before and after pregnancy. The initial visit to the midwife where a detailed medical history is taken should identify those women with pre-existing diabetes in order for a referral to be made to a specialist endocrine/obstetric clinic. Regular appointments at this clinic are usually at fortnightly intervals, where a multidisciplinary team of obstetrician, physician, dietician and specialist nurse/midwife will provide care. As this will be considered to be a high-risk pregnancy, the woman should *not* be assigned to low-risk schemes of care. Guidelines from NICE (2008) also recommend diabetes screening should be undertaken with women who present at the first appointment with the following risk factors for developing GDM:

- BMI >30 kg/m^2
- previous macrosomic baby ≥4.5 kg or above
- previous GDM
- first-degree relative with diabetes
- family origin with a high prevalence of diabetes, e.g. South Asian, African-Caribbean and Middle Eastern origin.

Newly diagnosed women will require education in monitoring their blood sugar glucose levels using the necessary equipment and reagent strips, which need prescribing. They will require education in self-administration of insulin and in balancing insulin requirements based on their blood glucose readings. Dietary assessment and advice is essential so that the insulin dose can be adjusted according to a woman's normal eating habits.

Medical management should achieve a delicate balance between preventing both hyperglycaemia and hypoglycaemia (de Valk and Visser 2011). Blood glucose target levels in pregnancy are likely to be a fasting blood glucose of between 3.5 and 5.9 mmol/l and one-hour postprandial blood glucose below 7.8 mmol/l (NICE 2008), which may be lower than the woman is used to. Qualitative research has shown that pregnant women are happier if their pre- and postprandial blood glucose levels are between 7 and 10 mmol/l with no hypoglycaemia (Richmond 2009), hence the midwife should stress to the woman the importance of complying with the prescribed levels and give advice to her and her family about recognizing the signs and symptoms of hypoglycaemia. However, the woman should be informed that her blood glucose levels will change throughout pregnancy due to altered hormone levels and the developing fetus having its own metabolic demands. Consequently, it is important that the woman carries glucose tablets/gel and a ready-to-use intramuscular device at all times in case of hypoglycaemic episodes. In addition, women should be advised that as most hypoglycaemia occurring during weeks 8–16 is attributed to nausea and vomiting of pregnancy, it is important they seek advice if this becomes a significant problem in maintaining diabetic control.

Key points to consider relating to the antenatal care of women presenting with/developing diabetes are detailed below:

- A supplement of 5 mg folic acid should be taken daily for the first 12 weeks of pregnancy to reduce the risk of congenital malformations in the fetus.
- Urinalysis should be undertaken at each visit to test for glucose, ketones as well as the protein.
- Women with type 1 diabetes should be offered ketone testing strips and be advised to test for ketonuria if they have symptoms of hyperglycaemia or become unwell.
- Blood pressure should be recorded at each visit with the midwife being alert for signs of pre-eclampsia, especially with GDM.
- Women should be discouraged from fasting, especially for long periods (e.g. as with religious observances).
- Women should test their blood glucose levels on waking and one hour postprandial after every meal during pregnancy.
- If taking insulin, women should also test their blood glucose level before going to bed.
- Women with type 2 diabetes are likely to be commenced on insulin: if taking metformin pre-pregnancy, some centres may decide to continue its use until 32 weeks due to emerging evidence of its safety (Gregory and Todd 2013).
- An ultrasonic scan is undertaken at 7–9 weeks' gestation to confirm viability and gestational age, followed by a further scan at 18–20 weeks to assess the four chambers of the fetal heart for any anomalies, estimate liquor volume and to ascertain fetal growth.
- Monthly scans are undertaken to assess fetal growth and their results recorded, observing for signs of macrosomia (dimensions above the 95th centile for the period of gestation).
- Weekly tests of fetal wellbeing, including CTG or biophysical profiles, should continue until labour commences or there is an indication to intervene earlier: e.g. induction at 38 weeks or caesarean section.

Intrapartum management

- If the labour is preterm, steroids are given to the woman to improve fetal lung maturation and additional insulin may be required.
- If the fetus is macrosomic, the woman should be informed of the risks and benefits of vaginal birth, induction of labour and caesarean section.
- Blood glucose levels should be monitored hourly through labour and birth, aiming to maintain them between 4 and 7 mmol/l.
- For women with type I diabetes an IVI of insulin and dextrose should be commenced from the onset of established labour.

- For women with type 2 and GDM an IVI of insulin and dextrose should be commenced if blood glucose levels cannot be maintained between 4 and 7 mmol/l.
- The neonatal team should be alerted that the woman is in labour, should their assistance be required when the baby is born.

Care of the baby at birth

- A paediatrician should be present at the birth if the woman is receiving insulin.
- The midwife should be alert for signs of respiratory distress, hypoglycaemia, hypothermia, cardiac decompensation and neonatal encephalopathy.
- A baby should be admitted to a neonatal intensive care unit (NICU) only if a significant complication is apparent.
- The woman should hold her baby as soon as is practical after the birth and prior to any transfer to the NICU.
- Blood glucose testing of the baby should be carried out after birth and at intervals according to local protocols.
- The baby should feed within 30 minutes of birth and then every 2–3 hours until pre-feed blood glucose levels are *at least* 2 mmol/l. If the blood glucose falls <1.5 mmol/l the paediatrician must be called and admission to the NICU is a possibility. (*NB: NICUs tend to set a higher baseline for neonatal hypoglycaemia, so local protocols should be consulted.*)
- Blood glucose levels should be assessed in babies who show signs of hypoglycaemia (abnormal muscle tone, level of consciousness, apnoea or seizures) with referral to the paediatrician, who is likely to treat with IV dextrose.
- The baby should not be transferred home until at least 24 hours old, is maintaining blood glucose levels and is feeding well.

Postnatal care of the woman with diabetes

- *Type 1 diabetes*: insulin should be reduced immediately after birth and blood glucose levels monitored with insulin adjusted until the appropriate dose is obtained.
- The woman should be observed for signs of hypoglycaemia.
- As placental hormone levels fall, the insulin sensitivity improves, such that the insulin infusion rate is likely to need reducing in the early postnatal period.
- The woman will usually return to her pre-pregnancy insulin levels, unless she is breastfeeding, when the insulin requirements are reduced by 30% (Gregory and Todd 2013).

- The woman should be advised that breastfeeding affects glycaemic control and there is the need for continued blood glucose monitoring and insulin adjustment.
- *For Type 2 diabetes:* insulin should cease immediately and the doctor should confer with the pharmacist as to which oral diabetic agents the woman may safely take if breastfeeding (otherwise she returns to her pre-pregnancy drug therapy).
- *For GDM*: insulin ceases immediately and blood glucose monitoring can stop.
- A fasting blood glucose test should be undertaken at 6 weeks and if there is a possibility that would indicate another form of diabetes, a GTT should be performed immediately.
- The woman should be advised of the risk of developing diabetes in future pregnancies and the need for pre-pregnancy screening.
- The woman should be informed of the importance of using contraception to prevent pregnancies in rapid succession and to seek pre-conception care prior to future pregnancies.
- A healthy lifestyle with regular exercise, smoking cessation and maintaining a BMI within normal limits should also be emphasized to the woman.
- A follow-up appointment at 6 weeks with the diabetes team or the local GP is also essential (Gregory and Todd 2013).

Thyroid disease

The thyroid gland is a highly vascular organ that is shaped like a butterfly and is situated at the front of the neck. Its main function is to produce the iodine-rich hormones tri-iodothyronine (T3) and thyroxine (T4). These hormones are secreted directly into the blood circulation in response to a negative feedback to the hypothalamus which secretes thyrotropin releasing hormone (TRH) that stimulate the anterior pituitary gland to secrete thyroid stimulating hormone (TSH) (Tortora and Derrickson 2010). TSH also initiates the uptake of iodine, which combines with an amino acid called tyrosine which enables synthesis of the thyroid hormones within the thyroid follicles (Dornhorst and Williamson 2012). Once in the blood circulation, 99% of T3 and T4 are bound to thyroxine-binding globulin (TBG) with the remaining 1% *unbound* or free: e.g. fT3 and fT4 (James et al 2011). It is fT3, fT4 and TSH that are measured in thyroid function tests.

Excess T4 is converted to the more potent T3 by deionization in the peripheral tissue (Dornhorst and Williamson 2012). Most body tissue has receptors for fT3, and once bound to the tissue, metabolic activities result. The thyroid hormones regulate the metabolic rate throughout all body tissue and influence growth and maturity.

In pregnancy, the circulating level of TBG enables increased levels of T3 and T4, so only fT3 and fT4 should be measured by laboratory testing (Dornhorst and Williamson 2012). The fetus cannot synthesize T3 and T4 until the 10th week of pregnancy and is dependent upon maternal thyroid hormones from placental transfer (Dornhorst and Williamson 2012). Normal development of the fetal brain is dependent upon maternally derived T4 which is converted intracellularly to T3 (Girling 2006).

Thyroid disease is the second most common cause of endocrine dysfunction in pregnancy and is difficult to recognize as the symptoms mimic pregnancy (Girling 2006; James et al 2011) indicated by Table 13.3. The most common thyroid disorders in pregnancy are *hypothyroidism* and *hyperthyroidism* (thyrotoxocosis), being of considerable significance due to their effect on both the woman and fetus.

Table 13.3 Similarities between clinical symptoms of thyroid disease and pregnancy

Pregnancy	Hyperthyroidism	Hypothyroidism
Heat intolerance	Yes	
Increased appetite	Yes	
Nausea	Yes	
Palpitations	Yes	
Tachycardia	Yes	
Tremor	Yes	
Sweating	Yes	
Warm palms	Yes	
Goitre	Yes	Yes
Amenorrhea	Yes	
Weight gain		Yes
Carpal tunnel syndrome		Yes
Fluid retention		Yes
Constipation		Yes
Loss of concentration	Yes	Yes
Tiredness	Yes	Yes

Reproduced from Girling J C 2006 Thyroid disorders in pregnancy, Current Obstetrics and Gynaecology 16: 47–53, with permission from Elsevier

Hypothyroidism

This is under-activity of the thyroid gland with absent or low levels of thyroid hormones T3 and T4 due to malfunctioning thyroid tissue, or secondary to pituitary or hypothalamic disease. The most common cause in pregnancy is autoimmune thyroiditis and goitre may or may not be present (Gregory and Todd 2013). Lack of dietary iodine can also cause goitre. Goitre is enlarged thyroid tissue due to infiltration of lymphocytes and increase of fibrous tissue; this condition is also known as *Hashimoto's disease*.

Hypothyroidism is familial and may be associated with other autoimmune disease such as type 1 diabetes (Gregory and Todd 2013). Symptoms include weight gain, intolerance to cold temperature, constipation, alopecia, dry skin, lethargy, hoarse voice, ataxia, bradycardia and cognitive impairment. Menstrual irregularities and infertility are common, because TRH stimulation induces hyperprolactinaemia which prevents ovulation. Not all women have symptoms and consequently the disease might be first recognized during infertility investigations. The most serious complication of untreated hypothyroidism is *myxoedema coma* which presents with hypothermia, hypoventilation and bradycardia, followed by unconsciousness (Gregory and Todd 2013).

Pregnancy complications of hypothyroidism are hypertension and low birth weight and psychomotor retardation in the fetus. Dornhorst and Williamson (2012) raise concern of the low Intelligence Quotient (IQ) of children born to mothers with untreated hypothyroidism and cretinism may result from severe maternal iodine deficiency associated with hypothyroidism (James et al 2011). Preconception care is therefore very important and fT4 and thyroxine levels should be measured and the dose of thyroxine adjusted until TSH reaches normal level (Gregory and Todd 2013).

During pregnancy the woman should be reviewed by an endocrinologist to measure fT4 and TSH levels at the outset in order to obtain a baseline measurement (Gregory and Todd 2013). The TSH level rises in pregnancy causing an increased demand for thyroxine and so the dose of therapeutic thyroxine is adjusted, usually increasing by 25–50% (Gregory and Todd 2013). Iron supplements should be taken at a different time to the thyroxine to maximize absorption (James et al 2011). Although a large goitre might cause complications for general anaesthesia (James et al 2011), there are otherwise no specific issues for labour and consequently intrapartum care may be provided by the midwife (Gregory and Todd 2013).

Postnatally, the thyroxine dose is reduced to the pre-pregnancy level and the fT4 and TSH levels should be measured at the 6-week follow-up or postnatal appointment. It is important that the neonatal bloodspot screening test is undertaken as the condition can be familial and thus the midwife should provide support to the parents, who are likely to be anxious (Gregory and Todd 2013). In addition, the woman needs to be observed for signs of thyroiditis and postnatal depression (James et al 2011).

Hyperthyroidism (thyrotoxicosis)

Hyperthyroidism is an overactivity of the thyroid gland that affects 0.2% of pregnant women (James et al 2011). It usually manifests as a clinical syndrome called *thyrotoxicosis* with signs and symptoms that include weight loss despite having a good appetite, intolerance to heat, sweating, tachycardia with *bouncing* pulse, insomnia, agitation, tremor, exophthalmos (protrusion of the eyeballs due to the tissue behind the eye becoming oedematous and fibrous), diarrhoea and menstrual irregularities (Gregory and Todd 2013). Non-pregnancy treatment is with *carbimazole* and *propylthiouracil*, which inhibit thyroid hormone synthesis (Dornhorst and Williamson 2012). *Thyroidectomy* is reserved for cases where there is excessively large goitre and drug therapy is ineffective. If radioiodine treatment has been used to destroy thyroid tissue to lower the thyroid levels, the woman should be counselled to delay conception for at least four months (James et al 2011).

The main complication of hyperthyroidism is the medical emergency of *thyroid crisis* (or thyroid storm) where there are exaggerated features of thyrotoxicosis with additional hyperpyrexia, cardiac dysrhythmias, congestive cardiac failure, altered mental state and ultimately coma. Goitre may also be present. Hyperthyroidism is treated with IV fluids, *hydrocortisone, propranolol, oral iodine, carbimazole* and *propylthiouracil* (Dornhorst and Williamson 2012). If the thyrotoxicosis is autoimmune, with antibodies to the TSH receptor, it is called *Graves' disease*, which accounts for 95% of hyperthyroidism in pregnancy (James et al 2011). Although the risk of miscarriage increases in early pregnancy, the disease otherwise tends to improve in pregnancy and women may go into remission in the latter half of pregnancy (Gregory and Todd 2013).

Care in pregnancy aims to *normalize* thyroid function and carbimazole and propylthiouracil are the drugs of choice with the dose adjusted after monthly measurements of fT4 and TSH. If the control is poor the fetus is at risk of fetal thyrotoxicosis which may necessitate cordocentesis to measure fetal fT4 and TSH (Gregory and Todd 2013). This is a high-risk pregnancy and the woman should consequently be referred to a specialist obstetric unit. The midwife should ensure monthly measurements of fT4 and TSH are undertaken and organize serial fetal growth ultrasound scans. There should also be regular assessment of the fetal heart rate to detect fetal tachycardia. As a result, continuous fetal heart monitoring during labour is required and the paediatrician should be informed when labour is established (Gregory and Todd 2013).

Labour can precipitate thyroid crisis/storm (James et al 2011) so meticulous monitoring and recording of maternal observations and wellbeing is vital. As with hypothyroidism, should goitre be present and is large, there may

be complications if general anaesthesia is warranted (James et al 2011).

Postnatally, the midwife should be alert for signs of thyrotoxicosis *flare* in the woman and extend the period of undertaking observations with emphasis on maternal pulse. Propylthiouracil is the drug of choice if the woman chooses to breastfeed her baby. The woman's thyroid hormone levels should also be measured 6 weeks following the baby's birth and the drug dose revised accordingly.

When examining the baby, the midwife should be alert for signs of neonatal goitre and thyrotoxicosis, referring promptly to the paediatrician if these are suspected. The baby might require temporary treatment with antithyroid drugs and propanolol necessitating admission to the NICU (Gregory and Todd 2013).

Prolactinoma

The pituitary gland increases in size by 50–70% in pregnancy due to normal lactotroph hyperplasia, which in rare cases causes symptoms in pregnancy (Dornhorst and Williamson 2012). The presence of an adenoma, called a *prolactinoma*, in the pituitary gland will further increase its size and cause symptoms. This adenoma, or cyst, increases the production of prolactin, which is the hormone that initiates lactation (Gregory and Todd 2013). There are two types of adenoma:

- *Microadenoma*: accounts for 90% of cases in pregnancy. They are <10 mm in diameter and rarely grow significantly, with some regressing spontaneously.
- *Macroadenoma*: accounts for 10% of cases in pregnancy. They are ≥10 mm in diameter and are more likely to expand and cause symptoms of headache and visual disturbance. Occasionally they may progress to pituitary apoplexy or diabetes insipidus (Dornhorst and Williamson 2012).

With both types of adenoma there is a risk of infertility and treatment is with dopamine agonists, which cause side-effects of nausea, vomiting, postural hypotension, constipation, nasal congestion and *Raynaud's phenomenon*. Pre-conception care is important and management depends upon the size of the adenoma which might involve a trial of discontinuing the dopamine agonist or changing to *bromocriptine*. In some cases, surgery might be attempted prior to conception to reduce the bulk size of the adenoma (Gregory and Todd 2013).

Once pregnant, the woman should be referred to a specialist unit as this is a high-risk pregnancy. Antenatal care, however, can be shared with the community midwife and medical/obstetric team. At the initial visit the midwife should take particular note of past surgery and current medication when undertaking the woman's history. At each subsequent visit the woman should be asked about headache and visual symptoms. It is the medical team who will determine the type and dose of dopamine agonist and perform monthly visual perimetry to detect early signs of compression on the optic chiasma (Gregory and Todd 2013). If there are indications of adenoma expansion, a magnetic resonance imaging (MRI) scan should be performed urgently and bromocriptine commenced.

In most cases the intrapartum care can be facilitated by the midwife, however if the adenoma is expanding the woman is likely to have a preterm induction of labour. The obstetric team may advise an elective instrumental birth to avoid a rise in intracranial pressure during the second stage of labour (Gregory and Todd 2013).

In the postnatal period the woman is advised to report any symptoms. An MRI scan might be ordered by the medical team and prolactin levels measured after 3 weeks, by which time the values should have returned to their pre-pregnancy levels. Follow-up appointments should be made with the specialist medical team who will evaluate the symptoms when determining the re-commencement of pre-pregnancy treatment with dopamine agonists. The midwife should consult with the doctor and pharmacist for suitable alternative medication if the woman wishes to breastfeed her baby as dopamine agonists are usually contraindicated. Furthermore, the woman will require specialist contraception advice as oestrogen contained within the oral contraceptive pill might further increase the size of the adenoma and consequently is contraindicated (Gregory and Todd 2013).

CARDIAC DISEASE

The chance of midwives caring for a woman with pre-existing cardiac disease, or developing cardiac disease in pregnancy, has increased over recent years due to many factors, including the increased age of childbearing women and the association it has with co-existing medical conditions such as diabetes, hypertension, as well as obesity, smoking and previous illicit drug use. Furthermore, improved life expectancy of women born with congenital cardiac disease and increased immigration revealing an increase in rheumatic heart disease adds to the prevalence. However, the majority of pregnancies complicated by maternal cardiac disease are expected to have a favourable outcome for both the woman and fetus.

Risk for morbidity and mortality depends on the nature of the cardiac lesion, its affect on the functional capacity of the heart and the development of pregnancy-related complications such as hypertensive disorders of pregnancy, infection, thrombosis and haemorrhage. Cardiac disease is the commonest cause of maternal death in the UK (Nelson-Piercy 2011), giving a maternal mortality rate of 2.31 per 100 000 maternities, with 53 women dying from heart disease associated with or exacerbated by

pregnancy in the triennium 2006–2008. Of these, *acquired heart disease* was the cause of the majority of deaths with sudden adult death syndrome (SADS) and ischaemic heart disease (IMD) being common causes of death in pregnancy. Women with *congenital heart disease* only accounted for one these deaths.

The majority of deaths secondary to cardiac causes occur in women with no previous history. It is vital that a midwife undertakes an accurate history from the woman at the first visit. Should any history of cardiac disease be revealed, a more detailed account should be elicited in order to ensure prompt and appropriate referral to an appropriately skilled and experienced multidisciplinary team, usually in regional centres. These women require an individualized midwifery approach to care to address the psychosocial concerns that may often get subsumed within a medical model of care. The midwife's role involves not only being astute to any deviation that may arise in the course of the woman's pregnancy, but also being supportive of the woman's individual needs as she may have the same pregnancy concerns as any other woman.

In a healthy pregnancy the haemodynamic profile alters in order to meet the increasing demands of the developing feto-placental unit. Healthy pregnant women are able to adjust to these physiological changes quite easily; for women with co-existing cardiac disease, however, the added workload can precipitate complications. The three sensitive periods of cardiovascular stress (28–32 weeks of pregnancy, during labour and 12–24 hours postpartum) are the most critical and life threatening for women with cardiac disease (Roberts and Adamson 2013). Understanding the changes in cardiovascular dynamics during pregnancy can support the midwife's recognition of key indicators and when limitations to cardiac function are occurring that require prompt referral (see Chapter 9).

Diagnosis of cardiac disease

Along with the signs and symptoms, physical assessment of functional capacity and laboratory tests can assist with the diagnosis of cardiac disease and determine the type of lesion. These may include:

- full cardiovascular examination, including personal history and assessment of lifestyle risk factors
- blood tests: full blood count, clotting studies and cardiac enzymes (Troponin)
- 12-lead electrocardiogram (ECG)
- echocardiogram: an ultrasound examination to examine cardiac structure and function
- chest X-ray to assess cardiac size and outline, pulmonary vasculature and lung fields (always undertaken when clinically indicated, e.g. in women presenting with chest pain)
- other imaging: computerized tomography (CT) scan or magnetic resonance imaging (MRI) scan of the chest.

Care of women with cardiac disease

Pre-conception care

Women with a pre-existing cardiac problem should receive pre-conception counselling to inform them of any potential risks that a pregnancy may have on their health and that of their unborn baby in terms of inheriting any congenital malformations. This will enable them to make informed decisions and plan their pregnancy monitoring more carefully to reduce any subsequent morbidity and mortality. The risk of inheriting cardiac disease varies between 3% and 50% depending on the type of maternal heart disease. Children of parents with a cardiovascular condition inherited in an autosomal dominant manner (e.g. *Marfan syndrome, hypertrophic cardiomyopathy*, or *long QT syndrome*) have an inheritance risk of 50%, regardless of gender of the affected parent.

For a steadily increasing number of genetic defects, genetic screening by chorionic villous biopsy (CVS) can be offered in the 12th week of pregnancy. All women with congenital heart disease should be offered fetal echocardiography between the 19th and 22nd week of pregnancy. Measurement of nuchal fold thickness around the 12th to 13th week of pregnancy is an early screening test for Down syndrome in women over 35 years of age. The sensitivity for the presence of a significant cardiac defect is 40–45%, while the specificity of the method is 99%. The incidence of congenital cardiac disease with normal nuchal fold thickness is 1/1000 (Eleftheriades et al 2012).

Antenatal care

The symptoms of physiological pregnancy can mimic the signs and symptoms of cardiac disease, e.g. dyspnoea on exertion, orthopnoea, palpitations, dizziness, fainting, a bounding pulse, tachycardia, peripheral oedema, distended jugular veins and alterations in heart sounds. Observations and investigations of the woman's health should be undertaken prior to and at the beginning of pregnancy to obtain baseline referral points. Adapted antenatal records that include triggers such as *shortness of breath, palpitations, pulse rate and rhythm* as well as *auscultation of the heart for any murmur and lung fields for signs of pulmonary oedema* are useful to prompt the midwife into early detection of subtle increases of any worsening symptoms. These observations should be undertaken alongside the usual antenatal examination, but the midwife also needs to be mindful that women with cardiac disease can also develop other complications such as pre-eclampsia or gestational diabetes (RCOG 2011b).

There should be frequent assessment of the woman with a multidisciplinary approach involving midwives, obstetricians, cardiologists and anaesthetists. The aim is to maintain a steady haemodynamic state and prevent complications, as well as promote physical and psychological wellbeing. In addition, the fetal wellbeing is assessed by the following means:

- ultrasound examination to confirm gestational age and any congenital malformation
- clinical assessment of fetal growth and amniotic fluid volume and by ultrasound
- monitoring of the fetal heart rate by CTG
- measurement of fetal and maternal placental blood flow indices by Doppler ultrasonography.

A care plan for pregnancy, labour and the early postnatal period should be informed by the individual woman's situation with a view to optimizing outcomes for her and her baby. Such a plan should be shared with the woman with copies being available in her own hand-held records and those held at a central point.

Potential interventions, such as attending parent education classes, can help in allaying the woman's general anxieties about motherhood alongside the antenatal care received from the midwife. This may involve advice regarding modifying and adjusting physical activity during pregnancy. Some women may need to commence maternity leave earlier than anticipated whereas others may require admission to hospital for rest and close monitoring. In addition, guidance about the constituents of a well-balanced diet with restricted intake of cholesterol, sodium-rich foods and salt should also be provided. Monitoring of weight gain should be undertaken as excess weight gain will place additional strain on the heart. Compliance with taking iron and folic acid supplementation is also important in preventing anaemia.

Antithrombotic therapy

The hypercoagulable state in pregnancy increases the risk of thromboembolic disease in women who have arrhythmias, mitral valve stenosis or who have had mechanical cardiac valve replacements. However, the treatment of women requiring antithrombotic therapy during pregnancy is challenging. *Warfarin* is commonly used as an antithrombotic, but as it is teratogenic to the developing embryo/fetus and associated with a high fetal loss rate, it is not used in pregnancy. Furthermore, warfarin also predisposes the woman and her fetus to haemorrhage when used in the third trimester. Subcutaneous low molecular weight heparins, such as *enoxaparin*, are useful for thromboprophylaxis but may not be suitable for women with mechanical heart valves. As a consequence, the advice of a haematologist should be sought. Full-length thromboembolism deterrent (TED) support stockings should be worn if the woman is admitted to hospital for rest and assessment, and should also be worn during labour and in the immediate postnatal period.

Intrapartum care: the first stage of labour

Many women with cardiac disease have an uncomplicated labour but it is good practice that there is effective communication among a dedicated multidisciplinary team of midwife, obstetrician, cardiologist, neonatologist, anaesthetist and the woman and her family to optimize birth outcome. Vaginal birth is preferred unless there is an obstetric indication for caesarean section as haemodynamic stability is greater and there is less chance of postoperative infection and pulmonary complications (RCOG 2011b).

Intrapartum care involves monitoring the maternal condition using the Modified Early Obstetric Warning Scoring (MEOWS) system that triggers any deviation in order to prompt timely intervention and maximize maternal and fetal wellbeing (McLean et al 2013). Continuous ECG is recommended in nearly all cases and pulse oximetry may be utilized to assess arterial haemoglobin saturation, which may be reduced in women with cardiac disease owing to disruption of normal gas exchange between the lungs and blood. Fluid balance should be recorded, and use of intravenous fluids may be limited. Routine antibiotic prophylaxis is not recommended. Continuous electronic fetal heart rate monitoring is usually recommended (Regitz-Zagrosek et al 2011).

Labour induction

If induction is indicated and the cervix is favourable (using the Bishop score: Chapter 19), artificial rupture of the membranes (ARM) is undertaken with an IVI of oxytocin should contractions not establish. A prolonged induction should be avoided. If the cervix is unfavourable, synthetic prostaglandin is used to soften/*ripen* it. While there is no absolute contraindication to *misoprostol* (prostaglandin E$_1$) or *dinoprostone* (prostaglandin E$_2$), there is a theoretical risk of coronary vasospasm and a low risk of arrhythmias. In addition, dinoprostone has more profound effects on BP than misoprostol and is therefore contraindicated in active cardiovascular disease.

Pain relief

The midwife should assist the woman to use the techniques that she has learned for coping with stress. Nitrous oxide and oxygen (Entonox®) and pethidine are usually considered safe means of intrapartum analgesia for women with cardiac disease, but it is important to review the labour plan with the multidisciplinary team before administration. In some situations, epidural anaesthesia may be the analgesia of choice for its effectiveness in relieving pain and decreasing cardiac output and heart rate (RCOG 2011b). It causes peripheral vasodilatation and decreases venous return, which alleviates pulmonary congestion. Furthermore, an effectively working epidural *in situ* may eliminate the need for emergency general anaesthesia.

Positioning

Cardiac output is influenced by the position of the woman during labour and consequently those with cardiac disease are particularly sensitive to aortocaval compression by the gravid uterus if adopting the supine position. It is recommended that midwives encourage an upright or left lateral position for women to adopt during labour and birth wherever possible (McLean et al 2013).

The second stage of labour

This should be short without undue exertion on the part of the woman. Prolonged pushing with held breath (the *Valsalva manoeuvre*) should be discouraged as it can further compromise the health of the woman with cardiac disease. Such a manoeuvre raises the intrathoracic pressure, forces the blood out of the thorax and impedes venous return, resulting in a fall in cardiac output. The midwife should therefore encourage the woman to breathe as normal and follow her natural desire to bear down giving several short pushes during each contraction.

An instrumental birth using forceps or ventouse may be undertaken to shorten the second stage of labour. Care should be taken, however, when the woman is in the lithotomy position, where the lower part of the body is higher than the trunk, as this produces a sudden increase in venous return to the heart, which may result in heart failure. A wedge should therefore be used to avoid aortocaval compression (McLean et al 2013).

The third stage of labour

An active third stage of labour is usually advocated with a slow IVI of 2 U/min oxytocin administered after the birth of the placenta to avoid systemic hypotension and prevent haemorrhage (see Chapter 18). Prostaglandin F analogues are useful to treat PPH, unless an increase in pulmonary artery pressure (PAP) is undesirable. *Ergometrine* is contraindicated in women with cardiac disease as it can cause vasoconstriction and hypertension (Regitz-Zagrosek et al 2011).

Postnatal care

The first 48 hours following the baby's birth are critical for the woman with significant cardiac disease. The heart must be able to cope with the extra volume of blood (*autotransfusion*) from the uterine circulation as well as the increased venous return following relief of aortocaval compression of the uterus. Conversely, the total blood volume may be diminished by the amount lost at birth and during the postnatal period. Furthermore, the heart will need to compensate should the blood flow be impaired due to PPH. Close monitoring of haemodynamic changes is required at this time and the midwife should identify early signs of infection, thrombosis or pulmonary oedema. Observation of the condition of the woman's legs, the use of antiembolic stockings and early ambulation are important strategies for the midwife to adopt in order to reduce the risk of thromboembolism.

Breastfeeding should be encouraged as cardiac output is not affected by lactation, although drug therapy for specific heart conditions may need to be reviewed for safety during breastfeeding. The midwife is required to provide the woman with support to successfully breastfeed her baby, emphasizing the importance of adequate rest and a dietary intake containing sufficient calories to sustain breastfeeding.

It is important that *prior* to transfer from hospital, the midwife explores the help and support available in the home for when the woman returns home with her baby. Relatives and friends often fulfil this need but community support services should also be considered if necessary. In addition, the midwife should offer appropriate contraceptive advice and the options available to the woman who has cardiac disease, considering their individual risks need to be balanced against the risk of pregnancy (RCOG 2011b).

Congenital heart disease

The most common congenital heart diseases (CHD) found in pregnancy are atrial septal defect (ASD), ventricular septal defect (VSD), patent ductus arteriosus (PDA), pulmonary stenosis, aortic stenosis and tetralogy of Fallot. The majority of these lesions should have been surgically corrected in childhood, resulting in a growing population of women with CHD achieving a pregnancy. Uncorrected lesions may cause pulmonary hypertension, cyanosis and severe left ventricular failure and are therefore present a greater risk in achieving successful pregnancy outcome. Congenital heart disease is also associated with increased fetal complications such as fetal loss, IUGR, pre-term birth and an increased risk of fetal CHD (Regitz-Zagrosek et al 2011). Particularly high-risk cardiac conditions for pregnancy include the following.

Eisenmenger's syndrome

A large left–right shunt of blood is apparent usually through a VSD, ASD or PDA, which is still patent. This results in an increase in the pulmonary blood flow, which over time leads to fibrosis and the development of pulmonary hypertension and cyanosis (Regitz-Zagrosek et al 2011). When the right-sided heart pressures exceed left heart pressures, the shunt reverses, with worsening cyanosis. Women with this condition are advised against pregnancy as maternal mortality lies in the region of 30–50%. Risk of prematurity contributes to the high perinatal mortality rate.

Marfan syndrome

This syndrome is caused by an autosomal dominant defect on chromosome 15. It is a connective tissue disease affecting the musculoskeletal system, the cardiovascular system and eyes. The cardiovascular abnormalities are the most life-threatening as the elastic fibres in the media of the blood vessels weaken. Dilatation of the ascending and descending aorta results, followed in some instances by dissection or rupture, or both. Pregnancy poses a significant risk because of the increased stress on the cardiovascular system. There is a 50% chance of a child inheriting Marfan syndrome if one parent is affected. Women who have minimal cardiovascular involvement and normal aortic root dimensions have a better pregnancy outcome. Careful monitoring is required throughout pregnancy, including the use of serial echocardiography to identify progressive aortic root dilatation. Prophylactic antihypertensive therapy using beta-blockers is recommended to reduce blood pressure and the rate of aortic dilatation (Roberts and Adamson 2013). Some individuals with Marfan syndrome also present with dural ectasia which, unless mild, presents an increased risk of a spinal cerebrospinal fluid (CSF) leak in the case of accidental dural puncture during epidural: consequently, epidural anaesthesia is not usually recommended. Whilst Marfan syndrome is a genetic condition, approximately 15% of cases are as a result of new mutation and thus some individuals remain undiagnosed and do not seek any preconception counselling. Pregnant women with Marfan syndrome should be referred to the specialist team containing a cardiologist for immediate assessment and investigation (RCOG 2011b).

Aortic dissection (acute)

Aortic dissection (acute) may occur in pregnancy in association with severe hypertension (systolic >160 mmHg) due to pre-eclampsia, coarctation of the aorta or connective tissue disease such as Marfan syndrome. The woman typically presents with severe chest or intrascapular pain. Early diagnosis using computed tomography chest scan, MRI or transoesophageal echocardiogram is critical, as maternal mortality is high.

Acquired heart disease

Rheumatic heart disease

Rheumatic heart disease causes inflammation and scarring of the heart valves and results in valve stenosis, with or without regurgitation. The mitral valve is most often affected with stenosis, occurring in two-thirds of cases. This condition is often diagnosed for the first time during pregnancy, presenting as severe breathlessness and tiredness. It tends to appear in immigrant or refugee women who have not had access to medical care. Most women with valvular heart disease can be treated medically, aiming to reduce the heart's workload.

During pregnancy, this involves bed rest, oxygen therapy and the use of cardiac drugs, e.g. *diuretics* (to reduce the fluid load), *digoxin* (to reduce and regulate the heart rate) and *heparin* (to reduce the risk of thromboembolic disease). Women with more severe symptomatic disease may require surgical intervention such as *balloon valvuloplasty* or *valve replacement*, although both of these procedures carry a degree of maternal and fetal mortality. Antibiotic prophylaxis is no longer recommended for all women with valvular lesions during labour although it may still be advisable for those who have mechanical valves.

Myocardial infarction and ischaemic heart disease

Myocardial infarction (MI) and ischaemic heart disease (IHD) are an increasing cause of maternal death in the UK. Identifiable risk factors include increasing maternal age, obesity, diabetes, pre-existing hypertension, smoking, family history and poor socioeconomic status. A myocardial infarction is most likely to occur in the third trimester of pregnancy and the peripartum period, when haemodynamic changes are at their optimum creating a higher risk of thrombotic events due to the hypercoagulability induced by hormonal changes. In the immediate postpartum period, spontaneous coronary artery dissection is the most common cause of MI. Typically, women present with ischaemic chest pain in the presence of an abnormal ECG and elevated cardiac enzymes, although these signs and symptoms may be masked during labour and birth (McLean et al 2013). Atypical features include abdominal or epigastric pain and vomiting. *Coronary angioplasty* is the fine line therapy to improve the patency of blocked arteries (Roberts and Adamson 2013).

Peripartum cardiomyopathy

Peripartum cardiomyopathy is relatively rare but is potentially fatal, with mortality rates ranging from 25% to 50%. A number of these deaths occur shortly after the onset of signs and symptoms. The incidence of this type of cardiac disease varies from $1:300$ to $1:4000$ pregnancies, with heart failure developing very rapidly in some cases. Predisposing factors to peripartum cardiomyopathy comprise of multigravidae, multiple pregnancies, family history, ethnicity, smoking, diabetes, hypertension, pre-eclampsia, malnutrition, pregnant teenagers or older pregnant women and prolonged use of beta-agonists (Mclean et al 2013).

Commonly women have no previous history of heart disease and diagnosis is usually made within a specific period of time between the last month of pregnancy and the first 5 months postpartum. Inflammation and enlargement of the myocardium (*cardiomegaly*) give rise to left ventricular heart failure and thromboembolic complications. Presenting features include orthopnoea and dyspnoea, chest pain and palpitations, new resurgent murmurs and pulmonary crackles, raised jugular pressure, ankle oedema and fatigue. Treatment involves the use of oxygen, diuretics, and vasodilators to decrease pulmonary congestion and fluid overload, followed by inotropic agents to improve myometrial contractility and anticoagulation therapy. As the cardiomegaly resolves there should be a corresponding improvement in the woman's condition but this process may take up to 6 months and there is a risk of recurrence in a subsequent pregnancy. In some women, left ventricular dysfunction persists and unless a heart transplant is performed mortality can be high (Regitz-Zagrosek et al 2011).

RESPIRATORY DISORDERS

Asthma

Asthma is a chronic disorder of the respiratory system entailing an inflammatory hyper-responsiveness of the airways to certain triggers (see Box 13.12). This causes episodic narrowing, resulting in obstruction of the airways and mucous production (Tortora and Derrickson 2010). Asthma is characterized by intermittent episodes of wheezing and shortness of breath as the individual attempts to inhale and exhale. These symptoms are variable and can be worse at night (Scullion et al 2013). The condition is under-diagnosed in female adolescents (Holmes and Scullion 2011). Key statistics reveal the extent of the problem in the UK:

- Asthma is the most common symptomatic long-term condition in the UK, affecting 5.4 million people, 1.1.million of whom are children (NICE 2013a)

> **Box 13.12 Triggers for asthma**
>
> - Pollen and house dust mite allergens
> - Chronic nasal rhinitis
> - Smoking: primary and passive
> - Infection
> - Occupational exposure
> - Pollution
> - Cold air and physical exercise
> - Food additives, e.g. monosodium glutamate, tartrazine and sulphites
> - Drugs, e.g. aspirin
> - Premenstrual conditions and pregnancy
>
> Source: Tortora and Derrickson 2010; Scullion et al 2013

- There are around 1000 deaths per year from asthma, about 90% of which are associated with preventable factors and 40% of these deaths being in individuals under 75 years of age.
- Of the nine maternal deaths attributed to respiratory disease in the triennium 2006–2008, there were five women dying from asthma (0.22/100 000 maternities), which is a similar rate to the two preceding reports (de Swiet et al 2011).

Investigations include:

- *peak expiratory flow measurements* using a small hand-held device (peak flow meter) to assess the speed by which air is exhaled
- *spirometry* via a spirometer to measure the volume and speed of air exhaled
- allergy testing
- chest X-ray to exclude other conditions
- steroid trial: 2 weeks of oral prednisolone or 6 weeks of an inhaled corticosteroid.

Treatment follows a *stepwise* approach and initial therapy will depend on the severity of the presentation. Some individuals may only require salbutamol for occasional symptoms, whereas others may commence on two inhalers (BTS [British Thoracic Society]/SIGN 2011):

- corticosteroid inhaler (e.g. *betclometasone dipropionate*), twice a day: usually colour-coded brown or orange and described as a *preventer inhaler*
- bronchodilator inhaler/beta-2 agonist (e.g. *salbutamol*), when required: colour-coded blue and described as a *reliever inhaler*.

Further treatment may involve long acting beta-2 agonists, theophyllines, leukotriene antagonists and, in extreme cases, oral corticosteroids (Holmes and Scullion 2011).

In pregnancy, women are at increased risk of delivering low birth weight and preterm babies and have a greater tendency to other medical complications such as pre-eclampsia (Scullion et al 2013). They should be advised of the importance of good control of their asthma to avoid problems for themselves and the baby and that medication used to control asthmatic symptoms is generally safe in pregnancy (Scullion et al 2013). These include:

- short- and long-acting beta-2 agonists
- inhaled steroids
- oral theophyllines
- leukotriene antagonists: if they are already being used, these should continue, but should not be commenced as a new therapy
- steroid tablets: indicated for severe asthma and exacerbations and should never be withheld because of pregnancy (BTS/SIGN 2011).

In addition, pregnant women should be encouraged to cease smoking and avoid passive cigarette smoke.

Severe acute asthma, also termed *status asthmaticus* or *asthma attack*, occurs when there is spasm of the smooth muscle in the walls of the smaller bronchi and bronchioles leading to partial or complete obstruction of the airways, known as *bronchoconstriction*. This manifests with periods of coughing, wheezing and difficulty with exhalation. Air may become trapped in the alveoli during exhalation. Excessive secretion of mucous may obstruct the bronchioles and worsen the attack. This is a medical emergency and pregnant women should be treated in hospital.

High flow oxygen should be administered immediately to maintain saturations between 94 and 98%, a systemic corticosteroid given and inhaled short-acting beta-2 agonists administered via a large volume spacer or nebulizer (BTS/SIGN 2011). If the response is poor, inhaled ipratropium bromide may be given and arrangements made to transfer the woman to the ICU/HDCU for ventilatory support.

The labour of a woman whose asthma is well controlled may progress physiologically, supported by the midwife. Those women who have been receiving oral steroids may require hydrocortisone during labour. If anaesthesia is required, epidural is preferable to general anaesthesia. If ergometrine and syntometrine are used to control blood loss following the birth of the placenta, extreme caution should be taken to reduce the risk of inducing bronchoconstriction (BTS/SIGN 2011; Scullion et al 2013). Breastfeeding should be encouraged and the woman should continue to take all prescribed medication for her asthma during lactation.

THROMBOEMBOLIC DISEASE

Thromboembolic disease is of considerable importance to midwifery practice because of the associated maternal mortality. Although maternal mortality attributed to thromboembolic disease has declined in the UK over recent years, it remains the third leading cause of direct maternal death with 18 deaths occurring in the last triennial report, 2006–2008 (Drife 2011). The pregnant woman has a ten-fold increased risk of developing venous thromboembolism (VTE) compared with the non-pregnant population, which rises to 25-fold in the puerperium (Clark et al 2012).

Thromboprophylaxis in pregnancy

This is the prevention of thromboembolic disease and is an important part of the midwife's role. There are additional risk factors for VTE in pregnancy and the RCOG (2009) provides a risk assessment scale, as summarized in Box 13.13.

Most UK NHS Trusts will have a risk assessment based on the criteria in Box 13.13. The midwife should perform and document this risk assessment on the following occasions:

Box 13.13 **Risk factors for venous thromboembolism**

Pre-existing factors

- Previous VTE
- Family history of VTE (e.g. deficiency of protein C or S, antithrombin deficiency, prothrombin gene variant, Factor V Leiden)
- Known thrombophilia
- Lupus anticoagulant
- Medical co-morbidities (e.g. sickle cell disease, cardiac disease, proteinuria >3 g/day)
- Age >35 years
- Obesity (BMI >30 kg/m^2)
- Parity >3
- Smoking
- Intravenous drug user
- Varicose veins

Obstetric factors

- Pre-eclampsia
- Dehydration/hyperemesis gravidarum
- Multiple pregnancy
- Caesarean section or forceps delivery
- Prolonged labour
- Postpartum haemorrhage

Transient factors

- Systemic infection
- Paraplegia or immobility
- Recent surgical procedure
- Ovarian hyperstimulation syndrome
- Travel >4 hours

Pregnant women with three or more risk factors should receive prophylactic low molecular weight heparin (LMWH).

Source: RCOG 2009, 2010a

- initial meeting with the woman (*booking visit*)
- any hospital admission
- following the birth of the baby.

If this assessment identifies women at risk of developing VTE, the midwife should promptly refer her to a consultant-led maternity unit with an expert in thrombosis in pregnancy (Elliott and Pavord 2013). The woman is likely to be commenced on subcutaneous injections of low molecular weight heparin (LMWH), as this does not cross the placental barrier with consequential effects on the fetus. The midwife, or specialist nurse, should educate the woman in self-administration of the heparin, alerting her to carry a medical alert card containing such details with

her at all times. The woman should be provided with a sharps bin for safe disposal of the injection devices.

Gradient compression stockings or TED stockings are likely to be prescribed. Such stockings are available in two lengths, below the knee or thigh, and are designed to give a pressure gradient from the ankle to the knee or thigh that mimics the pumping action of the deep leg vein calf muscles, with the highest pressure being at the ankle. It is important that the woman is measured correctly around the ankle and calf or thigh circumference depending upon the type of stocking prescribed (Llewelyn 2013). Midwives should be trained in their use to be able to instruct the woman how to wear them correctly and monitor their use (Elliott and Pavord 2013). For hygiene purposes, stockings should be removed daily, but this should be no more than 30 minutes. The legs should be inspected and measured by the midwife every three days to detect any changes in size or tissue damage (Llewelyn 2013).

The woman should be given advice about avoiding dehydration, ceasing smoking and eating a healthy diet (Copple and Coser 2013). If the pregnant woman is expecting to travel long distances, especially by air, she will benefit by wearing loose fitting clothing and flight socks (TED stockings), drinking plenty of water, avoiding alcohol and remaining ambulant for as long as possible/performing leg exercises when at rest (Elliott and Pavord 2013).

During labour, the midwife should encourage mobility with regular changes of position and passive leg exercises when the woman is at rest. It is important that hydration is maintained and regular observations are undertaken, including frequent examination of the woman's legs. If the woman has been prescribed LMWH in pregnancy, this should be omitted at the onset of contractions and regional anaesthesia avoided within 12 hours of the last administered dose. There should be active management of the third stage of labour with the oxytoxic drug being administered IV. If perineal suturing is required, the midwife should undertake this promptly to avoid the woman being in the lithotomy position for a prolonged time, as this further increases the risk for deep vein thrombosis (DVT). If surgery is necessary, intermittent calf compression will be required in theatre.

The postnatal period presents further risk to the woman for both DVT and pulmonary embolism (PE), and early mobilization should be encouraged. Routine postnatal observations are important, especially respiration rate and the development of any leg swelling. If either condition is suspected the woman must be referred urgently to a haematologist, or if at home she must be re-admitted to hospital.

Deep vein thrombosis

A blood clot formed within a blood vessel is termed a *thrombus*, which can become detached and lodge in

271

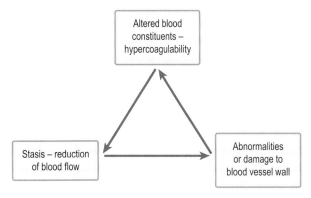

Fig. 13.1 Virchow's triad (after Bagot and Arya 2008).

another blood vessel and partially or wholly occlude it. *Virchow's triad* (see Fig. 13.1) outlines predisposing factors for thrombus formation (Bagot and Arya 2008).

In pregnancy, Virchow's triad is affected by the physiological changes to the haematological system (Greer et al 2007) (see Chapter 9). Despite pregnancy presenting a state of *hypervolaemia*, by term *hypercoagulability* also develops to compensate for the demands of the forthcoming labour and maintenance of haemostasis. In addition, there is relative venous stasis with a gradual 50% reduction in venous flow velocity, reaching its peak at 36 weeks and declining to pre-pregnancy values by 6 weeks following the baby's birth (Greer et al 2007). Furthermore, the physical effect of the gravid uterus exerts pressure on the pelvic veins and the inferior vena cava, increasing the woman's risk of developing a DVT in the veins of the calf, thigh and pelvis (Elliott and Pavord 2013).

In pregnancy, 90% of DVT occur in the left leg compared with 55% in the non-pregnant woman due to compression of the left iliac vein by the left iliac artery in pregnancy (Clark et al 2012). The ileofemoral veins are the most common location, having 70% of pregnancy occurrences versus 9% in the non-pregnant woman, and are more likely to result in pulmonary embolism (Clark et al 2012).

The complications of DVT are *pulmonary embolism* (PE) and *post-thrombotic syndrome* arising from damage to the venous valves that result in a backflow of blood, venous hypertension, oedema and tissue hypoxia (Elliott and Pavord 2013). The midwife needs to be aware of the signs of DVT (listed below) as she may be the first person to identify this when undertaking an antenatal or postnatal examination on the woman:

- pain in the area of the clot
- swelling (usually one-sided)
- red discoloration
- difficulty in weight-bearing on the affected leg
- low grade pyrexia
- lower abdominal or back pain.

If the leg appears swollen a tape measure should be used to assess the circumference of both legs at the affected area for comparison. A DVT is potentially life threatening and the midwife **must refer the woman immediately** to hospital for medical examination, investigation and treatment (RCOG 2010a). The classic diagnostic use of dorsiflexion of the foot (*Homan's sign*) is considered unreliable in pregnancy and the presence of severe lower back pain has greater significance (James et al 2011). Medical investigations involve Doppler ultrasound and serum investigations might be performed; however, Elliott and Pavord (2013) debate the usefulness of measuring D-dimers levels in pregnancy. Venography is generally avoided in pregnancy due to the small radiation risk to the fetus.

Treatment of DVT in pregnancy is with LMWH administered 12-hourly by subcutaneous injection to sustain the levels, and which should continue for at least 6 months after the diagnosis. Gradient compression stockings should be prescribed and the woman taught how to put them on. The woman will need to wear one on the affected leg for two years to reduce the risk of post-thrombotic syndrome (Elliott and Pavord 2013). Anticoagulation therapy should continue for at least 6 months after the diagnosis (RCOG 2010a).

The woman should be seen by the anaesthetist prior to labour to discuss the risks that thromboembolic disorders have on the administration of regional/general anaesthesia. As soon as labour commences, heparin should be omitted and compression stockings should be worn. As regional anaesthesia carries a risk of spinal bleeding, this should be avoided within 12 hours of administration of heparin. Although general anaesthetic is itself a thrombotic risk, it may have to be considered for caesarean section. The woman should be encouraged to remain mobile or undertake passive leg exercises and maintain hydration. An IVI should be sited, and drugs given IV instead of intramuscularly (IM). Prolonged use of the lithotomy position should be avoided, as this is a DVT risk. The third stage of labour should be actively managed with the oxytoxic drug being administered IV to prompt haemostasis. If perineal suturing is required, it should be undertaken promptly to limit the length of time the woman is in the lithotomy position (RCOG 2010a; Elliott and Pavord 2013).

The midwife should be aware that there is a 25-fold increased risk of DVT and the potential for PE during the postnatal period. As a consequence, the woman who has had a previous DVT is especially at high risk and thus the midwife is required to be particularly vigilant is assessing her condition, encouraging early ambulation and hydration. Heparin is recommended as directed by the medical team. This is usually 2 hours after a vaginal birth or longer if the woman had an epidural and/or caesarean section, and should continue until at least the 6-week postnatal appointment, at which point a decision to change to warfarin may be made (RCOG 2010b; Elliott and Pavord

2013). Oestrogen-based contraceptive pills are contraindicated so depo-provera or barrier methods of contraception should be discussed with the woman and her partner.

Pulmonary embolism

Pulmonary embolism (PE) occurs when a DVT detaches and becomes mobile, known as an *embolus*. A large embolus might lodge in the pulmonary artery and smaller ones can travel distally to small vessels in the lung periphery, where they may wholly or partially occlude the blood vessel (James et al 2011; Elliott and Pavord 2013). Initially the lung tissue is ventilated but not perfused, producing intrapulmonary dead space, and there is impaired gaseous exchange (Kumar and Clarke 2004). After some hours, surfactant production by the affected lung ceases, the alveoli collapse and hypoxaemia results. Pulmonary arterial pressure rises and there is a reduction in cardiac output. The area of the lung affected by the embolism may become infracted; however, in some instances, oxygenation of tissue continues to some extent from the bronchial circulation and airways (Kumar and Clarke 2004).

In the case of a small embolism, there is likely to be dyspnoea, discomfort or pain in the chest, haemoptysis and low grade pyrexia, all of which can be misdiagnosed as a chest infection. Cardiovascular examination is usually normal (Kumar and Clarke 2004; James et al 2011).

A larger embolism that occludes a major vessel will result in a more acute presentation, because of sudden obstruction of the right ventricle and its outflow (Kumar and Clarke 2004). There is severe central chest pain due to ischaemia, and pallor with sweating as shock develops. Tachycardia occurs and a *gallop rhythm* of the heart may be heard on examination. Hypotension develops as peripheral shutdown occurs. Syncope may result when cardiac output is suddenly reduced (Kumar and Clarke 2004). Admission to an intensive care unit is highly likely as there is a significant risk of death if treatment is delayed.

Pulmonary embolism is a medical emergency and urgent referral to hospital is indicated. Diagnosis is made from a combination of clinical probability score and radiological imaging. Heparin, usually LWMH, is commenced at presentation with subsequent anticoagulation treatment and management in labour and the postnatal period being similar to that for a woman presenting with DVT (Elliott and Pavord 2013).

Disseminated intravascular coagulation (DIC)

In DIC (also known as disseminated intravascular coagulopathy), damage to the endothelium (lining of blood vessel walls) arising from pre-eclampsia, placental abruption, major haemorrhage, embolism, intrauterine fetal death or retained placenta results in thromboplastins being released from the damaged cells, causing the extrinsic pathway to mount a coagulation cascade. Blood clotting occurs at the original site and then small clots (*micro-thrombi*) disperse throughout the rest of the vascular system. Large quantities of fibrinogen, thrombocytes (platelets) and clotting factors V and VIII are consumed. The micro-thrombi produced can occlude small blood vessels, resulting in ischaemia, hence some organ tissue dies and releases more thromboplastins and the cycle re-commences. All clotting factors and platelets are subsequently consumed and bleeding results. There is simultaneously widespread blood clotting *and* a clotting deficiency. Bleeding occurs, petechiae develop in the skin and, if untreated, major haemorrhage can result (Kumar and Clarke 2004; Craig et al 2006).

HAEMATOLOGICAL DISORDERS

Anaemia

Anaemia is a condition in which the number of red blood cells or their oxygen-carrying capacity is insufficient to meet the physiological needs of the individual, which consequently will vary by age, sex, altitude, smoking and pregnancy status (WHO 2013). In its severe form, it is associated with fatigue, weakness, dizziness and drowsiness, pregnant women and children being particularly vulnerable (WHO 2013). Anaemia in pregnancy is defined as a haemoglobin (Hb) concentration of less than 11 g/dl (James et al 2011).

Physiological anaemia of pregnancy

The increase of blood plasma in pregnancy causes a state of haemodilution (see Chapter 9). On laboratory testing, the Hb values decline, reaching the lowest in the second trimester followed by a gradual rise in the third trimester. This situation is not pathological unless the Hb reduces to such an extent that iron deficiency anaemia results.

Iron deficiency anaemia

Iron deficiency is thought to be the most common cause of anaemia globally and is defined by trimester, as shown in Table 13.4 (WHO et al 2001; NICE 2013b).

The daily iron requirement for a healthy woman is 1.3 mg, which can be acquired through a diet rich in iron and folate. In pregnancy this requirement rises to 3 mg per day, further increasing to 7 mg per day after 32 weeks (Addo et al 2013). Prophylactic antenatal iron supplementation is no longer administered routinely in the UK, unless the woman is at risk of developing iron deficiency anaemia.

Table 13.4 Anaemia defined by trimester

Trimester	Serum ferritin concentration	Haemoglobin
1	<30 µg/l	<11 g/dl
2 and 3	<30 µg/l	<10.5 g/dl

Iron deficiency is associated with:

- reduced intake of iron due to gastric malabsorption, gastric surgery or dietary deficiency
- short intervals between pregnancies
- chronic infection such as malaria or human immunodeficiency virus (HIV)
- chronic blood loss, e.g. menorrhagia or gastric ulcer
- haemorrhage
- secondary cause to medical disorders
- multiple pregnancy.

Iron deficiency interferes with body functions, leading to:

- tiredness
- irritability and depression
- breathlessness
- poor memory
- muscle aches
- palpitations
- cardiac failure
- maternal exhaustion in labour
- poor recovery from blood loss at the birth and during the postnatal period.

Routine serum blood samples should be taken from healthy pregnant women at intervals during the antenatal period according to local protocols for the early identification of anaemia. When anaemia is identified serum ferritin should be measured as an indication of the level of stored iron. It is recommended that women with known anaemia be screened at every antenatal appointment (Addo et al 2013). *Borderline anaemia* can be managed in the community setting, however severe or chronic cases should be referred to a consultant-led maternity unit as should those women who are symptomatic (Addo et al 2013).

The initial treatment is with iron tablets, such as Pregaday®, one tablet per day for 2 weeks. The woman should be advised to take the tablet 1 hour before food with orange juice, which contains ascorbic acid (vitamin C) to aid absorption of the iron. Unfortunately many brands of oral iron tablets have unpleasant gastric side-effects which reduce maternal compliance in taking them. Serum Hb estimation is undertaken after 2 weeks, and if the Hb appears to be rising, the woman should continue taking the iron tablets. However, if the Hb does not rise or there is intolerance or poor compliance, the woman should be referred to a haematology clinic for further management. Additional investigations may be undertaken to determine the cause of the anaemia and other oral iron, such as ferrous sulphate (200 mg 2–3 times daily) may be prescribed. If there is still intolerance to oral iron, then parenteral iron injections will be offered. These injections, however, are uncomfortable and can cause iron staining on the skin, so the *z-track injection method* should be used. Blood transfusion is used only in extreme cases during pregnancy (Addo et al 2013).

If the anaemia persists then the woman should be assessed regarding her risk for haemorrhage. An IVI should be sited in labour and blood samples taken for full blood count (FBC) and for group and save. The FBC results should be reviewed before the woman either eats or drinks. The midwife should be alert for signs of maternal exhaustion during labour with active management of the third stage of labour being undertaken, and all perineal trauma should be sutured to minimize the effects of blood loss at the time of the birth.

In the postnatal period the woman with anaemia is at risk of infection, postpartum haemorrhage, depression and poor wound healing. The midwife should observe and support her accordingly and ensure that a FBC blood sample is taken to identify further treatment requirements. Contraceptive advice should be given for adequate spacing of pregnancies along with dietary advice and a follow-up appointment. The FBC will also need repeating at the 6 week postnatal examination.

Folic acid deficiency

Folic acid is part of the vitamin B complex. In pregnancy it is necessary for effective cell growth and synthesis of ribonucleic acid (RNA) and deoxyribonucleic acid (DNA) especially the embryo, and a deficiency is associated with neural tube defects in the fetus. Deficiency can be due to multiple pregnancy, poor diet, adverse social circumstances and may arise secondary to drug therapy such as antiepileptic drugs (AEDs). The average daily folate requirements rise in pregnancy from 50 to 400 µg/day (Addo et al 2013). Although this can usually be met through a healthy diet, women are encouraged to take prophylactic folic acid 400 µg/day (0.4 mg) routinely in the first trimester, which should be increased to 5 mg if the woman is also taking AEDs or other drugs affecting folate metabolism. Chronic maternal folate deficiency can lead to megaloblastic anaemia (Greer et al 2007).

Megaloblastic anaemia

Megaloblastic anaemia refers to an abnormality of the erythroblasts in the bone marrow in which the maturation of the nucleus is delayed due to defective DNA synthesis resulting in the production of larger than normal red blood cells (*macrocytosis*). This arises from a deficiency of either of two B vitamins, *folic acid* and *cyanocobalmin* (B12), both of which are necessary for DNA synthesis (Kumar and Clark 2004). A deficiency of vitamin B12 alone is termed *pernicious anaemia*. One third of pregnancies worldwide are affected by megaloblastic anaemia, but the UK incidence is low at 0.5%. Megaloblastic anaemia is secondary to dietary deficiency (especially a vegan diet), alcoholism; gastrointestinal surgery, autoimmune disease, medical disorders, especially sickle cell disease, and drug therapy, e.g. azathioprine (Kumar and Clark 2004; NICE 2013).

Diagnosis is made through taking a detailed history from the woman, undertaking a physical examination and investigations including a FBC, blood film and assessing serum concentrations of vitamin B12 and folate. If vitamin B12 deficiency is evident, serum anti-intrinsic factor and antiparietal cell antibodies should be examined. If folate levels are low, tests for anti-endomysial or anti-transglutaminase antibodies are likely to be performed (NICE 2013). Treatment is determined according to the identity of the underlying cause. Supplements of *folic acid* and *cyanocobalmin* will be prescribed as necessary, and a referral to a dietician may be necessary.

The midwife has an important role in identifying at-risk women and referring them to appropriate personnel, encouraging compliance with medication and providing dietary advice.

Haemoglobinopathies

Haemoglobinopathies are a group of inherited conditions with abnormalities of the Hb. Haemoglobin consists of a group of four molecules, each of which as a *haem* unit made up of an iron porphyrin complex and a protein or *globin* chain. A total of 97% of adult Hb (HbA) has two α- and two β-chains and the remaining 3% is composed of two α- and two δ-chains. Fetal Hb (HbF) has two α- and two γ-chains, the latter being gradually replaced by the β-chain by around the age of 6 months. The type of globin chain is genetically determined and defective genes lead to the formation of abnormal haemoglobin. This may be as a result of impaired globin synthesis (*thalassaemia syndromes*) or from structural abnormality of globin (*haemoglobin variants* such as *sickle cell anaemia*). Haemoglobinopathies mainly affect people from Africa, West Indies, Asia, the Middle East and the eastern Mediterranean and the theory is that the carrier state offers some protection against malaria (Greer et al 2007).

Thalassaemia

There are different types of thalassaemia depending upon which haemoglobin chain has been affected: α-chains are formed by two genes from each parent whereas β-chains are formed by one gene from each parent. In α-thalassaemia, the production of α-globin is deficient and in β-thalassaemia the production of β-globin is defective. The classifications are:

α-thalassaemia

- *Normal:* genotype = α/α, α/α.
- α^+-*thalassaemia heterozygous:* genotype = $\alpha/-$, α/α. One defective α gene. Borderline Hb level and mean corpuscular volume (MCV), low mean corpuscular Hb (MCH): clinically asymptomatic.
- α^+-*thalassaemia homozygous:* genotype = $\alpha/-$, $\alpha/-$. Two defective α genes. Slightly anaemic, low MCV and MCH; clinically asymptomatic. This is known as *thalassaemia trait* and is associated with Africans.
- α^o-*thalassaemia heterozygous:* genotype = α/α, $-/-$. Two defective α genes. Slightly anaemic, low MCV and MCH; clinically asymptomatic. This is also known as *thalassaemia trait* and is associated with Asians.
- Haemoglobin H disease (HbH): genotype = $\alpha/-$, $-/-$. Three defective α genes. Mild to moderate anaemia with very low MCV and MCH; splenomegaly and variable bone changes.
- α-thalassaemia major: genotype = $-/-$, $-/-$. Four defective α genes. This type is also known as Hb Bart's. It presents as severe non-immune intrauterine haemolytic anaemia where the fetus has little circulating haemoglobin that is all tetrametric γ-chains. As a result the fetus becomes oedematous: known as *hydrops fetalis/Hb Bart's hydrops*, which is usually fatal (Addo et al 2013).

β-thalassaemia

- *Normal:* genotype = $\beta2$, $\beta2$.
- *β-thalassaemia trait:* genotype = $-$, $\beta2$. One defective β gene is inherited. HbA2 is >4% and the individual presents with mild anaemia, a low MCV and MCH, but is clinically asymptomatic.
- *β-thalassaemia intermedia:* genotype = $-$, βo or $\beta+$, $\beta+$. Both defective β genes are inherited. This type presents with high levels of HbF which can fluctuate, resulting in anaemia upon which symptoms usually develop when the haemoglobin level remains below 7.0 g/dl, a very low MCV and MCH, splenomegaly and variable bone changes. The dependency on blood transfusion to improve an individual's wellbeing is variable.
- *β-thalassaemia major:* genotype = $-$o/$-$o. In this type, both defective β genes are also inherited, but the Hb is comprised of >90% HbF (untransfused). As a result, the individual presents with severe haemolytic anaemia, a very low MCV and MCH, and hepatosplenomegaly, such that they are chronically dependent on frequent blood transfusions (Addo et al 2013).

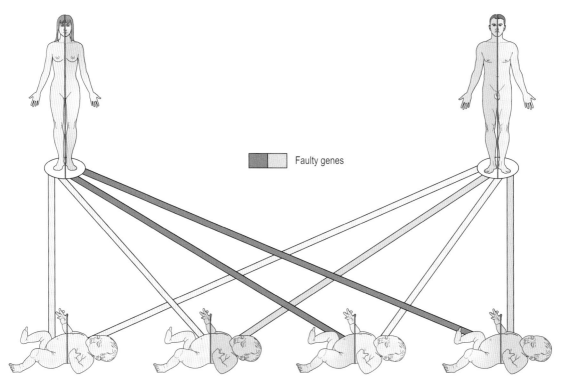

Fig. 13.2 The inheritance of a haemoglobinopathy when both parents are heterozygous.

Diagnosis is made by identifying those at high risk and performing the following:

- full blood count that would reveal a low mean corpuscular haemoglobin (MCH <27 pg) and a low mean cell volume (MCV <75 fl)
- bone marrow examination would reveal microcytic, hypochromic red blood cells
- haemoglobin analysis would reveal elevated HbA$_2$ levels (Addo et al 2013).

Pre-conception care is important and genetic counselling may be required, especially if there is inter-marriage of cousins. There is a 1 in 4 chance of a baby inheriting a major condition if both parents are carriers (see Fig. 13.2).

In early pregnancy diagnostic tests are offered to the woman, consisting of DNA analysis of chorionic villi and fetal blood sampling (Addo et al 2013) with termination of pregnancy being discussed should the fetus be adversely affected. Antenatal care should be provided within an obstetric unit where the woman can be assessed within a combined clinic with a haematologist in attendance. The treatment would entail regular assessment of FBC and serum ferritin. Iron is prescribed only if serum ferritin levels are low as there is a risk of iron overload, which may lead to congestive cardiac failure. Consequently, further investigations may be required to assess cardiac function.

Folic acid deficiency must be treated and dietary advice given by the midwife (Addo et al 2013).

If the woman has *thalassaemia major* she is at risk of pre-term labour, which might be iatrogenic, as well as both maternal and fetal hypoxia in labour. If the woman has any bone deformities, caesarean section may be necessary. There should be continuous fetal monitoring in labour and strict monitoring of blood pressure and fluid balance. Due to the risk of haemorrhage, it would be wise for the midwife to facilitate active management of the third stage of labour.

During the postnatal period, the woman should be observed for signs of infection and haemorrhage and any wound should be inspected for signs of poor healing. Furthermore, the anaemia might worsen following the birth and tiredness could also predispose to depression. The baby will require paediatric assessment prior to transfer home from hospital and any follow-up appointments should be made to monitor growth and development as well as determine the baby's thalassaemia status.

Sickle cell disease

Sickle cell disease refers to a group of disorders arising from defective genes that produce abnormal Hb molecules

(HbS). Defective genes produce abnormal haemoglobin α- or β-chains resulting in HbS. There are several variations and those of most significance to the midwife are the homozygous sickle cell anaemia/sickle cell disease (*HbSS*) and heterozygous sickle cell trait (*HbAS*).

Other variations can be summarized as follows.

- *Sickle cell HbC disease (HbSC)*: double heterozygote for HbS and HbC with intermediate clinical severity.
- *Sickle cell β⁰-thalassaemia (HbS/β⁰)*: severe double heterozygote for HbS and β⁰-thalassaemia with no normal β-chains produced. It is almost clinically indistinguishable from sickle cell anaemia.
- *Sickle cell β⁺-thalassaemia (HbS/β⁺)*: In this type a reduced amount of chains are made resulting in mild-to-moderate anaemia.

In sickle cell anaemia (HbSS) the erythrocytes are fragile, with a short life span of 17 days, compared with 120 days in a healthy individual. The erythrocytes have a characteristic crescent, or sickle, shape which blocks up the capillaries. This predisposes to clot formation in the capillaries. Diagnosis is by Hb electrophoresis, and identification of the abnormal sickle-shaped cells on a blood film. A bone marrow biopsy may also be required. Treatment outside of pregnancy includes the administration of 1 mg/day oral folic acid tablets, prophylactic penicillin, thromboprophylaxis, iron chelation agents and exchange blood transfusion.

A sickle cell crisis arises when the sickle cells form clots in the capillaries resulting in deoxygenation, and tissue death as a result of infarction. The crisis presents acutely with severe pain, breathlessness, pallor, fever, joint swelling and pain, and general weakness (Addo et al 2013). The crisis can be triggered, or exacerbated, by infection, cold temperature, dehydration, stress and exercise. Other complications are chronic anaemia, bone marrow suppression, thromboembolic disease, cardiac failure due to chronic hypoxaemia and aplastic anaemia, as well as sudden death (Addo et al 2013).

Pre-conception care is important to optimize the health of the woman, during which time the folic acid should be increased to 5 mg/day and iron chelation discontinued 3–6 months prior to conception due to possible teratogenicity (Addo et al 2013). If the woman has pulmonary hypertension, pregnancy is contraindicated due to the 50% maternal mortality risk (Oteng-Ntim et al 2006).

In pregnancy the woman's care should be shared between the obstetric and haematology team, with appointments being made for every 2–4 weeks to assess maternal and fetal wellbeing. The woman presenting with sickle cell anaemia is at risk of experiencing a sickle cell crisis secondary to infection, pre-eclampsia, miscarriage, IUGR, stillbirth and possible maternal death. Investigations include FBC, blood group and antibody screen, reticulocyte count, serum ferritin levels, HIV and hepatitis screening (because

of history of blood transfusions) renal and liver function tests. Folic acid should be increased to 5 mg/day if not done so pre-conceptually, and iron supplements only given if indicated by serum ferritin results. Antibiotic therapy may need to be continued. In the third trimester serial growth scans should be undertaken (RCOG 2011c; Addo et al 2013).

In labour an epidural is recommended for pain relief as opiates should be avoided. Blood should be taken for FBC, group and save. Graduated compression stockings are used to reduce the risk of VTE and the woman should be kept warm and hydrated to prevent any sickle cell crisis from occurring. Oxygen therapy might be required to maintain adequate oxygenation and improve cardiac function. Prophylactic antibiotics may be considered to reduce infection. A prolonged labour should be avoided and active management or caesarean section may be advised depending on the woman's health (RCOG 2011c; Addo et al 2013). Where there is IUGR, continuous fetal monitoring would also be recommended.

During the postnatal period, the midwife should be vigilant in her observations as the woman is at increased risk of sickle cell crisis, thromboembolism and postpartum haemorrhage. Prophylactic antibiotics and thromboprophylaxis should continue and early mobilization is encouraged. Four-hourly observations should be undertaken, including respiration rate. The woman should be advised about subsequent pregnancies and the risk they carry in increasing the frequency of crises. It is therefore important that the woman uses appropriate contraception in order to maximize her health as intrauterine contraceptive devices (IUCDs) are relatively contraindicated due to the risk of infection. Neonatal screening of babies must be undertaken by obtaining a capillary or venous sample of blood at birth. Those with a positive result require a follow-up appointment and electrophoresis at 6 weeks, including prophylactic antibiotic cover from 3 months of age (Addo et al 2013).

In sickle cell trait (HbAS) the individual is usually asymptomatic. Although the sickle screening test is positive, the blood appears normal. In pregnancy the woman may present with mild anaemia and so 5 mg/day folic acid is recommended to improve erythropoiesis.

NEUROLOGICAL DISORDERS

Epilepsy

Epilepsy is a common neurological disorder characterized by two or more seizures, with a UK prevalence of 9.7 per 1000 (0.97%) and a reduction in life expectancy of 2–10 years. It mainly presents in childhood, although there is a second peak of incidence in older years and women of childbearing age account for 23% of the population

Table 13.5 Categories of epileptic seizures

Category	Type	Characteristics
Partial	Simple	Remains conscious Experiences an aura (premonition) *Déjà vu* (experienced this previously) Pins and needles sensation in arms or legs Pallor, or alternatively a flushed face with sweating Muscle twitching in limbs with some stiffness
	Complex	Awareness of changes; loses memory of the event Rubbing of hands Chewing and smacking of lips Picking at clothes or fiddling Makes random noises Exhibits unusual posture
Generalized	Absence	Staring and blinking, day dreaming, loss of awareness for 5–20 seconds (*mainly affects children*)
	Myoclonic	Brief muscle jerking in an arm or leg. Lasts for a fraction of a second and individual remains conscious
	Tonic	All body muscles contract for <20 seconds, but there are no convulsions. The individual falls
	Tonic–clonic	The whole body contracts, then arms and legs convulse. Incontinence is possible. Lasts 1–2 minutes and the individual appears tired, wanting to sleep. The most common type of seizure (60% of cases)
	Atonic	All muscle tone is lost momentarily. The individual falls limply and head injury is probable, but gets up immediately with no confusion

Source: Adapted from McAuliffe et al 2013

affected by epilepsy, with a prevalence in pregnancy of 0.35%.

Seizures result from a sudden excess of electricity to the brain disrupting the normal message passing between the *cortical neurons* (brain cells). The messages become mixed or halted, and a seizure results. These seizures can be subcategorized as partial and generalized (McAuliffe et al 2013), as shown in Table 13.5.

Complications associated with epilepsy are:

- *Trauma* occurring during the seizure and include tongue biting and head or limb injury.
- *Status epilepticus:* a seizure lasting for >30 minutes, or a series of seizures without regaining consciousness in between.
- *Sudden Unexpected Death in Epilepsy (SUDEP)* of which there is no cause found for the sudden death.
- *Maternal death:* the risk of sudden maternal death in pregnancy remains higher in women with epilepsy than those with other long-term conditions. A number of these maternal deaths are classified as SUDEP.

Treatment is with antiepileptic drugs (AEDs) with monotherapy (one drug) or polytherapy (two or more) if seizure control is more problematic. In certain cases surgery or vagus nerve stimulation might be used (McAuliffe et al 2013).

Pre-conception care is of paramount importance as many AEDs are associated with folate deficiency and fetal abnormalities. The drug therapy may be changed to monotherapy after careful counselling about the risks of teratogenicity to the fetus and folic acid should be prescribed at an increased dose of 5 mg/day for 12 weeks prior to conception (McAuliffe et al 2013).

Management in pregnancy presents challenges and this is a high-risk pregnancy that requires referral and birth in a consultant obstetric unit. It is important to involve family and partners, as they may need to initiate first aid and safety measures as the seizure risk increases by 15–37% (McAuliffe et al 2013). Folic acid of 5 mg/day should be given throughout the first trimester, and if the woman is taking sodium valproate this should continue for all three trimesters. Women taking enzyme-inducing AEDs will require oral vitamin K for 4 weeks prior to the baby's birth to decrease the risk of fetal coagulopathy

(McAuliffe et al 2013). Antiepileptic drug levels should be monitored at regular intervals and the drugs and dosage reviewed by the obstetric team. The midwife should encourage the woman to comply with the pre-scribed medication. In addition advice should be given to avoid bathing alone and steamy environments, and to keep bathroom doors unlocked in case of a seizure. Screening for fetal anomalies should be discussed and then initiated after informed consent. A detailed struc-tural ultrasound scan is offered between 18 and 22 weeks of pregnancy.

For labour the midwife should discuss a realistic birth plan, and be aware that water birth is contraindicated on safety grounds (McAuliffe et al 2013). The risk of tonic–clonic seizure in labour is low at 1–2% but measures should be taken to react speedily should a seizure result. The management principles for an epileptic seizure are the same as for eclampsia (see Box 13.7). Anticonvulsant medication is continued throughout labour and regular review by the obstetric team is indicated. If seizures recur, short-acting benzodiazepines are administered (McAuliffe et al 2013). The woman should not be left alone in labour, and dehydration, hyperventilation and exhaustion should be avoided as they can all trigger a seizure. Should a seizure result, the differential diagnosis of eclampsia needs to be considered (Lowe and Sen 2005). Pethidine is contraindicated as it is metabolized to norpethidine which can also induce seizure, and either trans-electrical nerve stimulation (TENS) or epidural should be considered as an alternative. The birth can be spontaneously facilitated by the midwife. Following obtaining informed consent from the woman, vitamin K should be administered to the baby promptly after birth to protect against AED-induced haemorrhagic disease (McAuliffe et al 2013).

In the first 24 hours following the birth the woman has an increased risk of a seizure and so should remain in hospital. Breastfeeding is encouraged and the medical team and pharmacist should discuss suitable AEDs while lactating. The baby should be carefully observed and any concerns reported to the paediatrician immediately. Antiepileptic drugs affect hormonal contraceptives and alternative contraception such as barrier methods are rec-ommended (see Chapter 27). Advice should be given about safety when caring for the baby in case of mater-nal seizure. The midwife should encourage the woman to dress, change and feed the baby on a changing mat on the floor to prevent falling during a seizure while attend-ing to the baby. It is advisable that the baby is bathed by the mother in shallow water when someone else is around to assist if necessary and a carrycot or baby car seat should be used to carry the baby up and down stairs. When parents choose a pram/buggy for their baby, the midwife should advise them to ensure that they select one with brakes that initiate when the handle is released.

INFECTION/SEPSIS

Genital tract sepsis

Genital tract sepsis is a major cause of maternal morbidity and mortality and accounted for 29 deaths in the most recent triennial report, being the leading cause of direct maternal deaths in the UK (Harper 2011). Of these deaths, three were classified as *late* direct deaths occurring more than 6 weeks after the baby's birth, albeit the women became ill *before* or *soon after* they had given birth and so should be of great concern to all health professionals undertaking maternity care.

Genital tract sepsis arises from polymicrobial infections, usually from streptococcal bacteria, which can lead to overwhelming septicaemia that can affect not only the wellbeing of the pregnant woman but also the fetus. Signs and symptoms include pyrexia, swinging pyrexia and hypothermia, abdominal pain, diarrhoea, vomiting, tach-ycardia and tachypnoea. All childbearing woman should be advised of the possible signs and symptoms of infec-tion at all stages and be encouraged to seek advice promptly, to pay attention to effective hygiene and be aware of the risk from others , particularly any who have bacterial throat infections (Draycott et al 2011).

Bacterial Vaginosis (BV)

It is estimated that between 10%–30% of women will experience Bacterial vaginosis (BV) during their pregnancy, which is a common cause of abnormal discharge due to an imbalance of normal bacteria that inhabit the vagina. Typical symptoms are an offensive, fishy-smelling dis-charge. Although BV may regress spontaneously and even if treated with topical or oral metronidazole or clindamy-cin, it may recur. Whilst there is evidence that links BV with preterm labour, late miscarriage, and premature rupture of membranes, treatment studies have yielded inconsistent results. Consequently, current guidelines only recommends screening pregnant women identified as high risk of preterm birth (Hay 2012).

Candida albicans

Candida albicans is a yeast that causes itching, soreness and swelling of the genital area producing a creamy-white vaginal discharge. Candida albicans is not a Sexually Transmitted Infection (STI) as it commonly occurs during pregnancy, following antibiotic therapy and in individuals who have diabetes or a lowered immune system. It is easily diagnosed by a high vaginal swab (HVS) and treatment in pregnancy is via topical cream and/or vaginal pessaries, rather than via the oral route. Candida does not affect fertility or pregnancy outcome, but the baby may develop oral or genital thrush. This in turn may affect breastfeeding should candida be transferred to the breast while feeding (Francis-Morrill et al 2004; Weiner 2006).

Chlamydia trachomatis

Chlamydia is the most commonly diagnosed STI, especially in under 25-year-olds, and is caused by the bacterium *Chlamydia trachomatis*. Between 70 and 80% of women affected by chlamydia are asymptomatic. Signs and symptoms usually occur from 1 to 3 weeks following infection and include dysuria, vaginal discharge, lower abdominal pain, post-coital and inter-menstrual bleeding, anal discharge, conjunctivitis, eye infections and sore throats following anal or oral sexual practices. If left untreated, chlamydial infection can cause pelvic inflammatory disease (PID), which increases infertility and the risk of miscarriage and ectopic pregnancy.

Methods of testing are varied and can include urine testing, low vaginal swab (self-testing kits) and cervical swab. The NHS National Chlamydia Screening Programme (2012) recommends annual screening for under 25-year-olds if sexually active. Chlamydia can be transmitted to the neonate during vaginal birth and can result in neonatal eye infections and pneumonia. Treatment entails antibiotics such as azithromycin.

Cytomegalovirus

Cytomegalovirus (CMV) is a common viral infection from the *herpes family*, which may lie dormant and recur at a later time. It is estimated that 50% of the adult population has had the infection at some point in their lives. The virus causes a mild flu-like illness and pregnant women have an increased susceptibility to infection during pregnancy. However, primary infection in pregnancy is low, at around 1%. There is a 40% chance of transmission to the fetus causing congenital malformations such as hearing loss, learning difficulties and cerebral palsy. Around 5–10% of infected babies are symptomatic at birth and consequently their prognosis is poor. Furthermore, the risk relative to gestation is unclear. Although antiviral drugs have been used to treat CMV, there is currently no screening programme due to a lack of sensitivity in pregnancy or evidence-based effective treatment interventions (UK National Screening Committee 2012).

Gonorrhoea

Gonorrhoea is a common STI in the UK, affecting the genital tract (especially the cervix) and rectum. It is transmitted by sexual activity with an infected individual and is caused by the bacterium *Neisseria gonorrhoeae*. Although most individuals are often asymptomatic, signs and symptoms may occur 2–10 days after initial contact (Bignall and Fitzgerald 2011). Such symptoms include painful micturition, yellow/bloodstained vaginal discharge and post-coital bleeding.

If untreated, in women it can cause PID, giving rise to abdominal cramps, fever and inter-menstrual bleeding, with an increased risk of ectopic pregnancy. Individuals are also at a greater risk of acquiring HIV.

Testing for gonorrhoea is via urine and cervical swabs. More effective screening programmes detect the genes of the bacteria, rather than try to culture the bacteria. Treatment is with antibiotics, but drug resistance can be problematic. Gonorrhoea can be transmitted to the neonate during vaginal birth and can result in eye infections.

Hepatitis A, B and C

Hepatitis comprises a group of blood-borne viruses that cause hepatocellular inflammation and necrosis. They are found in bodily fluids, e.g. blood, saliva and semen, and are often transmitted via sexual activity, by sharing injecting equipment and via the placenta to the fetus during pregnancy. Vaccination for hepatitis A and B are available. Hepatitis B and C can lead to liver failure and death and are therefore notifiable diseases in the UK.

Pregnant women are offered routine screening for hepatitis B during early pregnancy and those at risk, e.g. sex workers, can be tested for hepatitis C. Any woman found to have hepatitis B virus (HBV) should have further tests to determine whether she is acutely or chronically infected; the presence of the e-antigen (HBeAg) denotes high infectivity, while the presence of antibodies (antiHBe) suggest a lower infectivity. During pregnancy women are counselled as to how they can reduce transmission and infants should be given hepatitis B immunization and immunoglobulin with their mother's consent, which can reduce vertical transmission by 90% (Watkins et al 2013). Breastfeeding is not contraindicated, although the presence of cracked nipples is a significant transmission risk.

Human immunodeficiency virus (HIV) and acquired immune deficiency syndrome (AIDS)

The human immunodeficiency virus (HIV) is a *retrovirus* that weakens an individual's immune system by invading the T4-helper cells making it difficult to mount an immune response to infection. There are two types of HIV which belong to the lentivirus subfamily of retroviruses that cause acquired immunodeficiency syndrome (AIDS). HIV-1 is the cause of the world pandemic of acquired immune deficiency syndrome (AIDS), whereas HIV-2 is largely confined to West Africa. HIV is transmitted through unprotected sexual activity with an infected person, contact with infected bodily fluids, e.g. blood, or perinatally via mother-to-fetus-transmission. Two to six weeks after exposure to HIV, 50–70% develop a transient non-specific illness (primary infection or seroconversion illness) with flu-like symptoms, e.g. pyrexia, rash and sore throat. This coincides with the development of serum antibodies to the core and surface proteins of the virus. The illness begins abruptly and usually lasts for 1–2 weeks, but may be more protracted.

Diagnosis is through an HIV test, where blood is examined for the presence of antibodies and/or antigens; this is known as the *combined test*. Pregnant women are offered an HIV test in early pregnancy (RCOG 2010b). Although there is no cure for HIV, antiretroviral (ART) therapy has significantly reduced the morbidity and mortality observed in previous decades. Without ART, seroconversion is followed by a clinically latent phase of about 10 years. During this time there is intense viral and lymphocyte turnover with worsening immunodeficiency and about one-third of infected individuals will experience persistent lymphadenopathy. The average time for progression from HIV to AIDS is between 5 and 20 years.

The prevalence of HIV in pregnancy is around 1 in 500 maternities and management aims to reduce the rate of transmission to the fetus, however, this is <2%, as most transmission occurs during birth or in the postnatal period through breastfeeding (RCOG 2010b). Highly active antiretroviral therapy (HAART) should continue, with elective caesarean section and the avoidance of breastfeeding. Fakoya et al (2008) reported that a planned vaginal birth should be considered for those women who have plasma viral loads of <50 copies/ml. As a result, this management regime has reduced the rates of HIV transmission to the fetus to <1% (RCOG 2010b).

Human papillomavirus

The human papillomavirus (HPV) is attributed to causing the second most common STI in the UK. It has over 100 strains, of which strains 6 and 11 are known to cause genital warts, which are more common in teenagers and young adults. They present as small, fleshy, painless growths, single or in clusters, appearing on the vaginal and anal regions following close genital contact or sexual activity with an affected person. The warts usually appear within 2–3 months of infection, but can take up to a year to become evident.

Treatment is either with topical lotions/creams or physical ablation, or a combination. Pregnancy may affect the size and number of warts and there is a small risk that they may affect progress in labour, as well as there being evidence of rare cases of transmissions to the baby during birth. Human papillomavirus strains 16 and 18 are associated with cervical cancer and vaccinations are available to all young women up to the age of 18 years. Emerging evidence from Ali et al (2013) would indicate that vaccination is reducing genital wart prevalence in young women.

Streptococcus A and B

Group A streptococcus (GAS) bacteria cause a variety of infections, such as acute pharyngitis, toxic shock syndrome, cellulitis and puerperal sepsis. Group B streptococcus (GBS) bacteria are commonly found in the vagina and lower bowel of around 40% of healthy adult women, where they remain dormant. GBS is not contagious, but it can cause neonatal GBS infection if the fetus comes into contact with the bacteria, usually during birth. However, GBS infection has been known to pass across the membranes and colonize the fetus *in utero*.

Women at higher risk of GBS include those in preterm labour, those with premature pre-labour rupture of membranes, prolonged rupture of membranes (>18 hr), and those with maternal pyrexia and a previous history of GBS. Screening is not currently offered routinely to all women but may be in the future, according to Plumb and Clayton (2013), and consists of lower vaginal swabs and rectal swabs in those at risk and IV antibiotics administered between 4 and 6 hours before birth (RCOG 2012).

GBS affects 1 in 1000 of all babies and has a mortality rate of 1 in 10, with survivors often having severe long-term disabilities (Plumb and Clayton 2013). There are two types of neonatal GBS. The most common type is *early onset GBS*, which is seen in 75% of cases and occurs within the first week of life, usually presenting within 24 hours of birth. The other type is *late onset GBS*, which presents in 25% of cases within the first 3 months of life. Signs and symptoms in an affected neonate may be vague and include problems maintaining their temperature, grunting, limpness, poor feeding behaviours and seizures. It is very important that midwives inform women of the signs and symptoms and promptly refer any ill baby.

Syphilis

Syphilis is a STI caused by the spirochete bacterium *Treponema pallidum*. Transmission occurs through contact with a syphilitic sore or chancre. Although the incidence of syphilis is low in the UK, worldwide the incidence in developing countries is 90%. There are four stages to the progression of the infection:

- *Primary*: occurring on average 21 days after exposure, where a single painless, firm, non-itchy ulcer or chancre appears.
- *Secondary*: occurs between 4 and 10 weeks after exposure, with the appearance of a non-itchy, diffuse rash with fever and sore throat evident. In the latent stage, the individual is generally asymptomatic, but still contagious to others.
- *Tertiary*: can occur between 3 to 15 years after the initial exposure. If the individual does not seek treatment, they will exhibit neurological symptoms such as general paresis and seizures, as well as cardiac symptoms including aneurysms.

The presence of syphilitic sores increases the transmission risk of HIV. Diagnosis is via a blood test and the treatment is penicillin. It is highly likely that transmission of syphilis will occur in pregnancy, causing preterm birth, stillbirth or perinatal death, thus screening for syphilis should be routinely offered to all pregnant women during the early antenatal period (NICE 2010c; Watkins et al 2013). The baby may be born with *congenital syphilis*, which is asymptomatic during infancy, but later in childhood they may develop multi-organ conditions such as deafness, seizures and cataracts.

Urinary tract infection

Urinary tract infection (UTI) is a common problem in pregnancy if pathogenic bacteria colonize the urinary tract. The bacteria originate from the bowel and the most commonly encountered is *Escherichia coli* (*E. coli*). Such an infection may be asymptomatic or present with symptoms of *dysuria* (a burning pain on micturition), *frequency* (small regular amounts of urine), *suprapubic discomfort* and *haematuria* (blood in the urine). If the infection is confined to the bladder it is termed *cystitis*, and in addition to these symptoms there may be *urgency* of micturition.

The infection can ascend to the kidneys and pyelonephritis develops. Acute pyelonephritis may present with nausea and vomiting, pyrexia, rigors and abdominal pain (James et al 2011). If inadequately treated, septicaemia may result, leading to acute renal failure, multiple organ failure and death (Brunskill and Goodlife 2013).

Asymptomatic bacteriuria (ABU), as the name implies, is an infection without symptoms and occurs in 2–10% of pregnancies (NICE 2010c). The presence of 10^5/ml of the same bacterial species in a midstream specimen of urine (MSSU) in the absence of symptoms confirms the diagnosis. This is of significance in pregnancy, as 25% of women will proceed to develop pyelonephritis and there is also risk of preterm labour (James et al 2011).

All pregnant women should have their urine tested for nitrates (which are produced by most urinary pathogens) at each antenatal visit. A mid-stream specimen of urine (MSSU) should be taken early in pregnancy (NICE 2010c), and repeated if there are symptoms of a UTI. Treatment is with antibiotics according to the culture and sensitivity from the MSSU results, and the MSSU should be repeated following treatment. If the causative organism is group B streptococcus, an alert note should be placed on the woman's maternity case notes. The midwife should encourage the woman to drink at least 2 litres of fluid per day, comply with antibiotic therapy, give advice on personal hygiene, especially following micturition, and recommend cranberry juice which may reduce infection and its symptoms (Brunskill and Goodlife 2013).

If the infection is still active when the woman commences labour she should be reviewed by the obstetrician and IV antibiotics may be commenced for the duration of labour and the immediate postnatal period. Urinary catheterization should be avoided. If the UTI persists into the postnatal period, then further investigations are indicated (Brunskill and Goodlife 2013).

REFERENCES

Addo A, Oppenheimer C, Robson S E 2013 Haematological disorders. In: Robson S E, Waugh J (eds) Medical disorders in pregnancy: a manual for midwives, 2nd edn. Wiley–Blackwell, Oxford, p 255–78

Ali H, Donovan B, Wand H et al 2013 Genital warts in young Australians five years into national human papillomavirus vaccination programme: national surveillance data. British Medical Journal 346:f2032

Amir L, Donath S 2007 A systematic review of maternal obesity and breastfeeding intention, initiation and duration. BMC Pregnancy and Childbirth 7:9 www.biomedcentral.com/1471-2393/7/9

Avery A, Allan J, Lavin J et al 2010 Supporting postnatal women to lose weight. Journal of Human Nutrition and Dietetics 23(4):439

Bagot C N, Arya R 2008 Virchow and his triad: a question of attribution. British Journal of Haematology 143(2):180–90

Baker J, Gamborg M, Heitmann B et al 2008 Breastfeeding reduces postpartum weight retention. American Journal of Clinical Nutrition 88:1543–51

Basaran A, Basaran M, Topatan B 2010 Combined vitamin C and E supplementation for the prevention of pre-eclampsia: a systematic review and metanalysis. Obstetrical and Gynecological Survey 65:653–67

Bellamy L, Casas J P, Hingorani A D et al 2009 Type 2 diabetes mellitus after gestational diabetes: a systematic review and meta-analysis. Lancet 373(9677):1773–9

Bignall C, Fitzgerald M 2011 [The British Association for Sexual Health and HIV (BASHH) Guideline Development Group] UK national guideline for the management of gonorrhoea in adults. International Journal of STD and AIDS 22:541–7. http://www.bashh.org/documents/3920.pdf (accessed 14 September 2014)

BTS (British Thoracic Society)/SIGN (Scottish Intercollegiate Guidelines Network) 2011 British Guideline on the Management of Asthma. BTS/SIGN, London, Edinburgh

Brunskill N J, Goodlife A 2013 Renal disorders. In: Robson S E, Waugh J (eds) Medical disorders in pregnancy: a manual for midwives, 2nd edn. Wiley-Blackwell, Oxford, p 91–104

Burrow G N, Duffey T P, Copel J A 2004 Hypertensive disorders in pregnancy. In: Medical complications during pregnancy, 6th edn. Elsevier, London, p 43–67

CMACE (Centre for Maternal and Child Enquiries) 2011 Saving mothers' lives: reviewing maternal deaths to make motherhood safer: 2006–08. The Eighth Report on Confidential Enquiries into Maternal Deaths in the United Kingdom. BJOG: An International Journal of Obstetrics and Gynaecology 118(Suppl 1): 1–203

Clark P, Thomson A J, Greer I A 2012 Haematological problems in pregnancy. In: Edmonds K (ed) Dewhurst's textbook of obstetrics and gynaecology, 8th edn. Wiley–Blackwell, Oxford, p 151–72

Clarke C E, Taylor R S, Shore A C et al 2012 The difference in blood pressure readings between arms and survival: primary care cohort study. British Medical Journal 344:e1327

Copple M, Coser P 2013 Stop the clot. Midwives 4:48–9

Craig J, McLelland D, Ludlam C 2006 Blood disorders. In: Boon N B, Colledge N R, Walker B R (eds) Davidson's principles and practice of medicine, 20th edn. Elsevier, London, p 1060–1

de Swiet M, Williamson C, Lewis G 2011 Other indirect deaths. In: CMACE (Centre for Maternal and Child Enquiries) 2011 Saving mothers' lives: reviewing maternal deaths to make motherhood safer: 2006–08. The Eighth Report on Confidential Enquiries into Maternal Deaths in the United Kingdom. BJOG: An International Journal of Obstetrics and Gynaecology 118(Suppl 1):119–31

de Valk H W, Visser G H A 2011 Insulin during pregnancy, labour and delivery. Best Practice & Research in Clinical Obstetrics and Gynaecology 25:65–76

de Vries J 2007 The obesity epidemic: medical and ethical considerations. Science and Engineering Ethics 13:55–67

Dornhorst A, Williamson C 2012 Diabetes and endocrine disease in pregnancy. In: Edmonds K (ed) Dewhurst's textbook of obstetrics and gynaecology, 8th edn. Wiley–Blackwell, Oxford, p 121–36

Doughty R, Waugh J 2013 Metabolic disorders. In: Robson S E, Waugh J (eds) Medical disorders in pregnancy: a manual for midwives, 2nd edn. Wiley–Blackwell, Oxford, p 241–54

Draycott T, Lewis G, Stephens I 2011 Centre for Maternal and Child Enquiries (CMACE) Executive Summary. BJOG: An International Journal of Obstetrics and Gynaecology 118(Suppl 1):E12–21

Drife J 2011 Thrombosis and thromboembolism. In: CMACE (Centre for Maternal and Child Enquiries) 2011 Saving mothers' lives: reviewing maternal deaths to make motherhood safer: 2006–08. The Eighth Report on Confidential Enquiries into Maternal Deaths in the United Kingdom. BJOG: An International Journal of Obstetrics and Gynaecology 118(Suppl 1): 57–65

Eleftheriades M, Tsapakis E, Sotiriadis A et al 2012 Detection of congenital heart defects throughout pregnancy: impact of first trimester ultrasound screening for cardiac abnormalities. Journal of Maternal–Fetal and Neonatal Medicine 25(12):2546–50

Elliott D, Pavord S 2013 Thrombo-embolic disorders. In: Robson S E, Waugh J (eds) Medical disorders in pregnancy: a manual for midwives, 2nd edn. Wiley–Blackwell, Oxford, p 279–97

England L J, Levine R J, Qian C et al 2004 Glucose tolerance and risk of gestational diabetes mellitus in nulliparous women who smoke during pregnancy. American Journal of Epidemiology 160(12):1205–13

Fakoya A, Lamba H, Mackie N 2008 British HIV Association, BASHH and FSRH Guidelines for the Management of the Sexual and Reproductive Health of People Living with HIV Infection. HIV Medicine 9:681–720

Foresight 2007 Tackling obesities: future choices. DH/Government Office for Science, London. www.bis.gov.uk/assets/bispartners/foresight/docs/obesity/17.pdf p34 (accessed 13 October 2013)

Francis-Morrill J, Heinig M, Pappagianis D 2004 Diagnostic value of signs and symptoms of mammary candidosis. Journal of Human Lactation 20(3):288–95

Gard M, Wright J 2005 The obesity epidemic: science, morality and ideology. Routledge Press, Oxford

Gardner B, Wardle J, Poston L et al 2011 Changing diet and physical activity to reduce gestational weight gain: a meta-analysis. International Association for the Study of Obesity 12:e602–e620

Girling J 2006 Thyroid disorders in pregnancy. Current Obstetrics and Gynaecology 16:47–53

Gluckman P, Hanson M 2012 Fat, fate and disease. Oxford University Press, Oxford

Greer I, Nelson-Piercy C, Walters B 2007 Maternal medicine: medical problems in pregnancy. Elsevier, London

Gregory R, Todd D 2013 Endocrine disorders. In: Robson S E, Waugh J (eds) Medical disorders in pregnancy: a manual for midwives, 2nd edn. Wiley–Blackwell, Oxford, p 105–24

Harper A 2011 Sepsis. In: CMACE (Centre for Maternal and Child Enquiries) 2011 Saving mothers' lives: reviewing maternal deaths to make motherhood safer: 2006–08. The Eighth Report on Confidential Enquiries into Maternal Deaths in the United Kingdom. BJOG: An International Journal of Obstetrics and Gynaecology 118(Suppl 1): 85–96

Hay P 2012 BASHH Guidelines, UK National Guideline for the management of Bacterial Vaginosis 2012. http://www.bashh.org/documents/4413.pdf (accessed 14 September 2014)

Heslehurst N, Rankin J, Wilkinson J R et al 2010 A nationally representative study of maternal obesity in England, UK: trends in incidence and demographic inequalities in 619,323 births, 1989–2007. International Journal of Obesity (London) 34:420–8

Holmes S, Scullion J 2011 Better asthma control could avoid majority of hospital admissions. Guidelines in Practice 14(7):1–8. Online at www.eguidelines.co.uk/eguidelinesmain/gip/vol_14/jul_11/holmes_asthma_jul11.php (accessed 23 October 2013)

Hughes C, Spence D, Holmes V A et al 2010 Pre-conception care for women with diabetes: the midwife's role.

British Journal of Midwifery 18(3):144–9

Hull J, Rucklidge M 2009 Management of severe pre-eclampsia and eclampsia. Update in Anaesthesia 25(2):49–54

Hutcheon J A, Lisonkova S, Joseph K 2011 Epidemiology of pre-eclampsia and the other hypertensive disorders of pregnancy. Best Practice in Research Clinical Obstetrics and Gynaecology 25:391–403

James D K, Steer P J, Weiner C P et al (eds) 2011 High risk pregnancy management options, 4th edn. Elsevier, London

Jevitt C, Hernandez I, Groer M 2007 Lactation complicated by overweight and obesity: supporting the mother and newborn. Journal of Midwifery and Women's Health 52(6):606–13

Johnson S, Burrows A, Williamson I 2004 Does my bump look good in this? The meaning of bodily changes for first-time mothers-to-be. Journal of Health Psychology 9(3):361–74

Kerrigan A M, Kingdon C 2010 Maternal obesity and pregnancy: a retrospective study. Midwifery 26:138–46

Khlat M, Jusot F, Ville I 2009 Social origins, early hardship and obesity: a strong association in women, but not in men? Social Science and Medicine 68:1692–9

Knight M 2007 Eclampsia in the United Kingdom 2005. BJOG: An International Journal of Obstetrics and Gynaecology 114:1072–8

Kumar P, Clarke M 2004 Clinical medicine, 5th edn. Saunders, London

Llewelyn C 2013 We've got it covered! Graduated compression stockings. The Practising Midwife 16(5):19–20, 22.

Lowe S A, Sen R 2005 Neurological disease in pregnancy. Current Obstetrics and Gynaecology 15:166–73

Marshall J E, Brydon S 2012 Case Study 2. Obesity: risk management issues. In: Raynor M D, Marshall J E, Jackson K (eds) Midwifery practice: critical illness, complications and emergencies case book. Open University Press, Maidenhead, p 19–40

McAuliffe F, Burns-Kent F, Frost D et al 2013 Neurological disorders. In: Robson S E, Waugh J (eds) Medical disorders in pregnancy: a manual for midwives, 2nd edn. Wiley–Blackwell, Oxford, p 125–52

McLean M, Bu'Lock F A, Robson S E 2013 Heart disease. In Robson S E, Waugh J (eds) Medical disorders in pregnancy: a manual for midwives, 2nd edn. Wiley–Blackwell, Oxford, p 43–74

Miller E, Mitchell A 2006 Metabolic syndrome: screening, diagnosis and management. Journal of Midwifery and Women's Health 51(3): 141–51

Modder J, Fitzsimons K S 2010 Management of women with obesity in pregnancy. Joint Guideline. CMACE/RCOG, London

Nash M (2012a) Weighty matters: negotiating 'fatness' and 'in-between-ness' in early pregnancy. Feminism and Psychology 22(3): 307–23

Nash M (2012b) Working out for two: performance of fitness and feminity in Australian prenatal aerobics classes. Gender, Place and Culture 19(4):449–71

National Health Service (NHS) National Chlamydia Screening Programme 2012 National Chlamydia Screening Programme Standards, 6th edn. Health Agency, London

NICE (National Institute for Health and Clinical Excellence) 2007 Intrapartum care: care of healthy women and their babies during childbirth. CG 55. NICE, London

NICE (National Institute for Health and Clinical Excellence) 2008 Diabetes in pregnancy: management of diabetes and its complications from pre-conception to the postnatal period. CG 63. NICE, London

NICE (National Institute for Health and Clinical Excellence) 2010a Hypertension in pregnancy: the management of hypertensive disorders during pregnancy. CG 107. NICE, London

NICE (National Institute for Health and Clinical Excellence) 2010b Weight management before, during and after pregnancy. PH 27. NICE, London

NICE (National Institute for Health and Clinical Excellence) 2010c Antenatal care: routine care for the healthy pregnant woman. CG 62. NICE, London

NICE (National Institute for Health and Clinical Excellence) 2011 Hypertension: clinical management of primary hypertension in adults. CG 127. NICE, London

NICE (National Institute for Health and Care Excellence) 2013a Quality standard for asthma. QS25. NICE, London. Online. www.nice.org.uk/ guidance/QS25 (accessed 13 October 2013)

NICE (National Institute for Health and Care Excellence) 2013b Anaemia B12 and folate deficiency. Clinical Knowledge Summary. Online. http:// cks.nice.org.uk/anaemia-b12-and-folate-deficiency (accessed 13 October 2013)

Neilson J 2011 Pre-eclampsia and eclampsia. In: CMACE (Centre for Maternal and Child Enquiries) 2011 Saving mothers' lives: reviewing maternal deaths to make motherhood safer: 2006–08. The Eighth Report on Confidential Enquiries into Maternal Deaths in the United Kingdom. BJOG: An International Journal of Obstetrics and Gynaecology 118(Suppl 1): 66–70

Nelson-Piercy C 2011 Cardiac disease. In: CMACE (Centre for Maternal and Child Enquiries) 2011 Saving mothers' lives: reviewing maternal deaths to make motherhood safer: 2006–08. The Eighth Report on Confidential Enquiries into Maternal Deaths in the United Kingdom. BJOG: An International Journal of Obstetrics and Gynaecology 118(Suppl 1):109–15

Nursing and Midwifery Council (NMC) 2012 Midwives rules and standards. NMC, London

Nyman V M K, Prebensen A K, Flensner G E M 2010 Obese women's experiences of encounters with midwives and physicians during pregnancy and childbirth. Midwifery 26(4):424–9

Oteng-Ntim E, Cottee C, Bewley S et al 2006 Sickle cell disease in pregnancy. Current Obstetrics and Gynaecology 16:353–60

Oteng-Ntim E, Varma R, Crocker H et al 2011 Lifestyle interventions for overweight and obese pregnant women to improve pregnancy outcome: systematic review and meta-analysis. BMC Medicine 10:47

Pallister C, Allan J, Lavin J et al 2010 Changes in well-being, diet and activity habits of pregnant women attending a commercial weight management organization. Journal of Human Nutrition and Dietetics 23(4):459

Pawelec M, Palczynski B, Karmowski 2012 HELLP syndrome in pregnancies below 26th week. Journal of Maternal–Fetal and Neonatal Medicine 25(5):467–70

Plumb J, Clayton G 2013 Group B Streptococcus infection: risk and prevention. The Practising Midwife (July/August):27–30

Redman C W G, Jacobson S L, Russell R 2010 Hypertension in pregnancy. In: Powrie R, Greene M, Camann W (eds) de Swiet's Medical disorders in obstetric practice, 5th edn. Wiley–Blackwell, Oxford, p 153–81

Reece E A, Leguizamón G, Wiznitzer A 2009 Gestational diabetes: the need for a common ground. Lancet 23(373):1789–97

Regitz-Zagrosek V, Blomstrom Lundqvist C, Borghi C et al 2011 ESC Guidelines on the management of cardiovascular diseases during pregnancy. European Heart Journal 32:3147–97

Richmond J 2009 Coping with diabetes in pregnancy. British Journal of Midwifery 17(2):84–91

Roberts W, Adamson D 2013 Cardiovascular disease in pregnancy. Obstetrics, Gynecology and Reproductive Medicine 23(7):195–201

RCOG (Royal College of Obstetricians and Gynaecologists) 2006 Exercise in pregnancy. Statement No. 4. RCOG, London

RCOG (Royal College of Obstetricians and Gynaecologists) 2009 Thrombosis and embolism during pregnancy and puerperium: reducing the risk. Green-top Guideline No. 37a. RCOG, London

RCOG (Royal College of Obstetricians and Gynaecologists) 2010a The acute management of thrombosis and embolism during pregnancy and the puerperium. Green-top Guideline No. 37b. RCOG, London

RCOG (Royal College of Obstetricians and Gynaecologists) 2010b Management of HIV in Pregnancy. Green-top Guideline No. 39. RCOG, London

RCOG (Royal College of Obstetricians and Gynaecologists) 2011a Obstetric cholestasis. Green-top Guideline No. 43. RCOG, London

RCOG (Royal College of Obstetricians and Gynaecologists) 2011b Cardiac disease and pregnancy: good practice guide. Green-top Guideline No. 13. RCOG, London

RCOG (Royal College of Obstetricians and Gynaecologists) 2011c Management of sickle cell disease in pregnancy. Green-top Guideline No. 61. RCOG, London

RCOG (Royal College of Obstetricians and Gynaecologists) 2012 The prevention of early onset neonatal Group B streptococcal disease. Green-top Guideline No. 36. RCOG, London

Saleh M M, Abdo K R 2007 Consensus on the management of obstetric cholestasis: National UK Survey. BJOG: An International Journal of Obstetrics and Gynaecology 114(1):99–103

Scanlon P, Harcombe J 2011 It's all in the eyes. Midwives 5:46

Scott-Pillai R, Spence D, Cardwell C R et al 2013 The impact of body mass index on maternal and neonatal outcomes: a retrospective study in a UK obstetric population, 2004-2011. BJOG: An International Journal of Obstetrics and Gynaecology 120(8):932–9

SIGN (Scottish Intercollegiate Guidelines Network) 2010 Management of diabetes: National Clinical Guideline 116. SIGN, Edinburgh

Scullion J, Brightling C, Goldie M 2013 Respiratory disorders, In: Robson S E, Waugh J (eds) Medical disorders in pregnancy: a manual for midwives, 2nd edn. Wiley–Blackwell, Oxford, p 75–90

Sellstrom E, Arnoldson G, Alricsson M et al 2009 Obesity: prevalence in a cohort of women in early pregnancy from a neighbourhood perspective. BMC Pregnancy and Childbirth 9:37

Shennan A H, Waugh J 2003 Pre-eclampsia. RCOG Press, London

Smith S, Hulsey T, Goodnight W 2008 Effects of obesity on pregnancy Journal of Obstetric, Gynecologic and Neonatal Nursing 37:176–84

Talaulikar V S, Manyonda I T 2011 Vitamin C as an antioxidant supplement in women's health: a myth in need of urgent burial. European Journal of Obstetrics, Gynecology and Reproductive Biology 157(1):10–13

Temple R 2011 Preconception care for women with diabetes: is it effective and who should provide it? Best Practice and Research Clinical Obstetrics and Gynaecology 25: 3–14

Tortora G, Derrickson B 2010 Essentials of anatomy and physiology, 8th edn. Wiley, Chichester

UK National Screening Committee (NSC) 2012 Review of screening for cytomegalovirus in the antenatal and/or postnatal periods. Policy Position Statement. UKNSC, London

Vijgen S M C, Koopmans C M, Opmeer B C et al 2010 An economic analysis of induction of labour and expectant monitoring in women with gestational hypertension or pre-eclampsia at term (HYPITAT trial). BJOG: An International Journal of Obstetrics and Gynaecology 117(13):1577–85

Villamor E, Cnattingius S 2006 Interpregnancy weight change and risk of adverse pregnancy outcomes: a population-based study. Lancet 368(9542):1164–70

Watkins K, Johnson-Roffey, Houghton J et al 2013 Infectious conditions. In: Robson S E, Waugh J (eds) Medical disorders in pregnancy: a manual for midwives, 2nd edn. Wiley–Blackwell, Oxford, p 215–40

Waugh J J S, Smith M C 2012 Hypertensive disorders. In: Edmonds K (ed) Dewhurst's textbook of obstetrics and gynaecology, 8th edn. Wiley–Blackwell, Oxford, p 101–10

Webb G 2008 Nutrition: a health promotion approach, 3rd edn. Hodder Arnold, London

Webster S, Dodd C, Waugh J 2013 Hypertensive disorders. In: Robson S E, Waugh J (eds) Medical disorders in pregnancy: a manual for midwives, 2nd edn. Wiley–Blackwell, Oxford, p 27–42

Weiner S 2006 Diagnosis and management of candida of the nipple and breast. Journal of Midwifery and Women's Health 51(2):125–8

Williams D, Craft N 2012 Pre-eclampsia. British Medical Journal 345; e4437.

doi: 10.1136/bmj.e4437 (accessed 11 January 2013)

WHO (World Health Organization) 2000 Obesity: preventing and managing the global epidemic: report of a WHO consultation. WHO Technical Report Series 894:i–253

WHO (World Health Organization) 2013 Anaemia. WHO, Geneva. www

.who.int/topics/anaemia/en/ (accessed 7 September 2013)

WHO (World Health Organization), United Nations Children's Fund [UNICEF], UN University 2001 Iron deficiency anaemia: assessment, prevention and control. A guide for programme managers. WHO, Geneva, p 15

FURTHER READING

Raynor M D, Marshall J E, Jackson K 2012 Midwifery practice: critical illness, complications and emergencies case book. Open University Press, Maidenhead

Part of a case book series, this text explores and explains the pathology, pharmacology and care principles of women presenting with, or who develop medical conditions and complications of pregnancy using test question and answers to assess learning.

Robson S E, Waugh J 2013 Medical disorders of pregnancy: a manual for midwives, 2nd edn. Wiley–Blackwell, Oxford

This second edition clearly outlines existing and pre-existing conditions that women can experience during pregnancy and explores possible complications, an outline of recommended treatment and the specific midwifery care. The text includes physiology, more illustrations and algorithms, and its accessible reference-style text enables information to be found quickly and easily.

USEFUL WEBSITES

Action on Pre-eclampsia: www.apec.org.uk

Association for the Study of Obesity: www.aso.org.uk

Asthma UK: www.asthma.org.uk

British Heart Foundation: www.bhf.org.uk

British Hypertension Society: www.bhsoc.org

British Society for Haematology: www.b-s-h.org.uk

British Thoracic Society: www.brit-thoracic.org.uk

British Thyroid Foundation: www.btf-thyroid.org.uk

Diabetes UK: www.diabetes.org.uk

Epilepsy Action (British Epilepsy Association): www.epilepsy.org.uk

Group B Strep Support: www.gbss.org.uk

Hepatitis Foundation: www.hepatitisfoundation.org

International Sepsis Forum: www.sepsisforum.org

National Chlamydia Screening Programme: www.chlamydiascreening.nhs.uk

National Institute for Health and Care (formerly Clinical) Excellence www.nice.org.uk

Obstetric Cholestasis Support: www.ocsupport.org.uk

Royal College of Obstetricians and Gynaecologists: www.rcog.org.uk

Scottish Intercollegiate Guidelines Network: www.sign.ac.uk

UK National Screening Committee: www.screening.nhs.uk

Chapter 14

Multiple pregnancy

Margie Davies

The term 'multiple pregnancy' is used to describe the development of more than one fetus *in utero* at the same time. Families expecting a multiple birth have different health needs, requiring extra practical support and understanding throughout pregnancy, the postnatal period and the early years. Information and support from well-informed healthcare professionals from the time the multiple pregnancy is diagnosed will help to prepare the parents and avoid potential problems.

THE CHAPTER AIMS TO:

- describe how types of multiple pregnancy may be distinguished
- consider the diagnosis and management of twin pregnancy, the labour and the care of the mother and babies after birth
- give an overview of the problems particularly associated with twins and higher order births and the fetal anomalies unique to the twinning process
- explain the special needs of the parents and identify the sources of help available.

INCIDENCE

The incidence of multiple births in England and Wales continues to rise. In 2012 there were 11 441 multiple births, a rate of 15.7 per 1000 maternities or 1 in 63 with 11 330 twins, 208 triplets and 5 quads (Table 14.1, Fig. 14.1) (ONS [Office of National Statistics] 2013).

In the 1940s and 1950s, the incidence of twins was 1 in 80 but then fell to 1 in 104 in 1979. The full explanation for the fall is unknown. The number of triplets born more than trebled in the 15 years up to 2001 (Blondel and Kaminski 2002). The highest number in any one year was 323 in 1998; this was due to the rise in treatments for infertility such as in vitro fertilization (IVF) and ovulation-stimulating drugs.

The single most important reason for the rise in multiple births is assisted conception (Black and Bhattacharya 2010), although women having children when they are older is a contributory factor though less significant. Multiple birth is the greatest single risk to the health and welfare of babies born after IVF due to the increased rates of stillbirth, preterm birth, neonatal death and disabilities. Maternal complications are also higher with a multiple pregnancy. Concern about the increased morbidity and mortality and high costs for health and social care led the Human Fertilisation and Embryology Authority (HFEA) to commission an expert group to review multiple births after IVF. The report 'One Child at a Time' (Braude 2006)

has led to significant changes in practice to reduce iatrogenic multiple births. Elective single embryo transfer in IVF cycles is the normal practice in the UK with spare good-quality embryos frozen for replacement in later cycles (Cutting et al 2008). The 'One at a Time' policy is supported by professional bodies and relevant organizations (Consensus Statement 2011).

TWIN PREGNANCY

Types of twin pregnancy

Twins will be either *monozygotic* (MZ) or *dizygotic* (DZ). Monozygotic or uniovular twins are also referred to as 'identical twins'. They develop from the fusion of one oocyte and one spermatozoon, which after fertilization splits into two (Chapter 5). These twins will be of the same sex and have the same genes, blood groups and physical features, such as eye and hair colour, ear shapes and palm creases. However, they may be of different sizes and often have very different personalities and characters.

Dizygotic or binovular twins develop when two separate oocytes are fertilized by two different spermatozoa; they are often referred to as fraternal or non-identical twins. They are no more alike than any brother or sister and can be of the same or different sex. In any multiple pregnancy there is a 50:50 chance of a girl or boy, half of dizygotic twins will be boy–girl pairs. A quarter of dizygotic twins will be both boys and a quarter, both girls. Of all twins born in the UK, two-thirds will be dizygotic and one-third monozygotic. Therefore, approximately one-third of twins are girls, one-third boys and one-third girl–boy pairs.

Determination of zygosity and chorionicity

Midwives must understand the differences between these two terms (Table 14.2) and why it is important.

Determination of zygosity means determining whether or not the twins are monozygotic (identical) or dizygotic (non-identical). In about one-third of all twins born, it will be obvious as the children will be of a different sex. Of the remaining same-sex twins, zygosity will usually be apparent from physical features by the time the children are 2 years old, although parents are not usually prepared to wait this long. By the age of 2, parents know their children so well and see their differences in character and personalities that they often find it difficult to believe they are identical. At birth, monochorionic twins can have a greater weight variation than dichorionic twins. In approximately two-thirds of monozygotic twins, a monochorionic diamniotic placenta (MCDA) will confirm monozygosity. If the babies have a single outer membrane, the chorion, they must be monochorionic and so monozygotic (Fig. 14.2).

Table 14.1 Multiple birth statistics, England and Wales 1985–2011

	1985	1986	1987	1988	1989	1990	1991	1992	1993	1994	1995	1996	1997
Total maternities	653 142	657 308	677 467	689 153	682 979	701 030	693 857	683 854	668 511	659 520	642 404	643 862	636 015
Twins	6700	6969	7186	7452	7579	7934	8160	8314	8302	8451	8749	8615	8899
Triplets	93	123	125	157	183	201	208	202	234	260	282	259	295
Quads						9	10	8	12	8	7	9	7
Quins	10	13	9	13	12	–	1	1	–	–	–	–	–
Sextuplets						–	–	–	1	–	–	–	–
Twinning rate/1000 maternities	10.3	10.6	10.6	10.8	11.1	11.3	11.7	12.2	12.4	12.8	13.6	13.4	14.0
Triplet rate/1000 maternities	0.14	0.19	0.18	0.23	0.27	0.29	0.30	0.30	0.35	0.39	0.44	0.40	0.46
Total maternities	10.40	10.80	10.80	11.10	11.40	11.60	12.10	12.50	12.80	13.20	14.10	13.80	14.50

Table 14.1 Continued

	1998	1999	2000	2001	2002	2003	2004	2005	2006	2007	2008	2009	2010	2011	2012
Total maternities	629926	615994	598580	588868	590453	615787	633728	639627	662915	682999	701297	698324	715467	716040	729674
Twins	8776	8636	8526	8484	8685	9001	9368	9396	9992	10334	10680	11301	11053	11330	11228
Triplets	297	267	262	211	172	127	148	146	138	135	174	153	169	172	208
Quads	7	4	4	4	4	3	5	1	7	1	1	5	6	3[a]	5
Quins	–	–	–	–	–	–	–	–	–	1	–	–	–	–	–
Sextuplets	–	–	–	1	–	–	–	–	–	–	–	–	–	–	–
Twinning rate/1000 maternities	13.9	14.0	14.2	14.4	14.70	14.61	14.78	14.68	15.07	15.13	15.22	16.2	15.4	15.8	15.4
Triplet rate/1000 maternities	0.47	0.43	0.43	0.43	0.29	0.20	0.23	0.22	00.21	0.19	0.24	0.23	0.2	0.24	0.29
Multiple birth rate/1000 maternities	14.40	14.46	14.68	14.77	15.00	14.82	15.02	14.91	15.29	15.3	15.5	16.4	15.7	16.0	15.9

NB: Figures include live and still births.

Source: Office of National Statistics, London (various years)

[a]For 2011 and 2012 this is a combined figure for quads and above.

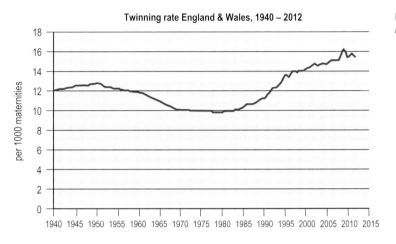

Fig. 14.1 Twinning rates, 1940–2012.
Data from Office of National Statistics.

Table 14.2 Relationship between zygosity and chorionicity	
Dichorionic	**Monochorionic**
Two placentae (may be fused)	One placenta
Two chorions	One chorion
Two amnions	Two amnions (one amnion in monoamniotic twins is very rare)
These twins can be either dizygotic or monozygotic	These twins can only be monozygotic

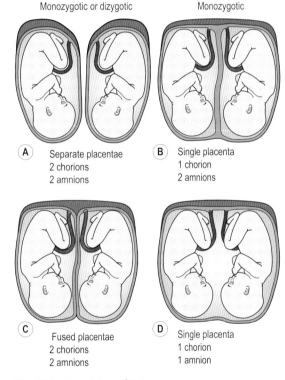

Fig. 14.2 Placentation of twins.
After Bryan 1984, with permission of Edward Arnold.

In one-third of monozygotic twins, the placenta will have two chorions and two amnions (DCDA), and either fused placentas (Fig. 14.2C) or two separate placentas (dichorionic) (Fig. 14.2A), which is indistinguishable from the situation in dizygotic twins.

With monozygotic twins the type of placenta produced is determined by the time at which the fertilized oocyte splits:

- 0–4 days: dichorionic diamniotic placenta DCDA (approx. 33% – 1/3 cases) (Fig. 14.2 A,C)
- 4–8 days: monochorionic diamniotic placenta MCDA (approx. 66% – 2/3 cases) (Fig. 14.2B)
- 8–12 days: monochorionic monoamniotic placenta MCMA (approx. 1% of cases) (Fig. 14.2D)
- 12–13 days: (very rare indeed) conjoined twins can develop when the division is incomplete (Bomsel-Helmreich 2005).

Despite the well-established facts about placentation and zygosity, professionals are still giving couples incorrect information. Same-sex dichorionic twins can be either non-identical or identical and it is only from either an amniocentesis whilst pregnant or deoxyribonucleic acid (DNA) testing after the birth that accurate zygosity can be known.

Chorionicity: why is it important to know?

This knowledge is important clinically because monochorionic twin pregnancies have a 3–5 times higher risk of perinatal mortality and morbidity than dichorionic twin pregnancies (Pasquini et al 2004).

Zygosity determination after birth

The most accurate method of determining zygosity is to compare DNA from each baby. The DNA can be extracted from cells taken from a cheek swab from inside the mouth. Specific genetic markers extracted from different chromosomes are compared and the results are up to 99.99% accurate. (For DNA testing, contact the Multiple Births Foundation [MBF].)

Zygosity determination should be routinely offered to all same-sex dichorionic twins for the following reasons:

- Most parents will want to know whether or not their twins are identical, so they can answer the most commonly asked question: 'Are they identical?' Also as the twins get older, they usually want to know.
- If couples are considering further pregnancies, the risk in DZ twin pregnancy increases approximately five-fold: these tend to run in families, usually on the female side. MZ twins do not run in families and the likelihood does not change (except in rare families who carry a dominant gene for monozygotic twinning). The chance of any fertile woman having MZ twins is approximately 1 in 350–400.
- It will help the twins in establishing their sense of identity; influence their life and family relationships.
- The information is important for genetic reasons, not just with monogenic disorders but with any serious illness later in life.
- Twins are frequently asked to be involved in research and for this knowledge of zygosity is essential.

Diagnosis of twin pregnancy

This is usually through ultrasound examination. Diagnosis can be made as early as 6 weeks, particularly for women who have had treatment for infertility, but usually at the early scan between 11 weeks and 13 weeks and 6 days (Chapter 11). If the pregnancy is diagnosed at 6 weeks, the woman should be told about the risk of 'vanishing twin syndrome' (Landy et al 1998).

The differences between the two types of placenta are more pronounced in the first trimester, so it is important to establish chorionicity at the early scan. The chorions forming the septum between the amniotic sacs can be seen more clearly and the membrane thickness measured, or by studying the septum at its base adjacent to the placenta where a tongue of placental tissue is seen ultrasonically between the two chorions; this is termed the lambda or T-sign (Wood et al 1996).

Once a multiple pregnancy has been diagnosed nomenclature should be assigned to each baby (e.g. A and B, or upper and lower).

The news that a woman is expecting a multiple pregnancy should be broken to the couple in a sensitive manner as it may be a huge shock. At diagnosis the mother must be given relevant information about the pregnancy, be referred to a specialist multiple pregnancy clinic, and given website addresses or telephone numbers of local and national support organizations (see Useful Websites).

Since the advent of routine ultrasound scanning, it is very rare for a woman to get to term with undiagnosed twins, but this will not apply in areas where this technology is unavailable, or where the mother declines.

THE PREGNANCY

A multiple pregnancy tends to be shorter than a single pregnancy. The average gestation for twins is 37 weeks, triplets 34 weeks and quadruplets 32 weeks.

Antenatal screening

- A healthcare professional experienced in twin and triplet pregnancies should offer information and counselling before and after every screening test.
- Screening for Down syndrome is by the combined test (see Chapter 11).
- Amniocentesis can be performed in twin pregnancies, usually between 15 and 20 weeks. It should be performed in a specialist fetal medicine unit. Most obstetricians prefer to do a dual needle insertion so there is no chance of contamination between the two sac.
- The role of chorionic villus sampling (CVS) with dichorionic placentas remains controversial because of a relatively high risk of cross-contamination of chorionic tissue, which may lead to false-positive or false-negative results. Such procedures should only be performed after detailed counseling (RCOG (Royal College of Obstetricians and Gynaecologists) 2010).

Ultrasound examination

- Monochorionic twin pregnancies should be scanned every 2 weeks from 16 to 24 weeks to check for discordant fetal growth and signs of twin-to-twin transfusion syndrome (TTTS). A detailed cardiac scan should be included with the anomaly scan due to increased incidence of cardiac problems with MZ twins; if uncomplicated after 24 weeks, then the same as dichorionic twins.
- Dichorionic twin pregnancies should be scanned monthly from 16 weeks, with the anomaly scan between $18+^0$ to $20+^6$ weeks.

Antenatal care and preparation

Early diagnosis of a twin pregnancy and of chorionicity is extremely important in order to give parents the specialist support and advice they will need.

Clinical care for women with twin and triplet pregnancies should be provided by a nominated multidisciplinary team consisting of: a core team of named specialist obstetricians, specialist midwives and ultrasonographers, all of whom have experience and knowledge of managing multiple pregnancies.

An enhanced team for referrals should include: a women's physiotherapist, an infant feeding specialist, a dietitian and a perinatal mental health professional. The type of care pathway the woman will follow for her antenatal care will depend on whether she is expecting monochorionic or dichorionic twins. Women expecting an uncomplicated monochorionic twin pregnancy should be offered at least nine antenatal appointments with healthcare professionals from the core team. At least two of these should be with the specialist obstetrician. Women with uncomplicated dichorionic twin pregnancies should be offered at least eight antenatal appointments with a healthcare professional from the core team, and two of these with the specialist obstetrician (NICE [National Institute for Health and Clinical Excellence] 2011).

Parent education

Routine parent education classes should be offered earlier for women expecting twins, ideally around 22–24 weeks' gestation. A specialist class for couples expecting a multiple birth would be the ideal (Owen et al 2004). When planning these classes, contact with a local twins club can provide a valuable source of practical information. Mothers from twins clubs are usually delighted to participate in the classes and talk on the practical issues such as coping with two or more babies, equipment and breastfeeding (Leonard and Denton 2006). Suggestions for class topics are listed in Box 14.1.

The news a multiple pregnancy is expected can come as a considerable shock and the midwife should give couples the opportunity to discuss any worries or problems they have, as two babies will add a considerable financial burden to any family's income (Denton and Bryan 1995).

Preparation for breastfeeding

Women will inevitably give a lot of thought to how they are going to feed their babies, not only from the nutritional but also from the practical point of view, as feeding will take up a large amount of their time during the first 6 months. Women should be encouraged right from the beginning that it is not only possible to breastfeed two, and in some cases three babies, but it is the best way for her to feed her babies nutritionally and it can be a very

---

Box 14.1 Topics for parent education classes

- Facts and figures on twins and twinning
- Diet and exercise
- Parental anxieties about obstetric complications
- Labour, pain relief and the birth
- Possibilities of premature labour and birth the outcome
- Visit to the special care baby unit
- Breastfeeding and bottle-feeding
- Zygosity
- Equipment (prams and buggies, car seats, layette, etc.)
- Coping with newborn twins or more
- Development of twins including individuality and identity
- Sources of help.

Box 14.2 Support needed by the breastfeeding mother of twins or more

- Consistent professional advice
- Reassurance of her ability to produce enough milk to satisfy her babies
- Encouragement from professionals and family in her ability to cope with feeding two or more
- Support from her partner
- Help at home with household chores
- Help with older siblings
- A high calorie and high protein diet

---

rewarding experience for her (see Fig. 14.6). Many sets of twins have been entirely breastfed, some beyond their first birthdays. Very few sets of triplets are totally breastfed (Leonard 2000), but many mothers manage to combine breast and bottlefeeding very successfully.

Early in the antenatal period the woman should be given full information and advice about both breast- and bottlefeeding, so she can make an informed choice on how to feed her babies. Both parents should have the opportunity to ask questions and be encouraged to meet another mother who is successfully breastfeeding her babies (Box 14.2). Introductions can usually be made through a local twins group (MBF 2011a, 2011b).

Abdominal examination

Inspection

On inspection, the size of the uterus may be larger than expected for the period of gestation, particularly after the

20th week. The uterus may look broad or round and fetal movements may be seen over a wide area, although the findings are not diagnostic of twins. Fresh striae gravidarum may be apparent. Up to twice the amount of amniotic fluid is normal in a twin pregnancy but polyhydramnios is not an uncommon complication of a twin pregnancy, particularly with monochorionic twins.

Palpation

On palpation, the fundal height may be greater than expected for the period of gestation. The presence of two fetal poles (head or breech) in the fundus of the uterus may be revealed on palpation and multiple fetal limbs may also be palpable. The head may be small in relation to the size of the uterus and may suggest that the fetus is also small and therefore there may be more than one present. Lateral palpation may reveal two fetal backs, or limbs on both sides. Pelvic palpation may give findings similar to those on fundal palpation, although one fetus may lie behind the other and make detection difficult. Location of three poles in total is diagnostic of at least two fetuses.

Auscultation

Hearing two fetal hearts is not diagnostic as one can often be heard over a wide area in a singleton pregnancy. If simultaneous comparison over one minute of the heart rates reveals a difference of at least 10 bpm, it may be assumed that two hearts are being heard beating.

Effects of pregnancy

Exacerbation of common disorders

The presence of more than one fetus *in utero* and the higher levels of circulating hormones often exacerbate the common disorders of pregnancy. Sickness, nausea and heartburn may be more persistent and more troublesome than in a singleton pregnancy.

Anaemia

Iron and folic acid deficiency anaemias are common in twin pregnancies. Early growth and development of the uterus and its contents make greater demands on the maternal iron stores; in later pregnancy (after the 28th week), fetal demands may lead to anaemia. Routine oral iron supplementation remains a controversial issue (Lassi et al 2013), but all pregnant women are advised to take folic acid daily (NICE 2008).

Polyhydramnios

This is also common and is particularly associated with monochorionic twins and with fetal abnormalities.

Polyhydramnios will add to any discomfort that the woman is already experiencing. If acute polyhydramnios occurs, it can lead to miscarriage or preterm labour.

Pressure symptoms

The increased weight and size of the uterus and its contents may be troublesome. Impaired venous return from the lower limbs increases the tendency to varicose veins and oedema of the legs. Backache is common and the increased uterine size may also lead to marked dyspnoea and indigestion.

Other

There can be an increase in complications of pregnancy such as obstetric cholestasis, and pelvic girdle pain (PGP) (see Chapters 12 and 13).

LABOUR AND THE BIRTH

Onset

The more fetuses the woman is carrying, the earlier labour is likely to start. Twins are usually born around 37 weeks rather than 40 weeks, and approximately 60% of twins are born spontaneously before 37 weeks' gestation. In addition to being preterm, the babies may be small for gestational age (SFGA) and therefore prone to the associated complications of both conditions. If spontaneous labour begins before 24 weeks, the chances of survival outside the uterus are very small, but it is possible the woman can be given drugs to inhibit uterine activity. Causes of preterm labour must, if at all possible, be diagnosed and treated quickly; for example, urinary tract infection should be treated with antibiotics. Antenatal corticosteroids are usually given to all women of multiple pregnancies before 36 weeks' gestation (NICE 2011).

Evidence shows that after 38 weeks' gestation there is increased risk of higher mortality in babies (Udom-Rice et al 2000), most obstetricians advise induction of labour by 38 weeks for dichorionic twins and between 36 and 37 weeks (Box 14.3) for monochorionic twins (RCOG 2006). In dichorionic pregnancies, if the first twin is a cephalic presentation, labour is usually allowed to continue to a vaginal birth, but if the first twin is presenting in any other way, an elective caesarean section (CS) is usually recommended (Fig. 14.3). For uncomplicated monochorionic twin pregnancies women are generally offered a vaginal birth, but for complicated monochorionic pregnancies birth is by elective CS. For triplets and above, the mode of birth is almost always by CS.

A 34-year-old primigravida was diagnosed with DCDA twins, no family history, so it was a complete shock. At the ultrasound department, a leaflet with local twin organizations and contacts was given to the mother. Through the hospital specialist, multiple birth midwife and twins club the mother started to come to terms with the prospect of twins. She knew she was expecting two boys and began to wonder if they were identical or not, but would have to wait until they were born and have DNA tests if they looked alike. She had a straightforward birth with her first child, so she was keen to have a vaginal birth again, but felt there was pressure on her to have an elective caesarean section. The pregnancy progressed normally and with support from the specialist midwife, she wrote her birth plan. The presenting baby was cephalic, and at 38 weeks labour was induced. The woman had an epidural and progressed to birth both babies vaginally after a short labour. Both babies were put to her breast in the labour suite; twin one sucked well but twin two was not interested. As establishing feeding was more problematic than she expected and she felt she needed a lot of help from the midwives, the mother stayed in hospital until day 5. Both babies were sucking well on return home, although twin two did occasionally need a 'top up' from the bottle.

Management of labour

During antenatal classes the couple must be warned that a multiple birth is less common and therefore, for educational purposes in the hospital setting, a number of professionals may ask to observe the birth. If the woman has any objection to this, her wishes must be respected and a record made in her notes that she wants only those concerned with her care to be present. Home births are not advisable with a multiple pregnancy, but some women may still request one, in which case every effort should be made to support her decision with an uncomplicated pregnancy. This will require meticulous risk assessment and planning, including the involvement of midwifery supervision in order that a plan of care for labour is clearly articulated and documented in the woman's records. A skilled team of midwives with confidence to deliver intrapartum care to women with twin pregnancies at home will need to be identified to be on call. It is good practice for the midwifery team to liaise with and communicate the plan of care to the paramedic team and local consultant-led unit.

The majority of women expecting twins will go into labour spontaneously. Theoretically the duration of the first stage of labour should be no different from that of a single pregnancy. However, there is an increased incidence

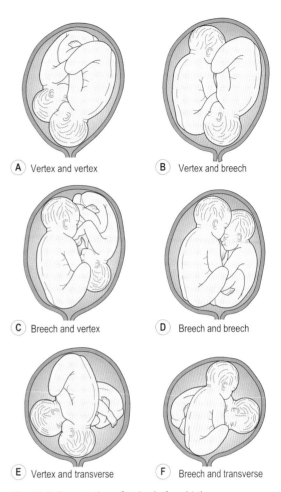

(A) Vertex and vertex   (B) Vertex and breech

(C) Breech and vertex   (D) Breech and breech

(E) Vertex and transverse   (F) Breech and transverse

Fig. 14.3 Presentation of twins before birth.
After Bryan 1984, with permission of Edward Arnold.

of dysfunctional labour in twin pregnancies, possibly because of overdistension of the uterus.

The presence of complications such as pregnancy-induced hypertension, obstetric cholestasis, intrauterine growth restriction (IUGR) or twin-to-twin transfusion syndrome may be reasons for earlier induction of labour.

Labour for women expecting twins must be recognized as high risk and continuous electronic fetal heart monitoring (EFM) of both fetuses is advocated. This can be achieved either with two external transducers or, once the membranes are ruptured, a scalp electrode on the presenting twin and an external transducer on the second. If a 'twin monitor' is available, both heartbeats can be monitored simultaneously to give a more reliable reading. Uterine activity will also need to be monitored.

If cardiotocography (CTG) is not available (e.g. a home birth), use of hand-held Dopplers may be more pragmatic for structured intermittent fetal heart rates (FHRs) auscultation than a Pinard's stethoscope. If the latter has to be used, two people must auscultate simultaneously, so that the two distinct FHRs are counted over the same minute.

While in labour, the woman should be encouraged to adopt whichever position she finds most comfortable. A foam rubber wedge under the side of the mattress will help to prevent supine hypotensive syndrome by giving a lateral tilt. It may be preferable for her to adopt a left lateral position, well supported by pillows or a beanbag. A birthing chair or a reclining chair, if available, may be more comfortable than a conventional labour suite birthing bed.

Regional epidural block provides excellent analgesia, and if necessary, allows easier instrumental births and also manipulation of the second twin. The use of Entonox analgesia may be helpful, either before the epidural is in situ or during the second stage, if the effect of the epidural is wearing off.

The woman should be encouraged to use whatever form of relaxation she finds helpful. If she chooses to use pharmacological means of analgesia only after non-pharmacological methods are no longer effective, her wishes should be respected. The midwife should explain that, if complications arise, intervention and the use of pharmacological analgesia might be necessary. Ideally this should be discussed with the woman antenatally so that the physiology of labour is not disturbed with new information (Chapter 16).

If fetal compromise occurs during labour, the birth will need to be expedited, usually by CS. Action may also need to be taken if the woman's condition gives cause for concern.

If uterine activity is poor, the use of intravenous oxytocin may be required once the membranes have been ruptured. Artificial rupture of the membranes (ARM) may be sufficient to stimulate good uterine activity but it may need to be used in conjunction with intravenous oxytocin. The CTG will give a good indication of the pattern of uterine activity, whether the labour is induced or spontaneous. The response of the fetal hearts to uterine contractions can be observed on the CTG.

If the babies are expected to be preterm, low birth weight, or known to have any other problems, the neonatal intensive care unit (NICU) must be informed that the woman is in labour so they can make the necessary preparations to receive the babies. When birth is imminent, the paediatric team should be summoned.

Throughout labour, the emotional and general physical condition of the woman must be considered. She requires the presence of her birthing partner and one-to-one care from the midwife.

Management of the birth

The onset of the second stage of labour should be confirmed by a vaginal examination. In the hospital setting, the obstetrician, paediatric team and anaesthetist should be present for the birth as there is a risk of complications.

Epidural analgesia may need to be 'topped up' prior to the birth. The possibility of emergency CS is ever present and the operating theatre should be ready to receive the mother at short notice. Monitoring of both FHRs should continue until birth. Provided that the first twin is presenting by the vertex, the birth can be expected to proceed normally, as with a singleton pregnancy. When the first twin is born, the time of birth and the sex are noted. This baby and cord must be labelled as 'twin one' immediately. The identity tags should be checked with the mother or father before they are applied to the baby in accordance with local policy. The baby may be given to the mother for skin-to-skin contact and encouraged to go to the breast as sucking stimulates uterine contractions (Chapter 34).

After the birth of the first twin, abdominal palpation is made to ascertain the lie, presentation (in the event of doubt a portable ultrasound machine should be available) and position of the second twin and to auscultate the FHR to ensure continuous EFM. An assistant may need to stabilize the lie of the second twin. If the lie is not longitudinal, an attempt may be made to correct it by external cephalic version (ECV) (see Chapter 17). ECV in this context in the UK should only be performed or supervised by a senior obstetrician (RCOG 2006). ECV is less invasive than internal podalic version, and will often be the default manoeuvre employed by obstetricians (RCOG 2006; Masson 2007).

If it is longitudinal, a vaginal examination is made to confirm the presentation. If the presenting part is not engaged it should be gently guided into the pelvis and kept in place until it firmly engages. ARM must not be performed on the second sac of membranes until the presenting part engages, as risk of cord prolapse is ever present. The FHR must be auscultated again; a scalp electrode might be required following ARM if external monitoring of the FHR is of poor quality If uterine activity does not recommence, intravenous oxytocin may be used.

When the presenting part becomes visible, the mother should be encouraged to birth her second twin with contractions. The midwife should always be aware there is a risk the placenta may start to separate before the birth of the second twin, causing oxygen deprivation. The birth will proceed as normal if the presentation is vertex, but if the fetus presents by the breech and the midwife is not experienced in breech births she will need a doctor's assistance.

The birth of the second twin should ideally be completed within 45 minutes of the first twin but, as long as there are no signs of fetal compromise in the second twin, it may be allowed to continue longer. If there are signs of compromise, the birth must be expedited and the second twin may need to be born by CS. An uterotonic drug (Syntometrine or oxytocin) is usually given intramuscularly or intravenously, depending on local policy, after the birth of the anterior shoulder as with a singleton pregnancy. This baby and cord are labelled as 'twin two'. The time of birth and sex of child must be noted. If either twin needs to be transferred to the NICU for observation, the mother should have a chance to see and hold the baby whenever possible.

Once the uterotonic drug has taken effect, controlled cord traction is applied to both cords simultaneously to aid birth of the placentas without delay. Emptying the uterus enables bleeding to be controlled and postpartum haemorrhage prevented.

The placenta(s) should be examined not only to check completion but the number of amniotic sacs, chorions and placentas noted (see Fig. 14.2). If the babies are of different sexes, they are dizygotic. If the placenta is monochorionic (MCDA), they must be monozygotic. If they are of the same sex and the placenta is dichorionic (DCDA), then further tests will be needed (see Zygosity). The umbilical cords should also be examined and the number of cord vessels and the presence of any abnormalities noted.

COMPLICATIONS ASSOCIATED WITH MULTIPLE PREGNANCY

The higher perinatal mortality associated with twinning is largely due to complications of pregnancy, such as the preterm onset of labour, IUGR and complications at birth. There is a six-fold increase in perinatal mortality comparing twins to singletons (CMACE [Centre for Maternal and Child Enquiries] 2011). The management of multiple pregnancy is concerned with the prevention, early detection and treatment of these complications.

Polyhydramnios

Mentioned earlier in the chapter, acute polyhydramnios may occur as early as 16 weeks. It may be associated with fetal abnormality but is more likely to be due to twin-to-twin transfusion syndrome (TTTS), which can also be known as feto-fetal transfusion syndrome (FFTS).

Twin-to-twin transfusion syndrome

Twin-to-twin transfusion syndrome (TTTS) can be acute or chronic. The acute form usually occurs during labour and is the result of blood transfusing from one fetus (donor) to the other (recipient) through vascular anastomosis in a monochorionic placenta. Both fetuses may die of cardiac failure if not treated urgently.

Chronic TTTS occurs in about 15% of monochorionic twin pregnancies (Dennes et al 2006) and accounts for

---

> **Box 14.4 Case history 2**
>
> A 26-year-old primigravida's early scan showed MCDA twins. The mother read on the Internet that problems can be associated with MCDA pregnancy and was very worried about TTTS.
>
> From 16 weeks, she had 2-weekly scans for signs of TTTS and growth discordancy. At 20 weeks, she noticed a rapid increase in abdominal size and her tummy was hard and uncomfortable. Her local hospital referred her to the Centre for Fetal Care (CFC) at a tertiary level hospital, where type 2 TTTS was diagnosed. Immediate treatment was amnio-reduction of over 2 litres and laser ablation of connecting blood vessels. Her care was transferred to CFC for weekly scans. Here she mainly saw doctors and felt she missed out on midwife contact. Unfortunately at 32 weeks she was diagnosed as type 3 TTTS, with very abnormal Dopplers in the donor twin. Steroid injections were given and an emergency caesarean section was performed at 33 weeks. Both babies were born in a fair condition and were admitted to the NICU. The mother was encouraged to hand express her milk as soon as she felt well enough, to continue 2–3-hourly during the day and on the 6th day she started expressing using an electric pump. The twins were able to go to the breast after 2 weeks and started sucking for very short periods. Progress continued and both babies were discharged home at 5 weeks of age, fully breastfeeding.

15% of perinatal mortality in twins (Yamamoto and Ville 2006). The placenta in TTTS transfuses blood from one twin fetus to the other. These cases are characterized by one or more deep unidirectional arteriovenous anastomoses. This results in anaemia and growth restriction in the donor twin (stuck twin) and polycythaemia with circulatory overload in the recipient twin (hydrops). The fetal and neonatal mortality is high but infants may be saved by early diagnosis and prenatal treatment with either amnioreduction, which may have to be repeated regularly as fluid can reaccumulate rapidly (Box 14.4), or laser ablation therapy of communicating placental vessels, or septostomy (MBF 2010).

The midwife should always be alert to the woman who complains of a rapid increase in her abdominal girth in the second trimester, as well as a uterus that feels hard and uncomfortable continuously. The skin over the uterus may look shiny and tight; this is usually due to polyhydramnios and if not treated urgently can cause preterm labour.

Fetal malformations

This is particularly associated with monochorionic twins.

Conjoined twins

This extremely rare malformation of monozygotic twinning results from the incomplete division of the fertilized oocyte; it occurs once in 50 000 births and over half the cases are stillborn. Birth has to be by CS. The site and extent of fusion of the fetuses are infinitely variable. Thoracopagus (conjoined twins united at the thorax) is the commonest form of fusion (over 70% of cases). The feasibility of separating conjoined twins depends on the site and extent of fusion and the degree to which organs are shared (Oleszczuk and Oleszczuk 2005). Many conjoined twins can now be successfully separated. Others pose major ethical dilemmas – particularly if one can be saved at the expense of the other (Mifflin 2001).

Twin reversed arterial perfusion

Twin reversed arterial perfusion (TRAP) occurs in about 1 in 30 000 births. In TRAP, one twin presents without a well-defined cardiac structure and is kept alive through placental anastomoses to the circulatory system of the viable fetus (Sebire and Sepulveda 2006).

Fetus-in-fetu

In fetus-in-fetu (endoparasite), parts of a fetus may be lodged within another fetus; this can happen only in MZ twins (Hoeffel et al 2000).

Malpresentations

Although the uterus is large and distended, the fetuses are less mobile than may be supposed. They can restrict each other's movements, which may result in malpresentations (Chapter 20), particularly of the second twin. After the birth of the first twin, the presentation of the second twin may change.

Preterm rupture of the membranes

Malpresentations due to polyhydramnios may predispose to preterm rupture of the membranes.

Cord prolapse

This too is associated with malpresentations and polyhydramnios and is more likely if there is a poorly fitting presenting part. The second twin is particularly at risk of cord prolapse.

Prolonged labour

Malpresentations are a poor stimulus to good uterine action and a distended uterus is likely to lead to poor uterine activity and consequently prolonged labour (Chapter 19).

Monoamniotic twins

Approximately 1% of MZ twins share the same amniotic sac. Monoamniotic (MCMA) twins risk cord entanglement with occlusion of the blood supply through the umbilical cords to one or both fetuses. In some centres this is treated with sulindac, which reduces the amniotic fluid levels, and birth is usually around 32–34 weeks and by elective CS.

Locked twins

This is a very rare but serious complication of twin pregnancy. There are two types. One occurs when the first twin presents by the breech and the second by the vertex; the other when both are vertex presentations (Fig. 14.4). In both instances, the head of the second twin prevents the continued descent of the first. Primigravidae are more at risk than multiparous women.

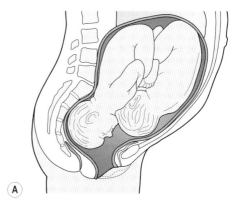

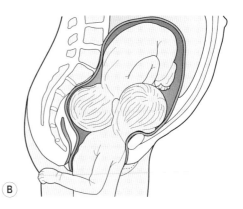

Fig. 14.4 Locked twins.

Delay in the birth of the second twin

After the birth of the first twin, uterine activity should recommence within 5 minutes. Ideally, as stated previously, the birth of the second twin should be completed within 45 minutes of the first twin being born but with close monitoring can be extended if there are no signs of fetal compromise. Poor uterine action as a result of malpresentation may be the cause of delay. The risks of such delay are intrauterine hypoxia, birth asphyxia following premature separation of the placenta and sepsis as a result of ascending infection from the first umbilical cord, which lies outside the vulva. After the birth of the first twin the lower uterine segment begins to reform and the cervical canal may have to dilate fully again.

The midwife may need to 'rub up' a contraction and put the first twin to the breast to stimulate uterine activity. If there appears to be an obstruction, medical aid is summoned and a CS may be necessary. If there is no obstruction, oxytocin infusion may be commenced or forceps-assisted birth considered.

Premature expulsion of the placenta

The placenta may be expelled before the birth of the second twin. In dichorionic twins with separate placentas, one placenta may be delivered separately; in monochorionic twins the shared placenta may be expelled. The risks of severe asphyxia and death of the second twin are very high. Haemorrhage is also likely if one twin is retained *in utero* as this prevents adequate retraction of the placental site.

Postpartum haemorrhage

Poor uterine tone as a result of overdistension or hypotonic activity is likely to lead to postpartum haemorrhage (Chapter 18). There is also a much larger placental site to contract down.

Undiagnosed twins

The possibility of an unexpected, undiagnosed second baby (in the UK this is unlikely with ultrasound scanning) should be considered if the uterus appears larger than expected after the birth of the first baby or if the baby is surprisingly smaller than expected. If an uterotonic drug has been given after the birth of the anterior shoulder of the first baby, the second twin is in great danger of birth asphyxia and birth should be expedited. The midwife must break the news of undiagnosed twins gently to the parents. These parents will require special support and guidance during the postnatal period.

Delayed interval birth of the second twin

There have been several reported cases where the first twin has been born, often very prematurely, and then a long gap before labour recommences; it can be days or even weeks before the second twin is born (Zhang et al 2004). This opportunity can be used to give antenatal corticosteroids to the mother to help mature the lungs of the second twin. Careful observations of the mother's condition must be made during this time for signs of infection and fetal compromise. The mother will need additional support from the midwives to cope with her anxieties for her preterm baby on the NICU, which may not survive, or time to grieve if the baby has died, as well as still being pregnant and her concerns for the outcome of her pregnancy.

POSTNATAL PERIOD

Care of the babies

Immediate care after the birth is the same as for a single baby. Maintenance of body temperature is vital, particularly if the babies are small; use of overhead heaters will help to prevent heat loss. Identification of the babies should be clear and the parents given the opportunity to check the identity bracelets and cuddle the babies. The babies may need to be admitted to the NICU from the labour suite, otherwise they can be encouraged to have skin-to-skin contact, and go to the breast if they are to be breastfed before being transferred to the postnatal ward with their mother.

Temperature control

Maintenance of a thermoneutral environment is essential, particularly for babies in the NICU. American studies have shown that a sick baby can benefit from sharing the incubator with its twin (Hedberg et al 1998). Clothing should be light but warm, and allow air to circulate.

Feeding

The mother may choose to feed her babies by breast or with formula milk, but whatever her choice, the midwife must support her in her decision. With breastfeeding, both babies may be breastfed separately or simultaneously. In the initial postnatal days, it is recommended she breastfeeds her twins separately, as this gives her time to get to know each baby individually and to feel confident in her ability to cope. If the babies are SFGA or preterm, the paediatricians may recommend that the babies be 'topped up' after a breastfeed. Expressed breastmilk is best for these babies. If the babies are not able to suck adequately at the breast the mother should be encouraged to express her milk regularly. Expressing should be initiated ideally within 6 hours of birth, then regularly every 2–3 hours during the day and once at night or on average 8 times per 24 hours. In some NICUs with a Millbank donor milk may be offered to preterm babies, this reduces the risk of necrotizing enterocolitis (NEC) (Patole and de Klerk 2005). As twin babies are more likely to be preterm or SFGA, their ability to coordinate the sucking and swallowing reflexes may be poor. If so, they may need to be fed intravenously or by nasogastric tube, depending on their size and general condition. The mother should be encouraged to participate in whatever method is used. Careful monitoring of weight gain is required. Hypoglycaemia may occur and regular capillary blood glucose estimations may be needed.

In the early postnatal days, mothers often worry that their milk supply is inadequate for two babies. The midwife should reassure her that lactation responds to the demands made by the babies sucking at the breast or expressing. The more stimulation the breasts are given, the more milk she will produce. At feeding times, the midwife must be with the mother to offer support and advice on positioning and fixing the babies (Fig. 14.5), as well as encouraging her in her ability to cope with breastfeeding two babies.

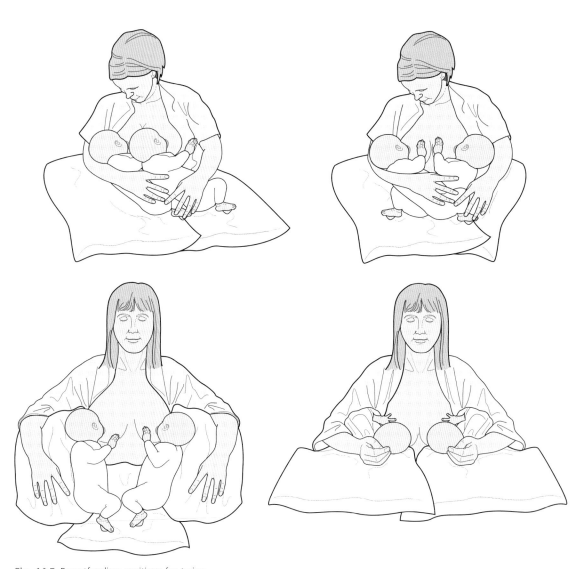

Fig. 14.5 Breastfeeding positions for twins.

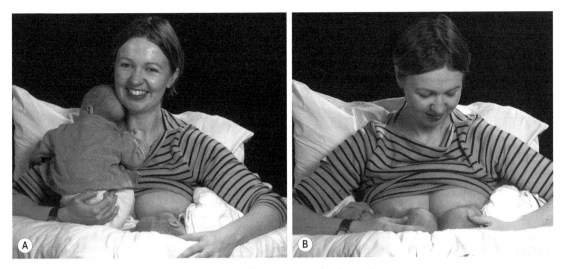

Fig. 14.6 Simultaneous feeding can be a very rewarding experience for the mother.

Breastfeeding

The advantages of breastfeeding twins are the same as for singletons (Chapter 34), but as twins have a higher tendency to be born preterm and SFGA, it is even more important that they should be breastfed. As well as the medical and nutritional advantages, there are practical reasons too, many of which are outlined in Chapter 34. Additionally, as time is limited for a mother of twins in the early days, twins can be breastfed together, when the feeds will take only a little longer than with a single baby. Some mothers will, however, prefer to feed separately.

Separate feeding

- It allows her to give one-to-one attention to each baby, something mothers of twins feel they have very little time for.
- It is easier for the mother, as she has both hands free to position and attach one baby at a time.
- If she does feed separately, it is recommended that she adopts a routine where whichever baby wakes first is fed and the second one is woken straight afterwards so keeping her feeds together.

Simultaneous feeding

- It saves time as both babies are feeding together, though the mother will need to be organized, and will need help in the early days to get both babies attached to the breast.
- If the mother does want to feed the babies together, it is advisable to try this before going home from hospital, where a midwife can stay with her throughout the entire feed, providing advice, support and an extra pair of hands.
- The woman will need additional pillows to support her back and take the weight of the babies, to avoid putting strain on her arms and back (Figs 14.5, 14.6).

Routine is the key to coping with two or more babies. It may take 4–6 weeks for a feeding routine to get established (MBF 2010).

Mother–baby relationships

Mothers with a multiple birth often worry they will find it more difficult to bond with each baby equally. This is a common concern and reassurance that their feelings are not unusual should be given. Once the mother gets to know her babies these feelings usually disappear. If, for example, they are of markedly different sizes, a mother may favour one over the other, or if one baby is in the NICU while the other is on the postnatal ward with her, she may find she bonds with the one on the ward much more quickly. In such cases the mother should be encouraged to spend as much time as possible with the baby on the NICU and to visit as soon after the birth as she feels able. If she has had an operative birth, she may find it difficult to care for two babies and extreme tiredness or anaemia will exacerbate the situation. She may have feelings of guilt if the birth and immediate postnatal period have not gone as she had planned. The midwife should be alert for such circumstances and help the mother to divide her attention between both babies and to give plenty of reassurance that she is not the first mother to feel the same way.

Mother–partner relationships

A mother who has had twins or more will inevitably turn to her partner for help with the care of the babies, and many families work well together in the care and upbringing of their children, despite the added strains and stresses a multiple birth puts on a family. In some cases her partner may feel that she is devoting too much time to the babies and not enough to him, thus making him feel excluded, especially if when he comes home from work she is too exhausted to take any interest in him. The strain on any relationship when a new baby is born can be quite difficult for the couple to adjust to, but with a multiple birth it is even worse. The midwife should always encourage the partner to be involved in the daily care of the babies, either in hospital or at home.

Care of the mother

Involution of the uterus will be slower because of its increased bulk. 'After pains' may be more troublesome and analgesia should be offered. A good diet is essential and if the mother is breastfeeding she requires a high protein, high calorie diet. It is quite common for breastfeeding mothers to feel hungry between meals and they should be encouraged to keep sensible snacks to hand for such times. A dietician may be able to offer help. The physiotherapist or midwife should instruct the mother in her postnatal exercises.

The midwife must give the mother of twins extra support. Teaching her simple parenting skills and encouraging her to carry them out with increasing assurance will build up her confidence.

The mother may feel 'in the way' if her babies are in a NICU and require a lot of intensive care. She may have feelings of guilt because of their prematurity and feel it was something she did or did not do that caused them to be born early. She should be given the opportunity to talk her feelings through. On the NICU she should always be kept up to date with the care and condition of her infants. Most NICUs now have a named nurse caring for each baby so parents know who to talk to. If one infant is very ill or dies, the parents will experience additional psychological problems. Some NICUs have psychologists as part of the team and parents can be referred to them.

Most units have a rooming-in policy so mothers can stay in the hospital with their babies for two or three nights before they are transferred home, to give them a chance to take over their total care and prepare them for coping at home.

Best practice is that twins or more should all be transferred home together from the NICU but this is not always possible. If they go home at different intervals, greater demands are placed on the mother, as she has to care for one baby at home and still visit the sick baby in hospital.

It is advisable for a mother of twins to organize help at home for the first 3–4 weeks after transfer. Initially, this may be in the form of her partner taking time off work. If relations or friends have offered to help, the mother should be sure to let them know what kind of help she is expecting from them before it is needed. If the parents are fortunate enough to be able to afford paid help, then they can say exactly what it is they expect to be done. There is no statutory help available for twins or triplets in England and Wales.

The community midwife will contact the mother after transfer home from hospital to arrange visits. The health visitor will also arrange to see the mother and her babies after the community midwife has transferred care to the health visitor.

At home the mother must be encouraged to rest and catch up on her sleep especially during the day, and eat a well-balanced diet. A good routine is the only way of coping with new babies and all mothers should be encouraged to establish one as soon as possible.

It may be wise to discourage visitors in the first week at home while the mother adjusts to the new circumstances. Her partner should be encouraged to help as much as possible.

Isolation can be a real problem for new mothers. The thought of getting two babies ready to go out can be quite fearful. Studies have shown the incidence of postnatal depression to be significantly higher in mothers of twins (Thorpe et al 1991). Stress, isolation and exhaustion are all significant precipitants of depression (Chapter 25); mothers of twins are therefore more vulnerable.

Development of twins

Twins in most respects will do as well as a single baby, but the one area they can fall behind is language development. With twins, the mother tends to talk to both of them together, so there is less one-to-one communication. Inevitably, she will be much busier and the temptation to leave the twins to amuse themselves is much greater. Talking to each other, the twins act as each other's role model for language (unlike the singleton baby, who has his or her mother). If one child speaks a word incorrectly the twin will copy it, reinforcing the mistake. This is how the so-called 'secret language' of twins develops, otherwise known as 'cryptophasia' or 'idioglossia'. It is essential that each twin is spoken to individually as much as possible. Eye contact is vital in any relationship but especially for language development. If one twin is more responsive and makes eye contact more easily than the other, the mother may respond much more readily to this twin without realizing it.

Identity and individuality

Parents of twins should be encouraged to think of their children as individuals. The distinction between twins can start in the postnatal ward with differently coloured blankets, or different small soft toys. As they grow up, dressing them in different style of clothes, giving them different hairstyles can make children individual. People should be encouraged to refer to the children by name, or 'the girls' or 'boys' and not 'the twins'. At birthdays or Christmas, separate cards and different presents help to retain individuality. The twins should be given the opportunity to spend time apart.

Siblings of multiples

An elder brother or sister of twins may find their arrival very difficult, especially if they have had a number of years of undivided parental attention. Parents must be alert to the feelings of their other children and include them as much as possible in all activities with the twins. A single older sibling may see the parents as a pair, the twins as a pair, while he or she feels isolated. It can be very helpful to find a 'special friend' for the older child, for instance a godparent, or other friend. A good idea is for the parents to arrange not only for the twins to have a present for the older child but for the older child to choose a present for each of the twins. Two different small cuddly toys as the first presents the twins receive can become very special gifts.

TRIPLETS AND HIGHER ORDER BIRTHS

The increasing number of surviving triplets and higher order births (Fig. 14.7) will produce many more families needing special advice and support from healthcare workers. In the 1980s the UK Triplet Study (Botting et al 1990) revealed the problems these families face are even greater than were previously realized.

A woman expecting three or more babies is at risk of all the same complications as one expecting twins, but magnified. She is more likely to have a period in hospital resting before the triplets' birth and they will almost certainly be born preterm. Perinatal mortality rates are higher for triplets than twins and the incidence of cerebral palsy is also increased (Pharoah et al 2002; CMACE 2011).

Triplets or more are almost always born by CS. The midwives must be prepared to receive several small babies within a very short time span. It is essential the paediatric team be present as specialist care may be required. The dangers associated with these births are asphyxia, intracranial injury and perinatal death.

The main difficulties these families experience are insufficient practical and financial help and the lack of awareness of their problems by professionals. The emotional stress and anxiety of the birth, having babies in the NICU and the worries of coping with the babies when they go home will seem overwhelming if no arrangements for extra help have been made before the babies are born. A mother should never be expected to manage by herself. Taking triplets out for a walk or any expedition can need major organization, even without the parents having to cope with uninvited comments from passers-by. Some of these can be insensitive and hurtful, making inferences about fertility and the parents bringing extra work on themselves.

The midwife must ensure that the mother's health visitor and, if necessary, a social worker are involved in her care. If the family needs extra outside help, this must be organized before the babies are born. Applications to the council for rehousing may also be needed.

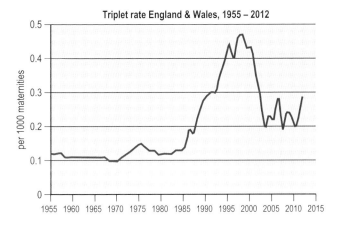

Triplet rate England & Wales, 1955 – 2012

Fig. **14.7** Triplet rates, 1955–2012. *Data from Office of National Statistics.*

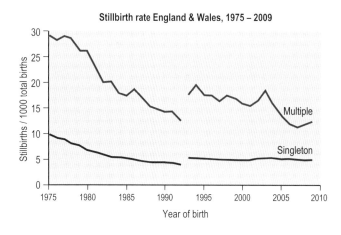

Fig. 14.8 Stillbirth rates, 1975–2009.
Data from Office of National Statistics 2011.

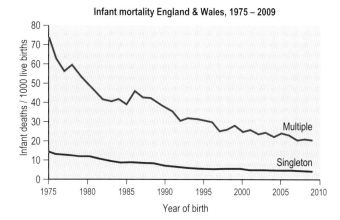

Fig. 14.9 Infant mortality, 1975–2009.
Data from Office for National Statistics 2011.

DISABILITY AND BEREAVEMENT

Perinatal mortality and long-term morbidity are both more common among multiple births than singletons. The perinatal mortality rate for twins is about four times that of singletons, and for triplets, 12 times (Figs 14.8, 14.9).

The grief of parents following the death of one of a multiple set is often underestimated. The specific problems they face are not understood and their needs poorly met. It often feels 'easier' to concentrate on the survivor(s), thus denying the parents essential time and space to grieve. All too often people say that they are lucky because they still have one healthy child (or more). No one ever says that to parents who lose one of their

two or three singleton children (Bryan 1986). The conflicting emotions the parents will feel and the need to grieve for the child who has died, while wanting to rejoice at the birth of the healthy twin, can be confusing. Birthdays and anniversaries and the constant presence of the survivor(s) are all reminders of the dead child. The parents may need help in relating to the survivor(s). Addresses of organizations that offer support should be made available to the parents. Where one or more of a multiple set has a disability it is often the healthy child who needs additional special attention. He or she may feel guilt that it was something they did that caused the twin's disability and may be resentful of the attention the other one needs, or of the loss of twinship. Any of these may lead to emotional and behavioral problems if not addressed early on.

MULTIFETAL PREGNANCY REDUCTION (MFPR)

This is the reduction of an apparently healthy higher-order multiple pregnancy down to two or even one embryo so the chances of survival are much higher. It may be offered to parents who have conceived triplets or more, whether spontaneously or as a result of assisted reproduction.

The procedure is usually carried out between the 10th and 12th week of the pregnancy. Various techniques may be used, either inserting a needle under ultrasound guidance via the vagina or, more commonly, through the abdominal wall into the fetal thorax. Potassium chloride is usually used, although some doctors prefer saline. Whichever technique is used, all embryos remain in the uterus until birth. Usually the pregnancy is reduced to two embryos, but in some cases to three or even one (Wimalasundera 2006). Any parents who have been offered this treatment must be given counselling, which should include:

- the advantages and disadvantages of reducing the pregnancy
- the risks of continuing with a higher multiple pregnancy
- the risks of MFPR
- the effects on the surviving children
- how the parents may feel afterwards
- help for the parents to reach the right decision for them
- organizations who can help them
- the offer of long-term support if and when required.

SELECTIVE FETICIDE

This may be offered to parents with a multiple pregnancy, where one of the babies has a serious abnormality. The affected fetus is injected as described in MFPR, but this is not usually performed until much later in the pregnancy so allowing the healthy fetus time to grow and develop normally. Counselling must again be offered to the parents. The full impact of either of these procedures and their bereavement will often not be felt until the birth of all their babies (including the dead baby) often many weeks later. Moreover, unlike the termination of a single pregnancy, the parents will be more aware of what could have been as they watch the survivor(s) grow up. When it comes to the labour, midwives must be ready to offer the appropriate care and understanding of the parents' bereavement. The bereavement should be clearly indicated in the notes so it is not forgotten when the mother comes back for her postnatal check and for future pregnancies.

SOURCES OF HELP

In the UK, there is at present no statutory obligation to provide any extra help for families with twins, triplets or more. The support provided by social services varies greatly so it is always advisable for families with triplets to apply. Healthcare workers should be prepared to write letters supporting any applications these families have made. In the UK child benefit is paid to all children whose parents have an individual income of less than £50,000. The first-born child receives a higher allowance than subsequent children. In multiple pregnancies, it is only the firstborn child that receives the higher allowance.

Parents should be advised to contact organizations such as Home Start (see Useful Websites), or local colleges with nursery training courses, both of which may be able to offer assistance.

The Multiple Births Foundation (MBF)

The MBF offers advice and support to families as soon as their multiple pregnancy is diagnosed, as well as to couples considering treatment for infertility. It offers information through its antenatal meetings for couples and professionals. The MBF also provides information and support to professionals through its education programme – study days, courses, lectures and publications.

Multiple births and their impact on families is a series of publications for professionals. It comprises a set of five books, which can be bought together or individually:

- *Facts about multiple births*
- *Multiple pregnancy*
- *Bereavement*
- *Special needs in twins*
- *Twins and triplets: the first five years and beyond*

See the MBF website for a complete list of the publications available.

TAMBA (Twins and Multiple Births Association)

This is the umbrella organization for the 150+ local twins clubs throughout the country. The clubs are run by parents of twins and are the best source of practical advice and support for parents expecting twins or more. TAMBA also runs a number of specialist groups.

TAMBA Twinline is a national, confidential listening and information telephone service for all parents of twins, triplets and more (see Useful Websites).

REFERENCES

Black M, Bhattacharya S 2010 Epidemiology of multiple pregnancy and the effect of assisted conception. Seminars in Fetal and Neonatal Medicine 15 (6):306–12

Blondel B, Kaminski M 2002 Trends in the occurrence, determinants, and consequences of multiple births. Seminars in Perinatology 26(4):239–49

Bomsel-Helmreich O, Al Mufti W 2005 Multiple pregnancy: epidemiology, gestation and perinatal outcome. Informa Healthcare, New York, p 94–100

Botting B, Macfarlane A J, Price F V 1990 Three, four and more: a study of triplets and higher order births. HMSO, London

Braude P 2006 One child at a time: reducing multiple births after IVF. Human Fertilisation & Embryology Authority, London

Bryan E M 1984 Twins in the family (a parent's guide). Constable, London

Bryan E M 1986 The death of a newborn twin. How can support for parents be improved? Acta Geneticae Medicae et Gemellologiae 5:166–70

CMACE (Centre for Maternal and Child Enquiries) 2011 Perinatal Mortality 2009: United Kingdom. CMACE, London. Accessed at www.hqip.org .uk/assets/NCAPOP-Library/ CMACE-Reports/35.-March-2011 -Perinatal-Mortality-2009.pdf (26 May 2013)

Consensus Statement 2011 Multiple births from fertility treatment in the UK. Human Fertility 14(3):151–3

Cutting R, Morroll D, Stephen A et al 2008 Elective single embryo transfer: guidelines for practice. British Fertility Society and Association of Clinical Embryologists Human Fertility 11(3): 131–46

Dennes W J B, Sullivan M F H, Fisk N M, 2006 Scientific basis of twin-to-twin transfusion syndrome In: Kilby M, Baker P, Critchley H et al (eds) Multiple pregnancy. RCOG Press, London, p 167–81

Denton J, Bryan E M 1995 Prenatal preparation for parenting twins, triplets or more: the social aspect. In: Whittle M, Ward R H (eds) Multiple

pregnancy. RCOG Press, London, p 119

Hedberg Nyquist K, Lutes L M 1998 Co-bedding twins: a developmentally supportive care strategy. Journal of Obstetrics, Gynecology and Neonatal Nursing 27(4):450–6

Hoeffel C C, Nguyen K Q, Phan H T et al 2000. Fetus-in-fetu: a case report and a literature review. Pediatrics 105:1335–44

Landy H J, Keith L G 1998 The vanishing twin. A review. Human Reproduction 4:177

Lassi Z S, Salam R A, Haider B A et al 2013 Folic acid supplementation during pregnancy for maternal health and pregnancy outcomes. Cochrane Database of Systematic Reviews, Issue 3. Art. No. CD006896. doi: 10.1002/14651858. CD006896.pub2

Leonard L G 2000 Breastfeeding triplets: the at-home experience. Public Health Nursing 17(3):211–21

Leonard L G, Denton J 2006 Preparation for parenting multiple birth children. Early Human Development 82:371–8

Masson G 2007 Twin pregnancy. In: Grady K, Howell C, Cox C (eds) The MOET course manual: managing obstetric emergencies and trauma, 2nd edition. RCOG, London, p 295–300

Mifflin P C 2001 Jodie and Mary: ethical and legal implications of separating conjoined twins. Practising Midwife 4(7):48–9

MBF (Multiple Births Foundation) 2010 Monochorionic pregnancy when twins share one placenta. Online. MBF, London

MBF (Multiple Births Foundation) 2011a Feeding twins, triplets and more. [A booklet for parents with advice and information.] MBF, London

MBF (Multiple Births Foundation) 2011b Guidance for health professionals on feeding twins, triplets and higher order multiples. MBF, London

NICE (National Institute for Health and Clinical Excellence) 2008 Antenatal care: routine care for the healthy

pregnant woman. CG62. NICE, London

NICE (National Institute for Health and Clinical Excellence) 2011 Multiple pregnancy: the management of twin and triplet pregnancies in the antenatal period. CG 129. NICE, London

ONS (Office of National Statistics) 2011 Childhood, infant and perinatal mortality in England and Wales 2011. www.ons.gov.uk/ons/ dcp171778_300596.pdf (accessed 12 June 2013)

ONS (Office of National Statistics) 2013 Births in England and Wales by characteristics of birth. www.ons.gov .uk (accessed 12 June 2013)

Oleszczuk J J, Oleszczuk A K 2005 Conjoined twins. In Keith L G, Blickenstein I (eds) Multiple pregnancy, 2nd edn. Parthenon, London, p 233–45

Owen D J, Wood L, Neilson J P 2004 Antenatal care for women with multiple pregnancies. The Liverpool approach. Clinical Obstetrics and Gynecology 47(1):263–71

Pasquini L, Wimalasundera R C, Fisk N M 2004. Management of other complications specific to monochorionic twin pregnancies. Best Practice and Research in Clinical Obstetrics and Gynaecology 18(4):577–99

Patole S K, de Klerk N 2005 Impact of standardised feeding regimens on incident of neonatal necrotising enterolitis: a systematic review and meta-analysis of observational studies. Archives of Disease in Childhood Fetal and Neonatal Edition 90(2):F147–F151

Pharoah P O D, Price T S, Plomin R 2002 Cerebral palsy in twins: a national study. Archives of Disease in Childhood Fetal Neonatal Edition 87(2):F122–4

RCOG (Royal College of Obstetricians and Gynaecologists) 2006 Multiple pregnancy. Consensus views arising from the 50th Study Group. RCOG, London, p 283–6

RCOG (Royal College of Obstetricians and Gynaecologists) 2010 Amniocentesis and chorionic villus sampling. Greentop guideline No 8. RCOG, London

Sebire N J, Sepulveda W 2006 Management of twin reversed arterial perfusion (TRAP) sequence. In: Kilby M, Baker P, Critchley H et al (eds) Multiple pregnancy. RCOG, London, p 199–222

Thorpe K, Golding J, MacGillivray I et al 1991 Comparisons of prevalence of depression in mothers of twins and mothers of singletons. British Medical Journal 302:875–8

Udom-Rice I, Inglis S R, Skupski D et al 2000 Optimal gestational age for twin delivery. Journal of Perinatalology 20(4):231–4

Wimalasundera R 2006 Selective reduction and termination of multiple pregnancies. In: Kilby M, Baker P, Critchley H et al (eds) Multiple pregnancy. RCOG, London, p 95–108

Wood S L, Onge R S, Connors G et al 1996 Evaluation of the twin peak or lambda sign in determining

chorionicity in multiple pregnancy. Obstetrics and Gynecology 88(1):6–9

Yamamoto M, Ville Y 2006 Twin-to-twin transfusion syndrome. In: Kilby M, Baker P, Critchley H et al (eds) Multiple pregnancy. RCOG, London, p 183–97

Zhang J, Hamilton B, Martin J et al 2004 Delayed interval delivery and infant survival: a population-based study. American Journal of Obstetrics and Gynecology 191(2):470–6

FURTHER READING

Cooper C 2004 Twins and multiple births. Vermilion, London
A GP and mother of twins gives practical advice on coping with twins and more. Suitable for parents and professionals alike.

Royal College of Obstetricians and Gynaecologists (RCOG) 2006 Multiple pregnancy. RCOG Press, London
Written by specialists in multiple pregnancy.

USEFUL WEBSITES AND CONTACT DETAILS

Homestart UK: www.home-start.org.uk
Multiple Births Foundation: www.multiplebirths.org.uk
Tel: 020 8383 3519 or 020 3313 3519. e-mail: mbf@imperial.nhs.uk

Twins and Multiple Births Association: www.tamba.org.uk
Tel: 01483 304442; TAMBA Twinline: 0800 138 0509

Section | 4 |

Labour

Chapter |15|

Care of the perineum, repair and female genital mutilation

Ranee Thakar, Abdul H Sultan, Maureen D Raynor, Carol McCormick, Kinsi Clarke

In the United Kingdom (UK), approximately 85% of women sustain some degree of perineal trauma following vaginal birth and it can be extrapolated that millions of women will be affected worldwide. Morbidity in the short and long term following trauma and repair can lead to major physical, psychological, sexual and social problems affecting the woman's ability to care for her newborn baby and other members of the family. Midwives should be aware that suturing is a major and sometimes traumatic event for women (Green et al 1998). The repair of the perineum is an important part of the continuing care of a woman during labour and birth (Kettle 2012). The permanent presence of midwives who are trained and continually developing expertise in perineal repair, minimizes the problems associated with the rotation of inexperienced junior medical staff (Draper and Newell 1996) and provides continuity of care for women.

This chapter presents an overview of key issues relating to perineal care during labour and childbirth. It is important that the reader has knowledge and understanding of the anatomy and physiology of the pelvic floor (see Chapter 3) prior to engaging with this chapter.

THE CHAPTER AIMS TO:

- draw on the evidence base to identify some of the factors associated with a reduced incidence of perineal trauma during the second stage of labour

- examine the standard classification used to describe the different types of perineal trauma
- discuss the systematic assessment necessary in order to accurately diagnose perineal trauma
- highlight the significance of female genital mutilation and the inherent consequences for birth and women's psychosexual wellbeing and health more broadly
- consider the basic principles involved in repairing perineal trauma
- examine the midwife's role and medicolegal considerations involved in perineal trauma.

FACTORS ASSOCIATED WITH REDUCED INCIDENCE OF PERINEAL TRAUMA

Many studies have compared interventions to prevent perineal trauma during the second stage of labour, starting with antenatal considerations such as diet and nutrition as well as the recommended antenatal perineal massage for nulliparous women (Beckmann and Garrett 2006). Coupled with this there are some well-documented risk factors associated with more complex perineal trauma (third- and fourth-degree tears) such as fetal macrosomia, Asian ethnicity, persistent occipitoposterior position, instrumental births and nulliparity (Groutz et al 2011; Chan et al 2012). Box 15.1 summarizes some of the factors that might lead to a reduction in perineal trauma.

DEFINITION OF PERINEAL TRAUMA

Perineal trauma may occur spontaneously during vaginal birth or when a surgical incision (episiotomy) is intentionally made to facilitate birth. It is possible to have an episiotomy and a spontaneous tear (e.g. extension of an episiotomy). Anterior perineal trauma is defined as injury to the labia, anterior vaginal wall, urethra or clitoris. Posterior perineal trauma is defined as any injury to the posterior vaginal wall or perineal muscles and may include disruption of the anal sphincters.

In order to standardize definitions of perineal tears, the classification outlined in Table 15.1 is recommended (Royal College of Obstetricians and Gynaecologists [RCOG] 2007; National Institute for Health and Clinical Excellence [NICE] 2007). (See Chapter 3 for details of pelvic floor anatomy) (Fig. 15.1.)

Box 15.1 Strategies to prevent/minimize perineal trauma during labour

Influencing factors	The evidence
Antenatal perineal massage but not perineal massage during the second stage of labour	Beckmann M M, Garrett A J 2006 (Cochrane review) and NICE 2007
Use of warm perineal compresses during the second stage of labour	Aasheim et al 2011 (Cochrane review)
Restricted use of episiotomy	Carroli and Mignini 2009 (Cochrane review)
Upright birth positions – freedom of woman to choose	Gupta et al 2004 (Cochrane review) and NICE 20007
Non-directed pushing (woman using her own urges to bear down without coaching from the midwife or doctor)	NICE 2007

Table 15.1 Classification of perineal trauma

First degree	Injury to perineal skin only
Second degree	Injury to perineum involving perineal muscles but not involving the anal sphincter
Third degree	Injury to perineum involving the anal sphincter complex: 3a: Less than 50% of external anal sphincter (EAS) thickness torn 3b: More than 50% of external anal sphincter thickness torn 3c: Both external anal sphincter and internal anal sphincter (IAS) torn
Fourth degree	Injury to perineum involving the anal sphincter complex and anal epithelium
Isolated button hole injury of rectum	Injury to the rectal mucosa without injury to the anal sphincters

Source: NICE 2007, RCOG 2007

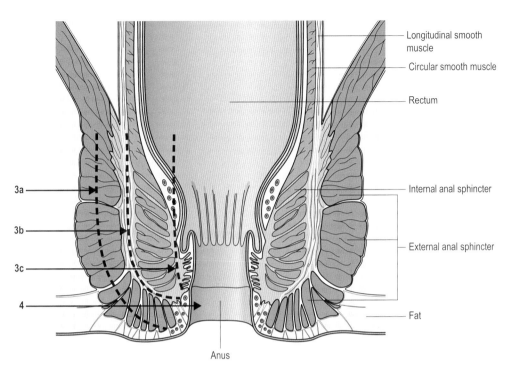

Longitudinal smooth muscle

Circular smooth muscle

Rectum

Internal anal sphincter

External anal sphincter

3a

3b

3c

4

Fat

Anus

Fig. 15.1 Classification of perineal trauma depicted in a schematic representation of the anal sphincters (modified from Sultan and Kettle 2007).

EPISIOTOMY

The traditional teaching that episiotomy is protective against more severe perineal lacerations has not been substantiated (Carroli and Mignini 2009), and therefore the liberal use of 'prophylactic' episiotomy is no longer recommended. However, there are still valid reasons to perform an episiotomy. A variety of episiotomy techniques are described in the literature (Kalis et al 2012), but two types of episiotomy are most frequently used:

- *Midline episiotomy*: Advantages of the midline episiotomy are that it does not cut through muscle, the two sides of the incised area are anatomically balanced, making surgical repair easier, and blood loss is less than with mediolateral episiotomy. A major drawback is that extension through the external anal sphincter and into the rectum can occur. For this reason midline episiotomy is not recommended in the UK.
- *Mediolateral episiotomy*: The right mediolateral episiotomy is the technique approved for use by midwives in the UK. The incision is made starting at the midline of the posterior fourchette and aimed towards the ischial tuberosity to avoid the anal

sphincter. In addition to the skin and subcutaneous tissues, the bulbospongiosus and the transverse perineal muscles are cut.

DIAGNOSIS OF PERINEAL TRAUMA

Following every vaginal birth a thorough assessment should be performed to exclude genital trauma. The healthcare professional should explain to the woman what they plan to do and why, offer inhalational analgesia and ensure that if there is pre-existing epidural analgesia, it is effective. There must be good lighting and the woman should be positioned so that she is comfortable and the genital structures can be seen clearly. If this is not possible then it is vital to explain to the woman the rationale for the examination and why it is necessary to place her in a comfortable position, i.e. lithotomy (NICE 2007). In the UK, modern birthing beds in the hospital setting mean that the use of lithotomy poles in midwifery practice to support women's legs during examination of the genital tract or to repair perineal trauma is not always warranted. However, supported lithotomy (i.e. use of poles) is necessary to aid the diagnosis and repair of complex trauma to the genital tract. When supported lithotomy position is to be employed, clear explanation should be provided to the woman in a sensitive manner. The midwife should be mindful that use of lithotomy poles may conjure up images associated with previous sexual abuse or female genital mutilation/female cutting (Kettle and Raynor 2010). Visualization, effective analgesia and systematic assessment of perineal trauma can be even more challenging at a homebirth, not least because of poor lighting and the use of settees or low bedroom furniture. When faced with such complexities it is perfectly acceptable for midwives attending home births to transfer women into the hospital setting for thorough assessment, especially if the repair is judged not to be straightforward or the midwife does not have the requisite skills/competence to perform the repair.

Importance of anorectal examination

Informed consent must be obtained for a vaginal and rectal examination. If the digital assessment is restricted because of pain, adequate analgesia must be given prior to examination. Following inspection of the genitalia, the labia should be parted and a vaginal examination performed to establish the full extent of the vaginal tear. When multiple or deep tears are present it is best to examine and repair in the supported lithotomy position, as previously stated.

A rectal examination should then be performed to exclude anal sphincter trauma. Figure 15.2 shows a partial tear along the external anal sphincter which would have been missed if a rectal examination was not performed. Every woman should have a rectal examination prior to suturing in order to avoid missing isolated tears such as a

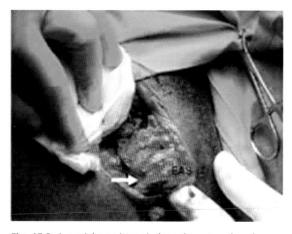

Fig. 15.2 A partial tear (arrow) along the external anal sphincter which would have been missed if a rectal examination was not performed (Sultan and Kettle 2007).

'button hole' of the rectal mucosa (NICE 2007). Furthermore, a third- or fourth-degree tear may be present beneath apparently intact perineal skin, highlighting the need to perform a rectal examination in order to exclude obstetric anal sphincter injuries (OASIS) following every vaginal birth (Sultan and Kettle 2007) (Fig. 15.3). Following diagnosis of the tear it should be graded according to the recommended classification (NICE 2007; RCOG 2007), as delineated earlier in Table 15.1.

In order to diagnose OASIS, clear visualization is necessary and the injury should be confirmed by palpation. By inserting the gloved index finger in the anal canal and the thumb in the vagina, the anal sphincter can be palpated by performing a pill-rolling motion. If there is still uncertainty, the woman should be asked to contract her anal sphincter (in the absence of an epidural) and if the anal sphincter is disrupted, there will be a distinct gap felt anteriorly. If the perineal skin is intact there will be an absence of puckering on the perianal skin anteriorly. This may not be evident under regional or general anaesthesia. As the external anal sphincter (EAS) is normally in a state of tonic contraction, disruption results in retraction of the sphincter ends. The internal anal sphincter (IAS) is a circular smooth muscle that appears paler (similar to raw fish) (Fig. 15.4) than the striated EAS (similar to raw red meat) (Sultan and Kettle 2007) (Fig. 15.5).

FEMALE GENITAL MUTILATION/ GENITAL CUTTING/FEMALE CIRCUMCISION

Background

Partly as a result of immigration and refugee movements, women who have undergone female genital mutilation (FGM) now present all over the world. Therefore healthcare professionals in all countries need to be familiar with the practice of genital cutting and its implications, particularly for childbirth and safeguarding of the next generation, as well as to be proactive in eradicating this harmful cultural practice altogether.

The language used by midwives and doctors when dealing with genital cutting is important as parents understandably resent the suggestion that they have mutilated their daughters. As a result, the word 'cutting' has increasingly come to be used to avoid alienating communities (World Health Organization [WHO] 2013).

There has been great debate amongst holy men as to whether, particularly type one, genital cutting (sometimes referred to as *Sunna* circumcision) is required in the Muslim faith, but it is clear that female genital cutting is not linked to the Bible or the Koran. It is in fact condemned by many Islamic scholars. Genital cutting predates both the Koran and the Bible, appearing in the 2nd

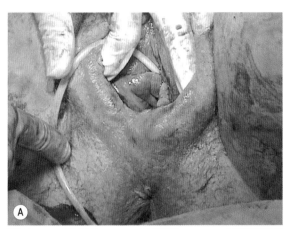

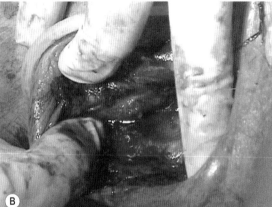

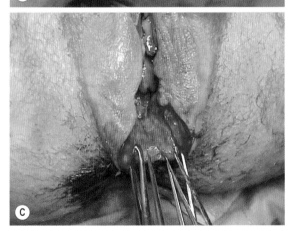

Fig. 15.3 A third- or fourth-degree tear may be present beneath apparently intact perineal skin highlighting the need to perform a rectal examination in order to exclude obstetric anal sphincter injuries (OASIS) following every vaginal delivery (Sultan and Kettle 2007). (a) An apparent intact perineum. (b) A 'bucket handle tear' is demonstrated behind the intact perineal skin. (c) The torn external anal sphincter.

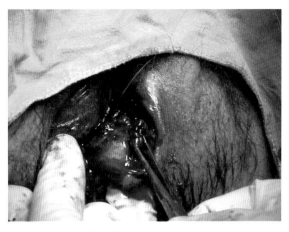

Fig. 15.4 The IAS is a circular smooth muscle that appears pale (similar to raw fish).

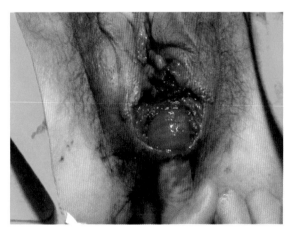

Fig. 15.5 The EAS is striated muscle and appears red in colour (similar to raw red meat).

century BC. It is a cultural practice, not a religious one. In countries when there is a mixture of Christians and Muslims it is practised by both faiths (WHO 2001, 2008, 2013).

What actually happens to the girls and women varies from ritualistic herbs rubbed into the genitalia to complete removal of the clitoris and labia minora, and stitching (or closing by other means, usually thorns) of the labia majora. The WHO (2001) define FGM as any procedure that intentionally alters or causes injury to the external female genital organs for non-medical reasons and describes four types, as depicted in Fig. 15.6.

Type 1: Clitoridectomy is partial or total removal of the clitoris and/or, in some cases, only the prepuce (the fold of skin surrounding the clitoris).

FGM I 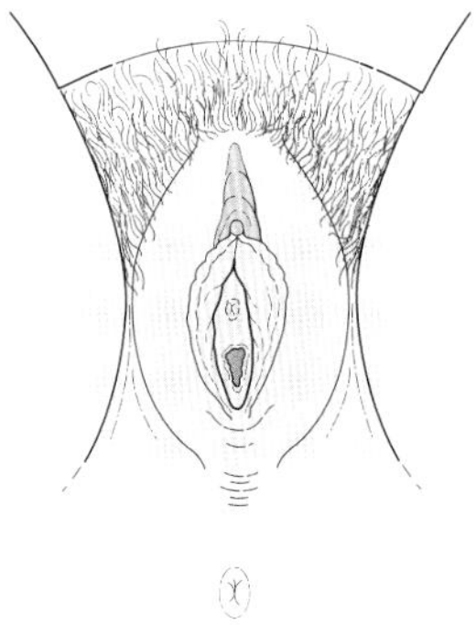		Partial or total removal of the clitoris and/or the prepuce **(clitoridectomy)**
FGM II 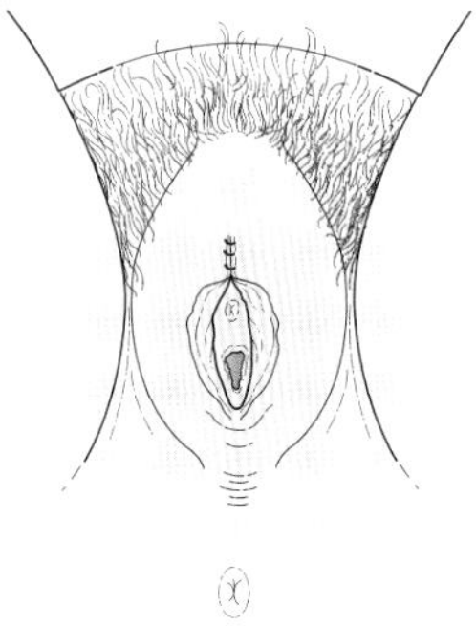		Partial or total removal of the clitoris and the labia minora, with or without excision of the labia majora **(excision)**
FGM III 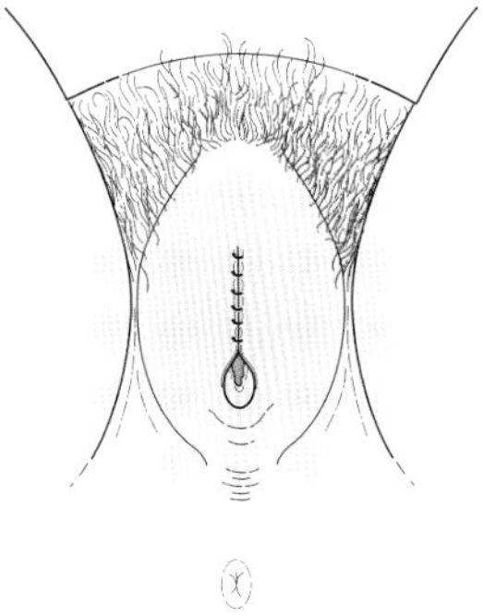		Narrowing of the vaginal orifice with creation of a covering seal by cutting and appositioning the labia minora and/or the labia majora, with or without excision of the clitoris **(infibulation)** **Source:** (UNICEF 2005)
FGM IV		All other harmful procedures to the female genitalia for non-medical purposes. This for example may include incising, scraping, pricking, piercing or other mutilating procedure.

Fig. 15.6 Types of female genital mutilation.

Type 2: Excision: partial or total removal of the clitoris and the labia minora, with or without excision of the labia majora (the labia are 'the lips' that surround the vagina).

Type 3: Infibulation: narrowing of the vaginal opening through the cutting of the labia minora and suturing or closing of the outer, labia majora, with or without removal of the clitoris.

Type 4: Other: all other harmful procedures to the female genitalia for non-medical purposes, e.g. pricking, piercing, incising, scraping and cauterizing the genital area.

In practice, however, it is often difficult to be clear about the classification. Uneven cutting, scarring and defects in suture lines are very common findings, therefore every woman who has undergone genital cutting should be assessed by an experienced practitioner and dealt with individually.

The age at which girls undergo genital cutting varies enormously according to their community. The procedure may be carried out when the girl is a newborn, during childhood, adolescence, at marriage or during the first pregnancy. Most commonly it is performed on girls between four and eight years of age (WHO 2001, 2008).

Girls are usually compliant when they have the procedure carried out as they believe they will be outcasts if they are not cut. Mothers and other family members believe they are doing the best for their children, as women are thought to be unclean and immoral unless they had been cut. In most cultures that practise FGM the girls/women would be unmarriageable if uncut. So deep-rooted is this cultural tradition that it is the opinion of some that a woman will not be promiscuous or unfaithful if she derives little or no pleasure from sexual intercourse (Elnashar and Abdelhady 2007). Despite being aware of the dangers associated with genital cutting, it is this very strong belief that makes parents ensure their daughters are cut in accordance with their cultural custom and tradition.

Anaesthetics and antiseptic treatment are not generally used and the practice is usually carried out using basic tools such as circumcision knives, scissors, scalpels, pieces of glass and razor blades. Often iodine or a mixture of herbs is placed on the wound to tighten the vagina and stop the bleeding.

Immediate complications include severe pain, shock, haemorrhage, tetanus, sepsis and urinary retention. Inexperienced or very old cutters may inadvertently cause injury to adjacent tissue. Late complications include sexual dysfunction with anorgasmia, keloid scar formation, dermoid cysts and psychological issues. There is an increasing trend for medically trained personnel to perform FGM in hospitals and institutions (Hassanin et al 2008). There are no known health benefits associated with FGM.

In the UK the Prohibition of Female Circumcision Act 1985 makes it an offence to carry out FGM or to aid, abet or procure the service of another person. The Female Genital Mutilation amendment to the Act 2003 makes it against the law for FGM to be performed anywhere in the world on UK permanent residents of any age and carries a maximum sentence of 14 years imprisonment (Home Office 2004). Europe and many other countries also have laws against FGM.

The role of the midwife

In order to have a robust plan of care during labour, identification of women from countries that practise FGM is essential antenatally. NICE (2008) highlights the importance of antenatal screening of these women. This should be performed in a timely manner so that referral and consultation with a practitioner who can address both the physical needs of the woman plus the safeguarding and legal issues for the unborn child in a sensitive manner can take place.

Antenatally, physical examination is necessary to assess the extent of genital cutting and make a birth plan, also to identify whether antenatal surgery (deinfibulation) would be beneficial before 20 weeks of pregnancy. Most women would prefer a deinfibulation in labour but a plan to deinfibulate during labour means all staff must have adequate training and experience in performing the procedure, which in most hospitals is an unrealistic expectation. Even women who have given birth before or have had a previous deinfibulation should be examined as they may have suffered trauma at the last birth and some women will have undergone a reinfibulation (being 'closed' again), usually in their country of origin.

There is contradicting evidence as to whether FGM is associated with prolonged or obstructed labour (De Silva 1989; Al-Hussaini 2003; Millogo-Traore et al 2007). However, during the second stage of labour the reduced labia and inelastic anterior tissue may be scarred and adherent to the labial vault and/or urethra, and therefore the birth process can cause significant anterior trauma to these structures. A low threshold for a right mediolateral episiotomy should be discussed with the woman antenatally, particularly if the type of cutting has left scar tissue that may prevent progress or cause additional trauma in the form of an anterior tear in the second stage of labour (RCOG 2009).

A proforma including a predrawn diagram, akin to that outlined in the RCOG (2009) guideline, should be completed for the identification of the type of FGM and the agreed birth plan as part of good note-keeping. The impact of FGM is very profound, as captured by the personal narrative at the end of the chapter (Box 15.2).

REPAIR OF PERINEAL TRAUMA

Basic principles prior to repairing perineal trauma (NICE 2007; Sultan and Thakar 2007)

The skills and knowledge of the operator are important factors in achieving a successful repair. Ideally the repair should be conducted in a timely manner by the same midwife who attended the woman in labour. This ensures seamless continuity of care, as the midwife would have established a good rapport and trust with the woman. The woman should be referred to a more experienced healthcare professional if uncertainty exists as to the nature or extent of trauma sustained. Having fully informed the woman why a detailed examination is required and to gain her consent, an initial systematic assessment of the perineal trauma must be performed including a sensitive rectal examination to exclude any trauma to the IAS/EAS is not missed (NICE 2007).

In order to reduce maternal morbidity, repair of the perineum should be undertaken as soon as possible to minimize the risk of bleeding and oedema of the perineum as this makes it more difficult to recognize tissue structures and planes when the repair eventually takes place. Perineal trauma should be repaired using aseptic techniques. Equipment should be checked and swabs and needles counted before and after the procedure.

A repair undertaken on a non-cooperative woman, due to pain, is likely to result in a poor repair. Ensure that the wound is adequately anaesthetized prior to commencing the repair. It is recommended that 10–20 ml of lidocaine 1% (maximum dose 3 mg/kg) is injected evenly into the perineal wound. If the woman has an epidural it may be 'topped-up' instead of injecting local anaesthetic.

The issue of obstetric anal sphincter injuries is addressed in more detail later in the chapter, but it is worth noting here that repair of such trauma should be undertaken in theatre, under general or regional anaesthesia. In addition to providing pain relief, this provides the added advantage of relaxing the muscles, enabling the operator to retrieve the ends of the torn sphincter and identify the full length of the anal sphincter prior to repair. An indwelling catheter should be inserted for at least 12 hours to avoid urinary retention.

In the case of FGM, if a woman undergoes a deliberate traumatic deinfibulation in labour without antenatal preparation she may ask to be reinfibulated (closed again), but any repair carried out after birth, whether following spontaneous laceration or deliberate defibulation, should be sufficient to oppose the raw edges of the perineal trauma and control bleeding. It must not result in a vaginal opening that makes intercourse difficult or impossible, as this would be in breach of the law. The WHO (2001, 2008, 2013) recommends suturing of raw edges to prevent spontaneous reinfibulation but an individual assessment should be made.

First-degree tears and labial lacerations

Women should be advised that, in the case of first-degree trauma, the wound should be sutured in order to improve healing, unless the skin edges are well opposed (NICE 2007). If the tear is left unsutured, the midwife or doctor must discuss the implications with the woman and obtain her informed consent. Details regarding the discussion and consent must be fully documented in the woman's case notes.

Labial lacerations are usually very superficial but may be very painful. Some practitioners do not recommend suturing, but if the trauma is bilateral the lacerations can sometimes adhere together over the urethra and the woman may present with voiding difficulties. It is important to advise the woman to part the labia daily during bathing to prevent adhesions forming. This is particularly important when caring for women with type 3 FGM.

Episiotomy and second-degree tears

Although the repair of these tears was previously carried out using the interrupted technique, the continuous suturing technique for perineal skin closure has been shown to be associated with less short-term pain. Moreover, if the continuous technique is used for all layers (vagina, perineal muscles and skin), the reduction in pain is even greater (Kettle et al 2007). The perineal muscles should be repaired using absorbable polyglactin material which is available in standard and rapidly absorbable forms. A recent Cochrane review has shown that there are few differences in short-term and long-term pain, between standard and rapidly absorbing synthetic sutures, but more women need standard sutures to be removed (Kettle et al 2010).

Technique for perineal repair

Technique is important, as is the suturing material used (Kettle and Fenner 2007).

Suturing the vagina (Fig. 15.7a)

Using 2/0 absorbable polyglactin 910 material (*Vicryl rapide®*), the first stitch is inserted above the apex of the vaginal skin laceration to secure any bleeding points.

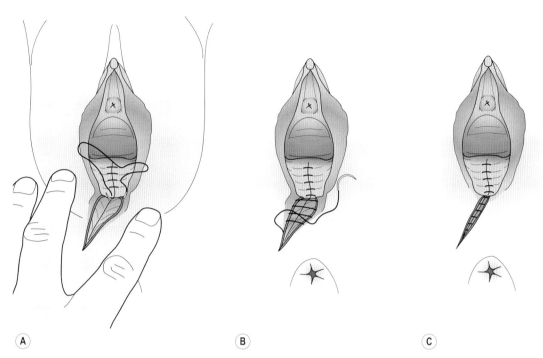

Fig. 15.7 Continuous suturing technique for mediolateral episiotomy (Kettle and Fenner 2007): (a) loose continuous non-locking stitch to the vaginal wall; (b) loose, continuous non-locking stitch to the perineal muscle; (c) closure of skin using a loose subcutaneous stitch.

The vaginal laceration is closed using a loose, continuous, non-locking technique ensuring that each stitch is inserted not more than 1 cm apart to avoid vaginal narrowing. Suturing is continued down to the hymenal remnants and the needle is inserted through the skin at the fourchette to emerge in the centre of the perineal wound.

Suturing the muscle layer (Fig. 15.7b)

The muscle layer is then approximated after assessing the depth of the trauma and the perineal muscles (deep and superficial) are approximated with continuous non-locking stitches. If the trauma is deep, two layers of continuous stitches can be inserted through the perineal muscles.

Suturing the perineal skin (Figure 15.7c)

To suture the perineal skin the needle is brought out at the inferior end of the wound, just under the skin surface. The skin sutures are placed below the skin surface in the subcutaneous tissue, thus avoiding the profusion of nerve endings. Bites of tissue are taken from each side of the wound edges until the hymenal remnants are reached. A loop or Aberdeen knot is placed in the vagina behind the hymenal remnants.

A vaginal examination is carried out to ensure that the vagina is not narrowed and a rectal examination carried out to ensure that sutures have not been inadvertently placed through the anorectal epithelium.

OBSTETRIC ANAL SPHINCTER INJURIES (OASIS)

The quoted rate of OASIS is 1% of all vaginal births (RCOG 2007), although a more recent analysis reveals the rate to be 3.2% in consultant-led units (unpublished data). However, 'occult' OASIS (i.e. defects in the anal sphincter detected only by anal endosonography) has been identified in 33% of primiparous women following vaginal birth (Sultan et al 1993). More recent work has shown that these defects were not really occult but could have been identified by an adequately trained doctor or midwife (Andrews et al 2006a). The most plausible explanation for what was previously believed to be an 'occult' OASIS is either an injury that has been missed, recognized but not reported, or, wrongly classified as a second-degree tear (Sultan and Thakar 2007).

Technique for OASIS repair
(Sultan and Thakar 2007)

In the presence of a fourth-degree tear, the torn anorectal epithelium is sutured with a continuous 3/0 Vicryl suture. When torn (Grade 3c tear/fourth-degree), the internal anal sphincter tends to retract and can be identified lateral to the torn anal epithelium. It should be repaired with mattress sutures using 3-0 PDS (Polydioxanone) or modern braided sutures such as 2/0 Vicryl (polyglactin – Vicryl®). To repair a torn external anal sphincter, the ends are grasped using Allis forceps and the muscle is mobilized. When the EAS is only partially torn (Grade 3a and some 3b) then an end-to-end repair should be performed using two or three mattress sutures. Haemostatic 'figure of eight' sutures must not be used to repair the mucosa or sphincter muscle. If there is a full-thickness EAS tear (some 3b, 3c or fourth-degree), either an overlapping or end-to-end method can be used with equivalent outcome. The limited data available from the Cochrane review on the topic showed that compared to immediate primary end-to-end repair of OASIS, early primary overlap repair appears to be associated with lower risks of faecal urgency and anal incontinence symptoms and deterioration of anal incontinence over time. However, as the experience of the surgeon was addressed in only one of the three studies reviewed, it would be inappropriate to recommend one type of repair over the other (Fernando et al 2006). After either technique of repairing the external sphincter the remainder of the tear is closed using the same principles and suture material outlined in the repair of episiotomy.

Basic principles after repair of perineal tears (NICE 2007; Sultan and Thakar 2007)

After repair, complete haemostasis should be achieved. A rectal and vaginal examination should be performed to confirm adequate repair, to ensure that no other tears have been missed and that a suture is not inadvertently placed through the rectal mucosa. Confirm that all tampons (if used) or swabs have been removed.

Detailed notes should be made of the findings and repair. Completion of a pre-designed proforma and a pictorial representation of the tears can prove very useful when notes are being reviewed following complications, audit or litigation. An accurate detailed account of the repair should be documented in the woman's case notes

following completion of the procedure, including details of suture method and materials used.

The woman should be informed regarding the use of appropriate analgesia, hygiene and the importance of a good diet and daily pelvic floor exercises. It is important that the woman is given a full explanation of the injury sustained and contact details if she has any problems during the postnatal period. In presence of OASIS women should be advised that the prognosis following EAS repair is good, with 60–80% being asymptomatic at 12 months (RCOG 2007). In the case of FGM, the woman and her partner must be advised about the legalities regarding reinfibulation and safeguarding issues if the baby is female.

POSTOPERATIVE CARE AFTER OASIS

Broad-spectrum antibiotics should be given intraoperatively (intravenously) and continued orally for 3 days. Severe perineal discomfort, particularly following instrumental delivery, is a known cause of urinary retention, and following regional anaesthesia it can take up to 12 hours before bladder sensation returns. A Foley catheter should be inserted for at least hours unless medical staff can ensure that spontaneous voiding occurs at least every 3–4 hours without undue overdistension of the bladder.

The degree of pain following perineal trauma is related to the extent of the injury and OASIS is frequently associated with other more extensive injuries, such as paravaginal tears. In a systematic review, Hedayati et al (2003) found that rectal analgesia such as diclofenac is effective in reducing pain from perineal trauma within the first 24 hours after birth and women used less additional analgesia within the first 48 hours after birth. Diclofenac is almost completely protein-bound and therefore excretion in breast milk is negligible. In women who had a repair of a fourth-degree tear diclofenac should be administered orally as insertion of suppositories may be uncomfortable and there is a theoretical risk of poor healing associated with local anti-inflammatory agents. Codeine based preparations are best avoided as they may cause constipation leading to excessive straining and possible disruption of the repair. It is of utmost importance that constipation is avoided as passage of constipated stool or indeed faecal impaction may disrupt the repair. Stool softeners (Lactulose) should be prescribed for the first 10–14 days postpartum and the dose titrated to keep the stools soft. The addition of isphagula husk (Fybogel) should be avoided as it has been shown to be non-beneficial (Eogan 2007). It is recommended that women with OASIS be contacted by a healthcare provider 24 or 48 hours after hospital discharge to ensure bowel evacuation has occurred (Sultan and Thakar 2007).

FOLLOW-UP

Special designated multidisciplinary clinics should be available for women with perineal problems to ensure that they receive appropriate, sensitive and effective management. All women who sustain OASIS should be assessed by a senior obstetrician at 6–12 weeks after birth (RCOG 2007). If facilities are available, follow-up of women with OASIS should be in a dedicated clinic with access to endo-anal ultrasonography and anal manometry, as this can aid decision on future mode of birth (RCOG 2007; Scheer et al 2009).

In the clinic a genital examination is performed looking specifically for scarring, residual granulation tissue and tenderness. Where facilities are available, women would undergo anal manometry and endosonography. The women are assessed by the physiotherapists and advised to continue pelvic floor exercises while others with minimal sphincter contractility may need electrical nerve stimulation.

If a perineal clinic is not available, women with OASIS should be given clear instructions, preferably in writing, before leaving the hospital. In the first six weeks following birth, they should look for signs of infection or wound dehiscence and call with any increase in pain or swelling, rectal bleeding, or purulent discharge. Any incontinence of stool or flatus should also be reported. Under such circumstances referral to a specialist gynaecologist or colorectal surgeon for endoanal ultrasound and manometry should be considered (RCOG 2007).

MEDICOLEGAL CONSIDERATIONS

Although creating a third- or fourth-degree tear is seldom found to be culpable, missing a tear is considered to be negligent. It is essential that a rectal examination is performed before and after any perineal repair and findings must be carefully documented in the notes. Delay in repairing in theatre, poor note-keeping, repair by untrained personnel, poor lighting and inadequate exposure, inadequate anaesthesia, failure to recognize extent of the tear, use of wrong suture material, forgotten swab in the vagina, deviation from recommended safe practice, failure to inform and counsel the woman, failure to inform the general practitioner, inappropriate follow-up and advice regarding subsequent pregnancy are common issues raised at litigation. In the UK a recent report by the National Health Service Litigation Authority (NHSLA 2012) demonstrated that during the review period, from 1 April 2000 to 31 March 2010, the NHSLA received 441 claims in which allegations of negligence were made arising out of perineal damage (principally third- and fourth-degree tears) caused

during labour. The total value of those claims, including both damages and legal costs, was estimated to be £31.2 million. Allegations of negligence included failure to consider a caesarean section or perform or extend the episiotomy, and failure to diagnose the true extent and grade of the injury including failure to perform a rectal examination. Failure to perform the repair and the adequacy of the repair itself were also raised as allegations in this cohort of claims (NHSLA 2012).

TRAINING

Throughout the centuries, midwives have received very little formal training in the art of perineal suturing. In June 1967, midwives working in the United Kingdom were permitted by their then regulatory body, the Central Midwives Board (CMB), to perform episiotomies, but they were not allowed to suture perineal trauma. In June 1970 the Chairman of the CMB issued a statement that midwives who were working in 'remote areas overseas' may be authorized by the doctor concerned to repair episiotomies, provided they have been taught the technique and were judged to be competent, but the final responsibility lay with the doctor. It was not until 1983, however, that perineal repair was included in the midwifery curriculum in the UK, when the European Community Midwives Directives came into force and the CMB issued the statement that midwives may undertake repair of the perineum provided they received the necessary instruction and are deemed competent to undertake the procedure (Thakar and Kettle 2010). Tohill and Kettle (2013) have provided evidence-based guidelines for midwives on how to suture correctly.

However, it has been reported that there is a lack of general knowledge on the agreed classification of perineal trauma and that midwives feel inadequately prepared to assess or repair perineal trauma (Mutema 2007). It has also been demonstrated that practitioners require more focused training relating to performing mediolateral episiotomies. Andrews et al (2006b) carried out a prospective study over a 12-month period of women having their first vaginal birth to assess positioning of mediolateral episiotomies. The depth, length, distance from the midline, the shortest distance from the midpoint of the anal canal, and the angle subtended from the sagittal or parasagittal plane were measured following suturing of the episiotomy. Results of the study demonstrated that no midwife and only 13 (22%) doctors performed a truly mediolateral episiotomy and that the majority of the incisions were in fact directed closer to the midline (Andrews et al 2006b). The current recommendation is that all relevant healthcare professionals should attend training in perineal/genital assessment and repair, and ensure that they maintain these skills (NICE 2007).

Box 15.2 **A personal perspective of FGM**

Kinsi Clarke

When I was asked if I minded sharing a short personal account on the effects of FGM for inclusion in a textbook for midwives, I was quite hesitant because the effects of FGM can be different for each woman and girl. But then I realized that is the whole point – *how it affected me* is what was asked.

I was born in one of the East African countries where the practice of FGM was, and still is, very prevalent; around 95 to 98 per cent. I remember very clearly the day I had to face my fate and join a long list of women (older sister, mother, grandmother, great grandmother, aunties, cousins, etc.) who went through the same process. There was never any doubt or question that I, along with all my sisters, would undergo FGM. It was always a matter of when, not if.

I was about 8 years old when the day arrived. A few days earlier I was told that I would be made clean, proper and a real girl going into womanhood. I was shown a little bag, containing a present for me, a new dress, which I would be allowed to wear on the day. The day before it happened, my mum said I would not need to do any household chores the following day and I could sleep longer in the morning, and enjoy a special breakfast, just for me. I was getting really excited about all these special treats and the promise of being the centre of attention all day. Little did I know what it all meant.

I woke up late that morning, had a full wash, which was itself a treat, put on my new dress and had a specially prepared breakfast including a small glass of milk. It must have been approaching midday when a strange looking old woman arrived with dusty and dirty looking sack of unknown contents. My mum, my aunty and a neighbour were already present. My family lived in the bush where water had to be fetched on the back of a camel once a fortnight from a village 20 miles away. We lived in a small hut made of straw and twigs in the middle of the open land. So there was no running water, no hygienic environment, and no sanitized equipment. I was told to empty my bladder (and bowels if necessary) and then join the ladies. I sat down in the middle, had my dress pulled up towards my shoulders and the first thing I can remember was a razor blade. I remember the old lady showing it to my mum, presumably reassuring her that it was clean and not too rusty. I remember feeling alarmed and frightened by the sight of the razor blade, and mum reassuring me and telling me to be a brave girl like so and so, and to fill my mouth with my dress and keep gripping it with my teeth all the time.

Things became rather too blurred too quickly. The first cut was so sharp and the pain so indescribable I remember my whole body convulsing violently and the women using all their strength to keep me still. I can't say how long it lasted. I think I might have fainted or was paralysed by the pain but I do not remember struggling too long. I had type III FGM where all the inner and external genitalia including major labia were removed and then sewn up. The gap that was left open for me to pass water was the size of the head of a cotton bud. I know this because I once went to see a doctor later, when I was growing up and had an infection, and I remember him struggling to put a cotton bud into the hole.

Recovery was very painful. I was 'stitched-up' using 16 long thorns, 8 in each direction in an alternate pattern. The tips of the thorns were broken off once they were in place to prevent them pricking my groin. However it was impossible not to feel the heads of the thorns whichever side I lay on. My legs were tied together and I was told to lie on my side, not on my back or front, to aid the process of the two edges sealing together. I was not allowed much food, just a very small amount of porridge and milk every other day. This was to prevent or minimize bowel movement which could put pressure in the sewn-up area and cause the sides to become undone. Passing water was unbearable and I remember how much I hated it and tried to avoid it by not drinking much. I was told to force myself to urinate once a day, otherwise the bladder (I was told) would eventually burst, open everything up, and I would have to go through the whole thing all over again.

The threat of undergoing the same thing again was so terrifying that I eventually had to let the water trickle through, stopping it every so often to catch my breath and bite my dress again. I was aware that a lot of girls didn't heal properly first time and they had to face being stitched-up again, but mine sealed up all the way and there was no need to repeat it. It was 8 days later when the old lady came back, inspected her handiwork and declared it a success. She took the thorns out and told me to start walking with very little steps. She also loosened the rope that was tied around my legs, from the hips to the toes, to stop my legs parting. I remember that so well because it was the first time in days that I slept a normal, full night's sleep. The removal of the thorns made sleeping not just possible but so peaceful and thoroughly enjoyable. Another week passed before I was allowed to remove the rope around my legs altogether and walk slowly with short steps on my own.

Box 15.2 **Continued**

As I said at the start, FGM probably affects every woman and girl differently. I am not medically trained but I heard many stories of girls dying during the operation. I have been lucky to the extent that I am alive and well.

I remember getting vaginal infections three or four times in my late teens and early 20s. It was always impossible for the doctor to see what was going on down there due to the almost total closure of the vagina but they used to give me oral antibiotics which did not always work. It used to itch like mad and smell too during those episodes and I wanted to rip it open so that I could wash and scratch it well!

When I was 18, I remember once asking my aunt who looked after me, if I could have it opened and leave it that way. She said it was possible if the hospital could give us a certificate stating I was opened on medical grounds necessitating internal treatment. However, said my aunty, my advice would be not to open yourself (literally and figuratively) to accusations which would damage your reputation irrevocably and would inevitably lessen your chances of a good marriage. I took her advice.

Nonetheless, in my case, I would say the effects have been more psychological than physical. Of course I have mutilated genitals, which is a daily reminder of the brutal way my clitoris and other parts were removed. It still takes me a lot longer to pass water than the average 'intact' woman, despite being fully 'opened-up' for 17 years. However, the greatest impact has been the loss of my childhood and the loss of my womanhood. Loss of a childhood because FGM ended who I was: a happy, carefree, playful and a popular *child* who was full of excitement and of the possibilities of what the future might bring. I emerged as traumatized, subdued, passive, docile, quiet and indifferent young person who was neither a child nor a woman. I do not remember playing or behaving like a child after that day. Nor was I expected to be one. This was the passage to womanhood, to prosperity, to a good marriage and motherhood.

The irony, for me, is that what should have completed me as a woman deprived me of the very thing.

In my country women are inspected and opened-up on their wedding night. It's every husband's duty to have intercourse with his new bride soon after the flesh is cut open, to prevent the raw edges sealing up again. I heard many horror stories from my friends of how painful having sex with their new husbands was. Those were girls who had no anaesthetic during the actual procedure of deinfibulation and who then had to face obligatory 'lawful' intercourse with their husbands soon after the flesh was sliced opened; in many cases, with another razor blade. Any husband who hesitated to carry out his duty would be considered weak and cowardly, given that an inspection would take place in the morning to prove that the groom had 'had his way', as indicated by the amount of fresh blood on the sheets.

Again I was lucky, or shall I say shrewd, in that I didn't face this second ordeal of bridal duty because, at the age 25, I married my husband who was from outside my culture and country. A kind, compassionate and understanding husband whose main concern was my welfare and comfort. I underwent deinfibulation by a qualified surgeon, under hygienic conditions, and I was allowed to heal naturally. Nonetheless, I found sexual intercourse extremely painful and unpleasant. Having lost all sensitive parts of my genitals, compounded by the tightness of shrunken muscles that had been sewn up for 17 years, made sex not an enjoyable experience, but an activity to be avoided. This aversion to intimacy naturally led to me not conceiving a child and thus not becoming a mother, the very thing FGM was supposed to prepare me for. Of course this had a significant impact on my relationship with my husband and my self-image as a woman, but we are fortunate in that sex is not an essential part of our relationship for either of us. On the plus side, I did not have to face further complications in connection with childbirth.

I would have done anything to have my body left intact as it was and to have experienced a normal sex life. For most women sex is probably a pleasurable part of a fulfilled life, but, for me, this was something I never had the chance to find out. It is difficult to quantify or to explain how FGM affected me; it has been a life-long physical and psychological pain which will remain with me for as long as I live. I made a conscious decision not to resent or hate my dear mum (who has now sadly passed away) and others who, I am sure, in their own minds, were doing me a good deed. And yet I cannot get the anger and the sense of being robbed of something precious, the sense of betrayal by the very people I trusted most, out of my head.

I could write a book on the visible and invisible damage caused to me by the imposition of type III FGM at such a tender age, so could every other victim; but, as midwives supporting women and girls living with the physical and mental scaring of FGM, I hope this short account will give you some sense of what it is like for us.

REFERENCES

Aasheim V, Nilsen A B V, Lukasse M et al 2011 Perineal techniques during the second stage of labour for reducing perineal trauma. Cochrane Database of Systematic Reviews 2011, Issue 12. Art. No. CD006672. doi: 10.1002/14651858.CD006672.pub2

Al-Hussaini T K 2003 Female genital cutting: types, motives and perineal damage in laboring Egyptian women. Medical Principles and Practice 12 (2): 123–8

Andrews V, Thakar R, Sultan A H 2006a Occult anal sphincter injuries. Myth or reality? BJOG: An International Journal of Obstetrics and Gynaecology 113: 195–200

Andrews V, Sultan A H, Thakar R et al 2006b Are mediolateral episiotomies actually mediolateral. BJOG: An International Journal of Obstetrics and Gynaecology 113:24–6

Beckmann M M, Garrett A J 2006 Antenatal perineal massage for reducing perineal trauma. Cochrane Database of Systematic Reviews 2006, Issue 1. Art. No. CD005123. doi: 10.1002/14651858.CD005123. pub2

Carroli G, Mignini L 2009 Episiotomy for vaginal birth. Cochrane Database of Systematic Reviews, Issue 1. Art. No. CD000081. doi: 10.1002/14651858.CD000081.pub2

Chan S S, Cheung R Y, Lee L L et al 2012 Prevalence of levator ani muscle injury in Chinese women after first delivery. Ultrasound in Obstetrics and Gynecology 36(6):704–9

De Silva S 1989 Obstetric sequelae of female circumcision. European Journal of Obstetrics, Gynecology and Reproductive Biology 32:233–40

Draper J, Newell R 1996 A discussion of some of the literature relating to history, repair and consequences of perineal trauma. Midwifery 12(3):140–5

Elnashar A, Abdelhady R 2007 The impact of female genital cutting on health of newly married women. International Journal of Gynaecology and Obstetrics 97:238–44. doi: 10.1016/j.ijgo.2007.03.008

Eogan M, Daly L, Behan M et al 2007 Randomised clinical trial of a laxative alone versus a laxative and a bulking agent after primary repair of obstetric anal sphincter injury. BJOG: An International Journal of Obstetrics and Gynaecology 114:736–40

Fernando R, Sultan A H, Kettle C et al (2006) Methods of repair for obstetric anal sphincter injury. Cochrane Database of Systematic Reviews 2006, Issue 3. Art. No. CD002866 doi: 10.1002/14651858. CD002866.pub2

Green J, Coupland V, Kitzinger J 1998 Great expectations: a prospective study of women's expectations and experiences of childbirth. Books for Midwives Press, Hale, Cheshire

Groutz A, Hasson J, Wengier A et al 2011 Third- and fourth-degree perineal tears: prevalence and risk factors in the third millennium. American Journal of Obstetrics and Gynecology 204 (4): 347.e1–4.

Gupta J K, Hoymeyr G J, Smyth R 2004 Position in the second stage of labour for women without epidural anaesthesia. Cochrane Database of Systematic Reviews 2004, Issue 1. Art. No. CD002006. doi: 10.1002/14651858.CD002006.pub2

Hassanin I M, Saleh R, Bedaiwy A A et al 2008 Prevalence of female genital cutting in Upper Egypt: 6 years after enforcement of prohibition law. Reproductive Biomedicine. Accessed online at www.rbmonline.com (1 February 2013)

Hedayati H, Parsons J, Crowther C 2003 Rectal analgesia for pain from perineal trauma following childbirth. Cochrane Database of Systematic Reviews, Issue 1. Art. No. CD004223. doi: 10.1002/14651858. pub2

Home Office 2004 Circular 10/2004: The Female Genital Mutilation Act 2003, Home Office, London. Accessed online at www.circulars. homeoffice.gov.uk (23 March 2013)

Kalis V, Laine K, de Leeuw J W et al 2012 Classification of episiotomy: towards a standardisation of terminology. BJOG: An International Journal of Obstetrics and Gynaecology 119(5):522–6.

Kettle C, Dowswell T, Ismail K 2010 Absorbable suture materials for primary repair of episiotomy and second degree tears. Cochrane Database of Systematic Reviews 2010, Issue 6. Art. No. CD000006. doi: 10.1002/14651858.CD000006.pub2

Kettle C, Fenner D 2007 Repair of episiotomy, first and second degree tears. In: Sultan A H, Thakar R, Fenner D (eds) Perineal and anal sphincter trauma. Springer, London, p 20–32

Kettle C, Hills R, Ismail K 2007 Continuous versus interrupted sutures for repair of episiotomy or second-degree tears. Cochrane Database of Systematic Reviews 2007, Issue 4. Art. No. CD000947. doi: 10.1002/14651858.CD000947. pub2

Kettle C, Raynor M D 2010 Perineal management and repair In: Marshall J E M, Raynor M D (eds) Advancing skills in midwifery practice. Churchill Livingstone, Edinburgh, p 104–20

Kettle C 2012 Evidence based guidelines for midwifery-led care in labour: suturing the perineum. London, Royal College of Midwives

Millogo-Traore F, Kaba S T, Thieba B et al 2007 Maternal and foetal prognostic in excised women delivery. [In French] Journal de Gynecologie, Obstetrique et Biologie de la Reproduction 36: 393–408

Mutema E K 2007 'A tale of two cities': auditing midwifery practice and perineal trauma. British Journal of Midwifery 15(8):511–13

NHSLA (National Health Service Litigation Authority) 2012 Ten years of maternity claims: an analysis of NHS Litigation Authority data. NHSLA, London, p 49–60

NICE (National Institute for Health and Clinical Excellence) 2007 Intrapartum care: care of healthy women and their babies, CG 55. NICE, London

NICE (National Institute for Health and Clinical Excellence) 2008 Antenatal care. Routine care for the healthy pregnant women, CG 62. NICE, London

RCOG (Royal College of Obstetricians and Gynaecologists) 2007 Management of third and fourth degree perineal tears following vaginal delivery. Guideline No. 29. RCOG, London

RCOG (Royal College of Obstetricians and Gynaecologists) 2009 Female genital mutilation and its management. Guideline No. 53. RCOG, London

Scheer I, Thakar R, Sultan A H 2009 Mode of delivery after previous obstetric anal sphincter injuries (OASIS) – a reappraisal. International Urogynecology Journal 20:1095–101

Sultan A H, Kamm M A, Hudson C N et al 1993 Anal sphincter disruption

during vaginal delivery. New England Journal of Medicine 329:1905–11

Sultan A H, Kettle C 2007 Diagnosis of perineal trauma. In: Sultan A H, Thakar R, Fenner D (eds) Perineal and anal sphincter trauma. Springer-Verlag, London, p 13–19

Sultan A H, Thakar R 2007 Third and fourth degree tears. In: Sultan A H, Thakar R, Fenner D (eds) Perineal and anal sphincter trauma. Springer-Verlag, London, p 33–51

Thakar R, Kettle C 2010 Episiotomy and perineal repair. In: Cardozo L and Staskin D (eds) Textbook of female urology and urogynecology, 3rd edn. Martin Dunitz, Hampshire, p 875–82.

Tohill S, Kettle C 2013 How to suture correctly. Midwives 1:31. Accessed online at www.rcm.org (25 February 2013)

WHO (World Health Organization) 2001 Management of pregnancy, childbirth and postpartum period in the presence of female genital mutilation. WHO, Geneva

WHO (World Health Organization) 2008 Eliminating female genital mutilation. WHO, Geneva

WHO (World Health Organization) 2013 Female genital mutilation. Fact sheet number 241. WHO, Geneva

FURTHER READING

Bick D E, Ismail K M K, Macdonald S et al 2012 How good are we at implementing evidence to support the management of birth related perineal trauma? A UK-wide survey of midwifery practice. BMC Pregnancy and Childbirth 12:57

An informative article, which identifies considerable gaps with implementation of evidence to support management of perineal trauma.

Chapman V 2009 Clinical issues: issues affecting the left-handed midwife. British Journal of Midwifery 17(9):588–92

This is a useful read for the left-handed practitioner.

HM Government 2011 Multi agency practice guidelines on female genital mutilation. London, HM Government. Available online at: www.dh.gov.uk

Kettle C 2012 Evidence based guidelines for midwifery led care in labour: care of the perineum. Royal College of Midwives, London

These guidelines summarize the evidence in an accessible way.

USEFUL WEBSITES

Female Genital Mutilation Clinical Group: www.fgmnationalgroup.org

The FGM National Clinical Group is a registered charity in England & Wales: 1125319.

Foundation for Women's Health Research and Development: www.forwarduk.org.uk

National Patient Safety Agency: www.npsa.nhs.uk

National Society for the Prevention of Cruelty to Children: www.nspcc.org.uk

World Health Organization: www.who.int

Chapter |16|

Physiology and care during the first stage of labour

Karen Jackson, Jayne E Marshall, Susan Brydon

CHAPTER CONTENTS

Birth is a dynamic and transforming experience, both on an individual and a societal level, and has the power to profoundly affect the lives of those involved. It is a physiological process characterized by non-intervention, a supportive environment and empowerment of the woman (Lavender et al 2009; Walsh 2012).

The midwife is a key figure in this process, supporting and assisting women safely through childbirth, recognizing the *woman's needs and wellbeing are central* rather than the needs of the maternity service. Consequently, the midwife is required to be a caring supporter, advocate, skilled practitioner, vigilant observer and an accurate recorder of facts. Women have differing needs and the way they approach and experience birth is unique and will depend on a number of factors, including cultural background, education, personal beliefs and previous life experience. In order to meet these varying needs, the midwife should possess wide-ranging skills and knowledge and have the willingness to place the woman at the centre of the care that is provided for her. Women and their chosen birth companion(s) should have an equal partnership with health professionals in all decision-making processes, so that they can make informed choices about their own labours and births.

THE CHAPTER AIMS TO:

- describe the physical changes taking place as labour progresses
- explore the factors that contribute to a positive birth experience for the woman, including communication, environment, support, assessment and monitoring
- reflect on the care and support that can optimize the wellbeing of the woman and her fetus during the course of labour
- consider the various ways in which midwives can support women to work with/relieve the pain of labour
- describe the principles in the assessment and care of labours presenting by the breech
- reflect on the midwife's role in caring for women who present with prelabour rupture of the fetal membranes.

DEFINING LABOUR

A human pregnancy is considered to last approximately 40 weeks, with labour usually occurring between 37 and 42 weeks' gestation (National Institute for Health and Clinical Excellence [NICE] 2007) (see Chapter 9). Complex physiological and psychological changes occur during the last few weeks of pregnancy, and also during the onset of labour, that prepare the woman for the process of labour and birth (Howie and Novak 2010; McNabb 2011; Walsh 2012) (see Chapter 9).

Labour, purely in the physical sense, may be described as the process by which the fetus, placenta and membranes are expelled through the birth canal; however, labour is much more than a purely physical event. What happens during labour can affect the relationship between the mother and baby and can influence the likelihood and/or experience of future pregnancies.

The World Health Organization (WHO) defines *normal* labour as one that is low risk throughout, spontaneous in onset with the fetus presenting by the vertex, culminating in the mother and infant being in good condition following birth (WHO 1999). However, a labour where the fetus is presenting by the *breech* with no other risk factors should also be considered *normal* (Burvill 2005). Furthermore, all definitions of labour appear to be purely physiological and do not encompass the psychological wellbeing of the woman.

Traditionally, three stages of labour are described: the *first*, *second* and *third stage*, but this is a rather pedantic view, as labour is obviously a continuous process. It has also been acknowledged that there are more than three stages of labour, namely the *latent*, *active* and *transitional phases*, and these not only encompass specific physical changes but should also account for the emotional effects observed in women during this time.

Labour for each woman has its own unique ebbs and flows. Walsh (2010a) describes this as *labour rhythms*. However, as labour tends to be described and recognized universally as having distinct *stages* of labour, this approach will be adopted for the purposes of this text. The *first stage of labour* is usually recognized by the onset of regular uterine contractions, an accompanying effacement and at least 4 cm dilatation of the cervix and finally culminates in full dilatation of the cervix (NICE 2007; Howie and Rankin 2010).

THE ONSET OF SPONTANEOUS PHYSIOLOGICAL LABOUR

The onset of labour is determined by a complex interaction of maternal and fetal hormones and is not fully understood. It would appear to be multifactorial in origin, being a combination of hormonal and mechanical factors. Levels of maternal oestrogen rise sharply during the last weeks of pregnancy, resulting in changes that overcome the inhibiting effects of progesterone. High levels of oestrogens cause uterine muscle fibres to display oxytocic receptors and form gap junctions with each other. Oestrogen also stimulates the placenta to release prostaglandins that induce a production of enzymes that will digest collagen in the cervix, helping it to soften (Tortora and Grabowski 2011). The process is unclear but it is thought that both fetal and placental factors are involved. There is no clear evidence that concentrations of oestrogens and progesterone alter at the onset of labour, but the balance between them does facilitate myometrial activity. Uterine activity may also result from mechanical stimulation of the uterus and cervix. This may be brought about by overstretching, as in the case of a multiple pregnancy, or pressure from a presenting part that is well applied to the cervix (Impey and Child 2012).

Recognition of the onset of labour

The onset of labour is a process, not an event; therefore it is very difficult to identify exactly when the painless (sometimes painful) contractions of prelabour develop into the progressive rhythmic contractions of established labour. Diagnosing the onset of labour is extremely important, since it is on the basis of this finding that decisions are made that will affect the intrapartum care and support subsequently provided (NICE 2007; Zhang et al 2010).

It is part of the role of the midwife to ensure that women have sufficient information to assist them in recognizing the onset of established labour. This information is also needed to enable women to make informed choices based on current and unbiased evidence. The complex physical, psychological and emotional experience of labour affects every woman differently and midwives must have sound knowledge and experience to enable the woman to maintain control over the birth of her baby. Women in labour should be encouraged to trust their own instincts, listen to their own body and verbalize feelings in order to receive the help and support they require. Anxiety can increase the production of adrenaline (epinephrine), which inhibits uterine activity and may in turn prolong labour (Simkin and Ancheta 2011).

Irrespective of whether they have given birth before, many women experience contractions before the onset of labour which may be painful and regular for a time, causing them to think that labour has started. Furthermore, some women's lived experiences of early labour report *prolonged contractions* or being *in labour for days* and thus it is important to note that the discomfort or even pain that the woman is conscious of is *genuine to her*. Although the contractions that the woman is experiencing are real, they have yet to settle into the rhythmic pattern of *established* labour, resulting in *effacement and dilatation*

of the cervix. Using terminology such as *spurious* or *false labour* is unhelpful and typically negative in terms of women's genuine experiences of early labour (Walsh 2012). Reassurance should be given and discussion of this potential situation earlier in the pregnancy can enable the woman and her partner to prepare for labour more effectively. Contact with the midwife should be made when **regular, rhythmic, uterine contractions are experienced**, and these are **perceived by the woman as uncomfortable or painful**.

Latent phase of labour

The *latent phase* of labour is *prior* to the active phase stage of labour and may last 6–8 hours in primigravidae when the cervix dilates from 0 cm to 4 cm dilated (Howie and Rankin 2010), although McDonald (2010) argues that the latent phase of labour is so subjective and poorly understood that a normal range is difficult to measure. According to Mukhopadhyay and Fraser (2009) the cervical canal shortens from 3 cm long to <0.5 cm in length during this time.

A woman may believe herself to be labouring, whereas sound midwifery judgement and understanding of the physiology of the first stage of labour may lead the midwife to the diagnosis of the *latent phase* of labour. Both the woman and midwife being aware of the latent phase of labour, and allowing this time to pass with no intervention, can prevent the medical diagnosis of *poor progress* or *failure to progress* later in labour. In a hospital setting, it is good practice not to commence the partogram until *active labour* has commenced. Assessing the active phase of labour has been highlighted as essential in reducing interventions in normal labour (Lauzon and Hodnett 2009).

Active phase of labour

The *active phase* within the first stage of labour is the time when the cervix usually undergoes more rapid dilatation. This begins when the cervix is at least 4 cm dilated and, in the presence of rhythmic contractions, progressively dilates to 10 cm or full dilatation.

When in labour, contractions will often be accompanied or preceded by a bloodstained mucoid *show*: that is, the release of the operculum from the cervical canal as effacement and dilatation progresses. Occasionally, the membranes will rupture, at which stage the midwife may seek assurance that there are no significant changes in the fetal heart rate due to the rare complication of cord prolapse and that meconium is not present in the liquor, indicating fetal compromise.

Transitional phase of labour

The *transitional phase* of the first stage of labour is from when the cervix is around 8 cm dilated until it is fully dilated or until expulsive contractions associated with the second stage of labour are felt by the woman. There is often a brief lull in the intensity of uterine activity at this time. Many women may feel the urge to push during transition. In addition to physiological responses, women can experience a range of experiences and emotions. Woods (2006) describes this as being from inner calm to acute distress. The woman may verbalize her distress, direct it at her birth partner(s), alternatively she may be quiet and contemplative.

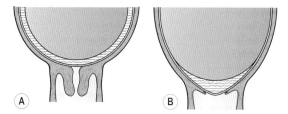

Fig. 16.1 (A) The cervix before effacement. (B) The cervix after effacement. The cervical canal is now part of the lower uterine segment.

PHYSIOLOGY OF THE FIRST STAGE OF LABOUR

Duration

The length of labour varies widely and is influenced by parity, birth interval, psychological state, presentation and position of the fetus. Maternal pelvic shape and size and the character of uterine contractions also affect timescale.

By far the greatest part of labour is taken up by the first stage and it is common to expect *the active phase* to be completed within 6–12 hours (Tortora and Grabowski 2011). Over the years there has been much debate surrounding the length of physiological active labour in low-risk populations of childbearing women to refute the original claim of Friedman (1954) that cervical dilatation occurred at the rate of 1 cm per hour (Albers 1999; Lavender et al 2006; Zhang et al 2010). A cervical dilatation rate of 0.5 cm per hour, however, has now been incorporated into the NICE (2007) intrapartum guidelines as being within the parameters of *normal* labour.

Cervical effacement

Effacement refers to the inclusion (*taking up*) of the cervical canal into the lower uterine segment. It is believed that this process takes place from above downward, meaning that the muscle fibres surrounding the internal os are drawn upwards by the retracted upper segment and the cervix merges into the lower uterine segment. The cervical canal widens at the level of the internal os, whereas the state of the external os remains unchanged (Cunningham et al 2010) (Fig. 16.1).

Effacement may occur late in pregnancy, or it may not take place until labour begins. In the nulliparous woman the cervix will not usually dilate until effacement is complete, whereas in the multiparous woman, effacement and dilatation usually occurs simultaneously and a small canal may be felt in early labour. This is often referred to by midwives as a *multips os* (Howie and Rankin 2010).

Cervical dilatation

Dilatation of the cervix is the process of enlargement of the os uteri from a tightly closed aperture to an opening large enough to permit passage of the fetus. Dilatation is assessed in centimetres and *full dilatation* at term equates to about 10 cm. However, acknowledging that all women are different sizes and shapes means that full cervical dilatation may be between 9 and 11 cm in individual women (Walsh 2012).

Dilatation occurs as a result of uterine action and the counter-pressure applied by either the intact bag of membranes or the presenting part, or both. A well-flexed fetal head closely applied to the cervix favours efficient dilatation. Pressure applied evenly to the cervix causes the uterine fundus to respond by contraction and retraction, often referred to as the *Ferguson reflex* (Howie and Rankin 2010).

Uterine action

Fundal dominance (Fig. 16.2)

Each uterine contraction commences in the fundus near one of the cornua and spreads across and downwards. The contraction lasts longest in the fundus, where it is also most intense, but the peak is reached simultaneously over the whole uterus and the contraction fades from all parts together. This pattern permits the cervix to dilate and the strongly contracting fundus to eventually expel the fetus at the end of labour (Howie and Rankin 2010).

Polarity

Polarity is the term used to describe the neuromuscular harmony that prevails between the two poles or segments of the uterus throughout labour. During each uterine contraction, these two poles act harmoniously. The upper pole contracts strongly and retracts to expel the fetus; the lower pole contracts slightly and dilates to allow expulsion to take place. If polarity is disorganized then the progress of labour is inhibited (Bernal and Norwitz 2012).

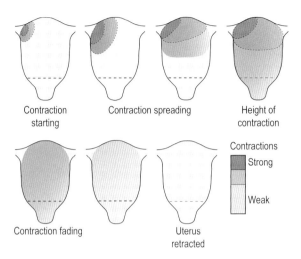

Fig. 16.2 Series of diagrams to show fundal dominance during uterine contractions.

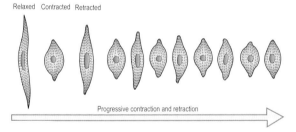

Fig. 16.3 Diagram to show how uterine muscle retains some shortening after each contraction.

Contraction and retraction

Uterine muscle has a unique property. During labour the contraction does not pass off entirely, as muscle fibres retain some of the shortening of contraction instead of becoming completely relaxed (Fig. 16.3). This is termed *retraction*. This process assists in the progressive expulsion of the fetus, such that the upper segment of the uterus becomes gradually shorter and thicker and its cavity diminishes.

Intensity and resting tone

Each labour is individual and does not always conform to expectations, but generally before labour becomes established, uterine contractions may occur every 15–20 minutes, lasting for about 30 seconds. They are often fairly weak and may even be imperceptible to the woman. The contractions usually occur with rhythmic regularity and the intervals between them where the muscle relaxes (*resting tone*) gradually lessen while the length and strength gradually intensifies through the latent phase and into the

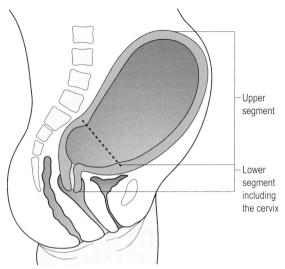

Fig. 16.4 Birth canal before labour begins.

active phase of the first stage of labour. By the end of the first stage, the contractions may occur at 2–3 minute intervals, last for 50–60 seconds and are very powerful (Cunningham et al 2010).

Formation of upper and lower uterine segments

By the end of pregnancy, the body of the uterus is described as having divided into two segments, which are anatomically distinct (Fig. 16.4). The upper uterine segment, having been formed from the body of the fundus, is mainly concerned with contraction and retraction, and is thick and muscular. The lower uterine segment is formed of the isthmus and the cervix, and is about 8–10 cm in length. The lower segment is prepared for distension and dilatation. Although there is no clear and strict division of these two segments, the muscle content reduces from the fundus to the cervix, where it is thinner. When labour begins, the retracted longitudinal fibres in the upper segment pull on the lower segment causing it to stretch. This is aided by the force applied by the descending presenting part (Howie and Rankin 2010; Impey and Child 2012).

The retraction ring

A ridge develops between the upper and lower uterine segments, known as the *retraction ring* (Fig. 16.5). The physiological retraction ring gradually rises as the upper uterine segment contracts and retracts and the lower uterine segment thins out to accommodate the descending fetus. Once the cervix is fully dilated and the fetus can leave the uterus, the retraction ring rises no further.

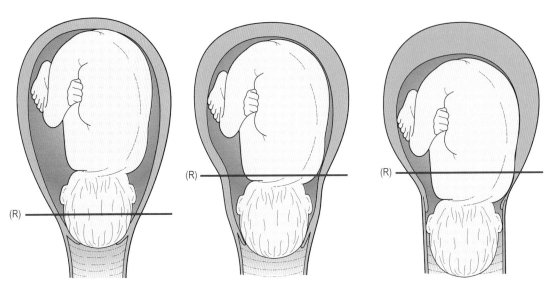

Fig. 16.5 Diagram showing the retraction ring (R) between the upper and lower uterine segments.

However, in extreme cases of *mechanically obstructed labour*, this physiological retraction ring becomes visible above the symphysis pubis and is described as *Bandl's ring*. A Bandl's ring may consequently be associated with fetal compromise (Lauria et al 2007).

Show

As a result of the dilatation of the cervix, the operculum, which formed the cervical plug during pregnancy, is released. The woman may observe a bloodstained mucoid discharge a few hours before, or within a few hours after, labour commences. The blood comes from ruptured capillaries in the parietal decidua where the chorion has become detached from the dilating cervix and should only be a staining (Impey and Child 2012). Frank, fresh bleeding is atypical at this stage, although during the transitional phase and as the first stage ends, there is often a *small* loss of bright red blood that heralds the second stage of labour. Both occurrences may be referred to as a *show*.

Mechanical factors

Formation of the forewaters and hindwaters

As the lower uterine segment forms and stretches, the chorion becomes detached from it and the increased intra-uterine pressure causes this loosened part of the sac of fluid to bulge downwards into the internal os, to the depth of 6–12 mm. The well-flexed fetal head fits snugly into the cervix and cuts off the amniotic fluid in front of the head from that which surrounds the body, forming two separate pools of fluid. The former is known as the *forewaters* and

the latter, the *hindwaters*. In early labour it is often possible to feel intact forewaters bulging even when the hindwaters have ruptured, making ruptured membranes a difficult diagnosis at times.

The effect of separation of the forewaters prevents the pressure that is applied to the hindwaters during uterine contractions from being applied to the forewaters. This may help keep the membranes intact during the first stage of labour and be a natural defence against ascending infection (Bernal and Norwitz 2012).

General fluid pressure

While the membranes remain intact, the pressure of the uterine contractions is exerted on the amniotic fluid and, as fluid is not compressible, the pressure is equalized throughout the uterus and over the fetal body, known as *general fluid pressure* (Fig. 16.6). When the membranes rupture and a quantity of fluid emerges, the fetal head, the placenta and umbilical cord are compressed between the uterine wall and the fetus during contractions with a consequential reduction in the oxygen supply to the fetus. Preserving the integrity of the membranes, therefore, optimizes the oxygen supply to the fetus and also helps to prevent intrauterine and fetal infection (Howie and Rankin 2010).

Rupture of the membranes

The optimum physiological time for the membranes to rupture spontaneously is at the *end of the first stage of labour*, after the cervix becomes fully dilated and no longer supports the bag of forewaters. The uterine contractions are also applying increasing expulsive force at this time.

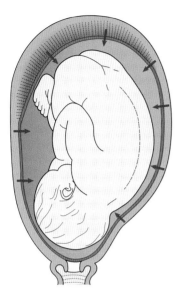

Fig. 16.6 General fluid pressure.

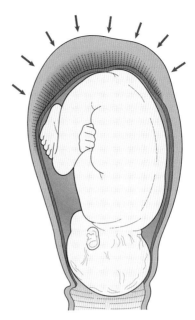

Fig. 16.7 Fetal axis pressure.

The membranes may sometimes rupture days before labour begins or during the first stage. If for any reason there is a badly fitting presenting part and the forewaters are not separated effectively then the membranes may rupture early. However, in most cases there is no apparent reason for early spontaneous membrane rupture. Occasionally the membranes do not rupture even in the second stage and appear at the vulva as a bulging sac covering the fetal head as it is born; this is known as the *caul*.

Early rupture of membranes may lead to an increased incidence of variable decelerations on cardiotocography (CTG), resulting in an increase in caesarean sections if fetal blood sampling is not available (Alfirevic et al 2013). A systematic review found that routine artificial rupture of membranes (ARM) does not significantly reduce the length of labour and thus routine amniotomy should not be performed (Smyth et al 2007). However, there was some evidence that ARM increased the rate of caesarean section but this finding did not reach significance. All women are required to give consent for this intervention and the midwife should have a clear indication for performing an ARM: details of which should be recorded in the woman's labour records (Nursing and Midwifery Council [NMC] 2009, 2012).

Fetal axis pressure

During each contraction, the uterus rises forward and the force of the fundal contraction is transmitted to the upper pole of the fetus, down the long axis of the fetus and applied by the presenting part to the cervix. This is known as *fetal axis pressure* (Fig. 16.7) and becomes much more significant after rupture of the membranes and during the second stage of labour.

RECOGNITION OF THE FIRST STAGE OF LABOUR

It is the woman herself who usually diagnoses the onset of normal labour and many women and their partners are apprehensive in case the labour is very quick, resulting in an unattended birth. Education during pregnancy is important to enable the woman to recognize the beginning of labour and understand the latent phase in order to consider possible strategies she may use for labour and birth.

Women should appreciate that in late pregnancy vaginal secretions *without* any bloodstaining increase. In addition, they should be aware that a *show*, which is usually a pink or bloodstained jelly-like loss, prior to the onset of labour or in early labour, is quite common. If a woman is examined vaginally in late pregnancy they should also be informed that there may be some slight blood loss after the procedure.

Braxton Hicks contractions are more noticeable in late pregnancy and some women experience them as painful. They are usually irregular or their regularity is not maintained for long spells of time, seldom lasting more than one minute. In active labour, contractions exhibit a pattern of rhythm and regularity, usually increasing in length, strength and frequency as time goes on. When the woman first feels contractions she may be aware only of backache, but if she places a hand on her abdomen she may perceive simultaneous hardening of the uterus. If the pregnancy has been problem-free, with a normal birth anticipated, the midwife should advise the woman to stay in her own surroundings, continue with her normal activities, to eat, be active and upright.

It is sometimes difficult to be certain whether or not the membranes have ruptured spontaneously prior to labour or in early labour. The woman may be experiencing some degree of stress incontinence, so she may be unsure if it is liquor or urine that she is passing. If there is any doubt, the woman should contact her midwife who may decide to insert a speculum into the vagina to observe for any amniotic fluid. Digital examination should be avoided if the woman is not in labour as it can increase the risk of ascending infection (Shepherd et al 2010).

INITIAL MEETING WITH THE MIDWIFE

Ideally, the woman should know her own midwife and be able to contact her when labour starts. Where this is not possible, it is crucial that the first meeting between the midwife, the labouring woman and her partner establishes a rapport, which sets the scene for the remainder of labour. If the woman is planning to birth in hospital, she may worry about the reception she and her companion will receive and the attitude of the people attending her. In addition, an unfamiliar environment may provoke feelings of vulnerability and undermine her confidence. Comfortable surroundings, a welcoming manner and a midwife who greets the woman as an equal in a partnership will engender feelings of mutual respect, thus enabling the woman to relax and respond positively to the amazing forces of labour and to her baby after it is born (Berry 2006; Fisher et al 2006; Raynor and England 2010).

The language of childbirth

It has been recognized that some of the childbirth terminology used when communicating with women appears medical, masculine and negative (Robertson 2003). The terms *pain* and *labour* are suggestive of *difficulty* and *trouble*. It is therefore vital the midwife observes what she says to women during childbirth and uses appropriate and adapted language which is woman-friendly. The word *delivery* has been replaced by the term *birthing* or *birth* as these appear more suitable when discussing the concept and practice of normality within midwifery.

Communication

The key issues for women relate to achieving a safe birth, feeling in control within the birth environment,

developing supportive relationships with their carers, and being treated with kindness, respect, dignity and cultural sensitivity if they are to realize a positive experience of birth (Helman 2007; Main and Bingham 2008; Redshaw and Heikkila 2010). Effective communication between the midwife and the woman and her partner, and with other clinicians in the multidisciplinary team, is essential to providing effective safe supportive care in labour and achieving the woman's objectives (Royal College of Obstetricians and Gynaecologists [RCOG] 2008). Communication does not consist only of the content of what is said, but also includes non-verbal communication and written records, such as the woman's birth plan.

Poor communication is the commonest cause of preventable adverse outcomes in hospitals and remains a significant cause of written complaints (Health and Social Care Information Centre 2012). An inquiry conducted by the Kings Fund into the safety of birth in England concluded that the overwhelming majority of births are safe but when there are increased risks to the woman or baby, that render some births *less* safe, *functioning teams* are the key to improving the outcome for the woman and baby (Kings Fund 2008).

Interpreting services

If the woman and midwife are unable to understand each other, communication will be ineffective and it is essential that adequate interpretation services are available when necessary. Although there is a tendency to rely on family members or friends to provide interpreting services, the use of such interpreters is deemed inappropriate when the midwife wishes to discuss sensitive issues such as past history, domestic abuse or the need for interventions. Wherever possible, professional interpretation services should be provided for all non-English-speaking women (Centre for Maternal and Child Enquiries [CMACE] 2011). If a face-to-face interpreter cannot be obtained, then the use of a telephone or Internet interpretation service should be considered.

Birth plan

Regardless of where the woman plans to give birth, a birth plan is a valuable tool for midwives to observe and use to facilitate the provision of holistic, individualized care. This is especially so in situations where the maternity care is fragmented and the woman first encounters the midwife who will be caring for her in labour when she attends the hospital to give birth. The birth plan therefore provides the opportunity for the midwife to discuss with each woman and her partner any plans about the type of birth they would like that they may have already prepared with support from their community midwife. An outline may be present in the case notes, or the couple may bring a birth plan with them. Frequently, the partner is involved in this forward planning, which should be a flexible proposal that can be reviewed and revised as labour progresses (Department of Health [DH] 2007). Some women, however, may not have prepared a birth plan and so the midwife should encourage them to consider any preferences that they may have, for example:

- her choice of birth companion(s)
- her choice of clothes for labour
- ambulation and fetal monitoring (intermittent, electronic or a combination)
- strategies for labour (water immersion, massage, pharmacological pain relief)
- position for labour and birth
- expectant or actively managed third stage of labour
- cutting of the umbilical cord
- skin-to-skin contact and feeding the baby after birth.

Having the opportunity to discuss such issues in early labour enables the establishment of a trusting relationship between the woman and the midwife to develop where the woman feels valued and involved in intrapartum decision-making: all details of which should be clearly documented in the intrapartum records (NMC 2009, 2012).

Emotional and psychological care

When a woman begins to labour, she may have a mixture of emotions. Most women anticipate labour with a degree of excitement, anxiety, fear and hope. Many other emotions are influenced by cultural expectations and previous life experiences. The state of the woman's knowledge, her fears and expectations are also influenced by her companions during labour, including the attitude and behaviour of the caregiver.

By the time labour starts, a decision will already have been reached about where the woman plans to give birth. Some women may choose to give birth at home, some in a midwife-led unit/birthing centre and others in hospital. Some women may also wish to labour as long as possible at home but give birth in hospital. Whatever choice the woman makes, she must be the focus of the care, able to feel she is in control of what is happening and contributing to the decisions made about her care (Sinivaara et al 2004; DH 2007). Hodnett et al (2012) assert that there is a powerful effect on maternal birth satisfaction and labour progress where women feel in control and involved in decision making.

Providing that there are no complications and labour is not well advanced, the woman may remain at home as long as she feels comfortable and confident. If labour commences prior to term, however, admission to hospital is always advised (Chapter 12).

Companion in labour

The fact that women should be encouraged to have support by birth partners of their choice is well recognized (NICE 2007; Midwives Information Resource Service [MIDIRS] 2008a). The woman herself is *central* to all the decisions made about care during labour and her chosen companion, whether sexual partner, friend or family member, should understand this. Ideally the companion should be involved in prelabour preparation and decision-making, have participated in compiling a birth plan and be aware of all the available options.

If the woman is giving birth in hospital, admission to a labour ward can be an alienating experience and the company of a supportive companion can help reduce anxiety. During labour, the companion should be made to feel useful and part of the team by the midwife, as they too may be feeling anxious (Longworth and Kingdon 2010). Such activities may include massaging the woman's back, offering drinks, assisting with breathing and relaxation awareness and supporting her decisions regarding her strategies for working with, or controlling, pain.

In some cases a midwife will be able to remain with one woman through her entire labour, but due to the unpredictable workloads and staffing levels this is not always possible. This can leave the woman feeling unsupported and processed, rather than cared for and can have profound negative effects on a woman's satisfaction and memory of the birth (Kirkham 2011). Despite such constraints it is not appropriate to use the birth partner as a substitute for close observation and attendance by the midwife. Equally so, the midwife should also recognize the need for the couple to have some personal space and leave them alone, albeit with the means to summon assistance should it be required. This would not be acceptable, however, when labour is well advanced, as being left alone could prove very frightening for the woman and her partner.

It would be a mistake to consider that all women have the same requirements, however, women have varying needs, with some preferring presence and others preferring complete privacy. The task for the midwife is to provide the individualized service that ensures that the woman feels safe and supported. Despite the aim to provide a good outcome for the woman, there is no doubt that a proportion of women are dissatisfied with the birthing experience and some are positively traumatized by their experience (Ayers et al 2008).

It is also important to ensure that support is available to the partner when it is needed if the woman is in significant pain or a sudden emergency develops and they are encouraged to take short breaks during a prolonged labour. If a caesarean section becomes necessary, the midwife should delegate someone to keep the partner informed so they are not left feeling abandoned or uncared for.

The concept of continuous support in labour

There is evidence that the presence of the midwife and one-to-one personal attention is positively associated with a woman's satisfaction with her care. Kennedy et al (2010) describe that the presence and demeanour of the midwife can enhance the woman's trust in her own ability to cope. In a systematic review by Hodnett et al (2011), the value of continuous support during labour and birth is clearly evident. The review, consisting of 21 randomized clinical trials, involving over 15 000 women, showed evidence that women who laboured *with* continuous support had shorter labours and were less likely to experience intrapartum interventions. These women were also less likely to have an epidural or other forms of pain medication, give birth by caesarean section, ventouse or forceps and consequently appeared more satisfied with their overall experience of childbirth (Hodnett et al 2011). These outcomes have been further strengthened by the results of Sandall et al (2013), who collected data from 13 trials culminating in the birth outcomes of 16 242 women. It was found that where women received midwife-led care throughout pregnancy and birth from a small group of midwives they were less likely to give birth prematurely or require interventions in labour than those women who received care based on a shared care model or medical model. Consequently Sandall et al (2013) affirm that all women should be offered *midwife-led continuity of care* unless they have serious medical or obstetric complications and women should be encouraged to ask for this option.

The essence of midwifery is to be *with woman*, providing comfort and support to women in labour. Although the midwife has an important role to play in providing support and care, there is evidence that a birth partner who is neither from the woman's social network or a member of the midwifery team, such as a doula, can provide the most effective continuous support during labour, resulting in less interventions and pain medication and an increase in positive childbirth experiences (Hodnett et al 2011).

The physical environment

In the developed world most births occur in hospital and therefore the atmosphere and environment of hospital birthing rooms are important (Sullivan and McCormick 2007). The clinical appearance of hospital birthing rooms, coupled with associated clinical regimes and loss of privacy, can alienate women and lead to feelings of loss of control (Marshall et al 2011). In turn, this loss of control can interfere with the normal physiological process of labour (Walsh 2010a, 2010b).

Whilst there has been an effort by hospitals to provide a less clinical and more *home-from-home* environment for birth, there has been some criticism in that such adaptations create an artificial situation whereby homeliness masks the unchanged clinical agenda and professional dominance found in traditional labour environments (Fannon 2003). Although evidence is limited, Hodnett et al (2009) found that efforts to make birthing rooms more homely are appreciated by women and can have a positive effect on them and their care providers. However, such an environment is unlikely on its own to improve birth outcomes or the birthing experience.

Reducing the risk of infection

In the latest Confidential Enquiries into Maternal Deaths report, the leading cause of *direct* deaths during the triennium 2006–2008, was *sepsis*, accounting for 26 deaths (Harper 2011). As a consequence, the prevention of infection was one of the top 10 recommendations from the report. In addition, health care-associated infections (HCAIs) have become the subject of considerable public interest as a consequence of the rise in methicillin-resistant *Staphylococcus aureus* (MRSA) and *Clostridium difficile* (*C. difficile*). With the introduction of a national strategy to reduce the rates of MRSA and *C. difficile*, there is evidence that the rates of both types of infection have more than halved (National Patient Safety Agency [NPSA] 2007a, 2007b; National Audit Office 2009).

Hand hygiene, the combination of processes including hand washing, the use of alcohol hand rub and carefully drying and caring for the skin and nails, is considered to be the single most important measure in preventing the spread of infection. Hand washing will remove transient microorganisms and render the hands socially clean, however, evidence suggests that the process of hand washing is poorly performed and therefore less effective than it otherwise could be. Prior to and immediately following any direct contact with the woman or baby and their immediate surroundings or after an exposure risk to any body fluids, effective hand hygiene practices as determined by WHO (2009) should be followed.

A clean environment is essential if infection rates are to be kept to a minimum and the midwife has an important role to play in ensuring that all equipment is cleaned according to local Trust guidelines and that there is adherence to all infection control measures. Rooms, birthing pools, beds and any equipment used by the midwife should be effectively cleaned before use.

When a woman is admitted to hospital, invasive procedures should be kept to a minimum as an intact skin provides an excellent barrier to organisms. Ideally, women should spend as little time in hospital as determined by their individual needs to minimize their exposure risk to infection. The fetal membranes should also be preserved intact unless there is a positive indication for their rupture that would outweigh the advantage of their protective functions (NICE 2007). Certain invasive techniques, such as the performance of vaginal examinations, may be deemed necessary during labour, however the midwife should ensure that she has a sound reason before embarking on any procedure. Women whose labour is prolonged are at particular risk of infection, often being subjected to a number of invasive procedures including the administration of intravenous fluids, repeated vaginal examinations, epidural analgesia and fetal blood sampling, all of which will increase the risk of infection. By adhering to infection control policies and minimizing interventions when required, the midwife should reduce the potential risk of infection to the woman and promote safety.

The midwife is encouraged to use personal protective equipment if she assesses that there is a risk of transmission of microorganisms to the woman, or the risk of contamination of her clothing and skin by the woman's body fluids (NICE 2007). This poses a difficulty for the midwife as every birth presents a risk of cross-contamination, but wearing a full gown, face masks and eye goggles can create an artificial barrier between herself and the labouring woman at a time when a relationship of trust is vital. Furthermore, face masks and eye goggles provide limited protection from spills or inhalation of spray. In most instances, appropriate hand hygiene and the use of single-use sterile gloves will be sufficient to reduce cross-contamination (NICE 2007).

The midwife's initial physical examination of the woman

The initial examination should include a discussion with the woman about when labour commenced, whether the membranes have ruptured and the frequency and strength of the contractions. The midwife should be aware that the woman will be very conscious of her body and may be unable to concentrate on the conversation or respond while experiencing a contraction. Since the woman has embarked on an intensely energy-demanding process, enquiry should be made about her ability to sleep and her most recent intake of food. If she is in early labour and there are no concerns about the pregnancy, the woman should be advised she can eat and drink as she wishes, remain mobile and maybe bathe if she would find this relaxing. Consideration should be given to the woman's social circumstances, including the care of other children and whether a birthing partner is available and has been contacted.

Past history

Of particular relevance at the onset of a woman's labour are:

- the contents of the birth plan
- her parity and age
- the gestational age and outcomes of previous labours
- the weights and condition of previous babies
- her blood results including grouping, Rhesus factor and haemoglobin

- her attendance at any specialist clinics
- evidence of any known problems: social or physical.

Consent

Prior to touching the woman, a sound explanation of the proposed examination and their significance should be given. Verbal consent should be obtained and recorded in the notes (NMC 2008, 2009). The midwife must be aware that a competent woman, with a capacity to make decisions, is within her rights to refuse any treatment regardless of the consequences to her and her unborn baby and does *not* have to give a reason (DH 2009). Should the midwife be providing care to a pregnant teenager under the age of 16 years, it is important to carefully assess whether there is evidence that she has sufficient understanding in order to give valid consent, i.e. complies with the Fraser guidelines, previously referred to as being *Gillick competent* (*Gillick* v *West Norfolk and Wisbech AHA* 1986; GMC 2013).

General assessment

Initial observations form a baseline for further examinations carried out throughout labour. Basic observations, including pulse rate, temperature and blood pressure, are assessed and recorded. The woman's hands and feet are usually examined for signs of oedema. Slight swelling of the feet and ankles is physiological, but pre-tibial oedema or puffiness of the fingers or face is not.

A detailed *abdominal examination* including symphysis fundal height and optimum position for auscultation of the fetal heart, as described in Chapter 10, should be undertaken and recorded. The abdominal examination may be repeated at intervals in order to assess descent of the presenting part, whether it be cephalic or breech. This is measured by the number of fifths palpable above the pelvic brim and should be recorded on the partogram.

The fetal heart rate should be auscultated for a minimum of *1 minute* immediately after a contraction using a Pinard stethoscope and the rate should be recorded as an average, in a single figure. The maternal pulse should be palpated to differentiate between maternal and fetal heart rates (NICE 2007). Although the Pinard stethoscope is recommended for the initial assessment of the fetal heart, this may not be suitable for use in women who are markedly obese or unable to remain still during auscultation. In such circumstances a hand-held Doppler may be used.

A *vaginal examination* (VE) may also be undertaken to help confirm the onset of labour and determine the extent of cervical effacement and dilatation (Fig. 16.8), with some women requesting it when seeking reassurance about the status of their labour. The procedure, however, is invasive, can be uncomfortable and also poses an infection risk.

337

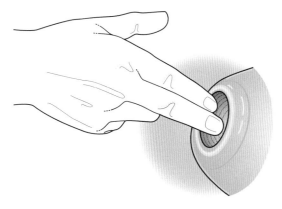

Fig. 16.8 Cervix 4 cm dilated.

Records

The midwife's record of labour is a legal document and must be kept meticulously. The records may be examined by any court for up to 25 years, or the Nursing and Midwifery Council's Professional Conduct Committee or Health Committee, and will be examined in the audit process of statutory supervision of midwifery or on behalf of the Clinical Negligence Scheme for Trusts (CNST) monitoring process. A summary of good record keeping is provided below (NMC 2009, 2012):

- Records should be as *contemporaneous* as possible.
- Each entry should be authenticated with the midwife's full signature with the name printed underneath.
- Records should be comprehensive but concise and consist of the woman's observations, her physical, psychological and sociological state, and any problem that arises as well as the midwife's response and any subsequent interventions.
- The records should be kept in chronological order as their accuracy provides the basis from which clinical improvements, progress or deterioration of the woman or fetus can be judged.
- The record is shared between the midwife and obstetrician and details of any consultation with other members of the multiprofessional team should be clearly documented by the midwife, including the time and nature of the consultation.
- The obstetrician is also responsible to record their findings, timing of visits and any prescriptions made as *the same standards apply to all practitioners*.
- The midwife usually enters in the records the summary of labour and initial details about the health of the baby.
- A midwife must ensure all records are stored securely and should not destroy or arrange for their destruction.

The partogram or partograph

In recent years the *partogram* or *partograph* has been widely accepted as an effective means of recording the progress of labour. It is a chart on which the salient features of labour are entered in a visual graphic form to provide the opportunity for early identification of deviations from normal (Fig. 16.9). However, Lavender et al (2008) found no evidence to support the routine use of the partogram in women who commenced labour spontaneously at term with regards to maternal and fetal outcomes in those labours where a partogram was used against those where there was no partogram. Nonetheless, the partogram remains an integral part of intrapartum record-keeping. The charts are usually designed to allow for recordings at 15-minute intervals and include:

- fetal heart rate
- maternal temperature, pulse and blood pressure
- frequency and strength of contractions every 10 minutes
- descent of the presenting part
- cervical effacement and dilatation
- colour of amniotic fluid
- degree of caput succedaneum/moulding
- fluid balance
- urine analysis
- drugs administered.

The cervicograph is the diagrammatic representation of the dilatation of the cervix charted against the hours in labour. Some initial studies (Friedman 1954; Pearson 1981) demonstrated that the cervical dilatation time of normal labour has a characteristic sigmoid curve. This curve can be divided into two distinct parts: the latent phase and the active phase. Women's progress in labour, however, does not fit neatly into predetermined criteria therefore rigid parameters of *normal* progress should not be adopted (Albers 1999; Lavender et al 2006). The rate of progress in labour must be considered in the context of the woman's total wellbeing and choice.

SUBSEQUENT CARE IN THE FIRST STAGE OF LABOUR

Assessing progress

Physical examination of the cervix is not the only way to assess labour. Midwives can use a range of skills, including visualization of the purple line, appearing from the woman's anal margin gradually extending to the nape of the buttocks (Hobbs 1998; Shepherd et al 2010), and observing the Rhombus of Michaelis, a kite-shaped area between the sacrum and ilea which becomes increasing visible as the fetal head descends in the pelvis (Shepherd et al 2010). In addition, the midwife should be vigilant in

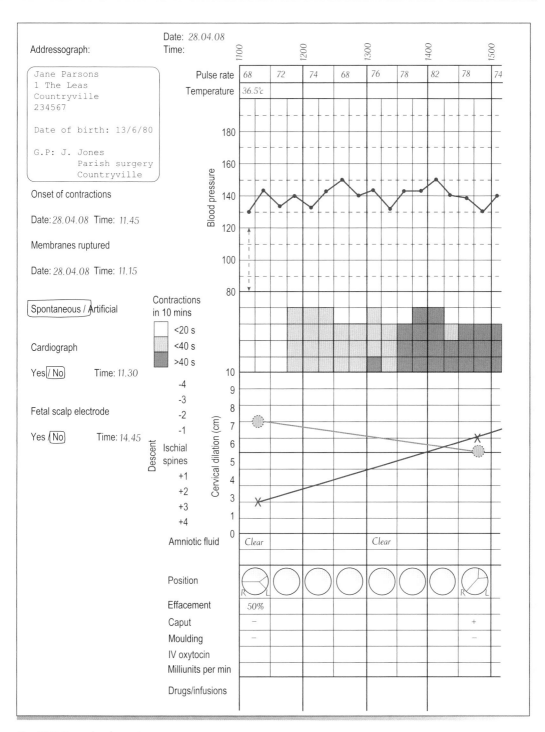

Fig. 16.9 Example of a partogram.

observing for changes in the woman's breathing, behaviour, noises, movements and posture alongside changes in the nature of contractions.

Abdominal examination

An abdominal examination should be repeated by the midwife at intervals throughout labour in order to assess the length, strength and frequency of contractions and the descent of the presenting part. Palpation is of benefit prior to undertaking a vaginal examination, as the findings will assist the midwife to be accurate when defining the position and station of the head/breech. It is also useful to record the position of the fetus contemporaneously during the labour, as this can assist with the analysis of events should a shoulder dystocia occur (Brydon and Raynor 2012).

Contractions

The frequency, length and strength of the contractions should be noted and recorded on the partogram, usually at 30 minute intervals. The uterus should always feel softer between contractions and failure to relax is evidence of hypertonicity. Hypertonicity is usually defined as a contraction lasting more than 2 minutes (NICE 2007). The contraction rate is usually assessed by counting the number of contractions in 10 minutes, over a 20-minute period. Evidence of five contractions or more in 10 minutes is evidence of *tachysystole* in spontaneous labour, or *hyperstimulation* in induced labour (Chapter 19). An excessive number of contractions or hypertonicity can result in fetal compromise as a result of prolonged cord compression or reduction in placental perfusion with consequent reduction in blood supply to the fetus.

Vaginal examination

Although vaginal examinations (VE) have become a routine procedure in labour there is very little evidence to support their efficacy. Dixon and Foureur (2010) state that vaginal examinations are arguably considered to be both an intervention and an essential clinical assessment tool in labour. Midwives should remember that to women who have survived sexual abuse, experienced female genital mutilation (FGM), or are extremely anxious, a vaginal examination can be very distressing and sometimes impossible. Vaginal examinations are undertaken using aseptic principles and should be used judiciously when more information is required if this cannot be gleaned from external observations of women in labour. Ideally the same person should perform the vaginal examinations to be in a better position to judge any changes. Observations and findings as detailed in Box 16.1 should be noted and recorded accordingly by the midwife.

Generally, the trend has moved away from routine 4-hourly VE and justification for each examination should always be recorded. An explanation of the procedure, obtaining of verbal consent from the woman and an abdominal examination should always precede the VE (DH 2009). The woman's bladder should be empty as the presenting part may be displaced by a full bladder as well as being very uncomfortable for the woman. In order to obtain the most information, the woman is usually asked to lie on her back but the technique can be easily adapted to accommodate other positions that suit the woman better. During the examination the woman's dignity and privacy need to be considered. In order to avoid unnecessary exposure, the woman can be asked to move and uncover herself when the midwife is ready to commence the examination. Tap water may be used to cleanse the vagina for this procedure (NICE 2007). With the combination of external and internal findings, the skilled midwife should gain a detailed account of the labour and its subsequent progress.

Indications for vaginal examination

There should be valid reasons to undertake a VE in labour, which are to:

- make a positive identification of the presentation
- determine whether the head is engaged in case of doubt
- ascertain whether the forewaters have ruptured, or to rupture them artificially
- exclude cord prolapse after rupture of the forewaters, especially if there is an ill-fitting presenting part or there are fetal heart rate changes
- assess progress or slow labour
- confirm full dilatation of the cervix (see Fig. 16.12)
- confirm the axis of the fetus and presentation of the second twin in a multiple pregnancy in order to rupture the second amniotic sac, if necessary.

Under no circumstances should a midwife make a vaginal examination if there is any frank bleeding unless the placenta is positively known to be in the upper uterine segment.

Assessing the wellbeing of the woman

Maternal observations

Pulse rate

A tachycardia can indicate pain or anxiety and is also associated with pyrexia, exhaustion and shock. The pulse rate should be recorded hourly (NICE 2007). If the rate increases to >100 bpm it may be indicative of anxiety, pain, infection, ketosis or haemorrhage. The pulse should also be assessed and recorded at any time that there is

> Box 16.1 **Vaginal examination observation and findings**
>
> | | |
> |---|---|
> | **Labia** | Varicosities/oedema/warts/other lesions |
> | **Perineum** | Scars from previous tears/episiotomies |
> | **Vaginal orifice** | Discharge/liquor/'show'/bleeding |
> | **Liquor** | Clear/bloodstained/offensive smell (indicating infection)/meconium staining |
> | **Rectum** | Loaded rectum may be felt on vaginal examination (can impede descent of presenting part) |
> | **Cervix** | *Position of cervix*: central/posterior/anterior/lateral
Consistency: hard, soft
Application to the presenting part: loose/well applied
Effacement: length of canal: may be effaced but closed in a primigravida
Dilatation: Approximate assessment (see Fig. 16.8): 10 cm equates to full dilatation or when no cervix can be felt (ensure no lips of cervix remain (Fig. 16.10)
Note in preterm labour, the smaller presenting part may pass through at a smaller cervical diameter |
> | **Membranes** | Intact/bulging/ruptured
Colour of liquor: clear/bloodstained (liquor/'show')/meconium
Following rupture of membranes, midwife needs to check that the cord has not prolapsed, listen to the fetal heart through contraction
Hindwaters may leak whilst forewaters remain intact |
> | **Presenting part (PP):** the part of the fetus lying over the cervical os (96% are cephalic) | *Identification*: cephalic/breech/footling/knee/compound (see Figs 16.31 and 16.32 below)
Level of bony part of PP in relation to the ischial spines, in cm *above*, *below* or *at the level* of the ischial spines (Fig. 16.11).
The fetus follows the curve of carus therefore it is impossible to judge the station precisely
Presence of *caput succedaneum* /*moulding*/*meconium (breech)* |
> | **Position of presenting part** | *Cephalic presentation:*
Sagittal suture: left or right oblique or transverse should rotate to anteroposterior diameter of the maternal pelvis (Fig. 16.12).
If *well flexed* the small triangular posterior fontanelle is felt: it has three sutures leaving it
The anterior fontanelle is diamond-shaped, has a membrane and four sutures leaving it
Landmarks of the fontanelles give information about the location of the fetal occiput
Breech presentation:
The sacrum is the diagnostic point in respect of its position with the maternal pelvis and the ischial spines |

concern about fetal wellbeing or if there is uncertainty about whether the maternal rather than the fetal pulse is being recorded (NICE 2007).

Temperature

A rise in temperature can be indicative of infection or dehydration. The temperature should be recorded 4-hourly (NICE 2007) and additionally when there is a clinical indication.

Blood pressure

Hypotension may be caused by the woman being in the supine position, by shock or as a result of vasodilation associated with epidural anaesthesia. *Hypertension* is an indicator of pre-eclampsia and in cases where a woman has pre-eclampsia or essential hypertension during pregnancy, labour may further elevate the blood pressure.

Blood pressure should be measured every 4 hours (NICE 2007) and additionally when there is a clinical

indication. It is usual practice to monitor the blood pressure at 5-minute intervals for 20 minutes following the administration of an epidural anaesthetic and following the administration of any bolus dose.

Fluid balance and urinalysis

A record should be kept of all urine passed in order to ensure that the bladder is being emptied. If an intravenous infusion is in progress, the fluids administered must be recorded accurately. It is particularly important to note how much fluid remains if a bag is changed when only partially used.

A trace of protein may be a contaminant following rupture of the membranes or a sign of a urinary tract infection, but more significant proteinuria may indicate pre-eclampsia. Urine passed during labour should be tested for ketones and protein. Ketones may occur in normal labour and a low level is very common and is not usually thought to be significant.

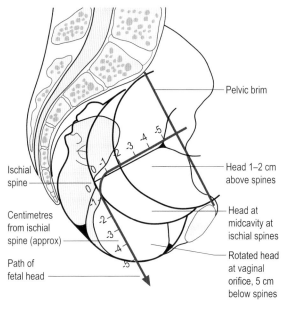

Fig. 16.10 Diagram to show stations of the fetal head in relation to the pelvic canal.

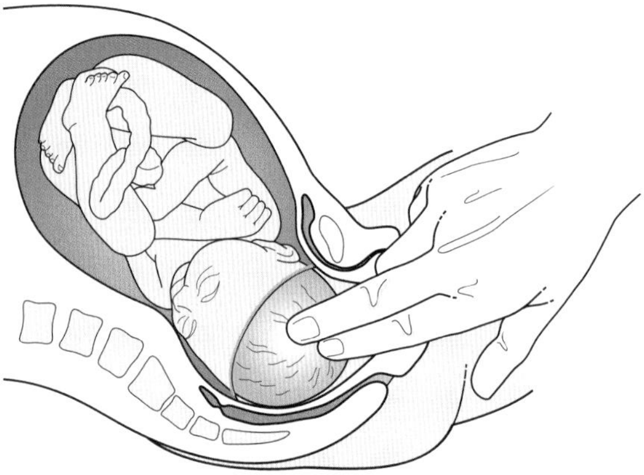

Pelvic brim

Head 1–2 cm above spines

Ischial spine

Head at midcavity at ischial spines

Centimetres from ischial spine (approx)

Rotated head at vaginal orifice, 5 cm below spines

Path of fetal head

Fig. 16.12 Cervix fully dilated.

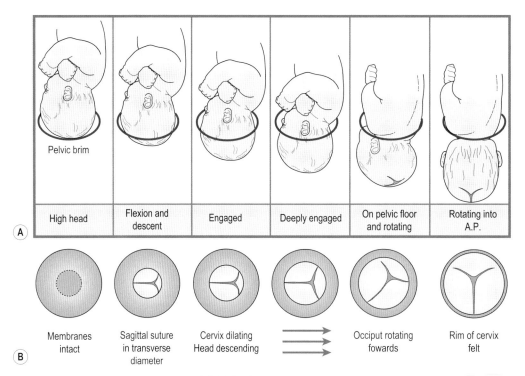

High head

Flexion and descent

Engaged

Deeply engaged

On pelvic floor and rotating

Rotating into A.P.

Pelvic brim

Membranes intact

Sagittal suture in transverse diameter

Cervix dilating Head descending

Occiput rotating fowards

Rim of cervix felt

Fig. 16.11 (A) Diagrams showing descent of the fetal head through the pelvic brim. (B) Diagrams showing dilatation of the cervix and rotation of the fetal head as felt on vaginal examination.

Cleanliness and comfort

Enemas and perineal shaving

There is no evidence to support the routine procedure of administering enemas or undertaking perineal shave to women in labour. However, if a woman reports constipation, or the midwife detects that the rectum is full on vaginal examination, or if the woman feels there would be benefit, an enema or glycerine suppositories can be offered. Sometimes for cultural reasons women will shave their own genital/perineal areas.

Bath or shower

Immersion in a warm bath or birthing pool can be an effective form of pain relief for labouring women that facilitates increased mobility with no increased incidence of adverse outcome for the woman or fetus (Da Silva et al 2009). The midwife should invite the woman who is mobile to have a bath or shower whenever she wishes during labour.

Clothing

It is entirely up to the individual woman what she wears in labour. If in hospital she may prefer to wear the loose gown offered or she may feel more comfortable wearing her own choice of clothing. As long as she is aware that the garment may become wet and bloodstained and that she may require more than one, there is no reason to restrict her choice.

Position and mobility

There are physical benefits if the woman maintains an upright position, including a shorter labour and a reduction in the need for analgesia (Lawrence et al 2009), fewer episiotomies and fewer abnormal fetal heart rate patterns (Gupta et al 2012). Other benefits include increasing the woman's sense of control (Coppen 2005), thus contributing to a positive birth experience. Lying on the bed during labour or birth does little to enhance the physiological birth process and has disadvantages, including a risk of aorto-caval compression and reduced interspinous diameter of the pelvic outlet, increased pain and slower descent of the presenting part.

The need to provide a continuous tracing of the fetal heart can inhibit maternal mobility and in some cases, such as with women who are significantly obese, have pre-existing mobility problems or have an epidural *in situ*, this cannot be avoided. Despite this, the majority of women, including some obese women, will be able to maintain an upright position, retain a degree of mobility and achieve birth away from a birthing bed if supported in doing so. A key factor in encouraging different labour positions and mobility is the environment (Royal College of Midwives [RCM] 2012a). The birthing room should contain equipment such as beanbags, birthing balls and chairs (Albers 2007) and the midwife should be proactive in encouraging the woman to remain active and to change her position. Although women should be encouraged to move and adopt whatever position they find most comfortable (NICE 2007), the midwife should be aware that the woman's choice of birth position may be influenced by what she thinks is expected of her rather than what is actually more comfortable.

Cultures where women are constrained and limited in their posture and positioning during labour are in fact the exception rather than the rule. Many cultures use movement, dance, physical contact and massage to encourage and sustain the process of labour. Henley-Einion (2007) discusses the value of the *Five Rhythms method*. Movements described as *flowing, staccato, chaos, lyrical* and *stillness*, which are a combination of expressive movements rather than a set of routine exercises, are employed to provide dance and the music defines, guides, inspires and prompts the body. Such a strategy would be a fitting one to use during the birthing process.

Pressure ulcer prevention

A pressure ulcer (*decubitus ulcer*) is a localized injury to the skin and underlying tissue that arises when an area of skin is placed under pressure. Where women have pre-existing mobility problems or an epidural in progress, they will be at increased risk of developing pressure ulcers during labour. In 2010 alone there were around 100 reports of women who had developed a pressure ulcer while in a maternity ward (NPSA 2010). All maternity areas should therefore have guidelines for the prevention of pressure ulcers and the midwife must take great care to ensure that the condition of the woman's skin is observed and described in the notes with details documented in the records at 2-hourly intervals.

Nutrition in labour

It has been estimated that in established labour a woman requires a calorie intake of 121 kcal/hour and that 47 kcal/hr is required to prevent ketosis (Hall Moran and Dykes 2006). Most women will be able to draw on glucose stores to provide energy but if insufficient carbohydrate is available energy will be obtained from body fat and this will release ketones, resulting in ketoacidosis.

Dietary care in labour is a controversial issue due to the dearth of good-quality evidence and as a result there is no universal consensus on management. Hospital policies are usually based on the need to restrict food intake in order to prevent gastric aspiration. However, the number of women experiencing gastric aspiration is extremely low and there is no evidence to support the view that starvation will guarantee an empty stomach or prevent gastric acidity (NICE 2007). Starvation in labour can also have psychosocial effects as the provision of food and drink can provide comfort and reassurance, whilst the denial can be seen as authoritarian, stressful and intimidating, which can increase feelings of apprehension (RCM 2012b). For many women in normal labour a low residue, low fat diet and freely available fluids will be appropriate. As there is evidence that the desire to eat is more common in women in early labour (Singata et al 2010) and most women do not want to eat in active labour, it is important that the woman is not encouraged to eat if she has no desire to do so.

Bladder care

Although frequent bladder emptying during labour is recommended, there is no evidence to support any particular regime of intervention. It is therefore reasonable to consider that the bladder should be emptied at least 4-hourly or more frequently if it is palpable abdominally. There is some evidence that infrequent bladder emptying in labour is associated with an increased risk of urinary incontinence in the postpartum period (Birch et al 2009). A full bladder may increase pain, reduce efficiency of uterine contractions and delay descent of the presenting part (Simkin and Ancheta 2011).

The woman's sensation to micturate during labour may be reduced by pressure of the presenting part during its descent through the pelvis, or by an effective epidural block. In all cases of delay in labour, the midwife should ascertain whether the bladder is full and encourage the woman to void regularly. Where possible the woman should be encouraged to use the toilet, and if this is not possible, the midwife should provide privacy and ensure maximum comfort by placing the bedpan on the chair, stool or bed and encouraging the woman to adopt a leaning forwards position. The sound or feel of water can also help to trigger the micturition reflex. If the bladder is incompletely emptied or the woman is unable to void for some hours, it may become necessary to introduce a catheter into the bladder. As the risk of infection is increased with the use of retaining catheters, it is generally recommended that an 'in-out' catheter is used.

Medicine records

Midwives have an exemption from requiring a prescription for specific medicines used in the care of women in physiological labour. In the UK, NHS Trusts also have locally agreed patient group directions to which the midwife should adhere, providing guidance as to which medicines are preferred and what doses and frequency should be used within that Trust. If the midwife is practising outside the area in which she has notified her intention to practise, she should consult the supervisor of midwives regarding any matters relating to the supply, administration, storage or surrender of controlled drugs or medicines (NMC 2010, 2012).

As well as being entered on the partogram, doses of drugs are recorded on the prescription sheet, in the summary of labour and, in the case of controlled drugs, in the Controlled Drugs Register.

ASSESSING THE WELLBEING OF THE FETUS

The aim of fetal monitoring in labour is to maintain wellbeing, detect fetal hypoxia and initiate appropriate intervention before the fetus becomes asphyxiated and neurological damage occurs. Despite the widespread practice of both intermittent and continuous fetal monitoring, there are no statistical differences in the rates of cerebral palsy, infant mortality or other standard measures of neonatal wellbeing with either form of monitoring (Alfirevic et al 2013). NICE (2007) recommend that in all low-risk established labours, *intermittent auscultation* should be practised. The midwife should discuss the recommendations for fetal monitoring and the available evidence with the woman in order that she can make an informed decision about how her baby's wellbeing will be monitored during labour.

Intermittent auscultation

Intermittent auscultation involves listening to the fetal heart rate at intervals using a Pinard stethoscope or a hand-held Doppler. The Pinard stethoscope will simply amplify the actual heart sound so that it can be heard and counted. However, it may be difficult to use when the woman is in certain positions, such as all-fours or squatting, and as the sound cannot be heard by the woman, this method may be less reassuring for her. The hand-held Doppler uses ultrasound to detect movement, either of the fetal heart muscle or valves, which are converted into a sound that can be heard and counted, such that the woman and her partner can also hear the fetal heart. It should be recognized that as the Doppler converts movement into sound it is possible for the maternal pulse to be detected and be mistaken for the fetal pulse. For this reason it is recommended that the Pinard stethoscope should be used to check the fetal heart when any concern arises (Medicines and Healthcare Products Regulatory Agency [MHPRA] 2010) and that the maternal pulse is also counted (NICE 2007). The normal fetal heart will have a rate of 110–160 bpm and there should be no audible decelerations (NICE 2007). If at any time a fetal heart rate abnormality is suspected or there is any concern about fetal wellbeing, such as following the detection of meconium staining of the liquor, electronic fetal monitoring (EFM) should be commenced following discussion with the woman and her companion (NICE 2007).

The current guidance is for intermittent auscultations to be performed in the active first stage of labour at least every 15 minutes for a full minute immediately following a contraction (NICE 2007). As with any observation, every recording should be documented in the labour records. In order to demonstrate compliance with the recommendation regarding the timing of auscultations, it is helpful at least once to provide a description in the intrapartum records of how and when auscultation is being performed.

Continuous electronic fetal monitoring

An admission cardiotocograph (CTG) is **not** recommended in low-risk labour (NICE 2007). Devane et al (2012) confirmed that such traces do not provide any benefit in terms of reducing perinatal morbidity or mortality but can increase the rate of caesarean section by approximately 20%.

Continuous electronic fetal monitoring (EFM) is recommended for any labour where there are risks to fetal well-being, including the use of oxytocin and epidural analgesia (NICE 2007; Afors and Chandraharan 2011). Whilst EFM will detect *suspect* pathology, as changes such as tachycardia or bradycardia can be seen, it has low specificity for identifying between the acidotic fetus and the fetus that is not compromised (Schiermeier et al 2008). Electronic fetal monitoring can detect changes in the pattern of the fetal heart that could indicate hypoxia but cannot provide a diagnosis as the CTG is a highly sensitive tool but the condition it is designed to detect is of low prevalence. This results in a high false-positive rate and a poor positive predictive value; consequently, EFM has shown an increase in the rate of operative and assisted birth without demonstrating a reduction in perinatal mortality, or the incidence of cerebral palsy (Ayres-de-Campos and Bernades 2010). For this reason, in the absence of a persistent bradycardia, any evidence of pathology should be further investigated by fetal blood sampling if this is feasible, otherwise birth should be expedited (NICE 2007). Decisions about the indications for fetal blood sampling and mode of birth will be made by an obstetrician.

Good practice points

- On admission an abdominal palpation should be performed to determine the optimal area for listening to the fetal heart.
- A Pinard or fetal stethoscope should be used at the initial assessment to establish the real sound of the fetal heart. Intermittent auscultation should be continued throughout established labour unless there is a reason for EFM.
- The maternal pulse should be palpated and recorded at the start of EFM and at any time that the trace is recommenced. If there is doubt about whether the maternal or fetal heart is being monitored, the maternal pulse should be palpated to differentiate between the two heart rates (NICE 2007).
- The term *fetal distress* should be avoided when describing the EFM trace as it can cause alarm to the woman and her companion(s) and is not helpful in the analysis of the trace.
- The trace should be systematically assessed and categorized and the findings described in the notes at least hourly. In maternity units where a *fresh eyes* approach has been adopted it is usual for this to take place every two hours.
- The CTG monitor clock should be periodically checked for accuracy.
- Significant events should be noted on the CTG, such as VE and mode of birth.
- Each clinician who is asked to review the CTG should sign the trace at the time of the review.
- EFM is **not** a substitute for, and should **not** interfere with, continuous care and support during labour (MIDIRS 2008a).
- Although EFM can interfere with maternal positioning, for most women it should be possible for the labour to be experienced out of bed and/or with the woman in an upright position.
- All staff who interpret CTG traces should receive up-to-date training and assessment (NICE 2007), and to fulfil CNST (2013) requirements, this should be every 6 months.
- When discontinued, the CTG trace should be systematically assessed, classified and the findings recorded on the trace which should be stored safely in the appropriate portion of the woman's records.

Interpretation of the cardiotocograph

When interpreting a CTG it is useful to perform a systematic assessment, identifying any existing risk factors for hypoxia, the reason for EFM and the stage of the labour. This will assist in the overall analysis of the CTG trace. The trace is then assessed to identify whether its features are *reassuring*, *non-reassuring* or *abnormal*, as shown in Box 16.2 (NICE 2007).

The four features of a CTG trace are:

Baseline rate

This is the *mean level* of the fetal heart rate between contractions, excluding accelerations and decelerations. A rising baseline rate may be of concern even if it remains within the normal range, if other non-reassuring or abnormal features are present.

Box 16.2 Classification of the fetal heart rate features

	Baseline (bpm)	Variability (bpm)	Decelerations	Accelerations
Reassuring	110–160	>5	None	Present
Non-reassuring	100–109 or 160–180	<5 for 40–90 minutes	Typical variable decelerations with over 50% of contractions for over 90 minutes Single prolonged deceleration for up to 3 minutes	The absence of accelerations in an otherwise *normal* trace is of uncertain significance
Abnormal	<100 >180	<5 for over 90 minutes	Either atypical variable decelerations with over 50% of contractions or late decelerations: both for over 30 minutes Single prolonged deceleration for over 3 minutes	

Source: NICE 2007

Baseline variability

This is the degree to which the *baseline varies over the period of a minute*. The baseline variability is under the influence of the autonomic nervous system and this produces an irregular jagged appearance on the CTG trace. However, if repeated accelerations are seen on a trace with *reduced* variability, the variability should **not** be assessed as non-reassuring.

Decelerations

These are reflected as a fall in the baseline rate of at least 15 bpm for at least 15 seconds. True uniform decelerations, usually referred to as *early*, are rare and benign, and are therefore not significant. Most decelerations in labour are variable, which means they are variable in presentation and appearance. There are two types of variable decelerations, *typical* and *atypical,* and it is important to distinguish between them.

Typical variable decelerations

Typical variable decelerations occur in response to intermittent cord compression and are commonly seen during the second stage of labour. They are quick to recover to the normal baseline, have normal variability, last less than 2 minutes and have evidence of *shouldering*, which is a normal physiological response to intermittent cord compression.

Atypical variable decelerations

These decelerations can be an indicator of hypoxia and have some or all of the following features:

- Loss of acceleration (shouldering) before and after deceleration
- Delayed recovery back to baseline
- Late component/biphasic deceleration

- Rebound tachycardia – caused by catecholamine release in response to stress
- Loss of variability/change in baseline rate.

Late decelerations

These decelerations are uncommon and are usually considered to be indicative of fetal hypoxia. The main features being:

- Reduced variability
- Repetitive and uniform shape
- Begin *at* or *after the peak* of the contraction
- Their lowest point is 20 seconds or more *after the peak* of contractions.

Accelerations

These particular features reflect an elevation in the baseline rate of 15 bpm for 15 seconds or more. The significance of the absence of accelerations in an otherwise *normal* trace is uncertain.

Overall classification of the fetal heart rate features

All four features of the fetal heart rate pattern are assessed and an overall classification of *normal, suspicious* or *pathological* is determined according to how many features are described as *reassuring, non-reassuring* and *abnormal,* as identified in Box 16.3.

It is important to record the classification of the trace at *each assessment* as the actions required will be informed by this.

Normal

If no other indication for CTG, discontinue and commence intermittent auscultation every 15 minutes (Fig. 16.13).

Suspicious

The trace should continue and the possible causes be considered. The woman's position should also be changed to the left lateral, her pulse and blood pressure assessed and fluids administered if appropriate. If the trace reverts to *normal* and there is no other indication for the CTG it could be discontinued; however review by an obstetrician may be required.

Should the trace remain *suspicious*, the appropriate level obstetrician should be consulted. Fetal blood sampling may be required (Fig. 16.14).

Pathological

The woman's position should be changed to the left lateral, her pulse and blood pressure assessed and fluids administered if appropriate. If there is a bradycardia in a hospital setting the emergency call bell should be used to summon assistance and referral to a Registrar or Consultant should be made immediately.

Fetal blood sampling or the need to expedite the birth may be necessary. If fetal blood sampling is performed this should be *prior* to the administration of pethidine, epidural or syntocinon, should the trace remain pathological (Fig. 16.15).

Fetal blood sampling

Maternity units that use electronic fetal monitoring should have 24 hours access to fetal blood sampling (FBS) facilities. When the fetal heart rate pattern is suspicious or pathological and fetal acidosis is suspected, then FBS should always be undertaken (NICE 2007) (Fig. 16.16). The procedure involves a small sample of blood being taken from the scalp of the fetal head with the woman in

---

Box 16.3 **Overall classification of the fetal heart trace**	
Normal:	**All four features** are classified as *reassuring* (please note comment about accelerations in Box 16.2)
Suspicious:	**One feature** is classified as *non-reassuring* and the remaining features are *reassuring*
Pathological:	**Two or more features** are classified as *non-reassuring* or **one or more** classified as *abnormal*
Source: NICE 2007	

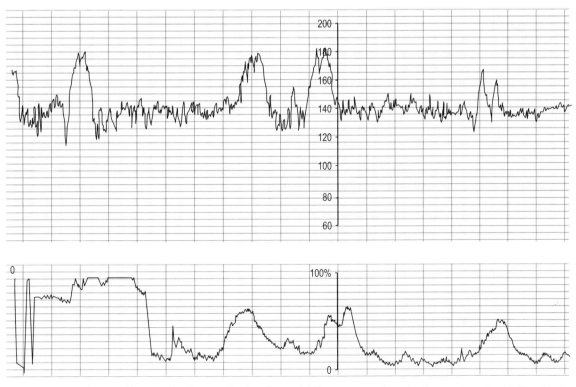

Fig. 16.13 Normal CTG with reassuring features (i.e. baseline variability, presence of accelerations and *no* decelerations here).

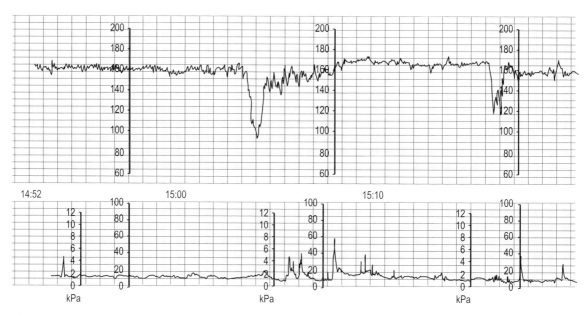

Fig. 16.14 Suspicious CTG with presence of one non-reassuring feature (i.e. *typical variable* decelerations).

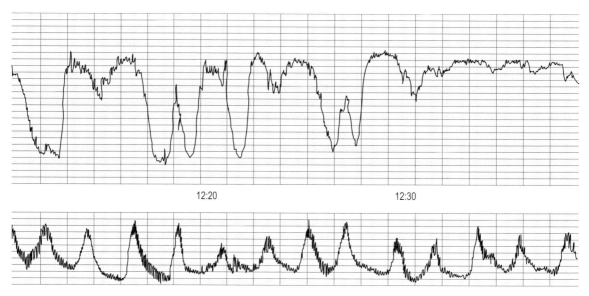

Fig. 16.15 Pathological CTG with abnormal features (i.e. *atypical variable* decelerations: note the biphasic pattern or *W* effect of the decelerations).

the left lateral position as the lithotomy position is more distressing for both the woman and fetus, causing supine hypotension which can increase fetal hypoxia. If the CTG trace is bradycardic or significantly pathological with no prospect of spontaneous birth, time should **not** be wasted performing a FBS. This would be the clinical decision of a senior obstetrician.

A normal fetal blood sample result should be repeated no more than an hour later if the trace remains pathological, or earlier if the heart rate pattern deteriorates. A fetal blood sample result of <7.25 should be repeated no more than 30 minutes later, whereas one that is <7.20 indicates that the baby requires immediate birth (NICE 2007).

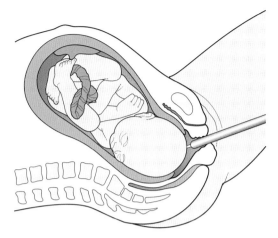

Fig. 16.16 Fetal blood sampling. Access to fetal scalp via amnioscope passed through the cervix.

WOMEN'S CONTROL OF PAIN DURING LABOUR

The relationship between the woman and the midwife is important and can also impact on how the woman perceives the pain of labour. Time, waiting and following the woman are important elements of care. The idea of patience and supporting the woman on her journey, giving meaning and sense to the pain of labour, is paramount.

The issue of pain during labour should be woman-centred, not medically oriented. A clear differentiation must be made between the traditional goal of pain relief and the control of pain in labour. Leap and Anderson (2008) proposed that midwives adopt one of two paradigms: *the pain relief* model and *the working with pain* model. In the *pain relief* model, midwives present a menu of pain-relieving options to the woman, but while this approach has the best of intentions, it inevitably undermines the woman's confidence in herself and her body to give birth without the aid of medication. However, in the *working with pain* model it is expected that most women in labour will experience some degree of pain that is fundamental to a physiological labour. Pain of normal labour is *positive* and has a purpose, and if this philosophy is embraced, midwives and women can work together to ensure labour is an enabling and ultimately uplifting experience.

It is appreciated that emotions such as fear, confidence and also cognition affect the person's perception of pain (Leap and Anderson 2008; Mander 2011). More than any other type of sensation, pain can be modified by past experience, anxiety, emotion and suggestion. Lack of food, rest and sleep also impact on the woman's perception of pain. The midwife must take into account not only the level or extent of the woman's pain, but also all other subjective or illusory aspects that may be contributing to the experience, and also to realize the importance of her own attitude to intrapartum *pain relief*, as this may be informed by the medical model.

The role of pain in labour is an important one. For some women it provides the dominant negative memory of the birth whilst for others it is viewed as empowering, bestowing a sense of triumphant achievement. As the pain of labour affects women in different ways, so then must the response of the midwife be tailored to the individual needs of the woman.

The physiology of pain

Pain stimulus and pain sensation

Unlike most pain, the pain experienced in labour is not caused by a pathological process or trauma and instead is the result of an interaction between physiological and psychological factors (Abushaikha and Oweis 2005). The discomfort or pain of labour is caused by the descent of the fetal head further into the pelvis. It is also caused by pressure on the cervix and the stretching of the vaginal walls and pelvic floor muscles, as descent of the presenting part occurs. The large uterine muscle contracts more strongly, more frequently and for a longer duration as labour progresses. This also increases the discomfort felt by the woman. It is not suitable to use pain-relieving measures used in other medical circumstances, as the purpose is not to stop or impair the birth process (or contractions), but to facilitate the labour progress normally, with the descent and rotation of the presenting part.

Pain is caused by a stimulus that may cause, or be on the verge of causing, tissue damage. Pain sensation may therefore be distinguished from other sensations, although emotions such as fear and anxiety are also experienced at the same time, thereby affecting the person's perception of pain. It must also be remembered that a painful stimulus may also induce such changes by the sympathetic nervous system as increased heart rate, a rise in blood pressure, release of adrenaline (epinephrine) into the bloodstream and an increase in blood glucose levels. There is also a decrease in gastric motility and a reduction in the blood supply to the skin, causing sweating. Thus, stimuli that cause pain result in a *sensory* incident or occurrence.

Pain transmission

The pain pathway or *ascending sensory tract* originates in the sensory nerve endings at the site of trauma. The impulse travels along the sensory nerves to the dorsal root ganglion of the relevant spinal nerve and into the posterior horn of the spinal cord. This is known as the *first neuron*. The *second neuron* arises in the posterior horn, crosses over within the spinal cord (the *sensory decussation*)

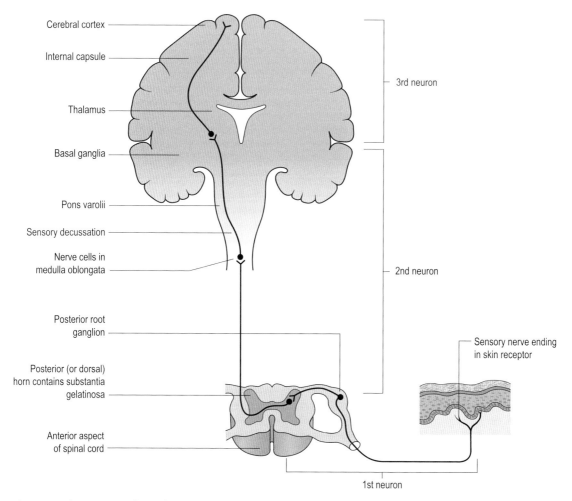

Cerebral cortex

Internal capsule

Thalamus

Basal ganglia

Pons varolii

Sensory decussation

Nerve cells in
medulla oblongata

Posterior root
ganglion

Posterior (or dorsal)
horn contains substantia
gelatinosa

Anterior aspect
of spinal cord

3rd neuron

2nd neuron

Sensory nerve ending
in skin receptor

1st neuron

Fig. 16.17 The sensory pathway showing the structures involved in the appreciation of pain.

and transmits the impulse via the *medulla oblongata, pons varolii* and the *mid-brain* to the *thalamus*. From here, it travels along the *third neuron* to the *sensory cortex* (Fig. 16.17).

In cases of *acute pain*, sensations are transmitted along Aδ *fibres*, which are large diameter nerve fibres. This type of pain is perceived as being a pricking pain that is readily localized by the sufferer. The pathway for *chronic pain* is slightly different as the nerve fibres involved are of smaller diameter and are called *C fibres*. Chronic pain is often described as a burning pain that is difficult to localize.

Somatosensory function

Somatic sensation refers to the sensory function of the skin and body walls. This is moderated by a variety of somatic receptors of which there are particular receptors for each sensation, such as heat, cold, touch, pressure, etc. On entering the central nervous system, the afferent nerve fibres from somatic receptors form synapses with interneurons that comprise the specific ascending pathways going to the somatosensory cortex via the brain stem and the thalamus.

An *afferent neuron*, with its receptor, makes up a sensory unit. Usually the peripheral end of an afferent neuron branches into many receptors. The receptors whose stimulation gives rise to pain are situated in the peripheries of small unmyelinated or slightly myelinated afferent neurons. These receptors are known as *nociceptors* because they detect injury (*noci*, being the Latin word for 'harm', 'injury'). The primary afferents coming from nociceptors form synapses with interneurons after entering the central nervous system. Substance P is a *neurotransmitter* that is liberated at some of these synapses when there is a pain impulse that facilitates information about pain which is then transmitted to the higher centres.

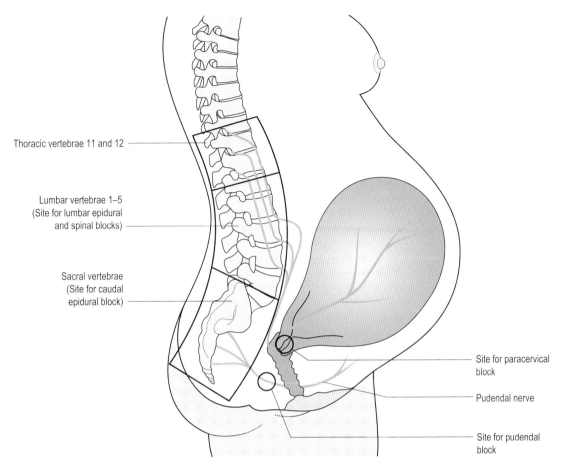

Thoracic vertebrae 11 and 12

Lumbar vertebrae 1–5
(Site for lumbar epidural
and spinal blocks)

Sacral vertebrae
(Site for caudal
epidural block)

Site for paracervical
block

Pudendal nerve

Site for pudendal
block

Fig. 16.18 Pain pathways in labour showing the sites at which pain may be intercepted by local anaesthetic techniques.

The stretching of the muscles and ligaments of the pelvic cavity and the pressure of the descending fetus during the birthing process causes pain in labour to varying degrees (Fig. 16.18). This sensation is transmitted by afferent or *visceral sensory neurons*, visceral pain being caused by the stretching or irritation of the viscera. Afferent neurons convey both autonomic sympathetic and parasympathetic fibres. Pain fibres from the skin and the viscera run adjacent to each other in the *spinothalamic tract*. Therefore pain from an internal organ may be perceived or felt as if it was coming from a skin area supplied by the same section or part of the spinal cord: for example, pain from the uterus may be perceived or felt by the woman as being in her back or labia. When this sort of pain occurs or is experienced, it is commonly called *referred pain*.

Martini et al (2011) suggest that the level of pain experienced can be disproportionate to the amount of painful stimuli due to the facilitation resulting from glutamate and substance P release. This effect can be one reason why women's perception of pain associated with childbirth differs so widely.

Endorphins and enkephalins

Endorphins are described as being opiate-like peptides, or *neuropeptides*, which are produced naturally by the body at neural synapses at various points in the central nervous system pathways. They modulate the transmission of pain perception in these areas. Endorphins are found in the limbic system, hypothalamus and reticular formation (Martini et al 2011). They bind to the presynaptic membrane, inhibiting the release of substance P, and therefore inhibit the transmission of pain. *Enkephalins* are also neuropeptides that have the ability to inhibit neurotransmitters along the pathway of pain transmission, thereby reducing it. These act like a natural pain relieving substance.

Theories of pain

Theories of pain include specificity, pattern, affect and psychological/behavioural theory (Mander 2011), however these are not always applicable to the pain experienced in childbirth. The most widely used and accepted theory is the *gate-control theory* of Melzack and Wall (1965), who established that gentle stimulation actually inhibits the sensation of pain. The *gate-control theory* declares that a neural or spinal gating mechanism occurs in the substantia gelatinosa of the dorsal horns of the spinal cord. The nerve impulses received by nociceptors, the receptors for pain in the skin and tissue of the body, are affected by the gating mechanism. It is the position of the gate that determines whether or not the nerve impulses travel freely to the medulla and the thalamus, thereby transmitting the sensory impulse or message to the sensory cortex. If the gate is closed, pain is blocked and does not become part of the conscious thought. If the gate is open, the impulses and messages pass through and are transmitted freely (Fig. 16.18), resulting in pain being experienced.

Physiological responses to pain in labour

Pain of labour is associated with an *increased respiratory rate*. This may cause a decrease in the $PaCO_2$ level, with a corresponding increase in the pH and a subsequent fall in the fetal $PaCO_2$ ensues. This may be suspected by the presence of late decelerations on the CTG if continuous monitoring is being employed during labour. The acid–base equilibrium of the system may be altered by hyperventilation and breathing exercises. Alkalosis may then affect the diffusion of oxygen across the placenta, leading to a degree of fetal hypoxia.

Cardiac output increases during the first and second stages of labour up to an extent of 20% and 50%, respectively. This increase is caused by the return of uterine blood to the maternal circulation, which constitutes about 250–300 ml with each contraction. Pain, apprehension and fear may also cause a sympathetic response, thereby producing a greater cardiac output.

Both the respiratory and cardiac systems are affected by catecholamine release. Adrenaline (epinephrine), which comprises about 80% of this release, has the effect of reducing the uterine blood flow, leading to a potential reduction in uterine activity.

Non-pharmacological methods for pain control in labour

Increasingly, non-pharmacological methods are being used by women during labour. In addition to the methods described below, there is some evidence that hypnosis, massage, acupuncture and acupressure reduce pain or decrease the need for pharmacological analgesia during labour (Tiran 2010a).

The midwife needs to be mindful that to administer any complementary therapy/

*alternative therapy to a woman in labour it is both essential **and** a professional requirement that an approved course of training is undertaken to be deemed knowledgeable and competent to practise such a skill. (NMC 2010, 2012)*

Aromatherapy

Aromatherapy is the use of essential oils for a range of purposes, for example to induce relaxation, reduction of pain or nausea and vomiting. These oils may be massaged into the skin, inhaled through diffusers or oil burners, or used in conjunction with hydrotherapy. This particular complementary therapy has become popular among childbearing women and midwives, with many maternity units in the UK providing this service for women during labour and birth (Smith et al 2011). Zahra and Leila (2013) conducted a randomized controlled trial (RCT) in Iran with women randomly assigned to either massage only or aromatherapy massage with lavender oil. Pain intensity was significantly lower in the aromatherapy massage group and first and second stages of labour were shorter. There were, however, only 30 women assigned to each group. Furthermore, the systematic review conducted by Smith et al (2011) on the efficacy of aromatherapy for pain management was also too small to draw any significant conclusions and thus there remains a need for more research in this area.

Homeopathy

Homeopathy uses small doses of natural medicines to stimulate the body's own physiological response to heal itself (Idarius 2010). Homeopathic remedies are prepared from plant extracts and from minerals. Professional advice is recommended during pregnancy as the holistic approach of this method entails a consideration of all the facets and the requirements of the individual. *Aconite* may be used to relieve fear and anxiety and *Kali Carbonate* to alleviate back pain during labour (Steen and Calvert 2006).

Hydrotherapy

Immersion in water during labour as a means of analgesia has been used for many years. Cluett and Burns (2009) cite that the effectiveness of hydrotherapy is due to heat-relieving muscle spasm, and therefore pain, and *hydrokinesis* eliminates the effects of gravity and also the discomfort and strain on the pelvis. Two studies comparing immersion in water during labour with land labour found that those immersed in water had significantly reduced duration of labour (Zanetti-Dallenbach et al 2007; Thoni et al 2010). Cluett and Burns (2009) found that immersion in water in the first stage of labour reduces the use of epidural/

spinal analgesia and no evidence of an increase in adverse effects on fetus/neonate or the woman. Water immersion is usually highly rated by both women and midwives, and the calming atmosphere of a pool room can benefit everyone as the woman appears less anxious and therefore feels less pain (Benjoya Miller 2006).

Music therapy

As well as at home, many birthing rooms are equipped with radio or CD apparatus and this is often a useful means to help women relax, be entertained and find some distraction during the early stages of labour. Many types of music are available for relaxation, some of which are specifically for childbirth. Henley-Einion (2007) recounts that music can have a positive effect on the woman's body, mind and spirit by providing empowerment and creating an enabling effect.

Transcutaneous electrical nerve stimulation (TENS)

Transcutaneous electrical nerve stimulation (TENS) is a widely used and well-appreciated method of pain relief. TENS stimulates the production of natural endorphins and enkephalins and impedes incoming pain stimuli. It consists of a small device that distributes low intensity electrical charges across the skin which is thought to prevent pain signals from the uterus, vagina and cervix arriving at the brain (de Ferrer 2006). The body's own pain relievers, the *endorphins*, are then released. TENS works by stimulating low threshold afferent fibres, such as the fibres of touch receptors which inhibit neurons in the pain pathways. As pathways activated by the touch receptors add a synaptic input into the pain pathways, the individual may massage a painful area to relieve the pain which is how TENS functions.

The apparatus consists of four electrodes and four flexes that connect these to the TENS unit, which has controls to alter the frequency and the intensity of the impulse (Fig. 16.19). The electrodes are positioned at the level of T10

and L1 on the woman's back and have been found to be effective in reducing pain during the first stage of labour. The remaining electrodes are placed between S2 and S4 and provide control of pain during the second stage of labour. The woman can use a boost control button to convey high intensity and high frequency patterns of stimulation of the dermatomes during the uterine contraction to provide additional relief, thus enhancing control over the birth process.

TENS is considered to be more effective when started in early labour (Juman Blincoe 2007). However, Dowswell et al (2011) found that women using TENs were less likely to rate their pain as severe and overall they did not find any overwhelming evidence that TENs significantly reduces pain in labour.

Pharmacological methods for pain control

Inhalation analgesia

A premixed gas made up of 50% nitrous oxide (N_2O) and 50% oxygen (O_2) administered via the Entonox apparatus is the most commonly used inhalation analgesia in labour. Nitrous oxide (also known as *laughing gas*), like many other forms of analgesia, acts by limiting the neuronal and synaptic transmission within the central nervous system. Evidence shows that N_2O induces opioid peptide release in *the periaqueductal* grey area of the mid-brain leading to the activation of the descending inhibitory pathways, resulting in modulation of the pain/nociceptive processing in the spinal cord (Fujinaga and Maze 2002). The mixture of gases is stable at normal temperature, but separates below $-7\,°C$. In many large obstetric units the gas is stored in a bank and piped to each birthing room or is available in cylinders. Midwives attending women at home births are responsible for the safe storage of the gas cylinders which should be on their side, rather than upright. This is because nitrous oxide is heavier than oxygen and the horizontal position reduces the risk of administering a severely hypoxic mixture. The cylinders

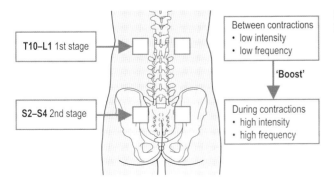

Fig. 16.19 TENS electrode positioning for use during labour.

must be brought into a warm room if they have been exposed to cold temperatures, and the gases remixed by inverting the cylinder at least three times before use.

Entonox apparatus is usually manufactured by the British Oxygen Company (BOC). Both the apparatus and the cylinder are made so that they do not fit on to other equipment. These fit together by a pin index system. The cylinder is blue with a blue and white shoulder. The one-way valve opens on inspiration and the woman should be advised that optimal analgesia is obtained by closely applying the lips around the mouthpiece or firmly applying the mask to the face. The gases take effect within 20 seconds and it is important that the woman uses it before a contraction commences. The maximum efficacy of the gases occurs after about 45–50 seconds which should coincide with the height of the contraction, providing maximum relief for the woman. This method of pain control is useful in that the woman is able to administer it herself, but its effectiveness is determined by the woman's ability to use the equipment as advised. A study by Teimoori et al (2011) showed that nitrous oxide and oxygen provided better analgesia and had more beneficial effects when compared to pethidine.

Exposure to high levels of nitrous oxide can cause teratogenic and other side-effects such as infertility among midwives and other staff. It is important that scavenging equipment to extract expired gases is installed in all birthing rooms to reduce such effects on staff (RCM 2012c).

Opiate drugs

Opiate drugs are frequently used during childbirth because of their powerful analgesic properties. The action of these drugs lies in their ability to bind with receptor sites which are mainly found in the *substantia gelatinosa* of the dorsal horn of the spinal cord (Anderson 2011). Others are located in the midbrain, thalamus and hypothalamus.

In the UK three systemic opioids are commonly used for pain relief in labour:

- pethidine (meperidine in the USA)
- diamorphine
- meptazinol (Meptid).

All have similar pain-relieving properties, but little evidence exists in relation to their effectiveness, maternal satisfaction of their use or their effect on the fetus/neonate in labour (Ullman et al 2010). There are numerous side-effects of opiate drugs and the extent to which they are experienced is influenced by the woman's metabolism of the drug, the degree and speed of transfer of the drug and metabolites from maternal to fetal circulation and the ability of the fetus to process and excrete both. Common side-effects of opiate drugs include:

- nausea and vomiting
- delayed emptying of the stomach

- drowsiness or sedation in the woman which may impair decision making
- reduction in fetal heart rate variability and depression of the baby's respiratory centre at birth
- a sleepy baby affecting the establishment of breastfeeding.

An anti-emetic agent is sometimes given to the woman at the same time to reduce the feeling of nausea. It is therefore important to ensure that the woman is fully informed during pregnancy of the effects of these drugs so that she can make informed decisions about methods of pain control.

Pethidine

Pethidine is a synthetic compound acting on the receptors in the body and is the most frequently used systemic narcotic analgesic in the UK. It is usually administered intramuscularly in doses of 50–150 mg, depending on the woman's size, and takes about 20 minutes to have an effect. Pethidine can be administered intravenously for a faster effect and some maternity units use a machine to enable the woman to control the administration: known as *patient-controlled analgesia* (PCA). Some reports show that opiates, especially pethidine, slow down the process of labour and are not significantly effective in relieving labour pain, as often sedation is confused with analgesia (Anderson 2011).

Diamorphine

Diamorphine has been found to provide effective analgesia for up to 4 hours in labour with the usual dose being 5 mg. It is more rapidly metabolized, accounting for its greater speed of effectiveness and consequently it is eliminated more readily from maternal and neonatal plasma (Fernando and Jones 2009). Diamorphine is used far less commonly than other opiates in labour, even though some claim it gives better pain relief and hence more comparative studies are needed (Jones et al 2012). It is possible that the lack of use of diamorphine in labour might be due to fears of its potentially addictive nature.

Meptazinol

Meptazinol is usually given in doses of 100–150 mg intramuscularly. It is fast-acting and is effective for about 4 hours. This opiate provides similar pain relief to pethidine and like other opiates, meptazinol is also associated with an increased incidence of nausea and vomiting (Ullman et al 2010).

Regional (epidural) analgesia

Epidurals are effective in relieving pain in labour and may be requested by women at any point during the first stage of labour. Women who have used other methods of pain relief on experiencing strong contractions may decide to request an epidural when labour is well advanced. This makes explanation of the benefits and risks of epidural analgesia *during pregnancy* even more important. The pain relief from an epidural is obtained by blocking the conduction of impulses along sensory nerves as they enter the spinal cord. It is an invasive procedure that requires informed consent from the woman and an experienced (obstetric) anaesthetist to initiate under strict aseptic conditions.

An intravenous infusion of crystalloid fluids is commenced prior to siting the epidural. The need for *preloading* has reduced since *low-dose epidural blockades* have been used, reducing the risk of hypotension (NICE 2007). The woman is either positioned in the left lateral position to reduce the risk of supine hypotension or in a sitting position to flex the spine, in an effort to separate the vertebrae, thus facilitating the management of the procedure. The fetal heart rate and the woman's blood pressure must be recorded throughout the procedure.

The skin is first cleansed followed by administration of local anaesthetic into the epidural space of the lumbar region, usually between L2 and L3, before the anaesthetist cautiously inserts a Tuohy needle (usually 16G) that has centimetre marking and a bevelled end to aid the insertion and positioning of a fine catheter, into the epidural space (Fig. 16.20). To locate the epidural space, the needle is first advanced until resistance of the *ligamentum flavum* is encountered. At this point a syringe is attached to the Tuohy needle and inserted further until it enters the epidural space. This is recognized by the loss of resistance when pressure is applied to the plunger of the syringe or loss of resistance to saline (Hawkins 2010). It is particularly important that the woman remains still at this stage as the subarachnoid space is only a few millimetres deeper and any slight movement could result in the Tuohy needle

puncturing the meninges and causing a *dural tap*. Smaller gauge needles are used for spinal anaesthesia reducing the risk of dural tap and have the advantage of relieving pain rapidly (Hawkins 2010).

Once the Tuohy needle is in the epidural space and there is no evidence of any leakage of blood or cerebrospinal fluid (CSF), a fine catheter is threaded through the needle and left *in situ* to facilitate bolus injections or continuous infusion of the local anaesthetic bupivacaine (marcain). The injection of bupivacaine into the epidural space bathes the nerves of the corda equina, blocking the autonomic nerve pathways supplying the uterus. The first dose is given by the anaesthetist to test for effect and observe for any adverse reactions. The needle is subsequently removed and an antibacterial filter is attached to the end of the catheter. The catheter is then secured to the woman's back with strapping and a syringe pump commenced if there is to be a continuous infusion.

Continuous infusion of dilute bupivacaine and opioids (usually fentanyl) has resulted in significant reductions in the amount of local anaesthetic used whilst ensuring rapid analgesia. In addition, because of the minimal motor block effect with this regime, the woman is able to move about more freely and bear down more effectively in the second stage of labour (Anim-Somuah et al 2011). The Comparative Obstetric Mobile Epidural Trial (COMET) Study Group UK (2001) found that low-dose infusion epidurals resulted in a lower incidence of instrumental vaginal births compared with traditional bolus epidurals.

Observations and care by the midwife

Each midwife is personally responsible for ensuring that they are competent to care for women who have epidural analgesia, including topping up the epidural block as specifically prescribed by the anaesthetist, being aware

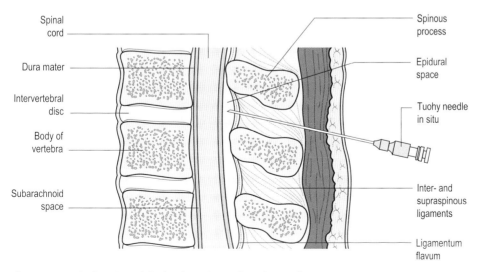

Fig. 16.20 Sagittal section of the lumbar spine with Tuohy needle in position.

Box 16.4 **Complications of epidural analgesia**

Complication	Cause	Treatment
Hypotensive incident	Affects the sympathetic nervous system by causing vasodilation and a fall in blood pressure	Assist woman into left lateral position, administer oxygen, call anaesthetist, rapidly infuse Hartmann's solution intravenously. Epinephrine, a vasopressor, may be given to raise the blood pressure
Dural puncture and consequent headache	Lowering of pressure/leakage of cerebrospinal fluid causing a stretching of brain tissue	Epidural injection of 10–20 ml of maternal blood (a *blood patch*), to seal the puncture and relieve the headache
Loss of bladder sensation	Poor intrapartum bladder care	Catheterization of the bladder
Total spinal leading to respiratory arrest	Induction of a high nerve block/injection of bupivacaine into a vein	Stop epidural and employ immediate resuscitation procedures
Local anaesthetic toxicity leading to cardiac arrest	Over infusion of local anaesthetic or too rapid administration	Stop epidural and employ immediate resuscitation procedures
Fetal compromise	Maternal hypotension or local analgesic toxicity	Stop epidural and assist woman into left lateral position
Increase in assisted vaginal births	Reduced muscle tone of the pelvic floor	Consider low dose infusion epidural Delay pushing if fetal condition is satisfactory
Neurological sequelae	Any of the above causes	Serious damage extremely rare; weakness/sensory loss is uncommon and soon resolves
Long-term backache	Common problem throughout childbirth due to the hormones of pregnancy softening the ligaments, BUT no evidence to suggest that epidurals cause long-term backache	Encourage mobility during labour so that pressure on the back is given relief

Source: NICE 2007; Hawkins 2010; Anim-Somuah et al 2011

of the possible complications and their immediate treatment.

After the administration of the first dose of bupivacaine and subsequent top-up doses of local anaesthetic the blood pressure and pulse should be measured and recorded every 5 minutes for 15 minutes and then every 30 minutes (NICE 2007). Temperature should also be recorded regularly. The woman may adopt any position she finds comfortable avoiding aorto-caval compression and encouraged to change position regularly to avoid soft tissue damage. The fetal heart is usually monitored electronically.

The spread of the block should be assessed hourly by the midwife using a cold object or ethyl chloride spray (NICE 2007). The sensation to void urine may be reduced so the midwife must ensure that the woman is encouraged to empty her bladder regularly to avoid postnatal urinary retention. Similarly the woman may not be as sensitive to feeling uterine contractions or the desire to bear down in the second stage of labour. This is due to the pelvic floor muscles being relaxed and affecting rotation of the fetal presenting part. The midwife therefore needs to be observant of these physiological changes.

Complications of epidural analgesia

The use of low-dose bupivacaine solutions for analgesia in labour has limited the risks of hypotension and local anaesthetic toxicity. Nevertheless, potential complications of epidurals still exist and these with their treatment are detailed in Box 16.4.

FIRST STAGE OF LABOUR: VAGINAL BREECH AT TERM

This section considers the physiology and intrapartum care in the first stage of labour of those term pregnancies presenting by the breech. In addition, the controversies surrounding the evidence of breech birth and the effect on women's choice for labour and birth are explored.

Incidence of breech presentation

Breech presentation involves a longitudinal lie of the fetus, with the buttocks in the lower pole of the maternal uterus. The presenting diameter is the bitrochanteric (10 cm) and the denominator is the sacrum. As pregnancy progresses, the incidence of breech presentation reduces: being around 15% at 28–32 weeks to around 3–4% by term as a result of spontaneous version (MIDIRS 2008b). It is worth considering, therefore, that a breech presentation at term is **not** an abnormality, it is just **unusual** and so a normal labour and spontaneous vaginal birth should not be excluded. Although in Western childbirth culture a breech birth has the status of **an emergency**, in many parts of the world a vaginal breech birth is part of normal practice (Burvill 2005). This used to be the case in the UK for most community midwives during the last century (Allison 1996). Following the Peel Report (Maternity Advisory Committee 1970) that gave rise to the transfer of childbirth from the home to the hospital environment, such skills of the midwife regarding vaginal breech births have been eroded as midwifery became subsumed into a medico-technocratic model, where obstetric intervention prevails.

Since the early 1990s, there has been much sociopolitical influence in the UK, aimed at improving childbirth choices and quality of maternity services for women. This has provided the opportunity for midwives to re-examine their role in providing a more holistic model of maternity care (DH 1993, 2004a, 2004b, 2007, 2008a, 2008b, 2010a, 2010b). The consequential reduction in junior doctors' hours (DH et al 2002) provided further opportunities for NHS Trusts to embrace collaborative working between health professionals (DH 2001), leading to a redefining of roles and responsibilities for midwives and their medical colleagues.

The clearly documented accounts from Cronk (1998a, 1998b), Reed (1999, 2003) and Evans (2007, 2012a, 2012b) provide first-hand detail of how midwives can support women with a breech presentation to give birth naturally other than by caesarean section and are an inspiration to other midwives seeking to develop or re-establish skills in this area. However, not all breeches can, or should be, born vaginally.

Types of breech presentation and position

There are six positions for a breech presentation, illustrated in Figs 16.21–16.26.

Breech with extended legs (frank breech)

The breech presents with the hips flexed and legs extended on the abdomen (Fig. 16.27). This type is particularly common in primigravidae whose efficient uterine muscle tone inhibits flexion of the legs and free turning of the mobile fetus. Consequently, this type of breech constitutes 70% of all breech presentations.

Complete breech

The fetal attitude is one of complete flexion (Fig. 16.28) with hips and knees both flexed and the feet tucked in beside the buttocks.

Footling breech

One or both feet present due to the fact that neither hip is fully flexed (Fig. 16.29). The feet are lower than the buttocks, distinguishing it from the complete breech. This type of breech is rare.

Knee presentation

This breech type is particularly rare and presents with one or both hips extended, with the knees flexed (Fig. 16.30).

Causes of breech presentation

Often there is no identifiable cause, but the following situations favour breech presentation:

- Extended legs
- Preterm labour
- Multiple pregnancy
- Polyhydramnios
- Hydrocephaly
- Uterine abnormalities such as a *septum* or a *fibroid*
- Placenta praevia

Diagnosis of breech presentation

In pregnancy

The woman may inform the midwife that she can feel something very hard and uncomfortable under her ribs that makes breathing uncomfortable at times. If the fetal feet are in the lower pole of the uterus, the woman is likely to experience some very hard kicks on her bladder. The use of ultrasound examination may be used to confirm a breech presentation where there is some uncertainty, however a decision on subsequent care, such as undertaking an external cephalic version (ECV), is usually deferred until nearer term. Some women may also attempt the use of moxibustion from 34 weeks' gestation to reduce the need for ECV (Tiran 2010b; Smith 2013).

Abdominal palpation

In primigravidae, diagnosis is more difficult because of the woman's firm abdominal muscles. The lie will be longitudinal with a *soft* presenting part felt in the lower part of the uterus. The head can usually be felt in the fundus as a round hard mass, which the midwife may be able to move independently of the back by balloting it with one or both hands. If the legs are extended, the feet may prevent such

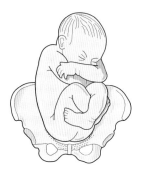

Fig. 16.21 Right sacroposterior.

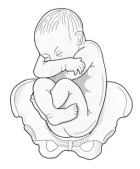

Fig. 16.22 Left sacroposterior.

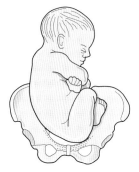

Fig. 16.23 Right sacrolateral.

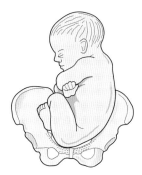

Fig. 16.24 Left sacrolateral.

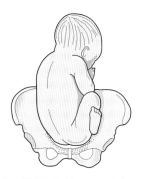

Fig. 16.25 Right sacroanterior.

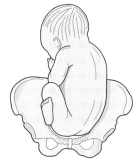

Fig. 16.26 Left sacroanterior.

Figs 16.21–16.26 Six positions in a breech presentation.

movement of the head. When the breech is anterior and the fetus well flexed it may be difficult to locate the head. However, the woman may complain of discomfort under her ribs, especially at night, owing to pressure of the head on the diaphragm, thus contributing to the diagnosis.

Auscultation

Prior to the breech passing through the pelvic brim, the fetal heart will be heard most clearly above the umbilicus. When the legs are extended, the breech descends into the pelvis easily such that the fetal heart is heard at a lower level.

During labour

Abdominal examination

A previously unsuspected breech presentation may not be diagnosed until the woman is in established labour. If the legs are extended, the breech may feel like a head on abdominal palpation and also on vaginal examination

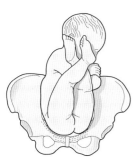

Fig. 16.27 Frank breech.

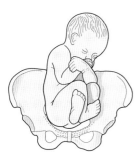

Fig. 16.28 Complete breech.

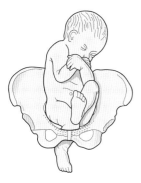

Fig. 16.29 Footling breech.

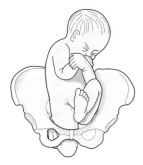

Fig. 16.30 Knee presentation.

should the cervix be less than 3 cm dilated and the breech is high.

Vaginal examination

The breech feels soft and irregular with no sutures palpable. On occasion the sacrum may be mistaken for a hard head and the buttocks for caput succedaneum. In addition, the anus may be felt and should the membranes have already ruptured, fresh meconium on the examining finger is diagnostic. If the legs are extended (Fig. 16.31) the external genitalia are very obvious, however, as these become oedematous, a swollen vulva can be mistaken for a scrotum.

If a foot is felt (Fig. 16.32) the midwife should differentiate from the hand. Toes are all the same length, are shorter than fingers and the big toe cannot be opposed to other toes. The foot is at right-angles to the leg and the heel has no equivalent in the hand.

Mode of birth: the evidence

The evidence regarding the safest mode for breech babies to be born has been somewhat controversial and misleading, with the randomized multicentre Term Breech Trial conducted by Hannah et al (2000) concluding the safest way to give birth was by planned caesarean section. This has had a major impact on the choices offered to women who may be presenting with a breech towards the end of their pregnancy regarding mode of birth, leading to a consequential increase in planned caesarean sections. By 2004 doubts had been cast on Hannah et al's (2000) research, with questions being raised over the validity and ethical basis of using a RCT for such a study and further research distrusting the results and recommendations (Alarab et al 2004; Háheim et al 2004; Kotaska 2004; Ulander et al 2004; Pradham et al 2005; Glezerman 2006; Fahy 2011). Furthermore, the two-year follow-up study by Whyte et al (2004) and Hannah et al (2004) did not show any differences in long-term outcomes between planned caesarean section or planned vaginal breech births.

Two further prospective trials undertaken by Goffinet et al (2006) and Maier et al (2011) clearly found that where planned vaginal breech birth is common practice and when strict criteria are met before and during labour, vaginal breech birth at term can still be a safe option. For a successful outcome, the evidence indicates that the most important factor is the presence of an experienced health professional, be it a midwife or obstetrician, facilitating the birth. As approximately one-third of all breech presentations are undiagnosed until labour and there is no evidence to support a caesarean section at this late stage, unless there is another clinical indication, it is important that midwives and obstetricians are competent to support vaginal breech birth. Consequently, the RCOG (2006) recommended that the most experienced available

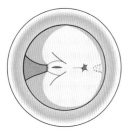

Fig. 16.31 No feet felt: the legs are extended.

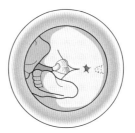

Fig. 16.32 Feet felt: complete breech presentation.

Figs 16.31–16.32 Vaginal touch pictures of left sacrolateral position.

practitioner should be present at a vaginal breech birth and that all maternity units have guidelines in place, including structured simulated training for all staff who may encounter vaginal breech births.

Place of birth

Vaginal birth should be presented to the woman as the norm for breech presentation (MIDIRS 2008b) provided there are no contraindications or complications. The woman should also be informed that there is an increase in the risk to the mother associated with Caesarean section births (Chapter 21). If a vaginal breech birth is planned for the home environment it is important that the midwife is competent to facilitate the birth and has clear lines of communication and support from her colleagues, including the Supervisor of Midwives, with a second midwife being present for the birth itself (NMC 2008, 2012). However, according to NICE (2007), a breech is considered to be a *malpresentation* indicative of risk, and recommends the labour and birth should be planned to take place in an obstetric unit. Outside of the hospital environment, any decision to transfer the woman from the home should be made promptly taking into consideration the time it would take to complete. An action plan for the labour and birth should be made with the woman that includes specifying those situations where midwives would make the decision to transfer to hospital, namely where there is a lack of progress or fetal compromise.

Posture for labour and birth

When women labour instinctively, without interruption or direction, they rarely choose to labour in a semi-recumbent position. In the campaign for normal birth, the RCM currently endorses an upright position for breech labour and birth as this aids descent of the presenting part, assisting the normal physiology of labour as well as reducing the risk of aorto-caval compression with subsequent improvement in placental blood flow (RCM 2005) (Chapter 17). However, as the upright position has not been fully evaluated, the RCOG (2006) still recommends the woman to be in a dorsal position for the actual birth.

Care in labour

Basic care during the first stage of labour is the same as those labours where the presentation is cephalic: minimizing intervention and enabling the normal physiology to progress. The breech with extended legs fits the cervix quite well, but with a less well applied presenting part as in the complete breech there is a tendency for the membranes to rupture early, increasing the risk of cord prolapse (Chapter 22). Should this occur, the midwife must undertake a vaginal examination to exclude cord prolapse and assess the fetal heart rate. It is not uncommon to find meconium staining of the amniotic fluid liquour with a breech presentation due to the compression of the fetal abdomen, and for this reason is *not* always a sign of fetal compromise.

PRELABOUR RUPTURE OF FETAL MEMBRANES AT TERM (PROM)

Prelabour rupture of membranes (PROM) at term (>37 weeks) complicates between 8 and 10% of all pregnancies and most women with PROM will labour spontaneously within 24 hours (NICE 2007). Following PROM with no signs of labour, regardless of whether or not liquor is draining, digital examination should be avoided owing to an increased risk of ascending infection (NICE 2007; NICE 2013). If there is doubt about whether the membranes have ruptured, a sterile speculum examination can be performed in order to observe whether there is pooling of liquor in the posterior fornix of the vagina (NICE 2013). If there are no facilities for this, the woman can be encouraged to wear a sanitary pad for an hour or two in order for the midwife to re-assess for signs of any liquor before a definite diagnosis can be made. The taking of low vaginal swabs is not recommended (NICE 2007). Initial assessment of the woman should include observation of her pulse, respiration rate, blood pressure, temperature, oxygen saturation and urinalysis. An abdominal examination should be undertaken and the fetal heart auscultated.

Following PROM the risk of serious neonatal infection is increased from 0.5% to 1%, compared with women whose membranes remain intact, and the woman should be advised of this (NICE 2007). In view of this, and in the absence of any clinical indication for immediate induction, such as Group B Streptococcus, maternal infection or meconium staining of the liquor, it is usual practice to advise the woman that if she does not go into spontaneous labour within 24 hours, labour should be induced after PROM (NICE 2007) (see Chapter 19). Women should be given adequate information to decide between expectant management and active management of labour following PROM. Hospital admission, in the absence of any other concerns, is not required whilst waiting for induction to take place.

Until the induction is commenced or if expectant management beyond 24 hours is chosen by the woman the following recommendations regarding advice to women and subsequent care should be followed (NICE 2007):

- Bathing or showering are **not** associated with an increase in infection, but having sexual intercourse may be.
- Body temperature should be recorded every 4 hours during waking hours and any change in the colour or smell of the vaginal loss should be reported to the midwife immediately.
- Fetal movements should be observed.
- In the absence of any risk indicators and with satisfactory evidence of fetal movements and a normal fetal heart rate, there is no reason for a CTG to be performed.

- Low vaginal swabs and blood samples to assess maternal C-reactive protein should not be taken.

PRETERM PRELABOUR RUPTURE OF THE MEMBRANES (PPROM)

Preterm prelabour rupture of the membranes (PPROM) occurs before 37 completed weeks' gestation, where the fetal membranes rupture without the onset of spontaneous uterine activity and the consequential cervical dilatation. It is discussed in Chapter 12.

THE RESPONSIBILITIES OF THE MIDWIFE

The midwife has an important enabling and facilitating role to support the woman during childbirth. It is vital that shared decision-making takes place between women and their caregivers at all times (Hodnett et al 2012). Accurate and detailed records of all care given during the first stage of labour, including the careful administration and monitoring of any medicines, is essential to the provision of quality care. These in turn will provide a good basis from which proper decisions may be made concerning the progress and the needs of the woman to optimize her labour experience and eventual birth outcome.

REFERENCES

Abushaikha L, Oweis A 2005 Labour pain experience and intensity: a Jordanian experience. International Journal of Nursing Practice 11(1):33–8

Afors K, Chandraharan E 2011 Use of continuous electronic fetal monitoring in a preterm fetus: clinical dilemmas and recommendations for practice. Journal of Pregnancy 84:87–94

Alarab M, Regan C, O'Connell M P et al 2004 Singleton breech delivery at term: still a safe option. Obstetrics and Gynecology 103(3):407–12

Albers L 1999 The duration of labor in healthy women. Journal of Perinatology 19(2):114–19

Albers L 2007 The evidence for physiologic management of the active phase of the first stage of labour. Journal of Midwifery and Women's Health 52:207–15

Alfirevic Z, Devane D, Gyte G 2013 Continuous cardiotocography (CTG) as a form of electronic fetal monitoring (EFM) for fetal assessment during labour. Cochrane Database of Systematic Reviews 2013 Issue 5. Art. No. CD006066. doi: 10.1002/14651858.CD006066.pub2

Allison J 1996 Delivered at home. Chapman and Hall, London

Anderson D 2011 A review of systemic opioids commonly used for labor pain relief. Journal of Midwifery and Women's Health 56(4):222–39

Anim-Somuah M, Smyth R, Jones L 2011 Epidural versus non epidural or no analgesia in labour. Cochrane Database of Systematic Reviews 2011, Issue 12. Art. No. CD000331. doi: 10.1002/14651858.CD000331.pub3

Ayers S, Joseph S, McKenzie-McHarg K et al 2008 Post-traumatic stress disorder following childbirth: current issues and recommendations for research. Journal of Psychosomatic Obstetrics and Gynecology 29(4):240–50

Ayres-de-Campos D, Bernades J 2010 Twenty-five years after the FIGO guidelines for the use of fetal monitoring: time for simplified approach? International Journal of Obstetrics and Gynaecology 110:1–6

Benjoya Miller J 2006 All women should have the choice of waterbirth. British Journal of Midwifery 14(8):484–5

Bernal A, Norwitz E 2012 The normal mechanism of labour. In: Edmonds K (ed) Dewhurst's textbook of obstetrics and gynaecology, 8th edn. Wiley–Blackwell, Chichester, p 245–68

Berry D 2006 Health communication: theory and practice. Open University Press, Maidenhead

Birch L, Doyle P, Ellis R et al 2009 Failure to void in labour: postnatal urinary and anal incontinence. British Journal of Midwifery 17:562–6

Brydon S, Raynor M 2012 Case Study 14: Shoulder dystocia. In: Raynor M, Marshall J, Jackson K (eds) Midwifery practice: critical illness, complications and emergencies case book. McGraw Hill/Open University Press, Maidenhead, p 227–46

Burvill S 2005 Managing breech presentation in the absence of obstetric assistance. In: Woodward V, Bates K, Young N (eds) Managing childbirth emergencies in community settings. Palgrave Macmillan, Houndsmill, Basingstoke, p 111–39

CMACE (Centre for Maternal and Child Enquiries) 2011 Saving mothers' lives: reviewing maternal deaths to make motherhood safer: 2006–2008. The Eighth Report on Confidential Enquiries into Maternal Deaths in the United Kingdom. BJOG: An International Journal of Obstetrics and Gynaecology 118(Suppl 1): 1–203

Clinical Negligence Scheme for Trusts (CNST) 2013 Standard 2 – Criterion 3: Continuous electronic fetal monitoring. Maternity clinical risk management standards. NHS Litigation Authority, London

Cluett E, Burns E 2009 Immersion in water in labour and birth. Cochrane Database of Systematic Reviews 2009, Issue 2. Art. No. CD000111. doi: 10.1002/14651858.CD000111. pub3

Comparative Obstetric Mobile Epidural Trial (COMET) Study Group UK 2001 Effect of low-dose mobile versus traditional epidural techniques on mode of delivery: a randomised controlled trial. Lancet 358:19–23

Coppen R 2005 Choice preference and control. In: Coppen R, Birthing positions. Do midwives know best?

MA Healthcare Limited, London, p 43–60

Cronk M 1998a Midwives and breech births. The Practising Midwife 1:7/8:44–5

Cronk M 1998b Hands off the breech. The Practising Midwife 1(6):13–15

Cunningham F G, Leveno K, Bloom S et al 2010 Williams obstetrics, 23rd edn. McGraw-Hill, New York

Da Silva F, de Oliveira S, Nobre M 2009 A randomized controlled trial evaluating the effect of immersion bath on labour pain. Midwifery 25(3):286–94

de Ferrer G 2006 TENS: non-invasive pain relief for the early stages of labour. British Journal of Midwifery 14(8):480–2

Devane D, Lalor J, Daly S et al 2012 Cardiotocography versus intermittent auscultation of fetal heart on admission to labour ward for assessment of fetal wellbeing. Cochrane Database of Systematic Reviews 2012, Issue 2. Art. No. CD005122. doi: 10.1002/14651858. CD005122.pub4

DH (Department of Health) 1993 Changing childbirth Part 1: Report of the Expert Maternity Group. HMSO, London

DH (Department of Health) 2001 Working together, learning together: a framework for lifelong learning in the NHS. TSO, London

DH (Department of Health) 2004a National Service Framework for children, young people and maternity services. DH, London

DH (Department of Health) 2004b The NHS Knowledge and Skills Framework (NHS KSF) and the development review process. TSO, London

DH (Department of Health) 2007 Maternity matters: choice, access and continuity of care in a safe service. DH, London

DH (Department of Health) 2008a High quality care for all: NHS next stage review final report (Darzi Report). TSO, London

DH (Department of Health) 2008b Framing the nursing and midwifery contribution: driving up the quality of care. TSO, London

DH (Department of Health) 2009 Reference guide to consent for

examination or treatment, 2nd edn. DH, London

DH (Department of Health) 2010a Equity and excellence: liberating the NHS. TSO, London

DH (Department of Health) 2010b Midwifery 2020: delivering expectations. TSO, London

DH (Department of Health), the National Assembly for Wales, the NHS Confederation and the British Medical Association 2002 Guidance on working patterns for junior doctors. TSO, London

Dixon L, Foureur M 2010 The vaginal examination during labour: is it of benefit or harm? New Zealand College of Midwives Journal. May. http://findarticles.com/p/articles/mi_6845/is_42_42/ai_n57137326/pg_6/?tag=content;col1 (accessed 20 July 2013)

Dowswell T, Bedwell C, Lavender T et al 2011 TENS (transcutaneous nerve stimulation) for pain management in labour. Cochrane Database of Systematic Reviews 2011, Issue 2. Art. No. CD007214. doi: 10.1002/14651858.CD007214.pub2

Evans J 2007 First do no harm. The Practising Midwife 10(8):22–3

Evans J 2012a The final piece of the breech jigsaw puzzle? Essentially MIDIRS 3(3):46–9

Evans J 2012b Understanding physiological breech birth. Essentially MIDIRS 3(2):17–21

Fahy K 2011 Is breech birth really unsafe? Treatment validity in the Term Breech Trial. Essentially MIDIRS 2(10):17–21

Fannon M 2003 Domesticating birth in the hospital: 'family-centred' birth and the emergence of 'homelike' birthing rooms. Antipode 35(3):513–35

Fernando R, Jones T (2009) Systemic analgesia: parenteral and inhalational. In: Chestnut D (ed), Chestnut's obstetric anaesthesia: principles and practice. Mosby Elsevier, Philadelphia, p 415–27

Fisher C, Hauck Y, Fenwick J 2006 How social context impacts on women's fears of childbirth: a Western Australian example. Social Science and Medicine 63(1):64–75

Friedman E 1954 The graphic analysis of labour. American Journal of

Obstetrics and Gynaecology 68:1568–75

Fujinaga M, Maze M 2002 Neurobiology of nitrous oxide-induced antinociceptive effects. Molecular Neurobiology 25(2):167–89

Glezerman M 2006 Five years to the term breech trial: the rise and fall of a randomized controlled trial. American Journal of Obstetrics and Gynecology 194(1):20–5

GMC (General Medical Council) 2013 Consent Guidance: *Gillick v West Norfolk and Wisbech AHA* [1986] AC 112. Children and young people's competence to consent to treatment. www.gmc-uk.org/guidance/ethical_guidance/consent_guidance_common_law.asp (accessed 23 September 2013)

Goffinet F, Carayol M, Foidart J et al, PREMODA Study Group 2006 Is planned vaginal delivery of breech presentation at term still an option? Results of an observational prospective survey in France and Belgium. American Journal of Obstetrics and Gynecology 194(4):1002–11

Gupta J, Hofmeyr G, Smith R 2012 Position for women during second stage of labour for women without epidural anaesthesia. Cochrane Database of Systematic Reviews 2012, Issue 5. Art. No. CD002006. doi: 10.1002/14651858.CD002006.pub3

Háheim L L, Albrechtsen S, Nordb Berge W et al 2004 Breech birth at term: vaginal delivery or elective caesarean section? A systematic review of the literature by a Norwegian review team. Acta Obstetrica et Gynecologica Scandinavica 83(2):126–30

Hall Moran V, Dykes F 2006 Maternal and infant nutrition and nurture. Controversies and challenges. MA Healthcare Limited, Malta

Hannah M E, Hannah W J, Hewson S A et al 2000 Term Breech Trial Collaborative Group. Planned caesarean section versus planned vaginal birth for breech presentation at term: a randomized multicentre trial. The Lancet 356(9239):1375–83

Hannah M E, Whyte H D, Hannah W J et al 2004 Term Breech Trial Collaborative Group. Maternal outcomes at two years after planned

caesarean section versus planned vaginal birth for breech presentation at term: the international randomized multi-centre trial. American Journal of Obstetrics and Gynecology 191(3):917–27

Harper A 2011 Sepsis. In: Centre for Maternal and Child Enquiries (CMACE) Saving mothers' lives: reviewing maternal deaths to make motherhood safer: 2006–2008. Eighth Report on Confidential Enquiries into Maternal Deaths in the United Kingdom. BJOG: An International Journal of Obstetrics and Gynaecology 118(Suppl 1): 85–96

Hawkins J 2010 Epidural analgesia for labor and delivery. New England Journal of Medicine 362(16):1503–10

Health and Social Care Information Centre 2012 Data on written complaints in the NHS 2011–2012. NHS Office of Statistics, Leeds

Helman G 2007 Culture, health, and illness, 5th edn. Hodder Arnold, London

Henley-Einion A 2007 The ecstasy of the spirit: Five Rhythms for healing. British Journal of Midwifery 10(3):20–3

Hobbs L 1998 Assessing cervical dilatation without VEs. The Practising Midwife 1(11):34–5

Hodnett E, Stremler R, Weston J et al 2009 Re-conceptualizing the hospital labor room: the PLACE (pregnant and labouring in an ambient clinical environment) pilot trial. Birth 36(2):156–66

Hodnett E, Gates S, Hofmeyr G et al 2011 Continuous support for women during childbirth. Cochrane Database of Systematic Reviews 2011, Issue 2. Art. No. CD003766. doi: 10.1002/14651858.CD003766.pub5

Hodnett E, Downe S, Walsh D 2012 Alternative versus conventional institutional settings for birth. Cochrane Database 2012, Issue 8. Art. No. CD000012. doi: 10.1002/14651858.CD000012.pub2

Howie L, Novak B 2010 The onset of labour. In: Stables D, Rankin J (eds), Physiology in childbearing, 3rd edn. Ballière Tindall, London, p 487–96

Howie L, Rankin J 2010 The first stage of labour. In: Stables D, Rankin J (eds), Physiology in childbearing,

3rd edn. Ballière Tindall, London, p 497–516

Idarius B 2010 The homeopathic childbirth manual, 2nd edn. Idarius Press, Ukiah, CA

Impey L, Child T 2012 Obstetrics and gynaecology, 4th edn. Wiley–Blackwell, Chichester

Jones L, Othman M, Dowswell T et al 2012 Pain management for women in labour: an overview of systematic reviews. Cochrane Database of Systematic Reviews 2012, Issue 3. Art. No. CD009234. doi: 10.1002/14651858.CD009234.pub2

Juman Blincoe A 2007 TENS machines and their use in managing labour pain. British Journal of Midwifery 15(8):516–19

Kennedy H P, Grant J, Walton C et al 2010 Normalizing birth in England: a qualitative study. Journal of Midwifery and Womens Health 55(3);262–9

Kings Fund 2008 Safe births: everybody's business. An independent inquiry into the safety of maternity services in England. Kings Fund, London

Kirkham M 2011 The role of the midwife with the woman in labour: to be with, to monitor or to wait on the landing. MIDIRS Midwifery Digest 21(4):469–70

Kotaska A 2004 Inappropriate use of randomized trials to evaluate complex phenomena: case study of vaginal breech delivery. British Medical Journal 329(7473):1039–42

Lauria M R, Barthold J, Zimmerman R et al 2007 Pathologic uterine ring associated with fetal head trauma and subsequent cerebral palsy. Obstetrics and Gynecology 109(2):495–7

Lauzon L, Hodnett E 2009 Antenatal education for the self diagnosis of the onset of active labour at term. Cochrane Database of Systematic Reviews 2009, Issue 1. Art. No. CD000935. doi:10.1002/14651858

Lavender T, Alfirevic Z, Walkinshaw S 2006 Effect of different partogram action lines on birth outcomes: a randomized controlled trial. Obstetrics and Gynaecology 108(2):295–302

Lavender T, Hart A, Smyth R 2008 Effect of partogram use on outcomes for women in spontaneous labour at term. Cochrane Database of Systematic Reviews, Issue 4. Art. No. CD005461. doi: 10.1002/14651858. CD005461.pub2

Lavender T, Hofmeyr G J, Neilson J P et al 2009 Caesarean section for non-medical reasons at term. Cochrane Database of Systematic Reviews 2006, Issue 3. Art. No. CD004660. doi: 10.1002/14651858. CD004660.pub2

Lawrence A, Lewis L, Hofmeyr G et al (2009) Maternal positions and mobility during the first stage of labour. Cochrane Database of Systematic Reviews 2009, Issue 2. Art. No. CD003934. doi: 0.1002/14651858

Leap N, Anderson P 2008 The role of pain in normal birth and empowerment of women. In: Downe S (ed.) Normal childbirth evidence and debate, 2nd edn. Churchill Livingstone, London, p 29–46

Longworth H, Kingdon C 2010 Fathers in the birth room: what are they expecting and experiencing? A phenomenological study. Midwifery 27(5):588–94

Maier B, Georgoulopoulos A, Jaeger T et al 2011 Fetal outcome for infants in breech by method of delivery experiences with a stand-by service system of senior obstetricians and women's choices of mode of delivery. Journal of Perinatal Medicine 39(4):385–90

Main E, Bingham D 2008 Quality improvement in maternity care: promising approaches from the medical and public health perspectives. Current Opinions in Obstetrics and Gynecology 20(6):574–80

Mander R 2011 Pain in childbearing and its control, 2nd edn. Blackwell Science, London

Marshall J, Fraser D, Baker P 2011 An observational study to explore the power and effect of the labour ward culture on consent to intrapartum procedures. International Journal of Childbirth 1(2):82–99

Martini F, Nath J, Bartholomew E 2011 Fundamentals of anatomy and physiology, 9th edn. Prentice Hall, London

Maternity Advisory Committee 1970 Domiciliary and maternity bed needs. Chairman Sir John Peel. HMSO, London

McDonald G 2010 Diagnosing the latent phase of labour: use of the partogram. British Journal of Midwifery 18(10):630–7

McNabb M 2011 Physiological changes from late pregnancy until the onset of lactation. In: Macdonald S, Magill-Cuerden (eds) Mayes Midwifery, 14th edn. Ballière Tindall, London, p 463–81

MHPRA (Medicines and Healthcare Products Regulatory Agency) 2010 Medicines and Healthcare Products Regulatory Agency Medical Device Alert. Fetal Monitor/ Cardiotocograph. Ref MDA/2010/054 [online] available at www.mhra.gov .uk/home/groups/dts-bs/documents/ medicaldevicealert/con085077.pdf (accessed 3 August 2013)

Melzack R, Wall P D 1965 Pain mechanisms: a new theory. Science 150:971–9

MIDIRS (Midwifery Information Resource Service) 2008a Informed choice for professionals Number 1: Support in labour. MIDIRS and the NHS Centre for Reviews and Dissemination, Bristol

MIDIRS (Midwifery Information Resource Service) 2008b Informed choice for professionals Number 9: Breech presentation: options for care. MIDIRS and the NHS Centre for Reviews and Dissemination, Bristol

Mukhopadhyay S, Fraser D 2009 The first stage of labour. In: Warren R, Arulkumaran S (eds), Best practice in labour and delivery. Cambridge University Press, Cambridge, p 14–25

National Audit Office 2009 Reducing healthcare associated infections in hospitals in England. TSO, London

NICE (National Institute for Health and Clinical Excellence) 2007 Intrapartum care: care of healthy women and their babies during childbirth. CG 55. NICE, London

NICE (National Institute for Health and Clinical Excellence) 2013 Vision Amniotic Leak detector to assess unexplained vaginal wetness in pregnancy. Medical Technology Guidance 15. NICE, London

NMC (Nursing and Midwifery Council) 2008 The Code: Standards of conduct, performance and ethics for nurses and midwives. London, NMC

NMC (Nursing and Midwifery Council) 2009 Record keeping. Guidance for nurses and midwives. London, NMC

NMC (Nursing and Midwifery Council) 2010 Standards for medicines management. London, NMC

NMC (Nursing and Midwifery Council) 2012 Midwives rules and standards. London, NMC

NPSA (National Patient Safety Agency) 2007a The national specifications for cleanliness in the NHS: a framework for setting and measuring performance outcomes. NPSA, London

NPSA (National Patient Safety Agency) 2007b Clean hands save lives: Patient Safety Alert, 2nd edn. NPSA, London

NPSA (National Patient Safety Agency) 2010 NHS to adopt zero tolerance approach to pressure ulcers. NPSA, London

Pearson J 1981 Partography. Nursing Mirror 153(2):xxv–xxix

Pradham P, Mohajer M, Deshpande S 2005 Outcome of term breech births: 10 year experience at a district general hospital. BJOG: An International Journal of Obstetrics and Gynaecology 112(2):218–22

Raynor M, England C 2010 Psychology for midwives. Open University Press, Maidenhead

RCM (Royal College of Midwives) 2005 Normal breech birth. www .rcmnormalbirth.org.uk/default .asp?sID=1099658440484 (accessed 1 August 2013)

RCM (Royal College of Midwives) 2012a Evidence based guidelines for midwifery-led care in labour. Positions in labour. RCM, London

RCM (Royal College of Midwives) 2012b Evidence-based guidelines for midwifery-led care in labour. Nutrition in Labour. RCM, London

RCM (Royal College of Midwives) 2012c Evidence-based guidelines for midwifery-led care in labour. Supporting women in labour. RCM, London

RCOG (Royal College of Obstetricians and Gynaecologists) 2006 The management of breech presentation. Green-top Guideline No. 20b. RCOG, London

RCOG (Royal College of Obstetricians and Gynaecologists) 2008 Standards for maternity care. RCOG, London

Redshaw M, Heikkila K 2010 Delivered with care: a national survey of women's experience of maternity care. National Perinatal Epidemiology Unit. University of Oxford, Oxford

Reed B 1999 Knee deep at a home birth. The Practising Midwife 2(8):46

Reed B 2003 A disappearing art: vaginal breech birth. The Practising Midwife 6(9):6–18

Robertson A 2003 The pain of labour: a feminist issue. www.acegraphics.com.au/articles/painlabour.html (accessed 4 August 2013)

Sandall J, Soltani H, Gates S 2013 Midwife-led continuity models versus other models of care for childbearing women. Cochrane Database of Systematic Reviews Issue 8. Art No. CD004667. doi: 10.1002/14651858.CD004667.pub3

Schiermeier S, Pildner von Steinburg S, Thieme A et al 2008 Sensitivity and specificity of intrapartum computerised FIGO criteria for cardiotocography and fetal scalp pH during labour: multicentre observational study. British Journal of Obstetrics and Gynaecology 115(12):1557–63

Shepherd A, Cheyne H, Kennedy S et al 2010 The purple line as a measure of labour progress: a longitudinal study. BMC Pregnancy and childbirth 10, Article 53. https://dspace.stir.ac.uk/handle/1893/2568 (accessed 19 August 2013)

Simkin P, Ancheta R 2011 The labor progress handbook: early interventions to prevent and treat dystocia, 3rd edn. Wiley–Blackwell, Chichester

Sinivaara M, Suominen T, Routasolo P et al 2004 How delivery ward staff exercise power over women in communication. Journal of Advanced Nursing 46(1):33–4

Singata M, Tranmer J, Gyte G 2010 Restricting oral fluid and food intake during labour. Cochrane Database of Systematic Reviews, Issue 1. Art. No. CD003930. doi: 10.1002/14651858.CD003930.pub2

Smith C A 2013 Moxibustion for breech presentation: significant new evidence. Acupuncture in Medicine 31(1):5–6

Smith C, Collins C, Crowther C 2011 Aromatherapy for pain management in labour. Cochrane Database of Systematic Reviews 2011, Issue 12. Art. No. CD009514. doi: 10.1002/14651858.CD009514

Smyth R, Alldred S, Markham C 2007 Amniotomy to shorten spontaneous labour. Cochrane Database of Systematic Reviews 2007, Issue 4. Art. No.: CD006167. doi: 10.1002/14651858.CD006167.pub2

Steen M, Calvert J 2006 Homeopathy for childbirth: remedies and research. Midwives. 9(11):438–40

Sullivan A, McCormick C 2007 The birthing environment. In: Liu D (ed) Labour ward manual, 4th edn. Churchill Livingstone, Edinburgh, p 19–22

Teimoori B, Sakhavar N, Mirteimoori M et al 2011 Nitrous oxide versus pethidine with promethesine for reducing labor pain. Gynaecology and Obstetrics 1(1):1–4

Thoni A, Mussner K, Ploner F 2010 Water birthing: retrospective review of 2625 water births. Contamination of birth pool water and risk of microbial cross infection. Minerva Ginecologica 62(3):203–11

Tiran D 2010a Complementary therapies in labour and delivery. In: Walsh D, Downe S (eds) 2010 Essential midwifery skills: intrapartum care. Wiley–Blackwell, Chichester, p 141–58

Tiran D 2010b Complementary therapies in midwifery: a focus on moxibustion for breech presentation. In: Marshall JE, Raynor MD (eds) Advancing skills in midwifery practice. Elsevier, Churchill Livingstone, Edinburgh, p 19–28

Tortora G, Grabowski S 2011 Introduction to the human body: the essentials of anatomy and physiology, 9th edn. John Wiley, New York

Ulander V M, Gissler M, Nuutila M et al 2004 Are health expectations of term breech infants unrealistically high? Acta Obstetrica et Gynecologica Scandinavica 83(2):180–6

Ullman R, Smith L, Burns E et al 2010 Parenteral opioids for maternal pain relief in labour. Cochrane Database of Systematic Reviews 2010, Issue 9. Art. No. CD007396. doi: 10.1002/14651858

Walsh D 2010a Labour rhythms. In: Walsh D, Downe S (eds) Essential midwifery practice: intrapartum care. Wiley–Blackwell, Chichester, p 63–80

Walsh D 2010b Birth environment. In: Walsh D, Downe S (eds) Essential midwifery practice: intrapartum care. Wiley–Blackwell, Chichester, p 45–62

Walsh D 2012 Normal labour and birth: a guide for midwives, 2nd edn. Routledge, London

WHO (World Health Organization), Department of Reproductive Health and Research 1999 Care in normal labour: a practical guide. WHO, Geneva

WHO (World Health Organization) 2009 Save lives: clean your hands. 'My five moments for hand hygiene': a user-centred design approach to understand, train, monitor and report hand hygiene. WHO, Geneva

Whyte H D, Hannah M, Saigal S et al 2004 Infant follow-up term breech trial collaborative group: outcomes of children at two years after planned caesarean birth versus planned vaginal birth for breech presentation at term: the international randomized Term Breech Trial. American Journal of Obstetrics and Gynecology 191(3):864–71

Woods T 2006 The transitional stage of labour. MIDIRS Midwifery Digest 16(2):225–8

Zanetti-Dallenbach R, Tschudin S, Zhong X et al 2007 Maternal and neonatal infections and obstetrical outcome in water birth. European Journal of Obstetrics and Gynecology and Reproductive Biology 134(2):37–43

Zahra A, Leila M 2013 Lavender aromatherapy massages in reducing labor pain and duration of labor. African Journal of Pharmacy and Pharmacology 7(8):426–30

Zhang J, Landy H, Branch W 2010 Contemporary patterns of spontaneous labor with normal neonatal outcomes. Obstetrics and Gynaecology 116(6):1281–7

FURTHER READING

Downe S (ed) 2008 Normal childbirth: evidence and debate, 2nd edn. Churchill Livingstone, London

This text explores contemporary issues in maternity care. It includes thought-provoking chapters by Nicky Leap and Tricia Anderson on 'the role of pain in normal birth', Soo Downe et al's chapters on 'rethinking risk and safety in maternity care' and on 'the early pushing urge'.

McCormick C, Cairns A 2010 Reducing unnecessary caesarean section by external cephalic version. In: Marshall J E, Raynor M D (eds) Advancing skills in midwifery practice. Elsevier, Churchill Livingstone, Edinburgh, p 47–55

This chapter examines the rationale for the procedure of external cephalic version (ECV). It discusses why and how midwives and obstetricians should acquire competency in such a skill to improve a woman's choice in achieving a vaginal birth should their baby be presenting by the breech.

National Institute for Health and Clinical Excellence NICE 2007 Intrapartum care: care of healthy women and their babies during childbirth. CG 55. NICE, London

This document contains evidence-based information for intrapartum care of women with uncomplicated pregnancies. The intention of the guidelines are to standardise practices among maternity units in the UK.

Walsh D (ed) 2012 Normal labour and birth: a guide for midwives, 2nd edn. Routledge, London

This textbook examines care during normal labour and birth, including excellent evidence-based guidance to normalize childbirth.

USEFUL WEBSITES

Royal College of Midwives: www.rcm.org.uk

National Childbirth Trust: www.nct.org.uk

Association of Radical Midwives: www.midwifery.org.uk

Midwives Information and Resource Service: www.midirs.org

National Institute for Health and Care [formerly Clinical] Excellence: www.nice.org.uk

Royal College of Obstetricians and Gynaecologists: www.rcog.org.uk

Chapter |17|

Physiology and care during the transition and second stage phases of labour

Soo Downe, Jayne E Marshall

When labour moves to the phase of active
maternal pushing, the whole tempo of activity
changes. The change in nature of uterine activity
can lead women to express confusion and loss of
control. Intense physical effort and exertion is
needed as the baby is finally pushed towards its
birth. The woman, her supporting companions
and her midwife all require stamina and courage.
Excitement and expectation mount as the birth
becomes imminent. A positive outcome will
depend upon mutual respect and trust between
all involved professional groups, and between
those groups and the labouring woman and her
companions. A woman will never forget a
midwife who positively supports her capacity to
give birth to her baby, as shown in Diane's story
(see Box 17.7).

- consider the nature of the transition and second stage phases of labour
- describe the usual sequence of events during these stages
- summarize signs of transition and of the expulsive phase of labour
- discuss the care of the mother, father and birth companions
- review the observations that should be carried out at this time
- discuss the physiology of birth and the role of the midwife when the term fetus is presenting by the breech.

The first section of this chapter is focused on labour where the presentation is cephalic. The special situation of the breech presentation at term is described in the second half of the chapter.

THE NATURE OF THE TRANSITION AND SECOND STAGE PHASES OF LABOUR

The second stage of labour has traditionally been regarded as the phase between full dilatation of the cervical os, and the birth of the baby. However, the physiological reality of stages and phases of labour has been questioned (Walsh 2010; Zhang et al 2010). See Box 17.1 for examples of other controversial issues at this point in labour. Most midwives and labouring women are aware of a transitional period between the period of cervical dilatation, and the time when active maternal pushing efforts begin. This is typically characterized by maternal restlessness, discomfort, desire for pain relief, a sense that the process is never-ending, and demands to attendants to end the whole process. Appropriate midwifery care encompasses both knowledge of the usual physiological processes of this phase and of the mechanism of birth, and insight into the needs and choices of each individual labouring woman.

The physiological changes are a continuation of the same forces that occurred in the earlier hours of labour, but activity is accelerated. This acceleration, however, does not occur abruptly. Some women may experience an urge to push before the cervical os is fully dilated, and others may experience a lull before the onset of strong expulsive second stage contractions. This latter phenomenon has been termed the *resting phase* of the second stage of labour. The formal onset of the second stage of labour is traditionally confirmed with a vaginal examination to check for full dilatation of the cervical os. However, a

---

Box 17.1 Examples of areas of controversy in labour transition and second stage

Discussion about the nature of normal physiological labour and birth has taken place for at least the last 50 years, with an increase in publications in this area over the last decade or so (Montgomery 1958; Crawford 1983; Downe 1994, 2004, 2006, 2008; Gould 2000; Anderson 2003 Downe et al 2013; Hannah et al 2013). These debates include:

- The utility of dividing labour into standard 'phases' or 'stages'.
- The need or otherwise for regular vaginal examinations to assess the progress of labour.
- The nature of transition.
- The nature and impact of the early pushing urge.
- Pushing in the context of epidural analgesia.
- The efficacy of signs of progress such as the anal cleft line and the appearance of the rhomboid of Michaelis.
- The significance, and optimum management, of the tight nuchal cord at the time of birth.
- The physiological limits to the length of the second stage of labour.
- Long-term outcome for the neonate relating to childbirth interventions.

---

finding of full cervical dilatation may occur some time after this stage has in fact been reached, and maternal behavioral changes may be a good indication that expulsive contractions are occurring (Baker and Kenner 1993; Dahlen et al 2013; Downe et al 2013).

Uterine action

Contractions become stronger and longer but may be less frequent, allowing both mother and fetus regular recovery periods. The membranes often rupture spontaneously towards the end of the first stage or during transition to the second stage. The consequent drainage of liquor allows the presenting part, either the hard, round fetal head or the buttocks, to be directly applied to the vaginal tissues. This pressure aids distension. Fetal axis pressure increases flexion of the presenting part, resulting in smaller presenting diameters, more rapid progress and less trauma to both mother and fetus. If the mother is upright during this time, these processes are optimized.

The contractions become expulsive as the fetus descends further into the vagina. Pressure from the presenting part stimulates nerve receptors in the pelvic floor. This phenomenon is termed the 'Ferguson reflex'. As a consequence, the woman experiences the need to push. This reflex may initially be controlled to a limited extent but becomes increasingly compulsive, overwhelming and involuntary.

The mother's response is to employ her secondary powers of expulsion by contracting her abdominal muscles and diaphragm.

Soft tissue displacement

As the fetal head descends, the soft tissues of the pelvis become displaced. Anteriorly, the bladder is pushed upwards into the abdomen where it is at less risk of injury during fetal descent. This results in the stretching and thinning of the urethra so that its lumen is reduced. Posteriorly, the rectum becomes flattened into the sacral curve and the pressure of the advancing head expels any residual faecal matter. The levator ani muscles dilate, thin out and are displaced laterally, and the perineal body is flattened, stretched and thinned. The fetal head becomes visible at the vulva, advancing with each contraction and receding between contractions until crowning takes place. The head is then born. The shoulders and body follow with the next contraction, accompanied by a gush of amniotic fluid and sometimes of blood. The second stage culminates in the birth of the baby.

RECOGNITION OF THE COMMENCEMENT OF THE SECOND STAGE OF LABOUR

Progress from the first to the second stage is not always clinically apparent.

Presumptive evidence

Expulsive uterine contractions

Some women feel a strong desire to push before full dilatation occurs. Traditionally, it has been assumed that an early urge to push will lead to maternal exhaustion and/or cervical oedema or trauma. More recent research indicates that the early pushing urge may in fact be experienced by a significant minority of women, and that, in certain circumstances, spontaneous early pushing may be physiological (Petersen and Besuner 1997; Roberts and Hanson 2007; Downe et al 2008; Borrelli et al 2013). It is not clear whether these findings are influenced by factors such as maternal or fetal position, or parity, and there is not enough evidence to date to determine the optimum response to the early pushing urge. The midwife needs to work with each individual woman in the context of each labour to determine the best approach in that specific case.

Rupture of the forewaters

Rupture of the forewaters may occur at any time during labour.

Dilatation and gaping of the anus

Deep engagement of the presenting part may produce this sign during the latter part of the first stage.

Anal cleft line

Some midwives have reported observing this line (also called 'the purple line') as a pigmented mark in the cleft of the buttocks which gradually ascends the anal cleft as the labour progresses (Hobbs 1998; Wickham 2007). There is some observational evidence from one study that this sign appears in the majority of women during labour, and that it is somewhat correlated to both cervical dilatation and position of the fetal head (Shepherd et al 2010). The efficacy of this observation in practice in large populations of women remains to be tested formally.

Appearance of the rhomboid of Michaelis

This is sometimes noted when a woman is in a position where her back is visible. It presents as a dome-shaped curve in the lower back, and is held to indicate the posterior displacement of the sacrum and coccyx as the fetal occiput moves into the maternal sacral curve (Sutton and Scott 1996). This seems to lead the labouring woman to arch her back, push her buttocks forward and throw her arms back to grasp any fixed object she can find. Sutton and Scott (1996) hypothesize that this is a physiological response, since it causes a lengthening and straightening of the curve of Carus, optimizing the fetal passage through the birth canal.

Upper abdominal pressure and epidural analgesia

It has been observed anecdotally that women who have an epidural in situ often have a sense of discomfort under the ribs towards the end of the first stage of labour. This seems to coincide with full cervical dilatation. The efficacy of these observations in predicting the onset of the anatomical second stage of labour remains to be researched.

Show

This is the loss of bloodstained mucus which often accompanies rapid dilatation of the cervical os towards the end of the first stage of labour. It must be distinguished from frank fresh blood loss caused by partial separation of the placenta or a ruptured vasa praevia.

Appearance of the presenting part

Excessive moulding of the fetal head may result in the formation of a large caput succedaneum which can protrude through the cervix prior to full dilatation of the os. Very occasionally, a baby presenting by the vertex may be visible at the perineum at the same time as remaining cervix. This is more common in women of high parity. Similarly a breech presentation may be visible when the cervical os is only 7–8 cm dilated.

Confirmatory evidence

In many midwifery settings, it is held that a vaginal examination must be undertaken to confirm full dilatation of the cervical os. This is both to ensure that a woman is not pushing too early, and to provide a baseline for timing the length of the second stage of labour. However, in some maternity settings, individual midwives do not always undertake this, unless there are observable maternal and/or fetal signs that the labour is not progressing as anticipated. Enkin et al (2000) noted that vaginal assessment of cervical dilatation is largely unevaluated, and a recent Cochrane review concludes that this lack of evidence persists (Downe et al 2013). Despite this, regular vaginal examinations are undertaken by most midwives and obstetricians, and expected by many women. Whether the midwife undertakes an examination or not, she should record all the signs she observes and all the measurements she takes, and she should advise and support the labouring woman on the basis of accurate observation and assessment of progress.

PHASES AND DURATION OF THE SECOND STAGE

Two distinct phases in second stage progress have been recognized in some women. These are the latent phase, during which descent and rotation occur, and the active phase, with descent and the urge to push.

The latent phase

In some women, full dilatation of the cervical os is recorded, but the presenting part may not yet have reached the pelvic outlet. Women in this situation may not experience a strong expulsive urge until the head has descended sufficiently to exert pressure on the rectum and perineal tissues. There is evidence from a study undertaken half a century ago that active pushing during the latent phase does not achieve much, apart from exhausting and discouraging the mother (Benyon 1990). More recent concerns over the impact of epidural analgesia on spontaneous birth have led to an increasing interest in the so-called passive second stage of labour, in which active pushing efforts are delayed until fetal descent and rotation have occurred (Simpson and James 2005; NICE 2007; Brancato et al 2008; Gillesby et al 2010). It is hypothesized that the prolongation of second stage progress when epidural

analgesia is used is due to the relaxation effect of epidural analgesia on the pelvic floor muscles, meaning that the fetal presenting part does not encounter the necessary resistant force from the pelvic floor to bring about the normal rotation process. This tends to be particularly evident in nulliparous women. Passive descent of the fetus can continue with good midwifery support for the woman until the head is visible at the vulva, or until the woman feels a spontaneous desire to push.

The active phase

Most women without epidural analgesia will experience a compulsive urge to push, or bear down, once the fetal head has rotated and started to descend. The phase of labour that involves active bearing down is termed the *active* second stage of labour.

Duration of the second stage

There is no good evidence about the absolute time limits of physiological labour (Downe 2004; NICE 2007; Zhang et al 2010). Most researchers who have examined this area have shown that, for healthy women and babies, the second stage of labour can last for up to three hours or so before the risk of maternal and/or fetal compromise begins to increase (Albers 1999; Allen et al 2009). In the presence of regular contractions, maternal and fetal well-being, and progressive descent, considerable variation between women is to be expected. While many maternity units do currently impose standardized limits on the second stage beyond which medical help should be called, these are not based on good evidence.

MATERNAL RESPONSE TO TRANSITION AND THE SECOND STAGE

Pushing

Traditionally, if the maternal urge to push occurs before confirmation of full dilatation of the cervical os, or the appearance of a visible vertex, the mother has been encouraged to avoid active pushing. This has been done to conserve maternal effort and allow the vaginal tissues to stretch passively. Techniques to avoid active pushing efforts in this situation include position change, often to the left lateral, using controlled breathing, inhalation analgesia, or even narcotic or epidural pain relief (Downe et al 2008). However, when mother and baby are well and labour has progressed spontaneously, anecdotally, an increasing number of midwives have adopted the practice of supporting the overwhelming urge to bear down without

Box 17.2 **Epidural analgesia and spontaneous vaginal birth**

Epidural analgesia provides optimal pain relief for women, but its use is associated with an increase in instrumental births (Anim-Somuah et al 2011). Women who use epidural analgesia are no more satisfied with their pain relief than those who do not, and their memories of labour as being extremely painful and therefore distressing may persist longer than for women with equal levels of pain in labour who do not receive epidural analgesia (Waldenstrom and Schytt 2009). Techniques for reducing the risk of instrumental births in this group have included:

- Minimizing the concentration of local anaesthetic (Stoddart et al 1994)
- Letting the block wear off towards the end of labour (Torvaldsen et al 2004)
- Using oxytocin in the second stage of labour (Costley and East 2012)
- Fundal pressure (Verheijen et al 2009)
- Delaying active pushing between the diagnosis of the onset of full dilatation of the cervix and a fixed point later in the labour (Roberts et al 2004)
- Using different positions (Downe et al 2004; Roberts et al 2005)
- Using combinations of anaesthetic that allow women to mobilize in labour (COMET Study Group UK 2001).

These techniques have had varying success rates, with most of them failing to show large differences in outcome.

confirming full dilatation of the cervical os, while paying close attention to the maternal and fetal condition (Downe et al 2008; Borrelli et al 2013). As stated above, the optimum response in this situation has not yet been established.

There has been convincing evidence for more than two decades that managed active pushing in the second stage of labour accompanied by breath holding (the Valsalva manoeuvre) has adverse consequences (Thomson 1993; Aldrich et al 1995; Enkin et al 2000; Yildirim and Beji 2008; Prins et al 2011). Whenever active pushing commences, the woman should be encouraged to follow her own inclinations in relation to expulsive effort. Few women need instruction on how to push unless they are using epidural analgesia (Box 17.2).

Spontaneous pushing efforts usually result in maximum pressure being exerted at the height of a contraction. In turn, this allows the vaginal muscles to become taut and prevents bladder supports and the transverse cervical ligaments from being pushed down in front of the baby's head. It is believed that this may help to prevent prolapse

and urinary incontinence in later life, although this belief has still not been formally tested (Benyon 1990).

Some mothers vocalize loudly as they push. This may aid in coping with the contractions, so women should feel free to express themselves in this way. Reassurance and praise will help to boost confidence, enabling the mother to assert her own control over events. The atmosphere should be calm and the pace unhurried.

Position

If the woman lies flat on her back, vena caval compression is increased, resulting in hypotension. This can lead to reduced placental perfusion and diminished fetal oxygenation (Humphrey et al 1974; Kurz et al 1982). The efficiency of uterine contractions may also be reduced. The semi-recumbent or supported sitting position, with the thighs abducted, is the posture most commonly used in Western cultures. While this may afford the midwife good access and a clear view of the perineum, the woman's weight is on her sacrum, which directs the coccyx forwards and reduces the pelvic outlet. In addition, the midwife needs to bend forward and laterally to support the birth, which may lead to injury.

Left lateral position

This position was widely used in the United Kingdom (UK) in the 20th century, although it is less common in current practice. The perineum can be clearly viewed and uterine action is effective, but an assistant may be required to support the right thigh, which may not be ergonomic. It provides an alternative for women who find it difficult to abduct their hips. It may also aid fetal rotation, especially in the context of epidural analgesia (Downe et al 2004).

Upright positions: squatting, kneeling, all-fours, standing, using a birthing ball

A review of studies examining upright versus recumbent positions during the second stage of labour showed there were clear advantages for women in adopting any position that was not horizontal, as shown in Figs 17.1 and 17.2 (Gupta et al 2012). These included reduced duration of second stage labour, fewer assisted births, fewer episiotomies, reduced severe pain in second stage labour, and fewer abnormal heart rate patterns. However, increased rates of perineal damage and of estimated blood loss >500 ml also occurred. The experimental group included women who used birthing chairs, a technique known to be associated with increased blood loss (Stewart and Spiby 1989; Turner et al 1988). It is not clear if this risk accrues to all upright positions. The 'upright position' group in this review included women who were in supported sitting positions on a bed, and in the lateral position. There are

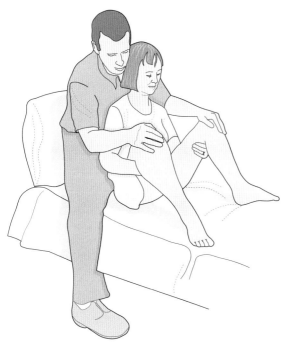

Fig. 17.1 Supported sitting position.
After Simkin and Ancheta 2006, with permission from Blackwell Science.

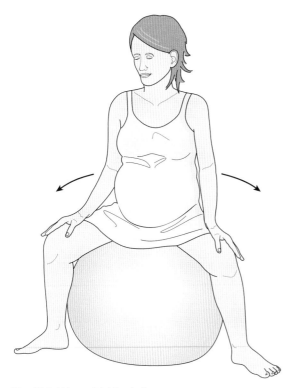

Fig. 17.2 Using a birthing ball.
After Simkin and Ancheta 2006, with permission from Blackwell Science.

a number of studies relating to positions and mobility for women using so-called 'walking epidurals', but recent data on the physiology of labour and birth for women in spontaneous labour who mobilize without the use of pharmacological pain relief do not seem to exist.

Radiological evidence demonstrates an average increase of 1 cm in the transverse diameter and 2 cm in the anteroposterior diameter of the pelvic outlet when the squatting position is adopted. This produces an average 28% increase in the overall area of the outlet compared with the supine position (Russell 1969). Some women find the all-fours position to be the optimum approach for all or part of their labours, especially in the case of an occipitoposterior position, due to relief of backache (Stremler et al 2005). In the case of a breech presentation, anecdotal evidence suggests that most women will spontaneously adopt an all-fours or forward-leaning position (see discussion below). It can, however, be tiring to maintain for a long period of time. A wide range of other standing and leaning positions can be experimented with to help the woman cope with her labour (Simkin and Ancheta 2006; Simkin 2010; Royal College of Midwives 2013). It is important not to insist on any position as the 'right' one. Positive and dramatic effects on labour progress can be achieved by encouraging the woman to change and adapt her position in response to the way her body feels.

The position the woman may choose to adopt is dictated by several factors:

- The woman's instinctive preference.
- The environment, which should not act as a constraint through lack of privacy or lack of supports such as cushions and chairs. In a hospital setting, it may help to move the labour bed from the middle of the room, and to provide other supports such as cushions and birthing balls, so that the woman can roam from one to another as the labour dictates. Low lighting and music of her choice may help the woman to see the room as a safe and secure place. Minimizing unnecessary intrusion by other members of staff is essential.
- The midwife's confidence. A full understanding of the mechanism of labour should enable the midwife to adapt to any position that the woman wishes to adopt, ensuring in the process that the postures adopted by the midwife are protective of her own health (and, specifically, of her back). One way of minimizing damage to the back is to refrain from placing the woman in a low supported sitting position with her feet resting on the midwife's hip. Minimizing vaginal examinations in labour will also reduce the risk of back injury. If the woman has an epidural in situ it is essential that help is called when the woman needs to be moved, and that ergonomic lifting positions are used.

Maternal and fetal condition

If the woman has had analgesia, or if there is any concern about her wellbeing or that of her baby, then more frequent or continuous monitoring may limit the choices available to her. However, there are often creative solutions to these situations, and good midwifery care involves finding these solutions where possible (RCM 2013).

THE MECHANISM OF NORMAL LABOUR (CEPHALIC PRESENTATION)

As the fetus descends, soft tissue and bony structures exert pressures that lead to descent through the birth canal by a series of movements. Collectively, these movements are called the *mechanism of labour*. There is a mechanism for every fetal presentation and position that can lead to a vaginal birth. Knowledge and recognition of the normal mechanism enables the midwife to anticipate the next step in the process of descent. Understanding and constant monitoring of these movements can help to ensure that normal progress is recognized, that the woman gives birth safely and positively, or that early assistance can be sought should any problems occur. The fetal presentation, position, and size relative to that of the woman will govern the exact mechanism as the fetus responds to external pressures. Principles common to all mechanisms are:

- descent takes place
- whichever part leads and first meets the resistance of the pelvic floor will rotate forwards until it comes under the symphysis pubis
- whatever emerges from the pelvis will pivot around the pubic bone.

It should be noted that, while the mechanism set out below is the most common, it is not an invariant blueprint, but a guide: each labour is unique.

During the mechanism of normal labour, the fetus turns slightly to take advantage of the widest available space in each plane of the pelvis. The widest diameter of the pelvic brim is the transverse: at the pelvic outlet the greatest space lies in the anteroposterior diameter.

At the onset of labour the most common presentation is the vertex and the most common position either left or right occipitoanterior; therefore it is this mechanism which will be described. In this instance:

- the lie is longitudinal
- the presentation is cephalic
- the position is right or left occipitoanterior
- the attitude is one of good flexion
- the denominator is the occiput
- the presenting part is the posterior part of the anterior parietal bone.

Main movements of the fetus

Descent

Descent of the fetal head into the pelvis often begins before the onset of labour. For a primigravid woman this usually occurs during the latter weeks of pregnancy. In multigravid women muscle tone is often more lax and therefore descent and engagement of the fetal head may not occur until labour actually begins. Throughout the first stage of labour the contraction and retraction of the uterine muscles reduces the capacity in the uterus, exerting pressure on the fetus to descend further. Following rupture of the forewaters and the exertion of maternal effort, progress speeds up.

Flexion

This increases throughout labour. The fetal spine is attached nearer the posterior part of the skull; pressure exerted down the fetal axis will be more forcibly transmitted to the occiput than the sinciput. The effect is to increase flexion which results in smaller presenting diameters that will negotiate the pelvis more easily. At the onset of labour the suboccipito-frontal diameter, which is approximately 10 cm, is presenting. With greater flexion, the sub-occipitobregmatic diameter, that is, approximately 9.5 cm, presents. The occiput becomes the leading part.

Internal rotation of the head

During a contraction, the leading part is pushed downwards onto the pelvic floor. The resistance of this muscular diaphragm brings about rotation. As the contraction fades, the pelvic floor rebounds, causing the occiput to glide forwards. As discussed above, resistance is an important determinant of rotation, as Fig. 17.3 demonstrates. This explains why rotation is often delayed following epidural analgesia, which causes relaxation of pelvic floor muscles. The slope of the pelvic floor determines the direction of rotation. The muscles are hammock-shaped and slope down anteriorly, so whichever part of the fetus first meets the lateral half of this slope will be directed forwards and towards the centre. In a well-flexed vertex presentation the occiput leads, and rotates anteriorly through ⅛ of a circle when it meets the pelvic floor. This causes a slight twist in the neck as the head is no longer in direct alignment with the shoulders. The anteroposterior diameter of the head now lies in the widest (anteroposterior) diameter of the pelvic outlet. The occiput slips beneath the sub-pubic arch and crowning occurs when the head no longer recedes between contractions and the widest transverse diameter (biparietal) is born. If flexion is maintained, the sub-occipitobregmatic diameter, approximately 9.5 cm, distends the vaginal orifice.

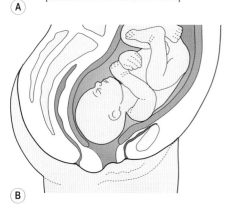

Fig. 17.3 (A) Internal rotation of the head begins. (B) Upon completion, the occiput lies under the symphysis pubis.

Extension of the head

Once crowning has occurred, the fetal head can extend, pivoting on the suboccipital region around the pubic bone. This releases the sinciput, face and chin, which sweep the perineum, and then are born by a movement of extension, as shown in Fig. 17.4.

Restitution

The twist in the neck of the fetus which resulted from internal rotation is now corrected by a slight untwisting movement. The occiput moves $\frac{1}{8}$ of a circle towards the side from which it started.

Internal rotation of the shoulders

The shoulders undergo a similar rotation to that of the head to lie in the widest diameter of the pelvic outlet, namely anteroposterior. The anterior shoulder is the first to reach the levator ani muscle and it therefore rotates anteriorly to lie under the symphysis pubis. This movement can be clearly seen as the head turns at the same time (external rotation of the head). It occurs in the same direction as restitution, and the occiput of the fetal head now lies laterally.

Lateral flexion

The shoulders are usually born sequentially. When the woman is in a supported sitting position, the anterior shoulder is usually born first, although midwives who encourage women to adopt an upright or kneeling positions have observed that the posterior shoulder is commonly seen first. In the former case, the anterior shoulder slips beneath the sub-pubic arch and the posterior shoulder passes over the perineum. In the latter the mechanism is reversed. This enables a smaller diameter to distend the vaginal orifice than if both shoulders were born simultaneously. The remainder of the body is born by lateral flexion as the spine bends sideways through the curved birth canal.

MIDWIFERY CARE IN TRANSITION AND THE SECOND STAGE

Care of the parents

The woman and her companions will now realize that the birth of the baby is imminent. They may feel excited and elated but at the same time anxious and frightened by the dramatic change in pace. They will need frequent explanations of events. The midwife's calm approach and information about what is happening can ensure the woman stays in control, and is confident. This is critical at the time of transition, when events can result in a sensation of panic. The midwife should praise and congratulate the woman on her hard work, recognizing that she is probably undertaking the most extreme physical activity she will ever encounter. Birth is an intimate act which often takes place in a public setting. The midwife should work hard to ensure that privacy and dignity are maintained.

Crucially, it is at the time of transition that a maternal request for analgesia may occur, even if she had stated antenatally that she did not want pain relief in labour. Such a request will need to be carefully assessed by the attending midwife. This is especially true when a supportive companion is not present. On the basis of her knowledge of the woman, the midwife may be able to help her over this transient phase with good midwifery support, and without utilizing pharmacological analgesia. The decision for or against pain relief at this stage must be made in partnership with the woman, recognizing that, particular for a nulliparous woman, a demand for pain relief may often be an unconscious proxy for a demand for labour support. In order to achieve the kind of supportive care that can help a woman over the uncertainties and distress of transition, it is eminently preferable that the woman should have continuous support throughout labour (Hodnett et al 2012). Ideally, the same midwife or small group of known midwives should attend the woman throughout (McLachlan et al 2012). Alternatives

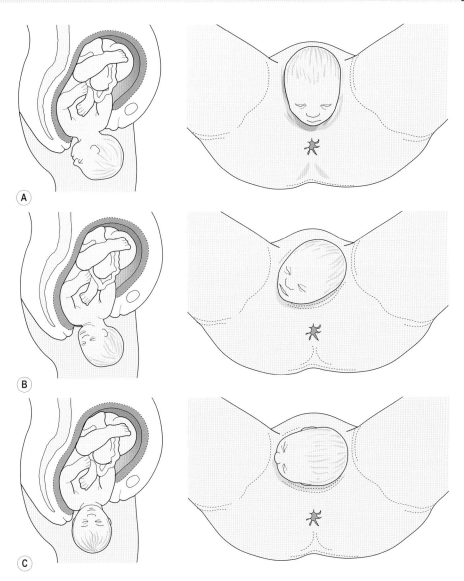

Fig. 17.4 (A) Birth of the head. (B) Restitution. (C) External rotation.

to pharmacological analgesia include praise and reassurance about progress, changes in position and scenery, massage and appropriate nutrition. Complementary therapies and optimal fetal positioning may also be offered if the midwife is competent to undertake them. Leg cramp is a common occurrence whichever posture is adopted. It can be relieved by massaging the calf muscle, extending the leg and dorsiflexing the foot. These measures may be crucial in re-energizing a labour that is beginning to flag in the second stage.

The midwife should also have regard to the wellbeing of the woman's partner and other companions as far as possible. Witnessing labour and birth is not easy,

especially for the woman's partner/birth companions. Indeed, recent qualitative research has indicated that birth companions can be profoundly affected by witnessing traumatic birth, and can even exhibit symptoms that appear to be similar to those of post-traumatic stress for years after the birth (White 2007; Steen et al 2012). The attitude of the midwife to the labour, to the woman, and to the partner/birth companions will have a profound effect on the labour (Halldorsdottir and Karlsdottir 1996; Lundgren 2004; El-Nemer et al 2006; Thomson and Downe 2008, 2010; Elmir et al 2010; Berg et al 2012), with possible consequences for the mother, her partner and the family after the birth (Thomson and Downe 2010). It is crucial to respect the woman and her partner/birth companions, and to respect the meaning that this birth will have for them, both on the day, and in the future.

Observations during the second stage

Four factors determine whether the second stage is continuing safely, and these must be carefully monitored:

* Uterine contractions
* Descent, rotation and flexion of the presenting part
* Fetal condition/suspicious or pathological changes in the fetal heart
* Maternal condition.

Uterine contractions

The strength, length and frequency of contractions should be assessed regularly by observation of maternal responses, and by uterine palpation during the second stage of labour. They are usually stronger and longer than during the first stage of labour, with a shorter resting phase. The posture and position adopted by the woman may influence the contractions.

Descent, rotation and flexion

Initially, descent may occur slowly, especially in primigravid women, but it usually accelerates during the active phase. It may occur very rapidly in multigravid women. If there is a delay in descent on abdominal palpation, despite regular strong contractions and active maternal pushing, a vaginal examination may be performed with maternal permission. The purpose is to confirm whether or not internal rotation of the head has taken place, to assess the station of the presenting part and to determine whether a caput succedaneum has formed. If the occiput has rotated anteriorly, the head is well flexed and caput succedaneum is not excessive it is likely that progress will continue. In the absence of good rotation and flexion, and/or a weakening of uterine contractions, change of position, nutrition and hydration, or use of optimal fetal positioning techniques maybe helpful (Simkin and Ancheta 2006). Consultation with a more experienced midwife may provide more suggestions to re-orientate the labour. However, if there is evidence that either fetal or maternal condition are compromised, an experienced obstetrician should be consulted.

Fetal condition/suspicious or pathological changes of the fetal heart

If the membranes are ruptured, the liquor amnii is observed to ensure that it is clear. While thin old meconium staining is not always regarded as a sign of fetal compromise, thick fresh meconium is ominous, and experienced obstetric advice must be sought if this sign appears (NICE 2007). It may, however, be the only indication of an undiagnosed breech presentation.

As the fetus descends, fetal oxygenation may be less efficient owing to either cord or head compression or to reduced perfusion at the placental site. A well-grown healthy baby will not be compromised by this transitory hypoxia. If continuous electronic fetal monitoring is being undertaken due to risk factors in the mother or baby, it is not unusual at this stage to see early decelerations of the fetal heart, with a swift return to the normal baseline after a contraction, and good beat-to-beat variation throughout. The midwife should learn to recognize the normal changes in fetal heart rate patterns during the second stage, both when monitored continuously (where there are specific risk factors) and when monitored intermittently. This will minimize the risk of iatrogenic intervention, and maximize a timely response to fetal compromise if it occurs. If the woman is labouring normally, NICE guidelines recommend that a Pinard's stethoscope or other hand-held system such as a Sonicaid should be used to monitor the fetal heart intermittently (NICE 2007). During the second stage this is usually undertaken immediately after a contraction, with some readings being taken through a contraction if the woman can tolerate this.

Late decelerations, and a lack of return to the normal baseline, a rising baseline or diminishing beat-to-beat variation, are signs of concern. While it is generally acknowledged that beat-to-beat variation is hard to identify in intermittent monitoring, the other characteristics can be identified. If these are heard for the first time in the second stage, they may be due to cord or head compression, which may be helped by a change in maternal position. However, if they persist, experienced obstetric aid must be sought. If the labour is taking place in a unit that is distant from an obstetric unit, an episiotomy may be considered – with maternal consent – if the birth is imminent, or midwives who are trained and experienced in ventouse birth may consider expediting the birth. Otherwise, with maternal consent, transfer to an obstetric unit should take place.

Maternal condition

The midwife's observation includes an appraisal of the woman's ability to cope emotionally as well as an assessment of her physical wellbeing. This includes close attention to what she says, as well as how she behaves, and a swift supportive response to any indication that she is losing belief in herself to accomplish the birth of her baby.

Maternal pulse rate is usually recorded half-hourly and blood pressure every few hours, provided that these remain within normal limits. If the woman has an epidural in situ, blood pressure will be monitored more frequently, and continuous electronic fetal monitoring will probably be in use.

Maternal comfort

As a result of her exertions the woman usually feels very hot and sticky, and she will find it soothing to have her face and neck sponged with a cool flannel. Her mouth and lips may become very dry. Sips of iced water or other fluids are refreshing and a moisturizing cream can be applied to her lips. Her partner may help with these tasks as a positive contribution to ease her discomfort.

The bladder is vulnerable to damage, due to compression of the bladder base between the pelvic brim and the fetal head. The risk is increased if the bladder is distended. The woman should be encouraged to pass urine at the beginning of the second stage unless she has recently done so.

Preparation for the birth

Once active pushing commences, the midwife should prepare for the birth. There is usually little urgency if the woman is primigravid, but multigravid women may progress very rapidly.

The room in which the birth is to take place should be warm with a spotlight available so that the perineum can be easily observed if necessary. A clean area should be prepared to receive the baby, and waterproof covers provided to protect the bed and floor. Sterile cord clamps, a clean apron, and sterile gloves are placed to hand. In some settings, sterile gowns are also used. An oxytocic agent may be prepared, either for the active management of the third stage if this is acceptable to the woman, or for use during an emergency. A warm cot and clothes should be prepared for the baby. In hospital a heated mattress may be used; at home, a warm (*not* hot) water bottle can be placed in the cot.

Neonatal resuscitation equipment must be thoroughly checked and readily accessible.

Birth of the baby

The midwife's skill and judgement are crucial factors in minimizing maternal trauma and ensuring an optimal birth for both mother and baby. These qualities are refined by experience but certain basic principles should be applied. They are:

- observation of progress
- prevention of infection
- emotional and physical comfort of the mother
- anticipation of normal events, and support for the normal processes of labour
- recognition of abnormal developments, and appropriate response to them.

During the birth, both mother and baby are particularly vulnerable to infection. While there is now evidence that strict antisepsis is unnecessary if the birth is straightforward (Keane and Thornton 1998; Lumbiganon et al 2004),

meticulous aseptic technique must be observed when preparing sterile surgical equipment that could be used for invasive techniques, such as episiotomy scissors. Surgical gloves should be worn during the birth for the protection of both woman and midwife. Goggles or plain glasses should be available to avoid the risk of ocular contamination with blood or amniotic fluid.

The equipment that is used during the birth of the baby includes the following items:

- warm swabbing solution or tap water
- cotton wool and pads
- sterile cord scissors and clamps
- sterile episiotomy scissors (these should be available in case they are needed).

Birth of the head

Once the birth is imminent, the perineum may be swabbed clean of any mucus should this be indicated (although no longer a common practice), and a clean pad is placed under the woman to absorb any faeces or fluids. If she is not in an upright position a pad is placed over the rectum on the perineum (but not covering the fourchette) and a clean towel is placed on or near the woman for receipt of the baby. Throughout these preparations the midwife observes the progress of the fetus. With each contraction the head descends. As it does so the superficial muscles of the pelvic floor can be seen to stretch, especially the transverse perineal muscles. The head recedes between contractions, which allows these muscles to thin gradually. The skill of the midwife in ensuring that the active phase is unhurried helps to safeguard the perineum from trauma, either observing the gradual advancement of the fetal head or controlling it with light support from her hand. One large study, the HOOP (Hands-Off Hands-Poised) trial, indicated that, compared with guarding the perineum, a hands-off technique was associated with slightly more maternal discomfort at 10 days postnatally (McCandlish et al 1998). The hands-off technique was also associated with a lower risk of episiotomy, but a higher risk of manual removal of placenta. There is some debate about the generalizability of this trial to all settings and positions in labour. However, account should be taken of these findings in working with individual women. Most midwives place their fingers lightly on the advancing head to monitor descent and prevent very rapid crowning and extension, which are believed to result in perineal laceration (see (Fig. 17.5). Excessive pressure on the head, however, may be associated with vaginal lacerations. Whatever technique the midwife adopts, it should be based on the assumption that it is the woman who is giving birth to her baby, and the midwife is there to add the minimum physical help necessary at any given time.

Once the head has crowned, the woman can achieve control by gently blowing or 'sighing' out each breath in order to minimize active pushing. Birth of the head in this

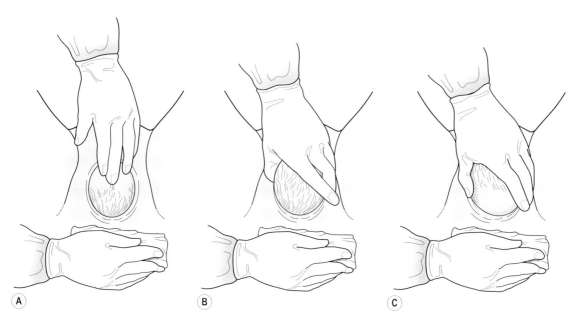

Fig. 17.5 Supporting the head. (A) Preventing rapid extension. (B) Controlling the crowning. (C) Easing the perineum to release the face.

way may take two or three contractions but may avoid unnecessary maternal trauma. The head is born by extension as the face appears at the perineum.

During the resting phase before the next contraction the midwife may check that the cord is not around the baby's neck. If found, it is usual to slacken it to form a loop through which the shoulders may pass. If the cord is very tightly wound around the neck, it is common practice in the UK to apply two artery forceps approximately 3 cm apart and to sever the cord between the two clamps (Jackson et al 2007). In the United States, the so-called 'somersault manoeuvre' is often performed, as shown in Fig. 17.6 (Mercer et al 2005, 2007). There has been controversy over early cord cutting for the healthy term baby, on the basis that, even if tightly around the neck, the cord is still supplying oxygen. Additionally, the blood volume model proposed by Mercer and Skovgaard (2004) suggests that the loss of blood volume occasioned by clamping and cutting the cord before it stops pulsating may be detrimental to the baby. This hypothesis has been supported by systematic reviews (Hutton and Hassan 2007; McDonald and Middleton 2008). However, these studies have not controlled for the possible adverse effects of a tight nuchal cord. If the cord is cut, the baby should be born very soon afterwards, as it now has no access to oxygen until it takes its first breath. For this reason, cutting of the nuchal cord should always be a last resort, if the cord cannot be freed or the baby born with the cord intact.

If the cord is clamped, great care must be taken that maternal tissues are not damaged. Holding a swab over

the cord as it is incised will reduce the risk of the attendants being sprayed with blood during the procedure. Once severed, the cord may be unwound from around the neck.

Birth of the shoulders

Restitution and external rotation of the head maximizes the smooth birth of the shoulders and minimizes the risk of perineal laceration. However, it is not uncommon for small babies, or for babies of multiparous women, to be born with the shoulders in the transverse, or even to have a twist in the neck opposite to that expected. While the hands-on technique in the HOOP trial included both perineal support and active birth of the trunk and shoulders (McCandlish et al 1998) it is not clear which component of this technique was beneficial for women and babies. If the position is upright, it is more common for the shoulders to be left to birth spontaneously with the help of gravity.

During a water birth, it is important not to touch the emerging fetus to avoid stimulating it to gasp underwater. If there is a problem with the birth in this circumstance, the woman should be asked to stand up out of the water before any manoeuvres are attempted.

If the midwife does physically aid the birth of the shoulders and trunk, she should be absolutely sure that restitution has occurred prior to trying to flex the trunk laterally. One shoulder is released at a time to avoid overstretching the perineum. A hand is placed on each side of the baby's

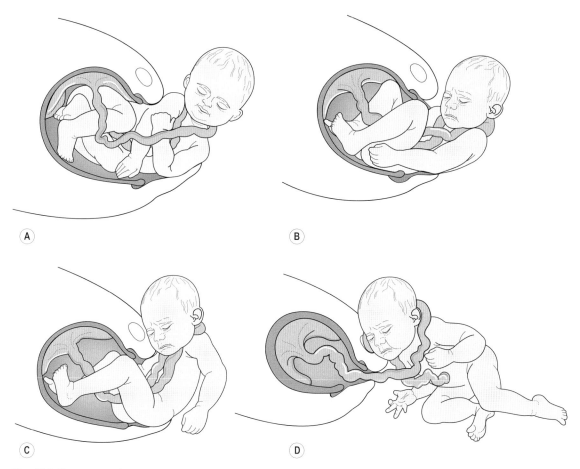

Fig. 17.6 The somersault manoeuvre.
From Mercer et al 2005.

head, over the ears, and gentle downward traction is applied (Fig. 17.7). This allows the anterior shoulder to slip beneath the symphysis pubis while the posterior shoulder remains in the vagina. If the third stage of labour is to be actively managed, the assistant will now give an intramuscular (IM) oxytocic drug. When the axillary crease is seen, the head and trunk are guided in an upward curve to allow the posterior shoulder to escape over the perineum. These manoeuvres are reversed if the mother is in a forward-facing position such as *all-fours*. The midwife or mother may now grasp the baby around the chest to aid the birth of the trunk and lift the baby towards the mother's abdomen. This allows the mother immediate sighting of her baby and close skin contact, and removes the baby from the gush of liquor which accompanies release of the body. If the midwife does not actively assist, she should be ready to support the head and trunk as the baby emerges. The time of birth is noted and recorded.

If this has not already been done, the cord is severed between two cord clamps placed close to the umbilicus at whatever time is considered appropriate, with due attention to the theories around the blood volume model set out above. The cord clamp is applied. The baby is dried and placed in the skin-to-skin position with the mother if she is happy with this (Moore et al 2007; Bystrova et al 2009). A warm cover is placed over the baby. Swabbing of the eyes and aspiration of mucus during and immediately following birth are not considered necessary providing the baby's condition is satisfactory. Oral mucus extractors should not be used because of the risks of mucus that is contaminated with a virus such as hepatitis or human immunodeficiency virus (HIV) entering the operator's mouth.

The moment of birth is both joyous and beautiful. The midwife is privileged to share this unique and intimate experience with the parents.

379

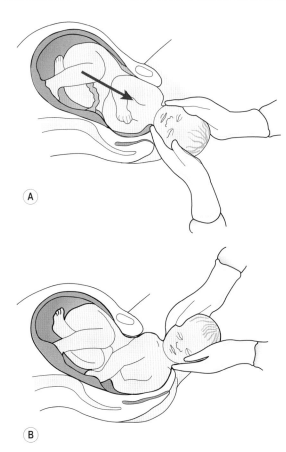

(A)

(B)

Fig. 17.7 (A) Downward traction releases the anterior shoulder. (B) An upward curve allows the posterior shoulder to escape.

VAGINAL BREECH BIRTH AT TERM

This section follows on from Chapter 16 regarding the physiology and management of the first stage of labour for women with term pregnancies where the fetus is presenting by the breech. The main aim for both chapters is to examine the knowledge and skills required to effectively facilitate *planned* vaginal breech births at term in both home and hospital settings. It is important that midwives are conversant with the controversies surrounding the Term Breech Trial (Hannah et al 2000) and the subsequent studies and guidance that are available to inform a woman's choice in mode of breech birth (Goffinet et al 2006; RCOG 2006; NICE 2007; Maier et al 2011) (see also Chapter 16). However, many midwives will, occasionally, find themselves in the situation of diagnosing a breech presentation in transition or the second stage of labour, sometimes while attending an out-of-hospital birth. For this reason, all midwives need to have the skills and

knowledge to support the woman in this situation, to make decisions, work with the normal physiology of the labour if the birth is proceeding spontaneously, to know how to recognize impending or actual problems, how when to undertake manoeuvres, and/or to transfer the woman to obstetric care in a hospital setting.

Mechanism of right sacro-anterior position

Similar to cephalic presentations that favour the left occipitoanterior position, breech presentations more commonly adopt the right sacro-anterior position, the mechanism of which is described below:

- The lie is longitudinal.
- The attitude is one of complete flexion.
- The presentation is breech.
- The position is right sacro-anterior.
- The denominator is the sacrum.
- The presenting part is the anterior (right) buttock.
- The bitrochanteric diameter (10 cm) enters the pelvis in the right oblique diameter of the maternal pelvic brim.
- The sacrum points to the right ilio-pectineal eminence.

Compaction

Descent takes place with increasing compaction owing to increased flexion of the limbs.

Internal rotation of the buttocks

The anterior (right) buttock reaches the pelvic floor first and rotates forward $\frac{1}{8}$ of a circle along the left side of the maternal pelvis to lie underneath the symphysis pubis. The bitrochanteric diameter is now in the anterioposterior diameter of the maternal pelvic outlet.

Lateral flexion of the body

The anterior buttock escapes under the symphysis pubis, the posterior buttock sweeps the perineum and the buttocks are born by a movement of lateral flexion: also known as 'rumping'.

Restitution of the buttocks

The anterior buttock turns slightly to the mother's left side.

Internal rotation of the shoulders

The shoulders enter the brim of the pelvis in the same oblique diameter as the buttocks: namely the right oblique diameter. The anterior shoulder rotates forward $\frac{1}{8}$ of a circle along the left side of the maternal pelvis and escapes under the symphysis pubis; the posterior shoulder sweeps the perineum and the shoulders are born.

Internal rotation of the head

The fetal head enters the maternal pelvis with the sagittal suture in the transverse diameter of the pelvic brim. The occiput rotates forwards ⅛ of a circle along the left side of the maternal pelvis and the suboccipital region (nape of the neck) impinges on the undersurface of the symphysis pubis.

External rotation of the head

At the same time the baby's body turns so that it lies parallel with the maternal body.

Birth of the fetal head

The chin, face and sinciput sweep the perineum, and the baby's head is born in a flexed attitude.

Undiagnosed breech presentation

It is still not uncommon for a breech presentation to be discovered for the first time during labour, often towards the end of labour, as the presenting part becomes more easily identified, or in the presence of fresh meconium. If the midwife attends a woman in labour at home with a breech presentation where a hospital birth had initially been planned, it is important to remain calm whilst undertaking a careful assessment of the risk to the woman and baby taking into consideration the parent's wishes before a decision to transfer to hospital is made. This will depend on the stage of labour, fetal position and maternal medical and obstetric history. If the woman is nearing the second stage of labour and the labour is progressing well, assistance should be promptly summoned while supporting her to give birth at home. Should a decision be made to transfer to hospital, the midwife must alert the hospital of the transfer and ensure that the paramedics are equipped for neonatal resuscitation. The fetal heart and maternal condition should be monitored and recorded throughout the journey to hospital. The midwife must always be prepared for the birth in transit as it may progress more rapidly than initially anticipated. In such a situation, the driver should be asked to stop the ambulance in order for the midwife to assist the birth, undertaking any necessary manoeuvres safely. If the baby is likely to be born in transit, it is useful to take a number of towels/blankets to wrap the baby, encouraging skin-to-skin contact and early breast feeding to maintain thermoregulation, i.e. warmth, and reducing the likelihood of hypoglycaemia and hypothermia.

Types of breech birth

Box 17.3 highlights the three types of vaginal breech birth.

Box 17.3 **Types of breech birth**	
Spontaneous	The birth occurs with little assistance from the attendant.
Assisted breech	The buttocks are born spontaneously, but some assistance is necessary for the birth of extended legs, arms and the head.
Breech extraction	This birth involves manipulating the fetal body by an experienced attendant (usually an obstetrician) in order to hasten the birth of the baby in an emergency situation, such as fetal compromise.

Position for breech birth

The woman's position can significantly affect the physiological labour and birth process and the one that is adopted should ideally be her choice. Many of the existing texts describing vaginal breech births tend to assume the woman should give birth in the hospital environment on the bed in a semi-recumbent, adapted lithotomy position (Chadwick 2002; Ndala 2005; Lewis 2011). Such a position affects the normal physiological process of labour, and may lead to malposition due to the reduction in gravitational force on the fetal mechanisms, consequently increasing the need for the midwife to undertake manoeuvres to assist the birth.

While gravity helps to expel the fetus, it is the expulsive contractions and angle of the pelvis that assist in facilitating a physiological breech birth if the woman adopts an upright forward-leaning position. Little assistance from the midwife is needed if these mechanisms are achieved spontaneously, except in the case of care with the birth of the after-coming head. Use of the birth pool is generally not advised, as the buoyancy of the water may work against gravity and thus impede the physiological mechanisms that effect a spontaneous breech birth. A *'hands off the breech'* approach is optimal when the woman either adopts a standing or an 'all-fours'/leaning forwards position (Cronk 1998a, 1998b; Reed 2003; Burvill 2005; Royal College of Midwives 2005; Evans 2012a).

Where the mother is on all-fours or leans upon the bed/settee or on her birth partner (see Fig. 17.8), the baby's trunk descends through the pelvis at 45° and is able to move more freely around the curve of Carus of the maternal pelvis. This position provides an excellent view of the birth process and access to the baby's face as it is born over the perineum, as well as ample space for the midwife to undertake any manoeuvres should they be necessary to assist the birth of the baby.

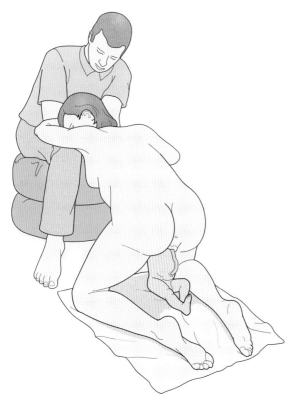

Fig. 17.8 The baby descending in the 'all-fours' position.

Facilitating a vaginal breech birth in an upright/kneeling position

Breech births can be as physiological as any other vaginal birth and a woman who has chosen to birth vaginally, or discovers in labour that her baby is presenting by the breech, requires calm support from skilled and confident midwives (Marshall 2010). The importance of not pushing until the cervix has been confirmed as fully dilated should be explained to the woman. In addition, the woman should be aware that other skilled attendants may need to be called to the birth.

At the start of the expulsive part of the second stage of labour, the woman tends to make pelvic rocking movements which facilitates the descent of the fetus and corrects positioning for further progress. As the woman commences pushing spontaneously, gradually the anterior buttock should descend, becoming visible at the introitus of the vagina, followed by the baby's anus, genitalia and posterior buttock. The bitrochanteric diameter is then born with lateral flexion, known as 'rumping'. While this is occurring, the baby's shoulders are entering the oblique diameter of the maternal pelvis.

Descent continues, the baby's thighs, popliteal fossa (back of the knee) and lower legs become visible and the pelvis is eventually born. The baby is then observed to arch its spine backwards, extending its pelvis causing its lower body to curl round the maternal symphysis pubis. As a result, the tension that this places on the baby's legs assists in their spontaneous release from the introitus, especially when the woman is in an upright, kneeling position, and the baby is born as far as the umbilicus. At this point, the woman may spontaneously lower her body so that the baby is sitting on the floor, further encouraging flexion of the baby. It is no longer common practice to pull down a loop of cord to avoid traction of the umbilicus unless there appears to be constriction of the blood vessels as manipulating the cord or stretching it can induce spasm of the vessels.

With further descent and continued anticlockwise rotation, the head enters the brim of the maternal pelvis as the shoulders rotate in the mid-cavity assisted by the pelvic floor muscles. Evans (2012b) emphasizes that this continued rotation of the baby's body assists in bringing the arms down using the pelvic floor muscles in a way that is very similar to the Løvset manoeuvre (used when the birth is delayed should the arms be extended). The anterior shoulder is released under the symphysis pubis and the posterior shoulder and arm pass over the perineum. At this point Evans (2012a) refers to the baby flexing its legs up towards its abdomen and its arms up towards its shoulders, similar to a sit-up or tummy scrunch. Such a movement, results in the baby flexing its head by bringing its chin down onto its chest and pivoting the occiput on the internal aspect of the symphysis pubis. This stimulates the woman to lower her body from an upright kneeling position to an all-fours or a knee–chest position, moving her pelvis round the baby's flexing head. This enables the baby's chin, face, sinciput and head to smoothly pass over the perineum. The midwife is only required to support the baby as the head is spontaneously born.

If a uterotonic is to be given to the woman as part of the third stage of labour management, it should be withheld until the baby's head is completely born.

The birth of the after-coming head

To avoid any sudden change in fetal intracranial pressure and subsequent cerebral haemorrhage it is vital the head is born in a steady and gradual fashion and often some assistance is given at this point. There are three methods used.

Burns Marshall manoeuvre

This particular manoeuvre facilitates movement of the baby's head through the maternal pelvic outlet, but is only possible when the woman is in a semi-recumbent, adapted lithotomy position. The baby is allowed to 'hang' until the head descends onto the perineum, when after about one to two minutes the nape of the neck becomes visible and the suboccipital region is born. The baby's ankles are grasped with forefinger between the two, maintaining sufficient traction to prevent the neck from extending and

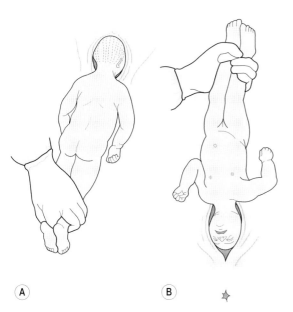

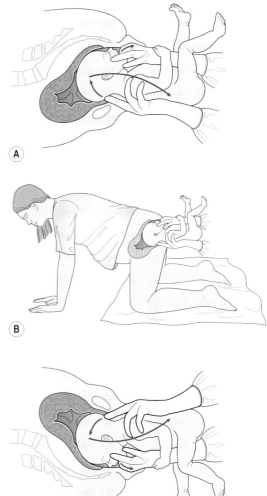

Fig. 17.9 Burns Marshall manoeuvre for the after-coming head. (A) Correct grasp around the fetal ankles. (B) The sub-occipital region pivots 180° under the pubic arch: the mouth and nose are free of the vulva.

resulting in possible cervical spine fracture (Fig. 17.9A). The feet are taken up through a 180° arc until the mouth and nose are free of the vulva. This should be undertaken slowly to prevent sudden changes in pressure to the baby's head and undue stretching of the perineum. The perineum can be guarded to prevent sudden escape of the head (Fig. 17.9B). It is imperative that the midwife observes the baby has descended sufficiently to ensure that it is the suboccipital region that pivots under the pubic arch and not the neck to avoid fracture of the cervical vertebra and crushing of the spinal cord.

Mauriceau–Smellie–Veit manoeuvre

Whilst the baby's head is facilitated through the same 180° arc as in the Burns Marshall manoeuvre, the Mauriceau–Smellie–Veit manoeuvre provides more control with the birth of the head and places less strain on the baby's back. This particular manoeuvre can be undertaken in a variety of positions that the woman may adopt for the birth: semi-recumbent, sitting, the adopted lithotomy position or the all-fours position. As this manoeuvre facilitates maximum flexion of the baby's head, it can be used to advantage when the head is extended and descent is delayed. Furthermore, it allows for slow birthing of the baby's head and thus reduces the risk of intracranial haemorrhage.

In an 'all-fours' position, the midwife supports the baby's back over her right arm and flexes the baby's head by tipping the occiput *forwards* with the middle finger of the right hand and by gentle pressure on the baby's malar bones (cheek bones) with the first and ring fingers

Fig. 17.10 Mauriceau–Smellie–Veit manoeuvre to assist the birth of the after-coming head in a breech presentation. (A and B) 'All-fours' position demonstrating how the occiput is tipped *forwards* to achieve flexion, pivoting *downwards* under the symphysis pubis to facilitate birth of the head. (C) In a semi-recumbent/sitting/adapted lithotomy position, showing position of hands and *downward* direction of flexion whilst pivoting *upwards* through a 180° arc under the pubic arch.

of the left hand (see Fig. 17.10A,B). It is important that the midwife avoids placing her finger in the baby's mouth to prevent fracture to the jaw or trauma to the mouth and gums, which can result in the baby having difficulties with feeding. The vault of the baby's head should be born slowly and gently to facilitate gradual adaptation of the head to the changing pressures imposed by the birth process. This should be in a *downwards* direction following the pelvic curve of Carus.

In the semi-recumbent position, the midwife should support the baby on one of her arms, with her first and ring fingers placed on the baby's malar bones, pulling the jaw down and increasing flexion. The other hand is placed across the baby's shoulders with the midwife's middle finger on the occiput to increase flexion. The outer fingers can apply gentle traction on the baby's shoulders. Maintaining flexion, the head is drawn out of the vagina until the suboccipital region appears and then the baby's head is slowly pivoted gently and slowly *upwards* around the symphysis pubis following the curve of Carus, delivering the chin and face first (see Fig. 17.10C).

Forceps birth

If an obstetrician is facilitating the vaginal breech birth, forceps may be applied to the after-coming head to ensure the birth is controlled.

Manoeuvres to assist the breech birth

If the midwife uses her professional judgement and decides to undertake a manoeuvre to assist the breech birth, as this will involve making some contact with the woman she must obtain the woman's consent in order to avoid the legal tort of trespass to the person (Dimond 2006; Nursing and Midwifery Council [NMC] 2008). If the fact that the baby is presenting by the breech is known before the onset of labour, it is recommended that the midwife and the woman discuss the reasons for any possible manoeuvres, including their benefit and risks. The midwife could seek consent to undertake any necessary manoeuvres prior to the labour.

The following manoeuvres were originally developed to facilitate a breech birth with the woman positioned on the bed, but can be utilized when the woman is on all fours or standing. With the benefits of gravity encouraging descent of the fetus in the latter positions, the likelihood of the midwife needing to adopt such measures is reduced. Nevertheless, as noted above, unexpected breech presentations in late labour still arise, so it is important that the midwife is both aware of, and skilled, in these manoeuvres and maintains her competence in these areas.

The birth of extended legs

If the fetal legs are not born spontaneously, it is likely they are extended, splinting the baby's body, which impedes lateral flexion of the spine and ultimately delays the birth. Gentle pressure, as shown in Fig. 17.11, can be applied in the popliteal fossa of one of the legs to encourage knee flexion. This assists in the birth of the leg by sweeping it to the side of the abdomen through abducting the hip. This can be repeated for the other leg if necessary. The knee is a hinge joint which bends in one direction only. If the knee is pulled forwards from the abdomen, severe injury to the joint can result.

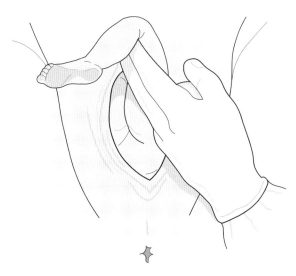

Fig. 17.11 Assisting the birth of extended leg by applying pressure in the popliteal fossa.

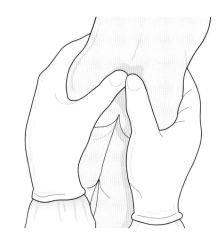

Fig. 17.12 Correct grasp for the Løvset manoeuvre for extended arms.

The birth of extended arms: the Løvset manoeuvre

This manoeuvre, which is a combination of rotation and downward traction, is used when the arms fail to appear during the birth of the baby's trunk and chest as a result of them being extended above the head. If the arms are not released then the birth will be delayed with increasing risk of hypoxia to the baby.

The baby is held at the iliac crests with thumbs over the sacrum and downward traction is applied whilst the baby is rotated 180° (Fig. 17.12). Care must be taken to always keep the baby's back towards the woman's front, i.e. the baby's *abdomen* must be *uppermost* in an all-fours position or the baby's *back* is *uppermost* in a semi-recumbent position. It is important that the baby is not grasped by the flanks or abdomen as this may cause intra-abdominal trauma resulting in kidney, liver or spleen injury.

To keep the baby's *abdomen* uppermost should the woman have adopted the all-fours position, if the baby's right arm is extended the baby should be rotated to the right by applying downward traction on the pelvic girdle in order to release the arm. This process is then repeated for the left arm if necessary.

The Løvset manoeuvre creates friction of the baby's posterior arm lying in the sacral curve against the pubic bone as the shoulder becomes anterior, sweeping the arm in front of the face (Fig. 17.13). The movement enables the shoulders to enter the maternal pelvis in the transverse diameter. The anterior arm is then born and the baby can be rotated back in the opposite direction in order for the other arm to be born. If the arm is not born spontaneously, it is usual to splint the humerus with two fingers, flex the elbow and sweep the arm across the face and downwards across the baby's chest ('cat-lick' manoeuvre).

Delay in the birth of the head

If the head is trapped in an incompletely dilated cervix, an air channel can be created to enable the baby to breathe pending intervention. This is done by inserting two fingers or a Sim's speculum in front of the baby's face and holding the vaginal wall away from the nose. Any mucus is wiped away and the airways are cleared. Attempts to release the head from the cervix result in high perinatal morbidity and mortality. Shushan and Younis (1992) have suggested the McRoberts manoeuvre as a method to facilitate the release of the fetal head. This requires the woman to lie flat on her back, bringing her knees up to her abdomen, and abducting the hips. More commonly this manoeuvre is used to relieve shoulder dystocia and is described in detail in Chapter 20.

Posterior rotation of the occiput is rare and usually results from mismanagement. If the woman is in a semi-recumbent position, the baby's back should always remain *uppermost* after the shoulders are born. To assist the birth should the head be in the occipitoposterior position, the baby's chin and face may pass under the symphysis pubis as far as the root of the nose and the baby is then lifted up towards the mother's abdomen to enable the occiput to sweep the perineum.

When facilitating the birth of a woman presenting with a breech at term, there are some important issues for the midwife to consider that are pertinent to the breech scenario. These have been summarized in the Second Stage of Labour Checklist, as detailed in Box 17.4.

Box 17.4 **Second stage of labour checklist for vaginal breech birth at term**

- **Regular fetal heart monitoring undertaken and documented:** Continuous electronic fetal heart monitoring *in hospital*. Pinard or sonicaid auscultation following every contraction in the second stage *at home* (NICE 2007 recommendations).
- **Check for cord prolapse if membranes rupture and buttocks are not engaged.**
- **Check for full dilatation before encouraging the woman to push:** The woman may experience a premature urge to push as the fetal body can pass through the cervix prior to full dilatation: the fetal head could become entrapped causing asphyxia increasing perinatal morbidity and mortality.
- **The umbilical cord may be loosened gently (*rarely required*):** This may be undertaken to prevent constriction of blood vessels as the baby's body is born. In the all-fours position, the condition of the baby can be easily monitored by observing the chest movements.
- **Encourage a physiological birth with minimum handling (*hands off the breech*):** To allow the baby to be born by gravity and propulsion and reduce trauma to the baby once the buttocks are distending the vulva.
- **Vault of the fetal skull should be born slowly:** To avoid rapid decompression resulting in intracranial haemorrhage.
- **Be aware and skilled in manoeuvres:** To assist the birth of the breech if problems arise with fetal descent and to control the birth of the baby's head.
- **DO NOT PERFORM BREECH EXTRACTION (routine use of manoeuvres/interventions to expedite birth):** This can cause delay and obstruction, e.g. fetal arms pulled upwards, head extended backwards.
- **Care of the baby following birth should include:** Appropriate resuscitation including suction of the oropharynx and inspection of the vocal cords (if thick meconium), maintaining the baby's body temperature, early feeding and paediatric assessment for signs of birth trauma.
- **Postnatal examination of the mother:** To assess the physical condition, including any birth trauma and discuss the birth and its outcome whilst assessing psychological wellbeing.
- **Documentation:** Is vitally important throughout the labour and birth, to include specific details of all discussions and referrals and the time they were initiated. As the breech is born, the time that each stage is reached and any manoeuvres undertaken should also be recorded. Additionally documentation should account for immediate condition of the baby, including any resuscitation measures taken, and the condition of the mother following the birth.

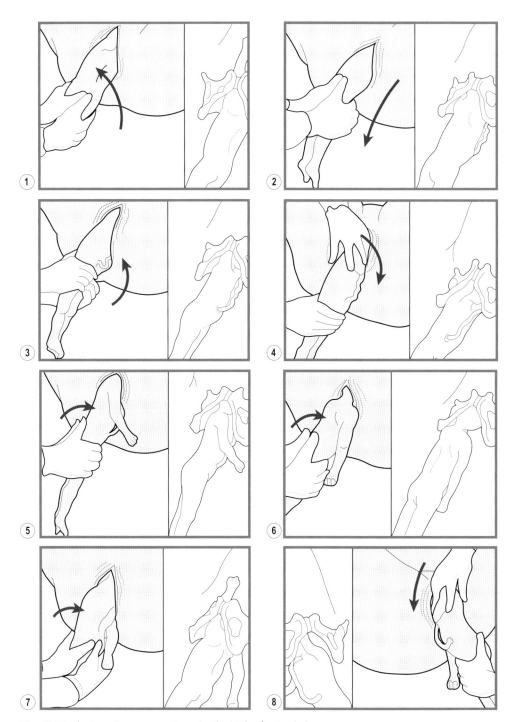

Fig. 17.13 The Løvset manoeuvre to assist the birth of extended arms.

Potential complications of breech birth

It is important that midwives are fully aware of the potential complications associated specifically with vaginal breech births at term, which are listed in Box 17.5. Many of these can be avoided by having an experienced and skilled attendant assisting at the birth. In the latest Centre for Maternal and Child Enquiries (CMACE) Report on Perinatal Mortality in 2009 there were eight intrapartum stillbirths at term (CMACE 2011): however, the mode of birth or place of birth were not articulated.

Professional responsibilities and term breech birth

As an autonomous, accountable practitioner, the midwife has responsibility to maintain skills in normal physiologi-

cal birth in relation to breech presentations at term in order to offer women real choice regarding mode of birth. This includes being familiar with the current evidence and re-developing the skills midwives once had to facilitate vaginal breech births at term where there are no contraindications. It is therefore essential that these skills are seen as part of the normal physiological birth process rather than viewed as a rare maternity *'emergency'*.

RECORD-KEEPING

It is the responsibility of the midwife assisting the birth to complete the labour record. This should include details of any drugs administered, of the duration and progress of labour, of the reason for performing an episiotomy, and of perineal repair. This information is recorded on the

---

Box 17.5 **Potential complications of breech birth**

Potential fetal/neonatal complication	Associated cause
Congenital abnormality, e.g. hydrocephaly.	A cause for the presentation. Mechanism of the birth itself poses risks.
Congenital dislocation of the hip ($\uparrow$ frank/extended breech).	Usually a complication of the presentation and *not* the birth process.
Fetal asphyxia.	Umbilical cord prolapse ($\uparrow$ preterm labour/footling breech/ ill-fitting presenting part). Cord compression. Premature placental separation due to uterine retraction once the baby's body has been born.
Intracranial haemorrhage.	Rapid decompression of the fetal skull causing tearing of the dura mater lining the brain and other major blood vessels.
Superficial tissue damage/bruising and oedema of baby's genitalia, feet.	Pressure on the cervix / prolapsed foot that lies in the vagina or at the vulva for some time.
Fractures of the femur, humerus, clavicle and spine/ spinal cord damage.	Incorrect or excessive handling during the birth.
Dislocation of the hip, shoulder, neck.	
Brachial nerve paralysis (Erb's palsy).	
Soft tissue damage/rupture to baby's liver, kidneys, spleen and adrenal glands.	Abdominal area is roughly squeezed.
Dislocation of fetal jaw/soft tissue damage to mouth and gums/feeding difficulties.	Baby's mouth incorrectly being used to create traction rather than the malar bones (cheekbones) in the Mauriceau–Smellie– Veit manoeuvre.
Cold injury/thermal shock and hypoglycaemia.	Ambient temperature too cool and baby loses heat during completion of the birth process.
Potential maternal complication	Associated cause
Urethral, vaginal and perineal trauma.	Rapid birth of the baby's head.
Effects of anaesthesia (local, regional general), infection, haemorrhage, thromboembolic disorders etc.	Risks of operative procedures.
Psychological distress, affecting attachment to baby, feeding difficulties and traumatic stress disorder.	Unexpected vaginal breech birth with lack of time to discuss options.

Box 17.6 **Dilemmas of practice**

- The contrast between the current evidence base and actual practices.
- The contrast between knowledge gained from experience (empirical knowledge) and that gained from evidence (authoritative knowledge).
- The problem of using guidelines and clinical risk assessments based on population evidence for individual women/babies.
- Balancing maternal choice, institutional demands, and midwifery expertise.

mother's notes (paper and/or computerized) and may be duplicated on her domiciliary record as well as in the birth register in some sites. Details of the baby's condition, including Apgar score, are also recorded. In some areas extra charts and monitoring processes are being introduced to respond to a range of imperatives. It is the professional responsibility of the midwife to remember that the primary purpose of record keeping is to ensure effective delivery and handover of care for each mother and baby, not to protect staff or the organization from the risk of litigation. As the Nursing and Midwifery Council Midwives Rules and Standards state: *'you must make sure the needs of the woman or baby are the primary focus of your practice'* (NMC 2012: 15). Midwives need to balance the need for complete and accurate record-keeping with the need to maintain a focus on the woman and her fetus and birth companions. If demands to complete duplicate or unnecessary records hinder this central activity, the midwife should bring the situation to the attention of her manager and/or supervisor of midwives. See Box 17.6 for other current dilemmas in practice as midwives negotiate around the various requirements of undertaking their vocation, being a professional, being an employee and practising competently and ethically.

New developments such as the All Wales Clinical Pathway for Normal Labour (NHS Wales 2006), which uses exception reporting, provide alternative approaches to record-keeping that may be useful for practitioners in the future. All data in the UK are subject to the Data Protection Act 1998.

Official notification of the birth must be completed within 36 hours. This may be undertaken by anyone present at the birth but is usually carried out by the midwife. The notification is sent to the Chief Medical Officer in the health district in which the baby was born.

CONCLUSION

The processes of transition and of second stage labour are likely to be very physically and emotionally intense,

Box 17.7 Diane's birth story

The birth of my first baby should have been one of the happiest days of my life. Instead, I felt I had failed; I was mentally and physically traumatized. Five years on, when I was eventually pregnant again, my fears started creeping back, and I considered having a caesarean section. I was referred to the local caseload midwifery team. When my midwife came to visit, I told her that my first birth had left me traumatized, confused and scared about everything. This was my big turn around: after talking to her I realized I did not want a caesarean section, and I started to feel confident about giving birth naturally.

The big day arrived. I was over the moon that I had started my labour naturally. After a few hours my midwife came to my house, just to check how everything was going. Eventually, we decided it was time to go to the hospital. When I arrived they organized an epidural for me, which I had discussed, and which was in my birth plan. I was getting excited, knowing I was going to meet my baby soon. My midwife supported me and encouraged me on everything I decided. She was there for me all the time, keeping me focused and positive about my birth. After about 3 hours, I started pushing hard with contractions. The epidural wore off enough for me to turn around on to my knees with my body upright, and I could feel the baby drop down. I gave it my all for two pushes, and out popped the head. I controlled my breathing, pushing slowly, and my beautiful baby girl came out. The midwife brought her through my legs so I could see her and that's when my husband cut her cord, which was memorable and overwhelming for him. I was the happiest person, I had the biggest smile on my face: to me this was a beautiful birth. Thanks to the wonderful midwives – it goes to show that with the right help and guidance you can overcome your fears and anxieties with positive thinking.

particularly for the woman, but also for her partner and other birth companions. If maternal behaviour and instinct are respected, in the context of skilled and watchful waiting, the vast majority of labours will progress physiologically. The skill of the midwife is to support the woman effectively, to guide her when her spirits or the labour are flagging, and to enable her to accomplish her birth safely and in triumph. Diane's story in Box 17.7 provides a personal account of how important this is for women.

Clear, comprehensive, proportionate record-keeping is essential. While much practice in this area is still not based on formal evidence (see Box 17.8), new observations about normal birth are beginning to be recorded, which will form the basis for future research.

Key issues in the management of the second stage of labour are summarized in Box 17.9.

Box 17.8 **Examples of areas in need of research in transition and second stage labour**

- The areas of controversy, as set out in Box 17.1.
- The nature of physiological fetal heart patterns, and variation and significance of variation in normal fetal heart tones and rhythms as heard with a Pinard's stethoscope.
- The physiological variation in mechanisms and patterns of labour in settings where no restrictions on positioning or length of labour are imposed as a matter of routine.
- Evaluation of maternal behaviours and other non-invasive techniques to assess progress in labour.
- The short-, medium- and long-term epigenetic consequences of physiological labour and birth for the mother and her baby.
- The optimum approach to supporting women who experience the early pushing urge.
- Tools and technologies (including e- and m-technologies) to enhance personalized approaches to tailoring maternity care provision for the specific needs and choices of individual women.

Box 17.9 **Key issues in the management of the second stage of labour**

- The transition and second stage phases of labour are emotionally intense and physically hard.
- The majority of labours will progress physiologically.
- Maternal behaviour is usually a good indication of progress during this time.
- The core midwifery skill is to support the woman in the context of a sound knowledge of the physiology and the mechanisms of this phase of labour.
- Support should be unobtrusive.
- The woman is the central player.
- Clear, comprehensive record keeping is essential.
- There are many gaps in the research evidence in this area.

REFERENCES

Albers L L 1999 The duration of labor in healthy women. Journal of Perinatology 19(2):114–19

Aldrich C J, D'Antona D, Spencer J A et al 1995 The effect of maternal pushing on fetal cerebral oxygenation and blood volume during the second stage of labour. British Journal of Obstetrics and Gynaecology 102(6):448–53

Allen V M, Baskett T F, O'Connell C M et al 2009 Maternal and perinatal outcomes with increasing duration of the second stage of labor. Obstetrics and Gynecology 113(6):1248–58

Anderson G 2003 A concept analysis of 'normal birth'. Evidence Based Midwifery 1(2):48–54

Anim-Somuah M, Smyth R M D, Jones L 2011 Epidural versus non-epidural or no analgesia in labour. Cochrane Database of Systematic Reviews 2011, Issue 12. Art. No. CD000331. doi: 10.1002/14651858.CD000331.pub3

Baker A, Kenner A N 1993 Communication of pain: vocalisation as an indicator of stage of labour. New Zealand Journal of Obstetrics and Gynaecology 33:385

Benyon C 1990 The normal second stage of labor: a plea for reform in its conduct In: Kitzinger S, Simkin P 1990 (eds) Episiotomy and the second stage of labor, 2nd edn. Penny-press, Seattle (Originally published in 1957 in the Journal of Obstetrics and Gynaecology of the British Empire 64:815–20)

Berg M, Asta Ólafsdóttir O, Lundgren I 2012 A midwifery model of woman-centred childbirth care in Swedish and Icelandic settings. Sexual and Reproductive Healthcare (2):79–87

Borrelli S E, Locatelli A, Nespoli A 2013 Early pushing urge in labour and midwifery practice: a prospective observational study at an Italian maternity hospital. Midwifery 29(8):871–5

Brancato R M, Church S, Stone P W 2008 A meta-analysis of passive descent versus immediate pushing in nulliparous women with epidural analgesia in the second stage of labor. Journal of Obstetric Gynecologic and Neonatal Nursing 37(1):4–12

Burvill S 2005 Managing breech presentation in the absence of obstetric assistance. In: Woodward V, Bates K, Young N (eds) Managing childbirth emergencies in community settings. Palgrave Macmillan, Houndsmill, p 111–39

Bystrova K, Ivanova V, Edhborg M et al 2009 Early contact versus separation: effects on mother–infant interaction one year later. Birth 36(2):97–109

Chadwick J 2002 Malpresentations and malpositions. In: Boyle M (ed) Emergencies around childbirth: a handbook for midwives. Radcliffe Medical Press, Oxford, p 63–81.

CMACE (Centre for Maternal and Child Enquiries) 2011 Perinatal mortality

2009: United Kingdom. CMACE, London

COMET (Comparative Obstetric Mobile Trial Study Group) UK 2001 Effect of low-dose mobile versus traditional epidural techniques on mode of delivery: a randomised controlled trial. The Lancet 358:19–23

Costley P L, East C E 2012 Oxytocin augmentation of labour in women with epidural analgesia for reducing operative deliveries. Cochrane Database of Systematic Reviews 2012, Issue 5. Art. No. CD009241. doi:10.1002/14651858.CD009241. pub2

Crawford J S 1983 The stages and phases of labour: outworn nomenclature that invites hazard. The Lancet ii: 271–2

Cronk M 1998a Midwives and breech births. The Practising Midwife 1(7/8):44–5

Cronk M 1998b Hands off the breech. The Practising Midwife 1(6):13–15

Dahlen H, Downe S, Duff M et al (2013) Vaginal examination dural normal labour: routine examination or routine intervention? International Journal of Childbirth 3(3):142–52.

Dimond B 2006 Legal aspects of midwifery, 3rd edn. Books for Midwives Press, Hale, Cheshire

Downe S 1994 How average is normality? British Journal of Midwifery 2(7):303–4

Downe S 2004 The concept of normality in the maternity services: application and consequences. In: Frith L (ed) Ethics and midwifery: issues in contemporary practice, 2nd edn. Butterworth Heinemann, Oxford

Downe S 2006 Engaging with the concept of unique normality in childbirth. British Journal of Midwifery 14(6):352–6

Downe S (ed) 2008 Normal birth, evidence and debate, 2nd edn. Elsevier, Oxford

Downe S, Gerrett D, Renfrew M J 2004 A prospective randomised trial on the effect of position in the passive second stage of labour on birth outcome in nulliparous women using epidural analgesia. Midwifery 20(2):157–68

Downe S, Gyte G M L, Dahlen H G et al 2013 Routine vaginal examinations

for assessing progress of labour to improve outcomes for women and babies at term. Cochrane Database of Systematic Reviews 2013, Issue 7. Art. No. CD010088. doi: 10.1002/14651858.CD010088.pub2

Downe S, Young C, Hall-Moran V, Trent Midwifery Research Group 2008 Multiple midwifery discourses: the case of the early pushing urge. In: Downe S (ed) Normal birth, evidence and debate. Elsevier, Oxford

Elmir R, Schmied V, Wilkes L et al 2010 Women's perceptions and experiences of a traumatic birth: a meta-ethnography. Journal of Advanced Nursing 66(10):2142–53

El-Nemer A, Downe S, Small N 2006 'She would help me from the heart': an ethnography of Egyptian women in labour. Social Science and Medicine 62(1):81–92

Enkin M, Keirse M J N C, Neilson J et al 2000 A guide to effective care in pregnancy and childbirth, 3rd edn. Oxford University Press, Oxford

Evans J 2012a The final piece of the breech jigsaw puzzle? Essentially MIDIRS 3(3):46–9

Evans J 2012b Understanding physiological breech birth. Essentially MIDIRS 3(2):17–21

Gillesby E, Burns S, Dempsey A et al 2010 Comparison of delayed versus immediate pushing during second stage of labor for nulliparous women with epidural anesthesia. Journal of Obstetric Gynecologic and Neonatal Nursing 39(6):635–44

Goffinet F, Carayol M, Foidart J M … PREMODA Study Group 2006 Is planned vaginal delivery of breech presentation at term still an option? Results of an observational prospective survey in France and Belguim. American Journal of Obstetrics and Gynecology 194(4):1002–11

Gould D 2000 Normal labour: a concept analysis. Journal of Advanced Nursing 31(2): 418–27

Gupta J K, Hofmeyr G J, Shehmar M 2012 Position in the second stage of labour for women without epidural anaesthesia. Cochrane Database of Systematic Reviews 2012, Issue 5. Art. No. CD002006. doi: 10.1002/14651858.CD002006. pub3

Halldorsdottir S, Karlsdottir S I 1996 Empowerment or discouragement: women's experience of caring and uncaring encounters during childbirth. Health Care for Women International 17(4):361–79

Hannah M E Hannah W J Hewson S A et al 2000 Term Breech Trial Collaborative Group. Planned caesarean section versus planned vaginal birth for breech presentation at term: a randomized multi-centre trial Lancet 356:1375–83

Hobbs L 1998 Assessing cervical dilatation without VEs: watching the purple line. The Practising Midwife 1(11):34–5

Hodnett E D, Gates S, Hofmeyr G J et al 2012 Continuous support for women during childbirth. Cochrane Database of Systematic Reviews 2012, Issue 10. Art. No. CD003766. doi: 10.1002/14651858.CD003766. pub4

Humphrey M D, Chang A, Wood E C et al 1974 A decrease in fetal pH during the second stage of labour when conducted in the dorsal position. Journal of Obstetrics and Gynaecology of the British Commonwealth 81:600–2

Hutton E K, Hassan E S 2007 Late vs early clamping of the umbilical cord in full-term neonates: systematic review and meta-analysis of controlled trials. Journal of the American Medical Association 297(11):1241–52

Jackson H, Melvin C, Downe S 2007 Midwives and the fetal nuchal cord: a survey of practices and perceptions. Journal of Midwifery and Women's Health 52:49–55

Keane H E, Thornton J G 1998 A trial of cetrimide/chlorhexidine or tap water for perineal cleaning. British Journal of Midwifery 6(1):34–7

Kurz C S, Schneider H, Hutch R et al 1982 The influence of maternal position on the fetal transcutaneous oxygen pressure. Journal of Perinatal Medicine 10(Suppl 2):74–5

Lewis P 2011 Malpositions and malpresentations. In: MacDonald S and Magill-Cuerden J (eds) Mayes midwifery, 14th edn. Balliere Tindall/Elsevier, Edinburgh, p 869–98

Lumbiganon P, Thinkhamrop J, Thinkhamrop B et al 2004 Vaginal chlorhexidine during labour for preventing maternal and neonatal infections (excluding Group B Streptococcal and HIV). Cochrane Database of Systematic Reviews 2004, Issue 4. Art. No. CD004070. doi: 10.1002/14651858.CD004070.pub2

Lundgren I 2004 Releasing and relieving encounters: experiences of pregnancy and childbirth. Scandinavian Journal of Caring Sciences 18(4):368–75

Maier B, Georgoulopoulos A, Zajc M et al 2011 Fetal outcome for infants in breech by method of delivery experiences with a stand-by service system of senior obstetricians and women's choices of mode of delivery. Journal of Perinatal Medicine 39(4):385–90

Marshall J E 2010 Facilitating vaginal breech at term. In: Marshall J E, Raynor M D Advancing skills in midwifery practice. Churchill Livingstone/Elsevier, Edinburgh, p 89–102

McCandlish R, Bowler U, van Asten H et al 1998 A randomised controlled trial of care of the perineum during second stage of normal labour. British Journal of Obstetrics and Gynecology 105(12):1262–72

McDonald S J, Middleton P 2008 Effect of timing of umbilical cord clamping of term infants on maternal and neonatal outcomes. Cochrane Database of Systematic Reviews 2008, Issue 2. Art. No. CD004074. doi: 10.1002/14651858.CD004074.pub2

McLachlan H L, Forster D A, Davey M A et al 2012 Effects of continuity of care by a primary midwife (caseload midwifery) on caesarean section rates in women of low obstetric risk: the COSMOS randomised controlled trial. British Journal of Obstetrics and Gynecology 119(12):1483–92

Mercer J, Skovgaard R 2004 Fetal to neonatal transition: first, do no harm. In: Downe S (ed) Normal birth, evidence and debate. Elsevier, Oxford

Mercer J, Skovgaard R, Peareara-Eaves J et al 2005 Nuchal cord management and nurse midwifery practice. Journal of Midwifery and Women's Health 50(5):373–9

Mercer J S, Erickson-Owens D A, Graves B et al 2007 Evidence-based practices

for the fetal to newborn transition. Journal of Midwifery and Women's Health 52(3):262–72

Montgomery T 1958 Physiologic considerations in labor and the puerperium. American Journal of Obstetrics and Gynecology Oct:706

Moore E R, Anderson G C, Bergman N 2007 Early skin-to-skin contact for mothers and their healthy newborn infants. Cochrane Database of Systematic Reviews 2007, Issue 3. Art. No. CD003519. doi: 10.1002/14651858.CD003519.pub3

Ndala R 2005 Breech presentation. In: Stables D and Rankin J 2005 Physiology of childbearing with anatomy and related biosciences. Elsevier, Edinburgh, p 541–51

NHS Wales 2006 All Wales Clinical Pathway for Normal Labour. Online. Available at www.wales.nhs.uk/sites3/page.cfm?orgid=327&pid=5786 (accessed 20 June 2013)

NICE (National Institute for Health and Clinical Excellence) 2007 Intrapartum care: management and delivery of care to women in labour. Online. Available at www.nice.org.uk/CG055 (accessed 20 June 2013)

NMC (Nursing and Midwifery Council) 2008 The Code: Standards of conduct, performance and ethics for nurses and midwives. NMC, London

NMC (Nursing and Midwifery Council) 2012 Midwives Rules and Standards. Available from www.nmc-uk.org/Documents/NMC-Publications/Midwives%20Rules%20and%20Standards%202012.pdf (accessed 20 June 2013)

Petersen L, Besuner P 1997 Pushing techniques during labor: issues and controversies. Journal of Obstetric, Gynecologic and Neonatal Nursing 26(6):719–26

Prins M, Boxem J, Lucas C et al 2011 Effect of spontaneous pushing versus Valsalva pushing in the second stage of labour on mother and fetus: a systematic review of randomised trials. BJOG: An International Journal of Obstetrics and Gynecology 118(6):662–70

Reed B 2003 A disappearing art: vaginal breech birth. The Practising Midwife 69:16–8

Roberts C L, Algert C S, Cameron C A et al 2005 A meta-analysis of upright positions in the second stage to

reduce instrumental deliveries in women with epidural analgesia. Acta Obstetricia et Gynecologica Scandinavica 84(8):794–8

Roberts C L, Torvaldsen S, Cameron C A et al 2004 Delayed versus early pushing in women with epidural analgesia: a systematic review and meta-analysis. BJOG: An International Journal of Obstetrics and Gynaecology 111(12):1333–40

Roberts J, Hanson L 2007 Best practices in second stage labor care: maternal bearing down and positioning. Journal of Midwifery and Women's Health 52(3):238–45

Royal College of Midwives 2005 Normal breech birth. Available at www.rcmnormalbirth.org.uk/default.asp?sID=1099658440484 (accessed 20 June 2013)

Royal College of Midwives 2013 'Getting off the bed'. Positions swatch. Available at www.rcmnormalbirth.org.uk/news/positions-swatch/. Videos at www.rcmnormalbirth.org.uk/news/positions-in-labour-and-birth-video-clips/ (accessed 20 June 2013)

RCOG (Royal College of Obstetricians and Gynaecologists) 2006 Clinical Green Top Guidelines for Management of Breech Presentation No. 20b. RCOG London

Russell J G B 1969 Moulding of the pelvic outlet. Journal of Obstetrics and Gynaecology 76:817–20

Shepherd A, Cheyne H, Kennedy S et al 2010 The purple line as a measure of labour progress: a longitudinal study. BMC Pregnancy and Childbirth 10:54

Shushan A, Younis J S 1992 McRoberts maneuver for the management of the aftercoming head in breech delivery. Gynecologic and Obstetric Investigation 34(3):188–9

Simkin P 2010 The fetal occiput posterior position: state of the science and a new perspective. Birth 37(1):61–71

Simkin P, Ancheta R 2006 Labor progress handbook, 2nd edn. Blackwell, Oxford

Simpson K R, James D C 2005 Effects of immediate versus delayed pushing during second-stage labor on fetal wellbeing: a randomized clinical trial. Nurse Researcher 54(3):149–57

Steen M, Downe S, Bamford N et al 2012 Not-patient and not-visitor: a metasynthesis of fathers' encounters with pregnancy, birth and maternity care. Midwifery 28(4):362–71

Stewart P, Spiby H 1989 A randomized study of the sitting position for delivery using a newly designed obstetric chair. British Journal of Obstetrics and Gynaecology 96(3):327–33

Stremler R, Hodnett E, Petryshen P et al 2005 Randomized controlled trial of hands-and-knees positioning for occipito-posterior position in labor. Birth 32(4):243–51

Stoddart A P, Nicholson K E, Popham P A 1994 Low dose bupivacaine/fentanyl epidural infusions in labour and mode of delivery. Anaesthesia 49(12):1087–90

Sutton J, Scott P 1996 Understanding and teaching optimal fetal positioning, 2nd edn. Birth Concepts, Tauranga

Thomson A M 1993 Pushing techniques in the second stage of labour. Journal of Advanced Nursing 18(2):171–7

Thomson G, Downe S 2008 Widening the trauma discourse: the link between childbirth and experiences of abuse. Journal of Psychosomatic Obstetrics and Gynaecology 29(4):268–73

Thomson G, Downe S 2010 Changing the future to change the past: women's experiences of a positive birth following a traumatic birth experience. Journal of Reproductive and Infant Psychology 28 (1): 102–12

Torvaldsen S, Roberts C L, Bell J C et al 2004 Discontinuation of epidural analgesia late in labour for reducing the adverse delivery outcomes associated with epidural analgesia. Cochrane Database of Systematic Reviews 2004, Issue 4. Art. No. CD004457. doi: 10.1002/14651858. CD004457.pub2

Turner M J, Sil J M, Alagesan K et al 1988 Epidural bupivacaine concentration and forceps birth in primiparae. Journal of Obstetrics and Gynecology 9(2):122–5

Verheijen E C, Raven J H, Hofmeyr G J. 2009 Fundal pressure during the second stage of labour. Cochrane Database of Systematic Reviews 2009, Issue 4. Art. No. CD006067. doi: 10.1002/14651858.CD006067. pub2

Waldenström U, Schytt E 2009 A longitudinal study of women's memory of labour pain – from 2 months to 5 years after the birth. BJOG: An International Journal of Obstetrics and Gynaecology 116(4):577–83

Walsh D 2010 Labour rhythms. In: Walsh D, Downe S (eds) Essential midwifery practice: intrapartum care. Wiley–Blackwell, Chichester

White G 2007 You cope by breaking down in private: fathers and PTSD following childbirth. British Journal of Midwifery 15(1):39–45

Wickham S 2007 Assessing cervical dilatation without VEs: watching the purple line. Practising Midwife 10(1):26–7

Yildirim G, Beji N K 2008 Effects of pushing techniques in birth on mother and fetus: a randomized study. Birth 35(1):25–30

Zhang J, Landy H J, Branch D W et al, Consortium on Safe Labor 2010 Contemporary patterns of spontaneous labor with normal neonatal outcomes. Obstetrics and Gynecology 116(6):1281–7

FURTHER READING

Davis E 2012 Heart and hands: a midwife's guide to pregnancy and birth, 5th edn. Ten Speed Press, New York

This is a manual of midwifery based on the skills and experiences gained by lay midwives working in America. If offers unique tips and insights.

Evans J 2005 Breech birth: what are my options? AIMS, Taunton

An informative and empowering text that discusses the major issues surrounding breech birth and explains the options for women and midwives to consider that are reinforced by the inclusion of poignant personal birth stories.

Floyd-Davis R, Sargent C F 1997 Childbirth and authoritative knowledge: cross-cultural perspectives. University of California Press, California

A seminal work, which explores how authority is given to certain kinds of knowledge, and how the knowledge and expertise of women and of less dominant cultures is not privileged, even in the area of childbirth, and even in the face of the evidence.

International Mother Baby Childbirth Initiative. Available at www.imbci. org/ (accessed 5 March 2013)

This international campaign is modelled on the Baby Friendly Initiative, and is based on 10 key steps which are believed to promote optimal births for mother and baby. The site includes inspirational material, and updates from demonstration sites across the world.

Leap N, Hunter B 1993 The midwife's tale: an oral history from handywoman to professional midwife. Scarlet Press, London

This is an historical account of trained midwives and laywomen practising in the 1950s. The stories of their experiences and responsibilities while attending women in labour are fascinating. The final chapter offers some accounts of labours from the point of view of women themselves.

Marshall J E 2010 Facilitating vaginal breech at term. In: Marshall J E, Raynor M D Advancing skills in midwifery practice. Churchill Livingstone/Elsevier, Edinburgh. pp 89–102

This chapter considers the midwife's professional, legal and ethical responsibilities in facilitating vaginal breech births at term within both the hospital and home environment.

Royal College of Midwives Campaign for Normal Birth. Online. Available at www.rcmnormalbirth.org.uk/ (accessed 5 March 2013)

The campaign was set up by the Royal College of Midwives to inspire and support normal birth practice in the midwifery

profession. It is a web-based initiative, using real stories and midwives' experiences, underpinned with a sound evidence base. The site includes top tips to maximize physiological childbirth. There are some excellent videos showing different *positions, and how to help women to adopt them.*

Walsh D 2007 Evidence based care for normal labour and birth. Routledge, London

A clearly written overview of both formal and informal evidence that effectively integrates narrative, evidence and experiential learning.

USEFUL WEBSITES

Campaign for Normal Birth: www.rcmnormalbirth.org.uk

The Breech Birth Network: www.breechbirth.org.uk

Midwifery Matters (Association of Radical Midwives): www.midwifery.co.uk

Chapter |18|

Physiology and care during the third stage of labour

Cecily Begley

The third stage of labour is a time of profound relief for most women, following on the exertions of labour and birth. During this stage, mother, baby and father come together as a family unit for the first time; parents explore and become familiar with their newborn, marvel at their baby's behaviour and relax. The physical mechanisms of birth continue almost unnoticed, and the placenta and membranes are expelled. Until the third stage is complete, continued vigilance on the part of the midwife is essential to ensure that postpartum haemorrhage (PPH) is prevented or treated early, and that the placenta and membranes are born intact. PPH is ranked among the top four major causes of maternal death globally (World Health Organization [WHO] 2012). Although the majority (99%) of deaths reported occur in developing countries, the risk of PPH should not be underestimated for any birth, and PPH is at present the sixth leading cause of direct maternal death in the United Kingdom (UK) (Centre for Maternal and Child Enquiries [CMACE] 2011). Maternal mortality rates in high resource countries are relatively low when compared to low resource countries; however, maternal morbidity is similar in significance and rates of PPH are increasing world-wide (Knight et al 2009). To facilitate a healthy, enjoyable outcome for mother and baby, good antenatal health plus preparation, coupled with skilled, evidence-based practice of the midwife are crucial.

- describe the normal physiological mechanism of placental separation, descent and expulsion, including factors that facilitate haemostasis
- present evidence on the types, use and side-effects of uterotonic drugs in active management of the third stage
- discuss the evidence relating to timing of clamping the umbilical cord, and controlled cord traction
- describe the risk factors most commonly associated with PPH and discuss the current evidence-based management strategies for prevention and treatment
- discuss the midwife's care of the mother and family unit, during and immediately after separation and expulsion of the placenta and membranes.

PHYSIOLOGICAL PROCESSES

The third stage can be defined as the period from the birth of the baby to complete expulsion of the placenta and membranes. It involves the development of the relationship between mother, baby and father, the separation, descent and expulsion of the placenta and membranes, the control of haemorrhage from the placenta site, and sometimes, the initiation of breast-feeding. Although traditionally labour is divided into three distinct component parts to aid comprehension, it should be viewed as one continuous process. With this in mind, it is important to understand that the physiology of the third stage depends, in part, on what has happened during pregnancy as well as during the first and second stage of labour, and on the woman's basic level of health and wellbeing. The midwife's knowledge and evidence-based skills play a crucial role in ensuring that the care received by the woman works with, not against, physiological processes.

The placenta may shear off during the final expulsive contractions accompanying the birth of the baby or remain adherent for some time. The third stage usually lasts between 5 and 15 minutes, but any period up to 1 hour may be considered normal.

Separation and descent of the placenta

Mechanical factors

The unique characteristic of uterine muscle lies in its power of retraction. During the second stage of labour, the uterine cavity progressively empties as the baby moves down, enabling the retraction process to accelerate. Thus, by the beginning of the third stage, the placental site has

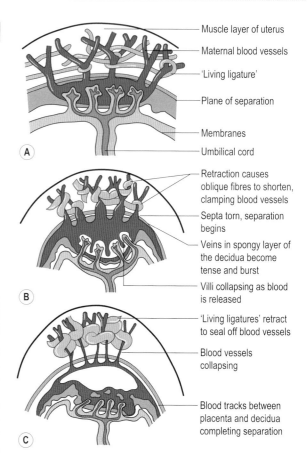

Muscle layer of uterus

Maternal blood vessels

'Living ligature'

Plane of separation

Membranes

Umbilical cord

Retraction causes oblique fibres to shorten, clamping blood vessels

Septa torn, separation begins

Veins in spongy layer of the decidua become tense and burst

Villi collapsing as blood is released

'Living ligatures' retract to seal off blood vessels

Blood vessels collapsing

Blood tracks between placenta and decidua completing separation

Fig. 18.1 The placental site during separation. (A) Uterus and placenta before separation. (B) Separation begins. (C) Separation is almost complete.

already diminished in area by about 75% (Baldock and Dixon 2006). As this occurs, the placenta becomes compressed and the blood in the intervillous spaces is forced back into the spongy layer of the decidua basalis. Retraction of the oblique uterine muscle fibres exerts pressure on the blood vessels so that blood does not drain back into the maternal system. The vessels during this process become tense and congested. With the next contraction the distended veins burst and a small amount of blood seeps in between the thin septa of the spongy layer and the placental surface, stripping it from its attachment (Fig. 18.1). As the surface area for placental attachment reduces, the relatively non-elastic placenta begins to detach from the uterine wall.

The majority of placentas are situated on the anterior or posterior wall of the uterus, and separation usually starts from the lower pole of the placenta and moves gradually upwards (Herman et al 2002). Fundal placentas separate first at both poles, followed by the fundal part. The length of the third stage may be approximately 2 minutes shorter

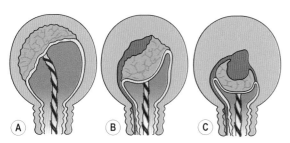

Fig. 18.2 The mechanism of placental separation.
(A) Uterine wall is partially retracted, but not sufficiently to cause placental separation. (B) Further contraction and retraction thicken the uterine wall, reduce the placental site and aid placental separation. (C) Complete separation and formation of the retroplacental clot. Note: The thin lower segment has collapsed like a concertina following the birth of the baby.

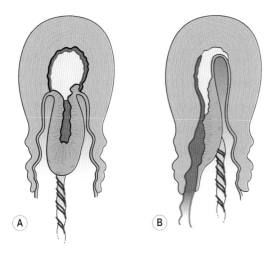

Fig. 18.3 Expulsion of the placenta. (A) Schultze method. (B) Matthews Duncan method.

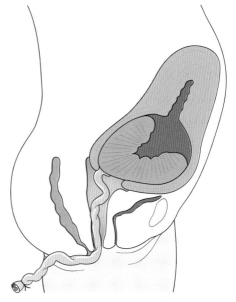

Fig. 18.4 Third stage: placenta in lower uterine segment.

when the placenta is located at the fundus (Altay et al 2007). If separation begins centrally, a retroplacental clot is formed (Fig. 18.2). This further aids separation by exerting pressure at the midpoint of placental attachment so that the increased weight helps to strip the adherent lateral borders and peel the membranes off the uterine wall so that the clot thus formed becomes enclosed in a membranous bag as the placenta descends, fetal surface first. This process of separation (first described by Schultze) is associated with more complete shearing of both placenta and membranes and less fluid blood loss (Fig. 18.3A). If the placenta begins to detach unevenly at one of its lateral borders, the blood escapes so that separation is unaided by the formation of a retroplacental clot. The placenta descends, slipping sideways, maternal surface first. This process (first described by Matthews Duncan in the nineteenth century) takes longer and is associated with ragged,

incomplete expulsion of the membranes and a higher fluid blood loss (Fig. 18.3B).

Once separation has occurred the uterus contracts strongly, forcing placenta and membranes to fall into the lower uterine segment (Fig. 18.4), and finally, into the vagina.

Haemostasis

The normal volume of blood flow through the placental site is 500–800 ml/min, but this is considerably reduced once the baby is born and the placental site on the uterine wall has diminished (Baldock and Dixon 2006). At placental separation, blood flow has to be arrested swiftly, or serious haemorrhage can occur. The interplay of four factors within the normal physiological processes that control bleeding are critical in minimizing blood loss and preventing maternal morbidity or mortality. They are:

1. Retraction of the oblique uterine muscle fibres in the upper uterine segment through which the tortuous blood vessels intertwine – the resultant thickening of the muscles exerts pressure on the torn vessels, acting as clamps, and preventing haemorrhage (see Fig. 18.1). It is the absence of oblique fibres in the lower uterine segment that explains the greatly increased blood loss usually accompanying placental separation in placenta praevia.
2. The presence of vigorous uterine contraction following separation – this brings the walls into apposition so that further pressure is exerted on the placental site.

3. The achievement of haemostasis – there is a transitory activation of the coagulation and fibrinolytic systems during, and immediately following, placental separation. It is believed that this protective response is especially active at the placental site so that clot formation in the torn vessels is intensified. Following separation, the placental site is rapidly covered by a fibrin mesh utilizing 5–10% of circulating fibrinogen.

4. Breast-feeding – the release of oxytocin from the posterior pituitary in response to skin-to-skin contact between mother and baby, and the baby's nuzzling at the breast, causes uterine contractions.

CARING FOR A WOMAN IN THE THIRD STAGE OF LABOUR

Two methods of care may be used during the third stage, expectant (physiological) care or active management. It is ultimately the woman's decision as to how she would, ideally, like her birth plan to be followed in the third stage. She may have philosophical, religious or cultural beliefs that influence her decision. The attending midwife may also have views, based on evidence, as to the ideal method of care for each particular woman. Midwives should ensure that, in order to facilitate informed decision-making by the woman, adequate time for deliberation and questions is made available, where possible, during the course of her routine antenatal consultations. The best available research information on care during the third stage of labour should be offered in an objective manner (Begley et al 2011), supported by written information on possible care options for the woman in keeping with the setting in which she intends to birth. Information on types of uterotonics, explanation of their different routes of administration, benefits, risks and side-effects involved, and timing and method of placental birth or delivery should be given.

The midwife's care of the mother should be based on an understanding of the normal physiological processes at work, including having access to as much information as possible about the woman's pregnancy and labour history. Progress of the first and second stages of labour are likely to impact on management of the third stage of labour and should not be reviewed in isolation. The midwife's actions can make the third stage a wonderful, relaxing time of birth and can reduce the risks of haemorrhage, infection, retained placenta and shock, any of which may increase maternal morbidity and even result in death. A mother's ability to withstand complications in the third stage depends, to a large degree, upon her general health and the avoidance of debilitating, predisposing problems, such as anaemia, ketosis, exhaustion and prolonged hypotonic uterine action. Factors that may influence the risk of haemorrhage are discussed in more detail later.

Detailed, accurate, written (contemporaneous wherever possible) documentation is extremely important in all aspects of care, particularly in areas where evidence-based information is relied upon to assess whether due care has been delivered. In the case of third stage management, two examples might be: where a woman requests expectant (physiological) management of the third stage of labour (EMTSL), the midwife should clarify the circumstances in which this decision may be reversed (e.g. if severe bleeding should occur); where a woman requests active management (AMTSL), the midwife should clarify the circumstances in which this decision may be reversed (e.g., if the baby requires attention and the placenta separates before a uterotonic has been given). The woman's preference for care must be recorded in her notes antenatally, and a record of the discussion may be signed by the woman. It would be prudent for midwives to notify their supervisor of midwives (SoM), clinical manager or the attending medical practitioner if any of the woman's requests are contrary to local guidelines.

Expectant (or physiological) care during the third stage of labour (EMTSL)

In expectant management, the normal, physiological mechanisms of labour are supported and no routine actions (such as administration of a uterotonic drug, or clamping of the umbilical cord) are carried out. A study of the reported actions of 27 expert midwives (who used EMTSL in at least 30% of births, and had recorded PPH rates of less than 4%) identified the key actions that they believed led to success when using EMTSL (Begley et al 2012). A synthesis of these actions, some of which are supported by other research also, provides the following instructions for best practice when using EMTSL:

1. Maintain a calm, quiet, warm environment. Use warmed sheets or blankets to wrap mother and baby together, skin-to-skin. This close contact, and the baby's eventual nuzzling at the breast, will stimulate oxytocin release, which may shorten the third stage and increase breast-feeding on discharge (Marín Gabriel et al 2010).

2. Maintain the woman in a comfortable, semi-upright position (at least a 45° angle) to encourage placental separation by maintaining a gentle downward weight.

3. Facilitate this time of parent–baby discovery and attachment by keeping quiet, observing from a distance and not interfering with the physiological processes.

4. Watch and wait. Take cues from the woman's behaviour; if she is alert and happy, examining the

baby and talking, she is not bleeding excessively or in need of any intervention. Reassurance can also be obtained from discretely checking the woman's pulse if there is any anxiety in, for example, a prolonged third stage.

5. Signs of placental separation:
   - The woman may fidget, make a face, or state that she has a contraction.
   - A large 'gush' of blood may follow, indicating partial or complete separation of the placenta. It usually ceases after 10–20 seconds, especially if the placenta has separated completely and the uterus has contracted well. This gush is larger than that seen when a uterotonic is given routinely, and midwives need to develop an understanding of this physiological blood loss and not rush to administer oxytocic treatment unnecessarily.

6. Signs of placental descent:
   - The woman may wriggle, change position, or complain of pressure, or a pain, in her back or bottom.
   - The cord may lengthen and/or the walls of the vulva may bulge as the placenta descends.
   - The uterus becomes hard, round and mobile (Fig. 18.5). This can be seen visually, or by the fact that the baby, resting on the mother's abdomen, has moved downwards. It is inadvisable to touch or manipulate the uterus at this stage, as this can prevent full contraction, disturb the fibrin mesh, and cause excessive bleeding. If there is concern that the uterus may be filling up with blood (a concealed haemorrhage), a gentle hand placed on the fundus will detect if there is a large, soft, uncontracted uterus.

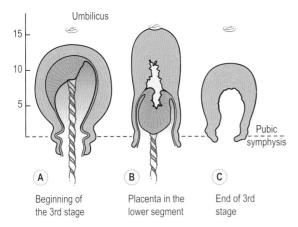

Fig. 18.5 Fundal height relative to the umbilicus and symphysis pubis.

7. Birthing the placenta:
   - Gravity should be used during the birth of the placenta by encouraging a truly upright position: sitting on a birthing stool, standing up in the birthing pool or on the birthing mat, walking out to the toilet, sitting on the toilet, kneeling upright or squatting over a bedpan. A basin, bin bag or disposable sheet can be placed strategically over, or in, the pan of the toilet to receive the placenta. It should be noted that such positions increase visible blood loss (Gupta and Nikodem 2002).
   - Maternal effort can be used to expedite expulsion, and most women will push the placenta out as soon as they feel pressure, with little effort.
   - The cord should be left unclamped until pulsation ceases (McDonald et al 2013), or until after the birth of the placenta, unless the mother wishes it to be cut earlier. Any mild resuscitation of the baby can be done at the site of birth, with the benefit of continued oxygen flow to the baby through the umbilical cord.
   - If the placenta is definitely separated and is sitting just inside the vagina (i.e., the insertion of the cord can be seen at the vulva, or the cord has lengthened and the vulval walls are bulging) the midwife may ease gently on the cord to help lift out the placenta. This is not controlled cord traction as no force is used, the placenta is separated and has left the uterus, therefore no counter-pressure is required on the abdomen as there is no risk of uterine inversion. *Controlled cord traction should NEVER be used in the absence of a well contracted uterus following uterotonic administration.*
   - Trailing membranes should be teased out gently, by turning the placenta around and twisting them into a 'rope', thus stripping the ends gently from the uterine wall.

8. At any time, a uterotonic may be administered to control haemorrhage, or if uterine tone is poor following placental birth. It is preferable to withhold administration until the placenta is delivered, if possible, to avoid the risk of a retained placenta when the uterus contracts strongly in response to the treatment.

This spontaneous process can take from 10 minutes to 1 hour to complete, with a median of 13 minutes (Begley 1990). If the placenta remains undelivered for a prolonged period, the risk of bleeding becomes greater because the uterus cannot contract down fully while the bulk of the placenta is in situ. Dombrowski et al (1995) found that the frequency of haemorrhage increased between 10 minutes and 40 minutes after the birth of the baby. However, patience and confidence not to interfere unnecessarily are required on the part of the midwife to secure a successful conclusion. Early attachment of the baby to the breast may enhance these physiological changes by stimulating the reflex release of oxytocin from the posterior lobe of the pituitary gland, which helps to secure good uterine action.

Active management of the third stage of labour (AMTSL)

An active management policy usually includes the routine prophylactic administration of a uterotonic agent, either intravenously, intramuscularly or (occasionally) orally, as a precautionary measure aimed at reducing the risk of postpartum haemorrhage. It is applied regardless of the assessed obstetric risk status of the woman, and is usually undertaken in conjunction with clamping of the umbilical cord shortly after birth of the baby and delivery of the placenta by the use of controlled cord traction. In situations where women may also be assessed as being at higher risk for PPH (e.g. multiple birth), a prophylactic infusion of larger doses of uterotonics diluted in intravenous solutions may be administered over several hours following the birth. This would also be considered to be part of an active management policy, as would routine uterine massage following delivery of the placenta in some countries (Jangsten et al 2011), although there is no evidence to support this practice once an oxytocic has been given (Hofmeyer et al 2013).

Active management in the third stage is the policy of third stage labour management most widely practised throughout the developed world. Like all interventions performed, skill in assisting the delivery of the placenta and membranes is extremely important to prevent complications. Whether women should routinely receive uterotonic drugs, have the umbilical cord clamped or be given assistance with placental delivery has been the subject of a great deal of debate and many research trials. These three aspects are considered separately here.

Administration of uterotonics

Uterotonics (also known as oxytocics, or ecbolics), are drugs (e.g. Syntometrine, Syntocinon, ergometrine and prostaglandins) that stimulate the smooth muscle of the uterus to contract. They may be administered with crowning of the baby's head, at the birth of the anterior shoulder of the baby, after the birth of the baby but prior to placental expulsion, or following the birth, or delivery, of the placenta and membranes.

In practice, one of the following uterotonic drugs is usually used.

Intravenous ergometrine 0.25–0.5 mg

This drug acts within 45 seconds, and is particularly useful in securing a rapid contraction where hypotonic uterine

action results in haemorrhage. If a doctor is not present in such an emergency, a midwife may give the injection, if it is within his/her scope of practice. There is no evidence for the continued *routine* use of intravenous ergometrine, which is associated with an increased risk of retained placenta (Prendiville et al 1988; Begley 1990), so this drug is more often used to treat a PPH rather than as a prophylactic drug. If an intravenous cannula is not already in situ, any difficulty encountered in locating a vein or sudden movement by the woman may result in failed venepuncture or at least a delay in administration. Ergometrine can cause headache, nausea, vomiting and an increase in blood pressure (Begley 1990) and it is contraindicated where there is a history of hypertensive disorder or cardiac disease (Dyer et al 2010). To decrease the chance of nausea and vomiting when the woman has had a caesarean section under epidural, it is advisable not to use ergometrine on its own (Balki and Carvalho 2005).

Combined ergometrine and oxytocin (a commonly used brand is Syntometrine)

A 1 ml ampoule contains 5 IU of oxytocin and 0.5 mg ergometrine and is administered by i.m. injection. The oxytocin acts within $2\frac{1}{2}$ min, and the ergometrine within 6–7 min (Fig. 18.6). Their combined action results in a rapid uterine contraction enhanced by a stronger, more sustained contraction lasting several hours. It can be administered as the anterior shoulder of the baby is born, or after the birth of the baby. The use of combined ergometrine/oxytocin or any ergometrine-based drug is associated with side-effects such as elevation of blood pressure, nausea and vomiting (Begley 1990). The most recent report on maternal deaths from the Centre for Maternal and Child Enquiries in the UK states that 'Syntometrine should be avoided as a routine drug completely' (CMACE 2011: 69).

CAUTION: No more than two doses of ergometrine 0.5 mg should be given, due to its side-effects.

Oxytocin

Oxytocin (a commonly used brand is Syntocinon) is a synthetic form of the natural oxytocin produced in the

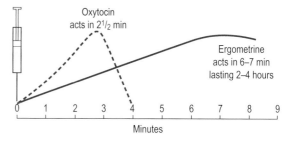

Fig. 18.6 The rapid action of oxytocin in comparison with ergometrine.

posterior pituitary, and is safe to use in a wider context than combined ergometrine/oxytocin agents. It can be administered as an intravenous and or intramuscular injection. However, an intravenous bolus of oxytocin can cause profound, fatal hypotension, especially in the presence of cardiovascular compromise. The recommendation of the Confidential Enquiry in Maternal Deaths (Lewis and Drife 2001: 21) is that 'when given as an intravenous bolus the drug should be given slowly in a dose of not more than 5 IU'.

Research evidence to date suggests that oxytocin is an effective uterotonic choice where routine prophylactic management of the third stage of labour is practised (Khan et al 1995; Cotter et al 2001; Choy et al 2002), more specifically in women who experience a blood loss exceeding 1000 ml. Two Cochrane reviews have suggested that it is probably better to use oxytocin rather than ergometrine, due to the side-effects of ergot (Cotter et al 2001; Liabsuetrakul et al 2007).

Carbetocin, originally developed for veterinary use and not widely employed for prophylactic use in management of the third stage, is a long-acting synthetic oxytocin analogue which can be administered as a single-dose 100 mg injection. Carbetocin has been shown in some trials to be as effective as oxytocin in preventing PPH (Reyes et al 2011; Su et al 2012); however, it does require refrigeration for stability.

Prostaglandins

The use of prostaglandins for third stage management has up until now been more often associated with the treatment of postpartum haemorrhage than with prophylaxis. This may be partly due to prostaglandin agents being more expensive and associated with side-effects, such as diarrhoea (Anderson and Etches 2007) and cardiovascular complications of increased stroke volume and heart rate (van Selm et al 1995).

In more recent years, a great deal of research time and investment has been invested in seeking alternate ways of implementing strategies to reduce the risk of PPH. Misoprostol (a prostaglandin E1 analogue) was first used to treat gastric ulcers, but when its potential as a uterotonic agent was discovered, optimism regarding its suitability in low resource settings was high. It is cheap, not prone to loss of potency, does not need to be sterile or refrigerated and can be administered vaginally, orally or rectally, negating the need for syringes. Misoprostol orally or sublingually (400–600 µg) appears to be a useful drug to prevent PPH, but is not as effective as Syntocinon (Ng et al 2007; Tunçalp et al 2012) and has unpleasant side-effects, such as severe shivering and higher temperature, both of which are transient but unacceptable to some women. Its use appears to be no more likely than Syntocinon to necessitate manual removal of the placenta. Even though the recommendation of the latest Cochrane review is that misoprostol should not replace other uterotonics, the

authors suggest that it may be useful in circumstances where nothing else is available (Tunçalp et al 2012).

Clamping of the umbilical cord

This may, necessarily, be carried out following birth of the baby's head if the cord is tightly around the neck; however, it is preferable, and usually possible, to loosen the loop and slip it over the baby's head, then allow the baby's body to slip out beside the loop. If the cord is looped several times around the neck it will be possible to gently tighten one, or more, of the loops of cord and then ease a looser loop over the baby's head. In this way, the baby's oxygen supply is not cut off prematurely, which could be very detrimental to their condition. If this is not successful, the midwife can be ready to clamp and cut the cord just as the woman starts a contraction, so that the oxygen supply is cut off only just before the birth.

Early clamping of the cord, as part of active management of the third stage of labour (AMTSL), is normally applied in the first 30 seconds to 3 minutes after birth, regardless of whether or not cord pulsation has ceased. It has been suggested that this practice may have the following effects:

- It may reduce the volume of blood returning to the fetus by an amount between 75 and 125 ml (van Rheenen and Brabin 2004; Farrar et al 2011), which is 30–40% of total potential blood volume (Farrar et al 2011).
- It may prematurely interrupt the respiratory function of the placenta in maintaining O_2 levels and combating acidosis in the early moments of life. This may be of particular importance in a baby who is slow to breathe.
- It may result in lower neonatal bilirubin levels, although the effect on the incidence of clinical jaundice is unclear (McDonald et al 2013).
- It may increase the likelihood of fetomaternal transfusion as a larger volume of blood remains in the placenta. Venous pressure is further increased as retraction continues and may be sufficiently high to rupture surface placental vessels, thus facilitating the transfer of fetal cells into the maternal system; this may be a critical factor where the mother's blood group is Rhesus negative (see Chapter 10).
- It results in the truncated umbilical vessels containing a quantity of clotted blood, which provides an ideal medium for bacterial growth; as this is near to, and has a patent opening into, the baby's abdomen there is potential for systemic infection (Mercer et al 2006).
- Heavier placental weight has also been associated with early cord clamping (Newton et al 1961), which may cause difficulty with delivery of the placenta, particularly when the cervix has contracted following administration of a uterotonic.

Proponents of late clamping suggest that no action be taken until cord pulsation ceases or the placenta has been completely delivered, thus allowing the physiological processes to take place without intervention. Suggested advantages of late clamping include:

- The route to the low resistance placental circulation remains patent, which provides the newborn with a safety valve for any raised systemic blood pressure. This may be critical when the baby is preterm or asphyxiated, as raised pulmonary and central venous pressures may exacerbate the difficulties in initiating respiration and accompanying circulatory adaptation (Dunn 1985).
- The transfusion of the full quota of placental blood to the newborn. This may constitute as much as 30–40% of the circulating volume (Farrar et al 2011), depending on when the cord is clamped and at what level the baby is held prior to clamping and may therefore be important in maintaining haematocrit levels.
- The neonatal effects associated with increased placental transfusion include higher mean birth weight by 87–116 g (Farrar et al 2011) and higher neonatal haematocrit accompanied by an increase in the incidence of jaundice in term (McDonald et al 2013) and preterm babies (Rabe et al 2012). There is growing evidence that delaying cord clamping confers improved iron status in infants up to 6 months post-birth (Chaparro et al 2006; Mercer 2006; Hutton and Hassan 2007; Rabe et al 2012; McDonald et al 2013).
- Delayed cord clamping in preterm babies (until at least 30–120 seconds) is associated with babies requiring fewer transfusions, and having a lower risk of developing necrotizing enterocolitis or intraventricular haemorrhage (Rabe et al 2012).
- Delayed cord clamping may decrease the risk of fetomaternal transfusion, which is important in women with Rhesus-negative blood (Wiberg et al 2008).

Given the benefits of delayed cord clamping and the documented harms caused by early clamping, many centres have now stopped using early cord clamping as part of their active management package (Afaifel and Weeks 2012).

The actual action to take when clamping the cord early is to place one clamp (usually a disposable plastic one) close to the baby's navel end. Care should be taken to apply the clamp 3–4 cm clear of the abdominal wall, to avoid pinching the skin or clamping a portion of gut, which, in rare instances, may be in the cord. A greater length of cord is left when umbilical vessels are needed for transfusion, for example in preterm babies and cases of Rhesus haemolytic disease. The second clamp is placed closer to the placental end of the cord, with approximately 2–4 cm between them. The cord between the two clamps is then cut, while shielding personnel from blood spurts with a gloved hand. The baby may then be placed on the mother's abdomen, put to the breast or be more closely examined on a warmed cot if resuscitation is required.

There is very little evidence concerning how much, if any, of a uterotonic agent the baby receives following birth, through an intact cord. In five documented cases of accidental administration of an adult dose of Syntometrine to a newborn infant, no long-term adverse effects were reported (Whitfield and Salfield 1980). If the cord is clamped and cut soon after birth, the midwife should release the second clamp and drain blood from the maternal end of the cord to simulate placental–fetal transfusion, as this may reduce maternal blood loss up to 77 ml and shorten the third stage by up to 3 minutes (Soltani et al 2011).

Delivery of the placenta and membranes

Controlled cord traction (CCT)

Recent research has shown that this manoeuvre has no effect on severe haemorrhage (>1000 ml) and little, if any, effect on mild PPH (>500 ml) in both high (Deneux-Tharaux et al 2013) and low income settings (Gülmezoglu et al 2012). It does, however, shorten the third stage of labour by 6 minutes (Gülmezoglu et al 2012). This means that, in developing countries in particular, oxytocin can be given by healthcare workers, without the need to train them in safe utilization of CCT (Gülmezoglu et al 2012), providing that they are taught to avoid manipulating the uterus or pulling on the cord.

If CCT is to be used successfully, the principles of placental separation described at the beginning of this chapter should be clearly understood. Before proceeding, the midwife should check:

- that a uterotonic drug has been administered
- that it has been given time to act
- that the uterus is well contracted
- that counter-traction is applied
- that signs of placental separation and descent are present.

At the beginning of the third stage, a strong uterine contraction results in the fundus being palpable below the umbilicus (see Fig. 18.5). It feels broad as the placenta is still in the upper segment. As the placenta separates and falls into the lower uterine segment there is a small fresh blood loss, the cord lengthens, and the fundus becomes rounder, smaller and more mobile as it rises in the abdomen above the level of the placenta.

It is important not to manipulate the uterus in any way as this may precipitate incoordinate action. No further step should be taken until a strong contraction is palpable. If tension is applied to the umbilical cord without this contraction, uterine inversion may occur. This is an acute

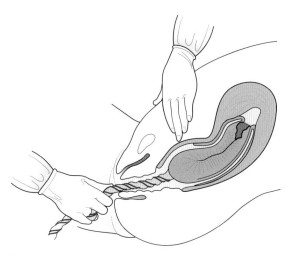

Fig. 18.7 Controlled cord traction.

obstetric emergency with life-threatening implications for the mother (see Chapter 22), and was implicated in one maternal death in the UK in the period 2006–2008 (CMACE 2011).

Once the uterus is found to be contracted, one hand is placed above the level of the symphysis pubis with the palm facing towards the umbilicus, exerting pressure in an upwards direction. This is counter-traction. The other hand, firmly grasping the cord, applies traction in a downward and backward direction following the line of the birth canal (Fig. 18.7). Some resistance may be felt but it is important to apply steady tension by pulling the cord firmly and maintaining the pressure. Jerky movements and force should be avoided. The aim is to complete the action as one continuous, smooth, controlled movement. However, it is only possible to exert this tension for a short time as it may be an uncomfortable procedure for the mother and the midwife's hand will tire.

Downward traction on the cord must be released before uterine counter-traction is relaxed as sudden withdrawal of counter-traction while tension is still being applied to the cord may also facilitate uterine inversion. If the manoeuvre is not immediately successful there should be a pause before the uterine contraction is again checked and a further attempt is made. Should the uterus relax, tension is temporarily released until a good contraction is again palpable. Once the placenta is visible it may be cupped in the hands to ease pressure on the friable membranes. A gentle upward and downward movement or twisting action will help to coax out the membranes and increase the chances of delivering them intact. Artery forceps may be applied to gradually ease the membranes out of the vagina. This process should not be hurried; great care should be taken to avoid tearing the membranes.

Is the timing of uterotonic administration, cord clamping and/or CCT clinically important in influencing the incidence of PPH?

Although active management leads to reduced risk of PPH, it is important to establish which of the components of this package lead(s) to this reduction. Given the difficulties of adhering to an active management policy, the absence of uterotonics in low resource countries, and the preferences of some women for physiological management, it is important to explore practice behaviours to clarify whether or not the policy, as it is currently practised, should continue.

Whether oxytocin is administered before or after the placenta is expelled does not appear to make any significant difference to the incidence of PPH (blood loss >500 ml and >1000 ml), maternal hypotension, retained placenta, length of third stage, mean blood loss, maternal haemoglobin, need for maternal blood transfusion or therapeutic uterotonics (Soltani et al 2010).

Similarly, CCT has no effect on severe haemorrhage (>1000 ml) and little, if any, effect on mild PPH (>500 ml) (Gülmezoglu et al 2012). Given the emerging evidence on the benefits of delaying cord clamping (McDonald et al 2013), it is now reasonable to suggest an active management package that includes cord clamping after 3 minutes, followed by administration of oxytocin (either before or after the birth of the placenta) and either maternal effort or controlled cord traction to expel the placenta once separation occurs. As AMTSL has not been implemented in that first 3 or more minutes, the principles of care described for expectant care during the third stage should be followed in that period.

Evidence for active versus expectant management

There is an increasing amount of appropriate, rigorously conducted research evidence available that suggests that the prophylactic administration of a uterotonic significantly reduces the risk of PPH, results in a lower mean blood loss, fewer blood transfusions are required and there is a reduced need for therapeutic uterotonics (Begley et al 2011). It has also been highlighted by the widely ranging 'risk status' of women included in several studies that it is in fact very difficult to define a group of women who are not at risk for PPH. However, women truly at 'low risk' for PPH do not appear to suffer undue harm from EMTSL (Begley et al 2011; Dixon et al 2011), and this should remain an option for care (NICE [National Institute for Health and Clinical Excellence] 2007). Midwifery students should be given the opportunity to assist at births using EMTSL, to learn and develop their skills, as 'knowledge of physiological management of the third stage of labour is considered a basic midwifery competency' by the International Confederation of Midwives (ICM 2008).

It should be noted that the care pathway, whether active or expectant, is reliant on all components of the pathway being carried out as recommended. For example, if management is expectant, then the introduction of a uterotonic drug, cord clamping or pulling on the cord will disrupt the intended sequence of the care process leading to what is often described as a fragmented approach. Once the sequence of the processes is altered, the clinician should commit to completing the process. That is, if the protocol for expectant management is interrupted the clinician should proceed to completing the process with an active management approach. This practice has been shown to reduce the incidence of PPH significantly in a birth centre setting (Patterson 2005).

Asepsis

The need for asepsis is even greater now than in the preceding stages of labour. Laceration and bruising of the cervix, vagina, perineum and vulva provide a route for the entry of microorganisms. At the placental site, a raw surface provides an ideal medium for infection. Strict attention to the prevention of infection is therefore vital.

Cord blood sampling

This may be required for a variety of conditions:
- when the mother's blood group is Rhesus negative or as a precautionary measure if the mother's Rhesus type is unknown;
- when atypical maternal antibodies have been found during an antenatal screening test;
- where a haemoglobinopathy is suspected (e.g. sickle cell disease);
- 'when there has been concern about the baby either in labour or immediately following birth' (NICE 2007:231).

The sample should be taken as soon as possible from the fetal surface of the placenta where the blood vessels are congested and easily visible. If the cord has not been clamped prior to placental birth the fetal vessels will not be congested, but a sample of sufficient volume may still be easily obtained, or can be taken by syringe prior to birth of the placenta. In the case of paired cord blood sampling being required for reasons outlined by NICE (2007), blood will be obtained from the umbilical cord. To achieve this, an additional clamp will need to be applied resulting in double-clamping of the cord. The appropriate containers should be used for any investigations requested. These may include the baby's blood group, Rhesus type, haemoglobin estimation, serum bilirubin level, cord blood analysis for acid base status, Coombs' test or electrophoresis.

Maternal blood for Kleihauer testing can be taken upon completion of the third stage.

COMPLETION OF THE THIRD STAGE

Once the placenta has spontaneously birthed, or has been delivered, the midwife must first check that the uterus is well contracted and fresh blood loss is minimal. Careful inspection of the perineum and lower vagina is important. A strong light is directed onto the perineum in order to assess trauma accurately prior to instigating repair. This should be carried out as gently as possible as the tissues are often bruised and oedematous. If perineal suturing (see Chapter 15) is required it should be carried out as expediently as possible to prevent unnecessary blood loss, increased risk of oedema at the site of trauma and perhaps unnecessary re-infiltration of additional local anaesthetics.

Blood loss estimation

Blood loss is difficult to measure and is frequently underestimated (Duthie et al 1990; Prastertcharoensuk et al 2000). Account must be taken of blood that has soaked into linen and swabs as well as measurable fluid loss and clot formation. The site of the blood loss does not necessarily alter the impact in terms of potential debility for affected women. Brandt (1966) believes that women can withstand perhaps a 1000–1500 ml blood loss. However, any further blood loss may not be tolerated so readily. Women who undergo elective caesarean section will for the most part have been adequately prepared. Women who undergo emergency caesarean section or vaginal birth who are dehydrated or anaemic may not withstand sudden large volumes of blood loss.

In his study of the importance and difficulties of precise estimation of PPH, Brandt (1967) calculated that 20% of women lose >500 ml of blood after a vaginal birth. It was estimated that 3940 ml of circulating blood volume were required to maintain the central venous pressure at 10 cmH$_2$O. Most measurement techniques are not sufficiently sensitive to detect a rapid volume change in the immediate setting when decisions need to be made.

Note: It should also be remembered that any amount of blood loss that causes a physical deterioration such as feeling faint, sudden onset of tachycardia, altered respirations or drop in blood pressure should be immediately investigated.

Examination of placenta and membranes

This should be performed as soon after birth as practicable so that, if there is doubt about their completeness, further

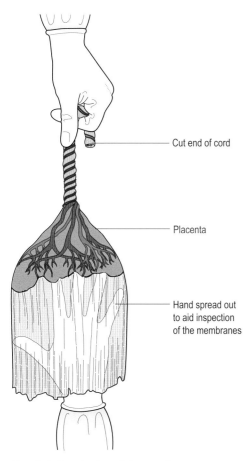

Cut end of cord

Placenta

Hand spread out
to aid inspection
of the membranes

Fig. 18.8 Examination of the membranes.

action may be taken before the woman leaves the birth room or the midwife leaves the home. A thorough inspection must be carried out in order to make sure that no part of the placenta or membranes has been retained. The membranes are the most difficult to examine as they become torn during the birth or delivery and may be ragged. Every attempt should be made to piece them together to give an overall picture of completeness. This is easier to see if the placenta is held by the cord, allowing the membranes to hang. The hole through which the baby was born can then usually be identified and a hand can be spread out inside the membranes to aid inspection (Fig. 18.8). The placenta should then be laid on a flat surface and both placental surfaces minutely examined in a good light. The amnion should be peeled from the chorion right up to the umbilical cord, which allows the chorion to be fully viewed.

Any clots on the maternal surface need to be removed and kept for measuring. Broken fragments of cotyledon must be carefully replaced before an accurate assessment is possible.

The lobes of a complete placenta fit neatly together without any gaps, the edges forming a uniform circle. Blood vessels should not radiate beyond the placental edge. If they do, this denotes a succenturiate lobe, which has developed separately from the main placenta (see Chapter 6). When such a lobe is visible there is no cause for concern, but if the tissue has been retained the vessels will end abruptly at a hole in the membrane. If there is any suspicion that the placenta or membranes are incomplete, they must be kept for inspection and a doctor informed immediately in case a PPH occurs or there is the possibility that a surgical intervention may be required.

Upon completion of the examination, the midwife should return her attention to the mother. The empty uterus should be firmly contracted and below the level of the umbilicus. If the fundus has risen in the abdomen a blood clot may be present. This should be expelled while the uterus is in a state of contraction by pressing the fundus gently in a downward and backward direction – with due regard to the risk of inversion and acute discomfort to the woman. Force should never be used.

Immediate care

It is advisable for mother and baby to remain in the midwife's care for at least 1 hour after birth, regardless of the birth setting. Much of this time will be spent in clearing up and completion of records but careful observation of mother and infant is very important. If an epidural catheter is in situ it is usually removed and checked at this time. Early physiological observations including ensuring a well-contracted uterus, assessment of vaginal blood loss and a gentle inspection of the genital tract to inspect for trauma should be undertaken (NICE 2007).

The woman should be encouraged to pass urine because a full bladder may impede uterine contraction. She may not actually feel an urge to do so, especially if she has passed urine immediately prior to giving birth or an effective epidural has been in progress, but she should be asked to try. Uterine contraction and blood loss should be checked on several occasions during this first hour. Once basic procedures to ensure the woman's and baby's safety and comfort have been completed, the woman may be offered a light meal such as tea and toast.

Most women intending to breastfeed will wish to put their babies to the breast during these early moments of contact. This is especially advantageous, as babies are usually very alert at this time and their sucking reflex is particularly strong. There is also evidence to suggest that women who breastfeed soon after birth successfully breastfeed for a longer period of time (Salariya et al 1979). An additional benefit lies in the reflex release of oxytocin from the posterior lobe of the pituitary gland, which stimulates the uterus to contract. This may result in the mother experiencing a sudden fresh blood loss as the uterus empties and she should be pre-warned and reassured that it is a normal response. The desire to feed a newborn baby is a warm, loving and instinctive response. While breastfeeding should be actively encouraged, a formula feed should be available for those who do not wish to breastfeed.

Record-keeping

A complete and accurate account of the labour, including the documentation of the administration of all medicines, physical examination and observations, is the midwife's responsibility. This should also include details of examination of the placenta, membranes and cord with attention drawn to any abnormalities. The volume of blood loss is particularly important. This record not only provides information that may be critical in the future care of both mother and infant but is a legal document that may be used as evidence of the care given. Signatures are therefore essential, with cosignatories where necessary. In the UK, many mothers now carry their own notes related to pregnancy and details of the birth. The completed records are a vital communication link between the midwife responsible for the birth and other caregivers, particularly those who take over care and provide ongoing community support services once the woman returns home.

It is usually the midwife who completes the birth notification form. Timely notification and referral may prevent delay in a woman receiving appropriate assistance should she need it.

Transfer from the birth room

The midwife is responsible for seeing that all observations are made and recorded prior to transfer of mother and baby to the postnatal ward, or home, or before the midwife leaves the home following the birth.

The postnatal ward midwife should verify these details prior to transfer of mother and baby. Following a domiciliary birth, the midwife should leave details of a telephone number where she may be contacted should the parents feel any cause for concern.

COMPLICATIONS OF THE THIRD STAGE

Postpartum haemorrhage

Primary postpartum haemorrhage is defined as bleeding from the genital tract in excess of 500 ml at any time following the baby's birth up to 24 hours postpartum (WHO 2003). A loss of 500–999 ml in a healthy woman is considered a mild PPH, and severe haemorrhage is deemed to be a loss of greater than 1000 ml (Bloomfield and Gordon 1990).

Postpartum haemorrhage (PPH) is one of the most alarming and serious emergencies a midwife may face and can occur following both traumatic and straightforward births. It is always a stressful experience for the woman and any support persons present and may undermine her confidence, influence her attitude to future childbearing and delay her recovery. Although the maternal mortality rate (MMR) in developed countries such as those of Western Europe, Australasia, North America and Japan is quoted as approximately 7, 6, 16 and 7 per 100 000 live births respectively (Hogan et al 2010), the reported MMR for lower resource countries is much higher; for example, southern Asia with 323 per 100 000 live births, and sub-Saharan Africa (west) with 629 per 100 000 live births (Hogan et al 2010). A significant number of the deaths recorded were due to PPH, often in the absence of a trained health professional. The midwife is often the first, and may be the only, professional person present when a haemorrhage occurs, so her prompt, competent action will be crucial in controlling blood loss and reducing the risk of maternal morbidity or even death.

Primary postpartum haemorrhage

Fluid loss is extremely difficult to measure with any degree of accuracy, especially when a mixture of blood and fluid has soaked into the bed linen and spilled onto the floor. It should also be remembered that measurable solidified clots represent only about half the total fluid loss. With these factors in mind, the best yardstick is that any blood loss, however small, that adversely affects the mother's condition constitutes a PPH. Much will therefore depend upon the woman's general wellbeing. In addition, if the measured loss reaches 500 ml, it must be treated as a PPH, irrespective of maternal condition; however, it should be noted that in high income countries, and in a woman who is otherwise healthy with a high haemoglobin, a blood loss of 500 ml is the equivalent of a routine blood donation and usually causes no ill effects.

Causes

There are several reasons why a PPH may occur, including atonic uterus, retained placenta, trauma and blood coagulation disorder.

Atonic uterus

This is a failure of the myometrium at the placental site to contract and retract and to compress torn blood vessels and control blood loss by a living ligature action. When the placenta is attached, the volume of blood flow at the placental site is approximately 500–800 ml/min. Upon separation, the efficient contraction and retraction of uterine muscle will staunch the flow and prevent a haemorrhage, which can otherwise ensue with horrifying speed (Box 18.1).

Box 18.1 **Causes of atonic uterine action**

- Incomplete separation of the placenta
- Retained cotyledon, placental fragment or membranes
- Precipitate labour
- Prolonged labour resulting in uterine inertia
- Polyhydramnios or multiple pregnancy causing overdistension of uterine muscle
- Placenta praevia
- Placental abruption
- General anaesthesia especially halothane or cyclopropane
- Episiotomy or perineal trauma
- Induction or augmentation of labour with oxytocin
- A full bladder
- Aetiology unknown

Incomplete placental separation

If the placenta remains fully adherent to the uterine wall, it is unlikely to cause bleeding. However, once separation has begun, maternal vessels are torn. If placental tissue remains partially embedded in the spongy decidua, efficient contraction and retraction are interrupted.

Retained placenta, cotyledon, placental fragment or membranes

These will similarly impede efficient uterine action (Sosa et al 2009).

Precipitate labour

When the uterus has contracted vigorously and frequently, resulting in a duration of labour that is less than 1 hour, then the muscle may have insufficient opportunity to retract.

Prolonged labour

In a labour where the active phase lasts >12 hours uterine inertia (sluggishness) may result from muscle exhaustion (Chapter 19).

Polyhydramnios, macrosomia or multiple pregnancy

The myometrium becomes excessively stretched and therefore less efficient (Sosa et al 2009).

Placenta praevia

The placental site is partly or wholly in the lower segment where the thinner muscle layer contains few oblique fibres: this results in poor control of bleeding.

Placental abruption

Blood may have seeped between the muscle fibres, interfering with effective action. At its most severe this results in a Couvelaire uterus (Chapter 12).

Induction or augmentation of labour with oxytocin

In some circumstances, the use of oxytocin during labour may result in hyperstimulation of the uterus and cause a precipitate, expulsive birth of the baby (Sosa et al 2009; Grotegut et al 2011). In this instance the uterus may still be responding in a stimulated, but ineffective manner in terms of contracting the empty uterus. In the case of induction or augmentation of labour, that continues over a prolonged period without establishing efficient uterine contractions, physical and emotional fatigue of the mother, and uterine fatigue or inertia may occur. This inertia inhibits the uterine muscle from providing strong, sustained contraction and retraction of the empty uterus that aids in the prevention of a postpartum haemorrhage.

Episiotomy, and need for perineal sutures

Blood loss from perineal trauma, in addition to even a normal blood loss from the uterus, can together equal a mild PPH (Sosa et al 2009). Poeschmann et al (1991) have shown that an episiotomy can cause up to 30% of postpartum blood loss.

General anaesthesia

Anaesthetic agents may cause uterine relaxation, in particular the volatile inhalational agents, for example halothane.

Mismanagement of the third stage of labour

'Fundus fiddling' or manipulation of the uterus may precipitate arrhythmic contractions so that the placenta only partially separates and retraction is lost.

A full bladder

If the bladder is full, its proximity to the uterus in the abdomen on completion of the second stage may interfere with uterine action. This also constitutes mismanagement.

Aetiology unknown

A precipitating cause may never be discovered.

There are in addition a number of factors that do not directly cause a PPH, but do increase the likelihood of excessive bleeding (Box 18.2).

Previous history of PPH or retained placenta

There may be a risk of recurrence in subsequent pregnancies, depending on the cause of the PPH in the previous birth. A detailed obstetric history taken at the first antenatal visit will ensure that optimum care can be given.

Fibroids (fibromyomata)

These are normally benign tumours consisting of muscle and fibrous tissue, which may impede efficient uterine action.

Anaemia

Women who enter labour with reduced haemoglobin concentration (below 10 g/dl) may feel a greater effect of any subsequent blood loss, however small. Moderate to severe anaemia (<9 g/dl) is associated with an increase in third stage blood loss and risk of postpartum haemorrhage (Kavle et al 2008; Soltan et al 2012).

HIV/AIDS

Women who have HIV/AIDS are often in a state of severe immunosuppression, which lowers the platelet count to such a degree that even a relatively minor blood loss may cause severe morbidity or death.

Ketosis

The influence of ketosis upon uterine action is still unclear. Foulkes and Dumoulin (1983) demonstrated that, in a series of 3500 women, 40% had ketonuria at some time during labour. They reported that if labour progressed well, this did not appear to jeopardize either the fetal or maternal condition. However, there was a significant relationship between ketosis and the need for oxytocin augmentation, instrumental delivery and PPH when labour lasted more than 12 hours. Correction of ketosis is therefore advisable and can be facilitated by ensuring women have an adequate intake of fluids and light solid nourishment as tolerated throughout labour. There is no evidence to suggest restriction of food or fluids is necessary during the normal course of labour (Singata et al 2010).

Caesarean section

It should be noted that, of the five women who died of postpartum haemorrhage in the UK in the period 2006–2008, four of them had had a caesarean section (the fifth concealed her pregnancy and died alone at home) (CMACE 2011). The report noted that in three of the four women (75%), a lack of routine observation of vital signs in the postoperative period, or failure on the part of staff to notice that bleeding was occurring, were key failures in care. Postoperative observations need to be recorded regularly, using a modified early obstetric warning score (MEOWS) chart, and abnormal findings acted upon (CMACE 2011).

Signs of PPH

Signs may be obvious, such as:
- visible bleeding
- maternal collapse.

However, more subtle signs may present, such as:
- pallor
- rising pulse rate
- falling blood pressure
- altered level of consciousness; the mother may become restless or drowsy
- an enlarged uterus as it fills with blood or blood clot; it feels 'boggy' on palpation (i.e. soft and distended and lacking tone); there may be little or no visible loss of blood.

Prophylaxis

By using the above list, it is possible for the midwife to apply some preventive screening in an attempt to identify women who may be at greater risk and to recognize causative factors. During the antenatal period a thorough and accurate history of previous obstetric experiences will identify possible risk factors. Arrangements for birth can be discussed with the woman, and the necessity for birth to take place in a unit where facilities for dealing with emergencies are available can be explained. The early detection and treatment of anaemia will help ensure that women enter labour with a haemoglobin level, ideally, in excess of 10 g/dl. The midwife should check that blood tests, if needed, are taken regularly and the results recorded and explained to the woman. If necessary, action can be taken to restore the haemoglobin level before birth. Women more prone to anaemia should be closely monitored, e.g. those with multiple pregnancies.

During labour, good management practices during the first and second stages are important to prevent prolonged labour and ketoacidosis. A mother should not enter the second or third stage with a full bladder. AMTSL is recommended for all women at high risk of PPH, and will reduce blood loss for women of mixed risk (Begley et al 2011). Two units of cross-matched blood should be kept available for any woman known to have a placenta praevia or other major predisposing risk factors for PPH.

Treatment of PPH

Whatever the stage of labour or crisis that may occur, the midwife should adhere to the underlying principle of always reassuring the woman and her support persons by continually relaying appropriate information and involving them in decision-making.

Three basic principles of care should be applied immediately upon observation of excessive bleeding, using the mnemonic ABC:

1. Call for medical **A**id.
2. Stop the **B**leeding by rubbing up a contraction, giving a uterotonic and emptying the uterus.
3. Resus**C**itate the mother as necessary.

Call for medical aid

This is an important initial step so that help is on the way whatever transpires. If the bleeding is brought under control before the doctor arrives, then no action by the doctor will be needed. However, the woman's condition can deteriorate very rapidly, in which case medical assistance will be required urgently. If the mother is at home or in a midwife-led unit, the emergency department of the closest obstetric unit should be contacted and, depending on the policy of the region, an obstetric emergency team summoned or ambulance transfer arranged.

Stop the bleeding

The initial action is always the same, regardless of whether bleeding occurs with the placenta in situ or later.

Rub up a contraction

The fundus is first felt gently with the fingertips to assess its consistency. If it is soft and relaxed, the fundus is massaged with a smooth, circular motion, applying no undue pressure. When a contraction occurs, the hand is held still.

Give a uterotonic to sustain the contraction

In many instances, oxytocin 5 units or 10 units, or combined ergometrine/oxytocin 1 ml, has already been administered and this may be repeated. Alternatively, ergometrine 0.25–0.5 mg may be injected intravenously (in the absence of contraindications), and will be effective within 45 seconds; vomiting may occur immediately. No more than two doses of ergometrine should be given (including any dose of combined ergometrine/oxytocin), as it may cause pulmonary hypertension. Several reports have described the dramatic haemostatic effects of prostaglandins used in cases of uterine atony. Misoprostol (Cytotec) or carboprost (Hemabate) are the most common prostaglandin drugs used to increase uterine contractility for the treatment of PPH. However, the side-effects (nausea, vomiting, pyrexia, hypertension, diarrhoea) associated with these drugs can make their use limited (Anderson and Etches 2007).

The baby may be put to the breast to enhance the physiological secretion of oxytocin from the posterior lobe of the pituitary gland, thus stimulating a contraction.

Empty the uterus

Once the midwife is satisfied that it is well contracted, she should ensure that the uterus is emptied. If the placenta is still in the uterus, it should be delivered; if it has been expelled, any clots should be expressed by firm but gentle pressure on the fundus.

Resuscitate the mother

An intravenous infusion should be commenced while peripheral veins are easily negotiated. This will provide a route for an oxytocin infusion or fluid replacement. As an emergency measure, the mother's legs may be lifted up in order to allow blood to drain from them into the central circulation. However, the foot of the bed should not be raised as this encourages pooling of blood in the uterus, which prevents the uterus contracting.

It is usually expedient to catheterize the bladder to ensure that a full bladder is not impeding uterine contraction and thus precipitating further bleeding, and to minimize trauma should an operative procedure be necessary.

On no account must a woman in a collapsed condition be moved prior to resuscitation and stabilization.

The flow chart in Fig. 18.9 briefly sets out the possible courses of action that may be taken depending on whether or not bleeding persists. If the above measures are successful in controlling any further loss, administration of oxytocin, 40 units in 1 litre of intravenous solution (e.g. Hartmann's or saline) infused slowly over 8–12 hours, will ensure continued uterine contraction. This will help to minimize the risk of recurrence. Before the infusion is connected, 10 ml of blood should be withdrawn for haemoglobin estimation and for cross-matching compatible blood. If bleeding continues uncontrolled, the choice of further action will depend largely upon whether the placenta remains undelivered.

Placenta delivered

If the uterus is atonic following birth of the placenta, light fundal pressure may be used to expel residual clots while a contraction is present. If an effective contraction is not maintained, 40 units of Syntocinon in 1 litre of intravenous fluid should be started. The placenta and membranes must be re-examined for completeness because retained fragments are often responsible for uterine atony and may need to be removed manually, under anaesthetic.

Bimanual compression

If bleeding continues, bimanual compression of the uterus may be necessary in order to apply pressure to the placental site. It is desirable for an intravenous infusion to be in

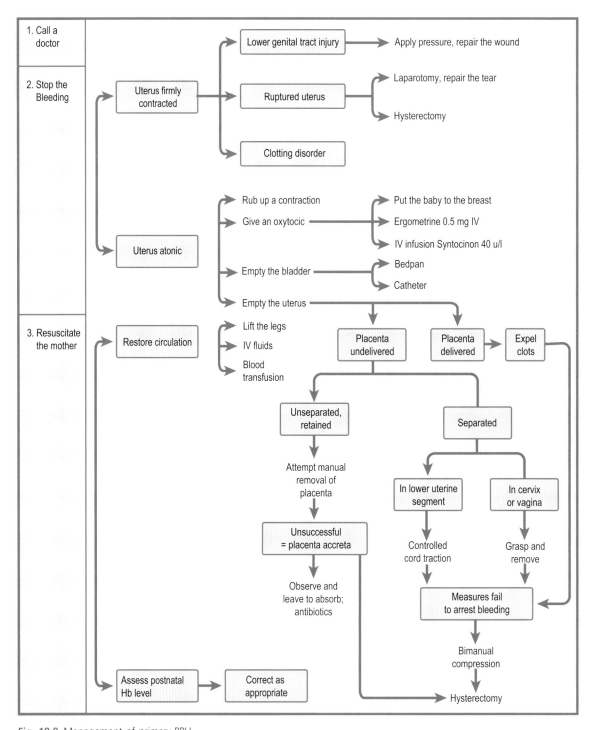

Fig. 18.9 Management of primary PPH.

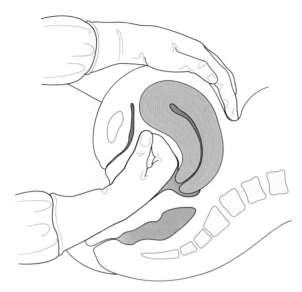

Fig. 18.10 Bimanual compression of the uterus.

progress. The fingers of one hand are inserted into the vagina like a cone; the hand is formed into a fist and placed into the anterior vaginal fornix, the elbow resting on the bed. The other hand is placed behind the uterus abdominally, the fingers pointing towards the cervix. The uterus is brought forwards and compressed between the palm of the hand positioned abdominally and the fist in the vagina (Fig. 18.10). If bleeding persists, a clotting disorder must be excluded before exploration of the vagina and uterus is performed under a general anaesthetic. Compression balloons may also be used to provide pressure on the placental site and if bleeding continues, ligation of the uterine arteries or hysterectomy may be considered.

Placenta undelivered

The placenta may be partially or wholly adherent.

Partially adherent

When the uterus is well contracted, an attempt should be made to deliver the placenta by applying CCT. If this is unsuccessful a doctor will be required to remove it manually.

Wholly adherent

Bleeding does not usually occur if the placenta is completely adherent. However, the longer the placenta remains in situ the greater is the risk of partial separation, which may give rise to profuse haemorrhage.

Retained placenta

This diagnosis is reached when the placenta remains undelivered after a specified period of time (usually 1 hour

following the baby's birth). The conventional treatment is to separate the placenta from the uterine wall digitally, effecting a manual removal.

Breaking of the cord

This is a not unusual occurrence during completion of the third stage of labour. Before further action, it is crucial to check that the uterus remains firmly contracted. If the placenta remains adherent, no further action should be taken before a doctor is notified. It is possible that manual removal may be indicated. If the placenta is palpable in the vagina, it is probable that separation has occurred and when the uterus is well contracted then maternal effort, with a fully upright posture, may be encouraged (see expectant management, above). If there is any doubt, the midwife applies fresh sterile gloves before performing a vaginal examination to ascertain whether this is so. As a last resort, if the woman is unable to push effectively then gentle fundal pressure may be used, following administration of a uterotonic drug. Great care is exercised to ensure that placental separation has already occurred and the uterus is well contracted. The woman should be relaxed as the midwife exerts downward and backward pressure on the firmly contracted fundus. This method can cause considerable pain and distress to the woman and result in the stretching and bruising of supportive uterine ligaments. If it is performed without good uterine contraction, acute inversion may ensue. This is an extremely dangerous procedure in unskilled hands and is not advocated in everyday practice when alternative, safer methods may be employed. It is very unlikely that this would be practised in the UK.

Manual removal of the placenta

This should be carried out by a doctor. An intravenous infusion must first be sited and an effective anaesthetic in progress. The choice of anaesthesia will depend upon the woman's general condition. If an effective epidural anaesthetic is already in progress, a top-up may be given in order to avoid the hazards of general anaesthesia. A spinal anaesthetic offers an alternative but where time is an urgent factor a general anaesthetic will be initiated.

Management

Manual removal is performed with full aseptic precautions and, unless in a dire emergency situation, should not be undertaken prior to adequate analgesia being ensured for the woman. With the left hand, the umbilical cord is held taut while the right hand is coned and inserted into the vagina and uterus following the direction of the cord. Once the placenta is located the cord is released so that the left hand may be used to support the fundus abdominally, to prevent rupture of the lower uterine segment (Fig. 18.11). The operator will feel for a separated edge of the placenta. The fingers of the right hand are extended and the border of the hand is gently eased between the

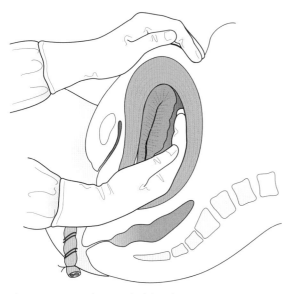

Fig. 18.11 Manual removal of the placenta.

placenta and the uterine wall, with the palm facing the placenta. The placenta is carefully detached with a sideways slicing movement. When it is completely separated, the left hand rubs up a contraction and expels the right hand with the placenta in its grasp. The placenta should be checked immediately for completeness, so that any further exploration of the uterus may be carried out without delay. A uterotonic drug is given upon completion.

In very exceptional circumstances, when no doctor is available to be called, a midwife would be expected to carry out a manual removal of the placenta. Once she has diagnosed a retained placenta as the cause of PPH, the midwife must act swiftly to reduce the risk of onset of shock and exsanguination. It must be remembered that the risk of inducing shock by performing a manual removal of the placenta is greater when no anaesthetic is given. In a developed country, the midwife is unlikely to find herself dealing with this situation.

At home

If the placenta is retained following a home birth, emergency obstetric help must be summoned. Under no circumstances should a woman be transferred to hospital until an intravenous infusion is in progress and her condition stabilized. It is best if the placenta can be delivered without moving the mother but if this is not possible, or if further treatment is needed, she should be transferred to a consultant unit, with her baby.

Morbid adherence of placenta

Very rarely, the placenta remains morbidly adherent; this is known as placenta accreta. If it is totally adherent, then

bleeding is unlikely to occur and it may be left in situ to absorb during the puerperium. If, however, only part of the placenta remains embedded then the risks of fatal haemorrhage are high and an emergency hysterectomy may be unavoidable.

Trauma as a cause of PPH

If bleeding occurs despite a well-contracted uterus, it is almost certainly the consequence of trauma to the uterus, vagina, perineum or labia, or a combination of these. As stated previously, Poeschmann et al (1991) cautioned that episiotomy may contribute up to 30% of total blood loss; in their study the severity of blood loss was linked to the length of time that elapsed between incision of the perineum and the commencement of repair. Predictably, the longer the wait the greater is the blood loss.

In order to identify the source of bleeding, the mother is placed in the lithotomy position under a good directional light. An episiotomy wound or tears to the anterior labia, clitoris and perineum often bleed freely. These external injuries are easily identified and torn vessels may be clamped with artery forceps prior to ligation. Internal trauma to the vagina, cervix or uterus more commonly occurs following instrumental or manipulative delivery. A speculum is inserted to enable the cervix and vagina to be clearly visualized and examined. Tissue or artery forceps may be used to apply pressure prior to suturing under general anaesthesia.

If bleeding persists when the uterus is well contracted and no evidence of trauma can be found, uterine rupture must be suspected. Following a laparotomy this is repaired, but if bleeding remains uncontrolled a hysterectomy may become inevitable.

Blood coagulation disorders causing PPH

As well as the causes already listed above, PPH may be the result of coagulation failure (see Chapters 12 and 13). The failure of the blood to clot is such an obvious sign that it can be overlooked in the midst of the frantic activity that accompanies torrential bleeding. It can occur following severe pre-eclampsia, antepartum haemorrhage, massive PPH, amniotic fluid embolus, intrauterine death or sepsis. Evaluation should include coagulation status and replacing appropriate blood components (Anderson and Etches 2007). Fresh blood is usually the best treatment, as this will contain platelets and the coagulation factors V and VIII. The expert advice of a haematologist will be needed in assessing specific replacement products such as fresh frozen plasma and fibrinogen.

Maternal observation following PPH

Once bleeding is controlled, the total volume lost must be measured and/or estimated as accurately as possible.

Large amounts appear less than they are in reality. A MEOWS chart should be maintained postpartum and abnormal scores should be reported and prompt action taken (CMACE 2011). Maternal pulse and blood pressure are recorded every 15 minutes and the temperature taken every 4 hours. The uterus should be palpated frequently to ensure that it remains well contracted and lochia lost must be observed. Intravenous fluid replacement should be carefully calculated to avoid circulatory overload. Monitoring the central venous pressure (see Chapter 22) will provide an accurate assessment of the volume required, especially if blood loss has been severe. Fluid intake and urinary output are recorded as indicators of renal function. The output should be accurately measured on an hourly basis by the use of a self-retaining urinary catheter.

The woman may need high dependency care if closer monitoring is required, until her condition is stable. All records should be meticulously completed and signed contemporaneously. Continued vigilance will be important for 24–48 hours. As this woman will need a period of recovery, she will not be suitable for early transfer home.

Secondary postpartum haemorrhage

Secondary postpartum haemorrhage is any abnormal or excessive bleeding from the genital tract occurring between 24 hours and 12 weeks postnatally. In developed countries, 2% of postnatal women are admitted to hospital with this condition, half of them undergoing uterine surgical evacuation (Alexander et al 2007). It is most likely to occur between 10 and 14 days after birth. Bleeding is usually due to retention of a fragment of the placenta or membranes, or the presence of a large uterine blood clot. Typically occurring during the second week, the lochia is heavier than normal and will have changed from a serous pink or brownish loss to a bright red blood loss. The lochia may also be offensive if infection is a contributory factor. Subinvolution, pyrexia and tachycardia are usually present. As this is an event that is most likely to occur at home, women should be alerted to the possible signs of secondary PPH prior to discharge from midwifery care.

Management

The following steps should be taken:

- call a doctor
- reassure the woman and her support person(s)
- rub up a contraction by massaging the uterus if it is still palpable
- express any clots
- encourage the mother to empty her bladder

- give a uterotonic drug either by the intravenous or intramuscular route
- keep all pads and linen to assess the volume of blood lost
- if bleeding persists, discuss a range of treatment options with the woman and, if appropriate, prepare her for theatre.

If the bleeding occurs at home and the woman has telephoned the hospital, midwife or her GP, she should be told to lie down flat until professional assistance arrives (the front door should be left unlocked if the woman is alone). On arrival, the doctor, midwife or paramedic will assess the amount of blood loss and the woman's condition and attempt to arrest the haemorrhage. If the loss is severe or uncontrolled, the nearest emergency obstetric unit will be called and the mother and baby prepared for transfer to hospital. The doctor, midwife or paramedic who attends will start an intravenous infusion and ensure that the mother's condition is stable first.

Careful assessment is usually undertaken prior to the uterus being explored under general anaesthetic. The use of ultrasound as a diagnostic tool is invaluable in minimizing the number of mothers who have operative intervention. If retained products of conception cannot be seen on a scan, the mother may be treated conservatively with antibiotic therapy and oral ergometrine. The haemoglobin should be estimated prior to discharge. If it is below 9 g/dl, options for iron replacement should be discussed with the woman. The severity of the anaemia will assist in determining the most appropriate care, which may be dependent on whether or not the woman is symptomatic (e.g. feeling faint, dizzy, short of breath). Management may vary from increased intake of iron-rich foods, iron supplements or, in extreme cases, blood transfusion. It is also important to discuss the common symptoms that may be experienced as a result of anaemia following PPH, including extreme tiredness and general malaise. Encourage the woman to seek assistance and stress the importance of making an appointment to see her GP to have her general health and haemoglobin levels checked.

Haematoma formation

PPH may also be concealed as the result of progressive haematoma formation. This may be obvious at such sites as the perineum or lower vagina, but it is more difficult to diagnose if it occurs into the broad ligament or vault of the vagina. A large volume of blood may collect insidiously (up to 1 litre). Involution and lochia are usually normal, the main symptom being increasingly severe maternal pain. This is often so acute that the haematoma has to be drained in theatre under a general anaesthetic. Secondary infection is a strong possibility.

Care after a postpartum haemorrhage

Whatever the cause of the haemorrhage, the woman will need the continued support of her midwife until she regains her confidence. Her partner may also be fearful of a recurrence and need much reassurance. If the mother is breastfeeding, lactation may be impaired but this will only be temporary and she should be reassured that persevering will result in a return to normal lactation.

CONCLUSION

Key issues in the management of the third stage of labour are summarized in Box 18.3.

REFERENCES

Afaifel N, Weeks A 2012 Editorial: Active management of the third stage of labour: oxytocin is all you need. British Medical Journal 345:e4546

Alexander J, Thomas P, Sanghera J 2007 Treatments for secondary postpartum haemorrhage. Cochrane Database of Systematic Reviews 2007, Issue 2. Art No. CD002867. doi: 10.1002/14651858.CD002867 (Level I)

Altay M M, Ilhan A K, Haberal A 2007 Length of the third stage of labor at term pregnancies is shorter if placenta is located at fundus: prospective study. Journal of Obstetrics and Gynaecology Research 33:641–4

Anderson J M, Etches D 2007 Prevention and management of postpartum hemorrhage. American Family Physician 75:875–82

Baldock S, Dixon L 2006 Physiological changes in labour and the postnatal period. In: Pairman S, Pincombe J, Thorogood C et al (eds) Midwifery: preparation for practice. Elsevier, Marrickville, Australia

Balki M, Carvalho J C A 2005 Intraoperative nausea and vomiting during cesarean section under regional anesthesia. International Journal of Obstetric Anesthesia 14:230–41

Begley C M 1990 A comparison of 'active' and physiological management of the third stage of labour. Midwifery 6:3–17

Begley C M, Guilliland K, Dixon L et al 2012 Irish and New Zealand midwives' expertise in expectant management of the third stage of labour: The 'MEET' study. Midwifery, 28:733–9

Begley C M, Gyte G M L, Devane D et al 2011 Active versus expectant management for women in the third stage of labour. Cochrane Database of Systematic Reviews 2011, Issue 11. Art. No. CD007412. doi: 10.1002/14651858.CD007412.pub3

Bloomfield TH, Gordon H 1990 Reaction to blood loss at delivery. Journal of Obstetrics and Gynaecology 10(Suppl 2): S13–S16

Brandt H A 1966 Blood loss at caesarean section. Journal of Obstetrics and Gynaecology of the British Commonwealth 73:456–9

Brandt H A 1967 Precise estimation of postpartum haemorrhage: difficulties and importance. British Medical Journal 1:398–400

Chaparro C M, Neufeld L M, Alavez G T et al 2006 Effect of timing of umbilical cord clamping on iron status in Mexican infants: a randomised controlled trial. Lancet 367:1997–2004

Choy C M Y, Lau W C, Tam W H et al 2002 A randomised controlled trial of intramuscular Syntometrine and intravenous oxytocin in the management of the third stage of labour. BJOG: An International Journal of Obstetrics and Gynaecology 109:173–7

CMACE (Centre for Maternal and Child Enquiries) 2011 Saving mothers' lives: reviewing maternal deaths to make motherhood safer: 2006–2008. The Eighth Report on Confidential Enquiries into Maternal Deaths in the United Kingdom. BJOG: An International Journal of Obstetrics and Gynaecology 118(Suppl 1): 1–203.

Cotter AM, Ness A, Tolosa JE 2001 Prophylactic oxytocin for the third stage of labour. Cochrane Database of Systematic Reviews 2001, Issue 4. Art. No. CD001808. doi: 10.1002/14651858.CD001808

Deneux-Tharaux C, Sentilhes L, Maillard F et al 2013 Effect of routine controlled cord traction as part of the active management of the third stage of labour on postpartum haemorrhage: multicentre randomised controlled trial (TRACOR). British Medical Journal 346:f1541

Dixon L, Fullerton J, Begley C et al 2011 Systematic review: The clinical effectiveness of physiological (expectant) management of the third stage of labour following a physiological labour and birth. International Journal of Childbirth 1:179–95

Dombrowski M P, Bottoms S F, Saleb A A A et al 1995 Third stage of labour: analysis of duration and clinical practice. American Journal of Obstetrics and Gynecology 172:1279–84

Dunn P M 1985 Management of childbirth in normal women: the third stage and fetal adaptation. In: Perinatal medicine. Proceedings of the IX European Congress on Perinatal Medicine, Dublin, September 1984. MTP Press, Lancaster, p 47–54

Duthie S J, Ven D, Yung G L K et al 1990 Discrepancy between laboratory determination and visual estimation of blood loss during normal delivery. European Journal of Obstetrics, Gynaecology and Reproductive Biology 38:119–24

Dyer R A, van Dyk D, Dresner 2010 A The use of uterotonic drugs during caesarean section. International Journal of Obstetric Anesthesia 19:313–19

Farrar D, Airey R, Law G R et al 2011 Measuring placental transfusion for term births: weighing babies with cord intact. BJOG: An International Journal of Obstetrics and Gynaecology 118:70–5

Foulkes J, Dumoulin J G 1983 Ketosis in labour. British Journal of Hospital Medicine 29:562–4

Grotegut C A, Paglia M J, Johnson L N C et al 2011 Oxytocin exposure in women with postpartum hemorrhage secondary to uterine atony. American Journal of Obstetrics and Gynecology 204:56.e1–56.e6.

Gülmezoglu A M, Lumbiganon P, Landoulsi S et al 2012 Active management of the third stage of labour with and without controlled cord traction: a randomised, controlled, non-inferiority trial. Lancet 379:1721–7

Gupta J K, Nikodem V C 2002 Position for women during second stage of labour. Cochrane Database of Systematic Reviews 2002, Issue 2. Art. No. CD002006. doi: 10.1002/14651858.CD002006.pub2

Herman A, Zimerman A, Arieli S et al 2002 Down–up sequential separation of the placenta. Ultrasound in Obstetrics and Gynecology 19:278–81

Hofmeyr G J, Abdel-Aleem H, Abdel-Aleem M A. Uterine massage for preventing postpartum haemorrhage. Cochrane Database of Systematic Reviews 2013, Issue 7. Art. No. CD006431. doi: 10.1002/14651858.CD006431.pub3

Hogan M C, Foreman K J, Naghavi M et al 2010 Maternal mortality for 181 countries, 1980–2008: a systematic analysis of progress towards Millennium Development Goal 5. Lancet 375:1609–23

Hutton E K, Hassan E S 2007 Late vs early clamping of the umbilical cord in full-term neonates: systematic review and meta-analysis of controlled trials. Journal of the American Medical Association 297:1241–52

ICM (International Confederation of Midwives) 2008 Role of the midwife in physiological third stage labour. The Hague: International Confederation of Midwives

Jangsten E, Mattsson L, Lyckestam I et al 2011 A comparison of active management and expectant management of the third stage of labour: a Swedish randomised controlled trial. BJOG: An International Journal of Obstetrics and Gynaecology 118:362–9

Kavle J A, Stolzfus R J, Witter F et al 2008 Association between anaemia during pregnancy and blood loss at and after delivery among women with vaginal births in Pemba Island, Zanzibar, Tanzania. Journal of Health Population and Nutrition 26:232–40

Khan Q K, John I S, Chan T et al 1995 Abu Dhabi third stage trial: oxytocin versus Syntometrine in the active management of the third stage of labour. European Journal of Obstetrics, Gynaecology and Reproductive Biology 58:147–51

Knight M, Callaghan W M, Berg C et al 2009 Trends in postpartum hemorrhage in high resource countries: a review and recommendations from the International Postpartum Hemorrhage Collaborative Group. BMC Pregnancy and Childbirth 9:

55. Available at www.biomedcentral.com/1471-2393/9/55

Lewis G, Drife J (eds) 2001 Why mothers die 1997–1999. The Fifth Report of the Confidential Enquiries into Maternal Deaths in the United Kingdom. RCOG Press, London

Liabsuetrakul T, Choobun T, Peeyananjarassri K et al 2007 Prophylactic use of ergot alkaloids in the third stage of labour. Cochrane Database of Systematic Reviews 2007, Issue 2. Art. No. CD005456. doi: 10.1002/14651858.CD005456.pub2

Marín Gabriel M A, Llana Martín I, López Escobar A et al 2010 Randomized controlled trial of early skin-to-skin contact: effects on the mother and the newborn. Acta Pædiatrica 99:1630–4

McDonald S J, Middleton P, Dowswell T et al Effect of timing of umbilical cord clamping of term infants on maternal and neonatal outcomes. Cochrane Database of Systematic Reviews 2013, Issue 7. Art. No. CD004074. doi: 10.1002/14651858.CD004074.pub3. [See more at: http://summaries.cochrane.org/CD004074/effect-of-timing-of-umbilical-cord-clamping-of-term-infants-on-mother-and-baby-outcomes#sthash.VnhmYz02.dpuf]

Mercer J S 2006 Current best evidence: a review of the literature on umbilical cord clamping. In: Wickham S (ed) Midwifery. Best practice, vol. 4. Elsevier, London

Mercer J S, Vohr B R, McGrath M M et al 2006 Delayed cord clamping in very preterm infants reduces the incidence of intraventricular hemorrhage and late-onset sepsis: a randomized, controlled trial. Pediatrics 117:1235–42

Newton M, Mosey L M, Egli G E et al 1961 Blood loss during and immediately after delivery. Obstetrics and Gynaecology 17:9–18

Ng P S, Lai C Y, Sahota D S et al 2007 A double-blind randomized controlled trial of oral misoprostol and intramuscular Syntometrine in the management of the third stage of labor. Gynecologic and Obstetric Investigations 63:55–60

NICE (National Institute for Health and Clinical Excellence) 2007 Intrapartum care: care of healthy women and their babies during childbirth, CG 55. NICE, London

Patterson D 2005 The views and experiences of childbirth educators providing a breastfeeding intervention during pregnancy. Proceedings of 27th Congress of the International Confederation of Midwives on 'Midwifery: Pathways to Healthy Nations', Brisbane, Australia

Poeschmann R P, Docsburg W H, Eskis T K 1991 Randomised comparison of oxytocin, sulprostone and placebo in the management of the third stage of labour. British Journal of Obstetrics and Gynaecology 98:528–30

Prastertcharoensuk W, Swadpanich U, Lumbiganon P 2000 Accuracy of the blood loss estimation in the third stage of labor. International Journal Gynecological Obstetrics 71:9–70

Prendiville W, Elbourne D, Chalmers I 1988 The effects of routine uterotonic administration in the management of the third stage of labour: an overview of the evidence from controlled trials. British Journal of Obstetrics and Gynaecology 95:3–16

Rabe H, Diaz-Rossello J L, Duley L et al 2012 Effect of timing of umbilical cord clamping and other strategies to influence placental transfusion at preterm birth on maternal and infant outcomes. Cochrane Database of Systematic Reviews 2012, Issue 8. Art. No. CD003248. doi: 10.1002/14651858.CD003248.pub3

Reyes O A, Gonzalez G M 2011 Carbetocin versus oxytocin for prevention of postpartum hemorrhage in patients with severe preeclampsia: a double-blind randomized controlled trial. Journal of Obstetrics and Gynaecology Canada 33:1099–104

Salariya E, Easton P, Cater J 1979 Early and often for best results. Nursing Mirror 148:15–17

Singata M, Tranmer J, Gyte G M L 2010 Restricting oral fluid and food intake during labour. Cochrane Database of Systematic Reviews 2010, Issue 1. Art. No. CD003930. doi: 10.1002/14651858.CD003930.pub2

Soltan M H, Ibrahim E M, Tawfek M et al 2012 Raised nitric oxide levels may cause atonic postpartum hemorrhage in women with anemia during pregnancy. International Journal of Gynecology and Obstetrics 116:143–7

Soltani H, Hutchon D R, Poulose T A 2010 Timing of prophylactic uterotonics for the third stage of labour after vaginal birth. Cochrane Database of Systematic Reviews 2010, Issue 8. Art. No. CD006173. doi: 10.1002/14651858.CD006173.pub2

Soltani H, Poulose T A, Hutchon D R 2011 Placental cord drainage after vaginal delivery as part of the management of the third stage of labour. Cochrane Database of Systematic Reviews 2011, Issue 9. Art. No. CD004665. doi: 10.1002/14651858.CD004665.pub3

Sosa C G, Althabe F, Belizan J M et al 2009 Risk factors for postpartum hemorrhage in vaginal deliveries in a Latin-American population. Obstetrics and Gynecology 113:1313–19

Su L L, Chong Y S, Samuel M 2012 Carbetocin for preventing postpartum haemorrhage. Cochrane Database of Systematic Reviews 2012, Issue 4. Art. No. CD005457. doi: 10.1002/14651858.CD005457.pub4

Tunçalp Ö, Hofmeyr G J, Gülmezoglu A M 2012 Prostaglandins for preventing postpartum haemorrhage. Cochrane Database of Systematic Reviews 2012, Issue 8. Art. No. CD000494. doi: 10.1002/14651858.CD000494.pub4

van Rheenen P, Brabin B J 2004 Late umbilical cord clamping as an intervention for reducing iron deficiency anaemia in term infants in developing and industrialized countries: a systematic review. Annals of Tropical Paediatrics 24:3–16

van Selm M, Kanhai H H H, Keiser M I N C 1995 Preventing the recurrence of atonic postpartum haemorrhage: a double-blind trial. Acta Obstetrica et Gynecologica Scandinavica 74:270–4

Whitfield M F, Salfield S A W 1980 Accidental administration of Syntometrine in adult dosage to the newborn. Archives of Disease in Childhood 55:68–70

WHO (World Health Organization) 2003 Managing complications in pregnancy and childbirth: a guide for midwives and doctors. Geneva: World Health Organization

WHO (World Health Organization) 2012 Maternal mortality. Fact sheet Number 348. Available from: www.who.int/mediacentre/factsheets/fs348/en/index.html (accessed 22 October 2012)

Wiberg N, Kallen K, Olofsson P 2008 Delayed umbilical cord clamping at birth has effects on arterial and venous blood gases and lactate concentrations. BJOG: An International Journal of Obstetrics and Gynaecology 115:697–703

FURTHER READING

Aflaifel N, Weeks A D 2012 The active management of the third stage of labour. BMJ; 345:e4546. doi: 10.1136/BMJ

A thought-provoking editorial.

Rogers C, Harman J, Selo-Ojeme D 2012 The management of the third stage of labour: a national survey of current practice. British Journal of Midwifery 20(12):850–7

This article debates the non-uniformity of third stage management in England in a variety of practice settings.

USEFUL WEBSITE

POPPHI: www.pphprevention.org (Prevention of Postpartum Hemorrhage Initiative)

Chapter |19|

Prolonged pregnancy and disorders of uterine action

Annie Rimmer

This chapter examines the evidence relating to prolonged pregnancy, induction of labour, prolonged labour and precipitate labour. Any decision with regards to the management of a pregnancy that continues beyond term is based on discussion between the woman and obstetrician, but the midwife is in a unique position to help the woman make sense of such discussions, thereby enabling her to make an informed decision based on informed choice.

When labour is induced, when there is failure to progress in labour or when labour is prolonged, with or without further complications, the midwife remains in a key position to ensure the woman is kept informed so that she is enabled to continue to exercise her ability to be autonomous in the plan of care of her own labour and birth and the execution of that plan.

The role of the midwife in the care of the woman will be discussed throughout.

THE CHAPTER AIMS TO:

- explore the issues relating to prolonged pregnancy with reference to research and other evidence
- outline the indications for the induction of labour and examine the methods used to induce labour in contemporary practice
- describe the process where there is perceived failure to progress in labour or labour is prolonged and review the current evidence used to support the management and care in such cases
- describe the serious complication that is obstructed labour and discuss the importance of competent

midwifery management and care of women during the antenatal and intrapartum period if such complications are to be avoided

- highlight the significant events in a precipitate labour.

PROLONGED PREGNANCY

Much of the confusion when exploring the research and other evidence on pregnancies that go beyond the expected date of birth (EDB) and more specifically beyond 42 weeks (294 days) lies in the terms used to describe such pregnancies such as post-term pregnancy, prolonged pregnancy and postdates. According to Hermus et al (2009) post-term pregnancy is defined as a pregnancy where the gestation exceeds 42 completed weeks (294 days). This definition is also used by others when referring to prolonged pregnancy (NICE [National Institute for Health and Clinical Excellence] 2008a; Simpson and Stanley 2011). Gülmezoglu et al (2012) refer to pregnancies that go beyond 294 days as both post-term and postdate.

What is clear is that all these terms refer to a specific gestation of the pregnancy and not the fetus or neonate. For the purposes of this chapter the term prolonged pregnancy will be used to describe a pregnancy equal to or beyond 42 weeks. Postmaturity refers to a description of the neonate with peeling of the epidermis, long nails, loose skin suggestive of recent weight loss and an alert face (Koklanaris and Tropper 2006). The relationship, if any, between prolonged pregnancy and postmaturity will be explored later in the chapter.

If prolonged pregnancy is defined by weeks of gestation, whether this is based on a calculation of the EDB using Naegele's rule or by ultrasound scan no later than 16 weeks, is to consider women as a homogenous group and neglects, among other things, the racial variations with shorter gestational age in South Asian and Black women (Balchin et al 2007). If the anxiety pertaining to prolonged pregnancy is possible adverse neonatal outcome then perhaps we need to consider how prolonged pregnancy is defined for these groups of women. Laursen et al (2004) suggest the notion of prolonged pregnancy as 'a normal variation of human gestation'. According to Hovi et al (2006) only a small proportion of prolonged pregnancies have babies that are postmature as described above.

INCIDENCE

According to NICE (2008a), the frequency or incidence of prolonged pregnancy is between 5% and 10%. The wide variation is a reflection of the disparate definitions as highlighted above, the number of women where EDB is uncertain and different induction policies (Simpson and Stanley 2011). Based on a definition of equal to or more than 42 weeks a true incidence of prolonged pregnancy is difficult to assess because in many cases women's labour is induced before reaching that time for specific complications in the pregnancy, for maternal request or because the pregnancy has gone beyond the EDB. According to the Department of Health (DH 2006), prolonged pregnancy was the most common indication given for induction of labour (IOL) in England, accounting for approximately 46% of inductions overall. Unfortunately the latest figures from the Health and Social Care Information Centre (HSCIC 2012) do not provide the same breakdown of statistics, only giving an overall induction rate for England for 2011–2012 of 22.1%. It is acknowledged that in this period in England 4.2% of women gave birth at 42 weeks and over (HSCIC 2012).

The use of an early ultrasound scan to date the pregnancy (Chapter 11), whether or not there is uncertainty with the last menstrual period (LMP), is thought by many to reduce the number of pregnancies categorized as prolonged (Ragunath and McKewan 2007; NICE 2008a; Simpson and Stanley 2011; Tun and Tuohy 2011; Oros et al 2012). Both accurately defining prolonged pregnancy and the accurate dating of a pregnancy is important if the woman is to be advised appropriately regarding the possible risks when discussing the options of expectant management or IOL where pregnancy is prolonged in order to avoid unnecessary intervention in an otherwise 'low-risk' pregnancy.

Possible implications for mother, fetus and baby

In exploring the research and other evidence, a number of studies suggest there is an increase in perinatal mortality and morbidity as the pregnancy goes beyond 41 weeks (Hermus et al 2009; Simpson and Stanley 2011; Cheyne et al 2012; Gülmezoglu et al 2012; Oros et al 2012). Whilst many authors acknowledge that the 'absolute risk is small' (NICE 2008a; McCarthy and Kenny 2010; Simpson and Stanley 2011; Cheyne et al 2012; Gülmezoglu et al 2012), this information almost appears as an afterthought and not worthy of further discussion. If prolonged pregnancy is to be perceived as a 'complication' the possible 'risks' need to be viewed from the perspectives of the mother, fetus and neonate with regards to morbidity and mortality.

Simpson and Stanley (2011) suggest that if a pregnancy continues beyond 41 completed weeks the risks for the mother are associated with a large for gestational age or macrosomic infant such as shoulder dystocia, genital tract trauma, operative birth and postpartum haemorrhage (PPH). In an otherwise low-risk pregnancy such risks must be balanced with the risks of IOL, such as increased need for epidural anaesthesia, uterine hyperstimulation, operative birth, PPH and failed induction (Ragunath and McKewan 2007; Hermus et al 2009; McCarthy and Kenny 2010; Bailit et al 2010; Gülmezoglu et al 2012; Jowitt 2012; Oros et al 2012).

According to Simpson and Stanley (2011), the possible risks for the fetus and neonate in a prolonged pregnancy appear to be two-fold: placental dysfunction linked to oligohydramnios, restricted fetal growth, meconium aspiration, asphyxia and still birth; conversely the cases where growth continues resulting in a macrosomic infant at risk of bony injury, soft tissue trauma, hypoxia and cerebral haemorrhage. The work of Fox (1997) suggests that the changes in the placenta over the course of pregnancy are part of a process of maturation and an increase in functional efficiency as opposed to a decrease in functional efficiency. Given that few post-term neonates exhibit signs of postmaturity, possible changes in placental function might be more appropriately linked to pregnancies where the neonate displays such characteristics rather than in prolonged pregnancies *per se* (Koklanaris and Tropper 2006).

Predisposing factors

Factors that might predispose a woman to a prolonged pregnancy include: obesity, nulliparity, family history of prolonged pregnancy, male fetus, fetal anomaly such as anencephaly (Olesen et al 2006; Biggar et al 2010; Arrowsmith et al 2011; Morken et al 2011; Simpson and Stanley 2011). Cardozo et al (1986) suggest there might be three sub-groups related to a prolonged pregnancy, which include those where the dates are incorrect, those with a normal prolonged gestation where physiological maturity is achieved after 42 weeks and those with correct dates and are functionally mature but who do not go into labour at term. Biggar et al (2010) looking at whether the spontaneous onset of labour is immunologically mediated found the risk of prolonged pregnancy is higher in first pregnancies and subsequently reduces with each following pregnancy, where the father is the same. If there is a different father the risk of prolonged pregnancy is as if it were a first pregnancy. Morken et al (2011) found there was a familial factor in relation to the recurrence of prolonged pregnancy across generations, which involves both the mother and the father. Laursen et al (2004) demonstrate a lower perinatal mortality rate in prolonged pregnancies where the mother has had a previous prolonged pregnancy, which would seem to support a possible genetic influence with a prolonged gestation as a normal variation on human gestation.

PLAN OF CARE FOR PROLONGED PREGNANCY

In previous editions of this book the subheading 'Management of prolonged pregnancy' has been used, which may give the impression that the woman has little to contribute to the pregnancy and how it should proceed once she has reached 42 weeks. This implies compliance with the 'choices' given by the healthcare professional rather than active participation in the discussion on the options and choices available which every woman is entitled to (Kirkham et al 2002; Cheyne et al 2012; Stevens and Miller 2012). The concept of 'plan of care' for prolonged pregnancy is perhaps less autocratic, the term implying an approach the purpose of which is for the healthcare professional to work with the woman to determine the most appropriate way forward with the pregnancy in order to ensure the optimum outcome for both mother and baby. In a prolonged pregnancy where there are any obstetric or medical complications the priority in the plan of care should, with maternal consent, follow the practice for the specific complication. If the pregnancy is otherwise low risk, the plan of care can follow an expectant or active approach, and the decision on which approach to take should be based on the woman (and partner) receiving the information on the possible benefits and risks of each to enable her to make an informed decision based on informed choice (NICE 2008a; Jowitt 2012).

If a woman chooses the expectant approach the recommendations from NICE (2008a) are increased antenatal surveillance which includes cardiotocography (CTG) at least two times a week, and an ultrasound scan to estimate the maximum amniotic fluid pool depth rather than a more complex approach to antenatal fetal surveillance which includes 'computerised CTG, amniotic fluid index, and assessment of fetal breathing, tone and gross body movements' (NICE 2008a: 279).

The use of a cervical membrane sweep (CMS) at 41 weeks' gestation has been shown to increase the spontaneous onset of labour before 42 weeks in some nulliparous and parous women (Mitchell et al 1977; de Miranda et al 2006). The purpose of CMS is to attempt to initiate the onset of labour physiologically thus avoiding the intervention of IOL using prostaglandin, artificial rupture of membranes (ARM) and oxytocin. CMS is designed to separate the membranes from their cervical attachment by introducing the examining fingers into the cervical os and passing them circumferentially around the cervix. The process of detaching the membranes from the decidua results in an increase in the concentration of circulating prostaglandins that may contribute to the initiation of the onset of labour in some individuals (Mitchell et al 1977). Massage of the cervix can be used when the cervical os remains closed and this process may also cause release of local prostaglandin. If after an appropriate time labour has not started spontaneously the process can be repeated. The practice of CMS is not associated with any increase in maternal or neonatal infection although women report more vaginal blood loss and painful contractions in the 24-hour period following the procedure. Simpson and Stanley (2011) state that to avoid IOL in one woman CMS would need to performed for seven women and suggest the benefit is therefore small. However, when one compares this to Stock et al (2012), who state that 1040 women would need to be induced to avoid one perinatal death, whilst leading to seven additional admissions to the special care baby unit, the 'odds' for CMS as a possible means to initiate labour seem extremely favourable.

Menticoglou and Hall (2002) argue that 'ritual induction' at 41 weeks is based on flawed evidence and interferes with a 'normal physiologic situation'. Heimstad et al (2007) compared IOL at 41 weeks' gestation with expectant management and found no difference between the two groups with regards to neonatal morbidity or mode of birth. A number of authors cite evidence that where there is an active approach and IOL is undertaken beyond 41 weeks there is a reduction in perinatal mortality (NICE 2008a; Simpson and Stanley 2011; Tun and Tuohy 2011). But as stated above, many authors acknowledge that the 'absolute risk of perinatal death is small' (NICE 2008a; McCarthy and Kenny 2010; Simpson and Stanley 2011; Cheyne et al 2012; Gülmezoglu et al 2012). Oros et al (2012) found that IOL at 41 weeks led to an increase in the length of hospital stay for the mother and an increase in the caesarean section rate.

The debate on the management of prolonged pregnancy centres on the disparate evidence with regards to fetal risk and neonatal outcome in terms of perinatal mortality and morbidity, and implementing a policy of 'management' rather than a 'plan of care' is designed to reduce these risks. When looking at the evidence surrounding post dates (40^{+0} weeks to 41^{+6} weeks) and prolonged pregnancy (42 weeks), what is clear is that nothing is clear. There is a plethora of evidence but much of it is contradictory and much of it is couched in emotive terms. Reference is consistently made to the 'risks of' prolonged pregnancy or the 'risk of' recurrence of prolonged pregnancy, which seems to imply that a poor outcome is inevitable. NICE (2008a) refers to the 'risks of' prolonged pregnancy against the harms and benefits of IOL to avoid prolonged pregnancy. The mechanisms leading to the onset of labour remain largely unknown and the possibility of a prolonged pregnancy being a variation on human gestation within normal parameters should be considered.

Like many authors, NICE (2008a) seem to imply, either implicitly or explicitly, there are no benefits to a prolonged pregnancy. Can nature really have got it so wrong? The emphasis appears to be that in human parturition an EDB is calculated, and it is downhill all the way from there; and whilst the EDB remains the focus, the debate and controversy will continue. A number of women will gladly accept, and may even request IOL once they go beyond their EDB and that decision must be respected, but the decision not to have labour induced *must* also be respected, rather than, as NICE (2008a: 29), suggest 'should' be respected.

The midwife's role

The woman and her partner must be given clear and unbiased information pertaining to the benefits and possible risks of any proposed plan of care to enable the woman to make an informed decision based on informed choice. It is clear from the literature that this is not always the case, and the woman is being directed towards IOL by over-emphasizing the risks of prolonged pregnancy whilst downplaying the risks associated with IOL (Gatward et al 2010; Cheyne et al 2012; Stevens and Miller 2012). Whilst the obstetrician will take the lead in such cases, the midwife has a key role in facilitating the woman's right to autonomy by ensuring she has been given clear and unbiased information, that she fully understands the options available to her, and in appropriate cases, acting as the woman's advocate (NMC [Nursing and Midwifery Council] 2012, 2008). Women are put in an unenviable situation at an extremely vulnerable time in their lives and they expect, quite rightly, that the experts will help them to make sense of the choices available to them. The midwife has a duty of care to assist women at this time. It is, however, important to understand that whatever plan of care is put in place in any pregnancy, it is not always possible to avoid a perinatal death.

See Box 19.1 for a summary of the key points relating to prolonged pregnancy.

INDUCTION OF LABOUR (IOL)

Labour is the process whereby the uterine muscle contracts and retracts leading to effacement and dilatation of the cervix, the birth of the baby, expulsion of the placenta and membranes, and the control of bleeding (see Chapters 16–18). It is only one part of the passage in the childbirth experience but for the majority of women and their partners it is the singular most important part and the care and management they receive will always be remembered.

IOL is an intervention to initiate the process of labour described above by artificial means and involves the use of prostaglandins, ARM (amniotomy), intravenous oxytocin, or any combination of these (WHO [World Health Organization] 2011). It is the term used when initiating this process in pregnancies from 24 weeks' gestation, the legal definition of fetal viability in the United Kingdom

(UK) (House of Commons Select Committee 2007). Where labour is being induced a full assessment must be made to ensure that any intervention planned will confer more benefit than risk for both mother and baby.

There has been a steady rise in IOL in recent years, the most recent statistics showing an IOL rate of 22.1% (HSCIC 2012). In the UK it is an intervention that has become routine practice in maternity units within the National Health Service (NHS). When comparing IOL to a spontaneous onset of labour, evidence demonstrates that it is more painful, that women are more likely to require epidural anaesthesia and an assisted mode of birth (NICE 2008a; WHO 2011). The decision therefore to induce labour should only be made when it is clear that a vaginal birth is the most appropriate outcome in this pregnancy, at this time, for that particular woman and her baby.

Indications for IOL

IOL is considered when the maternal or fetal condition suggests that a better outcome will be achieved by intervening in the pregnancy than by allowing it to continue. This most commonly applies to cases where there are deviations from the normal physiological processes of childbirth as a result of hypertension, diabetes, fetal growth restriction or macrosomia. A list of some of the indications for IOL can be seen in Box 19.2, although this should not be considered as a definitive list. The mother may also request to have labour induced, although NICE (2008a) state this should only be agreed in exceptional circumstances. Ultimately, the grounds on which the decision is made to induce labour must be sound enough to support the outcome whatever that outcome might be. There is no guarantee IOL will result in a vaginal birth or positive outcome for mother and/or her baby.

The contraindications for IOL are situations that preclude a vaginal birth in the best interests of the mother and/or baby. These are listed in Box 19.3.

Methods of induction

The cervix must maintain its integrity during pregnancy and then undergo remodelling prior to labour. For an induction to be successful the cervix needs to have undergone the changes that will ensure the uterine contractions are effective in the progressive dilatation and effacement of the cervix, descent of the presenting part and the birth of the baby.

The cervix is said to be ripe when it has undergone these changes. The Bishop score, devised in the 1960s (Bishop 1964), is the means by which the ripeness of the cervix is assessed using a scoring that examines four features of the cervix and the relationship of the presenting part to the ischial spines. Each of these five elements is scored between 0 and 3 on vaginal examination (VE). The scoring system has been modified and it is this version that is used in contemporary practice (see Table 19.1). Whilst a score of ≤6 is considered to be unfavourable, a score of 8 or more suggests a greater probability of a vaginal birth, similar to that when the onset of labour is spontaneous (NICE 2008a; Gülmezoglu et al 2012). A ripe or favourable cervix is one that for the purpose of IOL is more compliant, offering less resistance as the contraction and retraction of the myometrium forces the presenting part down (NICE 2008a).

> ### Box 19.3 Some contraindications for induction of labour
>
> - Placenta praevia
> - Transverse lie or compound presentation
> - HIV-positive women not receiving any anti-retroviral therapy or women on any anti-retroviral therapy with a viral load of 400 copies/ml or more (RCOG 2010; NICE 2011)
> - Active genital herpes
> - Cord presentation or cord prolapse when vaginal birth is not imminent
> - Known cephalo-pelvic disproportion (CPD)
> - Severe acute fetal compromise

A VE to assess the cervix and the likelihood of successful induction in this way is by nature a subjective examination and as such there will be inter-observer variations. Transvaginal ultrasound assessment of cervical length was found to be superior to the Bishop's score in predicting the success of IOL (Elghorori et al 2006), but currently VE remains the most common method of cervical assessment for IOL. Whilst it is acknowledged that a VE is a subjective means of assessment, if the same individual undertakes the assessment each time then inter-observer variation does not apply. This would also provide the woman with continuity of caregiver at an extremely vulnerable and anxious time for her, which is in the woman's best interest and a standard of care midwives should aim to meet.

Cervical membrane sweep

A cervical membrane sweep (CMS), as described previously, is considered by NICE (2008a) to be an addition to, rather than a method of IOL *per se*. They recommend it is offered to nulliparous women at the 40- and 41-week antenatal examination and to parous women at the 41-week review. It is commonly undertaken by a doctor or midwife experienced in the practice and has been shown to reduce the need for further methods to induce labour (Mitchell et al 1977; Boulvain et al 2005; McCarthy and Kenny 2010). However, Rogers (2010) suggests the evidence on this is inconclusive and both women and midwives need to be aware of this if the woman is to be able to make an informed choice. Some women may find the procedure uncomfortable or painful and they may experience vaginal spotting and abdominal cramps (McCarthy and Kenny 2010). Wong et al (2002) found that whilst the procedure was safe in that it did not lead to prelabour rupture of membranes, bleeding or maternal or neonatal infection, for some women it did cause significant discomfort and in their study was not found to reduce the need for IOL. Boulvain et al (2005) suggest the possible benefits in terms of a reduction in more formal induction methods need to be weighed against the discomfort of the VE and other adverse effects of bleeding and irregular contractions not leading to labour. The recommendation from NICE (2008a) to offer CMS at 40/41 weeks is to avoid prolonged

---

Table 19.1 Modified Bishop's pre-induction pelvic scoring system

Inducibility features	0	1	2	3
Dilatation of cervix in cm	<1	1–2	2–4	>4
Consistency of cervix	Firm	Firm	Med	Soft
Cervical canal length in cm	>4	2–4	1–2	<1
Position of cervix	Post	Mid	Ant	–
Station of presenting part in cm above or below ischial spine	−3	−2	−1, 0	+1, +2

pregnancy and is not meant for high-risk cases. Whilst the evidence on whether it leads to spontaneous labour is inconclusive, if the alternative is IOL for women whose only risk factor seems to be their EDB it is perhaps an 'intervention' that is worthy of consideration.

Prostaglandin E₂ (PGE₂) (Dinoprostone)

Prostaglandins are naturally occurring female hormones present in tissues throughout the body. Prostaglandin E_2 and F_2 are known to be produced by tissues of the cervix, uterus, decidua and the fetal membranes and to act locally on these structures. Dinoprostone is the active ingredient in PGE₂ vaginal tablets, gel and pessaries (BNF [British National Formulary] 2013). It replicates prostaglandin E_2 produced by the uterus in early labour to ripen the cervix and is seen as a more natural method than the use of oxytocin. PGE₂ placed high in the posterior fornix of the vagina, taking great care to avoid inserting it into the cervical canal (see Fig. 19.1) is absorbed by the epithelium of the vagina and cervix leading to relaxation and dilatation of the muscle of the cervix and subsequent contraction of uterine muscle. According to Blackburn (2013), the use of a prostaglandin greatly increases the probability of delivery occurring within 24 hours, and prior to the use of oxytocin potentiates the effects of the oxytocic agent (BNF 2013).

There are a number of preparations of PGE₂, which have been found to be clinically equivalent; but not bioequivalent. The current recommendation from NICE (2008a) is

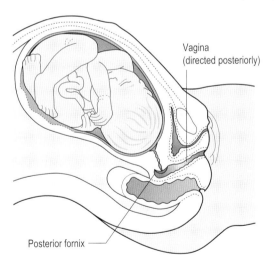

Fig. 19.1 Insertion of prostaglandins. The posterior fornix of the vagina is used to insert prostaglandins for ripening or induction of labour. The key point is that when undertaking a vaginal examination to assess the cervix midwives should follow the direction of the vagina, which will be directed posteriorly if the woman is semi-recumbent. The uterus is anteverted and anteflexed, creating the posterior fornix. The cervix may appear 'difficult to reach', particularly when unfavourable.

the use of gel, tablet or controlled release pessary. In a small study by Tomlinson et al (2001), the women receiving the slow release pessary gave a higher satisfaction score with regards to their perception of labour. Whilst the slow release preparation would appear to confer more benefit from the woman's perspective with regard to fewer vaginal examinations, the difference in cost between the gel, tablet and controlled release pessary, with currently the latter being marginally more expensive, may prohibit its use in some NHS Trusts for routine use in IOL.

Prior to the insertion of PGE₂, the midwife will carry out an abdominal examination to confirm fetal lie, presentation, descent of presenting part and fetal wellbeing by use of electronic fetal monitoring (EFM). All findings are clearly recorded in the woman's maternity records and if there is any doubt or concern in the findings the process must be stopped and the doctor informed (NMC 2012). Following insertion of PGE₂ the woman is advised to lie down for 30 minutes. When contractions begin continuous EFM is used to assess fetal wellbeing. If the CTG is confirmed to be normal, i.e. all four features are considered to be reassuring, the CTG can be discontinued and intermittent auscultation used unless there are any other clear indications for the use of continuous EFM (NICE 2007, 2008a). Currently the IOL process commonly takes place as an inpatient, either on the antenatal ward or labour suite depending on the reason for IOL. There is evidence to support starting the IOL process in the morning rather than the evening, citing increased maternal satisfaction with the process (NICE 2008a). Prior to the administration of the PGE₂ the midwife must confirm there is a bed available on the labour suite in the event there is a need to transfer the woman as a matter of urgency. For the safety of the woman and her baby any decision to proceed with IOL must take cognisance of the current situation on the labour suite because the woman's response to insertion of PGE₂ cannot be predicted. If there are any maternal or fetal risk factors in the pregnancy the IOL must take place on the labour suite.

Where the membranes are intact or ruptured the recommended initial dose for all women, whether it is a first or subsequent pregnancy, is one dose of PGE₂ tablet (3 mg) or gel (1–2 mg), re-assess in 6 hours and if labour is not established, and the woman has given consent, a second dose of tablet or gel is inserted into the posterior fornix of the vagina. This equates to one cycle. Alternatively one cycle of PGE₂ controlled-release pessary (10 mg) can be given over 24 hours, which is one pessary. The maximum recommended dose of PGE₂ tablet, gel or controlled-release pessary being one cycle (NICE 2008a). Side-effects of PGE₂ include nausea, vomiting and diarrhoea (BNF 2013). If labour is not established after one cycle of treatment the IOL is classed as having failed, and having established both mother and baby are in good health discussion must take place between the woman and doctor with regards to further options – these being another attempt to induce labour or elective caesarean section (NICE 2008a).

Vaginal PGE$_2$ is currently the only recommended route for the use of prostaglandins for IOL. Misoprostol (PGE$_1$) is not licensed for use in the UK. Whilst it is thought to be more effective and less expensive than PGE$_2$ and oxytocin for the IOL there remain questions about safety issues with regards to uterine hyperstimulation. Currently in the UK PGE$_1$ is recommended for IOL only where there is an intrauterine fetal death (IUFD).

With a caesarean section (CS) rate in excess of 25% (HSCIC 2012), it is inevitable that more and more women with a uterine scar will be faced with the decision regarding IOL. Whilst previously PGE$_2$ was not recommended where there was a scar on the uterus, women with a previous lower segment caesarean section (LSCS) may now be offered IOL using PGE$_2$. It is important for the midwife to understand the significance of a scarred uterus and choices with regards to IOL to ensure the woman is informed of the increased risk of requiring an emergency CS and increased risk of rupture of the uterus.

Risk associated with use of PGE$_2$

The use of PGE$_2$ can be unpredictable and may lead to uterine hyperstimulation, placental abruption, fetal hypoxia, pulmonary or amniotic fluid embolism (Kramer et al 2006). The risk of uterine rupture is rare, occurring in between 0.3% and 7% of labours.

Artificial rupture of membranes (ARM)

There are two layers of membrane surrounding the fetus: the amnion is closest to the fetus, and the chorion is nearest to the decidua. ARM is a relatively simple process that can be used in an attempt to induce labour if the cervix is favourable and the presenting part is fixed in the pelvis, particularly where the woman does not want to use drugs such as PGE$_2$ or oxytocin, or where there is a risk of hyperstimulation if using PGE$_2$. Prior to the procedure an abdominal examination is carried out and if the lie is longitudinal, the presenting part is engaged and the fetal heart rate is within normal limits, a VE is done to assess the cervix, confirm the presentation and station and to exclude possible cord presentation or vasa praevia. If these findings are satisfactory the bag of membranes lying in front of the presenting part (forewaters) is ruptured with the use of an amnihook or similar device to release the amniotic fluid. The fluid is assessed for colour and volume and following ARM it may be possible to distinguish other features on the presenting part to identify the position of the fetus. After the procedure the woman is made comfortable, the fetal heart is auscultated and all findings are recorded in the maternity notes. The longer the interval between ARM and birth increases the risk of the woman developing chorioamnionitis as a result of an ascending infection from the genital tract leading to an increased risk of perinatal mortality (Bricker and Luckas 2012; Blackburn 2013). For this reason if a decision has been made to induce labour for perceived risks it is common practice to start an oxytocin infusion within a few hours if labour has not been established following the ARM. In their review of two trials Bricker and Luckas (2012) found insufficient evidence to recommend amniotomy alone for the IOL.

Changes to ripen the cervix are thought to be in response to prostglandin produced by the amnion and cervix. In pregnancy the chorion provides a barrier to the amnion and fetus from the vagina and cervix. Prostaglandin dehydrogenase (PGDH) is an enzyme produced by the chorion that breaks down prostaglandin. As a result of the actions of this enzyme the changes in the cervix do not take place and pre-term labour is avoided (Smyth et al 2013). Mitchell et al (1977) found that VE in late pregnancy rapidly increases the concentration of circulating prostaglandins. This change occurs both in sweeping the membranes and with ARM. It is thought it is the disruption of the attachment of the membranes to the uterine wall that facilitates this change. In contrast, Van Meir et al (1997) found that in labouring women the part of the chorion that was in close contact with the cervical os released less PGDH allowing the prostaglandin from the amnion to come into contact with the cervix and facilitate ripening of the cervix. The theory is that if an ARM is performed too early the action of the amniotic prostaglandins on the cervix is lost.

Oxytocin

Oxytocin is synthesized in the hypothalamus and then transported to the posterior lobe of the pituitary gland from where it is episodically released to act on smooth muscle. The number of oxytocin receptors in the myometrium significantly increases by term increasing uterine oxytocin sensitivity (Blackburn 2013).

In its synthetic form, oxytocin (Syntocinon) is a powerful uterotonic agent that may be used as part of the process for IOL following ARM. NICE (2008a) do not recommend the use of oxytocin alone for IOL, or the use of ARM and oxytocin as a 'primary method' of IOL, unless the use of vaginal PGE$_2$ is specifically contraindicated. Oxytocin should be administered by slow intravenous infusion using an infusion pump or syringe driver with non-return valve. The infusion rate should follow NHS Trust protocol and the maximum rate of 0.2 units/minute should not be exceeded (BNF 2013). The dose is titrated against uterine activity, usually increasing the dose every 30 minutes with the aim of 3–4 contractions every 10 minutes with each contraction lasting approximately one minute, using the lowest possible dose. If contractions exceed this rate, or the contractions fail to establish, the infusion must be stopped and the case reviewed to determine the next step. There should be an interval of at least six hours between administration of prostaglandins and commencement of an oxytocin infusion.

When using an oxytocin infusion the fetal heart rate and uterine activity should be monitored using continuous EFM to ensure the fetus does not become compromised by the induced uterine contractions. There is a risk of hyperstimulation and hypertonic uterus leading to fetal compromise (Ragunath and McEwan 2007; McCarthy and Kenny 2010). In such cases the infusion is decreased or discontinued and medical aid summoned. Even with the use of the CTG the midwife still has an important role to play in assessing the woman's progress. The graphic representation on the CTG provides an indication of the frequency of the contractions but does not necessarily provide an accurate representation of the length and strength of the contractions, and for this reason it is important that the midwife continues to palpate the uterus to assess contractions for their length and strength. Whatever 'science' is being employed to assess maternal and fetal wellbeing the midwife has a valuable opportunity to be with the woman and to use her 'art' to make a more holistic assessment of the woman and how she is responding to the process and what she wants and needs at this time.

Risks associated with use of intravenous oxytocin include:

- Uterine hyperstimulation or hypertonus
- Fetal hypoxia and asphyxia
- Uterine rupture
- Fluid retention as a result of the antidiuretic effect of oxytocin
- Postpartum haemorrhage
- Amniotic fluid embolism (AFE)

Midwife's role when caring for the mother where labour is being induced

The midwife's responsibilities regarding IOL include care during the antenatal and intrapartum period. Where a decision has been made to induce labour it is important the midwife ensures the woman and her partner have been fully informed and understand the process and how it might be undertaken. As can be seen from above there are a number of ways that labour can be induced and the manner the induction will take will depend on the individual circumstances of each woman. All information should be given in an objective manner to ensure the woman and her partner understand the reason for the induction, any possible consequences or risks of having/ not having the procedure as well as any alternatives to IOL (NICE 2008a). It is important for the woman and her partner to understand that induction may be delayed if the labour suite is busy, that it might take some time for contractions to be initiated, and the possibility the induction

process will be unsuccessful. Whilst the assumption may be that this will already have been discussed, it is incumbent upon the midwife to ensure the woman is fully informed (NMC 2008, 2012). Time should be allowed for discussion with the midwife or obstetrician and it must be remembered that consent to a treatment can be withdrawn at any time and this decision by the woman must be respected (Griffith et al 2010). The midwife or doctor should record any discussion that takes place and any requests made in the maternity notes.

During the induction process all maternal and fetal observations will be recorded in the maternity notes. Until labour is established and the partogram is commenced the observation are normally recorded in the antenatal section of the notes. Because the layout is not as comprehensive and logical as the partogram it is important the midwife is clear and methodical in her documentation at this time (NMC 2012). The frequency and type of monitoring of the mother and fetus will depend on the reason for and method of induction. The midwife is advised to follow the local NHS Trust guidelines regarding IOL in each case, if this is what the woman wishes and has consented to. It is important when monitoring the wellbeing of the mother and fetus during the induction process that the midwife understands the possible risks associated with each method of induction and is confident and competent in recognizing and responding to any deviations from normal.

When the onset of labour is spontaneous it is a more insidious process and as such the woman has time to adjust to the changes in her body and is usually better able to cope with contractions. When labour is induced the sudden onset of strong painful contractions occurring every three to four minutes can be quite overwhelming and result in an early request for pain relief. As well as this the woman has to make a temporal shift from how she planned to birth her baby to what is now taking place. This can be extremely hard for the woman and her partner to come to terms with and can have a negative impact on this singularly important time in both their lives. Continuity of caregiver in labour is important in developing a rapport with the woman and her partner and in being able to make an assessment of her progress based on physical observations of abdominal examination and VE as well as less tangible observations of body language and behaviour (Lowe 2007; Laursen et al 2009; Hodnett et al 2012). In this way the midwife may be better able to advise the woman of her progress to help her in her decision as to how she would like her labour to proceed. IOL does not have to be a negative experience and the midwife is in a key position to use her 'art' to enable the woman to have a positive birthing experience, whatever the outcome.

It must be remembered that each woman's labour, whether it is spontaneous onset or induced, is their own individual experience, and what they wish for their labour may not always conform to NHS Trust guidelines. As in all care the midwife provides, valid consent must be obtained before any examination or intervention, and this requires taking time to give the woman the information so that she is fully informed and knows and understands what she is consenting to. When a woman is experiencing painful contractions in labour the information about any examinations or procedures that the midwife or doctor may wish to perform should be given between contractions.

Alternative approaches to initiating labour

For some women avoidance of any surgical or pharmacological intervention in an otherwise low-risk pregnancy is extremely important and they might seek advice from the midwife on this matter. Alternative approaches include the ingestion of castor oil, nipple stimulation, sexual intercourse, acupuncture and the use of homeopathic methods. Whilst some reviews, for example Kavanagh et al (2008) and Smith and Crowther (2012), have found insufficient evidence to recommend some of these as a method to initiate labour it is important for the midwife to understand how each of these are thought to work, and to be familiar with the wider literature on these subjects to develop a broad understanding to ensure that any advice given on alternative therapies is in line with her sphere of practice (NMC 2012). For the complete list of reviews on alternative approaches to initiating labour visit the Cochrane database online.

One alternative approach with more positive findings is that of stimulation of the breast. The findings of Kavanagh et al (2005) suggest stimulation of the breast either by massage or nipple stimulation 'appears beneficial in relation to the number of women not in labour after 72 hours, and reduced postpartum haemorrhage rates'. It appears to be less effective where the cervix is not ripe. Stimulation of the breast or more specifically the nipple appears to cause the release of endogenous oxytocin, the effect being to initiate a uterine response, but further studies are needed before it can be considered for use in high-risk groups.

FAILURE TO PROGRESS AND PROLONGED LABOUR

The physiology of labour encompasses effective uterine contractions and cervical changes leading to progressive effacement and dilatation of the cervix, rotation of the fetus and descent of the presenting part, the birth of the baby, and expulsion of the placenta and membranes and the control of bleeding. The psychology of labour encompasses the need for a safe and stress-free environment, one

in which the woman feels in control of events and has trust in those caring for her (Laursen et al 2009) and is an equally important part of the process of labour (see Chapter 1).

For many, the process of labour starts spontaneously and continues that way without the need to intercede. For others the process may falter and the caregiver must assess whether this is a temporary slowing down in progress as the woman's mind and body adjusts to what is happening, and to what has yet to happen, or whether it is the first signs of a delay in progress that may benefit from a change in the status quo. Historically, terms such as 'failure to progress', 'prolonged labour' and 'dystocia' have been used when labour is perceived not to be following a predetermined line of progress, whether that is the rate of cervical dilatation/hour or if the labour is considered to have exceeded a set number of hours. NICE (2007) do not specify these terms but refer to a change in progress in the first or second stage of labour as 'suspected delay' or 'delay' depending on the findings.

Prolonged labour is not easily defined, primarily because there is no consensus as to what constitutes a normal time limit for labour either in the latent or active part of the first stage or the passive or active part of the second stage. When labour is slow to progress or prolonged there is an increased risk of chorioamnionitis if there has been prolonged rupture of membranes, and an increased risk of postpartum haemorrhage as a result of an atonic uterus. Nonetheless it must also be remembered the interventions used to correct a dystocia, such as amniotomy, oxytocin infusion and instrumental or operative birth, are not risk-free and therefore any decision to intervene must take account of the full clinical picture and as importantly the wishes of the woman.

Delay in the latent phase of labour

In the first stage of labour, the latent phase is the period when structural changes occur in the cervix and it becomes softer and shorter (from 3 cm to less than 0.5 cm), its position is more central in relation to the presenting part and there are painful contractions (Chapter 16). According to NICE (2007), the dilatation of the cervix at this time is up to 4 cm. During this period the woman needs support and encouragement from those caring for her. The perceived result of painful contractions may be disappointing when hearing the cervix is 3 cm dilated after several hours. If progress in this phase of labour is considered to be slow the emphasis is on conservative management rather than intervention (Hayman 2004). The midwife must ensure the woman knows to keep eating and drinking if she feels able to as this will not only help maintain her energy levels but can also bring a sense of normality and comfort. It is important for the woman to rest at this time and not to feel that if she tries to sleep the contractions will cease. Advice on how to relieve pain might include simple back massage, changes of position, a warm bath or some simple analgesia; all are an important part of care at this time. Any intervention such as an ARM at this stage can interfere with the action of amniotic prostaglandin on the cervix and be counterproductive (Smyth et al 2013).

Delay in the active first stage of labour

NICE (2007) refers to the established first stage of labour rather than the active phase, and define this as the period when the uterine contractions are regular and painful and the cervix dilates progressively from 4 cm. Neal et al (2010) suggest that the active phase begins between 3 and 5 cm when there are regular uterine contractions.

For nulliparous women delay is suspected if their progress, in terms of cervical dilatation, is less than 2 cm in 4 hours. For parous women it is the same, or there is considered to be a 'slowing in progress' (NICE 2007: 40). This suggests the rate of cervical dilatation and duration of labour is measurable and such measurements can be applied to all nulliparous or multiparous women. It is, however, rather more complex and needs to take account of a wide range of variables in terms of maternal age, maternal size, fetal position etc. Such factors may mean labour does not conform to a pre-determined rate of progression whilst still being normal for that particular woman. Nonetheless, when caring for women in labour midwives do need some parameters to work within in order to better understand what is considered acceptable in terms of progress (Neal et al 2010). NICE (2007) acknowledges the active phase of labour does not follow the trajectory that Friedman (1954) put forward to suggest a rate of 0.5 cm/h. Although they suggest that consideration should also be given to the rotation, descent and station of the presenting part, these observations do not appear to merit the same importance as cervical dilatation. For some women good progress will be made in terms of rotation, descent and station of the presenting part, although such progress is not always reflected in a corresponding change in cervical dilatation. Neal et al (2010: 317) suggest that for low-risk, nulliparous women, with spontaneous onset of labour 'contemporary expectations of active labour are overly stringent'.

When there is 'suspected delay' the midwife needs to discuss with the woman how the situation might be best managed from this point onwards, with appropriate consideration of all the facts in the context of that particular woman. Alleviating anxiety by ensuring there is continuous support in labour, changing maternal position, alleviating pain using non-pharmacological means are some of the ways in which the midwife can help the woman at this time. Medical interventions to correct this include ARM or oxytocin or a combination of both, and the means to augment labour in this way has become common practice

in the UK, with as many as 50% of nulliparous women receiving an oxytocin infusion in labour (Hayman 2004). If these means fail, an instrumental or operative birth may be the only course of action depending on the stage of labour reached. The caesarean section rate in England is currently 25% with 14.8% being emergency caesarean sections (HSCIC 2012), and many of these will be for a diagnosis of failure to progress or prolonged labour.

The partogram or partograph is a graphical representation of the maternal and fetal condition in established labour and the dilatation of the cervix against time. Information on a number of findings that are important in making an appropriate assessment of the ongoing progress of labour are usually recorded on a single sheet. NICE (2007) recommends the use of a partogram once the woman is in established labour despite the only evidence to support its use being studies from low-income countries. In a recent review by Lavender et al (2012), the routine use of a partogram as part of the management of labour could not be recommended, suggesting that its use should be determined at a local level. Possibly one of the most debated issues in the use of a partogram is the plotting of cervical dilatation on a graph which has an 'alert line' and an 'action line'. The assumption is that the cervix dilates at a given rate in established labour, with the graph highlighting any perceived deviations from this pre-determined trajectory. Whilst a record of observations in labour on one sheet of paper might for example make for easier reading for anyone taking over care of a woman in labour, the plotting of cervical dilatation in this way suggest progress in labour can be assessed based on cervical dilatation alone.

The influence of the 3 'Ps'

Dystocia can be as a result of ineffective uterine contractions, malposition of the fetus leading to a relative or absolute CPD, malpresentation, or any combination of these. These may result in poor progress during the active phase or a cessation of cervical dilatation following a period of normal dilatation (Hayman 2004). An understanding of the role played by the 3 'Ps' – **p**assages, **p**assenger and **p**owers – will help in determining why there is a delay in progress in first or second stage of labour and what action might be taken.

In the developed world the majority of women have grown up well nourished, fit and healthy, and the passages the fetus must negotiate are unlikely to be seriously flawed, excluding possible trauma to the pelvis. Nonetheless the impact of a full rectum, full bladder and fibroids cannot be ignored in causing a delay in the progress of labour. A malpresentation such as shoulder, brow or face (mento-posterior) is one of the causes of poor progress or prolonged labour and this may occur as a result of a problem with the passage (Chapter 20). A brow might revert to a face (mento-anterior) or vertex presentation and the face

427

in mento-posterior position may rotate to mento-anterior at the pelvic floor and if so a vaginal birth may be possible (Singh and Paterson-Brown 2006). The shoulder, brow or face (mento-posterior) cannot be born vaginally but a carefully executed abdominal and vaginal examination will exclude or confirm this so that the necessary action can be taken to prepare the woman for caesarean section.

When the fetus is adopting an attitude where the head is deflexed or slightly extended and the occiput is posterior the presenting diameters are larger and there will be a degree of ascynclitism. This inevitably slows progress but does not necessarily mean progress is abnormal. This might be considered a relative CPD because with effective uterine contractions the fetus may adopt a more flexed attitude. On some occasions more time is needed to do this safely. El Halta (1998) suggests that rupturing the membranes when the fetus is an occipitoposterior position may result in a sudden descent of the fetal skull resulting in a deep transverse arrest whereby the occipito-frontal diameter (11.5 cm) is caught on the bi-spinous diameter of the outlet (10–11 cm). Epidural anaesthesia has been found to delay the progress of labour in the first and second stage (Lowe 2007; Cheng et al 2009), particularly so where there is an occipitoposterior position (Chapter 20). The musculature of the pelvic floor plays an important part in assisting the rotation of the presenting part and epidural anaesthesia causes the pelvic floor to relax inhibiting rotation. It also has an impact on the stretching of the birth canal that normally triggers the neuro-hormonal reflex (Ferguson's reflex). In some cases the head is simply (normally) large and any decision to intervene at this point with oxytocin may increase strength and frequency of uterine contractions in such a way as to unduly force this process with inevitable fetal heart rate changes prompting further intervention.

Although the uterus has prepared itself for the metabolic activity of labour, as labour continues the smooth muscle uses up its metabolic reserves and becomes tired. Any change to the strength, length or frequency of contractions will affect progress and is indicative of inefficient uterine action. Whilst some ketosis is considered normal in labour there remains a need for additional supplies of energy if the uterus is to continue contracting effectively and enable labour to progress without the need for medical intervention (Lowe 2007; Blackburn 2013). Women need to have adequate oral intake in order to cope with the very real demands that labour puts on their body.

The midwife's role in caring for a woman in prolonged labour

A prolonged labour leads to increased levels of stress, anxiety, fear and fatigue, and increases the risk of infection, PPH and emergency caesarean section (Svärdby et al 2006; Laursen et al 2009). The importance of effective antenatal education in developing a plan of care for labour should not be underestimated. Advice on suitable food and drink to eat in the early stages of labour to maintain energy levels, positions and activities to encourage a forward rotation where there is an occipitoposterior position are just some of the ways that might help to assist the woman in the normal progress of labour.

When the woman and her partner come into hospital, continuity of caregiver helps to create a sense of trust between the woman, partner and midwife but also allows for more accurate assessment over time to enable the midwife to suggest non-interventionist ways in which progress can be maintained if appropriate. An alternative position might help to facilitate more effective contractions or improve pelvic diameters when the position of the baby is posterior. At this stage it is also important to maintain hydration, to encourage voiding and to suggest non-pharmacological ways to relieve pain. Facilitating autonomy by keeping the woman and her partner informed of her progress and the choices she has is important in helping her to feel in control and to alleviate anxiety. Raised adrenalin levels as a result of fear, anxiety or pain can impact negatively on uterine activity and can slow progress in labour.

Accurate observations in labour are critical in assessing progress. Recognition and detection of abnormal progress in labour with appropriate clinical response will improve the outcome of labour for both mother and baby (Neilson et al 2003). An abdominal examination deftly undertaken can provide vital information about the labour with regard to the lie, presentation, position and descent of presenting part as well as the length, strength and frequency of contractions whereby any change in the pattern of the contractions can be picked up. If the woman consents to VE the findings can be compared to provide a more comprehensive picture of the progress of labour. On VE the midwife is assessing the presence and degree of moulding of the fetal skull, the presence and position of caput in relation to sutures and fontanelles, and the dilatation of the cervix noting any thickening and its application to the presenting part. Any changes to the colour of the liquor if the membranes have previously ruptured, or to the fetal heart rate will give some indication as to how the fetus is coping with the progress of labour. Continuity of caregiver at this time reduces the likelihood of interobserver variations whilst increasing the chance of spontaneous vaginal birth (Hodnett et al 2012).

When the decision to augment labour has been agreed by all parties, the woman and her partner will need additional support from the midwife, as the interventions necessary for this process may be very different from the birth they had previously imagined. Psychological as well as physical support is important at this time, as the control of the birth of their baby now appears to be in the hands of a third party and this can lead to negative feelings of the childbirth experience (Nystedt et al 2005, 2006).

The management of prolonged labour is a collaborative effort involving the woman and her partner, the midwife, obstetrician and anaesthetist. The normal pattern of observations and care in labour apply and any deviations from normal are reported to the obstetrician. When an ARM has been performed to augment labour an appropriate period of grace should be given for effective uterine contractions to resume before commencing an oxytocin infusion. The uterus responds with increased sensitivity to the oxytocin infused as the cervix dilates and it may be necessary to reduce the rate of the infusion as full dilatation is approached to avoid hyperstimulation of the uterus and the concomitant effects on mother and fetus. With the woman's consent, an assessment will be made 2–4 hours after ARM or after commencing oxytocin to ascertain the likelihood of a successful vaginal birth. If there is persistent poor progress in the active phase despite optimal contractions, 4 to 5 per 10 minutes lasting more than 40 seconds, and the woman is pain-free, well hydrated and with an empty bladder, it is unlikely that continuing with an oxytocin infusion will lead to a vaginal birth.

The decision to augment labour in parous women or in women with prior caesarean section must be made by an experienced obstetrician because of the very real risk of hyperstimulation and uterine rupture.

Delay in the second stage of labour

The second stage of labour can be divided into a passive (pelvic) phase and active (perineal) phase (Chapter 17). Delay in this stage of labour may be due to malposition causing failure of the vertex to descend and rotate; ineffective contractions due to a prolonged first stage; large fetus and large vertex; or absence of the desire to push with epidural analgesia. Assuming the woman is receiving active support and encouragement during the second stage, and has trust in those caring for her, some of these situations may be rectified with a change of position and further encouragement, or the judicious use of an oxytocin infusion to avoid the need for an instrumental or operative birth.

Time limits in second stage range from 30 minutes to 2 hours for parous women and 1 to 3 hours for nulliparous women (NICE 2007), but an understanding of the different phases as the head negotiates the birth canal can avoid the encouragement of premature bearing down efforts, which only serve to tire and demoralize the mother. The variation in time limits takes into consideration the impact of epidural analgesia on the desire to push in the second stage. The active phase when the mother is bearing down is the most critical time. When a diagnosis of delay in the second stage has been made the case is referred to the obstetrician for review and assessment. The impact on both mother and fetus if the second stage is allowed to exceed a pre-determined time limit must be weighed against the risks of any interventions at this critical time

in the childbirth experiences. Where there is any indication that the mother or the fetus is compromised the birth must be expedited as soon as possible but imposing an arbitrary time limit is felt by some to be unnecessary if both mother and fetus are doing well (Neilson et al 2003; Hayman 2004; Gilchrist et al 2010).

OBSTRUCTED LABOUR

Whilst obstructed labour is not uncommon in developing countries (Neilson et al 2003), in the UK it is only likely to be seen where a woman has laboured unattended at home for several hours and then seeks help at a hospital.

Obstructed labour occurs when despite good uterine contractions there is no advance of the presenting part. Possible causes of obstructed labour include absolute CPD, deep transverse arrest, malpresentation, lower segment fibroids, fetal hydrocephaly and multiple pregnancy with conjoined or locked twins. Because of the high presenting part if the woman goes into labour there may be spontaneous rupture of the membranes and cord prolapse with related risk to the fetus. If the condition is not recognized the mother's uterus will continue to contract to overcome the obstruction. She will become progressively more dehydrated, ketotic, pyrexial and tachycardic. The fetus will develop a bradycardia because of the relentless contractions. As the uterus continues to contract and retract the upper segment becomes progressively thicker, closely enveloping the fetus, and the lower segment becomes increasingly thinner. In nulliparous women the contractions may cease for a period before resuming again with increasing strength and frequency with little interval between contractions until the uterus assumes a state of tonic contraction. The difference between upper and lower segment may be seen as a ridge obliquely crossing the abdomen (Bandl's ring). The mother is in severe and unrelenting pain. If VE is possible the presenting part will be high with excessive moulding (Fig. 19.2). The uterus is in imminent danger of rupture and emergency measures must be taken if the situation has been allowed to get this far. Uterine rupture leads to maternal mortality and the tonic contractions and uterine rupture cause the hypoxia, asphyxia and subsequent perinatal mortality (Neilson et al 2003).

If the woman has been discovered in this condition at home a paramedic ambulance should be called for immediate transfer to hospital. The labour suite should be informed, which, in turn, should contact the senior obstetrician, anaesthetist, paediatrician, theatre staff and special care unit. Whilst waiting for the ambulance the midwife should cannulate, take blood for urgent cross-match and site an intravenous infusion. The woman's General Practitioner (GP) can be called if close by to provide additional

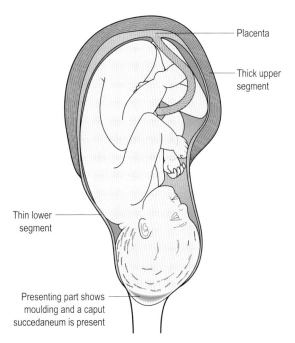

Placenta

Thick upper segment

Thin lower segment

Presenting part shows moulding and a caput succedaneum is present

Fig. 19.2 Obstructed labour. The uterus is moulded around the fetus; the thickened upper segment is obvious on abdominal palpation.

help and support until the ambulance arrives. Observations of mother and fetus, and any actions taken and by whom, are recorded in the maternity notes as soon as possible. If obstructed labour is diagnosed on admission to hospital an emergency caesarean section is performed.

In the UK obstructed labour is not something that is managed, in that when a woman is receiving skilled antenatal and intrapartum care it is not something that should occur. During antenatal care the midwife will highlight any predisposing maternal or fetal factors that might impact on normal progress in labour with appropriate referral to the obstetrician so that a full and frank discussion can take place and a decision made with the woman on the safest mode of birth. During labour, skilled observation and assessment of progress, particularly skilled abdominal examination, will alert the midwife to any malpresentation or failure of the presenting part to advance despite optimal uterine contractions. VE will confirm suspected malpresentation, and where the presentation is vertex, reveal increasing caput or moulding. With a high presenting part in labour cervical dilatation will be extremely slow and there will be little if any application to the presenting part. The obstetrician is informed as soon as possible so that the birth can be expedited. As for all women, despite the very real threat to maternal and perinatal wellbeing these procedures should only be undertaken with maternal consent.

PRECIPITATE LABOUR

Precipitate labour is defined as 'expulsion of the fetus within 3 hours of commencement of contractions' (NICE 2008a: 40). In some women the uterus is over-efficient and much or all of the first stage is not recognized because contractions are not painful and the realization of the birth of the head may be the first indication that labour has actually started. In women with spontaneous onset of labour the incidence of precipitate labour is approximately 2%, and women having a precipitate labour are at risk of placental abruption (NICE 2008a).

Other problems that may be associated with a precipitate labour include soft tissue trauma of the maternal genital tract due to sudden stretching and distension as the baby is born, fetal hypoxia as a result of the frequency and strength of the contractions, intracranial haemorrhage from the sudden compression and decompression of the fetal skull as it passes through the birth canal with speed, and possible injury as the head and body emerge rapidly and fall to the floor. The unexpected nature of the event means that the place of birth may be inappropriate and the baby may be further compromised if the importance of maintaining the baby's temperature is not recognized. The overefficient uterus may relax after the birth of the baby, resulting in retained placenta and/or PPH. The psychological impact of such a rapid birth must not be underestimated, and not surprisingly some women will be in a state of shock after the event.

Whilst precipitate labour will often recur in subsequent pregnancies there is no evidence to recommend IOL as a preventative measure. However, a woman who has experienced an unattended precipitate labour and birth may request IOL in order to ensure an attended birth in a safe environment (NICE 2008a)

MAKING BIRTH A POSITIVE EXPERIENCE

For the woman who has a spontaneous onset of labour at term, has a single fetus in a cephalic presentation and who has no underlying medical disorders, labour should be about the normal physiological event. The only intervention it requires on the part of the midwife is to be there to meet the needs of the woman and to offer continuous support and encouragement to enable her to feel secure and confident in those caring for her at this momentous time.

The views of midwives and doctors on childbirth are often considered to be diametrically opposite, with midwives looking on childbirth as normal until proved otherwise (RCM 2008) and obstetricians viewing it as normal retrospectively (El-Hamamay and Arulkumaran 2005).

Whatever the perspective taken, the primary outcome is the safety of the mother and baby. Whilst a high-risk pregnancy and labour cannot be made low-risk it can still be a positive birthing experience for the woman and her partner. Childbearing is a time of major life transition and each woman and partner deserve to have a positive birth experience whether labour is spontaneous or induced and the birth is vaginal or by caesarean section. Working together as a team cannot but help to contribute to that positive birth experience.

REFERENCES

Arrowsmith S, Wray S, Quenby S 2011 Maternal obesity and labour complications following induction of labour in prolonged pregnancy. BJOG: An International Journal of Obstetrics and Gynaecology 118(5):578–88

Bailit J L, Gregory K D, Reddy V M et al 2010 Maternal and neonatal outcomes by labour onset type and gestational age. American Journal of Obstetrics and Gynecology 202(3):245.e1–245.e12

Balchin I, Whittaker C, Patel R et al 2007 Racial variation in the association between gestational age and perinatal mortality: prospective study. British Medical Journal 334:833

Biggar R J, Poulsen G, Melbye M et al 2010 Spontaneous labor onset: is it immunologically mediated? American Journal of Obstetrics and Gynecology 202(3): 268.e1–268.e7

Bishop E H 1964 Pelvic scoring for elective induction Obstetrics and Gynecology 24(2):266–8

Blackburn S 2013 Maternal, fetal, and neonatal physiology: a clinical perspective, 4th edn. Elsevier Saunders, Philadelphia

BNF (British National Formulary) 2013 BNF 53, March. www.bnf.org

Boulvain M, Stan C M, Irion O 2005 Membrane sweeping for induction of labour. Cochrane Database of Systematic Reviews, Issue 1. Art. No. CD000451. doi: 10.1002/14651858. CD000451.pub2

Bricker L, Luckas M 2012 Amniotomy alone for induction of labour (Review). Cochrane Database of Systematic Reviews, Issue 8. Art. No. CD002862. doi: 10.1002/14651858 .CD002862

Cardozo L, Fysh J, Pearce J M 1986 Prolonged pregnancy: the management debate. British Medical Journal 293(6554):1059–63

Cheng Y, Nicholson J, Shaffer B et al 2009 The second stage of labor and epidural use: a larger effect than previously stated. American Journal of Obstetrics and Gynecology 201(6):S46

Cheyne H, Abhyankar P, Williams B 2012 Elective induction of labour: the problem of interpretation and communication of risks. Midwifery 28(4):412–15

de Miranda E, van der Bom J G, Bonsel G J et al 2006 Membrane sweeping and prevention of post-term pregnancy in low-risk pregnancies: a randomised controlled trial. BJOG: An International Journal of Obstetrics and Gynaecology 113(4A):402–8

DH (Department of Health) 2006 NHS Maternity Statistics, England: 2004–05. Department of Health, London

Elghorori M R M, Hassan I, Dartey W et al 2006 Comparison between subjective and objective assessments of the cervix before induction of labour. Journal of Obstetrics and Gynaecology 26(6):521–6

El Halta V 1998 Preventing prolonged labor. Midwifery Today Summer: 22–7

El-Hamamy E, Arulkumaran S 2005 Poor progress of labour. Current Obstetrics and Gynaecology 15(1):1–8

Fox H 1997 Aging of the placenta. Archives of Diseases in Childhood 77(3):171–5

Friedman E 1954 The graphic analysis of labor. American Journal of Obstetrics and Gynecology 68(6):1568–75

Gatward H, Simpson M, Woodhart L et al 2010 Women's experiences of being induced for post-date pregnancy. Women and Birth 23(1):3–9

Gilchrist L, Carrick-Sen D, Blott M et al 2010 Woman-centred second stage

guidelines compared to time-limited guidelines: evidence of benefit. Archives of Disease in Childhood. Fetal and Neonatal Edition 95 (Suppl 1).

Griffith R, Tengnah C A, Patel C 2010 Law and professional issues in midwifery. Learning Matters, Exeter

Gülmezoglu A M, Crowther C A, Middleton P et al 2012 Induction of labour for improving birth outcomes for women at or beyond term. Cochrane Database of Systematic Reviews 2012, Issue 6. Art. No. CD004945. doi: 10.1002/14651858. CD004945.pub3

Hayman R 2004 Poor progress in labour. In: Luesley D M, Baker P N (eds) Obstetrics and gynaecology. An evidence-based text for MRCOG. Arnold, London

HSCIC (Health and Social Care Information Centre) 2012 NHS Maternity Statistics 2011–2012 Summary Report. Available at www.hscic.gov.uk/ (accessed 12 June 2013)

Heimstad R, Skogvoll E, Mattsson L A et al 2007 Induction of labour or serial antenatal fetal monitoring in post term pregnancy: a randomised controlled trial. Obstetrics and Gynaecology 109(3):609–17

Hermus M A, Verhoeven C J, Mol B W et al 2009 Comparison of induction of labour and expectant management in postterm pregnancy: a matched cohort study. Journal of Midwifery and Women's Health 54(5):351–6

Hodnett E D, Gates S, Hofmeyr G J 2012 Continuous support for women during childbirth (Review). Cochrane Database of Systematic Reviews 2012, Issue 10. Art. No. CD003766. doi: 10.1002/14651858 .CD003766.pub4

House of Commons Select Committee on Science and Technology 2007

Twelfth Report: Scientific developments relating to the Abortion Act 1967. HC 1045-1. TSO, London

Hovi M, Raatikainen K, Heiskanen N et al 2006 Obstetric outcome in post-term pregnancies: time for reappraisal in clinical management. Acta Obstetricia et Gynecologica Scandinavica 85(7):805–9

Jowitt M 2012 Should labour be induced for prolonged pregnancy? Midwifery Matters 134(Autumn): 7–13

Kavanagh J, Kelly A J, Thomas J 2005 Breast stimulation for cervical ripening and induction of labour (Review). (Date of most recent substantive update: 10 March 2005). Cochrane Database of Systematic Reviews, Issue 3. Art. No. CD003392. doi: 10.1002/14651858 .CD003392.pub2

Kavanagh J, Kelly A J, Thomas J 2008 Sexual intercourse for cervical ripening and induction of labour (Review). Cochrane Database of Systematic Reviews, Issue 4. Art. No. CD003093. doi: 10.1002/14651858 .CD003093.

Kirkham M, Stapleton H, Thomas G 2002 Qualitative study of evidence based leaflets in maternity care. British Medical Journal 324:639–42

Koklanaris N, Tropper P 2006 Post term pregnancy. Female Patient: Ob/Gyn edition 31(6):14–18

Kramer M S, Rouleau J, Baskett T F et al 2006 Amniotic-fluid embolism and medical induction of labour: a retrospective, population-based cohort study. Lancet 368:1444–8

Laursen M, Bille C, Olesen A W et al 2004 Genetic influence on prolonged gestation: a population-based Danish twin study. American Journal of Obstetrics and Gynaecology 190:489–94

Laursen M, Johansen C, Hedegaar M 2009 Fear of childbirth and risk for birth complications in nulliparous women in Danish National Birth Cohort. BJOG: An International Journal of Obstetrics and Gynaecology 116(10):1350–5

Lavender T, Hart A, Smyth R M D 2012 Effect of different partogram use on outcomes for women in spontaneous labour at term (Review). Cochrane Database of Systematic Reviews, Issue 8. Art. No. CD005461. doi: 10.1002/14651858.CD005461.pub3

Lowe N K 2007 A review of factors associated with dystocia and cesarean section in nulliparous women. Journal of Midwifery and Women's Health 52(3):216–28

McCarthy F P, Kenny L C 2010 Induction of labour. Obstetrics, Gynaecology and Reproductive Medicine 21(1):1–6

Menticoglou S M, Hall P F 2002 Routine induction of labour at 41 weeks' gestation: nonsensus consensus. BJOG: An International Journal of Obstetrics and Gynaecology 109(5):485–91

Mitchell M D, Flint A P F, Bibby J et al 1977 Rapid increases in plasma prostaglandin concentrations after vaginal examination and amniotomy. British Medical Journal 2(6096):1183–5

Morken N H, Melve K K, Skjaerven R 2011 Recurrence of prolonged and post-term gestational age across generations: maternal and paternal contribution. BJOG: An International Journal of Obstetrics and Gynaecology 118(13):1630–5

Neal L, Lowe N K, Ahijevych K et al 2010 'Active labor' duration and dilation rates among low-risk, nulliparous women with spontaneous labor onset: a systematic review. Journal of Midwifery and Womens Health 55(4):308–18

NICE (National Institute for Health and Clinical Excellence) 2007 Intrapartum care. Care of healthy women and their babies during childbirth. Clinical Guideline 55. National Collaborating Centre for Women's and Children's Health. NICE, London

NICE (National Institute for Health and Clinical Excellence) 2008a Induction of labour. Clinical Guideline 70. National Collaborating Centre for Women's and Children's Health. NICE, London

NICE (National Institute for Health and Clinical Excellence) 2008b Diabetes in pregnancy. Clinical Guideline 63 National Collaborating Centre for Women's and Children's Health. NICE, London

NICE (National Institute for Health and Clinical Excellence) 2011 Caesarean section. Clinical Guideline 132. National Collaborating Centre for Women's and Children's Health. RCOG, London

Neilson J P, Lavender T, Quenby S et al 2003 Obstructed labour. British Medical Bulletin 67(1): 191–204

NMC (Nursing and Midwifery Council) 2008 The code: standards of conduct, performance and ethics for nurses and midwives. NMC, London

NMC (Nursing and Midwifery Council) 2012 Midwives rules and standards 2012. NMC, London

Nystedt A, Hogberg U, Lundman B 2005 The negative birth experience of prolonged labour: a case-referent study. Journal of Clinical Nursing 14:579–86

Nystedt A, Hogberg U, Lundman B 2006 Some Swedish women's experiences of prolonged labour. Midwifery 22(1):56–65

Olesen A W, Westergaard J G, Olsen J 2006 Prenatal risk indicators of a prolonged pregnancy. The Danish Birth Cohort 1998–2001. Acta Obstetricia et Gynecologica Scandinavica 85(11):1338–41

Oros D, Bejarano M P, Cardiel M R et al 2012 Low-risk pregnancy at 41 weeks: when should we induce labor? Journal of Maternal–Fetal and Neonatal Mdicine 25(6):728–31

Ragunath M, McEwan A S 2007 Induction of labour. Obstetrics, Gynaecology and Reproductive Medicine 18(1):1–6

Rogers H 2010 Does a cervical membrane sweep in term healthy pregnancy reduce the length of gestation? MIDIRS Midwifery Digest 20(3):315–19

Royal College of Midwives 2008 Campaign for normal birth: ten top tips for mothers and midwives. www.rcmnormalbirth.org.uk (accessed 12 May 2013)

RCOG (Royal College of Obstetricians and Gynaecologists) 2010 Management of HIV in pregnancy. Guideline No 39. www.rcog.org.uk (accessed 12 May 2013)

Simpson P D, Stanley K P 2011 Prolonged pregnancy. Obstetrics, Gynaecology and Reproductive Medicine 21(9):257–62

Singh S, Paterson-Brown S 2006 Malpresentations in labour. Current

Obstetrics and Gynaecology 16(4):234–41

Smith C A, Crowther C A 2012 Acupuncture for induction of labour (Review). Cochrane Database of Systematic Reviews, Issue 7. Art. No. CD002962. doi: 10.1002/14651858 .CD002962.pub2

Smyth R, Alldred S K, Markham C 2013 Amniotomy for shortening spontaneous labour (Protocol). Cochrane Database of Systematic Reviews, Issue 1. Art. No. CD006167. doi: 10.1002/14651858 .CD006167.pub3

Stevens G, Miler Y D 2012 Overdue choices: how information and role in decision-making influence women's preferences for induction for prolonged pregnancy. Birth 39(3):248–57

Stock S J, Ferguson E, Duffy A et al 2012 Outcomes of elective induction of labour compared with expectant management: population based study. BMJ 344(e2838):1–13

Svärdby K, Nordstrom L, Sellstrom E 2006 Primiparas with or without oxytocin augmentation: a prospective descriptive study. Journal of Clinical Nursing 16:179–84

Tomlinson A J, Archer P A, Hobson S 2001 Induction of labour: a comparison of two methods with particular concern to patient acceptability. Journal of Obstetrics and Gynaecology 21(3):239–41

Tun M, Tuohy J 2011 Rate of postdates induction using first-trimester ultrasound to determine estimated due date: Wellington Regional

Hospital Audit. Australian and New Zealand Journal of Obstetrics and Gynaecology 51(3):216–19

Van Meir C A, Ramirez M M, Matthews et al 1997 Chorionic prostaglandin metabolism is decreased in the lower uterine segment with term labour. Placenta 18:109–14

WHO (World Health Organization) 2011 WHO recommendations for induction of labour. World Health Organization, Geneva

Wong S F, Hui S K, Choi H et al 2002 Does sweeping of membranes beyond 40 weeks reduce the need for formal induction of labour? BJOG: An International Journal of Obstetrics and Gynaecology 109(6):632–36

FURTHER READING

Jukic A M, Baird D D, Weinberg C R et al 2013 Length of human pregnancy and contributors to its natural variation. Human Reproduction. doi: 10.1093/ humanrep/det297. http://humrep .oxfordjournals.org (accessed online 6 August 2013).
Although the study appears underpowered in its small sample size, it provides useful

nuggets of information, highlighting that healthy human pregnancy varies considerably by as much as 37 days for a number of reasons.

Mandruzzato G, Alfirevic Z, Chervenak F et al 2010 Guidelines for the management of post-term pregnancy. Journal of Perinatal Medicine 38 (2):111–19.

From an international perspective this is a useful resource that addresses a number of salient issues relating to prolonged pregnancy. It highlights that there is no unequivocal evidence that prolonged pregnancy is a major risk per se.

USEFUL WEBSITES

Cochrane Library of Systematic Reviews: http://onlinelibrary.wiley.com

Health and Social Care Information Centre: www.hscic.gov.uk/

National Institute for Health and Care [formerly Clinical] Excellence: www.nice.org.uk

Royal College of Midwives: www.rcm.org.uk

Royal College of Obstetricians and Gynaecologists: www.rcog.org.uk

World Health Organization: www.who.net

Chapter |20|

Malpositions of the occiput and malpresentations

Terri Coates

Malposition refers to any position other than occipitoanterior (OA) in a fetus with a vertex presentation. In a normal physiological labour, the fetal head presents with the occiput in lateral position in early stages of labour with anterior rotation as labour progresses.

Malpresentations are all presentations of the fetus other than the vertex. Malpresentations that occur due to extension of the fetal head, causing brow or face to present, are usually diagnosed during active labour. Prompt and appropriate referral must be made.

Both malpositions and malpresentations are associated with a difficult labour and an increased risk of operative intervention. The midwife must undertake regular clinical examinations to monitor the progress of labour to ensure fetal and maternal wellbeing. Effective communication and record keeping is crucial to provide safe care. The woman and her partner must be kept fully informed and supported throughout. Vaginal birth is possible in many cases, but intervention or operative birth become necessary when the malposition or malpresentation persist and labour fails to progress.

INTRODUCTION

Malpositions and malpresentations present the midwife with challenges of recognition and diagnosis both in the antenatal period and during labour. The midwife must ensure all examinations and discussions with the woman are documented and appropriate obstetric referral is made where a malpresentation or malposition has been found. The midwife should take time to discuss this with the women to ensure they understand what may happen and the activities that may help (Munro and Jokinen 2012).

The presenting diameters do not fit well onto the cervix and therefore do not produce optimal stimulation for uterine contractions and labour. Labour with a fetus in a malposition or a malpresentation can be long, tedious and painful, requiring empathy, sustained encouragement and support for the woman and her partner. All the usual care in labour is provided, paying particular attention to comfort and hydration (see Chapter 16). The woman should be encouraged to take an active part in decision-making and must be kept informed throughout.

In labour women should be encouraged to adopt postures and positions they find comfortable and encouraged to remain mobile. They should be supported to use coping methods to deal with their particular pattern of labour (Simkin 2010). The progress of labour may be slow so midwives should take care to avoid the use of language that may demoralize the woman and her partner. Any sign of fetal or maternal distress or delay in labour must be referred promptly to an obstetrician. Practices that are considered unhelpful include immobility and labouring on a bed, the setting of arbitrary time limits on the various stages of labour and the early use of epidural analgesia (Munro and Jokinen 2012).

OCCIPITOPOSTERIOR POSITIONS

Occipitoposterior (OP) positions are the most common type of malposition of the occiput and occur in approximately 10–30% of labours, but only around 5% of births (Pearl et al 1993; Ponkey et al 2003; Munro and Jokinen 2012). Women can be reassured that internal rotation to anterior positions can be expected in the majority of cases. A persistent OP position results from a failure of internal rotation or malrotation prior to birth (Gardberg et al 1998; Peregrine et al 2007). The vertex is presenting, but the occiput lies in the posterior rather than the anterior part of the pelvis. As a consequence, the fetal head is deflexed and larger diameters of the fetal skull present (Fig. 20.1).

Causes

The direct cause of the occipitoposterior position is often unknown, but it may be associated with an abnormally shaped pelvis. In an *android pelvis*, the forepelvis is narrow and the occiput tends to occupy the roomier hindpelvis. The oval shape of the *anthropoid pelvis*, with its narrow transverse diameter, favours a direct OP position.

Antenatal diagnosis

Abdominal examination

Listen to the woman, as she may complain of backache and report feeling that her baby's bottom is very high up against her ribs, as well as feeling movements across both sides of her abdomen.

On inspection

There is a saucer-shaped depression at or just below the umbilicus. This depression is created by the 'dip' between the head and the lower limbs of the fetus. The outline created by the high, unengaged head can look like a full bladder (Fig. 20.2).

On palpation

While the breech is easily palpated at the fundus, the back is difficult to palpate as it is well out to the maternal side, sometimes almost adjacent to the maternal spine. Limbs can be felt on both sides of the midline. The head is unusually high in an OP position which is the most common cause of non-engagement in a primigravida at term. This is because the large presenting diameter, the

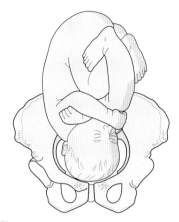

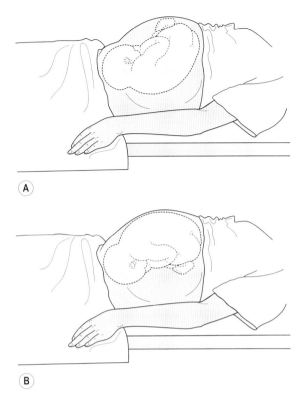

(A) Right occipitoposterior position

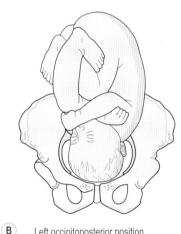

(A)

(B)

Fig. 20.2 Comparison of abdominal contour in (A) posterior and (B) anterior positions of the occiput.

(B) Left occipitoposterior position

Fig. 20.1 (A) Right occipitoposterior position. (B) Left occipitoposterior position.

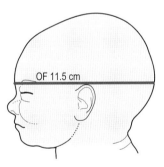

Fig. 20.3 Engaging diameter of a deflexed head: occipitofrontal (OF) 11.5 cm.

occipitofrontal (11.5 cm), is unlikely to enter the pelvic brim until labour begins and flexion occurs. The occiput and sinciput are on the same level (Figs 20.3 and 20.4). Flexion allows the engagement of the suboccipitofrontal diameter (10 cm).

The cause of the deflexion is a straightening of the fetal spine against the lumbar curve of the maternal spine. This makes the fetus straighten its neck and adopt a more erect attitude.

On auscultation

The fetal back is not well flexed so the chest is thrust forward, therefore the fetal heart can be heard in the midline. However, the fetal heart may be heard more easily at the flank on the same side as the back.

Antenatal preparation

There is no current evidence that suggests active changes of maternal posture will help to achieve an optimal fetal position before labour (Hunter et al 2007; Munro and Jokinen 2012). Research has shown that the woman adopting a knee–chest position several times a day may achieve temporary rotation of the fetus to an anterior position but has only a short-term effect upon fetal presentation (Kariminia et al 2004; Hunter et al 2007). There is

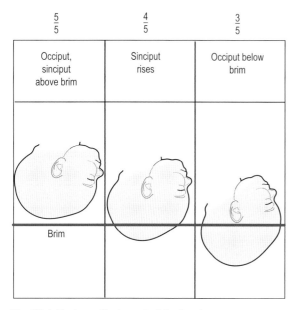

$\frac{5}{5}$	$\frac{4}{5}$	$\frac{3}{5}$
Occiput, sinciput above brim	Sinciput rises	Occiput below brim

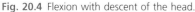

Brim

Fig. 20.4 Flexion with descent of the head.

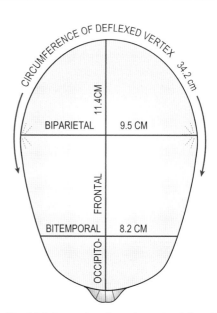

Fig. 20.5 Presenting dimensions of a deflexed head.

insufficient evidence to suggest that women should adopt the hands and knees posture, unless they find it comfortable (Simkin 2010; Munro and Jokinen 2012). Further research is needed to evaluate the effect of adopting a hands and knees posture on the presenting part during labour (Hunter et al 2007).

For customary antenatal assessment of fetal position Leopold's manoeuvres can be used during abdominal examination (see Chapter 10). These traditional methods of examination are only an assessment of the placement of the fetal spine and cannot estimate the direction of the fetal head. Peregrine et al (2007) used ultrasound scans to confirm abdominal palpation and found that the fetal head is often aligned differently within the pelvis than the fetal spine within the uterus. In other words, the fetus may have turned its head to the right or left and the head may be anterior within the pelvis but the fetal back may palpate as lateral.

A review of current techniques used to diagnose fetal position such as Leopold's manoeuvres, the location of fetal heart sounds, vaginal examinations and presence of back pain are often unreliable (Simkin 2010). Failure to identify fetal position accurately can impact on the ability of the midwife to offer appropriate care. Consequently it is considered that ultrasound is the most reliable way to accurately detect the fetal position (Munro and Jokinen 2012). More research studies are needed to examine the efficacy of midwifery skills in diagnosing fetal malpositions and non-technological approaches to improving the birth outcome for the woman and fetus.

Intrapartum diagnosis

The large and irregularly shaped presenting circumference (Fig. 20.5) does not fit well onto the cervix. This may hinder cervical ripening and predispose to a prolonged latent phase (Akmal and Paterson-Brown 2009). The contractions may also be in-coordinate. A high head predisposes to early spontaneous rupture of the membranes at an early stage of labour, which, together with an ill-fitting presenting part, may result in *cord prolapse* (see Chapter 22).

The woman may complain of continuous and severe backache, worsening with contractions. However, the absence of backache does not necessarily indicate an anteriorly positioned fetus. Descent of the head can be slow even with good contractions. The woman may have a strong desire to push early in labour because the occiput is pressing on the rectum.

Vaginal examination

The findings (Fig. 20.6) will depend upon the degree of flexion of the head. Locating the anterior fontanelle in the anterior part of the pelvis is diagnostic but this may be difficult if caput succedaneum is present. The direction of the sagittal suture and location of the posterior fontanelle will help to confirm the diagnosis. The position of the fetal head may be checked using ultrasound where reason for the delay in labour requires accurate diagnosis.

Anterior

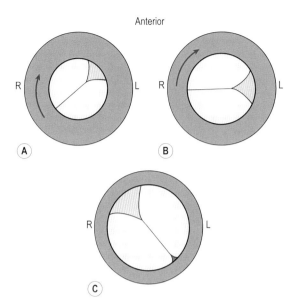

Fig. 20.6 Vaginal touch pictures in a right occipitoposterior position. (A) Anterior fontanelle felt to left and anteriorly. Sagittal suture in the right oblique diameter of the pelvis. (B) Anterior fontanelle felt to left and laterally. Sagittal suture in the transverse diameter of the pelvis. (C) Following increased flexion, the posterior fontanelle is felt to the right and anteriorly. Sagittal suture in the left oblique diameter of the pelvis. The position is now right occipitoanterior.

Midwifery care

First stage of labour

The woman may experience severe and unremitting backache, which is tiring and can be very demoralizing, especially if the progress of labour is slow. Continuous support from the midwife will help the woman and her partner to cope with the labour (Simkin 2010; Hodnett et al 2012) (see Chapter 16). The midwife can help to provide physical support such as massage and other comfort measures. Mobility should be encouraged with changes of posture and position and where possible, the use of a bath or birthing pool and other non-pharmacological measures such as transcutaneous electrical nerve stimulation (TENS) or aromatherapy. There is no evidence that the *all-fours position* either during pregnancy or in labour will rotate a malpositioned baby (Kariminia et al 2004; Munro and Jokinen 2012) but may help reduce persistent back pain. An *exaggerated Sims position* in labour may offer some relief, and anecdotal evidence suggests that it may also aid rotation of the fetal head.

The woman may experience a strong urge to push long before the cervix has become fully dilated. This is because of the pressure of the occiput on the rectum. However, if the woman pushes at this time, the cervix may become oedematous and this would further delay the onset of the

second stage of labour. The urge to push may be eased by a change in position and the use of breathing techniques, inhalational analgesia or other methods to enhance relaxation. The woman's partner and the midwife can assist throughout labour with massage and physical support. The woman may choose a range of pain control methods (see Chapter 16) throughout her labour depending on the level and intensity of pain she is experiencing at that time. The midwife must ensure that any delay in labour and fetal or maternal distress are promptly recognized and appropriate referrals made (Nursing and Midwifery Council [NMC] 2012).

Second stage of labour

Full dilatation of the cervix may need to be confirmed by a vaginal examination because moulding and formation of a caput succedaneum may be in view while an anterior lip of cervix remains. The second stage of labour is usually characterized by significant anal dilatation some time before the head is visible. The midwife can encourage the woman to adopt upright positions that may help to shorten the length of the second stage and reduce the need for operative assistance (see Chapter 17). Squatting may increase the transverse diameter of the pelvic outlet which may increase the chance of a vaginal birth.

The length of the second stage of labour is usually increased when the occiput is posterior, and there is an increased likelihood of an operative birth (Pearl et al 1993; Gimovsky and Hennigan 1995). In some cases where contractions are weak and ineffective an oxytocin infusion may be administered to stimulate adequate contractions and achieve advancement/descent of the presenting part.

Manual rotation

Manual rotation of the head from occipitoposterior (OP) or occipitotransverse (OT) positions to an anterior position has been shown to reduce the need for assisted birth and caesarean section by correcting the fetal malposition. This will facilitate the descent of the fetal head, to encourage a spontaneous vaginal birth (Shaffer et al 2011).

There are two techniques for undertaking manual rotation either by an obstetrician or an experienced and trained midwife. Both techniques require informed consent from the woman and adequate analgesia. The woman's bladder must be empty and the cervix should be fully dilated. Either, constant pressure is exerted with the tips of the fingers against the lambdoidal suture to rotate the fetal head into the occiput anterior position, or the whole hand is introduced into the birth canal and fingers and thumb positioned under the lateral posterior parietal bone and the anterior parietal bone (Phipps et al 2011): the head is then rotated to the anterior position. Using either method, the rotation may take two or three contractions to complete and then should be held for two contractions whilst the woman bears down to reduce the risk of the rotation reverting (Phipps et al 2011; Shaffer et al 2011). If a midwife is practising in a setting where operative birth is not readily available, such as in a birthing centre, this intervention may reduce maternal and neonatal morbidity and mortality (Shaffer et al 2011).

Malpositions and malpresentations are generally associated with a higher incidence of interventions in labour, complications and instrumental birth (Cheng et al 2006). Immediate and subsequent postnatal care of the woman and her baby following an instrumental birth are discussed in Chapter 21 and Chapter 31.

Mechanism of right occipitoposterior position (long rotation) (Figs 20.7–20.10)

- The lie is longitudinal.
- The attitude of the head is deflexed.
- The presentation is vertex.
- The position is right occipitoposterior.
- The denominator is the occiput.
- The presenting part is the middle or anterior area of the left parietal bone.

- The occipitofrontal diameter, 11.5 cm, lies in the right oblique diameter of the pelvic brim. The occiput points to the right sacroiliac joint and the sinciput to the left iliopectineal eminence.

Flexion

Descent takes place with increasing flexion. The occiput becomes the leading part.

Internal rotation of the head

The occiput reaches the pelvic floor first and rotates forwards ⅜ of a circle along the right side of the pelvis to lie under the symphysis pubis. The shoulders follow, turning ⅖ of a circle from the left to the right oblique diameter.

Crowning

The occiput escapes under the symphysis pubis and the head is crowned.

Extension

The sinciput, face and chin sweep the perineum and the head is born by a movement of extension.

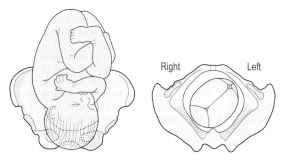

Fig. 20.7 Head descending with increased flexion. Sagittal suture in right oblique diameter of the pelvis.

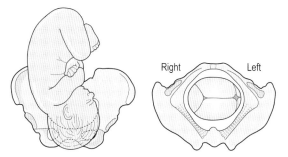

Fig. 20.8 Occiput and shoulders have rotated ⅛ of a circle forwards. Sagittal suture in transverse diameter of the pelvis.

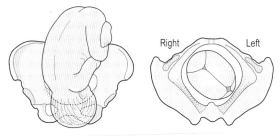

Fig. 20.9 Occiput and shoulders have rotated ⅖ of a circle forwards. Sagittal suture in the left oblique diameter of the pelvis. The position is right occipitoanterior.

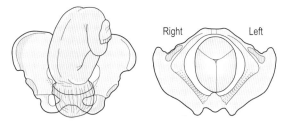

Fig. 20.10 Occiput has rotated ⅜ of a circle forwards. Note the twist in the neck. Sagittal suture in the anteroposterior diameter of the pelvis.

Figs 20.7–20.10 Mechanism of labour in right occipitoposterior position.

Restitution

The occiput turns $\frac{1}{8}$ of a circle to the right and the head realigns itself with the shoulders.

Internal rotation of the shoulders

The shoulders enter the pelvis in the right oblique diameter; the anterior shoulder reaches the pelvic floor first and rotates forwards $\frac{1}{8}$ of a circle to lie under the symphysis pubis.

External rotation of the head

At the same time the occiput turns a further $\frac{1}{8}$ of a circle to the right.

Lateral flexion

The anterior shoulder escapes under the symphysis pubis, the posterior shoulder sweeps the perineum and the body is born by a movement of lateral flexion.

Possible course and outcomes of labour

Long internal rotation

This is the commonest outcome. With good uterine contractions producing flexion and descent of the head, the occiput will rotate forward $\frac{3}{8}$ of a circle as described above.

Short internal rotation

The term persistent *occipitoposterior position* (Figs 20.11 and 20.12) indicates that the occiput fails to rotate forwards. Instead, the sinciput reaches the pelvic floor first and rotates forwards. As a result, the occiput goes into the hollow of the sacrum. The baby is born facing the pubic bone (*face to pubis*).

Cause

Failure of flexion: the head descends without increased flexion and the sinciput becomes the leading part. It

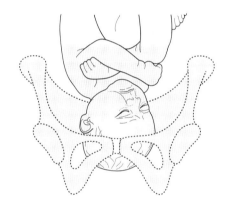

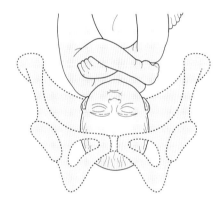

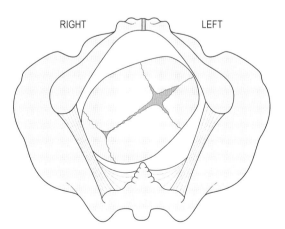

Fig. 20.11 Persistent occipitoposterior position before rotation of the occiput: position is right occipitoposterior.

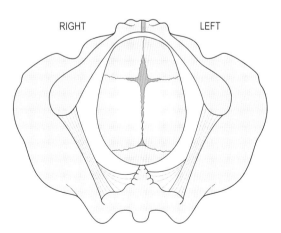

Fig. 20.12 Persistent occipitoposterior position after short rotation: position direct occipitoposterior.

reaches the pelvic floor first and rotates forwards to lie under the symphysis pubis.

Diagnosis

In the first stage of labour: signs are those of any posterior position of the occiput, namely a deflexed head and a fetal heart heard in the flank or in the midline. Descent is slow.

In the second stage of labour: delay is common. On vaginal examination the anterior fontanelle is felt behind the symphysis pubis, but a large caput succedaneum may mask this. If the pinna of the ear is felt pointing towards the woman's sacrum, this indicates a posterior position.

The long occipitofrontal diameter causes considerable dilatation of the anus and gaping of the vagina while the fetal head is barely visible, and the broad biparietal diameter distends the perineum and may cause excessive bulging. As the head advances, the anterior fontanelle can be felt just behind the symphysis pubis. Consequently the fetus is born facing the pubis. Characteristic upward moulding is present with the caput succedaneum on the anterior part of the parietal bone (Fig. 20.13).

The birth (Figs 20.14–20.17)

The sinciput will first emerge from under the symphysis pubis as far as the root of the nose and the midwife maintains flexion by restraining it from escaping further than the glabella, allowing the occiput to sweep the perineum and be born. She then extends the head by grasping it and bringing the face down from under the symphysis pubis. Perineal trauma is common and the midwife should watch for signs of rupture in the centre of the perineum (*button-hole* tear). An episiotomy may be required, owing to the larger presenting diameters.

Undiagnosed face to pubis

If the signs are not recognized at an earlier stage, the midwife may first be aware that the occiput is posterior

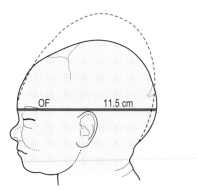

Fig. 20.13 Upward moulding (dotted line) following persistent occipitoposterior position. OF, occipitofrontal.

when the hairless forehead is seen escaping beneath the pubic arch. Any accidental extension of the fetal head should be corrected by flexion towards the symphysis pubis.

Deep transverse arrest

The head descends with some increase in flexion. The occiput reaches the pelvic floor and begins to rotate forwards. Flexion is not maintained and the occipito-frontal diameter becomes caught at the narrow bi-spinous diameter of the outlet. Arrest may be due to weak contractions, a straight sacrum or a narrowed pelvic outlet.

The sagittal suture is found in the transverse diameter of the pelvis and both fontanelles are palpable. Neither sinciput nor occiput leads. The head is deep in the pelvic cavity at the level of the ischial spines although the caput may be lower still. There is no advance and obstetric assistance will be required. Manual rotation may be attempted first, and then vaginal birth may follow with the woman's effort.

Management

The woman must be kept informed of progress and participate in decisions. Pushing at this time may not resolve the problem but the midwife and the woman's partner can help by encouraging 'sigh out slowly' (SOS) breathing. A change of position may help to overcome the urge to bear down (see Chapter 17).

Where assistance is needed for a safe birth the woman's informed consent is required. The procedure would be undertaken under local, regional or more rarely general anaesthesia (see Chapter 21) considering the choice of the woman, her condition and that of her unborn baby. The baby's head will be brought into an anterior position and the birth completed using forceps or vacuum extraction (see Chapter 21).

Conversion to face or brow presentation

When the head is deflexed at the onset of labour, extension occasionally occurs instead of flexion. If extension is complete then a *face presentation* results, but if incomplete, the head is arrested at the brim with the brow presenting. This is a rare complication of posterior positions, and is more commonly found in multigravidae.

Complications

Apart from prolonged labour with its attendant risks to the woman and fetus and the increased likelihood of instrumental birth, there are a number of complications that may occur which the midwife should consider.

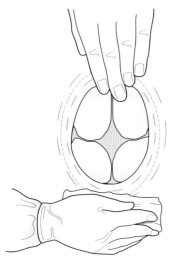

Fig. 20.14 Allowing the sinciput to escape as far as the glabella.

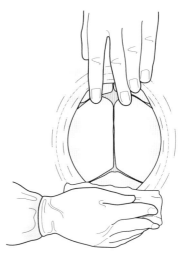

Fig. 20.15 The occiput sweeps the perineum, sinciput held back to maintain flexion.

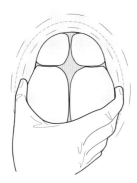

Fig. 20.16 Grasping the head to bring the face down from under the symphysis pubis.

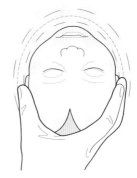

Fig. 20.17 Extension of the head.

Figs 20.14–20.17 Birth of head in a persistent occipitoposterior position.

Obstructed labour

This may occur when the head is deflexed or partially extended and becomes impacted in the pelvis (see Chapter 19).

Maternal trauma

A forceps birth will result in perineal bruising and trauma. Birth of a baby in the persistent occipitoposterior position, particularly if previously undiagnosed, may cause a third or fourth degree tear (Melamed et al 2013).

Neonatal trauma

The unfavourable upward moulding of the fetal skull, found in an occipitoposterior position, can cause intracranial haemorrhage, as a result of the falx cerebri being pulled away from the tentorium cerebelli. The larger presenting diameters also predispose to a greater degree of compression. Cerebral haemorrhage (see Chapter 31) may also result from chronic hypoxia, which may accompany prolonged labour.

Neonatal trauma occurring following birth from an occipitoposterior position has also been associated with forceps or ventouse births.

FACE PRESENTATION

When the attitude of the head is one of complete extension, the occiput of the fetus will be in contact with its spine and the face will present. The incidence is about ≤1:500 (Bhal et al 1998; Akmal and Paterson-Brown 2009) and the majority develop during labour from vertex presentations with the occiput posterior; this is termed *secondary face presentation*. Less commonly, the face presents before labour; this is termed *primary face presentation*. There are six positions in a face presentation; the denominator is the mentum and the presenting diameters are the submentobregmatic (9.5 cm) and the bitemporal (8.2 cm) (Figs 20.18–20.23).

Causes

Anterior obliquity of the uterus

The uterus of a multigravida with slack abdominal muscles and a pendulous abdomen will lean forward and alter the direction of the uterine axis. This causes the fetal buttocks to lean forwards and the force of the contractions to be directed in a line towards the chin rather than the occiput, resulting in extension of the head.

Contracted pelvis

In the flat pelvis, the head enters in the transverse diameter of the brim and the parietal eminences may be held up in the obstetrical conjugate causing the head to become extended such that a face presentation develops. Alternatively, if the head is in the posterior position with the vertex presenting, and remains deflexed, the parietal eminences may be caught in the sacrocotyloid dimension of the maternal pelvis so that the occiput cannot descend, and the head becomes extended resulting in a face presentation. This is more likely in the presence of an android pelvis, in which the sacrocotyloid dimension is reduced.

Hydramnios (polyhydramnios)

If the vertex is presenting and the membranes rupture spontaneously, the resulting rush of an excess of amniotic fluid may cause the head to extend as it sinks into the lower uterine segment.

Congenital malformation

Anencephaly can be a fetal cause of a face presentation. In a cephalic presentation, because the vertex is absent the face is thrust forward and presents. More rarely, a tumour of the fetal neck may cause extension of the head.

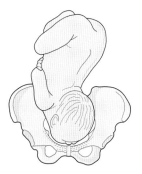

Fig. 20.18 Right mentoposterior.

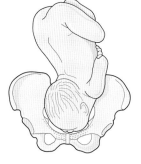

Fig. 20.19 Left mentoposterior.

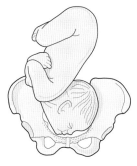

Fig. 20.20 Right mentolateral.

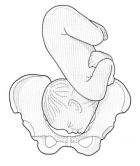

Fig. 20.21 Left mentolateral.

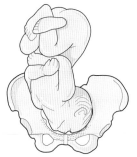

Fig. 20.22 Right mentoanterior.

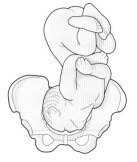

Fig. 20.23 Left mentoanterior.

Figs 20.18–20.23 Six positions of face presentation.

Antenatal diagnosis

Antenatal diagnosis is rare since face presentation develops during labour in the majority of cases. A cephalic presentation in a known anencephalic fetus may be presumed to be a face presentation.

Intrapartum diagnosis

Abdominal palpation

Face presentation may not be detected, especially if the mentum is anterior. The occiput feels prominent, with a groove between the head and back, but it may be mistaken for the sinciput. The limbs may be palpated on the side opposite to the occiput and the fetal heart is best heard through the fetal chest on the same side as the limbs. In a mentoposterior position the fetal heart is difficult to hear because the fetal chest is in contact with the maternal spine (Fig. 20.24).

Vaginal examination

The presenting part is high, soft and irregular. When the cervix is sufficiently dilated, the orbital ridges, eyes, nose and mouth may be felt. However, confusion between the mouth and anus could arise. The mouth may be open, and the hard gums are diagnostic with the possibility of the fetus sucking the examining finger. As labour progresses the face becomes oedematous, making it more difficult to distinguish from a breech presentation. To determine the position the mentum must be located. If it is posterior, the midwife should decide whether it is lower than the

sinciput, and if it can advance, it will rotate forwards. In a left mentoanterior position, the orbital ridges will be in the left oblique diameter of the pelvis (Fig. 20.25). Care must be taken not to injure or infect the eyes with the examining finger.

Mechanism of a left mentoanterior position

- The lie is longitudinal.
- The attitude is one of extension of the fetal head and neck.
- The presentation is the face (Fig. 20.26).
- The position is left mentoanterior.
- The denominator is the mentum.
- The presenting part is the left malar bone.

Extension

Descent takes place with increasing extension. The mentum becomes the leading part.

Internal rotation of the head

This occurs when the chin reaches the pelvic floor and rotates forwards $\frac{1}{8}$ of a circle. The chin escapes under the symphysis pubis (Fig. 20.27A).

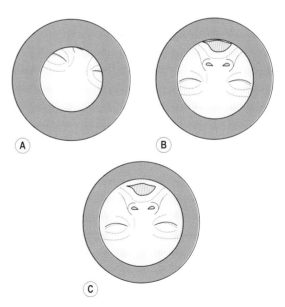

Fig. 20.25 Vaginal touch pictures of left mentoanterior position. (A) The mentum is felt to left and anteriorly. Orbital ridges in left oblique diameter of the pelvis. (B) Following increased extension of the head, the mouth can be felt. (C) The face has rotated $\frac{1}{8}$ of a circle forwards. Orbital ridges in transverse diameter of the pelvis. Position direct mentoanterior.

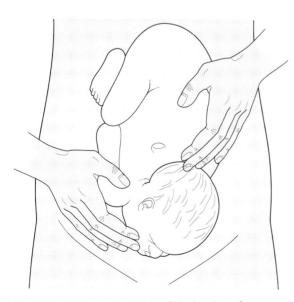

Fig. 20.24 Abdominal palpation of the head in a face presentation. Position right mentoposterior.

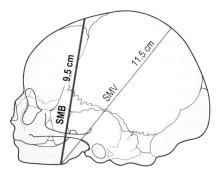

Fig. 20.26 Diameters involved in the birth of a face presentation. Engaging diameter, submentobregmatic (SMB) 9.5 cm. The submentovertical (SMV) diameter, 11.5 cm, sweeps the perineum.

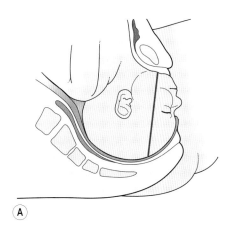

(A)

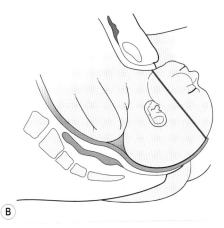

(B)

Fig. 20.27 Birth of head in mentoanterior position. (A) The chin escapes under symphysis pubis. Submentobregmatic diameter at outlet. (B) The head is born by a movement of flexion.

Flexion

This takes place and the sinciput, vertex and occiput sweep the perineum; the head is born (Fig. 20.27B).

Restitution

This occurs when the chin turns $\frac{1}{8}$ of a circle to the woman's left side.

Internal rotation of the shoulders

The shoulders enter the pelvis in the left oblique diameter of the maternal pelvis and the anterior shoulder reaches the pelvic floor first, rotating forwards $\frac{1}{8}$ of a circle along the right side of the pelvis.

External rotation of the head

This occurs simultaneously. The chin moves a further $\frac{1}{8}$ of a circle to the left.

Lateral flexion

The anterior shoulder escapes under the symphysis pubis, the posterior shoulder sweeps the perineum and the baby's body is born by a movement of lateral flexion.

Possible course and outcomes of labour

Prolonged labour

Labour is often prolonged because the face is an ill-fitting presenting part and does not therefore stimulate effective uterine contractions. The woman should be kept informed of her progress and any proposed intervention throughout labour.

In addition, the facial bones do not mould and, in order to enable the mentum to reach the pelvic floor and rotate forwards, the shoulders must enter the pelvic cavity at the same time as the head. The fetal axis pressure is directed to the chin and the head is extended almost at right-angles to the spine, increasing the diameters to be accommodated in the pelvis.

Mentoanterior positions

With good uterine contractions, descent and rotation of the head occur (Fig. 20.27) and labour progresses to a spontaneous birth as described below.

Mentoposterior positions

If the head is completely extended, so that the mentum reaches the pelvic floor first, and the contractions are effective, the mentum will rotate forwards and the position becomes anterior.

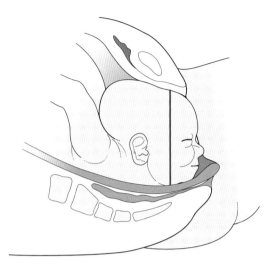

Fig. 20.28 Persistent mentoposterior position.

Persistent mentoposterior position

In this case, the head is incompletely extended and the sinciput reaches the pelvic floor first and rotates forwards $\frac{1}{8}$ of a circle, which brings the chin into the hollow of the sacrum (Fig. 20.28). There is no further mechanism. The face becomes impacted because, in order to descend further, both head and chest would have to be accommodated in the pelvis. Whatever emerges anteriorly from the vagina must pivot around the subpubic arch. When the chin is posterior this is impossible because the head can extend no further.

Reversal of face presentation

A face presentation in a persistent mentoposterior position may, in some cases, be manipulated to an occipito-anterior position using bimanual pressure (Neuman et al 1994; Gimovsky and Hennigan 1995). This method was developed to reduce the likelihood of an operative birth for those women who refused caesarean section. Using a tocolytic drug, such as terbutaline, to relax the uterus, the fetal head is disengaged using upward transvaginal pressure. The fetal head is then flexed with bimanual pressure under ultrasound guidance to achieve an occipitoanterior position.

Management of labour

First stage of labour

Upon diagnosis of a face presentation, the midwife should inform the doctor of this deviation from the normal. Routine observations of maternal and fetal conditions are made as in a normal physiological labour (see Chapter 16). A fetal scalp electrode must *not* be applied, and care

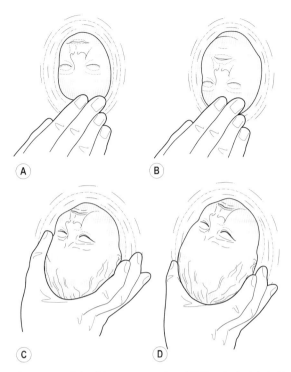

Fig. 20.29 Birth of face presentation. (A) The sinciput is held back to increase extension until the chin is born. (B) The chin is born. (C) Flexing the head to bring the occiput over the perineum. (D) Flexion is completed; the head is born.

should be taken not to infect or injure the eyes during vaginal examinations.

Immediately following rupture of the membranes, a vaginal examination should be performed to exclude cord prolapse which is more likely because the face is an ill-fitting presenting part. Descent of the fetal head should be assessed abdominally, and careful vaginal examination performed every 2–4 hours to determine cervical dilatation and descent of the head.

In mentoposterior positions the midwife should note whether the mentum is lower than the sinciput, since rotation and descent depend on this. If the head remains high in spite of good contractions, caesarean section is likely. The woman may be prescribed oral ranitidine, 150 mg every 6 hours throughout labour if it is considered that an anaesthetic may be necessary.

Birth of the head (Fig. 20.29)

When the face appears at the vulva, extension must be maintained by holding back the sinciput and permitting the mentum to escape under the symphysis pubis before the occiput is allowed to sweep the perineum. In this way, the submentovertical diameter (11.5 cm) instead of the mentovertical diameter (13.5 cm) distends the vaginal orifice. Because the perineum is also distended by the biparietal diameter (9.5 cm), an elective episiotomy may be performed to avoid extensive perineal lacerations.

If the head does not descend in the second stage of labour, the doctor should be informed. In a mentoanterior position it may be possible for the obstetrician to assist the baby's birth with forceps when rotation is incomplete. If the position remains mentoposterior, the head has become impacted, or there is any suspicion of disproportion, a caesarean section will be necessary.

Complications

Obstructed labour

Because the face, unlike the vertex, does not mould, a minor degree of pelvic contraction may result in obstructed labour (see Chapter 19). In a persistent mentoposterior position the face becomes impacted and caesarean section is necessary.

Cord prolapse

A prolapsed cord is more common when the membranes rupture because the face is an ill-fitting presenting part. The midwife should always perform a vaginal examination when the membranes rupture to rule out cord prolapse (see Chapter 22).

Facial bruising

The baby's face is always bruised and swollen at birth, with oedematous eyelids and lips. The head is elongated (Fig. 20.30) and the baby will initially lie with the head extended. The midwife should warn the parents in advance of the baby's *battered* appearance, reassuring them that this is only temporary as the oedema will disappear within 1 or 2 days, with the bruising usually resolving within a week. Trauma during labour may cause tracheal and laryngeal oedema immediately after the birth, which can result in neonatal respiratory distress. In addition, fetal anomalies or tumours, such as fetal goiters that may have contributed to fetal malpresentation, may make intubation difficult. As a result, a clinician with expertise in neonatal resuscitation should be present at the birth.

Cerebral haemorrhage

The lack of moulding of the facial bones can lead to intracranial haemorrhage caused by excessive compression of the fetal skull or by rearward compression, in the typical moulding of the fetal skull found in this presentation (Fig. 20.30).

Maternal trauma

Extensive perineal lacerations may occur at birth owing to the large submentovertical and biparietal diameters distending the vagina and perineum. There is an increased incidence of operative birth by either forceps or by caesarean section, both of which increase maternal morbidity.

BROW PRESENTATION

In the brow presentation the fetal head is partially extended with the frontal bone, which is bounded by the anterior fontanelle and the orbital ridges, lying at the pelvic brim (Fig. 20.31). The presenting diameter of 13.5 cm is the mentovertical (Fig. 20.32), which exceeds all diameters in an average-sized gynaecoid pelvis. This presentation is rare, with an incidence of approximately 1 in 1000 births (Bhal et al 1998).

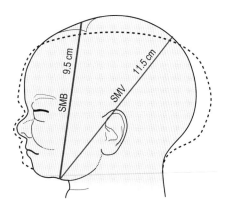

Fig. 20.30 Moulding in a face presentation (dotted line). SMB, submentobregmatic; SMV, submentovertical.

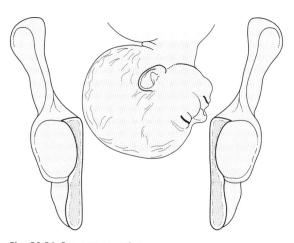

Fig. 20.31 Brow presentation.

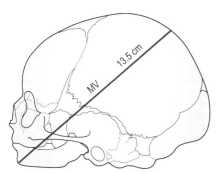

Fig. 20.32 Brow presentation. The mentovertical (MV) diameter, 13.5 cm, lies at the pelvic brim.

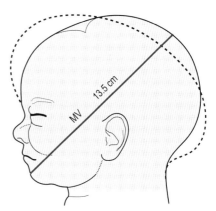

Fig. 20.33 Moulding in a brow presentation (dotted line). MV, mentovertical.

Causes

These are the same as for a secondary face presentation (see above); during the process of extension from a vertex presentation to a face presentation, the brow will present temporarily and in a few cases this will persist.

Diagnosis

Brow presentation is *not* usually detected before the onset of labour.

Abdominal palpation

The head is high, appears unduly large and does not descend into the pelvis despite good uterine contractions.

Vaginal examination

The presenting part is high and may be difficult to reach. The anterior fontanelle may be felt on one side of the maternal pelvis and the orbital ridges, and possibly the root of the nose, at the other (Fig. 20.33). A large caput succedaneum may mask these landmarks if the woman has been in labour for some hours.

Management

The doctor must be informed immediately this presentation is suspected. This is because vaginal birth is extremely rare and obstructed labour usually results. It is possible that a woman with a large pelvis and a small baby may give birth vaginally. When the brow reaches the pelvic floor the maxilla rotates forwards and the head is born by a mechanism somewhat similar to that of a persistent occipitoposterior position. However, the midwife should never expect such a favourable outcome. The woman should be warned about the possible course of labour and that a vaginal birth is unlikely.

If there is no evidence of fetal compromise, the doctor may allow labour to continue for a short while in case

further extension of the head converts the brow presentation to a face presentation. Occasionally spontaneous flexion may occur, resulting in a vertex presentation. If the head fails to descend and the brow presentation persists, a caesarean section is performed, with the woman's consent.

Complications

These are the same as in a face presentation, except that obstructed labour requiring caesarean section is the *probable* rather than a *possible* outcome.

SHOULDER PRESENTATION

When the fetus lies with its long axis across the long axis of the uterus (*transverse lie*) the shoulder is most likely to present. Occasionally the lie is oblique but this does not persist as the uterine contractions during labour make it longitudinal or transverse.

Shoulder presentation occurs in approximately 1 : 300 pregnancies near term. Only 17% of these cases remain as a transverse lie at the onset of labour of which the majority are multigravidae (Gimovsky and Hennigan 1995; Akmal and Paterson-Brown 2009). The head lies on one side of the abdomen, with the breech at a slightly higher level on the other. The fetal back may be anterior or posterior (Figs 20.34 and 20.35).

Causes

Maternal

Before term, transverse or oblique lie may be transitory, related to the woman's position or displacement of the

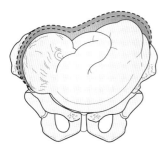

Fig. 20.34 Shoulder presentation, dorsoanterior.

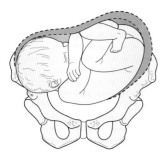

Fig. 20.35 Shoulder presentation, dorsoposterior.

presenting part by an overextended bladder prior to ultrasound examination. Other causes are described below.

Lax abdominal and uterine muscles

This is the most common cause and is found in multigravidae, particularly those of high parity.

Uterine malformation

A bicornuate or subseptate uterus may result in a transverse lie, as, more rarely, may a cervical or low uterine fibroid.

Contracted pelvis

Rarely, this may prevent the head from entering the pelvic brim.

Fetal

Pre-term pregnancy

The amount of amniotic fluid in relation to the fetus is greater, allowing the fetus more mobility than at term.

Multiple pregnancy

There is a possibility of hydramnios but the presence of more than one fetus reduces the room for manoeuvre when amounts of amniotic fluid are normal. It is the second twin that more commonly adopts a transverse lie after the birth of the first baby.

Hydramnios

The distended uterus is globular in shape and the fetus can move freely in the excessive amniotic fluid volume.

Macerated fetus

Lack of muscle tone causes the fetus to slump down into the lower pole of the uterus.

Placenta praevia

This may prevent the fetal head from entering the pelvic brim.

Antenatal diagnosis

Abdominal palpation

The uterus appears broad and the fundal height is less than expected for the period of gestation. On pelvic and fundal palpation, neither head nor breech is felt. The mobile head is found on one side of the abdomen and the breech at a slightly higher level on the other.

Antenatal management

A cause for the shoulder presentation must be sought before deciding on a course of management and requires a medical referral. Ultrasound examination can detect placenta praevia or uterine malformations, while X-ray pelvimetry will demonstrate a contracted pelvis (see Chapter 3). Any of these causes requires elective caesarean section. Once such causes have been excluded, external cephalic version (ECV) may be attempted. If this fails, or if the lie is transverse again at the next antenatal visit, the woman is admitted to hospital while further investigations into the cause are made. The woman frequently remains in hospital until labour commences because of the risk of cord prolapse if the membranes rupture.

Intrapartum diagnosis

The findings are as above but when the membranes have ruptured the irregular outline of the uterus is more marked. If the uterus is contracting strongly and becomes moulded around the fetus, palpation is very difficult. The pelvis is no longer empty as the shoulder is wedged into the brim.

Vaginal examination

In early labour the presenting part may not be felt. The membranes usually rupture early because of the ill-fitting presenting part, with a high risk of cord prolapse.

If the labour has been in progress for some time the shoulder may be felt as a soft irregular mass. It is sometimes possible to palpate the ribs, with their characteristic grid-iron pattern being diagnostic (Fig. 20.36). When the

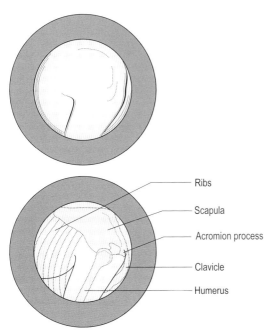

Fig. 20.36 Vaginal touch picture of shoulder presentation.

Ribs
Scapula
Acromion process
Clavicle
Humerus

shoulder enters the pelvic brim an arm may prolapse, which should be differentiated from a leg, i.e. the hand is not at right-angles to the arm, the fingers are longer than the toes and of unequal length, and the thumb can be opposed. No *os calcis* can be felt and the palm is shorter than the sole. If the arm is flexed, an elbow feels sharper than a knee.

Possible outcome

Whenever the midwife detects a transverse lie she must obtain medical assistance. There is no mechanism for the birth of a shoulder presentation.

If a transverse lie is detected in early labour while the membranes are still intact, the doctor may attempt an ECV. If this is successful, the doctor may then undertake a controlled rupture of the membranes. (This may be considered before labour in some cases [Hutton and Hofmeyr 2006]). If the membranes have already ruptured spontaneously, a vaginal examination must be performed immediately to detect possible cord prolapse.

If a shoulder presentation persists in labour, the birth of the baby must be by caesarean section to avoid obstructed labour and subsequent uterine rupture (see Chapter 22).

Immediate caesarean section must be performed:

- when ECV is unsuccessful
- when the membranes are already ruptured
- if the cord prolapses
- when labour has already been in progress for some hours.

Complications

Prolapsed cord

This may occur when the membranes rupture (see Chapter 22).

Prolapsed arm

This may occur when the membranes have ruptured and the shoulder has become impacted. Birth should be by immediate caesarean section.

Neglected shoulder presentation

With adequate supervision both antenatally and during labour, this should never occur.

The fetal shoulder becomes impacted, having been forced down and wedged into the maternal pelvic brim. The membranes have ruptured spontaneously and if the arm has prolapsed it becomes blue and oedematous. The uterus goes into a state of tonic contraction, the over-stretched lower segment is tender to touch and the fetal heartbeat may be absent. All the maternal signs of obstructed labour are present (see Chapter 19) and the outcome, if not treated in time, is a ruptured uterus and a stillbirth.

Management

An immediate caesarean section is performed regardless of whether the fetus is alive or dead, as attempts at manipulative procedures or destructive operations can be dangerous for the woman and may result in uterine rupture.

UNSTABLE LIE

The lie is defined as *unstable* when after 36 weeks' gestation, instead of remaining longitudinal, it varies from one examination to another between longitudinal and oblique or transverse.

Causes

Any condition in late pregnancy that increases the mobility of the fetus or prevents the fetal head from entering the pelvic brim may cause this.

Maternal

These include:

- lax uterine muscles in multigravidae
- contracted pelvis.

Fetal

These include:

- hydramnios
- placenta praevia.

Management

Antenatal

It may be advisable for the woman to be admitted to hospital to avoid unsupervised onset of labour with a transverse lie. Alternatively, the woman may admit herself to the hospital maternity unit as soon as labour commences. The risk associated with the possibility of rupture of membranes and cord prolapse should be emphasized if the woman chooses to remain at home.

Ultrasonography is used to exclude placenta praevia. Attempts will be made to correct the abnormal presentation by ECV. If unsuccessful, caesarean section is considered.

Intrapartum

Obstetricians may recommend induction of labour after 38 weeks' gestation, when the lie is unstable. Having first ensured that the lie is longitudinal, a controlled rupture of the membranes is performed so that the fetal head enters the pelvis and an intravenous infusion of oxytocin is commenced to stimulate contractions.

The midwife should ensure that the woman has an empty rectum and bladder before the procedure, as a loaded rectum or full bladder can prevent the presenting part from entering the pelvis. The abdomen should be palpated at frequent intervals to ensure that the lie remains longitudinal and to assess the descent of the fetal head. Labour is regarded as *a trial*.

If labour commences with the lie other than longitudinal, the complications are the same as for a transverse lie.

COMPOUND PRESENTATION

When a hand, or occasionally a foot, lies alongside the head, the presentation is said to be *compound*. This tends to occur with a small fetus or roomy maternal pelvis and seldom is difficulty encountered except in cases where it is associated with a flat pelvis. On rare occasions the head, hand and foot are felt in the vagina – a serious situation that may occur with a dead fetus.

If a compound presentation is diagnosed during the first stage of labour, medical aid must be sought. If diagnosis occurs during the second stage of labour and the midwife sees a hand presenting alongside the vertex, she should try to hold the hand back.

REFERENCES

Akmal S, Paterson-Brown S 2009 Malpositions and malpresentations of the foetal head. Obstetrics and Gynecology and Reproductive Medicine 199:240–6

Bhal P S, Davies N J, Chung T 1998 A population study of face and brow presentation. Journal of Obstetrics and Gynecology 18(3):231–5

Cheng Y W, Shaffer B L, Caughy A B 2006 The association between persistent occiput posterior and neonatal outcomes. Obstetrics and Gynecology 107(4):837–44

Gardberg M, Laakkonen E, Salevaara M 1998 Intra-partum sonography and persistent occiput posterior position: a study of 408 deliveries. Obstetrics and Gynecology 91(5):1746–9

Gimovsky M, Hennigan C 1995 Abnormal fetal presentations. Current Opinion in Obstetrics and Gynecology 7(6):482–5

Hodnett E D, Gates S, Hofmeyr G J et al 2012 Continuous support for women during childbirth. Cochrane Database of Systematic Reviews 2012, Issue 10. Art. No. CD003766. doi: 10.1002/14651858.CD003766.pub4

Hunter S, Hofmeyr G J, Kulier R 2007 Hands and knees posture in late pregnancy or labour for fetal malposition (lateral or posterior). Cochrane Database of Systematic Reviews 2007, Issue 4. Art. No. CD001063. doi: 10.1002/14651858.CD001063.pub3

Hutton E K, Hofmeyr G J 2006 External cephalic version for breech presentation before term. Cochrane Database of Systematic Reviews 2006, Issue 1. Art. No. CD000084. doi: 10.1002/14651858.CD000084.pub2

Kariminia A, Chamberlain M E, Keogh J 2004 Randomised controlled trial of effect of hands and knees posturing on incidence of occiput posterior position at birth. British Medical Journal 328(7438):490–3

Melamed N, Gavish O, Eisner M 2013 Third- and fourth-degree perineal tears – incidence and risk factors. Journal of Maternal–Fetal and Neonatal Medicine 26(7):660–4

Munro J, Jokinen M 2012 RCM evidence-based guidelines for midwifery-led care in labour. Persistent lateral and posterior fetal positions at the onset of labour. Royal College of Midwives Trust, London

Neuman M, Beller U, Lavie O 1994 Intrapartum bimanual tocolytic-assisted reversal of face presentation: preliminary report. Obstetrics and Gynecology 84(10):146–8

NMC (Nursing and Midwifery Council) 2012 Midwives Rules and Standards. NMC, London

Pearl M L, Roberts J M, Laros R K et al 1993 Vaginal delivery from the persistent occiput posterior position. Influence on maternal and neonatal morbidity. Journal of Reproductive Medicine 38(12):955–61

Peregrine E, O'Brian P, Jauniaux E 2007 Impact on delivery outcome of ultrasonographic fetal head position prior to induction of labor. Obstetrics and Gynecology 109(3):618–25

Phipps H, de Vries B, Hyett J et al 2011 Prophylactic manual rotation for fetal malposition to reduce operative delivery (Protocol). Cochrane Database of Systematic Reviews 2011, Issue 10. Art. No. CD009298. doi: 10.1002/14651858.CD009298

Ponkey S E, Cohen A P, Heffner L J et al 2003 Persistent fetal occiput posterior position: obstetric outcomes. Obstetrics and Gynecology 101(9):15–20

Shaffer B L, Cheng Y W, Vargas J E et al 2011 Manual rotation to reduce caesarean delivery in occiput posterior or transverse position. Journal of Maternal–Fetal and Neonatal Medicine 24(1):65–72

Simkin P 2010 The fetal occiput position: state of the science and a new perspective. Birth 37(1):61–71

FURTHER READING

Chapman K 2000 Aetiology and management of the secondary brow. Journal of Obstetrics and Gynaecology 20:(1)39–44

Six cases of vaginal birth from a brow presentation over a career of 39 years are recorded in this article. Most midwives will never see a brow presentation birth vaginally; this is a fascinating record from a long career.

Gardberg M, Tuppurainen M 1994 Anterior placental location predisposes for occiput posterior presentation near term. Acta Obstetrica et Gynecologica Scandinavica 73(2):151–2

In a series of 325 ultrasound examinations the authors demonstrated an association between an anteriorly situated placenta and OP position after 36 weeks of pregnancy.

Reichman O, Gdansky E, Latinsky B et al 2008 Digital rotation from occipito-posterior to occipito-anterior decreases the need for caesarean section. European Journal of Obstetrics and Gynecology and Reproductive Biology 136:25–8

The results of a prospective study suggest that digital rotation should be considered when managing the labour with a fetus in the OP position. The manoeuvre has been shown to have a high success rate, in experienced hands, reducing the need for vacuum extraction and caesarean section and so shortens the duration of hospital stay. The intervention has the potential to reduce maternal and neonatal morbidity and mortality.

Shaffer B I, Cheng Y W, Vargas J E et al 2011 Manual rotation to reduce caesarean delivery in persistent occiput posterior or transverse position. Journal of Maternal Fetal and Neonatal Medicine 24(1):65–72

Compared to expectant management manual rotation of the fetal head from OT or OP positions was associated with a reduction of caesarean sections and adverse maternal outcomes and no adverse neonatal outcomes. If a midwife is practising in a setting where operative birth is not readily available, this intervention may reduce maternal and neonatal morbidity and mortality.

Chapter |21|

Operative births

Richard Hayman

CHAPTER CONTENTS

This chapter describes the methods of operative birth that may be used when the mother is unable to give birth without medical or surgical assistance. The role of the midwife in these procedures will be explored, as will the principles of 'keeping the normal, normal'.

THE CHAPTER AIMS TO:

- identify the areas of midwifery care that relate to the preparation for an assisted vaginal birth (ventouse/forceps) or birth by caesarean section (CS)
- describe the role of the midwife in relation to the issues of informed consent and the management of complications following assisted birth
- consider the various techniques used for assisted vaginal birth (ventouse/forceps) and birth by CS, plus the skills required by the midwife to improve the experience for both the mother and her partner
- discuss the changing role of the midwife in relation to medical intervention.

ASSISTING A VAGINAL BIRTH

Assisted vaginal birth is a frequently and widely practised intervention in the provision of care to women during childbirth. In England during 2011–12, of the 668 936 births recorded, 85 009 (13%) were assisted with forceps or ventouse (Health and Social Care Information Centre, Hospital Episodes Statistics 2012). However, the incidence of instrumental intervention varies widely both between and within countries, and may be performed as infrequently as 1.5% or as often as 26%. Such differences may be linked to the alternative management strategies employed during labour in different units (Bragg et al 2010). Various techniques have been championed to help lower the rates of operative births. These are summarized in Box 21.1.

It should be noted, however, that other interventions, such as epidural analgesia, have been observed to be associated with an increased risk of instrumental vaginal birth and have been suggested to be linked to an increased risk of birth by caesarean section (CS) (Anim-Somuah et al 2011). However, such 'disadvantages' must be balanced against the higher rates of maternal satisfaction that this form of analgesia provides. It is up to the woman to make an informed choice as to which of the benefits and risks are most important, not up to the attending medical staff to make didactic decisions on her behalf. Indeed, whilst it has been commented (Johanson and Menon 1999) that, in general, maternal outcomes would be improved by lowering instrumental birth rates, no evidence to support such a statement has ever been forthcoming, as it is not easy to see what the alternatives are for a woman who, despite her own best efforts, has not been able to secure a 'normal birth'.

> ### Box 21.1 Useful techniques to help lower the operative birth rate
>
> - One-to-one care in labour (Hodnett et al 2011)
> - Active management of the second stage with Syntocinon (O'Driscoll et al 1993; Brown et al 2008)
> - Upright birth posture/mobilization (NICE 2007; Gupta et al 2012)
> - Delaying the onset of the active second stage by 1–2 hours in women with regional analgesia/anaesthesia (NICE 2007)
> - Fetal blood sampling rather than expediting birth when fetal heart rate abnormalities occur (NICE 2007)

INDICATIONS FOR VENTOUSE OR FORCEPS

The indications for assisted vaginal birth may be simply categorized into fetal and maternal. However, the reasons cited for intervention are frequently imprecise as multiple factors often interact.

Fetal

- Malposition of the fetal head (occipitolateral and occipitoposterior). Such positions occur more frequently in the presence of regional anaesthesia, as alterations in the tone of the pelvic floor may impede the spontaneous rotation to the optimal occipitoanterior position during the decent of the presenting part (vertex of the fetal head).
- Fetal 'distress' is a commonly cited indication for instrumental intervention; however, *'presumed fetal compromise'* is a more comprehensive term (unless a fetal blood sample has been obtained showing hypoxia and acidosis, in which case *'fetal hypoxia'* should be used) (NICE [National Institute for Health and Clinical Excellence] 2007).
- Elective instrumental intervention for infants of reduced weight. In infants weighing <1.5 kg, delivery with forceps does not confer an advantage over spontaneous birth and may increase the incidence of intracranial haemorrhage. Ventouse carries the same risks, but in addition should be avoided in infants of <34^{+6} weeks of gestation.
- Assisted vaginal breech birth. Forceps can be applied to the after-coming head to control the birth of the vertex, a situation where the ventouse is contraindicated.

Maternal

- The commonest maternal indications are those of maternal distress, exhaustion, or prolongation of the second stage of labour. This has been suggested as greater than 2 hours in a primigravida (3 hours if an epidural is in situ), or more than 1 hour in a multipara (2 hours if an epidural is in situ) (NICE 2007).
- Medically significant conditions such as: aortic valve disease with significant outflow obstruction; myasthenia gravis; significant antepartum haemorrhage due to placental abruption or vasa praevia; severe hypertensive disease; and previous CS (to minimize the risk of scar rupture).

CONTRAINDICATIONS TO AN INSTRUMENTAL VAGINAL BIRTH

Absolute

- The vertex is ≥1/5th palpable abdominally.
- The position as determined by a vaginal examination (occipitoanterior/posterior or lateral) of the fetal head is unknown.
- Before full dilatation of the cervix (although a possible exception occurs with the ventouse birth of a second twin).
- When the operator is inexperienced in instrumental vaginal birth.

In addition the ventouse *should not* be used:

- In gestations of <34^{+6} weeks because of the increased risk of intracranial haemorrhage in the fetus.
- With the fetus presenting by the face.
- If there is a significant degree of caput that may either preclude correct placement of the cup or, more sinisterly, indicate a substantial degree of cephalopelvic disproportion CPD).

Relative contraindications (for forceps or ventouse)

- Fetal bleeding disorders (e.g. alloimmune thrombocytopenia) or a predisposition to fractures (e.g. osteogenesis imperfecta) are relative contraindications specifically to an operative birth with the ventouse. However, the comparative risks of a birth by a difficult second stage caesarean section must also be considered and a discussion undertaken antenatally about the most appropriate plan for birth (it may be wiser to recommend that such women have an elective CS).
- There is minimal risk of fetal haemorrhage if the vacuum extractor is employed following fetal blood sampling or application of a scalp electrode.

PREREQUISITES FOR ANY OPERATIVE VAGINAL BIRTH

- Rupture of the membranes must be confirmed.
- The cervix must be fully dilated.
- Cephalic presentation with identification of the position (occipitoanterior/posterior or lateral).
- Adequate pelvis as ascertained by clinical pelvimetry.
- The fetal head must be <1/5th palpable *per abdomen*, with the presenting part at or below the ischial spines.

- Adequate analgesia/anaesthesia.
- Empty bladder/no obstruction below the fetal head (contracted pelvis/ovarian cyst).
- A knowledgeable and experienced operator with adequate preparation to proceed with an alternative approach if necessary.
- An adequately informed woman (with signed consent form detailing appropriate risks/benefits/complications as the situation demands).

BIRTH BY VENTOUSE

The ventouse is essentially a suction cup (made from plastic or metal) that is connected (via tubing) to a vacuum source. Following the placement of the cup onto the fetal head, traction can be applied to assist the birth.

There is no definitive guide as to which instrument to use on which occasion. However the ventouse cup may not be successful at securing birth and therefore obstetric forceps should be chosen if there is:

- suspected fetal macrosomia
- excessive caput or moulding
- poor maternal effort due to exhaustion (which may be compounded by epidural analgesia and poor sensation)
- gestation <34 completed weeks.

Types of ventouse

Until recently, the most commonly used ventouse in use in the United Kingdom (UK) was that of the 'soft' or silicone cup design (Fig. 21.1A). Whilst these cups have the undoubted advantages of being extremely malleable (reducing maternal trauma by being more easy to correctly place within the vagina) and having a reduced incidence of fetal scalp trauma when compared to other cup designs, soft cups have a poorer success rate than metal cups in achieving a vaginal birth (RCOG [Royal College of Obstetricians and Gynaecologists] 2011).

Metal cup ventouse designs are of the Bird or Malstrom types, which have a centrally placed traction chain with a laterally located vacuum conduit. They come in diameters of 4, 5 and 6 cm.

Both the standard soft and metal cup designs require the generation of an operating vacuum from an external source – and as such these pieces of equipment require two operators for their successful use (one to control the placement of the ventouse and assist the birth, the other (most commonly the attending midwife) to control the degree of vacuum that is generated.

More recent advances in design have removed the need for the external suction generators by incorporating the vacuum mechanism into 'hand-held' pumps (e.g. Kiwi OmniCup^{TM}) as illustrated in Fig. 21.1(B). Such devices are safe and may be useful for rotational births because they are low profile and are easily manoeuvered into the correct position. However, they have a significantly higher failure rate than the conventional metal cup ventouse, with cup detachments occurring more frequently.

The use of the ventouse

The ventouse is more frequently employed by obstetricians than the obstetric forceps due to its apparent ease of use and comparative safety. However, repeated meta-analyses have demonstrated that the ventouse is less likely to achieve a successful vaginal birth than forceps, although both types of instruments are associated with a lowering of the overall CS rate (Johanson and Menon 1999). Although the ventouse is associated with an increased risk of neonatal complications such as cephalohaematoma (Chapter 31), other facial (nerve palsies) and significant cranial injuries (fractures) are more common with forceps.

Procedure

- The rationale for the birth is discussed with the woman and her partner. The procedure is explained and consent obtained (written consent should be obtained if time allows).
- The woman's legs should be placed into the lithotomy position.
- Whilst inhalational analgesia may be sufficient (entonox – N_2O), more commonly a pudendal nerve block with perineal infiltration may be administered, or an epidural, if already in situ, may be topped up.
- Once adequate analgesia is assured, the maternal bladder is emptied.

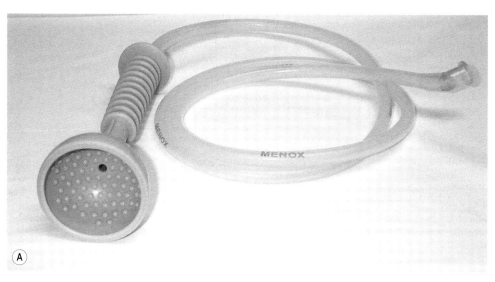

(A)

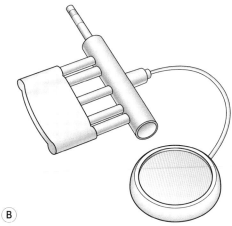

(B)

Fig. 21.1 (A) The soft cup ventouse. (B) The Kiwi OmniCup™.

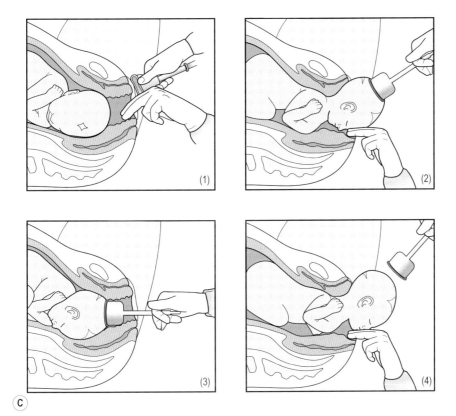

Fig. 21.1 *Continued* (C) Birth by ventouse.

- The fetal heart rate (FHR) must be continuously monitored (with a cardiotocograph – CTG).
- For the successful use of the ventouse, it is essential to determine the flexion point, which is located, in an average term infant, along the sagittal suture 3 cm anterior to the posterior fontanelle (and thus 6 cm posterior to the anterior fontanelle). The centre of the cup should be placed directly over this, as failure to adequately position the cup can lead to a progressive deflexion of the fetal head during traction.

The operating vacuum pressure for nearly all ventouse is between 0.6 and 0.8 kg/cm² (60–80 kPa/500–800 cmH₂O). No evidence exists that a stepwise reduction in pressure improves the rate of successful birth when compared with a linear reduction. Using the latter technique with a silastic cup, a caput succedaneum (Chapter 31) is formed instantly, and with the metal cup or OmniCup™, an adequate chignon is produced in <2 minutes. It is important to note that a cup of 5 cm diameter is suitable for nearly all births, even with larger babies.

When the vacuum is achieved, traction must be applied to coincide with a contraction and thus maternal expulsive efforts. Without both of these contributing factors, birth

with a ventouse will fail. Traction is provided along a track defined by the curve of Carus (Chapter 3): initially in a downwards and backwards direction, then in a forward and upward manner. Once the fetal head has crowned, the vacuum is released, the cup removed and with further maternal efforts the baby will be born. In addition to the relative ease of use and low risk of complications, it is undoubtedly this sense of contribution to the birth that makes the ventouse a more satisfactory birthing experience for the mother and her partner than an operative birth with obstetric forceps.

Precautions in use

With the ventouse, the operator should allow ≤2 episodes of breaking the suction in any vacuum assisted birth, and the maximum time from application to birth should ideally be ≤15 minutes. If there is no evidence of descent with the first pull, the woman should be reassessed to ascertain the reason for failure to progress. In addition, care should be taken to ensure that no vaginal skin is trapped in the edges of the cup as this can result in complex degrees of perineal trauma that can be extremely difficult to repair in a satisfactory fashion.

The midwife ventouse practitioner

Some midwives feel that women will be better served by a midwife ventouse practitioner rather than an obstetrician and embrace such innovations (Tinsley 2010). However, others see it as exceeding the limits of normal midwifery practice (Charles 1999). The fact is that midwifery care is changing and developing, specifically with the advancement of care within stand-alone midwife-led units.

Whilst the idea of reducing the psychological trauma to a woman during a birth by limiting the number of carers in attendance at this crucial and critical time is to be commended, it would be foolhardy to assume that the midwife ventouse practitioner would be the primary carer for every pregnant women on every occasion that required an assisted vaginal birth. As such it is likely that a midwife previously unknown to the labouring woman would be asked to assist at the moment when help is required, an event that would therefore be no less 'traumatic' for a woman or her partner than asking an obstetrician to attend. All accoucheurs, including midwife ventouse practitioners, must be well educated and trained before carrying out a ventouse birth – although it is highly unlikely that the more complex surgical skills required of a birth by forceps or CS would be mastered in addition. It should be remembered that as a ventouse will fail in up to 20% of cases, even in the most skilled hands, having no ability to change instruments or resort to birth by CS will place those midwives who work as ventouse practitioners in isolation in a most unenviable position.

BIRTH BY FORCEPS

Characteristics of the obstetric forceps

All obstetric forceps are composed of two separate blades (determined as right and left by reference to their insertion around the fetal head within the maternal vagina), two shanks (shafts) of varying length and two handles. Forceps are often described as non-rotational or rotational. Non-rotational forceps are 'held' together by either an English (non-sliding) lock on the shank or, in the case of rotational forceps, by a sliding lock on the shank. The blades have a cephalic curve to accommodate the form of the baby's head and are fenestrated (and not solid) to minimize the trauma to the baby's head during both placement and birth. They also have a pelvic curve to reduce the risks of trauma to the maternal tissues during the birth process.

When the blades are correctly positioned around the fetal skull, the handles will be neatly aligned in the hands of the doctor who applies them and will be noted to 'lock with ease'. Forceps that do not lock are most commonly incorrectly placed.

Classification of obstetric forceps

Forceps operations fall into two categories: mid- and low-cavity. Mid-cavity forceps are used when the leading part of the fetal head has reached below the level of the ischial spines; low-cavity forceps are used when the head has descended to the level of the pelvic floor. High-cavity forceps (with the leading part of the fetal head above the level of the ischial spines) are now considered unsafe and a CS will be the preferred method of birth in nearly all cases.

Types of obstetric forceps

Wrigley's forceps

These are designed for use in outlet lift-out when the head is on the perineum or to assist the birth of the fetal head at caesarean section. They have a short shank, fenestrated blades with both pelvic and cephalic curves, and an English lock (Fig. 21.2).

Neville–Barnes or Simpson's forceps

These are generally used for a low- or mid-cavity forceps birth when the sagittal suture is in the anteroposterior diameter of the cavity of the pelvis. Whilst they have cephalic and pelvic curves to the fenestrated blades, the handles are longer and heavier (Fig. 21.2) than those of the Wrigley's. Anderson's and Haig–Ferguson's forceps are also similar in shape and size.

Kielland's forceps

These were originally designed to deliver the fetal head at a station at, or above, the pelvic brim. They are now more commonly used for the rotation and extraction of a baby whose head is in the deep transverse or occipitoposterior malpositions. By comparison to the non-rotational forceps, the Kielland's forceps blades have fenestrated blades with a much-reduced pelvic curve (in order to allow for the safe rotation of the fetus), longer shanks (to enable rotation within the mid-cavity of the pelvis) and a sliding lock to allow for correction of any degree of asynclitism of the fetal head. These forceps (Fig. 21.2) should be used only by an obstetrician skilled in their application and use, and indeed in many units their use has been abandoned.

Procedure

In addition to the key points outlined for ventouse on page 458, i.e. rationale, consent, urinary bladder

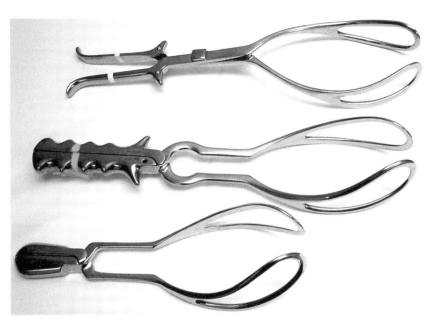

Fig. 21.2 Types of forceps. From above: Kielland's, Neville–Barnes and Simpson's. Note the difference in cephalic curve. The rotational forceps (Kielland's) have a long shaft and little pelvic curve. Wrigley's forceps have a shorter shank.

catheterization, FHR monitoring and position of the woman's legs, specific issues to consider are:

- Consideration should be given as to the location of the birth – in the birthing room (lift-out or low-cavity – non rotational deliveries) or in the obstetric theatre (all other forceps births).
- Unlike the ventouse, inhalational analgesia or a pudendal nerve block with perineal infiltration is unlikely to be sufficient for a forceps birth. In the majority of instances an epidural, if already in situ, may be topped up, or a spinal anaesthetic should be administered. These are mandatory before consideration is given to using Kielland's forceps.
- The forceps should be held discretely in front of the woman (to visualize how they will be inserted *per vaginum*) and placed around the fetal head. The left blade is inserted before the right blade, with the accoucheur's hand protecting the vaginal wall from direct trauma.
- The forceps blades come to lie parallel to the axis of the fetal head, and between the fetal head and the pelvic wall. The operator then articulates and locks the blades, checking their application before applying traction. The blades **must** be repositioned or the procedure abandoned if the application is incorrect.
- Traction should be applied in concert with uterine contractions and maternal expulsive efforts.

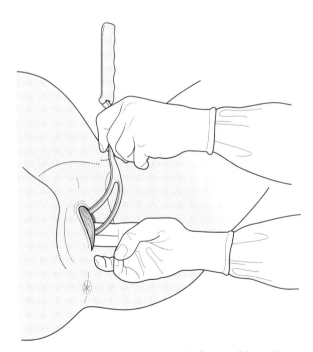

Fig. 21.3 Left blade being inserted. The fingers of the right hand guard the vaginal tissue.

- As with the ventouse, the axis of traction changes during the birth and is guided along the curve of Carus, the blades being directed to the vertical as the head crowns (see Figs 21.3–21.6).

461

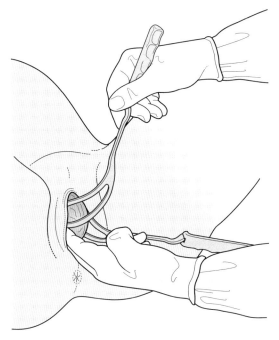

Fig. 21.4 Right blade being inserted.

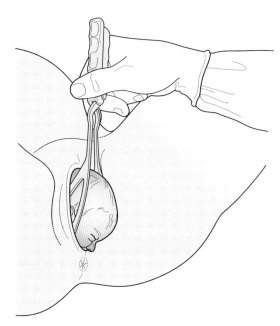

Fig. 21.6 As the head crowns it is lifted upwards.

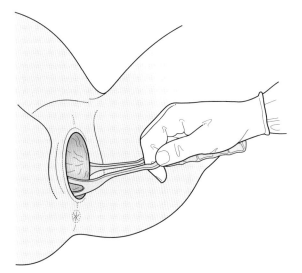

Fig. 21.5 Traction of the head is downwards until this point; when the head is low, the direction of pull is outward, towards the operator.

Complications of instrumental vaginal birth

Although forceps are less likely than the ventouse to fail to achieve a vaginal birth, they are significantly more likely to be associated with third- or fourth-degree tears (with or without the concurrent use of an episiotomy), vaginal trauma, use of general anaesthesia, flatal, faecal and urinary continence (Chapter 15).

Maternal complications

Complications may include:

- Trauma or soft tissue damage – occurring to the cervix, vagina or perineum.
- Dysuria or urinary retention, which may result from bruising or oedema to the tissues around the urethra.
- Perineal discomfort.
- Haemorrhage (both from tissue trauma and also uterine atony – the risk of which is always increased following an assisted vaginal birth).

Neonatal complications

Complications may include:

- Marks on the baby's face and bruising (commonly caused by the pressure from the forceps blades and around the caput succedaneum/chignon from the ventouse – nearly all of which resolve within 48–72 hours after birth; see Chapter 31).
- Facial palsy, which may result from pressure from a blade compressing a facial nerve (a transient problem in most instances).

■ Prolonged traction during a birth with a ventouse will increase the likelihood of scalp abrasions, cephalohaematoma or sub-aponeurotic bleeding (Chapter 31).

Some authors suggest that failure rates of <1% should be achieved using the correct technique and with well-maintained equipment. Many authors feel that this is an unrealistic target. Failure of the ventouse realistically arises in up to 20% of cases and indeed Johanson and Menon (1999) achieved vaginal birth with the first instrument in only 86% of assisted births.

The following as factors will often be found to have contributed to failure:

With the ventouse

- Failure to select the correct cup type – inappropriate use of the silastic cup – especially in the presence of deflexion of the fetal head, excess caput, 'dense' epidural block or fetal macrosomia (true CPD).
- Failure of the equipment to provide adequate traction as a consequence of a leakage of the vacuum.
- Incorrect cup placement – too anterior or lateral, with or without inclusion of maternal soft tissues within the cup.

With any instrument

- Inadequate initial case assessment – high head, misdiagnosis of the position and attitude of the head.
- Traction along the wrong plane (often too anteriorly and not along the curve of Carus).
- Poor maternal effort with inadequate use of syntocinon to maximize the contribution from coordinated uterine activity.

Whatever the outcome, the midwife in attendance is vital to the success of any manoeuvres undertaken, encouraging the mother to be an active participant in her birth, supporting the mother and her partner through what may be perceived to be a 'deviation from normal' and importantly, to support the clinician undertaking the assisted birth.

CAESAREAN SECTION

Caesarean section is an operative procedure, which is carried out under anaesthesia (regional or general), whereby the fetus, placenta and membranes are delivered through an incision made in the abdominal wall and uterus.

The RCOG (2001) National Sentinel Caesarean Section Audit reported that the overall CS rate was 21.5% (England and Wales), accounting for approximately 120 000 births per year. Whilst the CS rates for maternity units ranged from 10% to 65%, 10% of women had CS before labour (range between maternity units 4% to 59%), and 12% of women who went into labour had a CS (range between maternity units 2% to 22%).

It is believed that some of the differences in CS rates observed may be explained by differences in the demographic and clinical characteristics of the population, such as maternal age, ethnicity, previous CS, breech presentation, prematurity and induction of labour. However the exact reasons for these differences remains unclear.

Although there has been an increase in CS rates over the past 20 years, the four major clinical determinants of the CS rate have not changed. Common primary indications reported for women having a primary CS were: failure to progress in labour (25%), presumed fetal compromise (28%) and breech presentation (14%). The most common indications for women having a repeat CS were: previous CS (44%), maternal request as reported by clinicians (12%), failure to progress (10%), presumed fetal compromise (9%) and breech presentation (3%).

Currently in the UK, slightly more than one in seven women experience complications during labour that provide an indication for CS. These problems can be life-threatening for the mother and/or baby (e.g. eclampsia, abruptio placenta) and, in approximately 40% of such cases, a CS provides the safest route for birth. In all cases the principal aims must be to ensure that those women and babies who need birth by CS are so delivered, and that those who do not are saved from an unnecessary intervention.

In 1985, concern regarding the increasing frequency of caesarean section led the World Health Organization (WHO) to hold a Consensus Conference (Stephenson 1992). This conference concluded that there were no health benefits above a CS rate of 10–15%. The Scandinavian countries managed to hold CS rates at this level during the 1990s, with outcomes comparable to or better than those of countries with higher CS rates. However, this is no longer the case and CS rates in these countries have now increased towards those in the other developed nations.

Although many factors have been associated with an increase in the CS rate, not all have been to the detriment of the mother or baby. Interestingly, whilst the CS rate has risen over the two preceding decades, the instrumental vaginal birth rate has remained relatively constant.

Clarifying the indications for caesarean section

NICE (2011) recommends that the urgency of CS should be documented using the following standardized scheme in order to aid clear communication between healthcare professionals about the urgency of a CS:

1. Immediate threat to the life of the woman or fetus.
2. Maternal or fetal compromise which is not immediately life-threatening.

3. No maternal or fetal compromise but needs early delivery.
4. Delivery timed to suit woman or staff.

The need for birth by a category 1 ('crash') CS is fortunately a rare event as it can be a psychologically traumatic event for the woman and her partner. It is also extremely stressful for the clinical staff in attendance. Resources may have to be obtained from other areas of clinical care to facilitate such a birth and care standards risk being compromised in the rush to secure a 'safe' outcome. Care should therefore be exercised before making this decision, and *in utero* fetal resuscitation (fluids, tocolytics and oxygen) may give enough time for a more considered and careful approach.

Indications for which elective caesarean section would be the strongly recommended mode of birth:

- **Past obstetric history**
  - previous classical caesarean section
  - interval pelvic floor or anal sphincter repair
  - previous severe shoulder dystocia with significant neonatal injury.
- **Current pregnancy events**
  - significant fetal disease likely to lead to poor tolerance of labour
  - monoamniotic twins or higher-order multiple pregnancy
  - placenta praevia
  - obstructing pelvic mass
  - active primary herpes at onset of labour.
- **Intrapartum events**
  - presumed fetal compromise in the first stage
  - maternal disease for which delay in delivery may compromise the safety of the mother
  - absolute cephalopelvic disproportion (brow presentations etc).

These lists are not comprehensive and factors or other indicators may co-exist to influence the decision-making process.

The operative procedure

- The rationale for the intervention is discussed with the woman and her partner. The procedure is explained and consent obtained (written consent must be obtained in all cases other than a category 1 or 'crash section'). For elective procedures consent may be taken in a dedicated preoperative assessment (the decision having been previously discussed and agreed in the antenatal clinic by a senior clinician in consultation with the woman and her partner).

- A preoperative assessment includes: weight and observations of blood pressure, pulse and temperature. The woman is gowned, make-up, the presence of any nail varnish and jewellery removed (rings/ear-rings taped).
- The woman is visited by the anaesthetist and the operating department practitioner preoperatively, and assessed. An anaesthetic chart will be commenced.
- Results of any blood tests that have been requested are obtained (full blood count, group and save and cross match, if required).
- The woman will have fasted and have taken the prescribed antacid therapy.
- Many women prefer to have urinary catheterization in the theatre once the regional or general anaesthetic has been administered. However some women will prefer to have this procedure undertaken in the privacy of their room before entering the operating theatre.
- As the woman will need to lie flat, it is essential that a wedge or cushion is used, or the table is tilted, to direct the gravid uterus away from the inferior vena cava. The risks of supine hypotension syndrome will thus be reduced.
- The regional or general anaesthetics will be administered.
- A surgical 'time out' should be carried out on every woman entering the operating theatre prior to the preparation of the skin. In competent hands this takes a matter of seconds dramatically improving safety whilst not delaying the birth to any perceptible degree.
- The skin is prepared in accordance with local and national guidelines. Currently, it remains unclear what kind of skin preparation might be the most efficacious in the prevention of post CS surgical wound infection (Hadiati et al 2012).
- Intravenous antibiotics should be administered as surgical prophylaxis before the skin is incised. This reduces the risk of maternal infection more than prophylactic antibiotics given after skin incision, and no effect on the baby has been demonstrated.

The anatomical layers that need to be breached in order to reach the fetus are: skin, subcutaneous fat, rectus sheath, muscle (rectus abdominis), abdominal peritoneum, pelvic peritoneum and uterine muscle.

A transverse lower abdominal incision (bikini line incision) is usually performed with the skin and subcutaneous tissues incised using a transverse curvilinear incision at a level of two fingerbreadths above the symphysis pubis. The subcutaneous tissues are subsequently separated by blunt dissection and the rectus sheath incised transversely for 2 cm either side of the midline. This incision is then extended with scissors or blunt dissection before the facial sheath is separated from the underlying muscle. The recti are separated from each other, the peritoneum incised and the abdominal cavity entered.

The fold of the peritoneum over the anterior aspect of the lower uterine segment and above the bladder is incised and the bladder mobilized and reflected down. The uterus is incised transversely taking care not to cause surgical trauma to the fetus (a significant risk in the presence of low levels of amniotic fluid). The surgeon, with help from the surgical assistant (who must apply fundal pressure), will then secure the safe delivery of the baby.

The main reason for preferring the lower uterine segment technique is the reduced incidence of dehiscence of the uterine scar in any subsequent pregnancy and/or birth when compared to a classical or vertical incision (which may be the only surgical approach that is suitable in situations such as anterior wall placenta praevia, in extreme prematurity (where no lower uterine segment may be formed) or in the presence of dense adhesions from previous surgery.

Oxytocics (a bolus of 5 IU of Syntocinon) should be given by the anaesthetist after birth of the baby and clamping of the umbilical cord. When the baby and placenta have been delivered, the uterus is closed in two layers and the rectus sheath and skin sutured. Most surgeons use a braided polyglactin suture (Vicryl) for all layers. The wound is then dressed and the vagina swabbed to remove any clots. This also allows a final intraoperative assessment of any ongoing bleeding from within the uterus.

Women having a CS should be offered thromboprophylaxis because they are at increased risk of venous thromboembolism (Lewis 2007; CMACE [Centre for Maternal and Child Enquiries] 2011). The choice of method of prophylaxis (for example, graduated stockings, hydration, early mobilization, low molecular weight heparin) should take into account risk of thromboembolic disease, although in most cases it is simplest, and safest, to administer low molecular weight heparin to all women until they are fully mobile. Those with an increased risk (e.g. maternal obesity or concurrent maternal morbidity) should have a more formal assessment of risk and an individualized care plan put in place.

Early skin-to-skin contact between the woman and her baby should be encouraged and facilitated as it improves maternal perceptions of the infant, mothering skills, maternal behaviour, breastfeeding outcomes and reduces infant crying (Chapter 34). In addition, women who have had a CS should be offered additional support to help them to start breastfeeding as soon as possible after the birth of their baby. This is because women who have had a caesarean section are less likely to start breastfeeding in the first few hours after the birth, but, when breastfeeding is established, they are as likely to continue as women who have had a vaginal birth.

Women's request for caesarean section

The reasons behind the 'demands' for birth by CS are frequently complex. Despite the focus of attention in the media, evidence suggests that very few women actually request CS in the absence of medical indications and the 'too posh to push cohort' are in an extreme minority (Chaffer and Royle 2000; Weaver et al 2007). However, the accounts of women who have had difficult experiences of childbirth describe 'knowing something was wrong but believe that they were not listened to' are all too familiarly encountered. Such women frequently publicize their problems via Facebook or other social media networks, fuelling the idea of 'them against us', and the joys of any future pregnancy risk being overwhelmed by the focus for a birth by CS whatever the rationale behind their beliefs.

Psychological support and the role of the midwife

Choice is an important element in understanding this sequence. Women expect to be actively involved in their care and all staff involved must ensure that recent, valid and relevant information is provided in a comprehensible manner. This will help women to decide what is best for them, in relation to their own specific circumstances. The midwife, as an informed, confident and competent practitioner, will have a pivotal role in this process and be able to provide women with clear and unbiased information concerning the choices available (McAleese 2000). This will often relieve the stress of the situation and help women make a competent decision, supporting them in the midst of any misgivings.

One-to-one care from a support person during labour can influence the rate of birth by CS as a continual, supportive presence in labour is undoubtedly of considerable benefit, both to the woman and to her family (Walker and Golois 2001; Hodnett et al 2011). It is important that midwives recognize the positive impact on outcomes of their continuous presence during established labour (NICE 2007; Hodnett et al 2011).

Psychological support mechanisms may also help these women to overcome their fears and, as such, it may be appropriate to develop links with trained counsellors to enable women to explore their anxieties and reach a more informed and rational decision prior to electing to undergo major abdominal surgery. However, NICE (2011) recommends for women requesting a CS that if, after discussion and offer of support (including perinatal mental health support for women with anxiety about childbirth, see Chapter 25), a vaginal birth is still not an acceptable option, a planned caesarean section should be offered.

Vaginal birth after caesarean section (VBAC)

Ziadeh and Sunna (1995) reported that the widespread adoption of a policy whereby 80% of women with a prior CS should have a VBAC would potentially eliminate up to one-third of births by CS. This is still the target towards which those providing care to women in pregnancy strive.

When advising about the mode of birth after a previous CS it is important to consider the maternal preferences and priorities, the risks and benefits of repeat CS and the risks and benefits of planned VBAC, including the risk of unplanned (i.e. emergency) CS.

NICE (2011) recommends that women who have had up to and including four caesarean sections should be informed that the risks of fever, bladder injuries and surgical injuries do not vary with the planned mode of birth and that the risk of uterine rupture, although higher for planned vaginal birth, is rare. However it is a 'brave' clinician who would choose to recommend vaginal birth as a safe option in those women who have had two previous CS.

It is also important to remember that pregnant women with both a previous CS and a previous vaginal birth should be informed that they have an increased likelihood of achieving a vaginal birth than women who have had a previous CS but no previous vaginal birth.

Pare et al (2006) argued that the concerns around the safety of VBAC ignored the potential downstream consequences of a strategy whereby multiple elective repeat caesarean sections are considered to be the safer option. These include an increased length of stay in hospital and increased risks of placenta praevia and accreta in future pregnancies. They confirmed that for women who desire two or more additional children, the risks of multiple caesarean sections outweigh the risks of a VBAC attempt.

Criteria for a successful VBAC:

- Adequate supervision including continuous electronic fetal monitoring with CTG.
- All the facilities for assisted birth are readily available.
- Progress of the labour is sufficient, observed both in the descent of the presenting part and by the dilatation of the cervix.
- The woman and her partner are fully informed about the risks and benefits.

Postoperative care

After birth by CS women should be observed on a one-to-one basis by a properly trained member of staff until they have regained airway control, have observed cardiorespiratory stability and are able to communicate effectively. After recovery from anaesthesia, observations (respiratory rate, heart rate, blood pressure, pain and sedation) should be recorded every 15 minutes in the immediate recovery period (for the first 30 minutes) and thereafter every half-hour for 2 hours, and hourly thereafter provided that the observations are stable or satisfactory. If these observations are not stable, more frequent observations and medical review are recommended. In addition the wound and lochia must be inspected every 30 minutes to detect any ongoing blood loss. If the mother intends to breast-feed, the baby should be put to the breast as soon as possible, a process that can usually be achieved with minimal disturbance to the undertaking of these routine observations.

For women who have had intrathecal opioids, there should be a minimum hourly observation of respiratory rate, sedation and pain scores for at least 12 hours if diamorphine has been administered and for 24 hours in the case of morphine. For women who have had epidural opioids or patient-controlled analgesia (PCA) with opioids, there should be routine hourly monitoring of respiratory rate, sedation and pain scores throughout treatment and for at least 2 hours after discontinuation of treatment.

Postoperative analgesia

Postoperative analgesia should be given on a regular basis and may be given in a variety of ways:

- Ongoing epidural anaesthesia/analgesia. Women should have diamorphine (3 mg) or fentanyl (100 µg) administered into the epidural space for intra- and postoperative analgesia as it reduces the need for supplemental analgesia after a caesarean section. Intravenous or intramuscular administration of diamorphine (2.5–5 mg) is a suitable alternative. However, intramuscular or intravenous analgesia should never be given in conjunction with epidural opioids for at least the first 4 hours after administration of the epidural dose because of the cumulative effects and risks of respiratory depression.
- PCA using opioid analgesics may be offered after caesarean section as an alternative pain relief regimen.
- Antiemetics (e.g. cyclizine; prochlorperazine) are usually prescribed when opioids are required.
- Analgesia, such as diclofenac (oral or rectal) or paracetamol (oral, intravenous or rectal) are the mainstays of postoperative analgesia.
- Oral drugs (e.g. dihydrocodeine, codydramol, ibuprofen or paracetamol).

Providing there are no contraindications (history of kidney disease, sensitivity to nonsteroidal anti-inflammatory drugs [NSAIDs], peptic ulcer, severe brittle asthma), NSAIDs should be offered post-caesarean section as an adjunct to other analgesics, as they reduce the need for the administration of opioids.

Care following regional block

Following birth under epidural or spinal anaesthesia, the woman may sit up as soon as she wishes, provided her blood pressure is not low. All observations must be recorded as described above.

Women who are recovering well after CS and who do not have complications can eat and drink when they feel hungry or thirsty, at which point the intravenous fluid infusion can be discontinued.

The baby should remain with the mother unless there is a medical reason for care being provided elsewhere (e.g. on a special care or neonatal intensive care unit) and indeed they should be transferred to the postnatal ward together once it is safe to do so. Such care is undoubtedly of benefit to a woman's psychological health and long-term wellbeing.

Care in the postnatal ward

Once care is transferred to the postnatal ward, the blood pressure, temperature, respirations and pulse must be checked every 4 hours and recorded using a modified obstetric early warning score chart (MOEWS) (Lewis 2007). In addition, the wound and lochia should be inspected at the same time. Removal of the urinary bladder catheter should be carried out once a woman is mobile after a regional anaesthetic and not sooner than 12 hours after the last epidural 'top up' dose. Healthcare professionals caring for women who have had a CS and who have urinary symptoms should consider the possible diagnosis of: urinary tract infection, stress incontinence (which occurs in about 4% of women after CS) or urinary tract injury (which occurs in about 1 per 1000 women after birth by CS).

The mother should be encouraged to move her legs and to perform leg and breathing exercises, however routine respiratory physiotherapy does not need to be offered to women after a caesarean section under general or regional anaesthesia, as it does not improve respiratory outcomes such as coughing, phlegm, body temperature, chest palpation and auscultatory changes.

The woman should be helped to get out of bed as soon as possible following a CS, and should also be encouraged to become fully mobile. Prophylactic low molecular weight heparin and antiembolic or thromboembolic deterrent ('TED') stockings should be prescribed. However, the first dose of low molecular weight heparin should be delayed until 4 hours after the intrathecal injection or removal of the epidural catheter.

Women who have had a general anaesthetic for CS may feel very tired and drowsy for some hours. A woman may complain of a feeling of detachment and unreality and may feel that she does not relate well to the baby. The woman who is concerned should be reassured and be given the opportunity to talk freely.

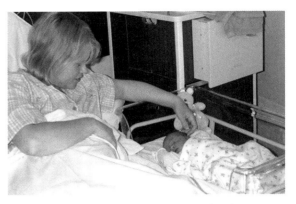

Fig. 21.7 Baby in clip-on cot, adjacent to and within easy reach of mother when in bed.

The mother must be encouraged to rest as much as possible and tactful advice may need to be given to her visitors. If the mother becomes too tired, help is needed with care for the baby. This should, preferably, take place at the mother's bedside and should include support with breast-feeding. The clip-on cots, which may be attached to the mother's bed, are invaluable in promoting good care (Fig. 21.7).

Caesarean section wound care should include: removing the dressing 24 hours after the delivery, assessing the wound for signs of infection (such as increasing pain, redness or discharge) separation or dehiscence, encouraging the woman to wear loose comfortable clothes and cotton underwear, gently cleaning and drying the wound daily if needed and planning the removal of sutures or clips if required.

Some women may have a lingering feeling of failure or disappointment at having had an emergency CS and may value the opportunity to talk this over with the midwife or other clinicians involved in her care. Indeed it is considered to be good practice for the obstetrician who undertook the CS to review the woman postpartum, not only in order to discuss the problems that necessitated the surgical intervention, but also to counsel about the options for any future pregnancy.

Healthcare professionals caring for women who have heavy and/or irregular vaginal bleeding following CS should be aware that this is more likely to be due to endometritis than retained products of conception. As a consequence, should this complication be suspected, first line treatment with broad spectrum antibiotics should be implemented rather than referral for ultrasound assessment. However, if there are any concerns about the completeness of the placental tissue or membranes, referral for senior review at an early stage should be the preferred course of action.

Whilst the length of hospital stay is likely to be longer after a caesarean section (an average of 3–4 days) than after a vaginal birth (average 1–2 days), women who are

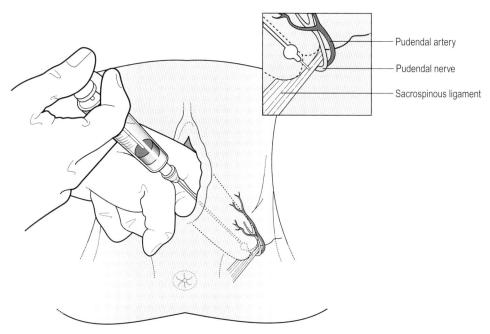

Pudendal artery
Pudendal nerve
Sacrospinous ligament

Fig. 21.8 Locating the pudendal nerve.

recovering well, are apyrexial and do not have complications following CS should be offered early transfer home (after 24 hours) from hospital and follow-up at home, as this is not associated with more infant or maternal readmissions compared with later transfer.

Analgesia/anaesthesia

Pudendal block

This is the procedure where local anaesthetic is infiltrated into the tissue around the pudendal nerve within the pelvis (Fig. 21.8). The pudendal nerve emerges from the spine at the level of the S2–S4 vertebrae and 'descends' into the pelvis crossing behind the ischial spine as it does so. The pudendal nerve supplies the levator ani muscles, the deep and superficial perineal muscles and the sensory nerves (pain/stretch and temperature) of the lower vagina and perineum. A pudendal needle (a specifically designed needle incorporating a sheath guard) is employed with up to 20 ml of local anaesthetic, usually 1% lidocaine (lignocaine), being injected into the region around and below the ischial spine. As both motor and sensory nerves are affected with this technique it may be used to provide analgesia for the lower vagina and perineum, and is therefore used during forceps and ventouse instrumental births.

Perineal infiltration

See Chapter 15 for infiltration and repair of episiotomy, as well as third- and fourth-degree perineal trauma.

Regional anaesthesia

The two most commonly employed regional anaesthetic techniques are those of epidural and intrathecal (spinal) anaesthetic.

The epidural space is the space located within the bony spinal canal just outside the dura mater. In contact with the inner surface of the dura is another membrane called the arachnoid mater. The cerebrospinal fluid (CSF) is contained between the arachnoid mater and the pia mater, another membrane that lies directly in contact with the spinal cord. In adults, the spinal cord terminates at the level of the lower border of the L2 vertebra below which lies a bundle of nerves known as the cauda equina ('horse's tail').

Insertion of an epidural needle involves threading a needle between the spinal vertebrae, through the ligaments and into the epidural potential space taking great care not to puncture the dura mater immediately below, which contains the CSF.

Techniques

Procedures involving injection of any substance into the epidural space require the operator to be technically proficient in order to avoid complications.

The subject is most commonly placed in the seated or lateral positions. Intravenous access is mandatory.

Following a standard aseptic technique protocol, the level of the spine at which the catheter/spinal needle is to be placed is identified.

Epidural

The iliac crest is a commonly used anatomical landmark for lumbar epidural injections, as this level roughly corresponds with the fourth lumbar vertebra, which is *usually* below the termination of the spinal cord. Following the infiltration of local anaesthetic, a Tuohy needle is usually inserted in the midline, between the spinous processes, passing below the vertebral lamina until reaching the ligamentum flavum and the epidural space. A slight clicking sensation may be felt by the operator as the tip of the needle breaches the ligamentum flavum and enters the epidural space.

A syringe containing saline is attached to the Tuohy needle – most practitioners using the loss of resistance to pressure to identify that the needle is correctly placed.

A catheter is then threaded through the needle (typically 3–5 cm into the epidural space), the needle withdrawn and the catheter secured to the skin with adhesive tape or dressings to prevent it becoming dislodged.

The catheter is a fine plastic tube, through which anaesthetic drugs may be injected into the epidural space. Many epidural catheters have three or more orifices along the shaft at the distal tip (far end) of the catheter to allow rapid and even dispersal of the injected agents more widely around the catheter and reduce the incidence of catheter blockage.

A person receiving an epidural for pain relief may receive local anaesthetic (most commonly levo-bupivacaine), with or without an opioid (most commonly fentanyl). These are injected in relatively small doses, compared to when they are injected intravenously or intramuscularly.

For a short procedure, the anaesthetist may introduce a single dose of medication (the 'bolus' technique), although the effects of this will eventually wear off. Thereafter, the anaesthetist or midwife may repeat the bolus provided the catheter remains undisturbed. For a prolonged effect, a continuous infusion of drugs may be employed. However there is evidence that patient controlled epidural analgesia (PCEA), whereby the administration of the boluses is controlled by the patient (up to a predetermined maximum dose) provides better analgesia than a continuous infusion technique, although the total doses received by the individual are often identical.

Typically, the effects of the epidural block are noted below a specific level on the body – a block at or below the T10 sensory level is ideal for women in labour or during birth. Nonetheless, giving very large volumes into the epidural space may spread the block higher.

The epidural catheter is usually removed prior to transfer to the postnatal ward.

Spinal anaesthesia

Intrathecal (spinal) anaesthesia is a technique whereby a local anaesthetic drug is injected into the cerebrospinal fluid through a fine (24–26 gauge) spinal needle. The technique has some similarity to epidural anaesthesia. However, important differences include:

- Intrathecal anaesthesia requires a lower dose of drug and has a faster onset than epidural anaesthesia.
- The block achieved with spinal anaesthesia is typically described as being more dense.
- A spinal anaesthetic block typically lasts for 2 hours, however it cannot be topped up, as no catheter is inserted.
- Intrathecal injections are performed below the second lumbar vertebral body to avoid damaging the spinal cord.

Complications

According to the Association of Anaesthetists of Great Britain and Ireland (AAGBI) (2002), these include:

- Failure to achieve analgesia or anaesthesia occurs in about 5% of cases, while another 15% experience only partial analgesia. If analgesia is inadequate, another epidural may be attempted.
- The following factors are associated with failure to achieve epidural analgesia/anaesthesia: obesity, history of a previous failure of epidural anaesthesia, history of substance abuse (with opiates), advanced labour (cervical dilatation of more than 7 cm at insertion) and previous history of spinal surgery.
- Accidental dural puncture with headache (common, about 1 in 100 insertions). The epidural space in the adult lumbar spine is only 3–5 mm deep. It is therefore comparatively easy to accidentally puncture the dura (and arachnoid) with the needle, causing cerebrospinal fluid (CSF) to leak out into the epidural space. This may, in turn, cause a post-dural puncture headache (PDPH). This can be severe and last several days, and in some rare cases weeks or months. It is caused by a reduction in CSF pressure and is characterized by postural exacerbation when the subject raises his/her head above the lying position. If severe it may be successfully treated with an epidural blood patch, however most cases resolve spontaneously with time.
- Bloody tap (about 1 in 30–50). It is easy to injure an epidural vein with the needle. In people who have normal blood clotting, it is extremely rare for significant complications to develop. However, people who have a coagulopathy may be at increased risk.
- Catheter misplaced into the subarachnoid space (rare, less than 1 in 1000). If the catheter is accidentally misplaced into the subarachnoid space (e.g. after an unrecognized accidental dural puncture), normally cerebrospinal fluid can be freely aspirated from the catheter (which would usually prompt the anaesthetist to withdraw the catheter and re-site it elsewhere). If, however, this is not

recognized, large doses of anaesthetic may be delivered directly into the cerebrospinal fluid. This may result in a high block, or, more rarely, a *total spinal*, where anaesthetic is delivered directly to the brain stem, causing unconsciousness and sometimes seizures.

- Neurological injury lasting less than 1 year (rare, about 1 in 6700).
- Death (very rare, less than 1 in 100 000).
- Epidural haematoma formation (very rare, about 1 in 168 000)
- Neurological injury lasting longer than 1 year (extremely rare, about 1 in 240 000).
- Paraplegia (extremely rare, 1 in 250 000).

General anaesthesia

Despite the increasing use of regional anaesthesia, general anaesthesia is required in up to 5% of women requiring anaesthesia during birth. General anaesthesia can usually be more rapidly administered than a regional block, and is therefore of value when speed is important (such as when the fetus is in serious jeopardy). Women are pre-oxygenated (they are given oxygen to breathe for several minutes) prior to the 'rapid sequence' induction of anaesthesia with the intravenous administration of anaesthetic (e.g. thiopentone or propofol) followed by a muscle relaxant (e.g. suxamethonium) and cricoid pressure is applied (essential to reduce the risks of aspiration of stomach contents). Maternal unconsciousness ensues within seconds and orotracheal intubation is secured with a cuffed tube. There are minimal side-effects and relatively little negative fetal consequence at the time of birth provided meticulous practices are in place.

Anaesthesia is sustained by inhalational anaesthetic means (commonly enflurane or sevoflurane) with an opioid administered intravenously after clamping the cord.

Difficult or failed intubation

This condition is more likely to occur in pregnant women, particularly with those who have pregnancy-induced hypertension or who are obese. Access to the larynx may be obstructed or difficult to view in these women and therefore anticipation of the disorder is the key to its management. Should difficulties be anticipated, anaesthetists should carry out the intubation using a well-lubricated stylet or bougie to aid the endotracheal intubation.

The management of a failed intubation is primarily to maintain adequate oxygenation via assisted ventilation of the woman until the effects of suxamethonium and thiopentone have worn off and the woman has regained consciousness. This is done through the continued application of cricoid pressure and ventilation via a face mask.

It is therefore imperative that surgery is not commenced until the anaesthetist has secured the airway and confirmed that the woman is adequately ventilated.

Complications

Although surgical and anaesthetic techniques have improved, women are still more liable to suffer from complications and to have increased morbidity following caesarean section under general anaesthetic when compared to regional blockade.

Mendelson's syndrome

This condition was described by Mendelson in 1946. It is a chemical pneumonitis caused by the reflux of gastric contents into the maternal lungs during a general anaesthetic. The acidic gastric contents damage the alveoli, impairing gaseous exchange. It may become impossible to oxygenate the woman and death may result. The predisposing factors are: the pressure from the gravid uterus when the woman is lying down, and the effect of the progesterone relaxing smooth muscle and the cardiac sphincter of the stomach. Analgesics administered during labour (e.g. pethidine) can cause significant delay in gastric emptying and will thereby exacerbate these risks.

Prevention of Mendelson's syndrome

Antacid therapy. Prophylactic treatment should be administered to all women in whom a caesarean is planned or anticipated. A usual regimen is for women having an elective operation to be given two doses of oral ranitidine 150 mg approximately 8 hours apart. If a general anaesthetic is anticipated, 30 ml of sodium citrate should be orally administered immediately before induction.

Cricoid pressure. This is a technique whereby pressure is exerted on the cartilaginous ring below the larynx, the cricoid, to occlude the oesophagus and prevent reflux (Fig. 21.9). This is the most important measure in preventing pulmonary aspiration. Cricoid pressure is administered during the induction of a general anaesthetic (most commonly by an operating department practitioner) and is maintained until the tracheal tube is confirmed as being correctly positioned and the seal of the cuff inflated.

In the UK the most recent review into anaesthetic complications during pregnancy and childbirth, for the 2006–2008 triennium, reviewed 127 cases in which anaesthetic services were involved in the care of women who died from either a direct or indirect cause of maternal death. This comprised 49% (127 of 261) of all the maternal deaths during that period. From these deaths the assessors identified seven (3%) women who died from problems directly associated with anaesthesia a rate of 0.31 deaths per 100 000 women who gave birth. However, in a further 18 deaths, anaesthetic management contributed to the outcome or there were lessons to be learned. There

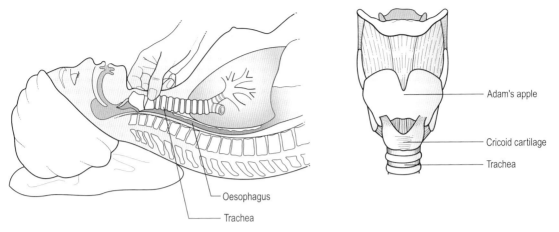

Fig. 21.9 Cricoid pressure showing occlusion of the oesophagus by pressure applied to the cricoid cartilage.

were also 12 women with severe pregnancy-induced hypertension or sepsis for whom obstetricians or gynae-cologists failed to consult with anaesthetic or critical-care services sufficiently early, which the assessors considered may have contributed to the deaths.

It was concluded that:

- The effective management of failed tracheal intubation is a core anaesthetic skill that should be rehearsed and assessed regularly.
- The recognition and management of severe, acute illness in a pregnant woman requires multidisciplinary teamwork. An anaesthetist and/or critical-care specialist should be involved early.
- Obstetric and gynaecology services, particularly those without an on-site critical-care unit, must have a defined local guideline to obtain rapid access to, and help from, critical-care specialists (CMACE 2011).

Research and the incidence of caesarean section: tackling high and rising caesarean section rates

Low CS rates are associated with low levels of intervention and high levels of psychological support. It is difficult to decipher whether caesarean section rates have been affected by interventions, such as proactive management of labour – that is, artificial rupture of membranes and use of oxytocin – or whether other factors have influenced these.

NICE (2011) guidelines recommend that the clinical interventions proven to reduce the rates of birth by CS include all the key points highlighted in Box 21.2.

While there is no accepted optimal rate for CS in the UK, some units manage to keep their CS rate below 20%.

> **Box 21.2 Cinical interventions proven to reduce the rates of birth by CS**
>
> - External cephalic version (ECV) at 36 weeks
> - Continuous support in labour
> - Induction of labour for pregnancies beyond 41 weeks
> - Use of a partogram with a 4 hour action line in labour
> - Fetal blood sampling before caesarean section for abnormal cardiotocograph in labour
> - Support for women who choose vaginal birth after caesarean section
>
> Source: NICE 2011

If reductions in the rate are to be achieved, efforts should focus on where there is the most potential for reduction: reducing primary CS, particularly in first-time mothers, and increasing rates of VBAC.

To provide more meaningful information to women when they are choosing their mode of birth, NICE has recommended that there is a pressing need to document the medium- to long-term outcomes in women and their babies after a planned CS or a planned vaginal birth. They note that it should be possible to gather data using stand-ardized questions (traditional paper-based questionnaires, face-to-face interviews and Internet-based questionnaires) about maternal septic morbidities and emotional well-being up to 1 year after a planned CS in a population of women who have consented for follow-up.

NICE (2011) also comment that it would be important to collect high-quality data on infant morbidities after a planned CS compared with a planned vaginal birth. A long-term morbidity evaluation (between 5 and 10 years after the CS) could use similar methodology to assess additional symptoms related to urinary and gastrointestinal function.

ACKNOWLEDGEMENT

The author would like to acknowledge the contribution of Adela Hamilton to this chapter.

REFERENCES

Anim-Somuah M, Smyth R M D, Jones L 2011 Epidural versus non-epidural or no analgesia in labour. Cochrane Database of Systematic Reviews, Issue 12. Art. No. CD000331. doi: 10.1002/14651858.CD000331.pub3

Association of Anaesthetists of Great Britain and Ireland (AAGBI) 2002 Immediate: Post anaesthetic recovery. AAGBI, London

Bragg F, Cromwell D A, Edozien L C et al 2010 Variation in rates of caesarean section among English NHS trusts after accounting for maternal and clinical risk: cross sectional study. British Medical Journal 341:c5065 (correction c65749).

Brown H C, Paranjothy S, Dowswell T et al 2008 Package of care for active management in labour for reducing caesarean section rates in low-risk women. Cochrane Database of Systematic Reviews, Issue 4. Art No. CD004907. doi:10.1002/14651858.CD004907.pub2

Chaffer D, Royle L 2000 The use of audit to explain the rise in caesarean section. British Journal of Midwifery 8(11):677–84

Charles C 1999 How it feels to be a midwife practitioner. British Journal of Midwifery 7(6):380–2

CMACE (Centre for Maternal and Child Enquiries) 2011 Saving mothers' lives: reviewing maternal deaths to make motherhood safer: 2006–08. The Eighth Report on Confidential Enquiries into Maternal Deaths in the United Kingdom. BJOG: An International Journal of Obstetrics and Gynaecology 118(Suppl 1):1–203

Gupta J K, Hofmeyr G J, Shehnmar M 2012 Position in the second stage of labour for women without epidural anaesthesia. The Cochrane Database of Systematic Reviews, Issue 5. Art No. CD002006. doi: 10.1002/14651858.CD002006.pub3

Hadiati D R, Hakimi M, Nurdiati D S 2012 Skin preparation for preventing infection following caesarean section. Cochrane Database of Systematic Reviews, Issue 9. Art. No. CD007462. doi: 10.1002/14651858.CD007462.pub2

Health and Social Care Information Centre, Hospital Episodes Statistics 2012 NHS maternity statistics 2011–2012 summary report. (Accessed online at www.data.gov.uk 14 May 2013)

Hodnett E D, Gates S, Hofmeyr G J et al 2011 Continuous support for women during childbirth. Cochrane Database of Systematic Reviews, Issue 2. Art No. CD003766. doi: 10.1002/1465/858.pub3

Johanson R B, Menon V 1999 Vacuum extraction versus forceps for assisted vaginal delivery. Cochrane Database of Systematic Reviews, Issue 2. Art. No. CD000224. doi: 10.1002/14651858.CD00022

Lewis G (ed) 2007 The Confidential Enquiry into Maternal and Child Health (CEMACH) Saving mothers' lives: reviewing maternal deaths to make motherhood safer – 2003–2005. The Seventh Report on Confidential Enquiries into Maternal Deaths in the United Kingdom. CEMACH, London

McAleese S 2000 Caesarean section for maternal choice? Midwifery Matters 84:1–7

NICE (National Institute for Health and Clinical Excellence) 2007 Intrapartum care. Care of healthy women and their babies during childbirth. CG 55. NICE, London

NICE (National Institute for Health and Clinical Excellence) 2011 Caesarean section. CG 132. NICE, London

O'Driscoll K, Meagher D, Boylan P 1993 Active management of labour, 3rd edn. Mosby, London

Pare E, Quiñones J, Macones G 2006 Vaginal birth after caesarean section versus elective repeat caesarean section: assessment of maternal downstream health outcomes. BJOG: An International Journal of Obstetrics and Gynaecology 113:75–85

RCOG (Royal College of Obstetricians and Gynaecologists) 2001 Clinical Effectiveness Support Unit. The National Sentinel Caesarean Section audit report. RCOG, London

RCOG (Royal College of Obstetricians and Gynaecologists) 2011 Operative vaginal delivery. Green-top Guideline No. 26. RCOG, London

Stephenson P A 1992 International differences in the use of obstetrical interventions. World Health Organization, Copenhagen, WHO EUR/ICP of MCH 112

Tinsley V 2010 Midwives undertaking ventouse births. In Marshall J E, Raynor M D (eds) Advancing skills in midwifery practice. Churchill Livingstone, Edinburgh, p 67–75

Walker R, Golois E 2001 Why choose caesarean section? Lancet 357:636–7

Weaver J, Stratham H, Richards M 2007 Are there 'unnecessary' cesarean sections? Perceptions of women and obstetricians about cesarean sections for nonclinical indications. Birth 34(1):32–41

Ziadeh S M, Sunna E I 1995 Decreased cesarean birth rates and improved perinatal outcome: a seven year study. Birth 22(3):144–7

FURTHER READING

CMACE 2011 (Centre for Maternal and Child Enquiries) Perinatal mortality 2009: United Kingdom. CMACE, London

A useful audit report on perinatal deaths in the UK.

James D K, Steer P J, Weiner C P et al 2010 High risk pregnancy: management options. Elsevier Health Sciences, London

This book examines the full range of challenges in general obstetrics, medical complications of pregnancy, prenatal diagnosis, fetal disease and management of labour and delivery. This comprehensive work features the fully searchable text online at www.expertconsult.com, as well as more than 100 videos of imaging and monitoring giving easy access to the resources needed to manage high-risk pregnancies. It is a reference book, but a thoroughly readable one.

Luesley D M, Baker P N (eds) 2010 Obstetrics and gynaecology: an evidence-based text for MRCOG, 2nd edn. Hodder/Arnold, London

This book, written by obstetricians approaching their Part 2 MRCOG examination, is a useful handbook for students of midwifery and midwives alike. The perspective is evidence-based and very woman-centred. Sections D and E focus on the first and second stages of labour, their complications and management. It contains useful references at the end of each chapter.

Simms R, Hayman R 2011 Instrumental vaginal delivery. Obstetrics, Gynaecology and Reproductive Medicine 21(1): 7–14

A general reference that informs the text of this chapter.

USEFUL WEBSITES

Mothers and Babies: Reducing Risk Through Audits and Confidential Enquiries Across the UK: www.mbrrace.ox.ac.uk

National Confidential Enquiry into Patient Outcome and Death: www.ncepod.org.uk

National Institute for Health and Care [formerly Clinical] Excellence: www.nice.org.uk

National Patient Safety Agency: www.npsa.nhs.uk

Royal College of Obstetricians and Gynaecologists: www.rcog.org.uk

Scottish Intercollegiate Guideline Network: www.sign.ac.uk

World Health Organization: www.who.net

Chapter 22

Midwifery and obstetric emergencies

Terri Coates

The emergency situations covered in this chapter are rare, but the communication and actions of the midwife are fundamental to the wellbeing of the woman, her baby and also her partner and family. Early detection of severe illness in childbearing women remains a challenge to all health professionals involved in their care. Awareness of local emergency procedures and knowledge of correct use of any supportive equipment are essential, and midwives in all practice settings must maintain skills that enable them to act appropriately in an emergency. The use of multiprofessional workshops to rehearse simulated situations can ensure that all members of the care team know exactly what is required when needed. Midwives need also to engage in reviews of practice to ensure that policies and protocols are regularly reviewed to incorporate best practice and current evidence.

THE CHAPTER AIMS TO:

- recognize the importance of effective communication between members of the multiprofessional team in critical clinical situations
- heighten awareness of sudden changes in maternal condition
- identify symptoms suggestive of serious illness
- discuss emergency situations with discussion of possible causes and the action to be taken
- consider the rare obstetric conditions of uterine rupture, acute inversion of the uterus and vasa praevia
- discuss amniotic fluid embolism and the prompt action required to preserve the woman's life
- review the treatment of hypovolaemic shock and septic shock in midwifery practice
- outline the drills for basic resuscitation.

INTRODUCTION

The immediate management of the emergencies discussed in this chapter is dependent on the prompt action of the midwife. Recognition of the problem and the instigation of emergency measures may determine the outcome for the mother or the fetus. The midwife should remain calm and attempt to keep the woman and her partner fully informed to obtain her consent and cooperation for procedures that may be needed.

It is recognized that pregnancy and labour are normal physiological events, however regular routine observations of vital signs must be an integral part of midwifery care. There is potential for pregnant women and those who have recently given birth to be at risk of physiological deterioration that is not always predicted or recognized (Centre for Maternal and Child Enquiries [CMACE] 2011). To improve recognition of women who are unwell before they become critically ill the modified early obstetric warning score (MEOWS) chart should now be used (CMACE 2011).

All midwifery and medical staff must be updated on the signs and symptoms of critical illness from both obstetric and non-obstetric causes. Regular drills should be held to maintain and improve these skills. All staff should be trained in basic life support to a nationally recognized level and emergency drills for maternal resuscitation should be regularly practised in all maternity units (CMACE 2011; National Health Service Litigation Authority [NHSLA]

2011). Furthermore, effective communication between members of the multiprofessional team is essential to ensure the optimum outcome for the childbearing woman who becomes unwell and her baby (National Health Service [NHS] Institute for Innovation and Improvement 2008).

COMMUNICATION

Health services are often criticized for poor communication among their staff, especially when the outcome does not go according to expectations. However, there are very few instruments that specifically focus on how to improve verbal communication. The SBAR: Situation, Background, Assessment and Recommendations tool developed by the NHS Institute for Innovations and Improvements (2008) is a framework that midwives can use to develop critical clinical conversations that require immediate attention and action.

Use of the SBAR tool

The tool consists of standardized prompt questions about the condition of an individual in four stages:

- Situation
- Background
- Assessment
- Recommendation.

These prompts can assist the midwife to assertively and effectively share concise and focused information about a woman's condition, reducing repetition. The SBAR tool can be used in *all* clinical conversations: face-to face, by telephone or through collaborative multiprofessional team meetings.

In each of the following midwifery and obstetric emergencies, the use of the SBAR tool should be paramount in facilitating appropriate action that is always in the best interest of the woman and her baby.

VASA PRAEVIA

The term *vasa praevia* is used when a fetal blood vessel lies over the cervical os, in front of the presenting part. This occurs when fetal vessels from a velamentous insertion of the cord or to a succenturiate lobe (Chapter 6) cross the area of the internal os to the placenta. The fetal life is at risk owing to the possibility of rupture of the vessels leading to exsanguination unless birth occurs within minutes. Good outcome depends on antenatal diagnosis and birth by caesarean section before the membranes rupture (Oyelese and Smulian 2006).

Diagnosis

Vasa praevia may be diagnosed antenatally using ultrasound scan. Sometimes vasa praevia will be palpated on vaginal examination when the membranes are still intact. If it is suspected, a speculum examination should be made. Fresh vaginal bleeding, particularly if it commences at the same time as rupture of the membranes, may be due to *ruptured* vasa praevia. Fetal distress disproportionate to blood loss may be suggestive of vasa praevia.

Management

The midwife should call for urgent medical assistance. The fetal heart rate should be monitored via cardiotocograph (CTG). If the woman is in the first stage of labour and the fetus is still alive, an emergency caesarean section is carried out. If she is in the second stage of labour, the birth should be expedited such that the baby may be born vaginally. Caesarean section may be carried out but the mode of birth will be dependent on parity and fetal condition.

There is a high fetal mortality associated with this emergency and a paediatrician should therefore be present for the birth. If the baby is born in poor condition, resuscitation, urgent haemoglobin estimation and a blood transfusion with O-negative blood may be necessary.

PRESENTATION AND PROLAPSE OF THE UMBILICAL CORD

Predisposing factors

These are the same for both presentation and prolapse of the cord (for definitions see Box 22.1). Any situation where the presenting part is neither well applied to the cervix nor well down in the pelvis may make it possible

---

Box 22.1 **Definitions**

Cord presentation

This occurs when the umbilical cord lies in front of the presenting part, with the fetal membranes still intact.

Cord prolapse

The cord lies in front of the presenting part and the fetal membranes are ruptured (see Fig. 22.1).

Occult cord prolapse

This is said to occur when the cord lies alongside, but not in front of, the presenting part.

---

for a loop of cord to slip down in front of the presenting part. Such situations include:

- high or ill-fitting presenting part
- high parity
- prematurity
- malpresentation
- multiple pregnancy
- hydramnios.

(Lin 2006; Holbrook and Phelan 2013)

High head

If the membranes rupture spontaneously when the fetal head is high, a loop of cord is able to pass between the uterine wall and the fetus resulting in its lying in front of the presenting part. As the presenting part descends, the cord becomes trapped and occluded.

Multiparity

The presenting part may not be engaged when the membranes rupture and malpresentation is more common.

Prematurity

The smaller size of the fetus in relation to the pelvis and the uterus allows the cord to prolapse. Babies of very low birth weight (<1500 g) are particularly vulnerable (Lin 2006; Holbrook and Phelan 2013).

Malpresentation

Cord prolapse is associated with breech presentation, especially complete or footling breech. This relates to the ill-fitting nature of the presenting parts and also the proximity of the umbilicus to the buttocks. In this situation, the degree of compression may be less than with a cephalic presentation, but there is still a danger of asphyxia.

Shoulder and compound presentation and transverse lie (Chapter 20) carry a high risk of prolapse of the cord, occurring with spontaneous rupture of the membranes.

Multiple pregnancy

Malpresentation, particularly of the second twin, is more common in multiple pregnancy with the consequences of possible cord prolapse.

Hydramnios

The cord is liable to be swept down in a gush of liquor if the membranes rupture spontaneously. Controlled release of liquor during artificial rupture of the membranes is sometimes performed to try to prevent this.

Cord presentation

This is diagnosed on vaginal examination when the cord is felt behind intact membranes. It may be associated with aberrations found during fetal heart monitoring such as decelerations, which occur if the cord becomes compressed.

Management

Under no circumstances should the membranes be ruptured. The midwife should discontinue the vaginal examination, in order to reduce the risk of rupturing the membranes. Medical aid should be summoned. To assess fetal wellbeing, continuous electronic fetal monitoring should be commenced or the fetal heart should be auscultated as frequently as possible. The woman should be assisted into a position that will reduce the likelihood of cord compression. Unless birth is imminent, caesarean section is the most likely outcome.

Cord prolapse

Diagnosis

Whenever there are factors present that predispose to cord prolapse (Fig. 22.1), a vaginal examination should be performed immediately on spontaneous rupture of the membranes.

Bradycardia and variable or prolonged decelerations of the fetal heart are associated with cord compression, which may be caused by cord prolapse. The diagnosis of cord prolapse is made when the cord is felt below or beside the presenting part on vaginal examination. The cord may be felt in the vagina or in the cervical os or a loop of cord may be visible at the vulva (Lin 2006).

Immediate action

Where the diagnosis of cord prolapse is made, the time should be noted and the midwife must call for urgent assistance. The midwife should explain to the woman and her birth partner her findings and any emergency measures that may be needed. If an oxytocin infusion is in progress this should be discontinued. If the cord lies outside the vagina, then it should be gently replaced to prevent spasm, to maintain temperature and prevent drying. Administering oxygen to the woman by face mask at 4 l/min may improve fetal oxygenation.

Relieving pressure on the cord

The risks to the fetus are hypoxia and death as a result of cord compression. The risks are greatest with prematurity and low birth weight (Holbrook and Phelan 2013). The midwife may need to keep her fingers in the vagina and hold the presenting part off the umbilical cord, especially during a contraction. The woman can be supported to change position and further reduce pressure on the cord. If the woman raises her pelvis and buttocks or adopts the knee–chest position, the fetus will be encouraged to gravitate towards the diaphragm (Fig. 22.2). The foot of the bed may also be raised (Trendelenburg position) to relieve compression on the cord. Alternatively, the woman can be helped to lie on her left side, with a wedge or pillow elevating her hips (exaggerated Sims' position) (Fig. 22.3). There is some evidence to suggest that bladder filling may also be an effective technique for managing

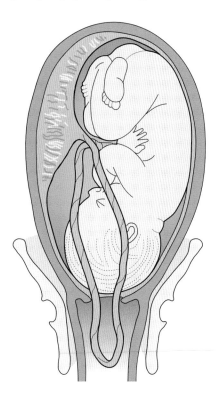

Fig. 22.1 Cord prolapse.

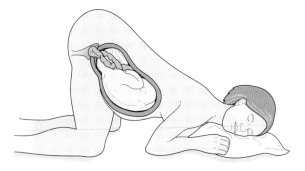

Fig. 22.2 Knee–chest position. Pressure on the umbilical cord is relieved as the fetus gravitates towards the fundus.

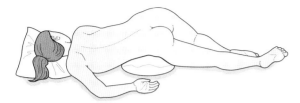

Fig. 22.3 Exaggerated Sims' position. Pillows or wedges are used to elevate the woman's buttocks to relieve pressure on the umbilical cord.

cord prolapse (Houghton 2006; Bord et al 2011). A self-retaining 16G Foley catheter is used to instill approximately 500–700 ml of sterile saline into the bladder. The full bladder can relieve compression of the cord by elevating the presenting part about 2 cm above the ischial spines until birth by caesarean section. The bladder would be drained in theatre immediately before the caesarean section commences.

Birth must be expedited with the greatest possible speed to reduce the mortality and morbidity associated with this emergency. Caesarean section is the treatment of choice in those instances where the fetus is still alive and vaginal birth is not imminent.

If a cord prolapse is diagnosed in the second stage of labour, with a multigravida, the midwife may perform an episiotomy to expedite the birth. Where the presentation is cephalic, assisted birth may be achieved through ventouse or forceps (Chapter 21).

If a cord prolapse occurs in the *community setting*, emergency transfer to a consultant-led maternity unit is essential. The midwife should carry out the same procedures to relieve the compression on the cord. Senior obstetric and anaesthetic staff should be informed and be prepared to perform an emergency caesarean section. An experienced paediatrician should be available to resuscitate the baby, should it be born alive.

SHOULDER DYSTOCIA

The term shoulder dystocia describes failure of the shoulders to traverse the pelvis spontaneously requiring additional manoeuvres after the birth of the head (Royal College of Obstetricians and Gynaecologists [RCOG] 2012). However, a universally accepted definition of shoulder dystocia has yet to be produced (RCOG 2012).

The anterior shoulder becomes trapped behind or on the symphysis pubis, while the posterior shoulder may be in the hollow of the sacrum or high above the sacral promontory (Fig. 22.4). This is, therefore, a bony dystocia, and traction at this point will further impact the anterior shoulder, impeding attempts to assist the baby's birth.

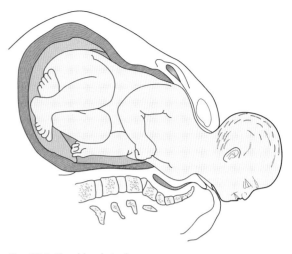

Fig. 22.4 Shoulder dystocia.

Incidence

Shoulder dystocia is not a common emergency: the incidence is reported as varying between 0.58% and 0.7% in collected data (RCOG 2012).

Risk factors

Although it would be useful to identify those women at risk from a birth complicated by shoulder dystocia, most risk factors can give only a high index of suspicion (Al-Najashi et al 1989). Antenatal risk factors include diabetes, post-term pregnancy, high parity, maternal age over 35 and maternal obesity (weight over 90 kg).

Fetal macrosomia (birth weight over 4000 g) has been associated with an increased risk of shoulder dystocia, the incidence increasing as birth weight increases (Delpapa and Mueller-Heubach 1991; Hall 1996). Ultrasound scanning for prediction of macrosomia to prevent shoulder dystocia still has a poor record of success though it is anticipated that ultrasound detection of macrosomia can be improved (Hall 1996; Siggelkow et al 2011). If a large baby is suspected then this fact must be communicated clearly to the team caring for the woman in labour (Confidential Enquiries into Stillbirths and Deaths in Infancy [CESDI] 1999).

Maternal diabetes and gestational diabetes have been identified as important risk factors (Athukorala et al 2007). In diabetic women, a previous birth complicated by shoulder dystocia increases the risk of recurrence to 9.8%; this compares with a risk of recurrence of 0.58% in the general population (Smith et al 1994; Ouzounian et al 2012). The National Institute for Health and Clinical Excellence (NICE) diabetes guideline currently recommends elective birth is offered at 38 weeks' gestation (NICE 2008).

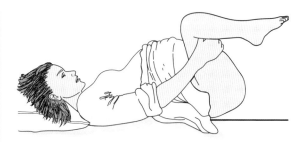

Fig. 22.5 The McRoberts manoeuvre position.

In labour, risk factors that have been consistently linked with shoulder dystocia include oxytocin augmentation, prolonged labour, prolonged second stage of labour and operative births (Benedetti and Gabbe 1978; Al-Najashi et al 1989; Keller et al 1991; Bahar 1996; Gupta et al 2010). For a clinically suspected large baby, the multiprofessional team must be alert for the possibility of shoulder dystocia (CESDI 1999).

Warning signs and diagnosis

The birth may have been uncomplicated initially, but the head may have advanced slowly, with the chin having difficulty in sweeping over the perineum. Once the head is born, it may look as if it is trying to return into the vagina (the turtle sign). Shoulder dystocia is diagnosed when manoeuvres such as gentle downward axial traction* on the head, that may normally be used by the midwife, fail to complete the birth (RCOG 2012). The woman should be discouraged from pushing and any further traction must be avoided.

Management and manoeuvres

The HELPERR Mnemonic (Box 22.2) devised to provide a systematic approach to the management of shoulder dystocia is limited and unhelpful as demonstrated by recent evidence. A study by Jan et al (2014) reported a poor correlation between healthcare professionals' knowledge of manoeuvres and their eponyms. They therefore concluded that any teaching of practical skills should not rely on mnemonics but should primarily be concerned with comprehension, learning and regular opportunities to practise skills and use clinical judgement e.g. mandatory 'skills and drills' training.

Upon diagnosing shoulder dystocia, the midwife must summon help immediately: the midwife coordinator, an experienced obstetrician, an anaesthetist and a person proficient in neonatal resuscitation. Stating the problem early

to the team has been associated with improvements in outcomes in shoulder dystocia (RCOG 2012).

Shoulder dystocia is a frightening experience for the woman, for her partner and for the midwife. The midwife should keep calm and explain as much as possible to the woman to ensure her full cooperation for the manoeuvres that may be needed to complete the birth.

The purpose of all these manoeuvres is to disimpact the shoulders. The principle of using the simplest manoeuvres first should be applied. The midwife will need to make an accurate and detailed record of the time help was summoned and those who attended, the type of manoeuvre(s) used and the time taken, the amount of force used and the outcome of each manoeuvre attempted (Nursing and Midwifery Council [NMC] 2012). It is also important to record which of the fetal shoulders was anterior.

Non-invasive procedures

Change in maternal position

Any change in the maternal position may be useful to help release the fetal shoulders as shoulder dystocia is a bony, mechanical obstruction. However, certain manoeuvres have proved useful and are described below. It is anticipated that following the use of one or more of these manoeuvres, the birth is likely to proceed.

The McRoberts manoeuvre

This manoeuvre involves assisting the woman to lie completely flat (pillows removed) with her buttocks at the edge of the bed and hyperflexing her hips to bring her knees up to her chest as far as possible (Fig. 22.5).

This manoeuvre will rotate the angle of the symphysis pubis superiorly and use the weight of the woman's legs to create gentle pressure on her abdomen, releasing the impaction of the anterior shoulder (Gonik et al 1983, 1989). The McRoberts manoeuvre is associated with the lowest level of morbidity and requires the least force to assist the birth (Bahar 1996; RCOG 2012).

Suprapubic pressure

Pressure should be exerted on the side of the fetal back and towards the fetal chest. This manoeuvre may help to

---

*Axial traction is traction in line with the fetal spine, i.e. no lateral deviation.

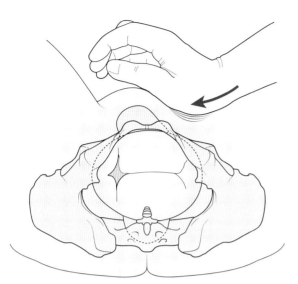

Fig. 22.6 Correct application of suprapubic pressure for shoulder dystocia.
After Pauerstein C (ed), Clinical obstetrics. Churchill Livingstone, New York, 1987, with permission.

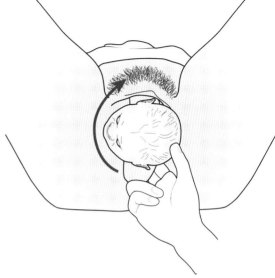

Fig. 22.7 The Rubin manoeuvre.

adduct the shoulders and push the anterior shoulder away from the symphysis pubis into the larger oblique or transverse diameter (Fig. 22.6). Suprapubic pressure can be employed together with the McRoberts manoeuvre to improve success rates (RCOG 2012).

All-fours position

The all-fours position (or *Gaskin manoeuvre*) is achieved by assisting the woman onto her hands and knees. The act of the woman turning may be the most useful aspect of this manoeuvre (Bruner et al 1998). In shoulder dystocia, the impaction is at the pelvic inlet and the force of gravity will keep the fetus against the anterior aspect of the mother's uterus and pelvis. However, this manoeuvre may be especially helpful if the posterior shoulder is impacted behind the sacral promontory as this position optimizes space available in the sacral curve and may allow the posterior arm/shoulder to be born first. Manipulative manoeuvres can be performed while the woman is on all fours but clear verbal communication is needed as eye contact is difficult.

Where non-invasive procedures have not been successful, direct manipulation of the fetus must be attempted, requiring the midwife to insert a whole hand into the vagina. The McRoberts position as detailed above can be used, or the woman could be placed in the lithotomy position with her buttocks well over the end of the bed so that there is no restriction on the sacrum.

Episiotomy

The problem facing the midwife is an obstruction at the pelvic inlet which is a bony dystocia, not an obstruction caused by soft tissue. Although episiotomy (Chapters 15 and 17) will not help to release the shoulders *per se*, the midwife should consider the need to perform one to gain access to the fetus without tearing the perineum and vaginal walls.

Rotational manoeuvres

The Rubin manoeuvre

Rubin (1964) advocated using suprapubic rocking to dislodge the anterior shoulder. If rocking alone proved unsuccessful, vaginal examination (inserting the whole hand) was suggested to identify the most accessible shoulder (usually the posterior shoulder), and push that shoulder in the direction of the fetal chest. This process adducts the shoulders and allows rotation away from the symphysis pubis. The manoeuvre reduces the 12 cm bisacromial diameter (Fig. 22.7).

The Woods manoeuvre

Woods' (1943) manoeuvre requires the midwife to insert a whole hand into the vagina and identify the fetal chest. Then, by exerting pressure on to the posterior fetal shoulder, rotation is achieved. Although this manoeuvre does abduct the shoulders, it will rotate the shoulders into a more favourable diameter and enable the midwife to complete the birth (Fig. 22.8).

Birth of the posterior arm

The midwife has to insert a hand into the vagina, making use of the space created by the hollow of the sacrum, as shown in Figs 22.9A,B. Then two fingers grasp the wrist of

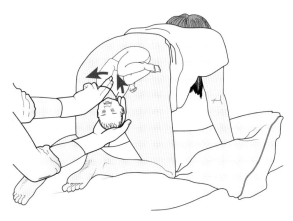

Fig. 22.8 The Woods manoeuvre.
After Sweet B R, Tiran D, Mayes' midwifery. Baillière Tindall, London, 1996: p 664, with permission.

the posterior arm (see Fig. 22.9C), to flex the elbow and sweep the forearm over the chest for the hand to be born, as shown in Fig. 22.9D (O'Leary 2009). If the rest of the birth is not then accomplished, the birth of the second arm is assisted following rotation of the shoulder using either the Woods or Rubin manoeuvre or by reversing the Løvset manoeuvre (Chapter 17).

Zavanelli manoeuvre

If the manoeuvres described above have been unsuccessful, the obstetrician may consider the Zavanelli manoeuvre (Sandberg 1985, 1999) as a last hope for birth of a live baby. The Zavanelli manoeuvre requires the reversal of the mechanisms of birth so far achieved and reinsertion of the fetal head into the vagina. The birth is then completed by caesarean section.

Method: The head is returned to its pre-restitution position (Fig. 22.10A). Pressure is then exerted onto the

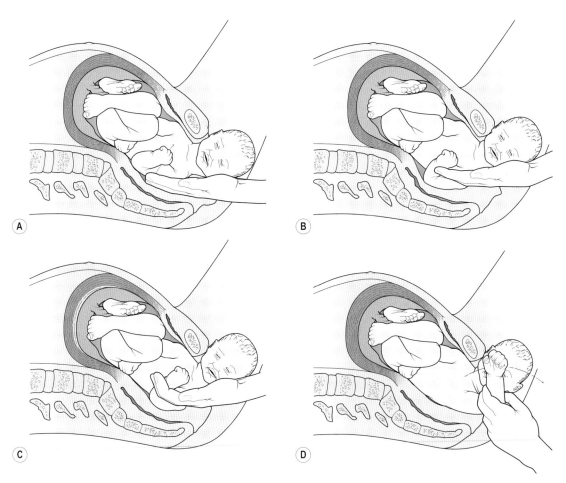

Fig. 22.9 Birth of the posterior arm. (A) Location of the posterior arm. (B) Directing the arm into the hollow of the sacrum. (C) Grasping and splinting the wrist and forearm. (D) Sweeping the arm over the chest and delivering the hand.

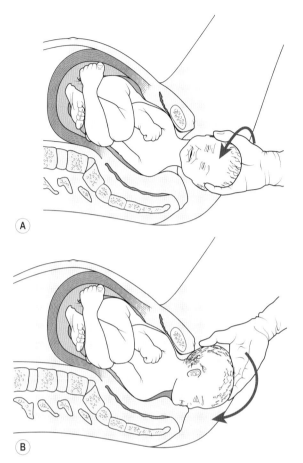

Fig. 22.10 The Zavanelli manoeuvre. (A) Head being returned to direct anteroposterior (pre-restitution) position. (B) Head being returned to the vagina.
After Sandberg 1985, with permission.

occiput and the head is returned to the vagina (Fig. 22.10B). Prompt birth of the baby by caesarean section is then required.

Symphysiotomy

Symphysiotomy is the surgical separation of the symphysis pubis and is used to enlarge the pelvis to enable the birth. It is usually performed in cases of cephalopelvic disproportion (CPD) and is used more routinely in the developing world. There are a few recorded cases where symphysiotomy has been used successfully to relieve shoulder dystocia (Wykes et al 2003), but the procedure has usually been associated with a high level of maternal morbidity. The rarity of reported cases makes it difficult to assess the technique for the relief of shoulder dystocia.

Outcomes following shoulder dystocia

Maternal

Approximately two-thirds of women will have a blood loss of >1000 ml from injury associated with the birth (O'Leary 2009). Maternal death from uterine rupture has been reported following the use of fundal pressure and from haemorrhage during and following the birth (O'Leary 2009).

Fetal

Neonatal asphyxia may occur following shoulder dystocia in 5.7–9.7% of cases and the attending paediatrician must be experienced in neonatal resuscitation (CESDI 1999; RCOG 2012). Brachial plexus injury is commonly associated with shoulder dystocia (Gurewitsch et al 2006; Sandmire and DeMott 2009). Damage to cervical nerve roots 5 and 6 may result in an Erb's palsy (Chapter 31).

Neonatal morbidity may be as high as 42% following shoulder dystocia and remains a cause of intrapartum fetal death (CESDI 1999). Fetal damage may occur even with excellent management using appropriate obstetric manoeuvres. Following shoulder dystocia, examination of the newborn should be carried out by a senior neonatal clinician (RCOG 2012).

The midwife must ensure that simulation training and practice drills are attended annually to maintain skills (Crofts et al 2006; RCOG 2012). Record keeping following shoulder dystocia should include identification of the anterior shoulder and the direction of the fetal head as shown in Box 22.3 (NMC 2012; RCOG 2012).

Box 22.3 Key points for record keeping following shoulder dystocia

- Time of birth of the head and time of birth of the body
- Anterior shoulder at the time of the dystocia
- Manoeuvres performed, their timing and sequence
- Maternal perineal and vaginal examination
- Estimated blood loss
- Staff in attendance and the time they arrived
- General condition of the baby (Apgar score)
- Umbilical cord blood acid–base measurements
- Neonatal assessment of the baby
- Time of completion of records

Adapted from RCOG (2012)

RUPTURE OF THE UTERUS

Rupture of the uterus is one of the most serious complications in midwifery and obstetrics. It is often fatal for the fetus and may also be responsible for the death of the mother. In the 2006–2008 triennial report, there were 111 cases of uterine rupture reported as causing morbidity in women, however, of the nine maternal deaths from haemorrhage, only *one* was associated with uterine rupture (Norman 2011). Nevertheless, uterine rupture remains a significant problem worldwide. With effective antenatal and intrapartum care, some cases of uterine rupture may be avoided.

Rupture of the uterus is defined as being complete or incomplete:

- *complete rupture* involves a tear in the wall of the uterus with or without expulsion of the fetus
- *incomplete rupture* involves tearing of the uterine wall but not the perimetrium.

Dehiscence of an existing uterine scar may also occur. This involves rupture of the uterine wall but the fetal membranes remain intact. The fetus is retained within the uterus and not expelled into the peritoneal cavity (Cunningham et al 2010; Landon 2010). The risk of uterine rupture is increased for those women who have a uterine scar. Studies cite figures of between 0.4 and 4% of labours following a previous caesarean section (Landon 2010).

Causes

Cases of spontaneous rupture of an unscarred uterus in primigravidae are reported in the literature (Roberts and Trew 1991; Uccella et al 2011), but are very rare in the developed world (Hofmeyr et al 2005).

Rupture of the uterus can be precipitated in the following circumstances:

- antenatal rupture of the uterus, where there has been a history of previous uterine surgery
- neglected labour, where there is previous history of caesarean section
- high parity
- use of oxytocin, particularly where the woman is of high parity
- use of prostaglandins to induce labour, in the presence of an existing scar (Lydon-Rochelle et al 2001; Landon 2010)
- obstructed labour: the uterus ruptures owing to excessive thinning of the lower segment (Bandl's ring)
- extension of severe cervical laceration upwards into the lower uterine segment – the result of trauma during an assisted birth
- trauma, as a result of a blast injury or an accident (Michiels et al 2007)

- perforation of the non-pregnant uterus can result in rupture of the uterus in a subsequent pregnancy (Usta et al 2007; Landon 2010).

Signs of intrapartum rupture of the uterus

Complete rupture of a previously non-scarred uterus may be accompanied by sudden collapse of the woman, who complains of severe abdominal pain. The maternal pulse rate increases and, simultaneously, alterations of the fetal heart may occur, including the presence of variable decelerations (Landon 2010). In the UK during the triennium 2003–2005 there were three intrapartum fetal deaths associated with ruptured uterus (Acolet 2007). There may be evidence of fresh vaginal bleeding. The uterine contractions may stop and the contour of the abdomen alters. The fetus becomes palpable in the abdomen as the presenting part regresses. The degree and speed of the woman's collapse and shock depend on the extent of the rupture and the blood loss (see Box 22.4).

Incomplete rupture may have an insidious onset found only after birth or during a caesarean section. This type is more commonly associated with previous caesarean section. Blood loss associated with dehiscence, or incomplete rupture, can be scanty, as the rupture occurs along the fibrous scar tissue, which is avascular (Landon 2010).

Whenever shock during the third stage of labour is more severe than the type of birth or blood loss would indicate, or the woman fails to respond to the treatment given, the possibility of incomplete rupture should be considered. Incomplete rupture may also be manifest as a cause of abdominal pain and/or postpartum haemorrhage following vaginal birth.

Management

All maternity units should have a protocol for dealing with uterine rupture. An immediate caesarean section is performed in the hope of procuring a live baby. Following the birth of the baby and placenta, the extent of the rupture can be assessed. Choice between the options to perform a hysterectomy or to repair the rupture depends on the

---

> ### Box 22.4 **Key signs of rupture of uterus**
>
> - Abdominal pain or pain over previous caesarean section scar
> - Abnormalities of the fetal heart rate and pattern
> - Vaginal bleeding
> - Maternal tachycardia
> - Poor progress in labour

extent of the trauma and the woman's condition. Further clinical assessment will include evaluation of the need for blood replacement and management of any shock.

The woman will be unprepared for the events that have occurred and therefore may be totally opposed to hysterectomy. Few reports of successful pregnancy following repair of uterine rupture are available (Landon 2010).

AMNIOTIC FLUID EMBOLISM

Amniotic fluid embolism (AFE) is rare, unpredictable and unpreventable. In the triennium 2006–2008, there were a total of 13 maternal deaths (0.57/100 000 maternities) resulting from AFE with the diagnosis having been confirmed clinically and by post-mortem examination (Dawson 2011). Although AFE has now fallen to fourth place among the leading causes of *direct* maternal deaths (Dawson 2011) and continues to be a significant factor in maternal mortality, it is no longer considered universally fatal through improvements in resuscitation.

Amniotic fluid embolism occurs when amniotic fluid enters the maternal circulation via the uterus or placental site such that maternal collapse can progress rapidly. The body responds to AFE in two phases. The initial phase is one of pulmonary vasospasm causing hypoxia, hypotension, pulmonary oedema and cardiovascular collapse. The second phase sees the development of left ventricular failure, with haemorrhage and coagulation disorder and further uncontrollable haemorrhage. Mortality and morbidity are high (Dawson 2011) though early diagnosis may lead to a better outcome (Knight et al 2010) and early transfer to an intensive care unit is associated with decreased morbidity (Dawson 2011).

When AFE occurs in a well-equipped unit, it should be considered a treatable and survivable event in the majority of cases (Knight et al 2010). Emergency drills for maternal resuscitation and peri-mortem caesarean section should be regularly practised in clinical areas in all maternity units (Dawson 2011).

Predisposing factors

Amniotic fluid embolism can occur at any gestation. Chance entry of amniotic fluid into the circulation under pressure may occur through the uterine sinuses of the placental bed. It is mostly associated with labour and its immediate aftermath, but cases in early pregnancy and postpartum have been documented (Knight et al 2010).

The barrier between the maternal circulation and the amniotic sac may be breached during periods of raised intra-amniotic pressure, such as termination of pregnancy or during placental abruption. Procedures such as artificial rupture of the membranes (ARM) and insertion of an

> Box 22.5 **Key signs and symptoms of amniotic fluid embolism**
>
> - Respiratory
>   - Cyanosis
>   - Dyspnoea
>   - Respiratory arrest
> - Cardiovascular
>   - Tachycardia
>   - Hypotension
>   - Pale clammy skin/shivering
>   - Cardiac arrest
> - Haematological
>   - Haemorrhage from placental site
>   - Coagulation disorders, DIC
> - Neurological
>   - Restlessness, panic
>   - Convulsions
> - Fetal compromise

intrauterine catheter, have been associated with AFE. Amniotic fluid embolism can also occur during an intrauterine manipulation, such as internal podalic version or during a caesarean section.

Clinical signs and symptoms

Premonitory signs and symptoms (restlessness, abnormal behaviour, respiratory distress and cyanosis) may occur before collapse (Knight et al 2010). There is maternal hypotension and uterine hypertonus. The latter will induce fetal compromise and is in response to uterine hypoxia. Cardiopulmonary arrest follows quickly. Only minutes may elapse before cardiac arrest. Blood coagulopathy develops following the initial collapse (Dawson 2011). The key signs and symptoms are summarized in Box 22.5.

Emergency action

Any one of the above symptoms is indicative of an acute emergency. As the woman is likely to be in a state of collapse, effective resuscitation needs to be commenced at once. An emergency team should be called since the midwife responsible for the care of the woman will require immediate assistance. If collapse occurs in a community setting, basic life support should be commenced prior to the arrival of emergency services.

Despite improvements in intensive care, the outcome of this condition is poor if AFE occurs outside a hospital setting. Specific management for the condition is life support, with high levels of oxygen being required.

Complications of amniotic fluid embolism

Disseminated intravascular coagulation (DIC) is likely to occur within 30 minutes of the initial collapse. In some cases the woman bleeds heavily prior to developing amniotic fluid embolism, which contributes to the severity of her condition. It has also been reported that the amniotic fluid has the ability to suppress the myometrium, resulting in uterine atony.

Acute renal failure is a complication of the excessive blood loss and the prolonged hypovolaemic hypotension. Prompt transfer to a critical care unit for specialized care improves the outcome in AFE (Knight et al 2010; Dawson 2011).

Midwifery support and advice should be continued for the family. The woman should be given the opportunity to talk about emergency treatment when she has recovered sufficiently (Mapp 2005; Mapp and Hudson 2005).

Effect of amniotic fluid embolism on the fetus

Perinatal mortality and morbidity are high where amniotic fluid embolism occurs before the birth of the baby. Delay in the time from initial maternal collapse to the baby's birth needs to be minimal if fetal compromise or death is to be avoided. However, maternal resuscitation may, at that time, be a priority. Box 22.6 summarizes the key points relating to amniotic fluid embolism.

All cases of suspected or proven amniotic fluid embolism, whether fatal or not, should be reported to the National Amniotic Fluid Embolism Register at the following address:

United Kingdom Obstetric Surveillance System [UKOSS]
National Perinatal Epidemiology Unit [NPEU]
University of Oxford (Old Road Campus)
Old Road
Headington
Oxford
OX3 7LF

Box 22.6 Key points for amniotic fluid embolism

- Major cause of maternal death worldwide
- Universal features: maternal shock, dyspnoea and cardiovascular collapse
- Fetal compromise
- Can occur at any time: most commonly immediately after labour
- Suspected in cases of sudden collapse or uncontrollable bleeding

---

ACUTE INVERSION OF THE UTERUS

This is a rare but potentially life-threatening complication of the third stage of labour. It occurs in approximately 1 in 20 000 births (Witteveen et al 2013). A midwife's awareness of the precipitating factors enables her to take preventive measures to avoid this emergency.

Classification of inversion

Inversion can be classified according to severity as follows:

- *first-degree:* the fundus reaches the internal os
- *second-degree:* the body or corpus of the uterus is inverted to the internal os (Fig. 22.11)
- *third-degree:* the fundus protrudes to or beyond the introitus and is visible
- *fourth degree*: this is *total* uterine and vaginal inversion where both the uterus and vagina are inverted beyond the introitus.

Inversion is also classified according to the timing of the event:

- *acute inversion:* occurs within the first 24 hours
- *subacute inversion:* occurs after the first 24 hours, and within 4 weeks
- *chronic inversion:* occurs after 4 weeks and is rare (Bhalia et al 2009).

It is the first of these, acute inversion, that the remainder of this section considers.

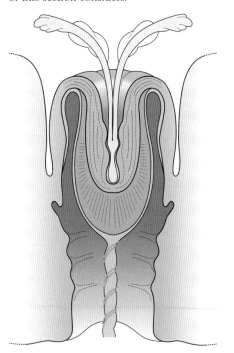

Fig. 22.11 Second-degree inversion of the uterus.

Causes

Causes of acute inversion are associated with uterine atony and cervical dilatation, and include:

- mismanagement in the third stage of labour, involving excessive cord traction to manage the birth of the placenta
- combining fundal pressure and cord traction to expel the placenta
- use of fundal pressure to expel the placenta while the uterus is atonic
- pathologically adherent placenta
- spontaneous occurrence, of unknown cause
- primiparity
- fetal macrosomia
- short umbilical cord
- sudden emptying of a distended uterus.

(Momin 2009; Witteveen et al 2013)

Careful management of the third stage of labour is needed to prevent inversion of the uterus. In active management of the third stage of labour, palpation of the fundus is essential to confirm that contraction has taken place, prior to undertaking controlled cord traction.

Warning signs and diagnosis

The major sign of acute inversion of the uterus is profound shock and usually haemorrhage. The blood loss is within a range of 800–1800 ml. Inversion of the uterus will cause the woman severe abdominal pain. On palpation of the uterus, the midwife may feel an indentation of the fundus. Where there is a major degree of inversion the uterus may not be palpable abdominally but may be felt upon vaginal examination or, in a severe case, the uterus may be seen at the vulva.

The pain is thought to be caused by the stretching of the peritoneal nerves and the ovaries being pulled as the fundus inverts. Bleeding may or may not be present, depending on the degree of placental adherence to the uterine wall. The cause of the symptoms may not be readily apparent and diagnosis may be missed if inversion is incomplete.

Management

Immediate action

A swift response is needed to reduce the risks to the woman. Throughout the events the woman and her partner should be kept informed of what is happening. Assessment of vital signs, including level of consciousness, is of utmost importance.

1. Urgent medical help is summoned.
2. The midwife in attendance should immediately attempt to replace the uterus. If replacement is delayed the uterus can become oedematous and replacement will become increasingly difficult. Replacement may be achieved by pushing the fundus with the palm of the hand, along the direction of the vagina, towards the posterior fornix. The uterus is then lifted towards the umbilicus and returned to position with a steady pressure known as *Johnson's manoeuvre*. If replacement cannot be achieved immediately the foot of the bed can be raised to reduce traction on the uterine ligaments and ovaries (Cunningham et al 2010; Witteveen et al 2013).
3. An intravenous cannula should be inserted and blood taken for cross-matching prior to commencing an infusion.
4. Analgesia such as morphine may be given to the woman.
5. If the placenta is still attached, it should be left *in situ* as attempts to remove it at this stage may result in uncontrollable haemorrhage.
6. Once the uterus is repositioned, the midwife or obstetrician should keep their hand *in situ* until a firm contraction is palpated. Oxytocics should be given to maintain the contraction (Cunningham et al 2010; Witteveen et al 2013).

Medical management

The hydrostatic method of replacement involves the instillation of several litres of warm saline infused through a giving set into the vagina. The pressure of the fluid builds up in the vagina and restores the uterus to the normal position, while the midwife or obstetrician seals off the introitus by hand or using a soft ventouse cup.

If the inversion cannot be replaced manually, a cervical constriction ring may have developed. Drugs can be given to relax the constriction and facilitate the return of the uterus to its normal position. Surgical correction via a laparotomy may be needed to correct inversion. Full support and explanation of the emergency should be offered to the woman in the postnatal period (Mapp 2005; Mapp and Hudson 2005; Witteveen et al 2013).

BASIC LIFE SUPPORT MEASURES

Cardiac arrests are rare in maternity units but they can occur and their management is sometimes suboptimal (CMACE 2011). The midwife must **undertake**, record and act on basic observations using the Modified Early Obstetric Warning Scoring (MEOWS) system that contain triggers to identify symptoms and recognize any deterioration in the woman's condition in order to prompt medical referral (CMACE 2011). All medical and midwifery staff should be trained to a nationally recognized level: Basic Life Support (BLS), Immediate Life Support (ILS) or Advanced Life Support (ALS), as appropriate (National Patient Safety

Agency 2007; Resuscitation Council UK [RCUK] 2010; CMACE 2011; RCOG 2011).

Emergency drills for maternal resuscitation should be regularly practised in clinical areas in all maternity units (NHSLA 2011). These drills should include the identification of the equipment required and appropriate methods for ensuring that cardiac arrest teams know the location of the maternity unit and theatres in order to arrive promptly. Specialized courses such as Advanced Life Support in Obstetrics (ALSO®) and Managing Obstetric Emergencies and Trauma (MOET) provide additional training for obstetric, midwifery and other staff employed in the area of midwifery and obstetric care.

Standards of basic life support have been agreed internationally for health professionals and lay people (RCUK 2010). Basic life support refers to the maintenance of an airway and support for breathing, without any specialist equipment other than possibly a pharyngeal airway. Recent guidelines place greater emphasis on high quality cardiopulmonary resuscitation (CPR) with minimal interruptions in chest compressions. The basic principles are as follows:

A   Airway
B   Breathing
C   Circulation
D   Disability: assess consciousness
E   Environment: keep safe
    (RCUK 2010)

1. Check the surroundings to establish it is safe to proceed.
2. Establish the level of consciousness by shaking the woman's shoulders and enquiring whether she can hear.
3. Summon urgent assistance by the most appropriate means if there is no response.
4. If the woman is already lying flat on her back, remove any pillows. A pregnant woman should be further positioned with a left lateral tilt to prevent aortocaval compression.
5. Tilt the woman's head back, lifting the chin upwards to open the airway (Fig. 22.12). Any obstruction, such as mucus or vomit, should be cleared away.
6. Observe for chest movements, listen and feel for breath.
7. Commence chest compressions, if the pulse is absent or the breathing is absent or abnormal.
8. Place the hands palm downwards one on top of the other with the fingers interlinked, with the heel of the lower hand positioned over the lower part of the sternum. With arms straight, compress the chest 100–120 times/min to a depth of 5 cm, releasing at the same rate as compression. The chest should recoil completely after each compression.
9. Consider kneeling over the woman or find something to stand on to ensure a suitable position

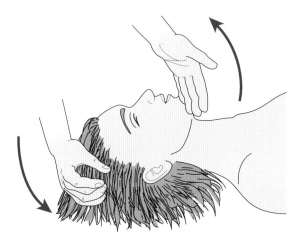

Fig. 22.12 The airway is opened by tilting the head backwards and lifting the chin upwards.

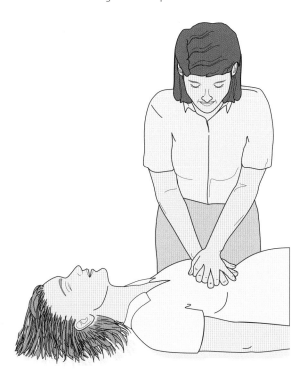

Fig. 22.13 Chest compression. The midwife leans well over the patient, with arms straight. Hands are one on top of the other with fingers interlinked. The heel of the hand is used to compress the chest.

to carry out resuscitation (Fig. 22.13). The surface under the woman must be firm for compressions to succeed.

10. Give two rescue breaths after 30 chest compressions, preferably by bag and mask but mouth-to-mouth if necessary. Each breath should last for only 1 second.

- Check safety of surroundings
- Gently shake the woman and shout
- Call for help
- Check the woman's breathing
- Check the woman's pulse
- Use 30 chest compressions to 2 breaths
- Continue resuscitative measures until help arrives

Adapted from RCUK (2010)

Ensure that the woman's chest rises with each breath and is seen to fall again. If unhappy to perform mouth-to-mouth breathing, continue chest compressions only.

11. Minimize any interruptions to chest compressions.
12. A change in rescuers should occur every 2 minutes where possible.

(RCUK 2010)

Chest compression and rescue breathing should be continued until help arrives when those experienced in resuscitation are able to take over (Grady et al 2007; RCUK 2010). The exact sequences of resuscitation will depend on the training of staff and their experience in assessment of breathing and circulation. These measures are summarized in Box 22.7.

SHOCK

Shock is a complex syndrome involving a reduction in blood flow to the tissues that may result in irreversible organ damage and progressive collapse of the circulatory system (Mulryan 2011; Chandraharan and Arulkumaran 2013). If left untreated it will result in death. Shock can be acute but prompt treatment results in recovery, with little detrimental effect on the woman. However, failure to initiate effective treatment, or inadequate treatment, can result in a chronic condition ending in multisystem organ failure, which may be fatal (NICE 2007).

Shock can be classified as follows:

- *hypovolaemic:* the result of a reduction in intravascular volume such as in severe haemorrhage during childbirth
- *septic or toxic:* occurs with a severe generalized infection
- *cardiogenic:* impaired ability of the heart to pump blood; in midwifery it may be apparent following a pulmonary embolism or in women with cardiac defects
- *neurogenic:* results from an insult to the nervous system as in uterine inversion

- *anaphylactic:* may occur as the result of a severe allergy or drug reaction.

This section deals with the principles of *hypovolaemic shock* and *septic shock*, either of which may develop as a consequence of childbirth.

Hypovolaemic shock

This is caused by any loss of circulating fluid volume as in haemorrhage, but may also occur when there is severe vomiting. The body reacts to the loss of circulating fluid in stages as follows.

Initial stage

The reduction in fluid or blood decreases the venous return to the heart. The ventricles of the heart are inadequately filled, causing a reduction in stroke volume and cardiac output. As cardiac output and venous return fall, the blood pressure is reduced. The fall in blood pressure decreases the supply of oxygen to the tissues and cell function is affected.

Compensatory stage

The fall in cardiac output produces a response from the sympathetic nervous system through the activation of receptors in the aorta and carotid arteries. Blood is redistributed to the vital organs. Vessels in the gastrointestinal tract, kidneys, skin and lungs constrict. This response is seen by the skin becoming pale and cool. Peristalsis slows down, urinary output is reduced and exchange of gas in the lungs is impaired as blood flow diminishes. The heart rate increases in an attempt to improve cardiac output and blood pressure. The pupils of the eyes dilate. The sweat glands are stimulated and the skin becomes moist and clammy. Adrenaline (epinephrine) is released from the adrenal medulla and aldosterone from the adrenal cortex. Antidiuretic hormone (ADH) is secreted from the posterior lobe of the pituitary. Their combined effect is to cause vasoconstriction, increased cardiac output and a decrease in urinary output. Venous return to the heart will increase but, unless the fluid loss is replaced, this will not be sustained.

Progressive stage

This stage leads to multisystem organ failure. Compensatory mechanisms begin to fail, with vital organs lacking adequate perfusion. Volume depletion causes a further fall in blood pressure and cardiac output. The coronary arteries suffer lack of supply and peripheral circulation is poor, with weak or absent pulses.

Final, irreversible stage of shock

Multisystem organ failure and cell destruction are irreparable and death ensues.

Effect of shock on organs and systems

The human body is able to compensate for loss of up to 10% of blood volume, principally by vasoconstriction. When that loss reaches 20–25%, however, the compensatory mechanisms begin to decline and fail. In pregnancy the plasma volume increases, as does the red cell mass. The increase is not proportionate, but allows a healthy pregnant woman to sustain significant blood loss at birth as the plasma volume is reduced with little disturbance to normal haemodynamics. In cases where the increase in plasma volume is reduced or there has been an antepartum haemorrhage, the woman is more susceptible to experience a pathological effect on the body and its systems following a much lower blood loss during childbirth. Individual organs are affected as below.

Brain

The level of consciousness deteriorates as cerebral blood flow is compromised. The woman will become increasingly unresponsive to verbal stimuli and there is a gradual reduction in the response elicited from painful stimulation.

Lungs

Gas exchange is impaired as the physiological dead space increases within the lungs. Levels of carbon dioxide rise and arterial oxygen levels fall. Ischaemia within the lungs alters the production of surfactant and, as a result of this, the alveoli collapse. Oedema in the lungs, due to increased permeability, exacerbates the existing problem of diffusion of oxygen. Atelectasis, oedema and reduced compliance impair ventilation and gaseous exchange, leading ultimately to respiratory failure. This is known as *adult respiratory distress syndrome* (ARDS).

Kidneys

The renal tubules become ischaemic owing to the reduction in blood supply. As the kidneys fail, urine output falls to less than 20 ml/hour. The body does not excrete waste products such as urea and creatinine, so levels of these in the blood rise.

Gastrointestinal tract

The gut becomes ischaemic and its ability to function as a barrier against infection wanes. Gram-negative bacteria are able to enter the circulation.

Liver

Drug and hormone metabolism ceases, as does the conjugation of bilirubin. Unconjugated bilirubin builds up and jaundice develops. Protection from infection is further reduced as the liver fails to act as a filter. Metabolism of waste products does not occur, so there is a build-up of lactic acid and ammonia in the blood. Death of hepatic cells releases liver enzymes into the circulation.

Management

Urgent resuscitation is needed to prevent the woman's condition deteriorating and causing irreversible damage (Chandraharan and Arulkumaran 2013). Women who decline blood products must have their wishes respected and a treatment plan in case of haemorrhage should be discussed with them before labour (CMACE 2011).

The priorities are to:

1. *Call for help:* shock is a progressive condition and delay in correcting hypovolaemia can lead ultimately to maternal death.
2. *Maintain the airway:* if the woman is severely collapsed she should be turned on to her side and 40% oxygen administered at a rate of 4–6 l/min. If she is unconscious, an airway should be inserted.
3. *Replace fluids:* two wide-bore intravenous cannulae should be inserted to enable fluids and drugs to be administered swiftly. Blood should be taken for cross-matching prior to commencing intravenous fluids. A crystalloid solution such as normal saline, Hartmann's, or Ringer's lactate is given until the woman's condition has improved. A systematic review of the evidence found that colloids were not associated with any difference in survival and were more expensive than crystalloids (Perel et al 2013). Crystalloids are, however, associated with loss of fluid to the tissues, and therefore to maintain the intravascular volume colloids are recommended after 2 l of crystalloid have been infused. No more than 1000–1500 ml of colloid such as Gelofusine or Haemocel should be given in a 24 hours period. Packed red cells and fresh frozen plasma are infused when the condition of the woman is stable and these are available.
4. *Arrest haemorrhage:* the source of the bleeding needs to be identified and stopped. Any underlying condition should be managed promptly and appropriately.
5. *Warmth:* it is important to keep the woman warm, but not over warmed or warmed too quickly, as this will cause peripheral vasodilatation and result in hypotension.

Assessment of clinical condition

An interprofessional team approach to management should be adopted to ensure that the correct level of expertise is available. A clear protocol for the management of shock should be used, with the midwife fully aware of key personnel required. Once the woman's immediate condition is stable, the midwife should continue to assess and record the woman's condition or liaise with staff on the critical care unit if the woman has been transferred there for subsequent care (Chandraharan and Arulkumaran 2013).

Hypovolaemic shock in pregnancy will reduce placental perfusion and oxygenation to the fetus, resulting in fetal distress and possibly death. Where maternal shock is caused by antepartum factors, the midwife should determine whether the fetal heart is present, but as swift and aggressive treatment may be required to save the woman's life, this should be *the first priority*.

Detailed MEOWS observation charts including fluid balance should be accurately maintained. The extent of the woman's condition may require her to be transferred to a critical care unit.

Observations and clinical signs of deterioration in hypovolaemic shock

1. Assess level of consciousness in association with the Glasgow Coma Score (GCS). This is a reliable, objective tool for measuring coma, using eye opening, motor response and verbal response. A total of 15 points can be achieved, and one of <12 is cause for concern. Any signs of restlessness or confusion should be noted (Dougherty and Lister 2011).
2. Assess respiratory status using respiratory rate, depth and pattern, pulse oximetry and blood gases. Humidified oxygen should be used if oxygen therapy is to be administered for any length of time.
3. Monitor blood pressure continuously, or at least every 30 minutes, with note taken of any fall in blood pressure.
4. Monitor cardiac rhythm continuously.
5. Measure urine output hourly, using an indwelling catheter and urometer.
6. Assess skin colour including core and peripheral temperature hourly.
7. If a central venous pressure (CVP) line has been sited, haemodynamic measures of pressure in the right atrium are taken to monitor infusion rate and quantities. The fluid balance should be maintained and recorded accurately.
8. Observe for further bleeding, including lochia, or oozing from a wound or puncture site.
9. Undertake venepuncture for haemoglobin and haematocrit estimation to assess the degree of blood loss.
10. The woman is likely to be nursed flat in the acute stages of shock. Clinical assessment will also include review and recording of pressure areas, with positional changes made as necessary to prevent deterioration. A lateral tilt should be maintained to prevent aortocaval compression if a gravid uterus is likely to compress the major vessels.

Box 22.8 summarizes the key points relating to the management of hypovolaemic shock.

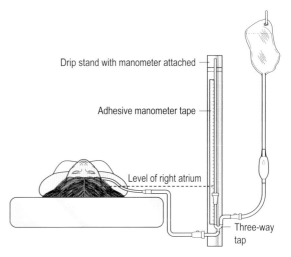

Fig. 22.14 Monitoring central venous pressure.

Drip stand with manometer attached

Adhesive manometer tape

Level of right atrium

Three-way tap

> Box 22.8 **Key points for managing hypovolaemic shock**
>
> - Call for help
> - Identify the source of bleeding and control temporarily if able
> - Gain venous access using two wide-bore cannulae
> - Rapidly infuse intravenous fluid to correct loss
> - Assess for coagulopathy and correct
> - Manage the underlying condition

Central venous pressure

It is unlikely that a midwife will experience central venous pressure (CVP) being measured outside of an intensive care unit (Fig. 22.14). CVP is the pressure in the right atrium or superior vena cava and is an indicator of the volume of blood returning to the heart, reflecting the competence of the heart as a pump and the peripheral vascular resistance. Normal CVP values will change with gestation, and can vary between +5 and +10 cmH$_2$O. Values within this range indicate that the vascular space is well filled and red cell transfusion would not be necessary. However, in the presence of acute peripheral circulatory failure, which accompanies severe shock, the monitoring of CVP aids assessment of blood loss with a negative value indicating the necessity for fluid replacement (Scales 2010). An isolated CVP recording is of little clinical value. Trends in CVP results are more useful clinically and are interpreted in conjunction with fluid balance and peripheral perfusion.

It is extremely dangerous to base an intravenous regimen on guesswork, as hypervolaemia or hypovolaemia, cardiac and renal failure may result.

Septic shock

Death and serious illness from pregnancy-related sepsis are rare. This means that many midwives will not have seen a case, and it is surprising and shocking when it does happen. The last Confidential Enquiry (CMACE 2011) reported a total of 26 women died over the triennium 2006–8 as a result of genital tract sepsis. Women and their families should be made aware of the importance of disclosing significant symptoms to enable earlier interventions in treatment of any underlying infection (Chapters 12 and 13).

Septic shock is a distributive form of shock, where an overwhelming infection develops. Certain organisms produce toxins that cause fluid to be lost from the circulation into the tissues. The commonest form of sepsis causing death in childbearing in the UK is reported to be that caused by beta-haemolytic *Streptococcus pyrogenes* (Lancefield Group A) (CMACE 2011). This is a Gram-positive organism, responding to intravenous antibiotics, specifically those that are penicillin-based. Gram-negative organisms such as *Escherichia coli*, *Proteus* or *Pseudomonas pyocyaneus* are common pathogens in the female genital tract.

The placental site and perineal wounds are the main points of entry for an infection associated with pregnancy and childbirth. This may occur following prolonged rupture of fetal membranes, birth trauma, septic abortion or in the presence of retained placental tissue.

Clinical signs

Sepsis is often insidious in onset but requires prompt recognition and immediate medical referral. Recognition is a particular challenge to the community midwife. The woman may present with tachypnoea, tachycardia, pyrexia or extremely low temperature, or rigors. However, a temperature recording may appear normal if the woman has taken paracetamol as this will reduce pyrexia. The woman may seem confused or anxious, exhibiting a change in her mental state. Abdominal pain and gastrointestinal symptoms are common in pelvic sepsis. Other symptoms, including hypotension, develop in septic shock as the condition progresses. Haemorrhage may be apparent, which could be a direct result of events due to childbearing, however, it occurs in septic shock due to disseminated intravascular coagulation (DIC) (Chapter 12). In hospital all observations should be recorded on a MEOWS chart to determine any further deterioration in the woman's condition and subsequent prompt action.

Management

The advice of an anaesthetist and the critical care team should be sought at an early stage.

Treatment is based on preventing further deterioration in the woman's condition by restoring circulatory volume and then eradication of the infection. Rigorous treatment with intravenous antibiotics is essential to halt the illness. Replacement of fluid volume will restore perfusion of the vital organs. Fluid balance is essential but difficult to manage in septic shock (especially when hourly urine output is low), as fluid overload may lead to fatal pulmonary or cerebral oedema. The midwife must maintain careful monitoring and clear, accurate documentation of the woman's condition throughout (NMC 2012).

Measures are needed to identify the source of infection and to protect the woman against re-infection by maintaining high standards of care in clinical procedures. A full infection screening should be undertaken, including a high vaginal swab, throat swab, midstream specimen of urine and blood cultures. Retained products of conception can be detected on ultrasound, and these can then be removed if they are apparent.

In all situations where the woman requires to be transferred to a critical care unit, relatives should be kept informed of her progress. The midwife may be the person with whom the relatives have formed a relationship and therefore is relied upon to give them information on the woman's condition and progress.

DRUG TOXICITY/OVERDOSE

Drug toxicity and illicit drug overdose should be considered as a cause in all cases of maternal collapse in any type of setting. The principals of observation and resuscitation already discussed in this chapter apply to such a scenario. Common sources of drug toxicity in midwifery and obstetric practice are local anaesthetic agents injected intravenously by accident and magnesium sulphate given in the presence of renal impairment (RCOG 2011).

REFERENCES

Acolet D (ed) 2007 Confidential Enquiry into Maternal and Child Health (CEMACH) Perinatal Mortality 2005: England, Wales and Northern Ireland. CEMACH, London. Available at www .hqip.org.uk/cmace-reports (accessed July 2013)

Al-Najashi S, Al-Suleiman S A, El-Yahia A et al 1989 Shoulder dystocia – a clinical study of 56 cases. Australian and New Zealand Journal of Obstetrics and Gynaecology 29:129–31

American Academy of Family Physicians (AAFP) 2004 Advanced life support in obstetrics (ALSO®): shoulder dystocia. AAFP, Kansas, USA

Athukorala C, Crowther C, Wilson K et al 2007 Women with gestational diabetes mellitus in the ACHOIS trial: risk factors for shoulder dystocia. Australian and New Zealand Journal of Obstetrics and Gynaecology 47:37–41

Bahar A M 1996 Risk factors and fetal outcome in cases of shoulder dystocia compared with normal deliveries of a similar birthweight. British Journal of Obstetrics and Gynaecology 103:868–72

Benedetti T J, Gabbe S G 1978 Shoulder dystocia: a complication of fetal macrosomia and prolonged second stage of labour with mid pelvic delivery. Obstetrics and Gynecology 52(5):526–9

Bhalia R, Wuntakal R, Odejinmi F et al 2009 Acute inversion of the uterus. The Obstetrician and Gynaecologist 11(1):13–18

Bord I, Gemer O, Anteby E Y et al 2011 The value of bladder filling in addition to manual elevation of presenting fetal part in cases of cord prolapse. Archives of Gynecology and Obstetrics 283(5):989–91

Bruner JP, Drummond SB, Meenan AL et al 1998 All-fours maneuver for reducing shoulder dystocia during labor. Journal of Reproductive Medicine 43(5):439–43

Chandraharan E Arulkumaran S (eds) 2013 Obstetric and intrapartum emergencies: a practical guide to management. Cambridge University Press, Cambridge

CMACE (Centre for Maternal and Child Enquiries) 2011 Saving mothers' lives: reviewing maternal deaths to make motherhood safer: 2006–08. The Eighth Report on Confidential Enquiries into Maternal Deaths in the United Kingdom. BJOG: An International Journal of Obstetrics and Gynaecology 118(Suppl 1): 1–203

Confidential Enquiries into Stillbirths and Deaths in Infancy (CESDI) 1999 Sixth annual report. Maternal and Child Health Research Consortium, London

Crofts J F, Bartlett C, Ellis D et al 2006 Training for shoulder dystocia. A trial of simulation using low-fidelity and high fidelity mannequins.

Obstetrics and Gynecology 108(6):1477–85

Cunningham F G, Leveno K J, Bloom S L et al 2010 Williams' obstetrics, 23rd edn. McGraw–Hill, New York

Dawson A 2011 Amniotic fluid embolism. In: Centre for Maternal and Child Enquiries (CMACE) 2011 Saving mothers' lives: reviewing maternal deaths to make motherhood safer: 2006–08. The Eighth Report on Confidential Enquiries into Maternal Deaths in the United Kingdom. BJOG: An International Journal of Obstetrics and Gynaecology 118(Suppl 1): 77–80

Delpapa E, Mueller-Heubach E 1991 Pregnancy outcome following ultrasound diagnosis of macrosomia. Obstetrics and Gynecology 78(1):340–3

Dougherty L, Lister S (eds) 2011 The Royal Marsden Hospital manual of clinical nursing procedures, 8th edn. Blackwell Science, Oxford

Gonik B, Allen R, Sorab J 1989 Objective evaluation of the shoulder dystocia phenomenon: effect of maternal pelvic orientation on force reduction. Obstetrics and Gynecology 74(1):44–8

Gonik B, Stringer C A, Held B 1983 An alternate maneuver for management of shoulder dystocia. American Journal of Obstetrics and Gynecology 145:882–3

Grady K, Howell C, Cox C 2007 Managing Obstetric Emergencies and Trauma: The MOET course manual, 2nd edn. RCOG, London

Gupta M, Hockley C, Quigley M A et al 2010 Antenatal and intrapartum prediction of shoulder dystocia. European Journal of Obstetrics and Gynecology and Reproductive Biology 151(2):134–9

Gurewitsch G T, Johnson E, Hamzehzadeh S et al 2006 Risk factors for brachial plexus injury with and without shoulder dystocia. American Journal of Obstetrics and Gynecology 2(194):486–92

Hall M 1996 Guessing the weight of the baby. British Journal of Obstetrics and Gynaecology 103:734–6

Hofmeyr G J, Say L, Gülmezoglu A M 2005 World Health Organization (WHO) systematic review of maternal mortality and morbidity:

the prevalence of uterine rupture. British Journal Obstetrics and Gynaecology 112(9):1221–8

Holbrook B D, Phelan S T 2013 Umbilical cord prolapse. Obstetrics and Gynecology Clinics of North America 40(1):1–14

Houghton G 2006 Bladder filling: an effective technique for managing cord prolapse. British Journal of Midwifery 14(2):88–9

Jan H, Guimicheva B, Gosh S, et al 2014 Evaluation of healthcare professionals'n understanding of eponymous maneuvers and mnemonics in emergency obstetric care. International Journal of Gynaecology and Obstetrics 125(3):228–31

Keller J D, Lopez J A, Dooley S L et al 1991 Shoulder dystocia and birth trauma in gestational diabetes: a five year experience. American Journal of Obstetrics and Gynecology 165:928–30

Knight M, Tuffnell D, Brocklehurst P et al 2010 Incidence and risk factors for amniotic-fluid embolism. UK Obstetric Surveillance System (UKOSS). Obstetrics and Gynecology 115(5):910–17

Landon M B 2010 Predicting uterine rupture in women undergoing trial of labor after prior cesarean delivery. Seminars in Perinatology 34(4):267–71

Lin M G 2006 Umbilical cord prolapse. Obstetrical and Gynecological Survey 61(4):269–77

Lydon-Rochelle M, Holt V L, Easterling T R et al 2001 Risk of uterine rupture among women with a prior cesarean delivery. New England Journal of Medicine 345(1):3–8

Mapp T 2005 Feelings and fears during obstetric emergencies 2. British Journal of Midwifery 13(1):36–40

Mapp T, Hudson K 2005 Feelings and fears during obstetric emergencies 1. British Journal of Midwifery 13(1):30–5

Michiels I, De Valck C, De Loor J et al 2007 Spontaneous uterine rupture during pregnancy, related to a horse fall 8 weeks earlier. Acta Obstetrica et Gynecologica Scandinavica 86(3):380–1

Momin A A, Saifi S G A, Pethani N R (2009) Sonography of postpartum uterine inversion from acute to chronic stage. Journal of Clinical Ultrasound, 37:53–6

Mulryan C 2011 Acute illness management. Sage, London

National Health Service Institute for Innovation and Improvement 2008 SBAR: Situation, Background, Assessment and Recommendation Tool. Available at www .improvement.nhs.uk (accessed 22 July 2013)

National Health Service Litigation Authority (NHSLA) 2011 Clinical Negligence Scheme for Trusts: Maternity Clinical Risk Management Standards, Version 1 2011/2012. NHSLA, London

NICE (National Institute for Health and Clinical Excellence) 2007 Acutely ill patients in hospital: recognition of and response to acute illness in adults in hospital. Clinical Guideline 50. NICE, London. Available at: www.nice.org.uk/cg50 (accessed 1 July 2013)

NICE (National Institute for Health and Clinical Excellence) 2008 Diabetes in pregnancy. Management of diabetes and its complications from pre-conception to the postnatal period. Clinical Guideline 63. NICE, London. Available at: www.nice.org .uk/cg63 (accessed 1 July 2013)

National Patient Safety Agency (NPSA) 2007 Safer care for the acutely ill patient: learning from serious incidents. NPSA, London

Norman J 2011 Haemorrhage. In: Centre for Maternal and Child Enquiries (CMACE) Saving mothers' lives: reviewing maternal deaths to make motherhood safer: 2006–08. The Eighth Report on Confidential Enquiries into Maternal Deaths in the United Kingdom. BJOG: An International Journal of Obstetrics and Gynaecology 118(Suppl 1):71–6

NMC (Nursing and Midwifery Council) 2012 Midwives Rules and Standards. NMC, London

O'Leary J A 2009 Shoulder dystocia and birth injury: prevention and treatment, 3rd edn. Humana Press, Totowa, NJ

Ouzounian J G, Gherman R B, Chauhan S et al 2012 Recurrent shoulder dystocia: analysis of incidence and risk factors. American Journal of Perinatology 29(7):515–18

Oyelese Y, Smulian J C 2006 Placenta previa, placenta accreta, and vasa previa. Obstetrics and Gynecology 107(4):927–41

Perel P, Roberts I, Ker K 2013 Colloids versus crystalloids for fluid resuscitation in critically ill patients. Cochrane Database of Systematic Reviews 2013, Issue 2. Art. No. CD000567. doi: 10.1002/14651858. CD000567.pub6

RCUK (Resuscitation Council UK) 2010 Resuscitation guidelines. RCUK, London. www.resus.org.uk/pages/ guide.htm (accessed 30 June 2013)

Roberts L, Trew G 1991 Uterine rupture in a primigravida. Journal of Obstetrics and Gynaecology 11(4):261–2

RCOG (Royal College of Obstetricians and Gynaecologists) 2011 Maternal collapse in pregnancy and the puerperium. Green-Top Guideline No. 56. RCOG, London

Royal College of Obstetricians and Gynaecologists (RCOG) 2012 Shoulder dystocia. Green-Top Guideline No. 42, 2nd edn. RCOG, London. www.rcog.org.uk/files/ rcog-corp/GTG%2042_Shoulder%20 dystocia%202nd%20edition%20 2012.pdf (accessed 30 June 2013)

Rubin A 1964 Management of shoulder dystocia. Journal of the American Medical Association 189:835

Sandberg E C 1985 The Zavanelli maneuver: a potentially revolutionary method for the resolution of shoulder dystocia. American Journal of Obstetrics and Gynecology 152:479–87

Sandberg E C 1999 The Zavanelli maneuver: 12 years of recorded experience. Obstetrics and Gynecology 93(2):312–17

Sandmire H F, DeMott R K 2009 Controversies surrounding the causes of brachial plexus injury. International Journal of Gynecology and Obstetrics 104(1):9–13

Scales K (2010) Central venous pressure monitoring in clinical practice. Nursing Standard 24(29):49–55

Siggelkow W, Schmidt M, Skala C et al 2011 A new algorithm for improving fetal weight estimation from ultrasound data at term. Archives of Gynecology and Obstetrics 283(3):469–74

Smith R B, Lane C, Pearson J F 1994 Shoulder dystocia: what happens at the next delivery? British Journal of Obstetrics and Gynaecology 101:713–15

Uccella S, Cromi A, Bogani G et al 2011 Spontaneous prelabor uterine rupture in a primigravida: a case report and review of the literature. American Journal of Obstetrics and Gynecology 205(5):e6–8

Usta I M, Hamdi M A, Abu Musa A A et al 2007 Pregnancy outcome in patients with previous uterine rupture. Acta Obstetrica et Gynecologica Scandinavica, 86(2):172–6

Witteveen T, van Stralen G, Zwart J et al 2013 Puerperal uterine inversion in The Netherlands: a nationwide cohort study. Acta Obstetricia et Gynecologica Scandinavica 92(3):334–7

Woods C E 1943 A principle of physics as applied to shoulder delivery. American Journal of Obstetrics and Gynecology 45:796–805

Wykes C B, Johnston T A, Paterson-Brown S et al 2003 Symphysiotomy: a lifesaving procedure. British Journal Obstetrics Gynaecology 110(2):19–21

FURTHER READING

Draycott T, Winter C, Crofts J et al (eds) 2008 PROMPT PRactical Obstetric Multi-Professional Training Course Manual Vol. 1. RCOG Press, London

Recommended training course for childbirth emergencies presenting current best practice.

Draycott T J, Crofts J F, Ash J P et al 2008 Improving neonatal outcome through practical shoulder dystocia training. Obstetrics and Gynecology 112(1):14–20

The introduction of shoulder dystocia training for all maternity staff was associated with improved management and

neonatal outcomes of births complicated by shoulder dystocia.

James A, Endacott R, Stenhouse E 2011 Identifying women requiring maternity high dependency care. Midwifery 27(1):60–6

Key issues in the management of women who become critically ill during pregnancy, labour and the postpartum period are discussed, with identification of recognition of signs of clinical deterioration with subsequent referral for appropriate care.

National Institute for Health and Clinical Excellence 2007 Acutely ill patients in hospital: recognition of and response to acute illness in adults in hospital. Clinical Guideline 50. NICE, London. http:// publications.nice.org.uk/acutely-ill -patients-in-hospital-cg50

Provides guidance on the care and management of the acutely ill patient.

Raynor M D, Marshall J E, Jackson K 2012 Midwifery practice: critical illness, complications and emergencies case book. Open University Press, Maidenhead

This text provides a case study approach to several critical conditions and emergencies that can prove a challenge to all healthcare professionals working in midwifery practice, with particular importance being placed on multiprofessional team working. Each case explores and explains the pathology, pharmacology and care principles and uses test questions and answers to assist learning.

Resuscitation Council UK 2010 Resuscitation guidelines. RCUK, London. www.resus.org.uk

Internationally agreed information and guidance on resuscitation and emergency life support. The website contains a range of publications, information and posters that can be downloaded to support clinical practice.

Robson S E, Waugh J J S (eds) 2013 Medical disorders in pregnancy: a manual for midwives, 2nd edn. John Wiley and Sons, London

The need for joint medical and midwifery care is stressed in the latest CMACE report, with a recommendation that contemporary midwifery education prepares midwives for problems in pregnancy and adverse pregnancy outcome.

Royal College of Obstetricians and Gynaecologists 2011 Maternal collapse in pregnancy and the puerperium. Green-Top Guideline No. 56. Royal College of Obstetricians and Gynaecologists, London. www.rcog.org.uk/files/ rcog-corp/GTG56.pdf

Provides up-to-date information and excellent reference material on maternal collapse in pregnancy and the puerperium.

USEFUL WEBSITES

Erb's Palsy Group, for parents and health professionals: www.erbspalsygroup.co.uk

National Amniotic Fluid Embolism Register: www.npeu.ox.ac.uk/ukoss/ current-surveillance/amf

National Institute for Health and Care (formerly Clinical) Excellence: www.nice.org.uk

NHS Improving Quality (formerly NHS Institute for Innovation and Improvement): www.nhsiq.nhs.uk/

Resuscitation Council UK: www.resus.org.uk

Royal College of Obstetricians and Gynaecologists: www.rcog.org.uk

Section | 5 |

Puerperium

Chapter |23|

Physiology and care during the puerperium

Mary Steen, Julie Wray

There is current evidence that postnatal care is often undervalued and under-resourced even though it is an important and challenging time for a mother who has recently given birth, her partner and family (Wray and Bick 2012). Current postnatal care in the United Kingdom (UK) can involve several healthcare practitioners. Midwives are the lead health professional, with support from maternity support workers, general practitioners, health visitors and other practitioners depending on the mother's individual needs and circumstances. Both public and voluntary services can work together to support the mother, father, baby and other family members to cope and adjust following the birth of a new baby (Department of Health [DH] 2005; National Institute for Health and Clinical Excellence [NICE] 2006; Nursing and Midwifery Council [NMC] 2012). This approach to postnatal care differs from that offered to women in most other developed countries where the provision for regular contact with midwives as the main healthcare professional responsible for postnatal care is less well defined. (Potential postnatal morbidity and in some cases mortality for the mother is discussed in Chapter 24.)

THE CHAPTER AIMS TO:

- review the historical background of postnatal care
- explore the role of the midwife in the assessment and care of women's postpartum health and wellbeing
- review the current evidence for women's general health and wellbeing after childbirth
- discuss the contemporary challenges for the provision of maternity care during the postnatal period
- explore women's and their partners views and experiences of postnatal care.

THE POSTNATAL PERIOD

Following the birth of a baby, placenta and membranes, the newly birthed mother enters a period of physical and emotional/psychological recuperation (Buckley 2006; Wray 2012). Skin-to-skin contact is advocated immediately following birth and during the postnatal period as there is clear evidence of benefit to the mother and father (Moore et al 2012). The *puerperium* starts immediately after birth of the placenta and membranes and continues for 6 weeks. In many cultures around the world 40 days for recuperation is a time-honoured practice (Hundt et al 2000; Waugh 2011). A general expectation is that by 6 weeks after birth a woman's body will have recovered sufficiently from the effects of pregnancy and the process of parturition. However, there has now been a recognition that the return to a non-pregnant state of health and wellbeing can take much longer (World Health Organization [WHO], 2010; Bick et al 2011). Some women continue to experience health problems related to childbirth that extend well beyond the 6-week period defined as the puerperium (WHO 2010). In some cases, healing and recovery can take up to a year following birth (Bedwell 2006; Wray and Bick 2012).

It has been customary to refer to the first weeks after the birth as the postnatal period, defined in the UK by the NMC as 'a period after the end of labour during which the attendance of a midwife upon a woman and baby is required, being not less than 10 days and for such longer period as the midwife considers necessary' (NMC 2012: 6).

By no longer stating an endpoint in time until which midwifery care can still be made available to women, it is envisaged that offering more flexibility to the provision of midwifery care will make a positive impact on the health and wellbeing of women (Cattrell et al 2005; Redshaw and Heikkila 2010).

The National Childbirth Trust (NCT) makes clear on its website that it is the quality of postnatal care provided to women and families in the first days and weeks after birth that can have a huge impact and affect mothers' and families' experiences of the transition to parenthood (NCT 2012).

However, in this present climate, when there is an ever-increasing birth rate, a shortage of midwives and ongoing financial constraints, this is an extremely challenging task for maternity service providers.

HISTORICAL BACKGROUND

Postnatal care in the UK has been an integral part of the midwife's role since the beginning of the last century following the introduction of the Midwives Act in 1902. This was instigated by the high maternal mortality rates. Despite a decline in death rates among all age groups in the general population, maternal mortality rates remained high. The majority of maternal deaths were caused by puerperal infection (interestingly, the latest triennial

report on the Confidential Enquiries into Maternal Deaths in the UK cites sepsis as currently the leading cause of maternal mortality [CMACE 2011]).

This had a marked effect on what constituted important aspects of postnatal care. Routine observations, such as temperature, pulse, respirations, blood pressure, breast examination, uterine involution and observation of lochia, were introduced as well as a set pattern of postnatal visits.

Midwives were expected to visit twice a day for the first three days and then daily until day 10, commonly referred to as the 'lying in period' (Leap and Hunter 1993). Two further Midwives Acts extended the regulatory maximum duration of postnatal care from 10 to 14 days in 1936 and then this was increased to 28 days in 1962. This approach to postnatal care was considered appropriate to meet the needs of women at that time. However, a considerable decline in maternal mortality rates began in the 1930s and has continued up to the present day. A traditional pattern and content of postnatal care continued until the 1980s. Then, two major changes happened that affected the pattern of postnatal care, those being the woman returning home much earlier following childbirth and the introduction of 'selective visiting' rather than specified days in 1986 by the former midwifery governing body, the United Kingdom Central Council (UKCC 1986). A postal survey undertaken in England in 1991 reported that most maternity services had changed from the daily home visits up to the tenth postnatal day to selective home visits, but there was wide variation in patterns of selective visiting (Garcia et al 1994). This may be due to the fact that little guidance was given on how to plan and implement this change and there was no evaluation with regard to the implications for women. A House of Commons Health Committee report (Winterton 1992) highlighted, among other things, that postnatal care was neglected and there was a lack of research in this area. This was followed by the establishment of the Expert Maternity Committee, whose remit was to examine policy and make recommendations for the maternity services in England and Wales. Their report 'Changing Childbirth' (DH 1993) recommended that the maternity services should offer women more choice, greater continuity of care, more involvement in the planning of their care and should be midwifery-led, and more recently the 'Maternity Matters' report (DH 2007a) reiterated these recommendations.

Today, a partnership approach, where the woman is encouraged to explore how she is feeling physically and emotionally and to seek the advice and support of the midwife, is advocated (Wray and Bick 2012). The importance of all newly birthed mothers having access to postnatal care that will meet their individual needs is underpinned by the NMC (2012) Midwives Rules and Standards and by a national guideline defining core care, and what should be provided for the mother and baby in the days and weeks following birth (NICE 2006).

FRAMEWORK AND REGULATION FOR POSTNATAL CARE

The initial framework for hospital postnatal care in the early 20th century involved a regimented approach, with the newly birthed mother being viewed as a patient; a period of prescribed bed rest, compliance with hospital regimens such as vulval swabbing, binding of legs and separation from her baby were thus routine procedures. A gradual shift in this 'sickness' framework of care as described by Parsons (1951) started to occur during the 20th century. Renfrew (2010) describes how mothers in the late 1970s and early 1980s were still kept in postnatal wards for a week or more after birth and their babies were kept in nurseries with their feeds timed and measured, regardless of whether they were being breastfed or formula-fed. In the 1990s the provision of postpartum care was reviewed with regard to its content, purpose or effectiveness (Marsh and Sargent 1991; Garcia and Marchant 1993; Twaddle et al 1993); this led to research that investigated and challenged regimented and ritual patterns of postpartum care (Bick et al 2002; Shaw et al 2006; Wray 2006).

Nowadays, mothers have the choice to return home in a few hours after the birth, as it is considered both safe and acceptable by society at large. The newly birthed mother can recuperate in her own familiar surroundings with the support of her family and friends.

The recent Health and Social Care Act 2012 will continue to support mothers to make their own choices about who and what services/care best meet their individual needs. Independent sector providers as well as National Health Service (NHS) maternity service providers will be free to innovate to deliver quality services.

MIDWIVES AND POSTPARTUM CARE

It is vitally important that midwives have the knowledge and skills to determine when to be proactive and undertake specific observations when there are indications to do so. Therefore, the midwife needs to be able to acknowledge and recognize what are normal expected outcomes following birth and also be able to identify signs of what is not normal and when to instigate care that will involve further investigation, tests and the support of other health professionals. It is the midwife's responsibility to ensure she is competent and to undertake any further necessary education and training if required to provide extended care (see Box 23.1).

Public health care

It has long been recognized that poverty and being socially disadvantaged is society leads to increased risk of poor

---

Box 23.1 The midwife's skills and knowledge

The UK's Nursing and Midwifery Council states in *The Code: Standards of Conduct, Performance and Ethics for Nurses and Midwives*:

Keep your skills and knowledge up to date:

- *You must have the knowledge and skills for safe and effective practice when working without direct supervision.*
- *You must recognise and work within the limits of your competence.*
- *You must keep your knowledge and skills up to date throughout your working life.*
- *You must take part in appropriate learning and practice activities that maintain and develop your competence and performance.*

Source: NMC 2008: 38–41

---

health and wellbeing (Hart 1971; Acheson 1998). In England, the Department of Health has acknowledged that 'Healthy mothers are key for giving healthy babies a healthy start in life' (DH 2004). It is important that mothers and their family receive information and advice about healthy lifestyles. Midwives have a vital role to address public health targets and are ideally situated to promote healthy lifestyles to the mother, her partner and extended family during the postnatal period. However, midwives cannot address public health issues alone and working collaboratively with other professionals and local communities and signposting to other services needs to occur. Models of care to give more intense care and support to disadvantaged groups have been developed. Sure Start centres were set up to provide accessible community-based services that would enable families with young children to improve their health and wellbeing (DH 1999). Targets were linked to public health issues such as smoking cessation, breastfeeding rates and reaching disadvantaged groups (National Evaluation of Sure Start [NESS] 2004). The government's *Every Child Matters: Change for Children* agenda (DfES 2004) supported the Sure Start goals and aimed to increase the support for children and young people up to the age of 19. These centres became Sure Start Children's Centres, where family healthcare and parenting skills from midwives and health visitors were delivered with support from other professionals (DCSF 2009).

Positive benefits for mothers and their families who live within the designated postcode for Children's Centre services have been reported (Tanner et al 2012). However, a sustained commitment to service provision and funding is essential for this to benefit mothers and their families. In 2009, Children's Centres became a statutory requirement under the Apprenticeships, Skills, Children and

Learning Act (HM Government 2009; DfE 2010). In 2010, the Coalition government offered protection from spending cuts to enable Children's Centres to continue to provide a range of services to local communities but at the time of writing there are concerns in the present economic climate with budget reductions; the government is interested in developing community management models such as cooperatives and social enterprises (DfE 2012).

Working in tandem with Children's Centres is the Family Nurse Partnership (FNP) Programme as developed in the USA and recently piloted in selected areas of high deprivation in England. It has been reported that teenage first-time mothers, their partners and family find this approach acceptable (Barnes et al 2011). Further work is being undertaken to see if a group approach is of any benefit to families who are not eligible for the FNP programme (Barnes and Henderson 2012). Early indications show that there are some benefits and peer support is valuable. An holistic maternal health and wellbeing programme, specifically designed to raise awareness of the general health and wellbeing of mothers, their babies and families also reported how beneficial group and peer support is to postnatal mothers (Steen 2007b) (see Box 23.2).

Recently, the Health and Social Care Act 2012 gives a new focus to public health (HM Government 2012). This Act provides the underpinnings for Public Health England, a new body to drive improvements in public health.

The provision of and need for postnatal care

The provision of midwifery care and support to newly birthed mothers needs to be woman-focused and family-orientated. Good communication to explain what is considered to be normal physical, emotional/psychological, occurrences during the postnatal period will reassure a mother that she is going through a normal physiological process. Building a trusting, caring relationship will give a mother confidence to ask questions when she has concerns and is anxious about her health and wellbeing.

A recent survey undertaken on behalf of the National Childbirth Trust (NCT 2010) involving 1260 first-time mothers reported that these mothers felt that midwives were always or mostly kind and understanding (80%) and treated them with respect (83%) . However, there were still gaps in the provision and satisfaction with regards to postnatal care reported. Only 4% of mothers reported being involved in the development of a postnatal care plan to meet their individual needs as recommended by NICE (2006). Mothers who had undergone either an operative or surgical procedure to aid their birth were reported to be the least satisfied with their postnatal care. Although this survey does not represent the whole of the UK maternal population and socially disadvantaged mothers' voices were not represented, it does give an insight into areas where improvements in postnatal care provision should be targeted.

Box 23.2 Examples of postnatal women's views

Postnatal workshops:

'I needed to talk about my birth as I was disappointed I had been induced, but I can understand why now.'

'I didn't know that most breast cancer is detected by the woman herself, I will start checking now.'

'I feel guilty about smoking and now I have my daughter to think about I will seriously think about stopping.'

'I'm finding being a mum hard. I'm always tired and feeling weepy but I feel a lot better once I have come to the class.'

Postnatal exercise classes:

'I couldn't do my pelvic floor exercises properly before. I can now.'

'I did some of the exercises in early labour and used the positions I was shown, it really helped.'

'I had a section in the end but I wasn't too disappointed as I coped really well during labour and used the Pilates and relaxation techniques.'

'I have a bit of weight to lose and this will help me get back into shape.'

'I'm steadily getting my figure back. The exercises appear to be helping.'

'I really enjoyed the exercises and intend to continue to do Pilates.'

Postnatal general comments:

'I always go home feeling good about myself and fit and healthy.'

'I love the company as well as being able to exercise.'

'It's great that you can bring your baby with you. I love being able to exercise with him on a mat next to me.'

'I bring my mum as well. We both have enjoyed it.'

'I'm going to come to the gym and get my boyfriend to come as well.'

'It will be difficult for me to attend classes when I go back to work but I intend to walk more and exercise on a weekend.'

'I have enjoyed coming to the sessions and I've loved being able to meet other mums.'

Source: Steen 2007b: 119

A social model of care that encompasses aspects of observing and monitoring the health and wellbeing of the mother, father and their baby initially, in a hospital and then home setting, will support both parents to adjust to their new parenting role. Guidance and reassurance is an important aspect of midwifery care. Working in partnership with the mother and father will assist them to develop confidence in their ability to be parents and care for their baby. There is growing evidence that when fathers are included this is beneficial to both the mother's and the baby's health and wellbeing (Flouri and Buchanan 2003; Bottorff et al 2006; Tohotoa et al 2009). For example, fathers can play an important role in breastfeeding support (Wolfberg et al 2004; Piscane et al 2005). Therefore, it is vital that they are included in discussions and pathways of care. Yet, there is also evidence that many fathers feel excluded unsure and fearful (Steen et al 2012). A recent publication entitled 'Reaching out: involving fathers in maternity care' (Royal College of Midwives [RCM] 2011: 3) has highlighted that 'to provide effective support fathers themselves need to be supported, involved and prepared'.

In the UK, it is still usual for a midwife to 'attend' a postpartum woman on a regular basis for the first few days regardless of whether the mother is in hospital or at home (NMC 2012). During the course of contact visits, midwifery practice has been to undertake a routine physical examination to assess the new mother's recovery from the birth (Rowan and Bick 2006; Bick 2012; Wray and Bick 2012). From an international perspective this practice is unusual; it is only comparatively recently that postpartum home visits, and postpartum support programmes, have been initiated in America, Canada and Australia (Boulvain et al 2004; Peterson et al 2005; Vernon 2007) and that women in these countries have recognized a need for and their satisfaction with current services (De Clerc 2006). In the UK, the role of maternity support worker (MSW) has been introduced to support midwives to provide care to mothers and their families. However, the development of MSWs can be inconsistent (Kings Fund 2011). The RCM (2010) Position Statement on maternity support workers reports that there should be a clear framework which defines their role, responsibility and arrangements for supervision. A study reviewed the involvement of maternity support workers in the community over an extended postnatal period and found no differences in health outcomes but reported that mothers found benefit in the extra support (Morrell et al 2000).

A common reference to postnatal services being the 'Cinderella' of the maternity service provision as a whole has led to repeated reports from women of poor support, disappointment in the services and in some cases evidence of negligence as a result of sub-standard care (Wray 2006; Lewis 2007; Redshaw and Heikkila 2010; WHO 2010).

The framework for assessing resources released from the NHS costs would appear to be based on a measurement of clinical need resulting in the main providers of health services having to make comparisons between postpartum women's needs and other members of the population who are suffering from acute or chronic illnesses (O'Sullivan and Tyler 2007). The birth of a baby does not attract the same level of funding as the needs of those with long-term conditions or terminal diseases. However, there has been an increasing awareness that there are important aspects around promoting good health and wellbeing of the newly birthed mother and baby as this has implications for the nation's healthcare costs (NICE 2006; NCT 2010). The postnatal care pathway recommended by NICE (2006) is divided into three 'time bands' which cover the postnatal period, these are:

- the first 24 hours after birth
- the first 2–7 days
- the period from day 8 to around 6–8 weeks.

During these postnatal time bands a midwife will need to advise women about some health problems that she may be at risk of developing and to discuss any symptoms or concerns she may have. Contact numbers and how to summon help and advice need to be made readily available and issuing regular reminders to encourage and enable a mother to do this if she has any concerns is paramount.

Midwifery postpartum contact and visits

The majority of postnatal care in the UK now occurs either in the family or a relative's home. Expectations of mothers about the purpose of home visits by the midwife may vary according to their cultural backgrounds and individual needs. Some faiths hold important ceremonies for the newborn baby and a home visit from a midwife will need to be mutually arranged to fit around these. Newly birthed mothers who have experienced motherhood before may feel that they need minimal support from a midwife and this can also be mutually arranged. In contrast, a first-time mother or a mother who has had complications will more likely need further support and contact. The concept of postpartum care is one that aims to assist the mother, her baby and family towards attaining an optimum health status. Where the visit from the midwife can be seen as supportive and useful to the mother and her family, this purpose is more likely to be achieved. Research that has explored the experiences of women from different ethnic backgrounds has demonstrated marked inequalities in both the provision of services as well as the actual direct contact with caregivers (Hirst and Hewison 2002). In contrast, where the timing of midwifery postpartum care is extended beyond 28 days, there is greater opportunity for midwives to continue midwifery support where this might be appropriate, and this has been welcomed as progress although the focus would appear to be more on social or psychological outcomes, or for breastfeeding support than overt clinical or physical morbidity (Winter et al 2001; Bick et al 2002). In the United States a woman can choose to employ a doula to help her during her transition to motherhood. A doula can provide physical, emotional and social support (Simkin 2008). This option is becoming more readily available in the UK (Gibbon and Steen 2012).

PHYSIOLOGICAL CHANGES AND OBSERVATIONS

Regardless of place of birth, the midwife is primarily concerned with the observation of the health of the postpartum mother and the new baby. As such, it has been common practice to have an overall framework upon which to base the assessment of the mother's state of health and for the observations contained within the examination to link with pre-stated categories in the postnatal midwifery records. This formalized approach to the postpartum review might be an appropriate tool to use if there is concern about a woman who is feeling unwell and there is a need for a comprehensive picture of the woman's state of health (see Chapters 13 and 24). Where this is not the case such an approach might be less useful from the viewpoint of the needs of a healthy woman who has recently given birth (Redshaw and Heikkila 2010). The concern focuses on whether in the time taken to complete a 'top to toe' examination as a thorough review of someone who is generally well, the midwife might ignore or give less attention to what the mother really wants to talk about (Ridgers 2007). However, Wray (2011: 158) highlights that women want to be 'checked over' (physically) as a means to obtain contact and feedback from the midwife about their bodies and recovery separate from their baby. As one new mother pointed out: 'it was only when she [the midwife] checked me over that you could think about yourself and talk about how you were healing and getting sorted'.

The skill of the midwife's care is to achieve a balance when deciding which observations are appropriate so that she does not fail to detect potential aspects of morbidity. The next part of this chapter identifies areas of physiology that are likely either to cause women the most anxiety or to have the greatest outcome with regard to morbidity. These descriptions relate to observations undertaken for women who have had vaginal births and uncomplicated pregnancies.

Returning to non-pregnant status

In the postnatal period, all of the mother's body systems have to adjust from the pregnant state back to the pre-pregnant state. Mothers go through a transitional period and the period of physiological adjustment and recovery following birth is closely related to the overall health status of the mother. The intricate relationships between physiological, emotional/psychological and cultural and sociological factors are all encompassed in the remit of caring for the postnatal woman and her newborn (MaGuire 2000; Wiggins 2000; Bick 2012).

Vital signs: general health and wellbeing

The following information is based on the premise that the midwife is exploring the health of the postpartum woman from a viewpoint of confirming normality. 'Common sense', although a concept that is very difficult to define, is probably a well-understood paradigm and taking such an approach is an important part of midwifery care with regard to addressing the issues that are visible before seeking out the less obvious. In this instance, an overall assessment of the woman's physical appearance will add considerably to the management of what will be undertaken prior to continuing any further investigation for either the woman or her baby.

Observations of temperature, pulse, respiration (TPR) and blood pressure (BP)

During the first 6 hours postnatal care observations to record vital signs will need to be taken and these should be within a normal range before a woman returns home if she has opted for an early transfer. An Early Warning Score has recently been introduced in some maternity units (Lewis 2007). If the woman has had a home birth the midwife must not leave the new mother's home until she is satisfied that vital signs are stable.

It is not necessary to undertake observations of temperature routinely for women who appear to be physically well and who do not complain of any symptoms that could be associated with an infection. However, where the woman complains of feeling unwell with flu-like symptoms, or there are signs of possible infection or information that might be associated with a potential environment for infection, the midwife should undertake and record the temperature. This will enhance the amount of clinical information available where further decisions about potential morbidity may need to be made.

Making a note of the pulse rate is probably one of the least invasive and most cost-effective observations a midwife can undertake. If undertaken when seated alongside or at the same level as the woman, it can create positive feelings of care while also obtaining valuable clinical information. While observing the pulse rate, particularly if this is done for a full minute, the midwife can also observe a number of related signs of wellbeing: the respiratory rate, the overall body temperature, any untoward body odour, skin condition and the woman's overall colour and complexion, as well as just listening to what the woman is saying.

Blood pressure

Following the birth of the baby, a baseline recording of the woman's blood pressure will be made. In the absence of any previous history of morbidity associated with hypertension, it is usual for the blood pressure to return to a normal range within 24 hours after the birth. Routinely undertaking observations of blood pressure without a clinical reason is therefore not required once a baseline recording has been taken. NICE (2006) suggest this should be within 6 hours of the birth.

Circulation

The body has to reabsorb a quantity of excess fluid following the birth and for the majority of women this results in passing large quantities of urine, particularly in the first day, as diuresis is increased (Cunningham et al 2005). Women may also experience oedema of their ankles and feet and this swelling may be greater than that experienced in pregnancy. These are variations of normal physiological processes and should resolve within the puerperal time scale as the woman's activity levels also increase. Advice should be related to taking reasonable exercise, avoiding long periods of standing, and elevating the feet and legs when sitting where possible. Swollen ankles should be bilateral and not accompanied by pain; the midwife should note particularly if this is present in one calf only as it could indicate pathology associated with a deep vein thrombosis.

Skin and nutrition

Women who have suffered from urticaria of pregnancy or cholestasis of the liver should experience relief once the pregnancy is over. The pace of life once the baby is born might lead to women having a reduced fluid intake or eating a different diet than they had formerly (Tuffery and Scriven 2005). This in turn might affect their skin and overall physiological state. Women should be encouraged to maintain a balanced fluid intake and a diet that has a greater proportion of fresh food in it (Tuffery and Scriven 2005; DH 2007b). This will improve gastrointestinal activity and the absorption of iron and minerals, and reduce the potential for constipation and feelings of fatigue.

Breast care

It is essential that midwives offer support and advice on common breast and breastfeeding problems. With a woman's permission a midwife needs to check for any physical problems such as engorgement, cracked or bleeding nipples, mastitis, or signs of thrush. Engorgement on postnatal day 3 and 4 is a common problem for most mothers regardless of whether they have chosen to breast- or formula-feed. It is important that mothers are aware of this and this needs to be discussed antenatally so it does not come as a complete surprise. If breastfeeding and engorged, advise the mother to feed on demand, perform breast massage from under her axilla and towards the nipple, to hand express, take analgesia if necessary, and to wear a well-fitting bra. For further content on complications see Chapters 24 and 34.

The uterus

After the birth, oxytocin is secreted from the posterior lobe of the pituitary gland to act upon the uterine muscle and assist separation of the placenta. Following the birth of the placenta and membranes, the uterine cavity collapses inwards; the now opposed walls of the uterus compress the newly exposed placental site and effectively seal the exposed ends of the major blood vessels. The muscle layers of the myometrium act like ligatures that compress the large sinuses of the blood vessels exposed by placental separation. These occlude the exposed ends of the large blood vessels and contribute further to reducing blood loss. In addition, vasoconstriction in the overall blood supply to the uterus results in the tissues receiving a reduced blood supply; therefore, de-oxygenation and a state of ischaemia arise. Through the process of autolysis, autodigestion of the ischaemic muscle fibres by proteolytic enzymes occurs resulting in an overall reduction in their size. There is phagocytic action of polymorphs and macrophages in the blood and lymphatic systems upon the waste products of autolysis, which are then excreted via the renal system in the urine. Coagulation takes place through platelet aggregation and the release of thromboplastin and fibrin (Cunningham et al 2005).

What remains of the inner surface of the uterine lining apart from the placental site, regenerates rapidly to produce a covering of epithelium. Partial coverage occurs within 7–10 days after the birth; total coverage is complete by the 21st day (Cunningham et al 2005).

Once the placenta has separated, the circulating levels of oestrogen, progesterone, human chorionic gonadotrophin and human placental lactogen are reduced. This leads to further physiological changes in muscle and connective tissues as well as having a major influence on the secretion of prolactin from the anterior lobe of the pituitary gland.

Abdominal palpation of the uterus is usually performed soon after placental expulsion to ensure that the physiological processes are beginning to take place (Chapter 18). On abdominal palpation, the fundus of the uterus should be located centrally, its position being at the same level or slightly below the umbilicus, and should be in a state of contraction, feeling firm under the palpating hand. The woman may experience some uterine or abdominal discomfort, especially where uterotonic drugs have been administered to augment the physiological process (Anderson et al 1998).

Uterine involution

The *process of involution* is essential background knowledge for midwives monitoring the physiological process of the return of the uterus to its non-pregnant state. Involution involves the gradual return and reduction in size of the uterus to a pelvic organ until it is no longer palpable above the symphysis pubis (Stables and Rankin 2011). This process is usually assessed by measuring the symphysio-fundal height (S-FD). This is the distance from the top of the uterine fundus to the symphysis pubis and is commonly assessed by anthropometry (abdominal palpation) (Bick et al 2009). NICE (2006) has concluded that there is insufficient evidence to recommend the routine measurement of fundal height and how often this should take place as the process of involution is highly variable between individual women. Therefore, involution of the uterus should be placed into context alongside the colour, amount and duration of the woman's vaginal fluid loss and her general state of health at that time. Uterine involution in combination with other observations such as a raised or lowered temperature abdominal tenderness and offensive lochia can be helpful to detect any maternal morbidity, e.g. sepsis (CMACE 2011).

Assessment of postpartum uterine involution

There are several aspects to the abdominal palpation of the postpartum uterus that contribute to the observation as a whole. The first is to identify height and location of the fundus (the upper parameter of the uterus). Assessment should then be made of the condition of the uterus with regard to uterine muscle contraction and finally whether palpation of the uterus causes the woman any pain. When all these dimensions are combined, this provides an overall assessment of the state of the uterus and the progress of uterine involution can be described. Findings from such an assessment should clearly record the position of the uterus in relation to the umbilicus or the symphysis pubis, the state of uterine contraction and the presence of any pain during palpation. A suggested approach to how this is undertaken in clinical practice can be found in Box 23.3.

'Afterpains'

'Afterpains' are caused by involutionary contractions and usually last for two to three days after childbirth. These cramping type of pains are more commonly associated with multiparity and breastfeeding. The production of the oxytocin in relation to the let-down response that initiates the contraction in the uterus and causes pain. Women have described the pain as equal to the severity of moderate labour pains and women require analgesia (Marchant et al 2002). A recent systematic analysis has concluded that non-steroidal anti-inflammatory drugs (NSAIDs) were better than placebo at relieving 'afterpains' and NSAIDs were better than paracetamol, but there were insufficient data to make conclusions regarding the effectiveness of opioids at relieving 'afterpains' (Deussen et al 2011).

> **Box 23.3 Suggested approach to undertaking postpartum assessment of uterine involution**
>
> - Discuss the need for uterine assessment with the woman and obtain her agreement to proceed. She should have emptied her bladder within the previous 30 min.
> - Ensure privacy and an environment where the woman can lie down on her back with her head supported. Locate a covering to put over her lower body.
> - The midwife should have clean, warm hands and should help the woman to expose her abdomen; the assessment should not be done through clothing.
> - The midwife places the lower edge of her hand at the umbilical area and gently palpates inwards towards the spine until the uterine fundus is located.
> - The fundus is palpated to assess its location and the degree of uterine contraction. Any pain or tenderness should be noted.
> - Once the midwife has completed the assessment she should help the woman to dress and to sit up.
> - The midwife should then ask the woman about the colour and amount of her vaginal loss and whether she has passed any clots or is concerned about the loss in any way.
> - Following the assessment, the woman should be informed about what has been found and any further action that is required, and then a record of the assessment is made in the midwifery notes.

It is helpful to explain the cause of 'afterpains' to women and that they might experience a heavier loss at this time, even to the extent of passing clots. Pain in the uterus that is constant or present on abdominal palpation is unlikely to be associated with 'afterpains' and further enquiry should be made about this. Women might also confuse 'afterpains' with flatus pain, especially after an operative birth or where they are constipated. Identifying and treating the cause is likely to relieve the symptoms or raise concern about a more complex condition that needs further attention.

Postpartum vaginal blood loss

Blood products constitute the major part of the vaginal loss immediately after the birth of the baby and expulsion of the placenta and membranes. As involution progresses the vaginal loss reflects this and changes from a predominantly fresh blood loss to one that contains stale blood products, lanugo, vernix and other debris from the unwanted products of the conception. This loss varies from woman to woman, being a lighter or darker colour, but for any woman the shade and density tends to be consistent (Marchant et al 2002).

Lochia is a Latin word traditionally used to describe the vaginal loss following the birth (Cunningham et al 2005). Medical and midwifery textbooks have described three phases of lochia and have given the duration over which these phases persist. Research has explored the relevance of these descriptions for women and raised questions about the use of these descriptions in clinical practice. Marchant et al (2002) reported that not all women are aware they will have a vaginal blood loss after the birth and that women experience a wide variation in the colour, amount and duration of vaginal loss in the first 12 weeks' postpartum. This suggests that, overall, descriptions of normality ascribed to the traditional descriptions of lochia are outdated and unhelpful to women and midwives in accurately describing a clinical observation.

Most women can clearly identify colour and consistency of vaginal loss if asked and will be able to describe any changes. It is important for a midwife to ask direct questions about the woman's vaginal loss: whether this is more or less, lighter or darker than previously and whether the woman has any concerns. It is of particular importance to record any clots passed and when these occurred. Clots can be associated with future episodes of excessive or prolonged postpartum bleeding (see Chapters 18, 24).

Assessment that attempts to quantify the amount of loss or the size of clot is problematic. However, the use of descriptions that are common to both woman and midwife can improve accuracy in these assessments – for example, asking the mother how often she has to change her maternity pad and describing her blood loss in her own words.

Continence after birth

The majority of women will revert back to their non-pregnant status during the puerperium without any major urinary or bowel problems. Any minor changes to women's urinary and bowel habits should resolve within the first few days of giving birth. Women suffering from perineal injury may need extra reassurance that having their bowels open may be uncomfortable but will not disrupt and dislodge any stitches in the perineal region (Chapter 15). A systematic review has reported that there is sufficient evidence to suggest that pelvic floor exercise training during pregnancy and after birth can prevent and treat urinary incontinence (Mørkved and Bø 2013). NICE (2006) recommends that pelvic floor muscle exercises should be taught as first line treatment for urinary incontinence.

It is important that women are given opportunities to discuss any urinary or bowel problems as it is often a taboo subject. Some women may find it embarrassing and will not seek help and advice whilst others may put up with urinary and bowel problems believing that it is an accepted outcome following childbirth. Therefore, it is essential that a midwife build a trusting, caring

relationship to encourage a woman to disclose any urinary or bowel problems.

Usually, urinary and bowel symptoms resolve within the first two weeks following birth but some problems do persist. If a woman continues to notice a change to her pre-pregnant urinary and bowel pattern by the end of the puerperal period, she should be advised to have this reviewed (Steen 2013). Initially, conservative management is advocated and then if the symptoms are persistent a referral to a specialist may be required (RCM/CSP 2013) (see Chapter 24).

Perineal trauma

Perineal and vaginal injury during childbirth continues to affect the majority of women (Albers et al 2006; East et al 2012b). Morbidity associated with perineal injury and repair is a major health problem for women throughout the world. The Royal College of Obstetricians and Gynaecologists (RCOG) (2004) reported that perineal trauma can have long-term social, psychological and physical health consequences for women. Perineal pain and discomfort associated with trauma may disrupt breastfeeding, family life and sexual relationships.

In the UK, it is estimated that 1000 women per day will require perineal repair (Kettle and Fenner, 2007). It is therefore important that midwives are firstly educated and trained to recognize the extent of perineal and vaginal trauma, and secondly, have gained the confidence and clinical skills to suture competently as failure to do so can contribute to negative consequences for women in both the short and long term (Steen 2010). In addition, it is important to consider how to alleviate the associated pain and discomfort attributed to perineal injuries following birth.

Up-to-date knowledge and an understanding of the negative consequences for women will help midwives to advise women on how to alleviate perineal pain, prevent further trauma and promote healing (Steen 2012).

Perineal pain

Regardless of whether the birth resulted in actual perineal trauma, women are likely to feel swollen and bruised around the vaginal and perineal tissues for the first few days after a vaginal birth. Women who have undergone any degree of actual perineal injury will experience pain for several days until healing takes place (East et al 2012b). It is essential that women are offered adequate pain relief initially following birth and then for them to be advised on how to alleviate the inflammation associated with perineal injuries and any pain felt during the postnatal period. In the first few days after the birth all women should be asked if they have any pain or discomfort in the perineal area regardless of whether there is a record of actual perineal trauma (Bick and Bassett 2013).

Where women appear to have no discomfort or anxieties about their perineum, it is not essential for the midwife to examine this area and arguably it is an intrusion on the woman's privacy to do so. The basic principles of morbidity or infection (Cunningham et al 2005) indicate that it is unusual for morbidity to occur without inflammation and pain although these factors are also integral to the healing process (Steen 2007a); therefore, although the area might be causing discomfort from the original trauma, where this is unchanged or absent a pathological condition should not be developing. There may be occasions, however, where the midwife might consider that the woman is declining this observation because she is embarrassed or anxious. In such cases, the midwife should use her skills of communication to explore whether there is a clinical need for this observation to be undertaken and, if so, to advise the woman accordingly. Examining the perineal area is undertaken to assess healing after birth. Standardized scales to assist the midwife are not readily available and formal evaluation appears to be an ongoing neglected area of women's health care (Steen 2010). Fortunately, for the majority of women, the perineal wound gradually becomes less painful and initial healing should occur by 10–14 days after the birth (Steen 2007a).

Alleviating perineal pain and discomfort

Evidence suggests that a combination of systemic and localized treatments may be necessary to achieve adequate pain relief which will meet individual women's needs (Steen and Roberts 2011).

There is some evidence that oral analgesia, bathing, diclofenac suppositories, lidocaine gel and localized cooling treatment can alleviate perineal pain. No adverse effects on healing have been reported when localized cooling is applied (East et al 2012a).

The treatments that appear to achieve pain relief are summarized in Box 23.4.

Box 23.4 Summary of evidence to alleviate perineal pain and discomfort

- **Oral analgesia**, self-administered, effective for mild to severe pain (Moffat et al 2006; Steen and Marchant 2007; Chou et al 2010).
- **Bathing** (Sleep and Grant 1988; Greenshields and Hulme 1993; Steen and Marchant 2007).
- **Voltarol suppositories** – effective in first 24–48 hr, some relief (Yoong et al 1997; Searles and Pring 1998; Hedayati et al 2005).
- **Lignocaine gel** – effective in first 48 hr (Harrison and Brennan 1987a, 1987b; Corkill et al 2001).
- **Localized cooling** (Steen et al 2000; Steen 2002; Steen and Marchant 2007; Navviba et al 2009; East et al 2012a)

Tiredness and fatigue

Most women will complain of tiredness and fatigue during the first few weeks following birth, and lack of sleep at the end of pregnancy, giving birth and establishing feeding can take its toll. It is therefore vitally important that a newly birthed mother is advised to consciously make time to rest and sleep during the postpartum period. For example, she should be advised to take the opportunity to have a 'nap' during the day when her baby is sleeping and not to feel guilty about doing this. A midwife may need to reassure a mother that household chores can wait and it takes time to adjust to caring for a newborn. Tiredness and fatigue can have an adverse effect on a mother's health and wellbeing status. Being tired and fatigued will inevitably have a negative effect on a woman's ability to care for her newborn (Troy and Dalgas-Pelish, 2003). Tiredness and fatigue can lead to maternal exhaustion and has been associated with maternal depression (Taylor and Johnson 2010) (see Chapter 25). However, it has been reported that the meaning of tiredness and fatigue are subjective and difficult to define and 'there is a lack of authoritative research on postnatal tiredness and fatigue' (McQueen and Mander 2003: 464). Nevertheless, midwives can play a vital role in supporting a woman to have realistic expectations about life after birth and advising her to nurture herself and on the importance of finding time to rest and recuperate.

Expectations of health

It is reasonable for women to look forward to regaining their body for themselves once the baby is born (MaGuire 2000; Steen 2007b). However, this is not the immediate outcome for many women and, once again, individual women will have their own expectations about the nature and speed at which they would like this recovery to occur. The role of the midwife at this point is to assist the woman to identify actual symptoms of disorder from the gradual process of reorder and advise what action the woman can do for herself in the way of progressive recovery. Advice for new parents in the matter of recovery from the birth is limited and often superficial; also women may feel they should know what to do, or have unrealistic expectations of motherhood and their ability to cope with these new experiences (Bartell 2004). This is one area where taking the time to talk about what might seem to the midwife a range of peripheral or even superficial issues that might be worrying the otherwise healthy new mother could be of more benefit that day than a range of routine clinical observations (Redshaw et al 2007).

Balancing exercise and healthy activity with rest and relaxation

Increasing the understanding in the general population about the value of different forms of exercise and health has been shown to be of psychological as well as physical benefit (Armstrong and Edwards 2004). There is substantial evidence that suggests exercising during the postnatal period has many positive effects (Goodwin et al 2000; Berk 2004; Steen 2007b). For example, women who exercise regularly are more likely to recover more quickly after the birth (Clapp 2001) (see Box 23.3).

Exploring each person's level of activity will encourage advice in relation to appropriate exercise and, by association, nutritional intake and rest or relaxation and sleep. Undertaking regular pelvic floor exercises is of benefit to women's long-term health (Mørkved and Bø 2013).

Future health, future fertility

Advice on managing fertility is within the sphere of practice of the midwife and it is an important aspect of postpartum care (see Chapter 27). Midwives need to be aware of a range of different needs with regard to women's sexuality and should be able to offer sensitive and appropriate advice on contraception where this is needed.

Record-keeping and documentation

A midwife has to provide high standards of practice and care at all times (NMC 2008). Clear and accurate records of any observations and discussions that have taken place during the postnatal period are a key tool in safeguarding the health and wellbeing of the mother and her baby. In its Code, the Nursing and Midwifery Council (NMC 2008) clearly states that a midwife must keep clear and accurate records (Box 23.5).

Box 23.5 **The midwife's record-keeping**

The UK's Nursing and Midwifery Council states in *The Code: Standards of Conduct, Performance and Ethics for Nurses and Midwives:*

Keep clear and accurate records:

- *You must keep clear and accurate records of the discussions you have, the assessments you make, the treatment and medicines you give and how effective these have been.*
- *You must complete records as soon as possible after an event has occurred.*
- *You must not tamper with original records in any way.*
- *You must ensure any entries you make in someone's paper records are clearly and legibly signed, dated and timed.*
- *You must ensure any entries you make in someone's electronic records are clearly attributable to you.*
- *You must ensure all records are kept securely.*

Source: NMC 2008: 42–7

Evidence and best practice

The midwife should gain a considerable amount of information during her contact with the mother and baby. The wide range for normality and the individuality within this can make it difficult for the midwife to decide whether an observation is related to morbidity. It is more likely to be the relationship between several observations that raises cause for concern and, where these appear to be more related to abnormality than normality, the midwife has a responsibility to make appropriate referral to a medical practitioner or other appropriate healthcare professional. In the UK the midwife's statutory framework (NMC 2012) is different from the overall guidance and frameworks for care provision developed under the auspices of various Departments of Health. This is an important distinction with regard to the professional accountability of the midwife and her obligation as an employee (NMC 2008).

TRANSITION TO PARENTHOOD

The transition to parenthood involves major adjustments within a family and some mothers will welcome and actively seek help and support from a midwife during the postnatal period, but some women, for a range of reasons, may not. Women from different cultural backgrounds may have traditions that conflict with the current management of postpartum care (Ockleford et al 2004), or consider that they already have sufficient skills and experience. Not being able to speak or understand English may also prevent a woman from seeking help.

Although a visit to the home might have been planned, there will also be times when women are not at home when the midwife visits. It is important to keep in mind individual circumstances and whether these might have any bearing on a no-access visit. For example, parents with a disability such as hearing loss or poor mobility might not hear a doorbell. It is, therefore, important to make arrangements for contact to be made by alternative means (e.g. using a visual alarm or telephone to alert the woman of the visit beforehand) (Disability Pregnancy and Parenthood International 2007).

The midwife needs to recognize situations where the mother perceives she has different priorities from those routinely provided by the healthcare services. The option of attending a postnatal clinic/drop-in centre has been introduced in some areas of the UK to meet maternity services local needs and offers some flexibility around postnatal follow-up care (Gibbon and Steen 2012).

A recent meta-synthesis has reported that fathers cannot support their partner effectively in achieving a positive parenthood experience unless they are themselves supported, included and prepared for parenthood (Steen et al

2012). A study has reported that inadequate preparation remains a concern to both women and their partners and concluded that there is an urgent need for an improvement in parents' preparation for parenthood (Deave and Johnson 2008). Becoming a parent is often a stressful event and can contribute to relationship difficulties and attachments within the family. Both parents have reported in studies that they would have benefited from some early warning and education (Deave and Johnson 2008; Steen et al 2011). The midwife has an important role in supporting both parents during the transition to parenthood as there are clear health and wellbeing benefits for the mother and baby (DfE 2010). In addition, the midwife may have an important role with regard to referral and support for women who are in abusive relationships (Steen and Keeling 2012).

Where there are concerns about the safety or protection of the newborn infant, the supervisor of midwives should be informed and advice sought from the local social services (the Safeguarding Children Board). Children's Centres offer a range of services to assist disadvantaged groups and local communities during the transition to parenthood. Family nurse practitioners (FNPs) can also offer further support. In addition, there is good evidence that new parents benefit from the support that their families, friends and other parents can offer.

REFERENCES

Acheson D 1998 Independent inquiry into inequalities in health. HMSO, London

Albers LL, Sedler KD, Bedrick EJ et al 2006 Factors related to genital tract trauma in normal spontaneous vaginal births. Birth 33:94–100

Anderson B, Torvin Anderson L, Sørensen T 1998 Methyl-ergometrine during the early puerperium; a prospective randomised double blind study. Acta Obstetrica et Gynecologica Scandinavica 77:54–7

Armstrong K, Edwards H 2004 The effectiveness of a pram-walking exercise programme in reducing depressive symptomatology for postnatal women. International Journal of Nursing Practice 10(4):177–94

Barnes J, Ball M, Meadows P et al 2011 The Family–Nurse Partnership Programme in England: Wave 1 implementation in toddlerhood and a comparison between Waves 1 and 2a of implementation in pregnancy and infancy. Department of Health, London

Barnes J, Henderson J 2012 Summary of the formative evaluation of the first phase of the group-based Family Nurse Partnership programme. Department of Health, London

Bartell S S 2004 Self-nurturance as a crucial element in mothering. International Journal of Childbirth Education 19(4):8–11

Bedwell C 2006 Are third degree tears unavoidable? The role of the midwife. British Journal of Midwifery 14(9):212

Berk B 2004 Recommending exercise during and after pregnancy: what the evidence says. International Journal of Childbirth Education. 19(2):18–22

Bick D 2012 Reducing postnatal morbidity. The Practising Midwife 15(6):29–31

Bick D, Bassett S 2013 How to provide postnatal perineal care. RCM Midwives Magazine 1:30–1

Bick D, MacArthur C, Knowles H et al 2002 Postnatal care. Evidence and guidelines for management. Churchill Livingstone, Edinburgh

Bick D, MacArthur C, Winter H et al 2009 Postnatal care: evidence and guidelines for management, 2nd edn. Churchill Livingstone, Edinburgh

Bick D E, Rose V, Weavers A et al 2011 Improving inpatient postnatal services: midwives views and perspectives of engagement in a quality improvement initiative. BMC Health Services Research 11:293

Bottorff J L, Oliffe J, Kalaw C et al 2006 Men's constructions of smoking in the context of women's tobacco reduction during pregnancy and postpartum. Social Science and Medicine 62:3096–108

Boulvain M, Perneger T V, Othenin-Girard V et al 2004 Home-based versus hospital-based postnatal care: a randomised trial. BJOG: An International Journal of Obstetrics and Gynaecology 111(8):807–13

Buckley S J 2006 Mother and baby – a good start. In: Wickham S (ed) Midwifery: best practice, 4. Elsevier, Edinburgh, p 201–6

Cattrell R, Lavender T, Wallymahmed A et al 2005 Postnatal care: what matters to midwives. British Journal of Midwifery 13(4):206–13

Chou D, Abalos E, Gyte G M L et al 2010 Paracetamol/acetaminophen (single administration) for perineal pain in the early postpartum period. Cochrane Database of Systematic Reviews, Issue 3. Art. No. CD008407. doi: 10.1002/14651858.CD008407

Clapp J F 2001 Recommending exercise during pregnancy. Journal of Paediatrics, Obstetrics and Gynaecology 27(4):21–8

CMACE (Centre for Maternal and Child Enquiries) (2011) Saving mothers' lives: reviewing maternal deaths to make motherhood safer: 2006–2008. The Eighth Report on Confidential Enquiries into Maternal Deaths in the United Kingdom. BJOG: An International Journal of Obstetrics and Gynaecology 118(Suppl 1):1–203

Corkill A, Lavender T, Wilinshaw S A et al 2001 Reducing postnatal pain from perineal tears by using lignocaine gel: a double-blind randomized trial. Birth 28(1):22–6

Cunningham F G, Leveno K J, Bloom S et al 2005 Williams obstetrics, 22nd edn. McGraw–Hill Medical, New York, ch 5, p 121–50; ch 30, p 695–710

DCSF (Department for Children, Schools and Families) 2009 About Sure Start Children's Centres. http://webarchive.nationalarchives.gov

.uk/20100202113922/http://dcsf.gov
.uk/everychildmatters/earlyyears/
surestart/aboutsurestart/
aboutsurestart/ (accessed 24 June
2013)

Deave T, Johnson D 2008 The transition
to parenthood: what does it mean
for fathers? Journal of Advanced
Nursing 63(6):626–33

De Clerc E, Sakal C, Corry M et al 2006
Listening to mothers II. Report of
the second National US survey of
Childbearing Women's Childbearing
Experiences. Childbirth Connections,
New York, p 45–8, 55–61

Deussen A R, Ashwood P, Martis R 2011
Analgesia for relief of pain due to
uterine cramping/involution after
birth. Cochrane Database of
Systematic Reviews, Issue 5. Art. No.
CD004908. doi: 10.1002/14651858.
CD004908.pub2

DfE (Department for Education) 2010
Sure Start Children's Centres
statutory guidance. http://
webarchive.nationalarchives.gov
.uk/20130401151715/https://www
.education.gov.uk/publications/
eOrderingDownload/SSCC%20
statutory%20guidance-2010.pdf
(accessed 24 June 2013)

DfE (Department for Education) 2012
Increasing parental and community
involvement in Sure Start Children's
Centre. http://media.education.gov
.uk/assets/files/pdf/i/increasing%20
parental%20and%20community%20
involvement%20in%20sure%20
start%20childrens%20centres%20
discussion%20paper.pdf (accessed
24 June 2013).

DfES (Department for Education and
Skills) 2004 Every child matters:
change for children. Nottingham:
DfES Publications. Available at
http://webarchive.nationalarchives
.gov.uk/20130401151715/https://
www.education.gov.uk/publications/
eOrderingDownload/DfES10812004
.pdf (accessed 1 May 2013)

DH (Department of Health) 1993
Changing childbirth. The Report of
the Expert Maternity Group. TSO,
London

DH (Department of Health) 1999
Making a difference: strengthening
the nursing, midwifery and health
visiting contribution to health and
healthcare. TSO, London

DH (Department of Health) 2004
National service framework for

children, young people and
maternity services. DH Publications,
London

DH (Department of Health) 2005
National service framework for
children, young people and
maternity services. Standard 11:
Maternity services. DH Publications,
London

DH (Department of Health) 2007a
Maternity matters: choice, access and
continuity of care in a safe service.
DH Publications, London

DH (Department of Health) 2007b The
early weeks: you. In: The pregnancy
book. DH Publications, London,
ch 15

Disability Pregnancy and Parenthood
International 2007 Working with
deaf parents: a guide for midwives
and other health professionals
www.dppi.org.uk/information/
publications/#goodpractice (accessed
1 May 2013)

East C E, Begg L, Henshall N E et al
2012a Local cooling for relieving
pain from perineal trauma sustained
during childbirth. Cochrane
Database of Systematic Reviews,
Issue 5. Art. No. CD006304. doi:
10.1002/14651858.CD006304.pub3

East C E, Sherburn M, Nagle C et al
2012b Perineal pain following
childbirth: prevalence, effects on
postnatal recovery and analgesia
usage. Midwifery 28(1):93–7

Flouri E, Buchanan A 2003 What
predicts fathers' involvement with
their children? A prospective study
of intact families. British Journal of
Developmental Psychology 21:81–97

Garcia J, Marchant S 1993 Back to
normal? Postpartum health and
illness. Research and the Midwife
Conference Proceedings 1992.
University of Manchester,
Manchester, p 2–9

Garcia J, Renfrew M, Marchant S 1994
Postnatal home visiting by midwives.
Midwifery 19(10):40–3

Gibbon K, Steen M (2012 Postnatal
care. Caring for women during a
homebirth. In: Steen M (ed)
Supporting women to give birth at
home. A practical guide for
midwives. Routledge, Abingdon,
p 148–54

Goodwin A, Astbury J, McKeen J 2000
Body image and psychological
well-being in pregnancy: a

comparison of exercisers and
non-exercisers. Australian and New
Zealand Journal of Obstetrics and
Gynaecology 40(4):442–7

Greenshields W and Hulme H (1993)
The perineum in childbirth: a survey
conducted by the National
Childbirth Trust. NCT, London

Harrison R F, Brennan M 1987a
Evaluation of two local anaesthetic
sprays for the relief of post-
episiotomy pain. Current Medical
Research Opinion 10(6):364–9

Harrison R F, Brennan M 1987b A
comparison of alcoholic and
aqueous formulations of local
anaesthetic as a spray for the relief of
post-episiotomy pain. Current
Medical Research Opinion
10(6):45–56

Hart J T 1971 'The inverse care law'. The
Lancet 297:405–12

Hedayati H, Parsons J, Crowther C A
2005 Topically applied anaesthetics
for treating perineal pain after
childbirth. Cochrane Database of
Systematic Reviews, Issue 2. Art. No.
CD004223. doi: 10.1002/14651858.
CD004223.pub2

Hirst J, Hewison J 2002 Hospital
postnatal care: obtaining the views
of Pakistani indigenous 'white'
women. Clinical Effectiveness in
Nursing 6(1):10–18

HM Government 2009 Apprenticeships,
Skills, Children and Learning Act
2009 c. 22. s. 198 Arrangements for
children's centres. www.legislation
.gov.uk/ukpga/2009/22/part/9/
crossheading/childrens-centres
(accessed 24 June 2013)

HM Government 2012 Health and
Social Care Act 2012 c 7. hwww
.legislation.gov.uk/ukpga/2012/7/
contents/enacted (accessed 24 June
2013)

Hundt G L, Beckerleq S, Kassem F et al
2000 Women's health custom made:
building on the 40 days postpartum
for Arab women. Health Care
Women International 21(6):529–42

Kettle C, Fenner D E 2007 Repair of
episiotomy, first and second degree
tears. In: Sultan A H, Thakar R,
Fenner D E (eds) Perineal and anal
sphincter trauma – diagnosis and
clinical management. Springer-
Verlag, London, ch 3, p 20–32

Kings Fund 2011 Staffing in maternity
units. Kings Fund, London

Leap N, Hunter B 1993 The midwife's tale. An oral history from handywoman to professional midwife. Scarlet Press, London

Lewis G (ed) 2007 Confidential Enquiry into Maternal and Child Health (CEMACH) Saving mothers' lives: reviewing maternal deaths to make motherhood safer – 2003–2005. The Seventh Report on Confidential Enquiries into Maternal Deaths in the United Kingdom. CEMACH, London

MaGuire M 2000 The transition to parenthood. In: Life after birth: reflections on postnatal care, report of a multi-disciplinary seminar, 3 July 2000. RCM, Cardiff

Marchant S, Alexander J, Garcia J 2002 Postnatal vaginal bleeding problems and general practice. Midwifery 18:21–4

Marsh J, Sargent E 1991 Factors affecting the duration of postnatal visits. Midwifery 7:177–82

McQueen A, Mander R 2003 Tiredness and fatigue in the postnatal period. Journal of Advanced Nursing 24(5):463–9

Moffat H, Lavender T, Walkinshaw S 2006 Comparing administration of paracetamol for perineal pain. British Journal of Midwifery 9(11):690–4

Moore E R, Anderson G C, Bergman N et al (2012) Early skin-to-skin contact for mothers and their healthy newborn infants. Cochrane Database of Systematic Reviews, Issue 5. Art. No. CD003519. doi: 10.1002/14651858.CD003519.pub3

Mørkved S, Bø K 2013 Effect of pelvic floor muscle training during pregnancy and after childbirth on prevention and treatment of urinary incontinence: a systematic review. British Journal of Sports Medicine 2013 Jan 30 [Epub ahead of print] doi:10.1136/bjsports-2012-091758

Morrell C J, Spiby H, Stewart P et al 2000 Costs and benefits of community postnatal support workers: randomised controlled trial. British Medical Journal 321:593–8

Navviba S, Abedian Z, Steen-Greaves M 2009 Effectiveness of cooling gel pads and ice packs on perineal pain. British Journal of Midwifery 17(11):724–9

NCT (National Childbirth Trust) 2010 Left to your own devices: the postnatal experiences of 1260 first-time mothers. NCT, London. www.nct.org.uk/sites/default/files/related_documents/PostnatalCareSurveyReport5.pdf (accessed 22 March 2013)

NCT (National Childbirth Trust) 2012 Postnatal care. NCT, London. www.nct.org.uk/professional/research/pregnancy-birth-and-postnatal-care/postnatal-care (accessed 29 December 2012)

NESS (National Evaluation of Sure Start) 2004 Towards understanding Sure Start local programmes: summary of findings from the national evaluation. DfES Publications, Nottingham. www.dcsf.gov.uk/everychildmatters/publications/0/937 (accessed 3 March 2013)

NICE (National Institute for Health and Clinical Excellence) 2006 Routine postnatal care of women and their babies. NICE, London

NMC (Nursing and Midwifery Council) 2008 The code: standards of conduct, performance and ethics for nurses and midwives. NMC, London

NMC (Nursing and Midwifery Council) 2012 Midwives rules and standards 2012. NMC, London

Ockleford E M, Berryman J C, Hsu R 2004 Postnatal care: what new mothers say. British Journal of Midwifery 12(3):166–71

O'Sullivan S, Tyler S 2007 Payment by results: speaking in code. RCM Midwives 10(5):241

Parsons, Talcott 1951 The social system. London: Routledge & Kegan Paul, p 436–7

Peterson W E, Charles C, DiCenso A et al 2005 The Newcastle satisfaction with nursing scales: a valid measure of maternal satisfaction with inpatient postpartum nursing care. Journal of Advanced Nursing 52(6):672–81

Piscane A, Continisio G I, Aldinucci M et al 2005 A controlled trial of the father's role in breastfeeding promotion. Pediatrics 116(4):494–8

RCM (Royal College of Midwives) 2010 The roles and responsibilities of the maternity support workers. Position statement. RCM, London. www.rcm.org.uk/college/your-career/maternity-support-workers/roles/(accessed 1 November 2012).

RCM (Royal College of Midwives) 2011 Reaching out: involving fathers in maternity care. Royal College of Midwives, London. www.rcm.org.uk/college/policy-practice/government-policy/fathers-guide/?utm_source=Adestra&utm_medium=email&utm_term= (accessed 19 July, 2013)

RCM/CSP (Royal College of Midwives and Chartered Society of Physiotherapists) 2013 RCM/CSP joint statement on pelvic floor muscle exercises: improving health outcomes for women following pregnancy and birth. RCM, London

RCOG (Royal College of Obstetricians and Gynaecologists) 2004 Methods and materials used in perineal repair. RCOG Guideline No. 23. Royal College of Obstetricians and Gynaecologists, London, p 3

Redshaw M, Heikkila K 2010 Delivered with care: a national survey of women's experience of maternity care 2010. National Perinatal Epidemiology Unit, Oxford

Redshaw M, Rowe R, Hockley C et al 2007 Recorded delivery – a national survey of women's experiences of maternity care in Oxford. National Perinatal Epidemiology Unit, Oxford

Renfrew M J 2010 Making a difference for women, babies and families. Evidence-based Midwifery 8(2):40–6

Ridgers I 2007 Passing through but needing to be heard. An ethnographic study of women's perspectives of their care on the postnatal ward. Unpublished PhD thesis. Bournemouth University, Bournemouth

Rowan C, Bick D 2006 Revising care to reflect CEMACH recommendations: issues for midwives and the maternity services. Evidence Based Midwifery 5(3):80–6

Searles J A, Pring D W 1998 Effective analgesia following perineal injury during childbirth: a placebo controlled trial of prophylactic rectal diclofenac. British Journal of Obstetrics and Gynaecology 105:627–31

Shaw E, Levitt C, Wong S et al 2006 Systematic review of the literature on postpartum care: effectiveness of postpartum support to improve maternal parenting, mental health, quality of life and physical health. Birth 33(30):210–20

Simkin P 2008 The birth partner. Boston, MA: Harvard Common Press

Sleep J, Grant A 1988 Effects of salt and Savlon bath concentrate post-partum. Nursing Times Occasional Paper 84:55–7

Stables D, Rankin J 2011 The puerperium. In: Stables D, Rankin J (eds) Physiology in childbearing with anatomy and related biosciences, 3rd edn. Baillière Tindall/Elsevier, London, p 757

Steen M P 2002 A randomised controlled trial to evaluate the effectiveness of localised cooling treatments in alleviating perineal trauma: The APT Study, MIDIRS Midwifery Digest 12(3):373–6

Steen M 2007a Perineal tears and episiotomy: how do wounds heal? British Journal of Midwifery 15(5):273–4, 276–80

Steen M 2007b Well-being and beyond. Midwives 10(3):116–19

Steen M 2010 Care and consequences of perineal trauma. British Journal of Midwifery 18(6):358–62

Steen M 2012 Risk, recognition and repair. British Journal of Midwifery 20(11):768–72

Steen M 2013 Continence in women following childbirth. Nursing Standard 28(1):47–55

Steen M, Cooper K, Marchant P et al 2000 A randomised controlled trial to compare the effectiveness of icepacks and Epifoam with cooling maternity gel pads at alleviating perineal trauma. Midwifery 16(1):48–55

Steen M, Downe S, Bamford N et al 2012 'Not-patient' and 'not-visitor': a metasynthesis of fathers' encounters with pregnancy, birth and maternity care. Midwifery 28(4):362–71

Steen M, Downe S, Graham-Kevan N 2011 Development of antenatal education to raise awareness of the risk of relationship conflict. Evidence-Based Midwifery 8(2):53–7

Steen M, Keeling J 2012 STOP! Silent screams. The Practising Midwife 15(2):28–30

Steen M, Marchant P 2007 Ice packs and cooling gel pads versus no localised treatment for relief of perineal pain: a randomised controlled trial. Evidence-Based Midwifery Journal 5(1):16–22

Steen M, Roberts T 2011 The consequences of pregnancy and birth for the pelvic floor. British Journal of Midwifery 19(11):692–8

Tanner E, Agur M, Hussey D et al 2012 Evaluation of Children's Centres in England. Research Report DFE-RR230. DfE, London

Taylor J, Johnson M 2010 How women manage fatigue after childbirth. Midwifery 26(3):367–75

Tohotoa J, Maycock B, Hauck Y L et al 2009 Dads make a difference: an exploratory study of paternal support for breastfeeding in Perth, Western Australia. International Breastfeeding Journal 29(4):15

Troy N A, Dalgas-Pelish P 2003 The effectiveness of a self care intervention for the management of postpartum fatigue. Applied Nursing Research 16(1):38–45

Tuffery O, Scriven A 2005 Factors influencing antenatal and postnatal diets of primigravid women. Journal of the Royal Society of Health 125(5):227–31

Twaddle S, Liao X H, Fyvie H 1993 An evaluation of postnatal care individualised to the needs of the woman. Midwifery 9(3):154–60

UKCC (United Kingdom Central Council for Nursing, Midwifery and Health Visiting) 1986 A midwife's code of practice. UKCC, London

Vernon D (ed) 2007 With women: midwives' experiences: from shiftwork to continuity of care. Australian College of Midwives, Canberra

Waugh L J 2011 Beliefs associated with Mexican immigrant families' practice of la cuarentena during postpartum recovery. Journal of Obstetric, Gynecologic and Neonatal Nursing 40(6):732–41

WHO (World Health Organization) 2010 WHO Technical Consultation on Postpartum and Postnatal Care. WHO Document Production Services, Geneva, Switzerland. http://whqlibdoc.who.int/hq/2010/WHO_MPS_10.03_eng.pdf (accessed 17 July 2013)

Wiggins M 2000 Psychosocial needs after childbirth. Life after birth: reflections on postnatal care, report of a multi-disciplinary seminar, 3rd July. RCM, Cardiff

Winter H R, MacArthur C, Bick D E et al 2001 Postnatal care and its role in maternal health and well-being. MIDIRS Midwifery Digest 11 (Suppl 1):S3–S7

Winterton N 1992 House of Commons Health Committee Second Report: Maternity services, vol 1. HMSO, London

Wolfberg A J, Michels K B, Shields W et al 2004 Dads as breastfeeding advocates: results of a randomized controlled trial of an educational intervention. American Journal of Obstetrics and Gynecology 191:708–12

Wray J 2006 Seeking to explore what matters to women about postnatal care. British Journal of Midwifery 14(5):246–54

Wray J 2011 Bouncing back? An ethnographic study exploring the context of care and recovery after birth through the experiences and voices of mothers. Unpublished PhD Thesis, University of Salford

Wray J 2012 Impact of place upon celebration of birth – experiences of new mothers on a postnatal ward. MIDIRS Midwifery Digest 23(3):357–61

Wray J, Bick D 2012 Is there a future for universal midwifery postnatal care in the UK? MIDIRS Midwifery Digest 22(4):495–8

Yoong W C, Biervliet F, Nagrani R 1997 The prophylactic use of diclofenac (Voltarol) suppositories in perineal pain after episiotomy: a random allocation double-blind study. Journal of Obstetrics and Gynaecology 17(1):39–44

FURTHER READING

Ball J 1994 Reactions to motherhood: the role of postnatal care. Books for Midwives Press, Hale, Cheshire

Baston H, Hall J 2009 Midwifery essentials: postnatal. Churchill Livingstone/Elsevier, Edinburgh

Brown S, Lumley J, Small R et al 1994 Missing voices: the experiences of motherhood. Oxford University Press, Melbourne

Byrom S, Edwards G, Bick D (eds) 2009 Essential midwifery practice: postnatal care. Wiley–Blackwell, Oxford

Choi P, Henshaw C, Baker S et al 2005 Supermum, superwife, supereverything: performing femininity in the transition to motherhood. Journal of Reproductive and Infant Psychology 23:167–80

Dykes F 2005 A critical ethnographic study of encounters between midwives and breast-feeding women in postnatal wards in England. Midwifery 21:241–52

Gibbon K, Steen M 2012 Postnatal care. Caring for women during a homebirth. In: Steen M (ed) Supporting women to give birth at home. A practical guide for midwives. Routledge, London, p 148–54

Lunt K 2013 How to undertake a postnatal examination. RCM Magazine, 4:32–3

Miller T 2005 Making sense of motherhood: a narrative approach. Cambridge University Press, Cambridge

USEFUL WEBSITES

Made for Mums: www.madeformums .com/breast-and-bottlefeeding/ how-to-breastfeed-your-baby/ 19342.html

Maternity Action: www.maternityaction.org.uk/

Mums net: www.mumsnet.com/

National Childbirth Trust: www.nct.org.uk/professional/ research/pregnancy-birth -and-postnatal-care/postnatal -care

National Institute for Health and Care [formerly Clinical] Excellence: http:// pathways.nice.org.uk/pathways/ postnatal-care

Royal College of Midwives: http:// www.rcm.org.uk/midwives/ by-subject/postnatal-care/

Chapter |24|

Physical health problems and complications in the puerperium

Julie Wray, Mary Steen

This chapter reviews the care of women who either entered the postpartum period having experienced obstetric or medical complications, including those who did not undergo a vaginal birth, or whose postpartum recovery, regardless of the mode of birth, did not follow a normal pattern. It includes the care for women with signs and symptoms of life-threatening conditions and those with obvious risks for increased postpartum physical morbidity. (The effects of morbidity related to psychological trauma are covered in Chapter 25.)

THE CHAPTER AIMS TO:

- discuss the role of midwifery care in the detection and management of life-threatening conditions and postpartum morbidity
- review best practice in the management of problems associated with trauma and pathology arising from pregnancy and childbirth
- review the role of the midwife (and family) where postpartum health is complicated by an instrumental or operative birth.

THE NEED FOR WOMEN-FOCUSED AND FAMILY-CENTRED POSTPARTUM CARE

A women-focused approach to care in the postpartum period alongside individualized care planning developed with the woman and her family will assist physical and psychological recovery (NICE [National Institute for Health and Clinical Excellence] 2006a). What is important is to focus upon the needs of women as individuals rather than fitting women into a routine care package (DH [Department of Health] 2004; Bick et al 2009; Wray and Bick 2012). The midwife needs to be familiar with the woman's background and antenatal and labour history irrespective of the care setting (NICE 2006a) when assessing whether or not the woman's progress is following the expected postpartum recovery pattern (Garcia et al 1998; DH 2004; Redshaw and Heikkila 2010).

All women should be offered appropriate and timely information with regard to their own health and wellbeing (and their babies) including recognition of, and responding to, problems (NICE 2006a; Bick et al 2011). The effects of obstetric or medical complications will be assessed for and reviewed within the context of the immediate and ongoing care by the midwife of the woman's health over the postnatal period. The role of the midwife in these cases is first to identify whether a potentially life-threatening condition exists and, if so, to refer the woman for appropriate emergency investigations and care (NMC (NICE 2006a, CMACE [Centre for Maternal and Child Enquiries] 2011; NMC [Nursing and Midwifery Council] 2012). Where the birth involves obstetric or medical complications, a woman's postpartum care is likely to differ from those women whose pregnancy and labour are considered straightforward. However, it must also be considered that some women have a perception of the whole birth experience as traumatic, although to the obstetric or midwifery staff no untoward events occurred (Singh and Newburn 2000; Marchant 2004).

POTENTIALLY LIFE-THREATENING CONDITIONS AND MORBIDITY AFTER THE BIRTH

Despite the apparent advances in medication and practice, women still die postpartum. The discovery of penicillin and the provision of a blood transfusion were major contributions to saving women's lives over the past century (Loudon 1986, 1987), and maternal death after childbirth where there has been no preceding antenatal complication is now a rare occurrence in the United Kingdom (UK) (Lewis 2007; CMACE 2011). Thrombosis or thromboembolism and haemorrhage were major causes of direct maternal deaths in the UK but these have declined (Lewis 2007). Cardiac disease is the most common cause of indirect death; the indirect maternal mortality rate has not changed significantly since 2003–2005 (CMACE 2011). However, sepsis is now the most common cause of direct maternal death in the triennium 2006–2008 associated with genital tract infection, particularly from community-acquired Group A streptococcal (GAS) infection (CMACE 2011). The mortality rate related to sepsis increased from 0.85 deaths per 100 000 maternities in 2003–2005 to 1.13 deaths in 2006–2008 (CMACE 2011).

Being aware of this information is vital for all those involved in giving postnatal care as good quality care can contribute to the prevention as well as the detection and management of potentially fatal outcomes (Wray and Bick 2012).

From research, it became clear that maternal morbidity after childbirth was typically under-reported by women (Bick and MacArthur 1995; Marchant et al 1999). The extent of postnatal morbidity was remarkable in the extensive nature of the problems and the duration of time over which such problems continued to be experienced by women (MacArthur et al 1991; Garcia and Marchant 1993; Glazener et al 1995; Brown and Lumley 1998; Glazener and MacArthur 2001; Waterstone et al 2003; Bick et al 2009).

The midwife has a duty to undertake midwifery care for at least the first 28 days, and according to NICE (2006a) all women should receive essential core routine care in the first 6–8 weeks after birth. The activities of the midwife are to support the new mother and her family unit by monitoring her recovery after the birth and to offer her appropriate information and advice as part of the statutory duties of the midwife (NMC 2012).

IMMEDIATE UNTOWARD EVENTS FOR THE MOTHER FOLLOWING THE BIRTH OF THE BABY

Immediate (primary) postpartum haemorrhage (PPH) is a potentially life-threatening event which occurs at the point of or within 24 hours of expulsion of the placenta and membranes and presents as a sudden, and excessive vaginal blood loss (see Chapter 18). Secondary, or delayed PPH is where there is excessive or prolonged vaginal loss from 24 hours after birth and for up to 6 weeks' postpartum (Cunningham et al 2005a). Unlike primary PPH, which includes a defined volume of blood loss (>500 ml) as part of its definition, there is no volume of blood specified for a secondary PPH and management differs according to apparent clinical need (Alexander et al 2002; Bick et al 2009).

Regardless of the timing of any haemorrhage, it is most frequently the placental site that is the source. Alternatively, a cervical or deep vaginal wall tear or trauma to the perineum might be the cause in women who have recently given birth. Retained placental fragments or other products of conception are likely to inhibit the process of involution, or reopen the placental wound. The diagnosis is likely to be determined more by the woman's condition and pattern of events (Hoveyda and MacKenzie 2001; Jansen et al 2005) and is also often complicated by the presence of infection (Cunningham et al 2005b; see Chapter 18). The recent CMACE (2011: 13) report states that, 'there remains an urgent need for the routine use of a national modified early obstetric warning score (MEOWS) chart in all pregnant or postpartum women who become unwell and require either obstetric or gynaecology services'. Usage of this score will help in providing timely recognition, treatment and referral of women who have or are developing a critical illness after birth and postnatal.

Maternal collapse within 24 hours of the birth without overt bleeding

Where no signs of haemorrhage are apparent other causes need to be considered (see Chapter 13). Management of all these conditions requires ensuring the woman is in a safe environment until appropriate treatment can be administered by the most appropriate health professionals, and meanwhile maintaining the woman's airway, basic circulatory support as needed and providing oxygen. It is important to remember that, regardless of the apparent state of collapse, the woman may still be able to hear and so verbally reassuring the woman (and her partner or relatives if present) is an important aspect of the immediate emergency and ongoing care.

POSTPARTUM COMPLICATIONS AND IDENTIFYING DEVIATIONS FROM THE NORMAL

Following the birth of their baby, women recount feelings that are, at one level, elation that they have experienced the birth and survived, and at another, the reality of pain or discomfort from a number of unwelcome changes as their bodies recover from pregnancy and labour (Gready et al 1997; Wray 2011a). Women may experience symptoms that might be early signs of pathological events. These might be presented by the woman as 'minor' concerns, or not actually be in a form that is recognized as abnormal by the woman herself. Where the postpartum visit is undertaken as a form of review of the woman's

physical and psychological health, led by the woman's needs, the midwife is likely to obtain a random collection of information that lacks a specific structure. Women will probably give information about events or symptoms that are the most worrying or most painful to them at that time. At this point the midwife needs to establish whether there are any other signs of possible morbidity and determine whether these might indicate the need for referral. Figure 24.1 suggests a model for linking together key observations that suggest potential risk of, or actual, morbidity.

The central point, as with any personal contact, is the midwife's initial review of the woman's appearance and psychological state. This is underpinned by an assessment of the woman's vital signs, where any general state of illness is evident, including signs of infection. It is suggested that a pragmatic approach be taken with regard to evidence of pyrexia as a mildly raised temperature may be related to normal physiological hormonal responses, for example the increasing production of breastmilk. However, infection and sepsis are important factors in postpartum maternal morbidity and mortality and the midwife should not make an assumption that a mildly raised temperature is part of the normal health parameters (Lewis 2007; CMACE 2011; Bick 2012). The accumulation of a number of clinical signs will assist the midwife in making decisions about the presence or potential for morbidity. Where there is a rise in temperature above 38 °C it is usual for this to be considered a deviation from normal and of clinical significance. If puerperal infection is suspected, the woman must be referred back to the obstetric services as soon as possible (CMACE 2011). Adherence to local infection control policies and awareness of the signs and symptoms of sepsis in postnatal women is important for all practitioners caring for women. This is particularly the case for community midwives, who may be the first to pick up any potentially abnormal signs during their routine postnatal observations for all women, not just those who have had a caesarean section (CS) (CMACE 2011).

The pulse rate and respirations are also significant observations when accumulating clinical evidence. Although there may be no evidence of vaginal haemorrhage, for example, a weak and rapid pulse rate (>100 bpm) in conjunction with a woman who is in a state of collapse with signs of shock and a low blood pressure (systolic <90 mmHg) may indicate the formation of a haematoma, where there is an excessive leakage of blood from damaged blood vessels into the surrounding tissues. A rapid pulse rate in an otherwise well woman might suggest that she is anaemic but could also indicate increased thyroid or other dysfunctional hormonal activity.

The midwife needs to be alert to any possible relationship between the observations overall and their potential cause with regard to common illnesses, e.g. that the woman has a common cold, and that the morbidity is

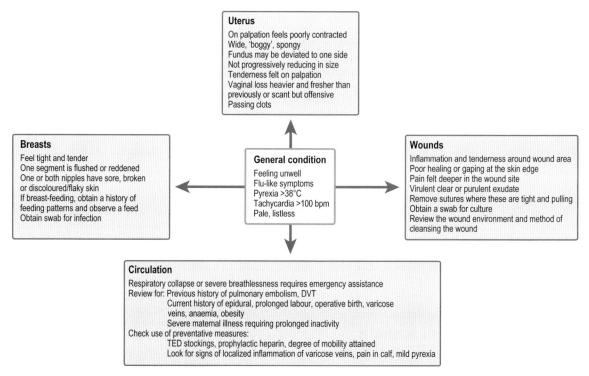

Uterus

On palpation feels poorly contracted
Wide, 'boggy', spongy
Fundus may be deviated to one side
Not progressively reducing in size
Tenderness felt on palpation
Vaginal loss heavier and fresher than
previously or scant but offensive
Passing clots

Breasts

Feel tight and tender
One segment is flushed or reddened
One or both nipples have sore, broken
or discoloured/flaky skin
If breast-feeding, obtain a history of
feeding patterns and observe a feed
Obtain swab for infection

General condition

Feeling unwell
Flu-like symptoms
Pyrexia >38°C
Tachycardia >100 bpm
Pale, listless

Wounds

Inflammation and tenderness around wound area
Poor healing or gaping at the skin edge
Pain felt deeper in the wound site
Virulent clear or purulent exudate
Remove sutures where these are tight and pulling
Obtain a swab for culture
Review the wound environment and method of
cleansing the wound

Circulation

Respiratory collapse or severe breathlessness requires emergency assistance
Review for: Previous history of pulmonary embolism, DVT
Current history of epidural, prolonged labour, operative birth, varicose
veins, anaemia, obesity
Severe maternal illness requiring prolonged inactivity
Check use of preventative measures:
TED stockings, prophylactic heparin, degree of mobility attained
Look for signs of localized inflammation of varicose veins, pain in calf, mild pyrexia

Fig. 24.1 Diagrammatic demonstration of the relationship between deviation from normal physiology and potential morbidity.

associated with or affected by having recently given birth. Where the midwife is in conversation with the woman as part of the postpartum assessment, if she receives information that suggests the woman has signs deviating from what is expected to be normal, it is important that a range of clinical observations are undertaken to refute or confirm this, followed by timely and appropriate referral.

Following an innovative research study into extended midwifery care of women beyond the conventional 10–14-day period, a set of guidelines were compiled to assist midwives make decisions about the need for referral (Bick et al 2009). As part of the NICE (2006a) process compiling guidelines for core care, it was recognized that midwives develop skills and processes from their experience to accumulate evidence from their observations and conversations about the overall wellbeing of the mother and the baby. However, this process was mainly covert and difficult to adapt in any formal way to help less experienced midwives or even explain the course of action to the women themselves (Marchant et al 2003; Marchant 2006). To clarify the actions necessary, when the NICE guidelines were published, a quick guide was also produced providing a table of the action required for possible signs/symptoms of complications and common health problems in women (NICE 2006a).

The uterus and vaginal loss following vaginal birth

It is expected that the midwife will undertake assessment of uterine involution at intervals throughout the period of midwifery care (see Chapter 23). It is recommended that this should always be undertaken where the woman is feeling generally unwell, has abdominal pain, a vaginal loss that is markedly brighter red or heavier than previously, is passing clots or reports her vaginal loss to be offensive (Hoveyda and MacKenzie 2001; Marchant et al 2006; Bick et al 2009; CMACE 2011).

Where the palpation of the uterus identifies that it is deviated to one side, this might be as a result of a full bladder. Where the midwife has ensured that the woman had emptied her bladder prior to the palpation, the presence of urinary retention must be considered. Catheterization of the bladder in these circumstances is indicated for two reasons: to remove any obstacle that is preventing the process of involution taking place and to provide relief to the bladder itself. If the deviation is not as a result of a full bladder, further investigations need to be undertaken to determine the cause.

Morbidity might be suspected where the uterus fails to follow the expected progressive reduction in size, feels wide or 'boggy' on palpation and is less well contracted than expected. This might be described as subinvolution of the uterus, which can indicate postpartum infection, or the presence of retained products of the placenta or membranes, or both (Khong and Khong 1993; Howie 1995).

Treatment is by antibiotics, oxytocic drugs that act on the uterine muscle, hormonal preparations or evacuation of the uterus (ERPC), usually under a general anaesthetic.

Vulnerability to infection, potential causes and prevention

Infection is the invasion of tissues by pathogenic microorganisms; the degree to which this results in ill-health relates to their virulence and number. Vulnerability is increased where conditions exist that enable the organism to thrive and reproduce and where there is access to and from entry points in the body. Organisms are transferred between sources and a potential host by hands, air currents and fomites (i.e. agents such as bed linen). Hosts are more vulnerable where they are in a condition of susceptibility because of poor immunity or a preexisting resistance to the invading organism. The body responds to the invading organisms by forming antibodies, which in turn produce inflammation initiating other physiological changes such as pain and an increase in body temperature.

Acquisition of an infective organism can be *endogenous*, where the organisms are already present in or on the body – e.g. *Streptococcus faecalis* (Lancefield group B), *Clostridium welchii* (both present in the vagina) or *Escherichia coli* (present in the bowel) – or organisms in a dormant state are reactivated, notably tuberculosis bacteria. Other routes are *exogenous*, where the organisms are transferred from other people (or animal) body surfaces or the environment. Other transfer mechanisms include *droplets* – inhalations of respiratory pathogens on liquid particles (e.g. β-haemolytic streptococcus and *Chlamydia trachomatis*), *cross-infection* and *nosocomial* (hospital-acquired) transfer from an infected person or place to an uninfected one (e.g. *Staphylococcus aureus*).

The bacteria responsible for the majority of puerperal infection arise from the streptococcal or staphylococcal species, with community acquired GAS infection causing most serious problems (CMACE 2011). The *Streptococcus* bacterium has a chain-like formation and may be haemolytic or non-haemolytic, and aerobic or anaerobic; the most common species associated with puerperal sepsis is the β-haemolytic *S. pyogenes* (Lancefield group A) although other strains of the streptococcal bacteria have also been identified as the source of serious morbidity (Muller et al 2006). The *Staphylococcus* bacterium has a grape-like structure, of which the most important species is *S. aureus* or *pyogenes*. Staphylococci are the most frequent cause of wound infections; where these bacteria are coagulase-positive they form clots on the plasma which can lead to more widely spread systemic morbidity. There is additional concern about their resistance to antibiotics and subsequent management to control spread of the infection. Regardless of the location of care, postpartum women and healthcare professionals should be aware of how infection can be acquired and should pay particular attention to effective hand-washing techniques. They should adhere to the accepted practice for aseptic technique such as local infection control policies when in contact with wound care, including the use of gloves for this, and where there is direct contact with areas in the body where bacteria of potential morbidity are prevalent. Avoiding the spread of infection is especially necessary when the woman or her family or close contacts have a sore throat or upper respiratory tract infection (CMACE 2011). Educating women and their family about the basic principles of good hand hygiene is a key public health role of the midwife in staving off infection.

The uterus and vaginal loss following operative birth

A lower segment caesarean section (CS) will have involved cutting of the major abdominal muscles and damage to other soft tissues. Palpation of the abdomen is therefore likely to be very painful for the woman in the first few days after the operation. The woman who has undergone a CS will have a very different level of physical activity from the woman who has had a vaginal birth. It may be some hours after the operation until the woman feels able to sit up or move about. Blood and debris will have been slowly released from the uterus during this time and, when the woman begins to move, this will be expelled through the vagina and may appear as a substantial fresh-looking red loss. Following this initial loss, it is usual for the amount of vaginal loss to lessen and for further fresh loss to be minimal. All this can be observed without actually palpating the uterus. For women who have undergone an operative birth, once 3 or 4 days have elapsed, abdominal palpation to assess uterine involution can be undertaken by the midwife where this appears to be clinically appropriate. By this time, the uterus or area around the uterus should not be overly painful on palpation.

Where clinically indicated, e.g. where the vaginal bleeding is heavier than expected, the uterine fundus can be gently palpated. If the uterus is not well contracted then medical intervention is needed. Uterine stimulants (uterotonics) are usually prescribed in the form of an intravenous infusion of oxytocin or an intramuscular injection of syntometrine/ergometrine, if not contraindicated (Chapter 18). If the bleeding continues where such treatment has been commenced, further investigations might include obtaining blood for clotting factors, or the woman might need to return to theatre for further exploration of the uterine cavity. The emergence of ultrasound scans (USS) in the postpartum period has led to some conflicting

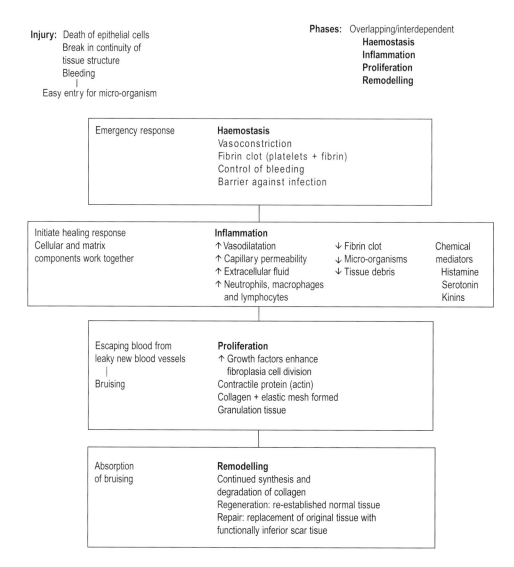

Fig. 24.2 The phases of wound healing.
Reproduced with permission from Steen 2007.

reports of the state of the normal postpartum uterus and the value of USS in distinguishing potentially pathological conditions (Hertzberg and Bowie 1991). More recent studies appear to support greater use of USS to assist diagnosis and clinical management of problems of uterine sub-involution (Shalev et al 2002; Deans and Dietz 2006).

Wound problems

Perineal problems

It is important that the midwife has an understanding of the effect of trauma as a physiological process and the

normal pattern for wound healing (Steen 2007). Knowledge and an understanding of the physiological process and the nutrients that are necessary to promote healing will assist a midwife to recognize when there is a delay in healing and also enable her to advise a woman on her dietary requirements. (See Fig. 24.2 and Table 24.1.)

Perineal pain is a result of perineal injury, which can be surgically or naturally induced. Women complain of varying degrees of severity of perineal pain. There is some evidence to suggest that the severity of the perineal injury is linked to the severity of perineal pain (Kenyon and Ford 2004). Perineal injury that requires suturing predisposes women to an increased risk of severe perineal pain

Table 24.1 Nutrients and their contribution to healing

Nutrient	Contribution
Carbohydrates	Energy for leucocyte, macrophage and fibroblast function
Proteins	Immune response, phagocytosis, angiogenesis, fibroblast proliferation, collagen synthesis, wound maturation
Fats	Provision of energy, formation of new cells
Vitamins	
Vitamin A	Collagen synthesis and cross-linking, tensile strength
Vitamin B (complex)	Immune response, collagen cross-linking, tensile strength
Vitamin C	Collagen synthesis tensile strength, neutrophil function, macrophage migration, immune response
Vitamin E	Reduce tissue damage from free radical formation
Minerals	
Copper	Collagen synthesis, leucocyte formation
Iron	Collagen synthesis, oxygen delivery
Zinc	Increases cell proliferation, epithelialization, collagen strength

(Chapter 15). This might be as a result of the analgesia no longer being effective, the presence of inflammation in the surrounding tissues or, more seriously, the formation of a haematoma. Haematoma usually develops deep in the perineal fascia tissues and may not be easily visible if the perineal tissues are already inflamed. Inadequate perineal repair or a traumatic vaginal birth can increase the risk of a haematoma. The blood contained within a haematoma can exceed 1000 ml and may significantly affect the overall state of the woman, who can present with signs of acute shock. Treatment is by evacuation of the haematoma and resuturing of the perineal wound, usually under a general anaesthetic.

Perineal pain that is severe and is not caused by a haematoma might arise as a result of inflammation causing the stitches to feel excessively tight. Local application of cold packs can bring relief as they reduce the immediate oedema and continue to provide relief over the first few days following the birth (Steen et al 2006). The use of oral analgesia as well as complementary therapies such as arnica and lavender oil is said to be beneficial, although the effectiveness of such therapies has to date not been confirmed by research findings (Bick et al 2009).

Midwives should undertake appropriate training in complementary therapies before advocating their use.

Factors that are associated with poor healing include poor diet, obesity, preexisting medical disorders and negative social conditions such as poor housing, increased stress and smoking (Steen 2007). Where pain in the perineal area occurs at a later stage, or re-occurs, this might be associated with an infection. The skin edges are likely to have a moist, puffy and dull appearance; there may also be an offensive odour and evidence of pus in the wound. A swab should be obtained for microorganism culture and referral made to a General Practitioner (GP). Antibiotics might be commenced immediately when there is specific information about any infective agent. Where the perineal tissues appear to be infected, it is important to discuss with the woman about cleaning the area and making an attempt to reduce constant moisture and heat. Women might be advised about using cotton underwear, avoiding tights and trousers and frequently changing sanitary pads. They should also be advised to avoid using perfumed bath additives or talcum powder.

If the perineal area fails to heal, or continues to cause pain, a referral should be made and resuturing or refashioning might be advised (a Cochrane Systematic Review on this topic is currently being undertaken to influence best practice guidelines). There is evidence to suggest that a substantial proportion of women continue to have problems during the first 12 months following birth and do not report these to healthcare professionals (Bedwell 2006). Therefore, it is important to advise women to seek help and encourage them to discuss any problems with their GP. Most women should be pain-free and be able to resume sexual intercourse within a few weeks after the birth; this will vary in individual women. Some women may still complain of discomfort, depending on the severity of trauma experienced and the healing process. Dyspareunia (painful sexual intercourse) can be related to perineal trauma (Chapter 15) and this can in the long-term affect the woman's relationship with her partner. In the first 3 months post-birth, approximately, 23% of women report dyspareunia (RCOG 2004). Although high levels of sexual morbidity after childbirth have been identified, the approach to discussion and management of this area appears to be problematic (Barrett et al 2000). When giving health advice and support, healthcare professionals are advised to identify an appropriate time, not to make assumptions with regard to sexual activity after childbirth and to be conversant with support agencies relevant to a range of cultural and sexual diversities and associated individual women's needs (Barrett et al 2000; NICE 2006a).

Caesarean section wounds

It is now common practice for women undergoing an operative birth to have prophylactic antibiotics at the time of the surgery (Smaill and Hofmeyr 2002). This has been

521

demonstrated to significantly reduce the incidence of subsequent wound infection and endometritis. In addition, it is now usual for the wound dressing to be removed after the first 24 hours, as this also aids healing and reduces infection. Advice needs to be offered to the woman about care of her wound and adequate drying when taking a bath or shower, or for more obese women where abdominal skin folds are present and are likely to create an environment that is constantly warm and moist. For these women, a dry dressing over the suture line might be appropriate.

A wound that is hot, tender and inflamed and is accompanied by a pyrexia is highly suggestive of an infection. Where this is observed, a swab should be obtained for microorganism culture and medical advice should be sought. Haematoma and abscesses can also form underneath the wound and women may identify increased pain around the wound where these are present. Rarely a wound may need to be probed to reduce the pressure and allow infected material to drain, reducing the likelihood of the formation of an abscess. With the hospital stay now being much shorter than previously, these problems increasingly occur after the woman has left hospital.

Circulation

Pulmonary embolism remains a major cause of maternal deaths in the UK and midwives and GPs need to be more alert to identify high-risk women and the possibility of thromboembolism in puerperal women with leg pain and breathlessness (Lewis 2007; CMACE 2011). Women who have a previous history of pulmonary embolism, a deep vein thrombosis (DVT), are obese or who have varicose veins have a higher risk of postpartum problems. Postpartum care of women who have preexisting or pregnancy-related medical complications relies on prophylactic precautions and should be undertaken for women who undergo surgery and have these preexisting factors. Thromboembolitic D (TED) stockings should be provided during, or as soon as possible after, the birth and prophylactic heparin prescribed until women attain normal mobility. All women who undergo an epidural anaesthetic, are anaemic, or have a prolonged labour or an operative birth are slightly more at risk of developing complications linked to blood clots. Women with preexisting problems are at higher risk because of their overall health status and environment of care postpartum. For example, women who undergo a CS as a result of maternal illness are more likely to spend longer in bed, thereby reducing their mobility and increasing their risk of morbidity.

Clinical signs that women might report include the following (from the most common to the most serious). The signs of circulatory problems related to varicose veins are usually localized inflammation or tenderness around the varicose vein, sometimes accompanied by a mild pyrexia. This is superficial thrombophlebitis, which is usually resolved by applying support to the affected area and administering anti-inflammatory drugs, where these are not in conflict with other medication being taken or with breastfeeding. Unilateral oedema of an ankle or calf accompanied by stiffness or pain and a positive Homan's sign might indicate a DVT that has the potential to cause a pulmonary embolism. Urgent medical referral must be made to confirm the diagnosis and commence anticoagulant or other appropriate therapy. The most serious outcome is the development of a pulmonary embolism. The first sign might be the sudden onset of breathlessness, which may not be associated with any obvious clinical sign of a blood clot. Women with this condition are likely to become seriously ill and could suffer a respiratory collapse with very little prior warning.

Some degree of oedema of the lower legs and ankles and feet can be viewed as being within normal limits where it is not accompanied by calf pain (especially unilaterally), pyrexia or a raised blood pressure.

Hypertension

Women who have had previous episodes of hypertension in pregnancy may continue to demonstrate this postpartum for several weeks after the birth (Tan and De Swiet 2002). There is still a risk that women who have clinical signs of pregnancy-induced hypertension can develop eclampsia in the hours and days following the birth although this is a relatively rare outcome in the normal population (Atterbury et al 1998; Tan and De Swiet 2002). In addition, some women appear to develop eclampsia postpartum where there has been no previous history of raised blood pressure or proteinuria (Chames et al 2002; Matthys et al 2004). Some degree of monitoring of the blood pressure should be continued for women who were hypertensive antenatally, and postpartum management should proceed on an individual basis (Tan and De Swiet 2002). For these women, the medical advice should determine optimal systolic and diastolic levels, with instructions for treatment with antihypertensive medication if the blood pressure exceeds these levels. As women can develop postnatal pre-eclampsia without having antenatal problems associated with this, because the symptoms can be fairly non-specific, such as a headache or epigastric pain or vomiting, the woman may delay or fail to contact a healthcare professional for advice. Where they do seek advice, the healthcare professional may not be alert to the possibility of the development of postpartum eclampsia (Chames et al 2002). Failure to detect symptoms at this initial stage may lead to more serious outcomes as the disease develops untreated (Chames et al 2002; Tan and De Swiet 2002; Matthys et al 2004). Therefore, if a postpartum woman presents with signs associated with pre-eclampsia, the midwife should be alert to this possibility and undertake observations of the blood pressure and urine and obtain medical advice.

For women with essential hypertension, the management of their overall medical condition will be reviewed postpartum by their usual caregivers. Undertaking clinical observation of blood pressure for a period after the birth is advisable so that information is available upon which to base the management of this for the woman in the future (Tan and De Sweit 2002).

Headache

This is a common ailment in the general population; concern in relation to postpartum morbidity should therefore centre around the history of the severity, duration and frequency of the headaches, the medication being taken to alleviate them and how effective this is. As this is also associated with hypertension, a recording of the blood pressure should be undertaken to exclude this as a primary factor. In taking the history, if an epidural analgesic was administered, medical advice should be sought. Headaches from a dural tap typically arise once the woman has become mobile after the birth and they are at their most severe when standing, lessening when the woman lies down. They are often accompanied by neck stiffness, vomiting and visual disturbances. These headaches are very debilitating and are best managed by stopping the leakage of cerebral spinal fluid by the insertion of 10–20 ml of blood into the epidural space; this should resolve the clinical symptoms. Where women have returned home after the birth, they would need to return to the hospital to have this procedure.

Headaches might also be precursors of psychological distress and it is important that other issues related to the birth event are explored, taking the time and opportunity to do this in a sensitive manner. Factors that might be overlooked include dehydration, sleep loss and a greater than usual stressful environment (see Chapter 25). However, the midwife should take time to discuss the woman's feelings and offer advice or reassurance about these where possible.

Backache

Many women experience pain or discomfort from backache in pregnancy as a result of separation or diastasis of the abdominal muscles (rectus abdominis diastasis [RAD]). Where backache is causing pain that affects the woman's activities of daily living, referral can be made to local physiotherapy services. Pelvic girdle pain experienced in pregnancy should resolve in the weeks after the baby is born but it may continue for a much longer period (Aslan and Fynes 2007).

Urinary problems

Urinary problems can have short- and long-term social, psychological and physical health consequences for women (WHO [World Health Organization] 2010). Approximately 19% of women will have urinary problems following birth (Laperriere 2000). Stress incontinence appears to be the most common form of urinary incontinence reported following birth but some women may also suffer from frequency, urgency and urge incontinence (Birch et al 2009). Some women who have had a complicated birth may be susceptible to the risk of urinary infections, which may lead to cystitis and in some severe cases pyelonephritis (Stables and Rankin 2010). Where a woman has undergone an epidural or spinal anaesthetic, this can have an effect on the neurological sensors that control urine release and flow, which may cause acute retention. The main complication of any form of urine retention is that the uterus might be prevented from effective contraction, which leads to increased vaginal blood loss. There is also increased potential for the woman to contract a urine infection with possible kidney involvement and long-term effects on bladder function.

In addition, women who have sustained pelvic floor damage during birth may suffer from continence problems in the short and long term. Stress and urge incontinence of urine, utero-vaginal prolapse, cystocele, rectocele and dyspareunia are associated with pelvic floor damage (Stables and Rankin 2010). Very rarely, urinary incontinence might be a result of a urethral fistula following complications from the labour or birth.

Management of urine output has been shown to lack consistency and recognition of its potential importance (Zaki et al 2004). A midwife will need to be alert to any urinary problems a woman may have as sometimes these can be missed. Being alert to the risks and being able to recognize ongoing urinary problems is an essential component of care (Steen 2013). Abdominal tenderness in association with other urinary symptoms, for example a poor output, dysuria or offensive urine and a raised temperature or general flu-like symptoms, might indicate a urinary tract infection (UTI). A mid-stream urine sample will be required to confirm a UTI and the infection can be treated with antibiotics (NICE 2006b).

Women might feel embarrassed about having urinary problems and midwives may need to consider appropriate ways of encouraging women to talk about any problems so that they can inform them about their future management. Specific enquiry about these issues should be made when women attend for their 6–8-week postnatal examination; further investigations should be made for women who are encountering these problems. Keeping a bladder diary can be a useful aid. NICE (2006b) have suggested that women should complete a bladder diary for three consecutive days to allow for variation in day-to-day activities to be captured.

Recently it has been reported that women with ongoing urinary incontinence following birth are nearly twice as likely to develop postnatal depression (Sword et al 2011). Therefore, it is essential that midwives have knowledge and an understanding of the risks and symptoms of urinary problems and are able to ask sensitive questions to identify women at risk as failure to do so can lead to poor mental health. These women will need additional social and psychological support (Steen 2013).

Bowel problems

Bowel problems can have short- and long-term social, psychological and physical health consequences for women (WHO 2010). It is estimated that about 3–10% of women will suffer from faecal incontinence (RCOG 2004; Van Brummen et al 2006). Faecal incontinence is associated with primiparity, instrumental birth and severe perineal injury (Thornton and Lubowski 2006; Guise et al 2007). Constipation and haemorrhoids can be a problem for some women. It is estimated that about 44% of women will suffer from constipation and 20–25% of women will suffer from haemorrhoids following birth. Symptoms such as flatus incontinence, passive leakage, urge and faecal incontinence can be caused by a neurological or muscular dysfunction or both (Pollack et al 2004) (see Chapter 15). The prevalence of bowel problems maybe higher as many women may suffer in silence and be too embarrassed to ask for help (Steen 2013).

Therefore, a midwife will need to be alert to any bowel problems and to ask a woman sensitively about her bowel habits. Being alert to the risks and being able to recognize ongoing bowel problems is an essential component of care. Enquiring about the pattern and frequency of bowel movements and comparing this to the woman's previous experience is likely to assist a midwife in identifying whether or not there is a problem. Factors such as dietary intake, a degree of dehydration during labour and concern about further pain from any perineal trauma can contribute to bowel problems. A diet that includes soft fibre, increased fluids and the use of prophylactic aperients that are non-irritant to the bowel can be prescribed to alleviate constipation, the most common and apparently effective of these being lactulose (Eogan et al 2007). Women need advice that any disruption to their normal bowel pattern should resolve within days of the birth, taking into consideration the recovery required by the presence of perineal trauma. They should also be reassured about the effect of a bowel movement on the area that has been sutured as many women may be unnecessarily anxious about the possibility of tearing their perineal stitches. Where women have prolonged difficulty with constipation, anal fissures can result (Corby et al 1997). These are painful and difficult to resolve and therefore advice about bowel management is important in avoiding this situation. Women who have haemorrhoids should also be given advice on following a diet high in fibre and fluids, preferably water and the use of appropriate aperients to soften the stools as well as topical applications to reduce the oedema and pain.

It is also of concern where women might experience loss of bowel control and whether this is faecal incontinence. It is important to determine the nature of the incontinence and distinguish it from an episode of diarrhoea. It might be helpful to ask whether the woman has taken any laxatives in the previous 24 hours and explore what food was eaten. Where the problems do not seem to be associated with other factors the woman should first be advised to see her GP.

The role of the midwife is to encourage women to talk about these problems by being proactive in asking women about any bowel problems. Where women identify any change to their pre-pregnant bowel pattern by the end of the puerperal period, they should be advised to have this reviewed further, whether it is constipation or loss of bowel control.

Anaemia

Iron-deficiency during pregnancy is extremely common even among well-nourished women and this can be a predisposing risk factor for anaemia in the postnatal period. The main cause of anaemia is iron deficiency and severe anaemia can have serious health and functional consequences (Goddard et al 2011). Whilst severe anaemia (haemoglobin <7 g/dl) is rare in resource-rich countries, it is a serious problem for many women in resource-poor countries. The impact, however, of the events of the labour and birth may leave many women looking pale and tired for a day or so afterwards. Where it is evident that a larger than normal blood loss has occurred, it can be valuable to obtain an overall blood profile within which the red blood cell volume, haemoglobin and ferritin levels can be assessed so as to provide appropriate treatment to reduce the effects of the anaemia; these include blood transfusions and iron supplements (Dodd et al 2004; Bhandal and Russell 2006). The degree to which the haemoglobin level has fallen should determine the appropriate management and this is particularly important in the presence of preexisting haemoglobinopathies, sickle cell and thalassaemia.

Where the haemoglobin level is <9 g/dl and women are symptomatic, a blood transfusion might be appropriate. Blood transfusions should be considered if a woman is at risk of cardiovascular instability because of their degree of anaemia (Goddard et al 2011). Body-store iron deficiency is diagnosed by a low serum ferritin level and this can indicate that the woman has a longstanding problem of iron deficiency. A cut-off ferritin level varies between 12 and 15 µg/l to confirm iron deficiency (Todd and Caroe 2007). However, ferritin levels can be raised if infection or inflammation is present, even if iron stores are low (Goddard et al 2011). Oral iron and appropriate dietary advice are advocated where the level is <11 g/dl. Usually, ferrous sulphate 200 mg twice daily is recommended; however, a lower dose may be effective and better tolerated. Alternatively, ferrous fumarate, ferrous gluconate or iron suspensions may be better tolerated and oral iron should be continued for 3 months after the iron deficiency is corrected to replenish the woman's stores of iron. Ascorbic acid (250–500 mg) twice daily may be prescribed to enhance iron absorption but to date there are no data to support its effectiveness (Goddard et al 2011). Women should be advised not to have milk (including hot beverages with milk added) at the time of having iron as it can interfere with its absorption.

Where the woman has returned home soon after the birth, the postpartum woman's haemoglobin values might not have been undertaken where there was no history of anaemia prior to labour and the blood loss at birth was not assessed as excessive. If there is no clinical information to hand, the midwife needs to rely on the woman's clinical symptoms; if these include lethargy, tachycardia and breathlessness as well as a clinical picture of pale mucous membranes, it would be prudent to arrange for the blood profile to be reviewed. Some researchers have questioned blood loss estimation after childbirth as well as the timing of blood tests taken to assess the physiological impact of this (Jansen et al 2007). Thus the postnatal day when the haemoglobin test is taken might have a clinically significant bearing on the subsequent management.

Breast problems

Regardless of whether women are breastfeeding, they may experience tightening and enlargement of their breasts towards the 3rd or 4th day as hormonal influences encourage the breasts to produce milk (see Chapter 34). For women who are breastfeeding the general advice is to feed the baby and avoid excessive handling of the breasts. Simple analgesics may be required to reduce discomfort. For women who are not breastfeeding, the advice is to ensure that the breasts are well supported but that this is not too constrictive and, again, that taking regular analgesia for 24–48 hours should reduce the discomfort. Heat and cold applied to the breasts via a shower or a soaking in the bath may temporarily relieve acute discomfort as well as the use of chilled cabbage leaves (Nikodem et al 1993; Roberts 1995).

PRACTICAL SKILLS FOR POSTPARTUM MIDWIFERY CARE AFTER AN OPERATIVE BIRTH

In the immediate period after an operative birth the attendant will be closely monitoring recovery from the anaesthetic used for CS (see Chapter 21). Regular observation of vaginal loss, leakage on to wound dressings and fluid loss in any 'redivac' drain system should also be undertaken.

Once the woman has fully recovered from the operation she should be transferred to a ward environment. Midwifery care involves the overall framework of core care (see Chapter 23). Appropriate care is to assess the needs of the individual woman and to formalize this within a documented postnatal care plan so that she and caregivers have a clear framework by which to promote recovery (DH 2004; NICE 2006a). Women who have undergone an operative birth need time to recover from a major physical shock to the systems of the body, for optimal conditions to allow tissue repair to take place as well as psychological adjustment to the events of the birth (Mander 2007).

Women who have undergone an operative birth will require assistance with a number of activities they would otherwise have done themselves. During their hospital stay, they will need help to maintain their personal hygiene, to get out of bed and mobilize and to start to care for their baby. The rate at which each woman will be able to regain control over these areas of activity is *highly individual*. It is strongly suggested that caregivers should not expect all women to have reached a certain level of recovery in line with their 'postnatal day'. Using such a framework to assess the degree to which a woman is recovering from a major operation leads to a tendency to become judgemental and unrealistic (Wray 2011a). Women may view undergoing a caesarean section or any complication in the birth in different ways depending on their social and cultural background and this might have associations to their ongoing psychological health and wellbeing (Chien et al 2006; McCourt 2006).

It is now common for women to have a much shorter period in hospital after birth; some women might return home 48–72 hours after a major operation with very minimal support (Wray and Bick 2012). Practical advice about the management of their recovery and self-care at home is also within the remit of midwifery postpartum care. For example; the midwife might suggest that the woman identifies the ways in which she could reduce the need to go upstairs. Alongside this, women can be encouraged to go out with their baby when someone is available to help with all the baby transportation equipment; this will encourage venous return and cardiac output at a level that is beneficial rather than exhausting. At the same time, getting 'out and about' can provide a sense of feeling good and improved wellbeing (Wray 2011b: 2).

The benefits of mobility after surgery are well known and although women may be supplied with thromboembolic stockings prior to the operation and be prescribed an anticoagulant regimen such as heparin, women need to be encouraged to mobilize as soon as practicable after the operation to reduce the risk of circulatory problems. Women need an explanation that mobility is of benefit soon after the birth, but it is also an important part of care to recognize when the woman has reached her limit with regard to physical activity and may need to rest (Wray 2011a). Regular use of appropriate analgesia should be made available to women where this is required (Mander 2007). Good information about self-care and recovery is important to every woman and the midwife has a key role to play in this process. Each woman is an individual and unique so her recovery from surgery alongside her adaptation to motherhood needs to be borne in mind and tailored to meet her own needs (Wray 2011a, 2011b).

EMOTIONAL WELLBEING: PSYCHOLOGICAL DEVIATION FROM NORMAL

Psychological distress and psychiatric illness in relation to childbirth are covered in depth in Chapter 25. However, it is relevant to reflect here on the possible importance of the relationship that develops between the woman and the midwife during their contact postpartum (Hunter 2004). Clearly, such relationships are enriched where there has been antenatal contact or a degree of continuity postpartum, or both, and women have commented positively where such continuity has been achieved (Singh and Newburn 2000; Bhavnani and Newburn 2010). This prior knowledge can mean that the midwife might detect or be concerned about a change in the woman's behaviour that has not been noticed by her family. Any initial concerns of the mother or the family should be explored by the midwife making use of open questions and listening skills during the postnatal contact either in the home or in the hospital setting (NICE 2007; Bick et al 2011). Behavioural changes may be very subtle, but, however small, they might be of importance in the woman's overall psychological state; it is the balance between the woman's physical condition and her psychological state that might influence an eventual decision to refer for expert advice.

Although the woman and her partner are likely to have an expectation of reduced sleep once the baby is born, the actual experience of this can have very varied effects on individual women (Wray 2012). The cause of the lack of sleep or tiredness is what is important – is the being unable to get to sleep a result of anxiety about the future and what is, as yet, unknown? This might include fears about the possibility of a cot death, or a lack of confidence in coping as a mother, financial or relationship worries. The opportunity to sleep might be reduced because the feeding is not yet established or the baby is not in a settled environment and so the mother is constantly disturbed when she tries to sleep. In addition, other people may not be allowing the mother to sleep when the baby does not need her attention. Tiredness and fatigue can adversely affect women's health and interfere with their adaptation to motherhood (Troy and Dalgas-Pelish 2003), however the terms fatigue and tiredness are subjective and difficult to define postnatally. Seeking to unravel the issues can help the midwife and the women to determine what is the underlying cause and whether simple interventions could improve the situation. As a result of this enquiry, women who come into the category where chronic fatigue or anxiety prevents them from sleeping when the opportunity arises may benefit from interagency referral and support. Alternatively, where there is a physiological reason for the tiredness, as a result of anaemia for example, the situation can be managed clinically (Jansen et al 2007). The midwife is an important member of the primary health care team and should practise within an interagency context (see Chapter 25). Enabling women to plan and set realistic goals as part of their own recovery from childbirth is ongoing and extends beyond 28 days and 6 weeks (Bick et al 2011; Wray 2012).

SELF-CARE AND RECOVERY

Self-care and managing one's own health following childbirth requires women to take some ownership of their own health and wellbeing (Wray 2011a). The pace at which women recover is highly variable, and notions of a set time period (6 weeks) do not apply to all women (NICE 2006a). Women need guidance and sound information to enable them to recover so that they are clear about what they can expect and what to do when they are concerned. Good rapport and positive feedback from midwives are known to help women in their recovery as well as support from partners, family and friends (Beake et al 2010; Wray 2011a). Central to self-care is robust information from the midwife from the outset, so that women can feel confident in their own assessments of themselves.

TALKING AND LISTENING AFTER CHILDBIRTH

The essence of the contact between the woman and the midwife after the birth event is to strive to maintain a therapeutic relationship – one of support and advice that builds on the relationship formed ideally antenatally. Within the current provision of care, it is not always possible to achieve the objective of continuity of carer postnatally, and some women will have postnatal home visits from several different midwives, possibly previously unknown to them. Indeed other healthcare workers such as maternity support workers (MSWs) may form part of the postnatal care-giving process under the supervision of midwives.

Once the birth is over and the woman has returned to her home environment there may be aspects of the birth that she does not understand or that even distress her to think about. Where appropriate, a midwife undertaking postnatal care in the woman's home might be able to help the woman review and reflect on the birth by talking about it and listening to her concerns. Where necessary, the midwife can facilitate referral to the key people involved in order that the woman can discuss the birth or see the records of the birth and clarify any outstanding issues

(Charles and Curtis 1994; Allen 1999; NICE 2006a). Other forms of support, for instance specific counselling for those with traumatic emotional experiences, might also be appropriate under professional guidance (NICE 2007) (see Chapter 25).

REFERENCES

Alexander J, Thomas P W, Sanghera J 2002 Treatments for secondary postpartum haemorrhage. Cochrane Database of Systematic Reviews 2002, Issue 1. Art. No. CD002867. doi: 10.1002/14651858.CD002867

Allen H 1999 Debriefing for postnatal women: does it help? Professional Care of Mother and Child 9(3): 77–9

Aslan E, Fynes M 2007 Symphysial pelvic dysfunction. Current Opinion in Obstetrics and Gynecology 19(2):133–9

Atterbury J L, Groome L, Hoff C et al 1998 Clinical presentation of women re-admitted with postpartum severe pre-eclampsia or eclampsia. Journal of Obstetrics, Gynecology and Neonatal Nursing 27(2): 134–41

Barrett G, Pendry E, Peacock J et al 2000 Women's sexual health after childbirth. BJOG: An International Journal of Obstetrics and Gynaecology 107(2):186–95

Beake S, Rose V, Bick D et al 2010 A qualitative study of the experiences and expectations of women receiving in-patient postnatal care in one English maternity unit. BMC Pregnancy and Childbirth 10:70

Bedwell C 2006 Are third degree tears unavoidable? The role of the midwife. British Journal of Midwifery 14(9):212

Bhavnani V, Newburn M 2010 Left to your own devices: the postnatal care experiences of 1260 first time mothers. NCT, London

Bhandal N, Russell R 2006 Intravenous versus oral iron therapy for postpartum anaemia. British Journal of Obstetrics and Gynaecology 113(11):1248–52

Bick D 2012 Reducing postnatal morbidity. The Practising Midwife 15(6):29–31

Bick D, MacArthur C 1995 The extent, severity and effect of health

problems after childbirth. British Journal of Midwifery 3:27–31

Bick D, MacArthur C, Knowles H et al 2009 Postnatal care: evidence and guidelines for management, 2nd edn. Churchill Livingstone, Edinburgh

Bick D E, Rose V, Weavers A et al 2011 Improving inpatient postnatal services: midwives' views and perspectives of engagement in a quality improvement initiative. BMC Health Services Research 11:293

Birch L, Doyle PM, Ellis R et al 2009 Failure to void in labour: postnatal urinary and anal incontinence. British Journal of Midwifery 17(9):562–6

Brown S, Lumley J 1998 Maternal health after childbirth: results of an Australian population based study. British Journal of Obstetrics and Gynaecology 105:156–61

Chames M C, Livingston J C, Ivester T S et al 2002 Late postpartum eclampsia: a preventable disease? American Journal of Obstetrics and Gynecology 186(6):1174–7

Charles J, Curtis L 1994 Birth afterthoughts: a listening and information service. British Journal of Midwifery 2(7):331–4

Chien L Y, Tai C J, Ko Y L et al 2006 Adherence to 'doing-the-month' practices is associated with fewer physical and depressive symptoms among postpartum women. Taiwan Research in Nursing and Health 29(5):374–83

CMACE (Centre for Maternal and Child Enquiries) 2011 Saving mothers' lives: reviewing maternal deaths to make motherhood safer: 2006–08. The Eighth Report on Confidential Enquiries into Maternal Deaths in the United Kingdom. BJOG: An International Journal of Obstetrics and Gynaecology 118(Suppl 1): 1–203

Corby H, Donnelly V S, O'Herlihy C et al 1997 Anal canal pressures are low in women with postpartum anal fissure. British Journal of Surgery 84(1):86–8

Cunningham F G, Leveno K J, Bloom S et al (eds) 2005a Maternal physiology. In: Williams' obstetrics, 22nd edn. McGraw Hill Medical, New York, p 121–50, 695–710

Cunningham F G, Leveno K J, Bloom S et al (eds) 2005b Puerperal infection. In: Williams' obstetrics, 22nd edn. McGraw Hill Medical, New York, p 710–24

Deans R, Dietz H P 2006 Ultrasound of the postpartum uterus. Australian and New Zealand Journal of Obstetrics and Gynaecology 46(4):345–9

DH (Department of Health) 2004 National Service Framework for Children, Young People and Maternity Services, Section 11. The Stationery Office, London

Dodd J M, Dare M R, Middleton P 2004 Treatment for women with postpartum iron deficiency anaemia. Cochrane Database of Systematic Reviews, Issue 4. Art. No. CD004222. doi: 10.1002/14651858. CD004222.pub2

Eogan M, Daly L, Behan M et al 2007 Randomised clinical trial of a laxative alone versus a laxative and a bulking agent after primary repair of obstetric anal sphincter injury. BJOG: An International Journal of Obstetrics and Gynaecology 114(6):736–40

Garcia J, Marchant S 1993 Back to normal? Postpartum health and illness. Research and the Midwife Conference Proceedings, 1992, University of Manchester, Manchester, p 2–9

Garcia J, Redshaw M, Fitzsimmons B et al 1998 First class delivery, a national survey of women's views of maternity care. Audit Commission, Abingdon

Glazener C M A, MacArthur C 2001 Postnatal morbidity. Obstetrician and Gynaecologist 3(4):179–83

Glazener C, Abdalla M, Stroud P et al 1995 Postnatal maternal morbidity: extent, causes, prevention and treatment. British Journal of Obstetrics and Gynaecology 102(4):282–7

Goddard A F, James M W, McIntyre A S et al 2011 Guidelines for the management of iron deficiency anaemia. Gut 60:1309–16

Gready M, Buggins E, Newburn M et al 1997 Hearing it like it is: understanding the views of users. British Journal of Midwifery 5(8):496–500

Guise J M, Morris C, Osterweil P et al 2007 Incidence of fecal incontinence after childbirth. Obstetrics and Gynecology 109 (2 Part 1):281–8

Hertzberg B, Bowie J 1991 Ultrasound of the postpartum uterus. Journal of Ultrasound Medicine 10:451–6

Hoveyda F, MacKenzie I Z 2001 Secondary postpartum haemorrhage: incidence, morbidity and current management. BJOG: An International Journal of Obstetrics and Gynaecology 108(9):927–30

Howie P W 1995 The puerperium and its complications. In: Whitfield C (ed) Dewhurst's textbook of obstetrics and gynaecology, 5th edn. Blackwell Science, Oxford, p 421–37

Hunter L 2004 The views of women and their partners on the support provided by community midwives during home visits. Evidence Based Midwifery 2(1):20–7

Jansen A J, Duvekot J J, Hop W C et al 2007 New insights into fatigue and health-related quality of life after delivery. Acta Obstetrica et Gynecologica Scandinavica 86(5):579–84

Jansen A J G, van Rhenen D J, Steegers E A P et al 2005 Postpartum hemorrhage and transfusion of blood and blood components. Obstetrical and Gynecological Survey 60(10):663–71

Kenyon S, Ford F 2004 How can we improve women's postbirth perineal health? MIDIRS Midwifery Digest. 14(1):7–12

Khong T Y, Khong T K 1993 Delayed postpartum haemorrhage: a morphologic study of causes and their relation to other pregnancy disorders. Obstetrics and Gynecology 82(1):17–22

Laperriere L 2000 Randomised trial of perineal trauma during pregnancy: perineal symptoms three months after delivery. Am J Obstet Gynecol. 182(1):76–80

Lewis G (ed) 2007 The Confidential Enquiry into Maternal and Child Health (CEMACH) Saving mothers' lives: reviewing maternal deaths to make motherhood safer – 2003–2005. The Seventh Report on Confidential Enquiries into Maternal Deaths in the United Kingdom. CEMACH, London

Loudon I 1986 Obstetric care, social class, and maternal mortality. British Medical Journal 293:606–8

Loudon I 1987 Puerperal fever, the streptococcus, and the sulphonamides, 1911–1945. British Medical Journal 295:485–90

MacArthur C, Lewis M, Knox G 1991 Health after childbirth: an investigation of long term health problems beginning after childbirth in 11,701 women. HMSO, London

Mander R 2007 Caesarean: just another way of birth? Routledge, London

Marchant S 2004 Transition to motherhood: from the woman's perspective. In: Stewart M (ed) Pregnancy, birth and maternity care: feminist perspectives. Elsevier, London

Marchant S 2006 The postnatal care journey – are we nearly there yet? MIDIRS Midwifery Digest 16(3):295–304

Marchant S, Alexander J, Garcia J 2003 Routine midwifery assessment of postpartum uterine involution. In: Wickham S (ed) Midwifery best practice. Elsevier, London

Marchant S, Alexander J, Garcia J et al 1999 A survey of women's experiences of vaginal loss from 24 hours to three months after childbirth (the BLiPP Study). Midwifery 15(2):72–81

Marchant S, Alexander J, Thomas P et al 2006 Risk factors for hospital admission related to excessive and/ or prolonged postpartum vaginal blood loss after the first 24 h

following childbirth. Paediatric and Perinatal Epidemiology 20(5):392–402

Matthys L A, Coppage K H, Lambers D S et al 2004 Delayed postpartum preeclampsia: an experience of 151 cases. American Journal of Obstetrics and Gynecology 190(5):1464–6

McCourt C 2006 Becoming a parent. In: Page L A, McCandlish R (eds) The new midwifery: science and sensitivity in practice, 2nd edn. Elsevier, Edinburgh, p 54–6

Muller A E, Oostvogel P M, Steegers E A P et al 2006 Morbidity related to maternal group B streptococcal infections. Acta Obstetrica et Gynecologica Scandinavica 85(9):1027–37

NICE (National Institute for Health and Clinical Excellence) 2006a Routine postnatal care of women and their babies. NICE, London

NICE (National Institute for Health and Clinical Excellence) 2006b Urinary incontinence: the management of urinary incontinence in women. NICE, London

NICE (National Institute for Health and Clinical Excellence) 2007 Antenatal and postnatal mental health: clinical management and service guidance. NICE, London

Nikodem V C, Danziger D, Gebka N et al 1993 Do cabbage leaves prevent breast engorgement? A randomized, controlled study. Birth 20(2):61–4

NMC (Nursing and Midwifery Council) 2012 Midwives Rules and Standards 2012. NMC, London

Pollack J, Nordenstam J, Brismar S et al 2004 Anal incontinence after vaginal delivery: a five year prospective cohort study. Obstetrics and Gynecology 104:1397–402

RCOG (Royal College of Obstetricians and Gynaecologists) 2004 Methods and materials used in perineal repair. Green-top Guideline No. 23. RCOG, London

Redshaw M, Heikkila K 2010 Delivered with care: a national survey of women's experience of maternity care 2010. National Perinatal Epidemiology Unit, Oxford

Roberts K L 1995 A comparison of chilled cabbage leaves and chilled gelpaks in reducing breast engorgement. Journal of Human Lactation 11(1):17–20

Shalev J, Royburt M, Fite G et al 2002 Sonographic evaluation of the puerperal uterus: correlation with manual examination. Gynecologic and Obstetric Investigation 53:38–41

Singh D, Newburn M (eds) 2000 Access to maternity information and support: the experiences and needs of women before and after giving birth. National Childbirth Trust, London

Smaill F, Hofmeyr G J 2002 Antibiotic prophylaxis for cesarean section. Cochrane Database of Systematic Reviews, Issue 3. Art. No. CD000933. doi: 10.1002/14651858. CD000933

Stables D, Rankin J 2010 The puerperium. In: Stables D and Rankin J (eds) Physiology in childbearing with anatomy and related biosciences, 3rd edn. Bailliere Tindall/Elsevier, London. ch 56

Steen M 2007 Perineal tears and episiotomy: how do wounds heal? British Journal of Midwifery Perineal Care Supplement 15(5):273–4, 276–80

Steen M 2013 Continence in women following childbirth. Nursing Standard 28(1):47–55

Steen M, Briggs M, King D 2006 Alleviating postnatal perineal trauma: to cool or not to cool? British Journal of Midwifery 14(5):304–6, 308

Sword W, Kurtz Landy C, Thabane L et al G 2011 Is mode of delivery associated with postpartum depression at 6 weeks? A prospective cohort study. BJOG: An International Journal of Obstetrics and Gynaecology 118:966–77

Tan L K, De Swiet M 2002 The management of postpartum hypertension. BJOG: An International Journal of Obstetrics and Gynaecology 109(7):733–6

Thornton M J, Lubowski D Z 2006 Obstetric-induced incontinence: a black hole of preventable morbidity. Australian and New Zealand Journal of Obstetrics and Gynaecology 46(6):468–73

Todd T, Caroe T 2007 Newly diagnosed iron deficiency anaemia in a premenopausal woman. BMJ 334(7587):259

Troy N A, Dalgas-Pelish P 2003 The effectiveness of a self care intervention for the management of postpartum fatigue. Applied Nursing Research 16(1):38–45

Van Brummen H J, Bruinse K W, van de Pol G et al 2006 Defecatory symptoms during and after the first pregnancy: prevalence and associated factors. International Urogynaecology Journal and Pelvic Floor Dysfunction 17:224–30

Waterstone M, Wolfe C, Hooper R et al 2003 Postnatal morbidity after childbirth and severe obstetric morbidity. BJOG: An International Journal of Obstetrics and Gynaecology 110(2):128–33

WHO (World Health Organization) 2010 WHO technical consultation on postpartum and postnatal care. WHO Document Production Services, Geneva. Available at http://whqlibdoc.who.int/hq/2010/WHO_MPS_10.03_eng.pdf (accessed 17 May 2013)

Wray J 2011a Bouncing back? An ethnographic study exploring the context of care and recovery after birth through the experiences and voices of mothers. Unpublished PhD thesis, University of Salford

Wray J 2011b Feeling cooped up after childbirth – the need to go out and about. The Practising Midwife 14:2

Wray J 2012 Impact of place upon celebration of birth – experiences of new mothers on a postnatal ward. MIDIRS Midwifery Digest 23(3):357–61

Wray J, Bick D 2012 Is there a future for universal midwifery postnatal care in the UK? MIDIRS Midwifery Digest 22(44):495–8

Zaki M M, Pandit M, Jackson S 2004 National survey for intrapartum and postpartum bladder care: assessing the need for guidelines. BJOG: An International Journal of Obstetrics and Gynaecology 111(8):874–6

FURTHER READING

Bhavnani V, Newburn M 2010 Left to your own devices: the postnatal care experiences of 1260 first-time mothers. NCT, London
A useful read to help inform postnatal care.

National Childbirth Trust 2010 Postnatal care – still a Cinderella story? NCT, London
An important insight into why postnatal care is still a neglected issue.

Romano M, Cacciatore A, Giordano R et al 2010 Postpartum period: three distinct but continuous phases. Journal of Prenatal Medicine 4(2):22–5. Available at www.ncbi.nlm.nih.gov/pmc/articles/PMC3279173/

USEFUL WEBSITES

National Childbirth Trust: www.nct.org.uk/parenting/you-after-birth

National Institute for Health and Care [formerly Clinical] Excellence: www.nice.org.uk
A new Quality Standard for postnatal care was introduced in July 2013 – see http://publications.nice.org.uk/postnatal-care-qs37

Postnatal Care HEAT module – Lab space, Open University: http://labspace.open.ac.uk/file.php/6632/HEAT_PNC_Final_Print_Output_cropped.pdf
Health Education and Training (HEAT) is an online educational series of modules launched in 2011 by the Open University with the aim to educate and train approximately 250 000 frontline healthcare workers across sub-Saharan Africa by 2016.

Royal College of Midwives (RCM): www.rcm.org.uk/midwives/by-subject/postnatal-care/

World Health Organization: www.who.int/maternal_child_adolescent/topics/newborn/postnatal_care/en/

Chapter |25|

Perinatal mental health

Maureen D Raynor, Margaret R Oates

In psychological terms, pregnancy, childbirth and the puerperium are major life events or life crises. Having children is associated with an immense increase in individual life changes that may lead to anxiety and chronic stressors, for example a new baby may result in a change of housing and brings increased financial demands. Pregnant women in employment will inevitably take maternity leave and may return to work in a different capacity or even on a part-time basis. A new baby may cause disruption to the family unit. Roles and responsibilities alter with changes to the dynamics of family relationships. Having a child may place strains on relationships and there is a higher rate of relationship discord and breakdown around this time. Many women find coping with the physiological adaptation to pregnancy, the plethora of antenatal screening tests and advice, issues around choice, control and communication emotionally draining. Therefore, while many women and their partners experience pregnancy and childbirth as a joyous, exciting and life-affirming event, the transition to parenthood is an emotionally charged time bringing common anxieties, a certain degree of loss and periods of self-doubt. This can culminate in pregnancy and postpartum being a fragile time of physical, psychological and social upheavals. Like other stressful life events childbirth can be associated with depression and anxiety. However, it is also known to be associated with an increased risk of serious psychiatric illness. Pregnancy provides a wealth of opportunities for promoting emotional health while predicting and preventing mental illness. It is important for midwives to be able to identify normal adjustment reactions to motherhood and distinguish them from the early warning signs of emotional distress or indeed mental illness.

This chapter is formed of two distinct but inter-related parts:

THE AIM OF PART A IS TO:

- explore the psychological context of pregnancy, childbirth and the puerperium by examining the full range of human emotions that may affect women as they adjust to change and make the transition to motherhood
- emphasize that awareness of the multiplicity of psychosocial factors and what constitutes normal emotions and behaviours are key components in enhancing understanding of perinatal mental health.

THE AIM OF PART B IS TO:

- explore the range of perinatal disorders, i.e. psychiatric conditions, that pre-exist or co-exist with pregnancy as well as those conditions presenting with the puerperium
- emphasize, by using a defined nomenclature, their recognition and management (including relevant pharmacology and the implications for breastfeeding and mother–baby relationship)
- highlight key recommendations from NICE and relevant triennial reports on the Confidential Enquiries into Maternal Deaths in the United Kingdom

Part A: Pregnancy, childbirth, puerperium: the psychological context

Maureen D Raynor

STRESS/ANXIETY

Pregnancy, labour and the puerperium are normal life events, yet they are periods in a woman's life when her vulnerability exposes her to a significant amount of stress and anxiety. Stress and anxiety are the psychopathology of humans' existence and a part of normal human emotion. A degree of stress during pregnancy is both essential and normal for the psychological adjustment of pregnant women. The 'worry work' that women encounter assists in their psychological adaptation to the emotional demands and changes of pregnancy. Conversely, elevated levels of stress hormones and unnecessary anxiety will stretch coping reserves, and could prove disabling. Stress is the body's psychophysical response to any type of demand or threat, whether good or bad. Anxiety on the other hand is a state of angst, worry or unease, often triggered by an element of perceived threat or an event where there is an uncertain outcome, such as a written examination or when important decisions have to be made. The brain plays a key role in how an individual responds and processes the perception of a threat. This is realized via a neurohormonal response by both the neocortex and limbic system. The 'fight or flight' reflex is produced when there is a threat to the self. Anxiety and fear causes the individual to become stressed, releasing stress response hormones namely catecholamines (adrenaline/noradrenaline) and cortisol. A host of psycho-physical symptoms can manifest, such as hyperalertness, tension, sense of unease, restlessness, insomnia, fear and forgetfulness. Gastrointestinal upset and marked changes in the cardiovascular system, e.g. sweating, palpitations, tachycardia, shortness of breath, dizziness, dry mouth and nausea, can also feature. Stress and anxiety therefore have a cognitive, somatic, emotional, physiological and behavioural component.

Anxiety disorders, on the other hand, are a group of mental illness that cause such marked distress that they disrupt normal function, overwhelm or impair the individual's ability to lead a normal life. Examples of anxiety disorders such as obsessional–compulsive and phobic anxiety states are discussed in more detail in Part B of the chapter.

Although many studies have raised the profile of elevated levels of stress hormones during the antenatal period having the potential to lead to deleterious effects on the fetus (Teixeira et al 1999; Evans et al 2001; Miller et al 2005; Glover and O'Connor 2006; Talge et al 2007;

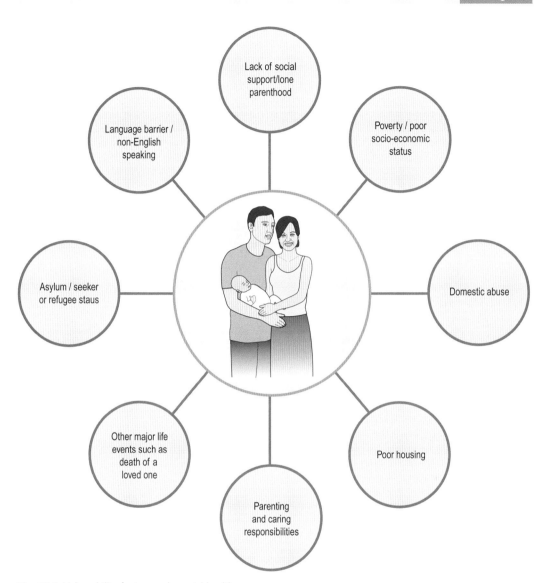

Fig. 25.1 Vulnerability factors and mental health.

O'Donnell et al 2009) or persistent antenatal anxiety acting as a possible precursor to maternal mental illness postpartum, this is still an emerging field. The mechanism by which raised levels of stress hormones may affect fetal development is not yet fully understood. Furthermore, the research studies have provided very little data to help guide midwifery practice on how antenatal stress can be alleviated in pregnant women.

Thus it can be concluded that there are many factors in women's lives that can impact on their happiness (Fig. 25.1) and affect their emotional health and wellbeing. Understanding the root cause and expression of anxiety, stress and mental distress in women is complex, as the social circumstances in which women live and into which

children are born play a major role in their health and wellbeing.

FEAR OF GIVING BIRTH (TOCOPHOBIA)

The fear of childbirth has grown in prominence over recent years, as demonstrated by the emergent studies mainly from Scandinavian countries. The exact incidence of this psychological condition is unknown but it is estimated that approximately 5–20% of pregnant women within Western society are fearful of childbirth

(Waldenstrom et al 2006; Rouhe et al 2009; Adams et al 2012). The picture within developing and more resource-poor countries is unreported. Understanding tocophobia is challenging as there is an array of complex social factors attributed to the roots of its expression, such as domestic abuse, communication difficulties, previous traumatic birth experience, poor socioeconomic status, lack of social support, nulliparity and pre-existing mental illness (Rouhe et al 2009, 2011). A study by Adams et al (2012) suggests that tocophobia might result in longer duration of labour and therefore more risk of obstetric intervention during childbirth. It is postulated that the fear and anxiety generated in the presence of tocophobia increases catecholamine levels, which can affect the frequency, strength and duration of uterine contractions. This can affect women's satisfaction with their birth experience and lead to maternal distress.

TRANSITION TO PARENTHOOD

Postnatally, parents may find coping with the demands of a new baby, e.g. infant feeding, financial constraints, the whole process of lifestyle adjustments and role changes, a real strain. For new mothers, this will involve diverse emotional responses ranging from joy and elation to sadness and utter exhaustion. Fatigue, pain and discomfort commonly result once the elation that follows the safe arrival of the baby wears off. Disturbed sleep is inevitable with a new baby. Mothers who are trying to establish breastfeeding, older women, women who are recovering from a caesarean section or those who have had a long and difficult labour/birth, twins or higher multiples, may feel wretched and constantly weary for months following childbirth. Soreness and pain being experienced from perineal trauma will affect libido, so too will feelings of exhaustion, despair and unhappiness that may be associated with the round-the-clock demands of caring for a new baby. Women may be left feeling bereft and quite miserable after giving birth.

Role change/role conflict

Having a baby, and particularly the transition to parenthood that accompanies the first child, leads to a significant shift in a couple's relationship; social networks are disrupted, especially those of the mother, and the quality and quantity of social support such networks can and do provide. There is a strong possibility that old relationships, particularly with those who are childless or single, may be weakened, leading to a sense of social isolation. However, some relationships are strengthened or even replaced gradually by new contacts established with other parents. The dynamics of relationships with family members are also altered during this process of transition and change.

The relationship with the woman's parents for example alters as the daughter becomes a mother herself and her parents develop new roles as grandparents. The competing demands on time of caring for a new baby may lead to role conflict and confusion for parents. Mothers may find that there is little time for them to pursue other activities, which can diminish any opportunity for contact with and support from others (Raynor and England 2010). Partners, especially young fathers, can also experience a sense of isolation as the dynamic within the couple's relation alters, becoming more baby-centred. Postnatal care is therefore essential to women's emotional wellbeing and should be a continuation of the care given during pregnancy. Its contribution plays a significant part in the positive adjustment to parenthood, as it assists in the acquisition of confident and well-informed parenting skills (DH [Department of Health] 2004; Barlow et al 2011).

Communication

Effective communication during pregnancy and the puerperium is essential. Yet poor communication is still the single most common factor that is associated with women's dissatisfaction with their care. A survey by the National Perinatal Epidemiology Unit (NPEU) reports that communication remains a matter of concern within the maternity service (Redshaw and Heikkila 2010). Being provided with adequate information will serve to:

- diminish women's anxiety levels and allay emotional distress
- facilitate choice
- enable women to maintain control over decision-making.

The ideology of motherhood

Motherhood, it is thought, ensures that a woman has fulfilled her biological destiny, confirms a woman's femininity and raises her status in society, but without financial gain (Crittenden 2001; Winson 2009). Instead of feeling elated by motherhood some women experience displeasure, harbour feelings of unhappiness and feel dismayed or even disappointed in their role as new mothers (Grabowska 2009). Many may be afraid to speak out about their feelings in case they are judged a 'bad' or not a 'good enough' mother. Painful emotions may be internalized, magnifying difficulties with coping and sleeping, leading many women to suffer in silence. Distress may then manifest as mothers rage against their impossible situation. Some women may even grieve for the loss of their former lifestyle, career or status. Nicholson (1998) contends that healthcare professionals have defined women's postnatal experience through proposing that well-adjusted, 'normal' and therefore 'good' mothers are those who are happy and fulfilled, but those who are unfulfilled, anxious or distressed are 'ill' and may be perceived as 'bad' mothers. This may lead to feelings of isolation, inadequacy and confusion. The ideology of motherhood is therefore an assumption and a paradox with inherent dichotomies as the woman strives to be 'super mum, super wife, super everything' (Choi et al 2005). Midwives have a pivotal role to play in assisting women and their partners to prepare for the physical, social, emotional and psychological demands of pregnancy, labour, the puerperium and, perhaps more importantly, parenthood (Barlow et al 2011; DH 2011).

Social support

During periods of stress, supportive and holistic care from midwives will not only assist in promoting emotional wellbeing of women, but will also help to ameliorate threatened psychological morbidity in the postnatal period (Oakley et al 1996; Webster et al 2000; Wessely et al 2000; Hodnett et al 2010). Women who are socially isolated or who have poor socioeconomic circumstances are particularly vulnerable to mental health problems and need additional help and support. This includes women from minority ethnic groups who do not speak English, and often have problems accessing health care (CMACE 2011). Bick et al (2009) provide evidence regarding the psychosocial benefits of midwifery care well beyond the historical boundaries of the traditionally defined postnatal period. The restructuring of postnatal care means there is now a social expectation that midwives will respond flexibly and responsively to women's emotional needs on an individual basis (Brown et al 2002; DH 2004, 2007a, 2007b; NICE [National Institute for Health and Clinical Excellence] 2006). This calls for skilled multidisciplinary and multi-agency collaboration as well as effective teamwork, taking into account the diversity within teams, for example the Department of Health (DH 2003a, 2003b) acknowledges the contribution of the maternity support worker in maternity care. Social support is further explored in Part B.

NORMAL EMOTIONAL CHANGES DURING PREGNANCY, LABOUR AND THE PUERPERIUM

Pregnancy

Since many decisions have to be made it is perfectly normal for women to have periods of self-doubt and crises of confidence. Box 25.1 outlines the many and varied emotions women may experience during the different trimesters of pregnancy. The reality for many women will encompass fluctuations between ambivalence to positive and negative emotions.

> **Box 25.1 Normal emotional changes during pregnancy**
>
> **First trimester**
> - pleasure, excitement, elation
> - dismay, disappointment
> - ambivalence emotional lability (e.g. episodes of weepiness exacerbated by physiological events such as nausea, vomiting and tiredness)
> - increased femininity
>
> **Second trimester**
> - a feeling of wellbeing, especially as physiological effects of tiredness, nausea and vomiting start to abate
> - a sense of increased attachment to the fetus; the impact of ultrasound scanning generating images for the prospective parents may intensify the experience
> - stress and anxiety about antenatal screening and diagnostic tests
> - increased demand for knowledge and information as preparations are now on the way for the birth
> - feelings of the need for increasing detachment from work commitments
>
> **Third trimester**
> - loss of or increased libido
> - altered body image
> - psychological effects from physiological discomforts such as backache and heartburn
> - anxiety about labour (e.g. pain)
> - anxiety about fetal abnormality, which may disturb sleep or cause nightmares
> - increased vulnerability to major life events such as financial status, moving house, or lack of a supportive partner

Labour

During labour, midwives must facilitate choice to help women maintain control. Factors that induce stress should be prevented, or at least minimized, as the woman's long-term emotional health may be severely compromised by an adverse birth experience (Lyons 1998; Redshaw and Heikkila 2010). Choice and control are important psychological concepts to mental health and wellbeing. Evidence from Green et al's (1998) prospective study of women's expectations and experiences of childbirth suggests that having choice in pregnancy and childbirth, and a sense of being in control, lead to a more satisfying birth experience. In England, the publication of 'Maternity Matters' (DH 2007a) epitomizes a real philosophical shift in maternity care in terms of the guaranteed choices for women.

Box 25.2 **Emotional changes during labour**

- Ranging from great excitement and anticipation, to utter dread
- Fear of the unknown
- Fear of technology, intervention and hospitalization
- Tension, fear and anxiety about pain and the ability to exercise control during labour
- Concerns about the wellbeing of the baby and ability of the partner to cope
- Fear of death: hospitals may be construed as places of illness, death and dying; the magnitude of such feelings may intensify if the woman experiences life-threatening complications or even an emergency caesarean section
- The process of birth thrusts a lot of private data into the realms of the public, so there could be a fear of lack of privacy or utter embarrassment

Box 25.3 **Normal emotional changes during the puerperium**

- Immediately following birth, the woman might experience relief. The woman might convey a cool detachment from events, especially if labour was protracted, complicated and difficult
- Contradictory and conflicting feelings ranging from satisfaction, joy and elation to exhaustion, helplessness, discontentment and disappointment as the early weeks seem to be dominated by the novelty and unpredictability of the new baby
- A feeling of closeness to partner or baby; equally the woman may feel disinterested in the baby
- Early skin-to-skin contact and breastfeeding will help to nurture the early stages of relationship building between mother and baby
- Being very attentive towards the baby; equally the woman may show disinterest in the baby
- Fear of the unknown and sudden realization of overwhelming responsibility
- Exhaustion and increased emotionality
- Pain (e.g. perineal, in nipples)
- Increased vulnerability, indecisiveness (e.g. in feeding), loss of libido, disturbed sleep and anxiety

Redshaw and Heikkila (2010) identify key factors related to women's perception of control during labour, these are:

- continuity of care with carer
- one-to-one care in labour
- not being left for long periods
- being involved in decision-making.

Ongoing research to determine the relationship between women's perception of control during childbirth and postnatal outcomes is needed in order to measure factors such as postnatal depression, positive parenting relationships and self-esteem. Common emotional responses during labour are detailed in Box 25.2.

The puerperium

The puerperium is hailed as the 'fourth trimester' – an emotionally complex transitional phase. By definition, it is the period from birth to 6–8 weeks postpartum, when the woman is readjusting physiologically, socially and psychologically to motherhood. Emotional responses may be just as intense and powerful for experienced as well as for new mothers. The major psychological changes are therefore emotional. The woman's mood appears to be a barometer, reflecting the baby's needs of feeding, sleeping and crying patterns. New mothers tend to be easily upset and oversensitive. A sense of proportion is easily lost, as women may feel overwhelmed and agitated by minor mishaps. The woman might start to regain a sense of proportion and 'normality' between 6 and 12 weeks. Exhaustion is also a major factor of women's emotional state. Perhaps the most important factor in regaining any semblance of normality is the mother's ability to sleep throughout the night. A woman's sexual urges, emotional stability and intellectual acuity may take months, if not

longer, to return. Normal emotional changes in the puerperium are summarized in Box 25.3.

POSTNATAL 'BLUES'

Childbirth is an emotionally intense experience. Mood changes in the early days postpartum are particularly common. The postnatal 'blues' is a transitory state, experienced by 50–80% of women depending on parity (Harris et al 1994). It has been identified as an antecedent to depression following childbirth (Gregoire 1995; Cooper and Murray 1997). The onset typically occurs between day 3 and 5 postpartum, but may last up to 1 week or more, though rarely persisting longer than 48 hours. The main features are mild and may include:

- a state whereby the woman experiences labile emotions (e.g. tearfulness, despair, irritability to euphoria and laughter)
- a state whereby the woman feels overwhelmed by the sudden realization of the relentless responsibility of the baby's 24-hour dependency and vulnerability.

The actual aetiology is unclear but hormonal influences (e.g. changes in oestrogen, progesterone and prolactin levels) seem to be implicated as the period of increased emotionality appears to coincide with the production of milk in the breasts. This state of heightened emotionality is self-limiting and will resolve spontaneously, assisted by support from loved ones. The midwife should be vigilant during this time as persistent features could be indicative of depressive illness.

DISTRESS OR DEPRESSION?

Repeated contact with women during pregnancy and puerperium afford a wealth of opportunity to explore feelings, experience and emotions, and for midwives to provide clear explanations to women about the differences between distress – a normal reaction to major life events – and depressive illness. However, midwives should be mindful of over-reliance on the medical model to describe women's moods as such an approach may serve to pathologize or medicalize normal emotional changes (Nicholson 1998).

Emotional distress associated with traumatic birth events

Understanding the root cause and expression of mental distress associated with pregnancy and childbirth is complex. It is important to recognize the inter-relationship between traumatic life events and women's mental health. Vulnerability factors such as a history of childhood sexual abuse or a morbid fear of childbirth can negate a woman's experience of childbirth. What is intended to be one of the happiest days in a woman's life can quickly turn into anguish and distress. Furthermore, environmental factors may lead to a sense of loss of control, for example effects of intense pain, use of technological interventions, insensitive and disrespectful care or an emergency caesarean section (CS) may prove very distressing and frightening. Post-traumatic stress disorder (PTSD), a term most commonly associated with individuals who have suffered the onslaught of war, has emerged in the literature around maternity care (Lyons 1998). Obstetric PTSD occurs when women feared they or their baby were in danger of dying. Not surprisingly it is commonest after emergency CS or obstetric emergencies, particularly involving intensive care. It is estimated 6% of emergency CS are followed by obstetric PTSD (Beck 2009). Box 25.4 highlights some of the reported symptoms of obstetric PTSD.

Unlike mild to moderate depression in the postpartum period, which seems to have its roots in the biophysical and psychosocial domains, obstetric distress after childbirth appears to be directly linked to the stress, fear and trauma of birth, yet its prevalence is unrecognized (Lyons 1998). Psychological interventions such as 'debriefing' have been suggested to manage immediate symptomatology but there is no reliable evidence that it is a useful intervention in reducing psychological morbidity (Alexandra 1998; Wessely et al 2000; Bick et al 2009). Moreover, clinical guidelines from NICE (2007) have stated that following a traumatic birth, women should not routinely be

---

Box 25.4 Reported symptoms of obstetric PTSD

Features of obstetric PTSD – applies where symptoms are present for more than 1 month (Lyons 1998; Beck 2009)
- Intrusive thoughts or images resulting in nightmares, panic attacks or 'flashbacks' about the birth
- Detachment from loved ones and difficulty with mother–baby relationship (attachment)
- Avoidance especially of issues relating to pregnancy/ birth
- Hypervigilance/increased arousal – having a sense of imminent disaster
- Sleep disturbances
- Irritability or angry outbursts
- Anxiety/depression

Other features are not dissimilar to those previously discussed in the text relating to stress and anxiety.

Box 25.5 Summary of key points

- In the UK pregnancy and the postnatal period are unparalleled periods when women engage with health care and have repeated contact with healthcare professionals
- Women during pregnancy, labour and puerperium are in a state of transition punctuated by heightened emotions and anxiety. Family life and daily routines become disrupted by the arrival of a new baby
- Vulnerability factors such as domestic abuse, poverty and social isolation, can impact on the mother–baby relationship with consequences for child development
- Risk identification of vulnerable groups of women antenatally presents a unique opportunity for multidisciplinary and multi-agency collaboration in promoting mental health and wellbeing

---

offered 'single-session formal debriefing focused on the birth'. Instead midwives and other healthcare professionals should support women who wish to talk about their experience and draw on the love and support of family and friends. Neither should midwives overlook the impact of birth on the partner.

CONCLUSION

A plethora of significant social and health policies and clinical guidelines have resulted in wider consideration being given to the social and psychological context of pregnancy and the puerperium. Midwives need to have knowledge and understanding of how they influence care provision. Box 25.5 provides a summary of key points.

Part B: Perinatal psychiatric conditions

Margaret R Oates

INTRODUCTION

Perinatal psychiatric disorder is now an accepted term used both nationally and internationally. It emphasizes the importance of psychiatric disorder in pregnancy as well as following childbirth and the variety of psychiatric disorders that can occur at this time, not just the ubiquitously known postnatal depression (PND). It also places emphasis on the significance of psychiatric disorders that were present before conception as well as those that arise during the perinatal period (Box 25.6).

The emotional wellbeing of women is of primary importance to midwives. Not only can mental illness affect obstetric outcomes but also the transition to parenthood and emotional wellbeing and health problems in the infant. Over the last 15 years psychiatric disorder in pregnancy and the postpartum period has been a leading cause of maternal mortality, as highlighted in the 'Why Mothers Die in the UK' (Oates 2001, 2004) and 'Saving Mothers' Lives' (Oates 2007; Oates and Cantwell 2011) reports. These reports of the Confidential Enquiry into Maternal Deaths recommend that midwives routinely ask at early pregnancy assessment about previous mental health problems, their severity and care. These recommendations have also been made by the Royal College of Psychiatrists (RCPC 2000), the Women's Mental Health Strategy (part of the Mental Health National Service Framework; DH 1999), Maternity Standard 11 of the Children, Young Peoples and Maternity National Service Framework (DH 2004), the NICE Guidelines (2007) on the management of antenatal and postnatal mental health and the Clinical Negligence Standards for Trusts (NHSLA [National Health Service Litigation Authority] 2011). In addition, NICE (2007) recommends that midwives should ask questions (the Whooley questions) on at least two occasions – antenatally and following birth – about women's current mental health. Systems should be in place locally to ensure that women with mental health problems and those at risk of developing them receive the appropriate care.

It is therefore essential that all midwives have education and training to be familiar with normal emotional changes, commonplace distress and adjustment reactions as well as the signs and symptoms of more serious psychiatric illnesses.

TYPES OF PSYCHIATRIC DISORDER

The term 'mental health problem' is commonly used to describe all types of emotional difficulties from transient and temporary states of distress, often understandable, to severe and uncommon mental illness. It is also used frequently to describe learning difficulties, substance misuse problems and difficulties coping with the stresses and strains of life. It is therefore too general and too nonspecific to be of use to the midwife. The term does not discriminate between severity and need and does not help the midwife distinguish between those conditions that she can manage and those that require specialist attention. For this reason, in this chapter, the term 'psychiatric disorder' is preferred as it can be further categorized and the different types can be described aiding recognition and the planning of care.

Psychiatric disorders are conventionally categorized into:

Serious mental illnesses

These include schizophrenia, other psychotic conditions, bipolar illness and severe depressive illness. Previously, these conditions were called psychotic disorders.

Mild to moderate psychiatric disorders

These were previously known as 'neurotic disorders'. These include non-psychotic mild to moderate depressive illness, mixed anxiety and depression, anxiety disorders including phobic anxiety states, panic disorder, obsessive–compulsive disorder and post-traumatic stress disorder.

Adjustment reactions

These would include distressing reactions to life events, including death and adversity.

Box 25.6 **What is perinatal psychiatric disorder?**

- Psychiatric disorders that complicate pregnancy, childbirth and the postnatal period
- Includes not only those illnesses that develop at this time but also pre-existing disorders such as schizophrenia, bipolar illness and depression
- Care involves consideration of the effects of the illness itself and of its treatment on the developing fetus and infant
- Care involves multidisciplinary and multi-agency working, especially close relationships with Maternity Mental Health and Children's Services

---

Substance misuse

This includes those who misuse or who are dependent upon alcohol and other drugs of dependency, including both prescription and legal/illegal drugs.

Personality disorders

This is a term that should be used only to describe people who have persistent severe problems throughout their adult life in dealing with the stresses and strains of normal life, maintaining satisfactory relationships, controlling their behaviour, foreseeing the consequences of their own actions and which persistently cause distress to themselves and other people.

Learning disability

This is a term used to describe people who have a lifetime evidence of intellectual and cognitive impairment, developmental delay and consequent learning disabilities. This is usually graded as mild, moderate or severe.

Overall psychiatric disorders are very common in the general population. The General Household Survey 2000, as reported by the Office of National Statistics (ONS 2002), reveals a prevalence of over 20% of these disorders. Recent figures from ONS (2012) have shown little change in this trend in the adult population in the UK, reporting that in 2007, approximately 1 : 6 adults had a common mental disorder such as anxiety or depression.

They are commoner in women than in men with the exception of substance misuse problems. However, the majority of psychiatric disorders in the community are mild to moderate conditions, particularly general anxiety and depression. Mild to moderate depressive illness and anxiety disorders are at least twice as common in women than in men, and are particularly common in young women with children under the age of 5. The majority of these disorders are managed in primary care and do not require the attention of specialist psychiatric services. Mild to moderate depressive illness and anxiety states respond to psychological treatments. Despite this, perhaps because of shortage of such treatments, prescription of antidepressants is widespread in the community, particularly among women.

Serious mental illnesses are less common. Both schizophrenia and bipolar illness affect approximately 1% of the population. Bipolar illness affects men and women equally. However, schizophrenia, particularly the more severe chronic forms, is commoner among men. These conditions require the attention of specialist psychiatric services and require medical treatments as well as psychological care.

In the UK psychiatric services are usually organized separately for adult mental health (serious mental illnesses), substance misuse (drug and alcohol treatment services) and learning disability. There are also, but not relevant to this chapter, separate services for psychiatric disorders in the elderly.

PSYCHIATRIC DISORDER IN PREGNANCY

In general, psychiatric disorder is not associated with a decrease in fertility. Therefore all the previously described psychiatric disorders can and do complicate pregnancy and the postpartum period. The prevalence of psychiatric disorder in young women means that at least 20% of women will have current or previous psychiatric disorder in early pregnancy, many of whom will be taking psychiatric medication at the time of conception. However, it can be seen that only a small number will have a past history of a serious mental illness and an even smaller number will be currently suffering from such an illness. Pregnancy is not protective against a recurrence or relapse of a previous psychiatric disorder, particularly if the medication for these disorders is stopped when pregnancy is diagnosed. Women with a previous history of serious illness are at increased risk of a recurrence of that illness following birth. It is for these reasons that it is so important for midwives to enquire into women's current and previous mental health at early pregnancy assessment. Table 25.1 highlights the incidence of perinatal psychiatric disorders.

Mild–moderate conditions

The incidence (new onset) of psychiatric disorder in pregnancy is mostly accounted for by mild depressive illness, mixed anxiety and depression or anxiety states. These disorders present most commonly in the early weeks of pregnancy, becoming less common as the pregnancy progresses.

Table 25.1 Incidence of perinatal psychiatric disorders	
Psychiatric disorder	**(%)**
'Depression'	15–30
PND (postnatal depression)	10
Moderate/severe depressive illness	3–5
Referred psychiatry	2
Admitted to hospital	0.4
Admitted psychosis	0.2
Births to schizophrenic mothers	0.2

They are probably predominantly of psychosocial aetiology, and for some women they will represent a recurrence of a previous episode, of depression, anxiety, panic or obsessional disorders particularly if they have suddenly stopped their antidepressant medication. Women may also be vulnerable at this time because of:

- previous fertility problems
- previous obstetric loss
- anxieties about the viability of their pregnancy
- social and relationship problems
- ambivalence towards the pregnancy
- other reasons for personal unhappiness.

In the past, it was often assumed that hyperemesis gravidarum (severe vomiting) was a psychosomatic manifestation of personal unhappiness and psychological disturbance. This condition is less common than in the past and usually resolves by 16 weeks of pregnancy. Psychological factors, anxiety and cognitive misattribution remain a significant factor in some women.

Prognosis and management

Most of the conditions are likely to improve as the pregnancy progresses. Psychological treatments and psychosocial interventions are effective for these conditions and caution needs to be exercised before pharmacological interventions are initiated during pregnancy, although medication may be necessary for the more severe illnesses.

For others, particularly those who develop a psychiatric illness in the later stages of pregnancy, their condition is likely to continue and worsen in the postpartum period.

Serious conditions

This term refers to schizophrenia, other psychoses, bipolar illness (manic depressive illness) and severe depressive illness.

Incidence

Women are at a lower risk of developing a serious mental illness for the first time during pregnancy than at other times in their lives. This is in marked contrast to the elevated risk of suffering from such a condition in the first few months following childbirth (Kendell et al 1987). While these conditions are uncommon, they require urgent and expert treatment, particularly as an acute psychosis in pregnancy can pose a risk to the mother and developing fetus, both directly because of the disturbed behaviour and indirectly because of the treatments. There is a possibility that such an illness can interfere with proper antenatal care.

Prevalence

While new onset psychosis in pregnancy is relatively rare, the prevalence of these illnesses (pre-existing) at the beginning of pregnancy will be the same as at other times. Women suffering from schizophrenia or bipolar illness are as likely to become pregnant as the rest of the general population. This means that approximately 2% of women in pregnancy will either have had such an illness in the past or be currently suffering from one. It is important to realize that these women may range from women who are well and stable, leading normal lives through to those who are disabled, chronically symptomatic and on medication. The management of these women in pregnancy therefore has to be individualized and plans made on a case-by-case basis. Nonetheless, there are three broad groups of women.

Group 1

The first group includes women who have had a previous episode of bipolar illness or a psychotic episode earlier in their lives. They are usually well, stable not on medication and may not be in contact with psychiatric services. These women, if their last episode of illness was more than 2 years ago, may not be at an increased risk of a recurrence of their condition during pregnancy but face at least a 50% risk of becoming psychotic in the early weeks postpartum. The most important aspect of their management is therefore a proactive management plan for the first few weeks following birth.

Group 2

The second broad group of women are those who have had a previous and/or recent episode of a serious mental illness, who are relatively well and stable but whose health is being maintained by taking medication. This may be antipsychotic medication or in the case of bipolar illness, a mood stabilizer (lithium or an anticonvulsant). These women are at risk of a relapse of their condition during pregnancy. This risk is particularly high if they stop their medication at the diagnosis of pregnancy. As some of these medications may have an adverse effect on the development of the fetus and yet an acute relapse of the illness also is hazardous, it is important that these women have access to expert advice on the risks and benefits of continuing the treatment or changing it as early as possible in pregnancy.

Group 3

The third broad category includes women who are chronically mentally ill with complex social needs, persisting symptoms and on medication. These women will usually be in contact with psychiatric services. Midwifery and obstetric care needs to be closely integrated into the case management of these women and there needs to be a close working relationship between maternity, psychiatric and social services.

Ideally, all women who have a current or previous history of serious mental illness should have advice and counselling before embarking upon a pregnancy. They should be able to discuss the risk to their mental health of becoming pregnant and becoming a parent as well as the risks to the developing fetus of continuing with their usual medication and perhaps the need to change it. However, in the general population, at least 50% of all pregnancies are unplanned at the point of conception. Midwives should therefore enquire at early pregnancy assessment about the women's previous and current psychiatric history and alert psychiatric services as soon as possible about the pregnancy so that relapses of the psychiatric illness during pregnancy and recurrences postpartum can be avoided wherever possible.

PSYCHIATRIC DISORDER AFTER BIRTH

The majority of postpartum onset psychiatric disorders are affective (mood) disorders. However, symptoms other than those due to a disorder of mood are frequently present. Conventionally three postpartum disorders are described:

- the 'blues'
- puerperal (postpartum) psychosis
- postnatal depression.

The 'blues' is a common dysphoric, self-limiting state, occurring in the first week postpartum (see Part A).

Puerperal (postpartum) psychosis

Globally, puerperal psychosis, the most severe form of postpartum affective (mood) disorder has been recognized and described since antiquity. It leads to 2 in 1000 women being admitted to a psychiatric hospital following childbirth, mostly in the first few weeks postpartum. Although a relatively rare condition, there is a marked increase in the risk of suffering from a psychotic illness following childbirth (Kendell et al 1987; Munk-Olsen et al 2012). It is also remarkably constant across nations and cultures.

Risk factors

Most women who suffer from this condition will have been previously well, without obvious risk factors, and the illness comes as a shock to them and their families. However, some women will have suffered from a similar illness following the birth of a previous child, some may have suffered from a non-postpartum bipolar affective disorder from which they have long recovered or they may

have a family history of bipolar illness. For others there may be marked psychosocial adversity. It is generally accepted that biological factors (neuroendocrine and genetic) are the most important aetiological factors for this condition. This implies that puerperal psychosis can and does strike without warning, women from all social and occupational backgrounds – those in stable marriages with much-wanted babies as well as those living in less fortunate circumstances.

Clinical features

Puerperal psychosis is an acute, early onset condition. The overwhelming majority of cases present in the first 14 days postpartum. They most commonly develop suddenly between day 3 and day 7, at a time when most women will be experiencing the 'blues'. Differential diagnosis between the earliest phase of a developing psychosis and the 'blues' can be difficult. However, puerperal psychosis steadily deteriorates over the following 48 hours while the 'blues' tends to resolve spontaneously.

During the first 2–3 days of a developing puerperal psychosis there is a fluctuating rapidly changing, undifferentiated psychotic state. The earliest signs are commonly of perplexity, fear – even terror – and restless agitation associated with insomnia. Other signs include: purposeless activity, uncharacteristic behaviour, disinhibition, irritation and fleeting anger, and resistive behaviour and sometimes incontinence.

A woman may have fears for her own and her baby's health and safety, or even about its identity. Even at this early stage, there may be, variably throughout the day, elation and grandiosity, suspiciousness, depression or unspeakable ideas of horror.

Women suffering from puerperal psychosis are among the most profoundly disturbed and distressed found in psychiatric practice (Dean and Kendell 1981). In addition to the familiar symptoms and signs of a manic or depressive psychosis, symptoms of schizophrenia (delusions and hallucinations) may occur. Depressive delusions about maternal and infant health are common. The behaviour and motives of others are frequently misinterpreted in a delusional fashion. A mood of perplexity and terror is often found, as are delusions about the passage of time and other bizarre delusions. Women can believe that they are still pregnant or that more than one child has been born or that the baby is older than it is.

Women often seem confused and disorientated. In the very common mixed affective psychosis, along with the familiar pressure of speech and flight of ideas, there is often a mixture of grandiosity, elation and certain conviction alternating with states of fearful tearfulness, guilt and a sense of foreboding. The sufferers are usually restless and agitated, resistive, seeking senselessly to escape and difficult to reassure. However, they are usually calmer in the presence of familiar relatives.

The woman may be unable to attend to her own personal hygiene and nutrition and unable to care for her baby. Her concentration is usually grossly impaired and she is distractible and unable to initiate and complete tasks. Over the next few days her condition deteriorates and the symptoms usually become more clearly those of an acute affective psychosis. Most women will have symptoms and signs suggestive of a depressive psychosis, a significant minority a manic psychosis and very commonly a mixture of both – a mixed affective psychosis.

Relationship with the baby

Some women are so disturbed, distractible and their concentration so impaired that they do not seem to be aware of their recently born baby. Others are preoccupied with the baby, reluctant to let it out of their sight and forever checking on its presence and condition. Although delusional ideas frequently involve the baby and there may be delusional ideas of infant ill health or changed identity, it is rare for women with puerperal psychosis to be overtly hostile to their baby and for their behaviour to be aggressive or punitive. The risk to their baby lies more from an inability to organize and complete tasks, and to inappropriate handling and tasks being impaired by their mental state. These problems, directly attributable to the maternal psychosis, tend to resolve as the mother recovers.

Management

Most women with psychotic illness following childbirth will require admission to hospital, which should be to a specialist mother and baby unit, the only setting in which the physical needs of the mother who has recently given birth can be met and where specialist psychiatric nursing is available. This ensures that the physical and emotional needs of both mother and baby are met and the developing relationship with the baby promoted.

Prognosis

In spite of the severity of puerperal psychoses, they frequently resolve relatively quickly over 2–4 weeks. However, initial recovery is often fragile and relapses are common in the first few weeks. As the psychosis resolves, it is common for women to pass through a phase of depression and anxiety and preoccupation with their past experiences and the implications of these memories for their future mental health and their role as a mother. Sensitive and expert help is required to assist women through this phase, to help them understand what has happened and to acquire a 'working model' of their illness. The overwhelming majority of women will have completely recovered by 3–6 months postpartum. However, they face at least a 50% risk of a recurrence should they have another

child and some may go on to have bipolar illness at other times in their lives (Robertson et al 2005).

Postnatal depressive illness

Approximately 10% of all postnatal women will develop a depressive illness. The studies, from which this figure is derived, are usually community studies using the Edinburgh Postnatal Depression Scale (EPDS) either as a diagnostic tool or as a screen prior to the use of other research tools. Studies using a cut-off point of 14 usually give an incidence of 10%; those using lower scores will give a higher incidence. A score on a screening instrument is not the same as a clinical diagnosis. Nonetheless a score of 14 is said to correlate with a clinical diagnosis of major depression and the lower scores with that of major and minor depression (Elliot 1994). The incidence of women who would meet the diagnostic criteria for moderate to severe depressive illness is lower, probably between 3% and 5% (Cox et al 1993). Depression following childbirth has the same range of severity and subtypes as depression at other times. According to the symptomatology, duration and severity, they may be graded as mild to moderate or severe, and subtypes may have prominent anxiety and obsessional phenomena.

Postnatal depressive illness of all types and severities is therefore relatively common and represents a considerable burden of disability and distress in these women. Although postnatal depressive illness is popularly accepted, with the exception of the most severe forms, it is no more common than during pregnancy or in non-childbearing women of the same age (O'Hara and Swain 1996). However, this does not detract from its importance. Depressive illness of any severity occurring at a time when the expectation is of happiness and fulfillment and when major psychological and social adjustments are being made together with caring for an infant, creates difficulties not found at other times in the human lifespan.

The term 'postnatal depression' is often used as a generic term for all forms of psychiatric disorder presenting following birth. While in the past this has undoubtedly been helpful in raising the profile of postpartum psychiatric disorders, improving their recognition and reducing stigma, it has also become problematic. Use of the term in this way can diminish the perceived seriousness of other illnesses, and has led to a 'one size fits all' view of diagnosis and treatments (Oates 2001). The term postnatal depression should only be used for a non-psychotic depressive illness of mild to moderate severity which arises within 3 months of childbirth.

Severe depressive illness

Severe depressive illness affects at least 3% of all women who have given birth, with a seven-fold increase in risk in the first 3 months (Cox et al 1993). Again, the majority of women who suffer from this condition will have been previously well. However, women with a previous history of severe postnatal depressive illness or severe depression at other times or a family history of severe depressive illness or postnatal depression are at increased risk. Psychosocial factors are more important in the aetiology of this condition than in puerperal psychosis, although biological factors play an important role in the most severe illnesses. Nonetheless, severe postnatal depression can affect women from all backgrounds not just those facing social adversity.

Like puerperal psychosis, severe depressive illness is an early onset condition in which the woman commonly does not regain her normal emotional state following birth. However, unlike puerperal psychosis, the onset tends not to be abrupt; rather, the illness develops over the next 2–4 weeks. The more severe illnesses tend to present early, by 4–6 weeks postpartum, but the majority present later, between 8 and 12 weeks postpartum. These later presentations may be missed. This is partly because some of the symptoms may be misattributed to the adjustment to a new baby and partly because the mother may 'put on a brave face', concealing how she feels from others.

Risk factors

A variety of risk factors for postnatal depressive illness have been identified and include those associated with depressive illness at other times. To these can be added ambivalence about the pregnancy, high levels of anxiety during pregnancy and adverse birth experiences, previous perinatal death to name but a few. Many of these risk factors, though statistically significant are so common as to have little positive predictive value. However a clustering of these risk factors might lead to those caring for the woman to be extra vigilant. Of more use are those risk factors that have a higher positive predictive value. These include a family history of severe affective disorder, a family history of severe postnatal depressive illness, developing a depressive illness in the last trimester of pregnancy and the loss of the previous infant (including stillbirth). There may also be an increased risk in those women who have conceived through IVF.

Clinical features

The familiar symptoms of severe depressive illness are often modified by the context of early maternity and the relative youth of those suffering from the condition:

The 'somatic syndrome' (biological features) of broken sleep and early morning wakening, diurnal variation of mood, loss of appetite and weight, slowing of mental functioning, impaired concentration, extreme tiredness and lack of vitality can easily be misattributed to a crying baby, understandable tiredness and the adjustment to new routines.

The all-pervasive anhedonia or loss of pleasure in ordinary everyday tasks, the lack of joy and fearfulness for the future may be misattributed by the woman herself to 'not loving the baby' or 'not being a proper mother' and all too easily described as 'bonding problems' by professionals. Anhedonia is a particularly painful symptom at a time when most women would expect to feel overwhelmed with joy and happiness and in turn contributes to feelings of guilt, incompetence and unworthiness that are very prominent in postnatal depressive illness. These overvalued ideas can verge on the delusional.

It is also common to find overvalued morbid beliefs and fears for the woman's own health and mortality and that of her baby. She may misattribute normal infant behaviour to mean that the baby is suffering or does not like her. A baby that settles in the arms of more experienced people may confirm the mother's belief that she is incompetent. Commonplace problems with establishing breastfeeding may become the subject of morbid rumination.

Some women with severe postnatal depressive illness may be slowed, withdrawn and retreat easily in the face of offers of help, avoid the tasks of motherhood and their relationship with the baby. Others may be agitated, restless and fiercely protective of their infant, resenting the contribution of others.

Anxiety and obsessive–compulsive symptoms

Although women with pre-existing anxiety and panic disorder or obsessional–compulsive disorder (OCD) frequently experience relapses or recurrences postpartum, it is not known whether there is an increase in incidence (new onset) of these conditions following birth. Nonetheless, severe anxiety, panic attacks and obsessional phenomena are common following birth. These symptoms may dominate the clinical picture or accompany a postnatal depressive illness. They frequently underpin mental health crises, calls for emergency attention and maternal fears for the infant. Repetitive intrusive, and often deeply repugnant, thoughts of harm coming to loved ones, particularly the infant, are commonplace, often leading to repetitive doubting and checking. The woman may doubt that she is safe as a mother and believe that she is capable of harming her infant. Crescendos of anxiety and panic attacks may result from the baby's crying or being difficult to settle and may lead the mother to be frightened to be alone with her child. This is easily misinterpreted by professionals who may fear that the child is at risk.

Obsessional, vacillating indecisiveness is also common and contributes to an overwhelming sense of being unable to cope with everyday tasks in marked contrast to premorbid levels of competence. While complex obsessive–compulsive behavioural rituals are relatively rare, obsessive cleaning, housework and checking are common. Intrusive obsessional thoughts and the typical catastrophic cognitions associated with panic attacks frequently lead to a fear of insanity and loss of control.

Relationship with the baby

Severe depressive symptomatology, particularly when combined with panic and obsessional phenomena, can have a profound effect on the relationship with the baby, in many, but by no means all women. Most women who suffer from severe postnatal depressive illness maintain high standards of physical care for their infants. However, many are frightened of their own feelings and thoughts and few gain any pleasure or joy from their infant. They may find smiling and talking to their babies difficult. Most affected women feel a deep sense of guilt and incompetence and doubt whether they are caring for their infant properly. Normal infant behaviour is frequently misinterpreted as confirming their poor views of their own abilities. While a fear of harming the baby is commonplace, overt hostility and aggressive behaviour towards the infant is extremely uncommon. It should be remembered that the majority of mothers who harm small babies are not suffering from a serious mental illness. The speedy resolution of maternal illness usually results in a normal mother–infant relationship. However, prolonged chronic depressive illness can interfere with attachment, social and cognitive development in the longer term, particularly when combined with social and mental problems (Cooper and Murray 1997).

Management

These conditions need to be speedily identified and treated, preferably by a specialist perinatal mental health team. The value of early contact with professionals who recognize and validate the symptoms and distress, and can re-attribute the overvalued ideas of the mother and instill hope for the future cannot be underestimated. The treatment of the depressive illness is the same as the treatment of depressive illness at other times. The use of antidepressants together with good psychological care should result in an improvement of symptoms within 2 weeks and the resolution of the illness between 6 and 8 weeks.

Prognosis

With treatment, these women should fully recover. Without, spontaneous resolution may take many months and up to one-third of women can still be ill when their child is 1 year old.

Women who have had a severe depressive illness face a 1:2 to 1:3 risk of a recurrence of the illness following the birth of subsequent children (Cooper and Murray 1995). They are also at elevated risk from suffering from a depressive illness at other times in their lives. However, the long-term prognosis would appear to be better than when the first episode is in non-childbearing women, both in terms of the frequency of further episodes and in their overall functioning (Robling et al 2000).

Mild postnatal depressive illness

This is the commonest condition following childbirth, affecting up to 10% of all women postpartum. It is in fact no commoner after childbirth than among other non-childbearing women of the same age.

Risk factors

Some women who suffer from this condition will be vulnerable by virtue of previous mental health problems or psychosocial adversity, unsatisfactory marital or other relationships or inadequate social support. Others may be older, educated and married for a long time, perhaps with problems conceiving, previous obstetric loss or high levels of anxiety during pregnancy. Unrealistically high expectations of themselves and motherhood and consequent disappointment are commonplace. Also common are stressful life events such as moving house, family bereavement, a sick baby, experience of special care baby units and other such events that detract from the expected pleasure and harmony of this stage of life.

Clinical features

The condition has an insidious onset in the days and weeks following childbirth but usually presents after the first 3 months postpartum. The symptoms are variable, but the mother is usually tearful, feels that she has difficulty coping and complains of irritability and a lack of satisfaction and pleasure with motherhood. Symptoms of anxiety, a sense of loneliness and isolation as well as dissatisfaction with the quality of important relationships are common. Affected mothers frequently have good days and bad days and are often better in company and anxious when alone. The full biological (somatic subtype) syndrome of the more severe depressive illness is usually absent. However, difficulty getting to sleep and appetite difficulties, both over-eating and under-eating, are common.

Relationship with the baby

Dissatisfaction with motherhood and a sense of the baby being problematic are often central to this condition, particularly when compounded by difficulty in meeting the needs of older children. Lack of pleasure in the baby, combined with anxiety and irritability, can lead to a vicious circle of a fractious and unsettled baby, misinterpreted by its mother as critical and resentful of her and thus a deteriorating relationship between them. However, it should also be remembered that the direction of causality is not always mother to infant. Some infants are very unsettled in the first few months of their life. A baby who is difficult to feed and cries constantly during the day or is difficult to settle at night can just as often be the cause of a mild postnatal depressive illness as the result of it. Even mild illnesses, particularly when combined with socioeconomic deprivation and high levels of social adversity, can lead to longer-term problems with mother–infant relationships and subsequent social and cognitive development of the child (Cooper and Murray 1997). A very small minority of sufferers from this condition may experience such marked irritability and even overt hostility towards their baby that the infant is at risk of being harmed.

Management

Early detection and treatment is essential for both mother and baby. For the milder cases, a combination of psychological and social support and active listening from a health visitor will suffice. For others, specific psychological treatments, such as cognitive behavioural psychotherapy and interpersonal psychotherapy, are as effective, if not more than, antidepressants as outlined in Antenatal and Postnatal Mental Health guidelines (NICE 2007).

Prognosis

With appropriate management, postnatal depression should improve within weeks and recover by the time the infant is 6 months old. However, untreated there may be prolonged morbidity. This, particularly in the presence of continuing social adversity, has been demonstrated to have an adverse effect not only on the mother–infant relationship but also on the later social, emotional and cognitive development of the child.

Breastfeeding

There is no evidence that breastfeeding increases the risk of developing significant depressive illness, nor that its cessation improves depressive illness. Continuing breastfeeding may protect the infant from the effects of maternal depression and improve maternal self-esteem.

TREATMENT OF PERINATAL PSYCHIATRIC DISORDERS

The role of the midwife

Midwives need knowledge and understanding of the different management strategies for perinatal psychiatric disorder and of the use of psychiatric drugs in pregnancy and lactation. This knowledge is required because the women themselves may wish for advice, because the midwife may have to alert other professionals, for example general practitioners and psychiatrists, to ask for a review of the woman's medication and because in case of serious mental illness, the midwife will be part of a multiprofessional team caring for the women.

Midwives should routinely ask all women at antenatal booking clinic whether they have had an episode of serious mental illness in the past and whether they are currently in contact with psychiatric services. Those women who have a previous episode of serious mental illness (schizophrenia, other psychoses, bipolar illness and severe depressive illness) should be referred to a psychiatric team during pregnancy even if they have been well for many years. This is because they face at least a 50% risk of becoming ill following birth. The midwife should also urgently inform the psychiatric team if the woman is currently in contact with psychiatric services. The psychiatric team may not be aware of the pregnant woman who is taking psychiatric medication at the time when the midwife first sees her should be advised not to abruptly stop her medication. The midwife should urgently seek a review of the woman's medication from the general practitioner, obstetrician or psychiatrist as appropriate. This may result in the woman being advised to reduce, change or undertake a supervised withdrawal of her medication.

There are three components to the management of perinatal psychiatric disorder: psychological treatments and social interventions, pharmacological treatments and the skills, resources and services needed.

Those who are seriously mentally ill will require all three. Those with the mildest illnesses may require only psychological and social interventions, which can be carried out in primary care (NICE 2007).

Psychological treatments

All illnesses of all severities and indeed those who are not ill but experiencing commonplace episodes of distress and adjustment need good psychological care. This can only be based upon an understanding of the normal emotional and cognitive changes and common concerns of pregnancy and the puerperium. It also requires a familiarity with the symptoms and clinical features of postpartum illnesses.

For most women with mild depressive illness or emotional distress and difficulties adjusting, extra time given by the midwife or health visitor, 'the listening visit', will be effective. For others, particularly those with more persistent states associated with high levels of anxiety, brief cognitive therapy treatments and brief interpersonal psychotherapy are as effective as antidepressants and may confer additional benefits in terms of improving the mother–infant relationships and satisfaction. Similar claims have been made for infant massage and other therapies that focus the mother's attention on enjoying her baby. It is particularly important during pregnancy to use psychological treatments wherever possible and avoid the unnecessary prescription of antidepressants.

Social support

Lack of social support, particularly when combined with adversity and life events, has long been implicated in the aetiology of mild to moderate depressive illness in young women. Social support not only includes practical assistance and advice but also having an emotional confidante, female friends and people who improve self-esteem. There is evidence that organizations that are underpinned by social support theory, such as Home Start and Sure Start, can have a beneficial effect on maternal and infant well-being and perhaps on mild postnatal depression (Oakley et al 1996; Barlow et al 2007).

Pharmacological treatment

In general, psychiatric illnesses occurring during the perinatal period respond to the same treatments as at other times. There are no specific treatments for perinatal psychiatric disorder. Moderate to severe depressive illnesses respond to antidepressants, psychotic illnesses to antipsychotics and mood stabilizers may be needed for those with bipolar illnesses. However, the possibility of adverse consequences on the embryo and developing fetus and via breastmilk on the infant makes the choice and dose of the drug important.

The evidence base for the safety or adverse consequences of psychotropic medication is constantly changing both in the direction of increased concern and of reassurance. Any text detailing specific advice is in danger of being quickly out of date and the reader is directed to the regularly updated information published by the National Teratology Information Service (NTIS) – via Toxbase website: www.toxbase.org/ – and to NICE (2007) Guidelines on Antenatal and Postnatal Mental Health or Drugs and Lactation Database (LactMed).

No matter what the changing evidence is, some general principles apply:

- The absence of evidence of harm is not the same as evidence of safety.
- It may take 20–30 years after the introduction of a drug for its adverse consequences to be fully realized. An example of this is sodium valproate in pregnancy.
- In general there is more evidence on older than on newer drugs although this does not necessarily mean they are safer.
- All psychotropic medication passes across the placenta and into the breastmilk.
- Both the architecture and function of the fetal central nervous system continues to develop throughout pregnancy and in early infancy. Concern should not be confined to the adverse effects in the first 3 months of pregnancy.
- The threshold for initiating medication in pregnancy and breastfeeding should be high. If there is an alternative, non-pharmacological treatment, of equal efficacy then that should be the treatment of choice.
- Serious mental illness requires robust treatment. In all cases of illness, occurring in a pregnant or breastfeeding mother, the clinician must endeavour to balance the risk of not treating the mother on both mother and baby against the risk to the fetus or infant of treating the mother. The more serious the illness is, the more likely it is that the risks of not treating outweigh the risks of treating.
- The risks to both mother and baby of a serious maternal mental illness are greater than the risks of medication.
- The fetus and baby is no less likely to suffer from the side-effects of psychotropic medication than an adult. Fetal and infant elimination of psychotropic medication is slower and less than adults and their central nervous systems more sensitive to the effects of these drugs.
- Adverse consequences of medication on the fetus and infant are dose-related. If medication is used it should be used in the lowest effective dose and given in divided dosage throughout the day.
- The exposure of the baby to psychotropic medication in breastmilk will depend on the volume of milk, the frequency of feeding, weight and age. A totally breastfed baby under 6 weeks old will receive relatively more psychotropic medication than an older baby who is partially weaned.

Antidepressants

Tricyclic antidepressants

Pregnancy

Tricyclic antidepressants (e.g. imipramine, lofepramine, amitriptyline and dosulepin) have been in use for 40 years. Tricyclic antidepressants are not associated with an increased risk of fetal abnormality, early pregnancy loss or growth restriction when used in later pregnancy. However clomipramine (Anaframil) has been linked to cardiac abnormalities. Newborn babies of mothers who were receiving a therapeutic dose of tricyclic antidepressants at the point of birth are at risk of suffering from withdrawal effects (jitteriness, poor feeding and on occasion fits). Consideration should therefore be given to a gradual tapering and reduction of the dose prior to birth.

Breastfeeding

The excretion of tricyclic antidepressants in breastmilk is very low. However doxepin should not be used because it has been reported to cause sedation in babies. Any adverse effects in the fully breastfed newborn baby can be minimized by dividing the dose, e.g. 50 mg of imipramine t.d.s.

Selective serotonin reuptake inhibitors

Pregnancy

Selective serotonin reuptake inhibitors (SSRIs) (e.g. fluoxetine, paroxetine, citalopram) have been in use for approximately 15 years and are now the antidepressants most used in the treatment of depressive illness at other times.

There has been some concern about the possible adverse effects of certain SSRIs in early pregnancy. The evidence continues to emerge and the risks are therefore difficult to quantify. There may be an increased risk of miscarriage associated with the use of all SSRIs. It is likely that there is an increased risk of cardiac abnormalities related to first trimester exposure to SSRIs, particularly ventricular septal defects (VSD) with paroxetine (Seroxat). This has led to both the manufacturer and the drug regulation authorities in the USA and the UK advising against the use of paroxetine in pregnancy. At the moment, this restriction does not apply to fluoxetine (Prozac) and sertraline (Lustral) but it remains to be seen whether this adverse effect is related to all SSRI medications. The NICE (2007) guidelines recommend that either tricyclic antidepressants or sertraline should be the treatment of choice if antidepressants are required during pregnancy. They also recommend that antidepressants should not be used for mild to moderate illness and that psychological treatments should be used wherever possible. However, the withdrawal of SSRI antidepressants in early pregnancy, particularly if the woman has been receiving them for some time, is often associated with a withdrawal syndrome or the recurrence of her condition. In such circumstances, consideration should be given to changing the woman to a 'safer' alternative or reducing the dose and supervised withdrawal.

Continued use of SSRI medication during pregnancy has been associated with pre-term birth, reduced crown–rump measurement and lower birth weight. Babies born to mothers receiving SSRI medication at the point of birth are likely to experience withdrawal effects, particularly those babies who are preterm. SSRIs, such as citalopram and fluoxetine that have a long half-life, are also associated with a serotonergic syndrome in the newborn (jitteriness, poor feeding, hypoglycaemia and sleeplessness). Consideration should therefore be given to reducing and withdrawing this medication before birth.

Breastfeeding

The excretion of SSRIs in breastmilk is higher than that of tricyclic antidepressants. The fully breastfed newborn may be vulnerable to serotonergic side-effects. Those SSRIs with a long half-life (fluoxetine and citalopram) should be avoided when breastfeeding the newborn. Venlafaxine and paroxetine are not recommended for use in breastfeeding mothers. However, in older and larger-weight infants, particularly those who are partially weaned, other SSRIs, particularly sertraline, may be less problematic.

Tricyclic antidepressants or sertraline should be the antidepressants of choice in breastfeeding.

Antipsychotics

There are two groups of antipsychotic medications, the older 'typical' antipsychotics (e.g. trifluoperazine, haloperidol, chlorpromazine) and the newer *atypical antipsychotics* (e.g. risperidone, olanzapine, clozapine).

Typical antipsychotics

Pregnancy

Typical antipsychotics have been in use for 40 years. There is no evidence that their use in early pregnancy is associated with an increased risk of fetal abnormality nor that their continuing use in pregnancy is associated with growth restriction or pre-term birth. However, antipsychotic medication freely passes to the developing fetus and its brain and the dose should be reduced to that which is the minimum for clinical effectiveness. Babies born to mothers receiving relatively high doses of typical antipsychotics may experience a withdrawal syndrome and extrapyramidal symptoms (muscle stiffness, rigidity, jitteriness and poor feeding). Consideration therefore should be given to a reduction of the dose before birth and a possibility of induction at term. Withdrawal of medication at any stage in pregnancy may be associated with a risk of a relapse of the maternal condition.

Breastfeeding

Typical antipsychotics are present in breastmilk, although the amount to which the infant is exposed is likely to be very small. The added benefits of breastfeeding to the infant probably justify the continuation of breastfeeding providing that the dose required is small and divided. Drugs such as procyclidine, given to prevent extrapyramidal side-effects, are not recommended.

Atypical antipsychotics

The manufacturers advise against the use of atypical antipsychotics in pregnancy and breastfeeding but this reflects lack of data rather than evidence of harm. The use of olanzapine in pregnancy has been associated with an increased risk of gestational diabetes. Women who become pregnant while taking these newer antipsychotics should be urgently reviewed. In some cases, it may be possible to change their medication to the older type of antipsychotic. In others, because of the substantial risk of relapse of their condition, it may be necessary to continue with their medication. Again this should be reduced to the lowest possible dose and consideration given to a further reduction immediately prior to birth and, if necessary, a managed delivery. Clozapine should not be used in pregnancy and breastfeeding because of the risk of blood dyscrasias in the infant.

Mood stabilizers

This is a group of drugs used to treat the manic component of bipolar illness and, long term, to prevent relapses of the condition. The drugs used as mood stabilizers are lithium carbonate (Priadel) and various anti-epileptic drugs, commonly sodium valproate and carbamazepine but also on occasion lamotrigine.

Pregnancy

Lithium carbonate in pregnancy is associated with a risk of developing a rare, serious cardiac condition, Ebstein's anomaly. Although the relative risk is large, the absolute risk is low, being 2 in 1000 exposed pregnancies. However, there is also an increased risk of a range of cardiac abnormalities, including milder and less serious conditions. The absolute risk of all types of cardiac abnormality is 10 per 100 exposed pregnancies. Lithium in early pregnancy is not associated with an increased risk of neural tube abnormalities.

The continued use of lithium throughout pregnancy is associated with an increased risk of fetal hypothyroidism, diabetes insipidus, fetal macrosomia and the 'floppy baby' syndrome (neonatal cyanosis and hypotonia). These risks are difficult to quantify. An additional problem is that the woman will require increasing doses of lithium in later pregnancy to maintain a therapeutic serum level because of the increased maternal clearance of lithium. However, the fetal clearance does not increase. Women receiving lithium in pregnancy therefore require frequent estimations of their serum lithium and close monitoring of their condition. During labour and immediately following birth, physiological diuresis can result in toxic levels of maternal lithium. The woman therefore requires frequent estimations of her serum lithium throughout labour and in the early postpartum days.

Women who are taking lithium carbonate should be advised to carefully plan their pregnancies and to seek medical advice. Abrupt cessation of lithium is associated with a substantial risk of a recurrence of their condition. These women will usually be advised to either slowly withdraw their lithium prior to conception or consider changing to another medication. However, there will be rare occasions when it is necessary to continue lithium throughout pregnancy. Such a pregnancy will need to be managed by an obstetrician working closely with psychiatric services and a fully compliant, well-informed woman.

Breastfeeding

Lithium should not be used in breastfeeding as it is present in substantial quantities in breastmilk and can result in infant lithium toxicity, hypothyroidism and 'floppy baby' syndrome.

Anticonvulsants

Anticonvulsants have been used as mood stabilizers for 30 years. Carbamazepine was first used in this way, sodium valproate is now increasingly the mood stabilizer of choice and recently the newer anticonvulsants such as lamotrigine and topiramate are being used.

Pregnancy

All anticonvulsants are associated with a doubling of the base-line risk of fetal abnormality if used in the first trimester of pregnancy. A total of 4 in 100 infants exposed to carbamazepine will have a major congenital malformation. The risk of cleft lip and palate is further increased with exposure to lamotrigine. The risks are highest with sodium valproate: 8 per 100 exposed pregnancies. The use of folic acid reduces but does not eliminate the risk of neural tube abnormalities. Continued use of anticonvulsants throughout pregnancy is associated with an increased risk of neurodevelopmental problems in the child. This is particularly high with sodium valproate. For this reason, NICE (2007) guidelines advise against the use of sodium valproate in pregnancy. Women receiving these medications should carefully plan their pregnancies with expert advice. They should, wherever possible, either have a supervised withdrawal of their medication or change to a 'safer' alternative. They should also take folic acid. If a woman becomes pregnant while still taking these medications, she should be urgently referred for expert advice and for an early fetal anomaly scan. As all harm is dose-related, the woman should be advised wherever possible to reduce her sodium valproate to below 1000 mg daily.

Breastfeeding

The advantages of breastfeeding probably outweigh the risks of taking carbamazepine or sodium valproate during breastfeeding. However, the infant should be monitored for excessive drowsiness and, in the case of sodium valproate, rashes. Lamotrigine should not be used in breastfeeding because of the increased risk of severe skin reactions in the infant.

Service provision

There are a number of national recommendations for the needs of women with perinatal psychiatric disorders Box 25.7. The distinctive clinical features of the conditions, their physical needs and the professional liaison with maternity services all require specialist skills and knowledge (Oates 1996). The frequency of the serious conditions at locality level makes it difficult for general adult psychiatric services to manage the critical mass of patients required to develop and maintain their experience and skills. It is difficult for maternity services to relate to multiple psychiatric teams. However, at supra-locality (regional) level, the frequency of serious perinatal psychiatric disorder is sufficient to justify the joint commissioning and provision of specialist services. Mothers, who require admission to a psychiatric hospital in the early months postpartum should, unless it is positively contraindicated, be admitted to a mother and baby unit. This is not only humane but also in the best interests of the infant and cost-effective as it shortens inpatient stay and

Box 25.7 **Perinatal mental health: national documents (regularly updated)**

Royal College of Psychiatrists CR88
SIGN Guidelines – postnatal and puerperal psychosis
CNST 2004
National Screening Committee
NICE guidelines on antenatal care: routine care for the healthy pregnant woman
NICE guidelines on antenatal and postnatal mental health
NICE guidelines on postnatal care: routine postnatal care of women and their babies
Department of Health Reports:
    Children's, young person and maternity NSF. Maternity Standard 11
    Women's mental health into the mainstream
    Responding to domestic abuse
CEMACH/CMACE 'Why mothers die' triennial reports

prevents re-admission. There should be specialist perinatal community outreach services available to every maternity service, to deal with psychiatric problems that arise postpartum but also to see women in pregnancy who are at high risk of developing a postnatal illness.

The majority of women suffering from postnatal mental illness will not require to be seen by specialist psychiatric services. However, there is a need for integrated care pathways to ensure that women are effectively identified and managed in primary care and, if necessary, referred on to specialist services. There is a need to enhance the skills and competencies of health visitors, midwives, obstetricians and GPs to deal with the less severe illnesses themselves.

PREVENTION AND PROPHYLAXIS

Prevention

The National Screening Committee (2001) and NICE (2007) guidelines do not recommend routine screening using the EPDS and other 'paper and pen' scales in the antenatal period for those at risk of postnatal depression. They also find that there is a lack of evidence to support antenatal interventions to reduce the risk of non-psychotic postnatal illness. In contrast, these and other bodies (DH 2004; NICE 2008; CMACE 2011) all recommend that women should be screened at early pregnancy assessment for a previous or family history of serious mental illness, particularly bipolar illness, because they face at least a 50% risk of recurrence of that condition following birth. Those who undertake early pregnancy assessment will need training to refresh their knowledge of psychiatric disorder.

There is little point in screening for women at high risk of developing severe postnatal illness if systems for the pro-active peripartum management of these conditions are not in place and if appropriate resources are not available. It is recommended that all women who are at high risk of developing a severe postpartum illness by virtue of a previous history are seen by a specialist psychiatric team during the pregnancy and a written management plan placed in the maternity records in late pregnancy and shared with the woman, her partner, her GP, midwife, obstetrician and psychiatrist.

Prophylaxis

If a woman has a previous history of bipolar illness or puerperal psychosis, consideration should be given to starting medication on day one postnatally. For bipolar illness the use of lithium carbonate has been shown to reduce the risk of a recurrence. It is plausible that the use of antipsychotic medication may also reduce the risk of recurrence. However, lithium is not compatible with breastfeeding. Some women will not wish to take medication when they perceive there is a 50% chance of them remaining well. They may also place a priority on continuing to breastfeed. Breastfeeding mothers at risk of developing a bipolar or mixed affective illness may take carbamazepine or sodium valproate. The evidence that antidepressants taken prophylactically may prevent the onset of a depressive psychosis is lacking. Antidepressants should be used with great caution in any woman who has bipolar disorder in her personal or family history because of the propensity of antidepressants to trigger a manic illness.

Hormones

There is no evidence that progesterone, natural or synthetic, prevents or treats postnatal depression or puerperal psychosis. Indeed there is evidence to suggest they may cause depression. While there is some evidence that transdermal oestrogens are effective in treating postnatal depression, the potential adverse physical effects (Dennis et al 1999) and the known efficacy of antidepressants mean this should not be the treatment of choice.

The most important aspect of preventative management and one that will promote early identification and the avoidance of a life-threatening emergency is close surveillance, contact and support in the early weeks, the period of maximum risk. A specialist community perinatal psychiatric nurse together with the midwife should visit on a daily basis for the first two weeks and remain in close contact for the first six. The local mother and baby unit should be aware of the woman's expected date of birth and systems put in place for direct admission if necessary.

The Confidential Enquiries into Maternal Deaths: psychiatric causes of maternal death

Confidential Enquiries into Maternal Deaths (Oates 2001, 2004, 2007, 2011) have found that suicide and other psychiatric causes of death are a leading cause (indirect) of maternal death in the UK, between 1997 and 2008, contributing to over 15% of maternal deaths.

Maternal suicide is more common than previously thought. Overall, the maternal suicide rate appears to be equivalent to that of the general rate in the female population. Suicide in pregnancy is less common. The majority of suicides took place in the year following birth, most in the first 3 months. Not only is the assumption of the 'protective effect of maternity' called into question but also the relative risk of suicide for seriously mentally ill women following childbirth is elevated. An elevated standardized mortality ratio (SMR) of 70 for women with serious mental illness in the postpartum year has previously been reported (Appleby et al 1998) and further confirmed by evidence from the Enquiries with improved case ascertainment.

In contrast to other causes of maternal death, suicide was not associated with socioeconomic deprivation. The majority of suicides were older, married and relatively socially advantaged and seriously ill. A worrying number were health professionals. This underlines the error of merging issues of maternal mental health with those of socioeconomic deprivation.

The majority of the suicides occurred violently by jumping from a height or by hanging. This stands in contrast to the commonest method of suicide among women in general (self-poisoning), and underlines the seriousness of the illness from which the women died.

Half of the suicides had a previous history of admission to a psychiatric hospital. In few cases had this risk been identified at booking and in even fewer had any proactive management been put into place. Had these women's illnesses been anticipated, a substantial number of these deaths might have been avoided.

Women also died from other consequences of psychiatric disorder. Some of these were due to accidental overdoses of illicit drugs. However, deaths also occurred from physical illness that would not have occurred in the absence of a psychiatric disorder. Some of these were the physical consequences of alcohol or illicit drug misuse, others from side-effects of psychotropic medication. However, a worrying number of deaths, some of which took place in a psychiatric unit, were due to physical illness being missed because of the psychiatric disorder or mistakenly attributed to a psychiatric disorder. These findings underline the importance of remembering that physical illness can present as or complicate psychiatric disorder. Suicide is not the only risk associated with perinatal psychiatric disorder. Box 25.8 identifies the four main categories of psychiatric deaths emerging from 'Saving Mothers' Lives' (Oates and Cantwell 2011).

These findings have major implications for psychiatric and obstetric practice. If psychiatrists discussed with women plans for parenthood prior to conception; if obstetricians and midwives detected those at risk of serious mental illness; if psychiatric and maternity professionals communicated freely with each other and worked together; if specialist perinatal mental health services were available for those women who needed them; and if all had a greater understanding of perinatal mental illness, then not only would a substantial number of maternal deaths be avoided but also the care and outcome of other mentally ill women would be greatly improved.

> **Box 25.8 The four main categories of psychiatric deaths emerging from 'Saving Mothers' Lives' (Oates 2007; Oates and Cantwell 2011)**
>
> - Suicide
> - Overdose of drugs abuse
> - Medical conditions caused by or mistaken for psychiatric disorder
> - Violence and accidents related to psychiatric disorders
>
> Note: New themes are included, concerning child protection and termination of pregnancy.

CONCLUSION

The full range of psychiatric disorders can complicate pregnancy and the postpartum year. The incidence of affective disorder, particularly at the most severe end of the spectrum, increases following birth. The familiar signs and symptoms of psychiatric disorder are all present in postpartum disorders as well, but the early maternity context and the dominance of infant care and mother–infant relationships exert a powerful effect on the content, if not the form, of the symptomatology. Early maternity is a time when there is an expectation of joy, pleasure and fulfillment. The presence of psychiatric disorder at this time, however mild, is disproportionately distressing. No matter how ill the woman feels, there is still a baby and often other children to be cared for. She cannot rest and is reminded on a daily basis of her symptoms and disability. Compassionate care and understanding and skilled care aimed at speedy symptom relief and re-establishing maternal confidence are thus essential.

REFERENCES

Adams S S, Eberhard-Gran M, Eskild A (2012) Fear of childbirth and duration of labour: a study of 2206 women with intended vaginal delivery. BJOG: An International Journal of Obstetrics and Gynaecology 119(10):1238–46

Alexandra J 1998 Confusing debriefing and defusing postnatally: the need for clarity of terms, purpose and value. Midwifery 14(2):122–4

Appleby L, Mortenson P B, Faragher E B 1998 Suicide and other causes of mortality after postpartum psychiatric admission. British Journal of Psychiatry 173(9):209–11

Barlow J, Kirkpatrick S, Wood D et al 2007 Family and parenting support in Sure Start Local Programmes. NESS: London

Barlow J, Smailagic N, Bennett C et al (2011) Individual and group based parenting programmes for improving psychosocial outcomes for teenage parents and their children. Cochrane Database of Systematic Reviews, Issue 3. Art. No. CD002964. doi: 10.1002/14651858

Beck C T 2009 Birth trauma and its sequelae. Journal of Trauma Dissociation 10(2):189–2003

Bick D, MacArthur C, Knowles H et al 2009 Postnatal care: evidence and guidelines for management. Churchill Livingstone, Edinburgh

Brown J, Small R, Faber B et al 2002 Early postnatal discharge from hospital for healthy mothers and term infants. Cochrane Library of Systematic Reviews, Issue 3. Update Software, Oxford

Choi P, Henshaw C, Baker S et al 2005 Supermum, superwife, super everything: performing femininity in the transition to motherhood. Journal of Reproduction and Infant Psychology 23(2):167–80

CMACE 2011 Saving mothers' lives: reviewing maternal deaths to make motherhood safer: 2006–2008. The Eighth Report of the Confidential Enquiries into Maternal Deaths in the United Kingdom. BJOG: An International Journal of Obstetrics and Gynaecology 118(Suppl 1): 1–203

Cooper P J, Murray L 1995 The course and recurrence of postnatal depression. British Journal of Psychiatry 166:191–5

Cooper P J, Murray L 1997 Effects of postnatal depression on infant development. Archives of Disease in Childhood 77:97–101

Cox J L, Murray D, Chapman G (1993) A controlled study of the onset, duration and prevalence of postnatal depression. British Journal of Psychiatry 163:27–31

Crittenden A 2001 The price of motherhood: why the most important job in the world is still least valued. Metropolitan Books, New York

Dean C, Kendell R E 1981 The symptomatology of puerperal illnesses. British Journal of Psychiatry 139:128–33

Dennis C L, Ross L E, Herxheimer A 1999 Oestrogens and progestins for preventing and treating postpartum depression. Cochrane Database of Systematic Reviews, Issue 3. Art. No. CD001690. doi: 10.1002/14651858

DH (Department of Health) 1999 National Service Framework for Mental Health: modern standards and service models. DH, London

DH (Department of Health) 2003a Mainstreaming gender and women's mental health. DH, London

DH (Department of Health) 2003b Choosing the best: choice and equity in the NHS. DH, London

DH (Department of Health) 2004 National Service Framework for children, young people and maternity services. Maternity services, Standard 11. DH, London

DH (Department of Health) 2007a Maternity matters: choice, access and continuity of care in a safe service. DH, London

DH (Department of Health) 2007b Our health, our care, our say: one year on. DH, London

DH (Department of Health) 2011 Preparation for birth and beyond: a resource pack for leaders of community group activities. DH, London

Elliot S 1994 Uses and misuses of Edinburgh Postnatal Depression Score in primary care: a comparison of models developed in health visiting. In: Cox J L, Holden J M (eds) Perinatal psychiatry: use and misuse of the Edinburgh Postnatal Depression Scale. Gaskell, London, p 221–8

Evans J, Heron J, Francomb H et al 2001 Cohort study of depressed mood during pregnancy and childbirth. British Medical Journal 323:257–60

Glover V, O'Connor T (2006) Maternal anxiety: its effect on the fetus and the child. British Journal of Midwifery 14(11):663–7

Grabowska C 2009 Unhappiness after childbirth. In: Squire C (ed) The social context of birth. Radcliffe Press, Oxford, p 236–50

Green J M, Coupland V A, Kitzinger J V 1998 Great expectations: a prospective study of women's expectations and experiences of childbirth. Books for Midwives, Hale, Cheshire

Gregoire A 1995 Hormones and postnatal depression. British Journal of Midwifery 3(2):99–104

Harris B, Lovett L, Newcombe R G 1994 Maternity blues and major endocrine changes: Cardiff puerperal mood and hormone study 2. British Medical Journal 308:949–53

Hodnett E D, Fredericks S, Weston J 2010 Support during pregnancy for women at increased risk of low birth weight babies. Cochrane Database of Systematic Reviews, Issue 2. Art No. CD000198. doi: 1002/14651858

Kendell R E, Chalmers J C, Platz C 1987. Epidemiology of puerperal psychoses. British Journal of Psychiatry 150:662–73

Lyons S 1998 A prospective study of post-traumatic stress symptoms 1 month following childbirth in a group of 42 first time mothers. Journal of Reproduction and Infant Psychology 16:91–105

Miller N M, Fisk N M, Modi N et al 2005 Stress at birth: determinants of cord arterial cortisol and links with cortisol response in infancy. BJOG: An International Journal of

Obstetrics and Gynaecology 112(7):921–6

Munk-Olsen T, Munk-Laursen T, Meltzer-Brody S et al 2012 Psychiatric disorders with postpartum onset: possible early manisfestations of bipolar affective disorders. Archives of General Psychiatry 69(4):428–34. doi:10.1001/archgenpsychiatry.2011.157

National Screening Committee 2001 A screening for postnatal depression. Department of Health, London

NHSLA (National Health Service Litigation Authority) 2011 Clinical Negligence Scheme for Trusts: Maternity Clinical Risk Management Standards Version 1 2011/12, London, NHSLA

NICE (National Institute for Health and Clinical Excellence) 2006 Postnatal care: routine postnatal care of women and their babies. CG 37. NICE, London

NICE (National Institute for Health and Clinical Excellence) 2007 Antenatal and postnatal mental health: clinical management service guidance. CG 45. NICE, London

NICE (National Institute for Health and Clinical Excellence) 2008 Antenatal care: routine care for the healthy pregnant woman. CG 62. NICE, London.

Nicholson P 1998 Postnatal depression: psychology, science and the transition to motherhood. Routledge, London

Oakley A, Hickey D, Rajan L et al 1996 Social support in pregnancy – does it have long term effects? Journal of Reproduction and Infant Psychology 14:7–22

Oates M R 1996 Psychiatric services for women following childbirth. International Review of Psychiatry 8:87–98

Oates M R 2001 Deaths from psychiatric causes. In: Lewis G, Drife J (eds) Why mothers die 1997–1999. The Fifth Report of the Confidential Enquiries into Maternal Deaths in the United Kingdom. RCOG Press, London

Oates M R 2004 Deaths from psychiatric causes. In: Lewis G, Drife J (eds) Why

mothers die 2000–2002. The Sixth Report of the Confidential Enquiries into Maternal Deaths in the United Kingdom. RCOG Press, London

Oates M R 2007 Deaths from psychiatric causes. In: Lewis G (ed) Confidential Enquiry into Maternal and Child Health (CEMACH) Saving mothers' lives: reviewing maternal deaths to make motherhood safer – 2003–2005. The Seventh Report on Confidential Enquiries into Maternal Deaths in the United Kingdom. CEMACH, London

Oates M R Cantwell R 2011 Deaths from psychiatric causes. In: Centre for Maternal and Child Enquiries (CMACE) Saving mothers' lives: reviewing maternal deaths to make motherhood safer: 2006–2008. The Eighth Report on Confidential Enquiries into Maternal Deaths in the United Kingdom. BJOG: An International British Journal of Obstetrics and Gynaecology 118(Suppl 1):1–203

O'Donnell K, O'Connor TG, Glover V (2009) Prenatal stress and neuro-development of the child: focus on the HPA axis and the role of the placenta. Development Neuroscience 31(4):285–92

O'Hara M W, Swain A M 1996 Rates and risk of postpartum depression – a meta-analysis. International Review of Psychiatry 8:87–98

ONS (Office for National Statistics) 2002 Living in Britain. General Household Survey No. 31. Office for National Statistics, London

ONS (Office for National Statistics) 2012 General lifestyle survey overview: a report on the general lifestyle survey. Office for National Statistics, London

Raynor M, England C 2010 Psychology for midwives: pregnancy, childbirth and puerperium. Open University Press, Maidenhead

RCPC (Royal College of Psychiatrists Council) 2000 Perinatal maternal mental health services. Report CR88. RCPC, London

Redshaw M, Heikkila K (2010) Delivered with care: a national survey of women's experience of maternity care 2010. National Perinatal Epidemiology Unit, Oxford

Robertson E, Jones I, Hague S et al 2005 Risk of puerperal and non-puerperal recurrence of illness following bipolar affective puerperal (postpartum) psychosis. British Journal of Psychiatry 186(6):258–9

Robling S A, Paykel E S, Dunn V J et al 2000 Long-term outcome of severe puerperal psychiatric illness: a 23 year follow-up study. Psychological Medicine 30:1263–71

Rouhe H, Salmela-Aro K, Gissler M et al (2011) Mental health problems common in women with fear of childbirth. BJOG: An International Journal of Obstetrics and Gynaecology 118(9):1104–11.

Rouhe H, Salmela-Aro K, Halmesmaki E et al (2009) Fear of childbirth according to parity, gestational age, and obstetric history. BJOG: An International Journal of Obstetrics and Gynaecology 116(7):67–73

Talge N M, Neal C, Glover V (2007) Antenatal maternal stress and long-term effects on child neuro-development: how and why? Journal of Child Psychology and Psychiatry 48:245–61

Teixeira J M A, Fisk N M, Glover V 1999 Association between anxiety in pregnancy and increased uterine artery resistance index: cohort based study. British Medical Journal 318:153–7

Waldenstrom U, Hildingsson I, Ryding E L (2006) Antenatal fear of childbirth and its association with subsequent caesarean section and experience of childbirth. BJOG: An International Journal of Obstetrics and Gynaecology 113(6):638–46

Webster J, Linnane J W J, Dibley L M et al 2000 Measuring social support during pregnancy: can it be simple and meaningful? Birth 27(2):97–103

Wessely S, Rose S, Bisson J 2000 Brief psychological interventions ('debriefing') for treating immediate trauma related symptoms and prevention of post traumatic stress disorder. The Cochrane Library of Systematic Reviews, Issue 3. Update Software, Oxford

Winson N 2009 Transition to motherhood. In: Squire C (ed.) The social context of birth. Radcliffe, Oxford, p 145–60

FURTHER READING

DiPietro J A (2012) Maternal stress in pregnancy: considerations for fetal development. Journal of Adolescent Health 51:S3–S8

Considers a number of methodological issues in strengthening understanding of the effects of stress/anxiety on fetal neuro-behaviour and possible consequences for the developing nervous system.

National Institute for Health and Clinical Excellence 2010 Pregnancy and complex social factors (CG 110). NICE, London

Addressing a variety of social complexities that may affect a woman's emotional wellbeing such as poverty, homelessness, domestic abuse, communication difficulties, refugee or asylum status, young teenage mother, substance misuse etc.

Shaw R L, Giles D C 2009 Motherhood on ice? A media framing analysis of older mothers in the UK news. Psychology and Health 24(2):221–36

An interesting discourse about how older mothers are portrayed in the popular media.

USEFUL WEBSITES

Department of Health: www.dh.gov.uk

Fathers Institute: www.fatherhoodinstitute.org/

Midwifery 2020: www.midwifery2020.org

Mothers and Babies: Reducing Risk Through Audits and Confidential Enquiries across the UK: www.mbrrace.ox.ac.uk

National Institute for Health and Care [formerly Clinical] Excellence: www.nice.org.uk

Perinatal Illness UK: www.chimat.org.uk (from April 2013 this charity has become part of Public Health England and the URL address is likely to change in the near future).

Scottish Intercollegiate Guideline Network: www.sign.ac.uk

Chapter |26|

Bereavement and loss in maternity care

Rosemary Mander

This chapter introduces the reader to issues relating to bereavement and loss in the maternity area. The intention is to facilitate better coping among staff and, thus, care for those affected. Throughout the chapter, particular attention is paid to the knowledge on which practice is based, such as research, evidence or personal experience.

THE CHAPTER AIMS TO:

- consider the meaning of bereavement and loss in maternity and childbearing
- contemplate the significance of bereavement and loss in maternity and childbearing
- discuss forms of loss
- draw on research evidence and other knowledge to review the care of those affected by loss.

INTRODUCTION

In 21st-century Western society, bereavement is closely linked with loss through death. In this chapter, to increase the relevance of these concepts, the focus is broadened to include other sources of grief that are likely to affect midwifery care. In widening the topic, the original meaning of 'bereavement' is reflected, which implies plundering, robbing, snatching or otherwise removing traumatically and, crucially, without consent. This meaning may conflict with the other part of the title – 'loss' – which is also widely used in this context. But any inconsistency is fallacious because, although bereavement involves 'taking' in various ways, the unspoken hopes and expectations invested in that which is lost remain irretrievable.

In many ways, loss in childbearing is unique, which is due to the awful contrast between the sorrow of death and the mystical joy of a new life. Additionally, the cruel paradox of the 'juxtaposition' of birth and death aggravates responses (Howarth 2001: 435). We tend to assume that birth and death are separated by a lifetime; this means that the experience becomes incomprehensible when they are unified (Bourne 1968). Although any childbearing loss is unique, the uniqueness of both the individual's experience and the phenomenon itself must be contrasted with the frequency with which 'lesser' childbearing losses happen. Such lesser losses include the reduction of the parents' independence, the woman's loss of her special relationship with her fetus at birth, or the family loss of the expected idealized baby when they recognize that the actual baby is all too real (Atkinson 2006). Central to this chapter is the woman losing a baby and her care by the midwife. The midwife draws on theory which, as in any care, is grounded in firm knowledge, such as research evidence. Such knowledge is utilized in skilled care to facilitate adjustment to these greater and lesser losses. Thus, as well as loss through death, other forms of childbearing-related loss are also considered.

GRIEF AND LOSS

Grief, like death and other fundamentally important matters, is a fact of life. All human beings invariably face grief in some form, possibly when young. Despite its universality, a woman in a higher income country experiencing childbearing loss may be too young to have previously encountered the grief of death. This is a further reason for the uniqueness of childbearing loss.

Attachment

Limited understanding of mother–baby attachment, or 'bonding', long prevented our recognition of the significance of perinatal loss. The strength of the growing relationship between the woman and her fetus emerged in a research project involving bereaved mothers (Kennell et al 1970). This relationship develops with feeling movement and experiencing pregnancy, including investigations such as ultrasound scans. Ordinarily, attachment continues to develop beyond the birth (Bowlby 1997). Attachment during pregnancy means that, should the relationship not continue, it must be ended as with any parting. Thus, the reality of the mother–baby relationship needs to be recognized before the loss can be accepted. These processes are crucial for the initiation of healthy grieving.

Grief

Through grieving we adjust to more serious, and lesser, losses throughout life. Healthy grief means that we can move forward, although probably not directly, from the initial distraught hopelessness. We eventually achieve some degree of resolution, or perhaps integration, which permits ordinary functioning much of the time. Through grief we learn something about both ourselves and our resources (Vera 2003).

Grief has been viewed historically as apathetic passivity, but it is really a time when the bereaved person actively struggles with the emotional tasks facing her; the term 'grief work' summarizes this struggle (Engel 1961). The stages of grief through which the person works have been described in various ways, but Kübler-Ross's (1970) account is memorable. These stages (Box 26.1) are not necessarily negotiated in sequence; individual variations cause the person to move back and forth between them before reaching a degree of resolution.

The initial response to loss comprises a defence mechanism protecting the individual from the full impact of the news or realization. This reaction comprises shock or denial, which insulates the bereaved person from the unbearably unthinkable reality. Facilitating coping with impending realization, this initial response allows some 'breathing space', during which the person marshals their emotional resources.

Denial soon becomes ineffective and awareness of the reality of loss dawns. Awareness brings powerful emotional reactions, together with physical manifestations. Sorrowful feelings emerge but, less acceptably, other emotions simultaneously overwhelm the bereaved person. These include guilt and dissatisfaction, as well as compulsive searching and, disconcertingly, anger. Realization dawns in waves as the bereaved person tries coping strategies to 'bargain' with herself to delay accepting the grim reality.

Box 26.1 **Stages of grief**

- **Shock and denial**
- Increasing awareness
  - Emotions: sorrow – guilt – anger
  - Searching
  - Bargaining
- **Realization**
  - Depression
  - Apathy
  - Bodily changes
- **Resolution**
  - Equanimity
  - Anniversary reactions.

When such fruitless strategies are exhausted, the despair of full realization materializes, bringing apathy and poor concentration, together with bodily changes. At this point, the bereaved person may show anxiety and physical symptoms, like depression.

When the loss is eventually accepted, it starts to become integrated into the person's life (Walter 1999). As mentioned already, this is not straightforward and may involve slow progress and many setbacks, with oscillation and hesitation. Although the person may never 'get over' the loss, it should eventually be integrated. This ultimate degree of 'resolution' is recognizable in the bereaved person's contemplation with equanimity of the strengths, and weaknesses, of the lost person and relationship.

Significance

Healthy grieving matters because it contributes to balance or homeostasis in the bereaved person's life. Grief helps people deal with the wounds inflicted by the greater and lesser losses of life. The hazards of being unable to grieve healthily have long been recognized in emotional terms, but there may be an association between perinatal loss and physical illness (Boyce et al 2002). This research suggested the woman's need for support regardless of the nature of the loss or the extent to which it is recognized, or her grief sanctioned, by society.

Culture

A general picture of healthy grieving, and individual variation, common to people of different ethnic backgrounds, has been described (Katbamna 2000). The manifestations of grief, and accompanying mourning rituals, vary hugely. These variations are influenced by many factors. Cecil (1996) shows the massive differences between ethnic groups in attitudes towards childbearing loss. A midwife may encounter difficulty understanding the different attitudes to loss in cultures other than her own (Mander 2006). Whether the midwife is able to work through such feelings, to support the woman with different attitudes, is uncertain. Closely bound up with culture, and influencing mourning, are the grieving person's religious beliefs, or lack thereof. These aspects, however, are difficult to separate from social class and prevalent societal attitudes.

Despite huge variations in its manifestation, mourning has a universal underlying purpose. It establishes support for those closely affected, by strengthening links between the people who remain. In perinatal loss the midwife initially provides this support. The midwife's role is to be with the woman when she begins to realize the extent of her loss and to prevent interference in the woman's healthy initiation of grieving.

FORMS OF LOSS

The terms 'loss' and 'bereavement' apply to a range of experiences, varying hugely in severity and effects (Despelder and Strickland 2001). We must be careful, however, to avoid assumptions about the meaning of loss to a particular person. It is difficult, even impossible, for anybody to understand the significance of a pregnancy or a baby to someone else. This is because childbearing carries a vast range of profound feelings, including unspoken hopes and expectations based on personal and cultural values. We should accept that grief in childbearing, like pain, is what the person who is going through it says it is (McCaffery 1979).

Some situations in which we encounter grief are mentioned. Some situations of childbearing grief are not included here, while some situations listed here may not engender grief.

Perinatal loss

When loss in childbearing is mentioned, loss in the perinatal period comes quickly to mind, which includes the stillborn baby and the baby dying in the first week. Attempts have been made to compare the severity of grief of loss at different stages, perhaps to demonstrate that certain women deserve more sympathy. A classic study investigating severity, however, showed no significant differences in the grief response between mothers losing a baby by miscarriage, stillbirth or neonatal death (Peppers and Knapp 1980). This study emphasized the crucial role of the developing mother–baby relationship – the understanding of which has facilitated changes in care.

Stillbirth

A retrospective Swedish study focused on the mother's long-term recovery from stillbirth. Rådestad and colleagues (1996a) compared the recovery of 380 women who had given birth to a stillborn baby with 379 women who birthed a healthy child. The 84% response rate shows the mothers' perception of the importance of this study. These researchers found that the mother recovered better if she could decide how long to keep her baby with her after the birth and if she could keep birth mementoes. The mother whose recovery was more difficult was the one where the birth of the baby was delayed after realization of fetal demise. Clearly, these findings have important implications for midwifery care (see section on The Mother, below). Additionally, the researchers discuss the 'known' stillbirth, when the mother knows before labour that her baby has died, previously termed 'intrauterine death' or 'IUD'. Alternatively, the loss is unexpected. While avoiding comparisons, it is understandable that the mother aware of carrying a dead baby bears particular emotional burdens. These burdens, compounded by the baby's changing appearance, may impede her grieving.

Early neonatal death

Grieving a liveborn baby who dies may be facilitated by three factors. First, the mother has seen and held her real live baby; giving her genuine memories. Second, United Kingdom (UK) legislation requires the registration of both the birth and death of a baby dying neonatally, providing written evidence of the baby's life. Third, staff investment in the care of this dying baby increases the likelihood of effective parental support (Singg 2003). Even for the mother whose preterm baby survives, though, there may still be elements of grief (Shah et al 2011).

Accidental loss in early pregnancy: miscarriage

Early pregnancy loss may be due to various pathological processes, such as ectopic pregnancy or spontaneous abortion. The word 'abortion' is better avoided in this context, because it carries connotations of deliberate interference, which are unacceptable to a grieving mother. The term 'miscarriage' is preferable, to include all accidental losses. The grief of miscarriage has long been ignored, because of its frequency. This has been estimated to be about one-third of pregnancies, although the figure may be higher (Oakley et al 1990).

Understanding the woman's experience of miscarriage has been sought through qualitative research, which shows miscarriage to be far from an insignificant event, with some mothers so ill that they fear for their lives. Although mothers find reassurance in the conception of the pregnancy that was lost, some come to doubt their fertility. As in other forms of loss, the mother finds difficulty in locating support and encounters comments denigrating her loss (Simmons et al 2006). It may be necessary to seek the cause of a woman's miscarriage, especially if it happens repeatedly (Hyer et al 2004). Although miscarriage has been linked with stressful life events, Nelson et al (2003) found no link between psychosocial stress and miscarriage. Limited recognition of miscarriage is now being addressed, and women are encouraged to create their own rituals to assist grieving. Brin (2004) showed the helpful nature of a religious service, of photographs or of communicating sorrow through writing a poem or letter.

Infertility

Grief associated with involuntary infertility is less focused than when grieving for a particular person (Lau 2011). In this situation the couple grieve for the hopes and expectations integral to the conception of a baby. Realization of their infertility, and the associated grief, is aggravated by the widespread assumption that conception is easy, which is sufficiently prevalent for the emphasis, in society generally and healthcare particularly, to be on preventing conception. Complex investigations and prolonged infertility treatment result in a 'roller-coaster' of hope and despair.

As with any grief, the couple in an infertile relationship grieve differently from each other, engendering tensions. Being told the diagnosis or cause of their infertility resolves some uncertainty, but raises other difficulties. These include one partner being 'labelled' infertile and, hence, 'blamed' for the couple's difficulty. A complex spiral of blame and recrimination may escalate to damage an already vulnerable relationship (Allen 2009). Clearly, counselling an infertile couple differs markedly from counselling those bereaved through death.

Relinquishment for adoption

Although long accepted that relinquishment is followed by grief (Sorosky et al 1984), the view persists that, because relinquishment is voluntary, grief is unlikely. Each mother in the study conducted by Mander (1995) was clear that her relinquishment was definitely involuntary and she had no alternative to relinquishment. These mothers really were 'bereaved' in the original sense (see Introduction, above).

The grief of relinquishment differs crucially from grief following death. First, after relinquishment grief is delayed. This is partly because of the woman's lifestyle and partly because of the secrecy imposed on the woman who does not mother her baby as is usual. Secondly, the grief of relinquishment is not resolved in the short or medium term. This is because, ordinarily, acceptance of loss is crucial to resolving grief. After relinquishment, such acceptance is impossible due to the likelihood that the one who was relinquished will make contact when legally able. Being reunited with the relinquished one was fundamentally important to the mothers interviewed. 'Rosa's' words reflect many mothers' hopes: 'I'd be delighted if she would turn up on the doorstep' (Mander 1995).

Termination of pregnancy (TOP)

Grief associated with termination of an uncomplicated pregnancy is problematic and for this reason it tends not to be included in the literature on grief. The experience of grief following TOP for fetal abnormality and of guilt following TOP do, however, tend to be recognized and accepted. In view of the frequency of TOP and the grief engendered, this deserves more attention.

TOP for fetal abnormality (TFA)

The package of investigations known as 'prenatal diagnosis' (see Chapter 11) may ultimately lead to the decision to undergo TFA. Although it may be assumed that the mother's reaction is solely one of relief at avoiding giving birth to a baby with a disability, Iles (1989) suggests reasons for a mother in this situation experiencing conflicting emotions that impede grieving:

- the pregnancy was probably wanted;
- the TFA is a serious event in both physiological and social terms;
- the reason for TFA may arouse guilty feelings;
- the recurrence risk may constitute a future threat;
- the woman's biological clock is ticking away;
- her failure to achieve a 'normal' outcome may engender guilt.

Interventions have been introduced to facilitate the grieving of the mother who has undergone TFA, which involve counselling and the creation of memories, as in other forms of child-bearing loss (see section on The Baby, below). A randomized controlled trial to study the effectiveness of psychotherapeutic counselling in such mothers with no other risk factors was undertaken by Lilford et al (1994). This study suggested that bereavement counselling makes no difference to the difficulty or duration of grieving. Additionally, the researchers concluded that mothers attending for counselling would probably have resolved their grief more satisfactorily than the control group anyway.

TOP for other reasons

The non-recognition of grief associated with TOP may be because the mother whose pregnancy is ended may be considered 'undeserving' of the luxury of grief. Further, this may be aggravated by her being blamed for her situation. Research on the psychological sequelae of TOP has focused on the guilt of having decided to end the pregnancy, as opposed to grief reactions; it may be that this focus is associated with the acrimonious abortion debate that continues in some countries. Thus, the grief and depression, presenting as tearfulness, were thought normal after termination of pregnancy (Wahlberg 2006). Perhaps these reactions could be prevented by counselling before, as well as after, the TOP.

The baby with a disability

For various reasons a baby may be born with a disability, which may or may not be anticipated. Disabilities vary hugely in severity and their implications for the baby. The mother may have to adjust to the possibility of her baby dying, but many conditions permit the continuation of a healthy life.

The mother's reaction to a baby with a disability will involve some grief. This is particularly true if the condition was unexpected, as the mother must grieve for her expected baby before relating to her real baby. The mother may be shocked to find herself thinking that her baby might be better off not surviving (Lewis and Bourne 1989). Although the mother may be reassured that such thoughts are not unique, she may still find it difficult to begin her grieving.

If a baby is born with an unexpected disability, the problem of breaking the news emerges. There are no easy answers to how this can be done to reduce the trauma, but clear, effective and honest communication is crucial (Farrell et al 2001).

The midwife's experience

The emotional reaction that may sometimes be experienced by the midwife may come as a surprise to her. Considering herself to be a professional person, she may be taken aback by the strength and complexity of her feelings when caring for a bereaved mother. This aspect has now begun to be addressed by research and to be opened up to debate (Kenworthy and Kirkham 2011; see Box 26.2).

LOSS IN HEALTHY CHILDBEARING

It may be hard to understand that, even in uncomplicated, healthy childbearing, grief may still present as a feature.

The 'inside baby'

The woman's grief may be because, despite obstetric technology, the mother is unable to view her baby before birth. Inevitably the real baby differs from the one whom she came to love during pregnancy. These differences may be minor, such as the amount of hair or crying behaviour. Lewis (1979) coined the term 'inside baby' to denote the one whom she came to love during pregnancy and who was perfect. The 'outside baby' is the real one, for whom she will care and who may have some imperfections, such as the wrong colour of hair. Clearly the mother may have moments of regret, during which she grieves the loss of her fantasy 'inside' baby, before being able to begin her relationship with her real baby.

The mother's birth experience

A further form of loss, over which the mother may need to grieve, is her loss of her anticipated birth experience. If she hoped for an uncomplicated birth, even some of the more common interventions may leave her feeling like a failure (Green and Baston 2003). Thus, in the same way as the woman may need to grieve her 'inside baby', even though all appears satisfactory, this disappointed mother has some grief work to complete.

Box 26.2 That sad day

This is a summary of feelings and thoughts when I discovered an intrauterine death at 41 weeks' gestation. The woman involved had been admitted for induction of labour and neither of us was prepared for this.

My heart sank when on initial palpation her abdomen felt cold and then the electronic fetal monitor did not detect the heart beat (I had just used the machine earlier). I knew, although it would be difficult, that I had to try and prepare her. I stayed later to try and give some continuity of care and support for her and her husband. After the scan confirmed the death I hugged her and her husband and cried with them. After this happened, I had a day off work with a severe migraine caused by stress. I felt very nervous and sick about going back to work, this was compounded when I discovered that the woman had been admitted to Intensive Care and was very ill. However, I did go back to work, visited the woman and sat holding her hand. We talked about her sadness and she said she had been worried about me leaving work late and wondered how I had coped getting home and facing my two children. I couldn't believe that she was concerned about me! She remembered every word I had said to her and praised my honesty. I had told her before the scan that I was sure that the baby had not survived. Two weeks later I attended the funeral in order to seek closure and to demonstrate my sympathy and sadness for the parents.

I have been a midwife for over 12 years and this has NEVER happened to me before. The whole event was very traumatic and upsetting for me. Some colleagues told me not to be upset, cry and/or get involved, but this was ineffective advice. I was so determined that my experience should not be in vain that I wrote this reflective piece. In total I have experienced the loss of over nine friends and relatives including my parents when I was fairly young. However, nothing can prepare someone (even a professional) for discovering that a baby has died and having to prepare the parents for this. Without the love and support of my family, friends and colleagues I would not have coped. As healthcare professionals we should be empathic and display understanding towards our colleagues in similar situations.

As Rosemary Mander [2004b] writes in 'When the professional gets personal':

for professional staff who provide effective care, there is likely to be a personal cost. These are the 'costs of caring', which may be regarded as the negative side of engaging with patients and clients and with one's work.

The whole experience will have a huge effect on my practice in various ways. I will encourage midwives to be honest with the clients. This will ensure that words are carefully chosen and also sensitively put, because they will be clearly remembered in years to come. I will not try to smooth over colleagues' feelings when they are involved in issues like this.

I am also going to liaise with the Local Supervising Authority to look at guidance for other midwives in situations like this. The success of the 'Birth Afterthoughts Service' within the Trust has led me to identify the need for a service for midwives dealing with bereavement and perhaps morbidity as well. Therefore, as a Supervisor of Midwives I aim to promote separate sessions for midwives – even if the midwife says she is unaffected. This will not be blame-based but will simply allow the members of staff to come to terms with their emotions and feelings by helping them to move on in a positive way.

To summarize, writing about this episode has been a catharsis for me and hopefully my experience will have a positive outcome for other staff who find themselves in the same sad and extremely difficult situation, and therefore benefit the parents as well.

Source: Reproduced with the kind permission of *The Practising Midwife*

CARE

In considering the care that midwives provide in the event of loss, there are difficulties in deciding where to begin. Thus, I have organized this section by focusing first on those who are involved or affected and then on other crucial issues. From this material will emerge the principles of midwifery care. While recognizing the artificiality of distinguishing care for the individuals involved in this complex situation, this approach helps us to consider the different needs among the people affected by the loss.

The baby

It is particularly hard to separate the care of the baby from the care of those who are grieving, because much of our care comprises the creation of memories of the baby, which will facilitate their grieving (Box 26.3). Midwives may think of the care of the baby before the birth by considering the cot in the labour room (Mander 2006). Although the cot's presence may cause the staff some discomfort, it reminds everybody of the baby's reality. If possible, that is if the baby's demise is known in advance, the midwife discusses with the parents prior to the birth their contact with the baby. This contact takes any of a number

---

Box 26.3 **Creating memories**

- Midwifery activities
  - Information-giving
  - Arranging for/taking photographs*
  - Cutting a lock of hair*
  - Taking a footprint*
  - Giving a cot card and/or name-band
- Parental activities
  - Naming baby
  - Seeing baby
  - Holding baby
  - Caring for baby: bathing – dressing
  - Taking photographs
- Other activities
  Writing in a book of remembrance
  Service/funeral/burial/cremation
  Tree planting
  Writing a letter and/or poem

*Parents' informed consent will be needed.

---

of forms, beginning with just a sight of the wrapped baby. Contact with the baby has been said to resolve some of the confusion surrounding the birth; but the benefits of such care have also been called into question (Hughes et al 1999).

The midwife faces the quandary of whether, and how much, she will encourage the mother to make contact with her baby, drawing on her understanding of its beneficial effect on grief (Mander 2006). This quandary is difficult, but midwives tend to be overcautious in encouraging the mother to have contact. This was an important finding from a study of 380 mothers who had experienced perinatal loss (Rådestad et al 1996b). These researchers found that one-third of the mothers would have appreciated more encouragement to have contact with their babies.

The mother may choose to have considerable contact with her baby, perhaps keeping the baby with her for some time. During this time, the mother may wish to have her baby baptized which, as well as its religious significance, emphasizes the baby's reality. This simple act, possibly undertaken by the midwife, additionally presents an opportunity to name the baby. The mother may also during this time have other opportunities to create memories of her experience; these include doing some of the things a mother ordinarily does for a baby, such as bathing and dressing him or her.

Irrespective of whether the mother chooses to have contact with her baby immediately, it is usual to collect certain mementoes at the time of the birth, such as a lock of hair, a footprint or photographs. If the mother chooses to have no contact at the birth she may later ask for these mementoes. Taking photographs of a suitable quality may present a challenge to the midwife who is not skilled in using a camera, causing dissatisfaction (Rådestad et al 1996b). Figure 26.1 shows the sensitive way in which a photograph may be used to help create memories of the birth.

In the hope of preventing a future loss, the parents may be advised that the baby should have a post mortem examination. This raises difficult issues for parents who consider that their baby has already suffered enough. In the UK there are guidelines providing information for the parents prior to seeking their consent for the post mortem. These guidelines aim to prevent certain abuses, which have previously caused anguish to bereaved parents (Dimond 2001; Royal College of Pathologists [RCP] 2000).

The funeral serves a multiplicity of purposes, including a demonstration of general support as well as establishing the reality of the loss. A young woman with no experience of death may have difficulty imagining how such a ritual could ever be beneficial. She may be helped, though, by being reminded how cemetery and crematorium staff are sensitive to the need to provide a suitable ceremony and a congenial environment in which the child may subsequently be remembered. In some situations, such as early miscarriage, a funeral is inappropriate. The mother may find that an impromptu service is helpful near the time of her loss or, later, she may create her own memorial by writing a letter to her lost baby or planting a tree. The care of this mother is particularly important if and when she decides to embark on another pregnancy (Reid 2007; Armstrong et al 2009).

The mother

Much of the midwife's care of the grieving mother comprises helping her to make sense of her mystifying experience. As mentioned already, the mother needs help to recognize that she has given birth, even though she no longer has her baby. Integral to this is assisting her realization that she is a mother, through midwifery care.

The mother may start to make sense of her loss by talking about it. Although this sounds simple enough, 'opening up' presents the mother with certain challenges. For example, she may be inexperienced and uncomfortable in talking about profound feelings. Further, she may have difficulty finding a suitable and willing listener precisely when she feels ready. The problem of her finding a listener was identified in a research project showing that senior hospital staff appear too busy, and other staff insufficiently experienced, for her to unburden herself. Family members, who might listen, have their own difficulties to face, making them less receptive to the mother's needs (Rajan 1994).

In a situation of loss, any of us may feel that our control over our lives is slipping away. Such feelings of losing

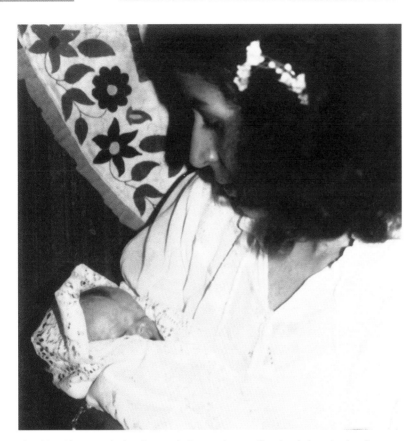

Fig. 26.1 Photograph showing a grieving mother cradling her baby, who has been named Baby Shane.

control are exacerbated when the loss involves a physiological process such as childbearing, which many people achieve successfully and effortlessly. Midwives should be able to help the mother to retain some degree of control. They can do this is by giving her accurate information about the choices open to her and on which she is able to base decisions. In this way, the midwife may be able to empower the woman and the two may form a partnership together.

The reality of the grieving mother's control over her care was the subject of research by Gohlish (1985). She interviewed 15 mothers of stillborn babies and asked them to identify the 'nursing' behaviours they considered most helpful. This study showed the importance to the grieving mother of assuming control over her environment. While the midwife may be keen to share many aspects of control in the form of decision-making with the grieving mother, there are some decisions that midwives consider unsuitable for the mother to make (Mander 1993). The suitable decisions include the contact that the mother has with her baby; whereas the unsuitable decisions may include the environment in which she is cared for during her hospital stay.

The support offered to the woman was the subject of a systematic review, which found that there is little evidence to indicate the effectiveness of psychological support at this time (Flenady and Wilson 2008). A randomized controlled trial by Forrest et al (1982) investigated the effects of support following perinatal loss. The experimental group, comprising 25 bereaved mothers, received ideal supportive midwifery care together with counselling; the control group comprised another 25 bereaved mothers who received standard care. Unlike the more psychotherapeutically oriented study by Lilford et al (1994), Forrest et al (1982) found that the well-supported and counselled group recovered from their grief more quickly than the control group. Unfortunately, both studies had difficulty retaining contact with the grieving mothers.

The mother may find helpful support in a number of people, who provide support on a more or less formal basis (Forrest et al 1982). Although we may assume that identifying support is easy, research by Rådestad et al (1996b) has shown that, like finding a suitable listener, locating support may be problematic for the mother. These researchers found that for just over one-quarter of bereaved mothers the support lasted for under 1 month;

while for just over another quarter the support was non-existent.

Of particular significance to midwives is the contribution of the lay support and self-help groups. Research by Mander (2006) showed that midwives are happy to recommend that a mother may find a support group, such as the Stillbirth and Neonatal Death Society (SANDS), helpful. Unfortunately, little is known about their effectiveness or the experiences of those who attend.

If the loss occurs while the woman is in hospital, her transfer home is crucially important, due to the likelihood of other agencies becoming involved. At this point good inter-agency communication ensures that the woman's healthy grieving is not jeopardized. In her large study, Moulder (1998) identified the quality of the help provided for the grieving mother by community agencies. She found that women experience very different standards of care from the various professionals, such as health visitors, general practitioners, community midwives and counselling personnel. Similarly, the 6-week follow-up presents an opportunity, not only to check the woman's physical recovery, but also to discuss important outstanding issues. These include the couple's emotional recovery from their loss, the post mortem results (if relevant), any questions arising or remaining, as well as plans for the future. The research by Moulder (1998) found that this follow-up visit is often handled appropriately sensitively, in a suitable environment, with appropriate personnel present and adequate time to address matters of concern. Unfortunately, though, some women's appointments were delayed and staff were condescending.

The family

The mother is clearly most intimately involved with, and affected by, a perinatal loss. To a greater or lesser extent, those close by will share her grief. In this context, the chapter includes, as well as conventional family members, a range of non-blood and non-marital relationships.

The father

The effect of the loss on the father may previously have been underestimated (Mander 2004a). This is partly because men tend to show their grief differently from women and partly because they are socialized into supporting their womenfolk, possibly at the cost of their own emotional well-being. Further, men are stereotypically unlikely to avail themselves of the therapeutic effects of crying and articulating sorrow. Men's coping mechanisms also involve less healthy grieving strategies, including returning early to work and using potentially harmful substances such as nicotine or alcohol.

Possibly in association with their different patterns of grieving (Samuelsson et al 2001), the parental relationship is likely to change following perinatal loss. Whether the couple find their relationship strengthened or threatened is unpredictable.

Other family members

Perhaps because they are less closely involved, grandparents may be disproportionately adversely affected by the loss, possibly due to their inability to protect their children (the bereaved parents) from painful loss. Inevitably and additionally they experience their own sense of loss at the threat to the continuity of their family and what that means to them.

The effects of perinatal loss on a sibling may be problematic because of uncertainty about the child's understanding of the event (Hayslip and Hansson 2003; Dyregrov 2008). This difficulty is compounded by the parents' difficulty in articulating their pain in a suitable form. The parents may seek to 'solve' these problems by 'protecting' their other child(ren) from the truth. They little know that 'protection' creates a pattern of unhealthy grieving, leaving a family legacy of dysfunctional relationships (Dyregrov 2008).

Whilst midwives often assume that family are best at supporting a grieving mother (Mander 1996), family responses may not always be healthy or helpful (Kissane and Bloch 1994).

The formal carers

The difficulty that staff face in caring for a grieving mother has been linked with their personal reactions to the loss of a baby (Bourne 1968). This may be the reason for the historical neglect of such mothers in particular and this topic in general. Furthermore, loss of a baby represents all too clearly the failure of the healthcare system, and those who work in it, to ensure a successful outcome to the pregnancy. The fear of failure in turn engenders a cycle of avoidance, which perpetuates neglect of the mother.

This vicious cycle has been interrupted so that as the care of the mother has been changed, it is necessary to question whether the care of staff has kept pace (Clarke and Mander 2006). The emotional costs of providing care are now being recognized (Kenworthy and Kirkham 2011). The devaluation of the emotional component of care is associated with increasing use of the medical model and contributes to the increasing recognition of 'burnout'. The need for extra support is particularly important for less experienced staff when providing care for grieving families (Mander 2000). The education of staff for their counselling role is another solution, which is enhanced by supervision for the counsellors. The role of the midwife manager in creating a supportive environment for staff in stressful situations should not be underestimated. The midwife may also be able to locate support in others alongside whom she works, such as the hospital minister or chaplain or her named Supervisor of Midwives. Additionally, there are helpful agencies which may be located within or outwith the healthcare system (see Useful Websites, below).

The involvement of staff in the mother's grief raises some difficult questions. First there is the helpfulness or otherwise of the midwife sharing the bereaved mother's tears. Although some midwives are prepared to cry alongside the mother, others feel that crying is 'unprofessional' and would not be comfortable shedding even a few tears. The midwives in Mander's (2006, 2009) research said that, generally, crying was not a problem; but any loss of control that impeded their ability to provide care must be avoided at all costs. Another difficult decision is whether staff should attend the baby's funeral. Some of the midwives interviewed found this helpful and they had not been uncomfortable attending. In some circumstances, however, this might not apply.

Other aspects of care

Not least because of their effect on grieving, other aspects of care assume greater importance.

Record-keeping and documentation

Record-keeping in this context becomes even more significant. This is because communication is vital in ensuring consistent care, which will facilitate the mother's grieving. Although not ideal, it may be difficult to avoid this care being provided by different personnel. Thus, each midwife must be able to learn from the mother's records about decisions and actions already taken (Horsfall 2001).

The cremation or burial

The documents required for the 'disposal' of the baby differ according to whether the baby was born before or after 24 weeks' gestation (the current legal limit of viability in the UK), according to whether the baby was born alive or not, and according to where the baby was born. If the baby was pre-viable, there is no legal requirement for the baby to be buried or cremated. It is, however, essential to ensure that the baby's remains are removed according to the mother's wishes. If she decides not to participate in the removal of the baby's remains, they should still be removed sensitively (Royal College of Obstetricians and Gynaecologists [RCOG] 2006). A book of remembrance in the maternity unit is available to parents to record their names, their baby's details and thoughts about the baby.

For a baby born after 24 weeks, burial or cremation may be arranged by the hospital, with the parents' permission, or by the parents. Cemeteries and churchyards are subject to individual regulation, but the local cemetery is likely to have a special plot for babies to be buried individually and a religious or other service may be available. There is also the possibility that the parents may erect a headstone, although the design may be subject to approval.

The statutory documentation is specific to each of the countries of the UK. Details of the registration requirements in each of the four countries of the UK are provided on the websites listed at the end of this chapter.

The mother's choices

If she loses her baby, as well as her grief work, the mother has certain choices. In terms of how the baby's body should be buried or cremated, the mother decides whether to arrange this privately or allow the hospital to organize it. The mother also needs to decide the extent to which she would like to be involved in planning the funeral, the blessing or the memorial ceremony. In some hospitals, services of remembrance are held on a regular basis, and bereaved parents choose whether to attend. As mentioned above, the mother needs appropriate information to decide about the funeral and post mortem.

THE DEATH OF A MOTHER

A form of loss that happens even less frequently than the death of a baby is when the mother dies; this is usually known as maternal death. In the UK, the rate of maternal death is approximately 1 in 10,000 births (Lewis 2011: 48). This means that in a medium-sized maternity unit a mother is likely to die about once every 3 years.

Although the obstetric and epidemiological aspects of maternal death have been well addressed (Maclean and Neilson 2002; Edwards 2004; Lewis 2011), the more personal aspects tend to be avoided (Mander 2001a). There is, however, little understanding of the family's experience, or the life of the motherless child. Palliative care principles may be appropriately applied to the care of the childbearing woman with or dying from an incurable condition (Mander 2011). The care of this woman and the implications for her baby and the other family members are likely to become increasingly important as women choose to delay child-bearing into their mature years. This childbearing woman's care has yet to be subjected to serious research attention.

However, the experience of the midwife providing care around the time of the death of a mother has begun to be addressed (Mander 2001b, 2004b). This research shows the dire implications for the midwife of attending a mother who dies, to the extent that the experience assumes the proportions of a disaster. The midwife's desperate need for support may be met by midwifery colleagues who either shared her experience or have been through a similar one. The midwife's family also plays a fundamentally important role in supporting her (Mander 1999).

CONCLUSION

This chapter has shown that, for the midwife's care of the mother grieving a loss in childbearing to be of a suitably high standard, there needs to be a suitably strong knowledge base. Although obtaining such knowledge is not easy, it is only by obtaining and using it that midwives are able to give this mother and family the high standard of care which they deserve and need. In this way, the midwife facilitates healthy grieving in the mother, having avoided the impediments that interfere with or complicate her grief and prevent its resolution. In this most human of situations, midwives must remember that 'being nice' is not enough; they need to ensure that midwifery care is based on a firm knowledge base if the woman is to come to terms with her loss. Other, less widely recognized or discussed forms of loss in childbearing have also been addressed.

REFERENCES

Allen H T 2009 Managing intimacy and emotions. In: Advanced fertility care. M&K Publishing, Keswick

Armstrong D S, Hutti M H, Myers J 2009 The influence of prior perinatal loss on parents' psychological distress after the birth of a subsequent healthy infant. Journal of Obstetric, Gynecologic and Neonatal Nursing 38(6):654–66

Atkinson B 2006 Gaining motherhood, losing identity? MIDIRS Midwifery Digest 16(2):170–4

Bourne S 1968 The psychological effects of stillbirth on women and their doctors. Journal of the Royal College of General Practitioners 16:103–12

Bowlby J 1997 Attachment and loss, vol 1: Attachment. Pimlico, London

Boyce P M, Condon J T, Ellwood D A 2002 Pregnancy loss: a major life event affecting emotional health and well-being. Medical Journal of Australia 176(6):250–1

Brin D J 2004 The use of rituals in grieving for a miscarriage or stillbirth. Women and Therapy 27(3/4):123–32

Cecil R 1996 The anthropology of pregnancy loss: comparative studies in miscarriage, stillbirth and neonatal death. Berg, Oxford

Clarke J, Mander R 2006 Midwives and loss: the cost of caring. The Practising Midwife 9(4):14–17

Despelder L A, Strickland A L 2001 Loss. In: Howarth G, Leaman O (eds) Encyclopedia of death and dying. Routledge, London, p 288–90

Dimond B 2001 Alder Hey and the retention and storage of body parts. British Journal of Midwifery 9(3):173–6

Dyregrov A 2008 Grief in children: a handbook for adults, 2nd edn. Jessica Kingsley, London

Edwards G 2004 Adverse outcomes in maternity care. Books for Midwives, Edinburgh

Engel G C 1961 Is grief a disease? A challenge for medical research. Psychosomatic Medicine 23: 18–22

Farrell M, Ryan S, Langrick B 2001 'Breaking bad news' within a paediatric setting: an evaluation report of a collaborative education workshop to support health professionals. Journal of Advanced Nursing 36(6):765–75

Flenady V, Wilson T 2008 Support for mothers, fathers and families after perinatal death. Cochrane Database of Systematic Reviews, Issue 1. Art. No. CD000452. doi: 10.1002/14651858.CD000452.pub2

Forrest G, Standish E, Baum J 1982 Support after perinatal death: a study of support and counselling after perinatal bereavement. British Medical Journal 285:1475–9

Gohlish M C 1985 Stillbirth. Midwife Health Visitor and Community Nurse 21(1):16–22

Green J M, Baston H A 2003 Feeling in control during labor: concepts, correlates, and consequences. Birth 30(4):235–47

Hayslip B, Hansson R O 2003 Death awareness and adjustment across the life span. In: Bryant C D (ed) Handbook of death and dying. Sage, Thousand Oaks, CA, vol 1, part IV, p 437–47

Horsfall A 2001 Bereavement: tissues, tea and sympathy are not enough.

Royal College of Midwives Journal 4(2):54–7

Howarth G 2001 Stillbirth. In: Howarth G, Leaman O (eds) Encyclopedia of death and dying. Routledge, London, p 434–5

Hughes P M, Turton P, Evans C D 1999 Stillbirth as risk factor for depression and anxiety in the subsequent pregnancy: cohort study. British Medical Journal 318:1721–4

Hyer J S, Fong S, Kutteh W H (2004) Predictive value of the presence of an embryonic heartbeat for live birth: comparison of women with and without recurrent pregnancy loss. Fertility and Sterility 82(5):1369–73

Iles S 1989 The loss of early pregnancy. In: Oates M R (ed) Psychological aspects of obstetrics and gynaecology. Baillière Tindall, London, p 769–90

Katbamna S 2000 'Race' and childbirth. Open University Press, Buckingham

Kennell J, Slyter H, Klaus M 1970 The mourning response of parents to the death of a newborn infant. New England Journal of Medicine 283(7):344–9

Kenworthy D, Kirkham M 2011 Midwives coping with loss and grief: stillbirth, professional and personal losses. Radcliffe Publishing, London

Kissane D, Bloch S 1994 Family grief. British Journal of Psychiatry 164:728–40

Köbler-Ross E 1970 On death and dying. Tavistock Publications, London

Lau A K L 2011 The experience of being treated for infertility in Hong Kong. Unpublished PhD thesis, University of Edinburgh

Lewis E 1979 Mourning by the family after a stillbirth or neonatal death. Archives of Disease in Childhood 54:303–6

Lewis E, Bourne S 1989 Perinatal death. In: Oates M (ed), Psychological aspects of obstetrics and gynaecology. Baillière Tindall, London, p 935–54

Lewis G 2011 The women who died 2006–2008. In: CMACE (Centre for Maternal and Child Enquiries) Saving mothers' lives: reviewing maternal deaths to make motherhood safer: 2006–08. The Eighth Report on Confidential Enquiries into Maternal Deaths in the United Kingdom. BJOG: An International Journal of Obstetrics and Gynaecology 118(Suppl 1): 1–203 (ch 1)

Lilford R, Stratton P, Godsil S et al 1994 A randomised trial of routine versus selective counselling in perinatal bereavement from congenital disease. British Journal of Obstetrics and Gynaecology 101(4):291–6

Maclean A B, Neilson J P 2002 Maternal morbidity and mortality. RCOG, London

Mander R 1993 Who chooses the choices? Modern Midwife 3(1):23–5

Mander R 1995 The care of the mother grieving a baby relinquished for adoption. Avebury, Aldershot

Mander R 1996 The grieving mother: care in the community? Modern Midwife 6(8):10–13

Mander R 1999 Preliminary report: a study of the midwife's experience of the death of a mother. RCM Midwives Journal 2(11):346–9

Mander R 2000 Perinatal grief: understanding the bereaved and their carers. In: Alexander J, Levy V, Roth C (eds) Midwifery practice: core topics 3. Macmillan, London, p 29–50

Mander R 2001a Death of a mother: taboo and the midwife. Practising Midwife 4(8):23–5

Mander R 2001b The midwife's ultimate paradox: a UK-based study of the death of a mother. Midwifery 17(4):248–59

Mander R 2004a Men and maternity. Routledge, London

Mander R 2004b When the professional gets personal – the midwife's experience of the death of a mother. Evidence Based Midwifery 2(2): 40–5

Mander R 2006 Loss and bereavement in childbearing, 2nd edn. Routledge, London

Mander R 2009 Good grief: staff responses to childbearing loss. Nurse Education Today 29(1):117–23

Mander R 2011 'Being with woman': the care of the childbearing woman with cancer. In: Fawcett T F and McQueen A (eds) Perspectives on cancer care. Wiley–Blackwell, London

McCaffery M 1979 Nursing management of the patient with pain. Lippincott, Philadelphia

Moulder C 1998 Understanding pregnancy loss: perspectives and issues in care. Macmillan, London

Nelson D B, Grisso J A, Joffe M M et al 2003 Does stress influence early pregnancy loss? Annals of Epidemiology 13(4):223–9

Oakley A, McPherson A, Roberts H 1990 Miscarriage. Penguin, Harmondsworth

Peppers L, Knapp R 1980 Maternal reactions to involuntary fetal/infant death. Psychiatry 43:55–9

Rådestad I, Steineck G, Nordin C et al 1996a Psychological complications after stillbirth. British Medical Journal 312:1505–8

Rådestad I, Nordin C, Steineck G et al 1996b Stillbirth is no longer managed as a non-event: a nationwide study in Sweden. Birth 23(4):209–16

Rajan L 1994 Social isolation and support in pregnancy loss. Health Visitor 67(3):97–101

RCOG (Royal College of Obstetricians and Gynaecologists) 2006 The management of early pregnancy loss. RCOG, London

RCP (Royal College of Pathologists) 2000 Guidelines for the retention of tissues and organs at post-mortem examination. RCP, London

Reid M 2007 The loss of a baby and the birth of the next infant: the mother's experience. Journal of Child Psychotherapy 33(2):181–201

Samuelsson M, Rådestad I, Segesten K 2001 A waste of life: fathers' experience of losing a child before birth. Birth 28(2):124–30

Shah, P E, Clements M, Poehlmann J (2011) Resolution of grief following preterm birth: implications for early dyadic interactions and attachment security. Pediatrics 127:284–92

Simmons R K, Singh G, Maconochie N et al 2006 Experience of miscarriage in the UK: qualitative findings from the National Women's Health Study. Social Science and Medicine 63(7):1934–46

Singg S 2003 Parents and the death of a child, Part 7. In: Bryant C D (ed) Handbook of death and dying. Sage, Thousand Oaks, CA, p 880–8

Sorosky A D, Baran A, Pannor R 1984 The adoption triangle. Anchor Books, New York

Vera M 2003 Social dimensions of grief, Part 7. In: Bryant C D (ed) Handbook of death and dying. Sage, Thousand Oaks, CA, p 838–46

Wahlberg V 2006 Memories after abortion. Radcliffe, Oxford

Walter T 1999 On bereavement: the culture of grief. Open University Press, Philadelphia, PA

FURTHER READING

Dickenson D, Johnson M, Samson Katz J 2000 Death, dying and bereavement, 2nd edn. Sage and The Open University, London
An easily readable examination of a wide range of issues.

Field D, Hockey J, Small N 1997 Death, gender and ethnicity. Routledge, London
The politics of loss.

Jones A 1996 Psychotherapy following childbirth. British Journal of Midwifery 4(5):239–43
An in-depth exploration of relevant psychoanalytical issues.

Kenworthy D, Kirkham M 2011 Midwives coping with loss and grief. Radcliffe, London

A thought-provoking, yet accessible, analysis of the midwife's experience of caring for a grieving woman.

Mander R 2006 Loss and bereavement in childbearing, 2nd edn. Routledge, London

A wide-ranging exploration of issues relating to childbearing loss, using research and other knowledges.

Schott J, Henley A 1996 Childbearing losses. British Journal of Midwifery 4(10):522–6

The implications of cultural and religious variations in the context of childbearing loss.

Thompson N 2002 Loss and grief: a guide for human services practitioners. Palgrave Macmillan, Basingstoke

Very relevant for midwives.

Walter T 1999 On bereavement: the culture of grief. Open University Press, London

A scientific examination of the social aspects of bereavement in general.

Wimpenny P, Costello J (eds) 2012 Grief, loss and bereavement: evidence and practice for health and social care practitioners. Routledge, London

Some up-to-date ideas and recent developments.

USEFUL WEBSITES

Registration and other statutory documentation of a stillborn baby

England & Wales: www.gro.gov.uk/gro/content/certificates/default.asp

Scotland: www.gro-scotland.gov.uk/regscot/registering-a-stillbirth.html

Northern Ireland: www.belfastcity.gov.uk/deaths/stillbirths.asp?menuitem=registering-a-stilldeath

Support groups

The Miscarriage Association: www.miscarriageassociation.org.uk/

SANDS (Stillbirth and Neonatal Death Society): http://uk-sands.org/

CRUSE Bereavement Care: www.crusebereavementcare.org.uk/

BLISS – The Premature Baby Charity: www.bliss.org.uk/

TCF – The Compassionate Friends (UK): www.tcf.org.uk/

Support for bereaved parents and their families.

Born with Wings: www.bornwithwings.co.uk/

Support for parents from parents.

EPT Ectopic Pregnancy Trust: www.ectopic.org.uk/

NORCAP: www.norcap.org.uk/

Support for adults affected by adoption.

Infertility Network UK: www.infertilitynetworkuk.com/

Advice, support and understanding.

SOFT UK: www.soft.org.uk/

Support organization for trisomy 13/18 and related disorders.

ARC Antenatal Results & Choices: www.arc-uk.org/

Incorporating SATFA (Support Around Termination for Abnormality).

Support for the Midwife

AIMS – Association for Improvements in Maternity Services: www.aims.org.uk/

Midwifery Supervisor and Local Supervising Authority

RCM – Royal College of Midwives: www.rcm.org.uk/

The Local Steward or Regional Officer can be contacted via the website.

Chapter |27|

Contraception and sexual health in a global society

Karen Jackson

Contraception and sexual health are important considerations for women of childbearing age. There are numerous ways in which women can control their fertility, but the choice of contraception will depend on a multitude of factors, including: method of infant feeding, age, culture, religion, access to contraception and previous experience. Women with additional challenges such as physical, sensory or cognitive needs, or those who do not speak or read English, may need extra support and information to enable them to make informed decisions about postpartum contraception.

THE CHAPTER AIMS TO:

- provide up-to-date knowledge of all forms of contraception
- emphasize the role of the midwife in providing contraceptive information and advice for women in their care.

THE ROLE OF THE MIDWIFE

The midwife has a unique and pivotal role in discussing contraception and sexual health. The Nursing and Midwifery Council (NMC) in the United Kingdom (UK) states that one of the activities of a midwife is to provide sound family planning information and advice (NMC 2012). Midwives are encouraged to take on a wider public health role and are in a key position to create and use opportunities to enable women to express their needs in respect of choice of contraception.

The most appropriate time to discuss sexual health, resumption of sexual activity and contraception will, in some respect, be dependent on the individual woman. Some midwives may feel that any encounter with post-natal women, even soon after giving birth, will capitalize on contraceptive and sexual health education opportunities. The National Institute for Health and Clinical Excellence (NICE) (2006) recommends that contraception advice should be imparted within a week of the birth. Issues such as loss of libido, adjustment to motherhood, breastfeeding, discomfort of the perineum, vaginal dryness and body image may also influence choice and use of a particular method of contraception (Faculty of Sexual and Reproductive Healthcare Clinical Effectiveness Unit [FSRH] 2009a). The use of a leaflet from the Family Planning Association (FPA) can be helpful as such leaflets are clear to understand in both text and illustration, and are in a variety of languages. The midwife should be familiar with the contraception and sexual health services available in the area in which she practises and know the system of referral to these specialist services.

For contraceptive methods discussed in this chapter, the efficacy rate is given as a percentage. This rate does not reflect the fact that fertility decreases with age and may be suppressed during lactation, or that the success of a method is partially dependent on motivation, experience of using the method and the teaching received on its use. It is recognized that if 100 sexually active women do not use any contraception, 80–90 of them will become pregnant within a year (FPA 2012). Sexual intercourse following childbirth is a hitherto seldom discussed issue. McDonald and Brown (2013) found in their study of 1507 primigravidae that almost 60% of the women had not resumed intercourse six weeks following the birth. Discussions need to take place well before this time to ensure no unintended pregnancies occur. Some women may even appreciate information on contraception in the antenatal period, to give them plenty of time to decide which contraceptive method would be right for them. Partnership working between the new mother and midwife is essential and conversations regarding contraception should take place in a quiet, relaxed setting, with the midwife having up-to-date knowledge on all methods available.

In the UK, all contraception is available free of charge from the National Health Service (NHS). This is different in other parts of the world, with a range of charges for certain methods of contraception.

HORMONAL CONTRACEPTIVE METHODS

The combined hormonal contraceptive pill

The combined oral contraceptive pill (COC or 'the pill') (Fig. 27.1) came as a breakthrough, in 1960, in terms of women being in a better position to control their fertility. This method has subsequently proven to be both effective and safe. The overall use varies greatly between countries but it is estimated to be used by approximately 1% of Japanese women who are married or in a union, 53% in Germany, 28% in the UK and 50% of women in Western Europe (Guillebaud and MacGregor 2013). In the UK, approximately 95% of women under the age of 30 have used oral contraceptives at some time. Around 100 million women rely on the pill worldwide (Guillebaud and MacGregor 2013).

The combined pill contains the synthetic steroid hormones *oestrogen* and *progestogen*. All COCs available in the UK contain ethinyl oestradiol, with the exception of Norinyl-1, which contains mestranol and Qlaira which contains estradiol valerate. There are a variety of COCs available containing different progestogens. This accounts for subtle differences in their biological effects and provides women with a wide choice. The most commonly used pills in the UK are *monophasic* pills, which deliver a constant dose of steroids throughout the packet. 'Everyday' pills contain 28 pills in each packet, 21 of which are active monophasic pills while the seven remaining pills contain no hormones (FPA 2012).

Also available are *biphasic* and *triphasic* pills, in which the dose of steroids administered varies in two or three phases throughout the packet to mimic the natural fluctuations of the hormones during the menstrual cycle. These pills are less commonly used in the UK. A relatively new pill, called Qlaira, is licensed in the UK; it is a complex *quadraphasic* pill designed to give optimal cycle control. It is taken every day but has two placebo tablets.

The first generation COC pills contained large doses of oestrogen and were associated with a high risk of deep vein thrombosis. They were replaced in the late 1960s with pills that had lower doses of oestrogen and progestogen. They were equally as effective as the earlier pills, being much safer and better tolerated. The progestogens in these second generation pills were norethisterone and levonorgestrel. The third generation pills, which came along in the mid-1980s, contained a variety of new synthetic progestogens,

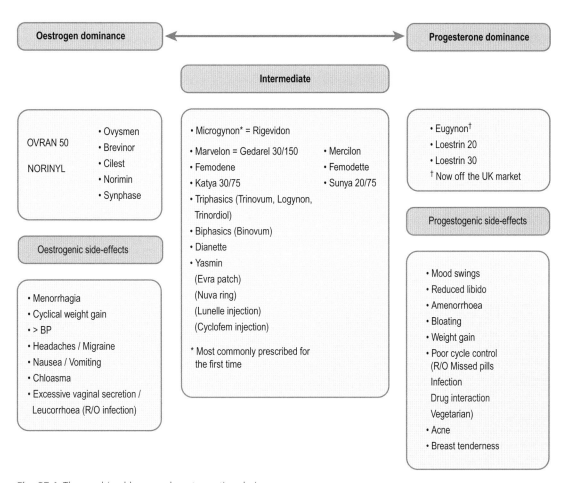

Fig. 27.1 The combined hormonal contraceptive choices.

that appeared to have better effects on serum lipid profiles. Among these were desogestrel and norgestimate, which were also less androgenic; gestodene, which was the most potent, achieving the best cycle control; and cyproterone acetate, which was anti-androgenic but licensed only as a treatment for acne. Drospirenone has been available from the late 1990s, with mild antimineralocorticoid activity to counteract oestrogen-induced water retention. It is also anti-androgenic.

Mode of action

Combined oral contraceptives work primarily by preventing ovulation. The first seven active pills in a packet inhibit ovulation and the remaining pills maintain anovulation (FSRH 2011a).

Oestrogen and progestogen suppress follicle stimulating hormone (FSH) and luteinizing hormone (LH) production causing the ovaries to go into a resting state; the ovarian follicles do not mature and ovulation does not normally take place. Progestogen also causes the cervical mucus to thicken, making penetration by spermatozoa difficult. The pill renders the endometrium unreceptive to implantation by the blastocyst. These actions provide additional contraception in the event of breakthrough ovulation occurring.

Efficacy

Provided that the pill is taken correctly and consistently, and that it is absorbed normally and interaction with other medication does not affect its metabolism, its reliability with *consistent perfect use* is almost 100% (Guillebaud and MacGregor 2013).

Important considerations

The combined oral contraceptive pill is a reliable contraceptive, which is independent of sexual intercourse and has many advantages. Healthcare providers should manage consultations for contraceptive pills with due regard for the woman's personal context and contraception experience.

Additional benefits of taking the COC pill, in the short term, are regular, lighter, less painful periods, possible reduction in premenstrual symptoms, reduction in acne, protection against pelvic inflammatory disease (PID) (because of the thickened cervical mucus), decreased incidence of ectopic pregnancy and reduced risk of benign breast disease. Taken long term, COC pills offer protection against ovarian and endometrial cancers and reduction in the incidence of ovarian cysts and benign ovarian tumours (FSRH 2011a).

Use of the COC pill may lead to side-effects such as irregular bleeding, headaches, nausea and breast tenderness; there is little evidence to support the association of weight increase, depression and COC use (FSRH 2011a). These effects often diminish with continued use or may improve with a change of pill. A basic knowledge of the side-effects attributable to the components of the COC pill is helpful when making decisions about changing pills.

Oestrogen dominance in a pill may cause water retention, resulting in breast tenderness, mild headaches, elevated blood pressure and cyclical weight gain. It may also be responsible for nausea and vomiting, excessive vaginal secretion (*leucorrhoea*) and skin pigmentation similar to chloasma. The progestogens may lower mood and libido, provoke acne and seborrhoea and cause mastalgia.

The vast majority of women experience no adverse effects. Every woman is unique in their biological response and also in their perception and tolerance of side-effects. The metabolic effects of the COC pill can occasionally result in major side-effects. The risks of venous thromboembolism (VTE) with the COC pill, in absolute terms, show a rarity of VTE in women of reproductive age (see Table 27.1). The risk of VTE is higher in women with a Body Mass Index (BMI) over 30, heavy smokers, those with a previous history of deep vein thrombosis or a family history of venous thrombosis and those who are immobile.

Allan and Koppula (2012) concluded that the risks of VTE when comparing all COCs appear to be unclear, but if there are differences they are likely to be very small and similar, therefore, any of the COCs may be considered for prescription if this method has been chosen for contraception.

Some women may develop a significantly high blood pressure, which could increase the potential for haemorrhagic stroke and myocardial infarction. Hypertension with a blood pressure (BP) between 141/91 mmHg and 159/94 mmHg is considered to be at a level of risk that outweighs the benefits of using the COC. Hypertension with BP of 160/95 mmHg or higher poses an unacceptable health risk with COC use (FSRH 2011a).

Cigarette smoking is known to potentiate most of the risks associated with COC pill use such as ischaemic and haemorrhagic stroke and myocardial infarction (FSRH 2011a).

The research surrounding the risk of developing breast cancer for COC users is largely contradictory, but it is widely acknowledged that there is a small increase in this risk (FPA 2012). Any excess risk of breast cancer associated with COC use declines in the first ten years after discontinuing the pill.

Studies show a small increase in the relative risk of cervical cancer, which is associated with a long duration of use (Guillebaud and MacGregor 2013). However, the effects of confounding factors such as sexually transmitted infections (STI), non-use of barrier methods and a high number of sexual partners may distort an accurate understanding of the influence of the COC pill.

Contraindications to COC pill use are pregnancy, undiagnosed abnormal vaginal bleeding, history of arterial or venous thrombosis (or predisposing factors such as immobility), hypertension, focal migraines, current liver disease, trophoblastic disease (until serum human chorionic gonadotrophin [hCG] is no longer detectable), smoking (if the woman's age is over 35 years) and a BMI over 39. This is not an exhaustive list. As the pill is not suitable for everyone, women wishing to consider using this form of contraception should have a full history recorded and be fully informed and counselled regarding possible side-effects.

Using the COC pill

When initially commencing the pill, the very first pill is usually taken on the first day of the menstrual period (for *postpartum use*, see later). Starting on any day up to the fifth day is just as effective, provided the first seven pills are taken correctly. If a 21-day pill has been prescribed, the contraceptive effect is immediate, provided that the remainder of pills in the packet are taken correctly. If the pill is initially commenced on any day beyond the fifth day of the cycle, additional contraception (such as a condom) should be used in conjunction with the pill for the first **seven** days. It is recommended that Qlaira is taken

Table 27.1 Risks of venous thromboembolism	
	Risk of VTE per 10 000 woman years
Not using COC	4–5
COC users (risk depends on type of COC)	9–10
In pregnancy	29
Immediate postpartum	300–400
Adapted from FSRH 2011a	

on the first day of the menstrual cycle, and if taken on any other day, additional contraception should be used for **nine** days. One pill is taken every day for 21 days, then no pills for the next seven days. Vaginal bleeding usually occurs within the seven day break, before the next packet of pills is commenced (FPA 2012).

When commencing the *'Everyday'* (ED) COC pill, the active pills are taken first. One pill is taken daily, with care to take the pills in the correct order. Vaginal bleeding will usually occur when the inactive pills are taken, which are usually denoted by a different coloured section on the pill packet. If two or more pills have been missed, or the next pack of pills is two or more days late, the advice given in Fig. 27.2 should be followed. If a pill is forgotten from the beginning or end of a packet, the pill-free interval is lengthened and ovulation may be more likely to occur (FSRH 2011a). If a woman is concerned about a missed or late pill, she can contact the local contraception clinic or General Practitioner (GP) for reassurance or advice, as emergency contraception may be indicated (see later).

Other factors that may render the pill less effective include interaction with other medication, vomiting within 2 hours of taking a pill and severe diarrhoea. Medications that may hinder the effectiveness of the pill include liver-enzyme-inducing drugs such as rifampicin, some anticonvulsants and some herbal remedies, for example St John's wort. After absorption, synthetic oestrogen and progestogen are transported to the liver via the portal vein. Liver-enzyme-inducing drugs reduce the efficacy of the pill by increasing the metabolism, and

subsequent elimination of oestrogen and progestogen in the bile. Some newer antiepileptics are not enzyme inducers but the COC pill may reduce seizure control with lamotrigine.

Please note that additional precautions are no longer required when taking antibiotics (non-enzyme inducing) (FSRH 2011a).

The advice to be given in cases of an illness with severe vomiting and diarrhoea is to follow the missed pill rules. It is important that women are made aware of possible drug interactions and inform their medical practitioner/GP that the COC pill is being taken whenever other medications are prescribed.

Preconception considerations

It is useful to wait for one natural period after discontinuing the pill before trying to conceive as dating the pregnancy can be more accurate and pre-pregnancy care can begin.

Postpartum considerations

The combined oral contraceptive pill reduces milk supply, particularly if lactation is not well established, and is therefore not recommended for use in the early months in lactating women. If the mother is bottle-feeding her baby, the COC pill may be commenced 21 days postpartum. This allows the high oestrogen levels of pregnancy to decrease before introducing the pill (Guillebaud and MacGregor 2013), thus reducing the risk of thromboembolism, but

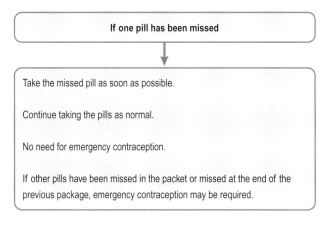

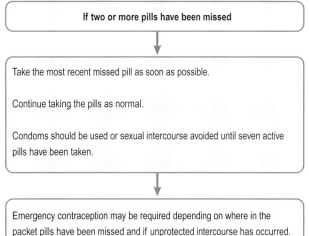

Fig. 27.2 Missed pill rule (FSRH 2011b).

allowing the contraceptive effect to be initiated before ovulation resumes. Women who have experienced pregnancy-induced hypertension should be assessed on an individual basis with regard to recommencing COC use (Guillebaud and MacGregor 2013).

The COC pill can be commenced immediately following spontaneous miscarriage or therapeutic termination of pregnancy. Due to the risk of thromboembolism, the COC pill should be discontinued 4 weeks before major surgery and a progestogen-only method of contraception used. If this is not possible, then thromboprophylaxis and compression hosiery are advised. Women who have minor surgery do not need to discontinue taking the pill.

Further postpartum considerations for discussion with the mother may include whether remembering to take the pill will fit into her current lifestyle and if she can easily access a clinic or doctor's surgery. Appropriate follow-up, including blood pressure assessments, should be conducted. Following the first prescription, follow-up is usually at 3 months postpartum and thereafter it may be annually.

The combined hormone injectable (Lunelle)

Lunelle contains 25 mg medroxyprogesterone acetate and 5 mg estradiol cypionate. It is not yet licensed in the UK due to its poor uptake and subsequent withdrawal from the market in the United States of America (USA), but it is popular in South America and Asia (Guillebaud and MacGregor 2013). Lunelle is commenced on the first day or within five days of a menstrual period, and given every 28–33 days. It is both effective and reversible. Side-effects include breakthrough bleeding and weight gain. The efficacy is comparable with perfect use of the COC pill. Cyclofem and Mesigyna are similar monthly injections also available to women in many countries outside of the USA, mainly in South America and Asia.

The combined hormone patch

The combined hormone patch (EVRA) was licensed in the UK in 2003. One patch is used weekly for three weeks followed by one week patch-free. It is particularly suitable for women who are unable to tolerate oral medications and those with malabsorption syndrome. It releases 20 mg of ethinyl oestradiol and 150 mg of norelgestromin every 24 hours. Compliance and cycle control may be improved. The efficacy of the combined hormone patch is comparable with the COC pill. The patch may be worn on most places on the body except the breasts. It is extremely sticky and should stay on during showering or swimming.

The FPA (2011a) suggest it may be used from day 21 in the postnatal period. However, if the mother is breastfeeding her baby, the patch should not be recommended as it will reduce breast milk production.

The combined hormone vaginal ring

The combined hormone vaginal ring (NuvaRing) is inserted into the vagina on the first day of the menstrual cycle. If inserted at any other time additional contraception such as condoms should be used for seven days. It is then used continuously for three weeks followed by one week free of its use. It releases 15 mg of ethinyl oestradiol and 120 µg of etonogestrel per 24 hours. The NuvaRing appears to be acceptable to many women and well tolerated, with studies finding that compliance and cycle control are also remarkably good (Roumen et al 2006; Brucker et al 2008). The efficacy of the NuvaRing is comparable with the COC pill.

The progestogen-only pills

Progestogen-only pills (POP) were introduced partly to avoid the side-effects of oestrogen in the combined pill, as discussed earlier. They also offer increased choice for women. Currently available in the UK are the older preparations, which contain norethisterone (Noriday, Micronor), etynodiol diacetate (Femulen) and levonorgestrel (Norgeston) and the new anovulant progestogen-only pills containing desogestrel (Cerazette). All have lower doses of progestogen compared with the COC pill.

Mode of action

The POP exerts its contraceptive effects at different levels. The cervical mucus is viscid, making it impenetrable to spermatozoa and the endometrium is modified to prevent implantation. The older POPs have been shown to suppress ovulation in up to 60% of women. The new POP Cerazette is anovulant and also suppresses FSH and LH consistently such that it is effective in about 97% of women (FSRH 2008a).

Limitations to POP use include menstrual disturbances, encompassing unpredictable and quite often prolonged bleeding, oligomenorrhoea or amenorrhoea. Little is understood about the mechanism of erratic uterine bleeding, which most women experience to some degree. The menstrual disruption is the most common reason for discontinuation of progestogen-only methods. This indicates the need for careful explanation of the limitations to potential users.

An increased prevalence of functional ovarian cysts has been demonstrated in women using progestogen-only pills. These may settle with continuation of use and will resolve if the POP is discontinued.

Contraindications to the use of progestogen-only-pills are pregnancy, undiagnosed abnormal vaginal bleeding, severe arterial disease and hydatidiform mole (until serum hCG is no longer detectable). The rate of ectopic pregnancy in women using the progestogen-only pill is no higher than in women using no contraception; however, the POP prevents uterine pregnancy more effectively than tubal pregnancy. This is not a problem with the anovulant POP Cerazette.

Antibiotics do not adversely affect progestogen-only methods of contraception but women should be advised to consult the doctor/GP regarding possible interactions if any other medications (especially enzyme inducers such as rifampicin) are prescribed.

Preconception considerations

There is no evidence of a teratogenic effect with the POP.

Postpartum considerations

Progestogen-only-pills may be commenced 21 days postpartum for contraception. These pills have no adverse effect on lactation. Secretion of the hormone in breast milk and absorption by the neonate is minimal and does not affect the short-term growth and development of infants. The POP can be used immediately following spontaneous miscarriage or therapeutic termination of pregnancy.

Using the POP

The POP is taken every day as there are no pill-free days and thus tablets are taken throughout the menstrual period. If the first tablet is taken on the first to fifth day of the menstrual cycle, the contraceptive effect is immediate. If the POP is started on any other day of the cycle then additional contraception, such as a condom, should be used for the first two days (FSRH 2008a).

If a pill is *forgotten*, the woman has only 3 hours in which to remember to take it. If the woman is over 3 hours late in taking a pill, she should continue taking her pills and use additional contraception for the next two days. However, with the anovulant POP Cerazette, the woman has up to 12 hours in which to remember to take the forgotten pill.

Following vomiting or severe diarrhoea, additional contraception should be used until two days after the illness ceases. Women concerned about missed or late pills should be advised to contact their contraception and sexual health clinic or GP, as emergency contraception may be indicated (see later). The effects of broad-spectrum antibiotics on the gut flora do not affect the action of the POP.

Efficacy

The effectiveness of the older POP is dependent upon meticulous compliance. With perfect use, the POP is more than 99% effective (FSRH 2008a).

LONG ACTING REVERSIBLE CONTRACEPTION (LARC)

Contraceptives that are used daily or weekly sometimes fail because of non-adherence or incorrect use. A LARC is defined by NICE (2005) as contraceptive methods that require administration less than once per menstrual cycle or month. These guidelines recommend giving women wider access to long acting reversible contraceptive (LARC) methods, as a feasible way to reduce unintended pregnancy (NICE 2005). Long acting reversible contraceptive methods are considered to be more reliable and cost-effective than other methods.

Long acting reversible contraceptive methods include injectable progestogen contraceptives, intrauterine contraceptive devices (IUCD), intrauterine hormonal systems and subdermal contraceptive implants. These are all available in the UK but usage remains low due to inadequate awareness of their availability and access as most GPs and practice nurses do not fit implants and intrauterine methods of contraception.

For a long acting method to be initiated, informed choice is crucial because only women who have realistic expectations may tolerate protracted side-effects. The implants and intrauterine systems are expensive, therefore a reasonable continuation rate is pertinent.

Progestogen injections

The two contraceptive progestogen injections currently available in the UK are Depo-Provera, or depot medroxyprogesterone acetate (DMPA), and Noristerat (norethisterone enanthate). Both methods are given by deep intramuscular injection.

DMPA is the method of choice for many women, not simply those for whom other methods are contraindicated. Over 6 million women use this method in 130 countries worldwide, and in some countries, for example South Africa, it is the most commonly used reversible method. In the UK, less than 2% of women attending contraception clinics use injectables. The progestogen injections prevent ovulation, thicken cervical mucus and cause atrophy of the endometrium.

Depot medroxyprogesterone acetate

This is the most commonly used injectable and is given in a 150 mg dose at 12 week intervals. It is released slowly from the injection site into the circulation. DMPA is more than 99% effective. Prolonged spotting, however, is a common side-effect in the first year but amenorrhoea often prevails in long-term use. Some DMPA users experience other side-effects such as breast discomfort, nausea, vomiting, weight gain, seborrhoea, acne and mood swings. It is now recognized that amenorrhoea for more than two years with DMPA is associated with chronic low serum oestrogen and reduced bone density. All women choosing DMPA should be aware of this information. Teenagers, who will not have attained peak bone mass, should be advised to use other methods. The peak bone mass is attained around the age of 30 years. Women who have been amenorrhoeic for more than three years receiving DMPA should have their bone density assessed with dual X-ray absorptiometry (DEXA) scan. It may be reassuring to learn that reduced bone mineral density (BMD) when using DMPA does not progress indefinitely but usually stabilizes after about five years. The BMD returns to normal after discontinuation (Scholes et al 2005).

Depot medroxyprogesterone acetate can offer additional health benefits for women with homozygous sickle cell haemoglobinopathy by reducing haemolytic and bone pain crises (Guillebaud and MacGregor 2013).

After discontinuation of DMPA, there may be a delay in the return of fertility for up to 18 months.

Norethisterone enanthate (NET-EN)

Marketed as Noristerat, this injectable contraceptive is given intramuscularly in a 200 mg dose at 8 week intervals. It is used more commonly in Germany and many developing countries. Noristerat is more than 99% effective and its side-effects are similar to DMPA.

Using injectable progestogens

If the initial injection is given within the first five days of the menstrual period (preferably days 1 to 3), the contraceptive effect is immediate. If given at any other time, the practitioner must ensure that there is no likelihood of pregnancy already and advise that additional contraceptive cover is required for the next seven days (Guillebaud and MacGregor 2013).

Specific considerations

This method is irreversible from the time of action, therefore any side-effects may be present until the injection wears off. The efficacy of DMPA and NET-EN is not affected by concurrent use of liver enzyme-inducing medications.

Preconception considerations

Injectable progestogen is not recommended as contraception for women who plan to conceive soon.

Postpartum considerations

Injectable progestogen contraceptives can be given prior to the 21st day postpartum, thus preventing the earliest ovulation; however, the woman must be warned about the increased risk of bleeding. It can be used by women who are breastfeeding their baby but delaying commencement until 6 weeks postpartum is often advised to ensure lactation is well established and reduce bleeding problems.

Subdermal contraceptive implants

Contraceptive implants have been used internationally for several years. Norplant was used in the UK from 1993 and replaced by Implanon from 1999. Nexplanon, however, replaced Implanon in 2010. The differences in the more recent implant are that the rod is radio-opaque, containing barium in order to locate it on X-ray if necessary, and it has a pre-loaded applicator which has been designed to reduce insertion errors.

Using implants

Implants are capsules containing progestogen, which are inserted under local anaesthetic into the inner aspect of the non-dominant upper arm (Fig. 27.3). The steroid is released into the circulation, producing a change in the cervical mucus which prevents spermatozoa penetration, disturbance of the maturation of the endometrium and suppression of ovulation.

Norplant, which had six capsules containing levonorgestrel, has been replaced by Norplant 2 (also marketed as Jadelle), which has two capsules. Jadelle is effective for 5 years and still available in many developing countries. Nexplanon and Implanon are single contraceptive rods containing 68 mg of etonogestrel. These single contraceptive rod devices should be inserted during the first five days of the menstrual cycle and no additional contraceptive cover is required. Ovulation is suppressed within 24 hours. They are effective for 3 years but can be removed at any time if the woman wishes. After removal, the serum

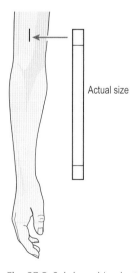

Actual size

Fig. 27.3 Subdermal implant.

is cleared of etonogestrel within 1 week and fertility is promptly regained.

Efficacy

Norplant is more than 99% effective. Nexplanon and Implanon have practically zero failure rates if instructions are carefully followed (Guillebaud and MacGregor 2013). Reported implant failures are often due to interaction with enzyme-inducing medications used concurrently, failing to recognize that the implant has been incorrectly inserted and failing to recognize the woman is pregnant before the fitting.

Specific considerations

Irregular bleeding is the most common problem for women using subdermal contraceptive implants. Only 20–30% of users become amenorrhoeic, however headache, seborrhoea, acne and mood swings have also been reported as side-effects. Insertion and removal require a minor surgical procedure, with accompanying risks of bleeding and infection. These aspects should be discussed prior to the woman making her decision. Counselling before fitting and during use appears to be the only way to reduce premature discontinuation due to the side-effects.

Preconception considerations

The action of the implant is quickly reversible and ovulation can return within 21 days of removal in 94% of women (FSRH 2008b). This makes it suitable also for women wishing to 'space' pregnancies.

Postpartum considerations

If the implant is inserted up to or at 21 days postpartum it is effective immediately; however, if it is inserted after the 21st day postpartum, additional contraception, such as a condom, should be used. The implant is safe for women who are breastfeeding their babies. The implant can also be inserted immediately after miscarriages or induced terminations of pregnancy. No extra contraceptive precautions need to be taken.

Intrauterine contraceptive device (IUCD)

These devices are inserted into the uterus, as illustrated in Fig. 27.4. They contain copper, which increases contraceptive efficacy. There seems to be an aversion for the use of IUCDs and progestogen-releasing intrauterine systems (IUS) in the UK, where only 6% of women use them (Guillebaud and MacGregor 2013). The IUCD is the most popular method in some countries and 150 million women worldwide use IUCDs, of which 60 million are in China.

Mode of action

The IUCD creates an inflammatory response in the endometrium. Leucocytes are capable of destroying spermatozoa and ova. Gamete viability is also impaired by alteration of uterine and tubal fluids. Copper affects endometrial enzymes, glycogen metabolism and oestrogen uptake, thus rendering the endometrium hostile to implantation, consequently IUCDs are more than 99% effective (see Fig. 27.4A).

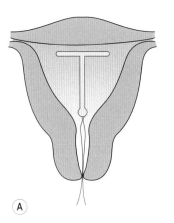 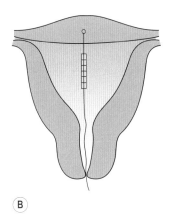 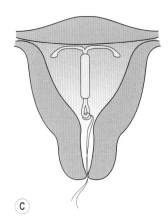

(A) (B) (C)

Fig. 27.4 Intrauterine contraceptive devices (IUDs). After insertion through the cervix, the framed devices assume the shape shown; the threads attached to it protrude into the vagina. (A) Copper-carrying device. (B) Frameless copper device. (C) Levonorgestrel-releasing system.

Using the IUCD

A copper IUCD can be inserted any time during the menstrual cycle if it is certain that the woman is not pregnant, or up to 5 days following the earliest estimated date of ovulation: that is, day 19 in a 28-day cycle, when it will be effective immediately. The woman may experience some discomfort during the procedure, which should be performed using aseptic techniques. Depending upon the type of IUCD used, it may be left in place from 5–10 years and longer in some instances; e.g. if a woman aged 40 years or over has an IUCD fitted, it may remain in place until one year after the menopause, if this occurs after the age of 50. Once *in situ*, the device requires no action of the user and it does not interfere with sexual intercourse. Women are usually taught to feel the threads attached to the IUCD on a regular basis as reassurance that it remains in place. A follow-up appointment in 3–6 weeks following insertion is recommended to assess for any infection, translocation or expulsion. Subsequently the woman requires further follow-up appointments only if she has any concerns. The traditional routine annual review is no longer recommended (NICE 2005).

Side-effects of using the IUCD include menorrhagia, dysmenorrhoea, bacterial vaginosis and colonization by *Actinomycetes*-like organisms. When the latter is reported in a routine cervical smear, the woman should be counselled about the options of either changing the IUCD or retaining it and being reviewed periodically to ensure there is no pelvic infection. Removal of the IUCD whenever desired is easy and painless, and fertility is promptly restored.

The suggestion that IUCDs promote pelvic inflammatory disease (PID) has been refuted. Clinical risk assessment for sexually transmitted infection (STI) is recommended (Guillebaud and MacGregor 2013). Routine or selective screening for chlamydia and gonorrhoea may be appropriate in some cases, where prompt treatment and contact tracing will be offered. Intrauterine contraceptive devices are associated with a decreased risk of ectopic pregnancies because of their effectiveness. However, in the unlikely event that a pregnancy should occur, the ratio of ectopic to intrauterine pregnancies is greater among women using IUCDs, as in general the device prevents more intrauterine pregnancies than ectopic pregnancies. Thus a woman who has an IUCD fitted should be advised to seek early medical advice, should she suspect that she is pregnant.

If uterine pregnancy occurs, there is an increased risk of spontaneous miscarriage, therefore gentle removal of the device is preferred, to prevent infection and premature labour. If removal is not possible, it is reassuring to know there is no evidence of teratogenicity in the fetus.

A newer frameless device, GyneFix, as shown in Fig. 27.4(B), comprising six copper sleeves crimped onto a polypropylene monofilament thread, is fitted with one end embedded into the fundal myometrium of the uterus. This device is associated with lower expulsion rates and less dysmenorrhoea.

Progestogen-releasing intrauterine system (IUS)

The intrauterine system was developed to overcome some of the problems associated with conventional IUCDs and heavy menstrual bleeding. The progestogen-releasing intrauterine system in current use consists of a small plastic T-shaped frame carrying a Silastic sleeve loaded with 52 mg of levonorgestrel (see Fig. 27.4C). It is inserted into the uterus and the steroid hormone is released steadily at 20 µg/day. The hormone prevents endometrial proliferation, thickens the cervical mucus and may suppress ovulation in some cycles. The frame, by inducing a sterile inflammatory reaction, may also contribute to the contraceptive effect. The system is fitted within the first seven days of the menstrual period, when the contraceptive effect is immediate. It is licensed for 5 years of use and is more than 99% effective. A new frameless device containing progestogen has already been developed (Fibroplant-LNG) and has been trialled in several countries, including Belgium. In addition, a lower dose T-frame IUS called Femilis (Femilis Slim for nulliparae) have been developed with trials also being undertaken in Belgium regarding its use and efficacy. It is not known, however, if these products will be introduced into the UK market in the near future.

Specific considerations

Irregular vaginal bleeding is common initially with the IUS, and then it gradually ceases. The uterine bleeding associated with the IUS is lighter than the menstrual period experienced when using a copper IUCD, with possible amenorrhoea in the long term. The failure rates of both intrauterine methods compare favourably with female sterilization.

Postpartum considerations

The IUS and copper IUCD have no adverse effect on lactation. They can be inserted 4 weeks after vaginal birth or Caesarean section (FSRH 2009b). Following miscarriage or induced termination of pregnancy, immediate insertion is safe.

BARRIER METHODS OF CONTRACEPTION (MALE AND FEMALE METHODS)

Barrier methods of contraception prevent the sperm coming into contact with the oocyte. These methods include male and female condoms, caps and diaphragms which can be used in conjunction with spermicidal preparations to further increase their efficacy.

Some of the advantages of using condoms are that they are easily available at many outlets in the UK and using them does not require medical intervention. They offer some protection against STIs (FPA 2011b) and cervical cancer and can be used with another method of contraception. This is often called '*double Dutch method*'. One of the main disadvantages of using barrier methods of contraception is the possible interruption to sexual intercourse, which may be off-putting for some couples.

It is good practice to ensure that anyone choosing a barrier method is also aware of emergency contraception and how to access it, should it be required.

Male condom

Some 4.4 billion couples worldwide use the male condom (Fig. 27.5) for contraception, with 6 billion couples using it for Human Immunodeficiency Virus (HIV) prevention. However, there are striking geographical differences. Japan accounts for more than one-quarter of all condom users in the world, being used by 75% of the contraception-using population. By contrast, and despite the substantial

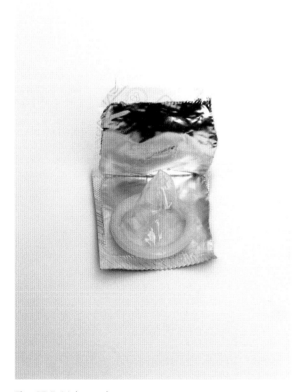

Fig. 27.5 Male condom.
Photograph K Jackson.

problem of HIV, the use of this method of contraception remains remarkably low in Africa, the Middle East and Latin America (Guillebaud and MacGregor 2013).

Guillebaud and MacGregor (2013) state that recent studies show approximately 25% of all couples in the UK use condoms but this may be occasional use or in addition to other methods. There are many varieties of condoms on the market, including latex, hypoallergenic and polyurethane. Polyurethane condoms are less sensitive to heat and humidity and not affected by oil-based lubricants (FPA 2011b).

Correct use of condoms is essential. Only condoms with a CE (European standard) mark should be used and the expiry date should be checked on the condom's package. Condoms should be stored away from extremes of heat, light and damp and care should be taken when handling the condom to prevent it from tearing. The condom is rolled on to the *erect penis before* any genital contact is made, as it is possible for some sperm to be present in the pre-ejaculate (Guillebaud and MacGregor 2013). About 1 cm of air-free space must be left at the tip of the condom for the ejaculate, otherwise the condom may burst. Some condoms are designed with a teat end for this purpose. The penis should be withdrawn very soon after ejaculation before it reduces in size and the condom becomes loose. The condom should be held in place during withdrawal of the erect penis so that it does not slip off. The condom should only be used once, and then disposed of in a waste bin: it should not be flushed down the toilet.

Oil-based lubricants can damage rubber condoms but not polyurethane types. Water-based lubricants are not known to cause damage and are therefore recommended.

The efficacy of the condom if used correctly is 98% but is dependent on experience and age of the user.

Female condom

The female condom consists of a polyurethane sheath that is inserted into the vagina (Fig. 27.6). The closed inner end is anchored in place by a polyurethane ring, while the outer edge lies flat against the vulva. It is available free from contraception clinics and may be purchased from selected chemists. Great care has to be taken to ensure that the penis is inserted *inside* the polyurethane sheath and not incorrectly positioned between the condom and the vaginal wall.

The efficacy depends on age and experience of the user, as with the male condom; however, the FPA (2011b) states that if it is used correctly it is 95% effective.

Diaphragm

A diaphragm consists of a thin rubber dome with a metal circumference to help maintain its shape (Fig. 27.7). A range of types and sizes are available and, in the UK,

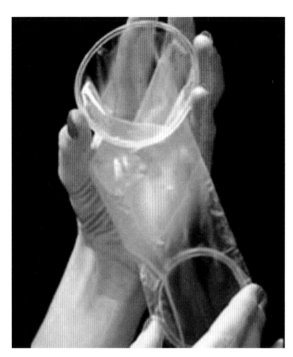

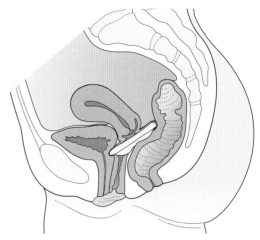

Fig. 27.8 The diaphragm in place.

Fig. 27.6 Female condom.
Image reproduced courtesy of Sciencephoto, with permission.

diaphragms are individually fitted at contraception clinics and some GP practices. Less than 1% of women use this method of contraception in the UK (Guillebaud and MacGregor 2013). It is not used widely in developing countries and Guillebaud and MacGregor (2013) believe this may be due to the fact that the device requires medical fitting.

When in place, the rim of the diaphragm should lie closely against the vaginal walls and rest between the posterior fornix and the symphysis pubis. Before insertion, a spermicide should be applied. After insertion, the woman has to check that her cervix is covered by the diaphragm (see Fig. 27.8). In order to preserve spontaneity during sexual intercourse, the diaphragm can be inserted every evening as a matter of routine.

If sexual intercourse occurs more than 3 hours after insertion of the diaphragm, then additional spermicide is required. The diaphragm must be left in place for at least 6 hours after the last intercourse, to ensure any sperm cannot reach the cervix. Once removed, the diaphragm should be washed with a mild soap, dried and inspected for any damage. A new diaphragm should be fitted annually or following a loss or gain in weight of more than 3 kg.

Efficacy depends on the age and experience of the user and the FPA (2010a) quote that it is between 92% and 96% effective if used according to their guidance.

Cultural beliefs may affect use of this method, for example in Judaism, where it is viewed as unacceptable to use any method of contraception that prevents the sperm from reaching its intended goal (Jogee 2004).

Postnatal considerations

The size of diaphragm should be reassessed at the 6th week postpartum, when the vagina and pelvic floor muscles will have regained some of their tone and

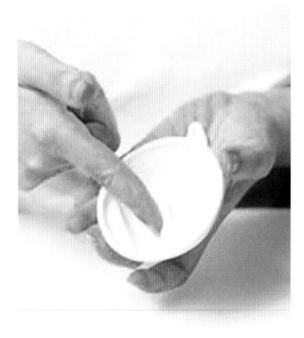

Fig. 27.7 The diaphragm.
Image reproduced courtesy of Sciencephoto, with permission.

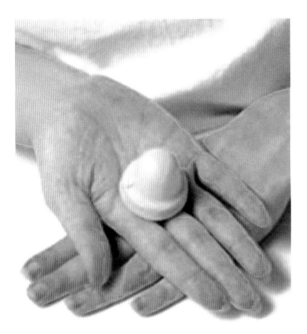

Fig. 27.9 The cervical/vault cap.
Image reproduced courtesy of Sciencephoto, with permission.

any tissue injury sustained from the birth will have healed.

Cervical and vault caps

Cervical and vault caps cover only the cervix, adhering to it by suction. They are made of rubber and look smaller in diameter than the diaphragm (Fig. 27.9). They require fitting at a contraception clinic. Only one cervical cap, the FemCap, is now available in the UK (Guillebaud and MacGregor 2013).

Spermicidal products

Spermicidal agents have not been shown to increase efficacy of condoms and because they can cause irritation to genitalia, may in fact increase the risk of HIV transmission. Use of Nonoxinol-9 lubricated condoms is no longer generally recommended. However, current advice is still to use this spermicide with the female barrier methods – diaphragms and caps – as this has been shown to be beneficial (Guillebaud and MacGregor 2013). Up until recently, a range of spermicidal products were available for use in the UK. However, the only product now available is Gygel, a clear gel containing Nonoxinol-9. Spermicidal pessaries are no longer available in the UK. Foams and aerosols are yet to be introduced into the UK market, but may well be available in other countries (Guillebaud and MacGregor 2013).

Efficacy

General teaching in the UK is that spermicidal products are not effective when used alone.

EMERGENCY CONTRACEPTION

Emergency contraception is required when contraception has not been used before, or during sexual intercourse, used incorrectly or when there is perceived to have been a failure in the contraception used, e.g. a condom mishap such as breaking, tearing or coming off. There are three types of emergency contraception:

- emergency hormonal contraception (EHC)
- selective progesterone receptor modulator (SPRM)
- copper intra-uterine contraceptive device (IUCD).

Emergency hormonal contraception (EHC)

EHC is a progestogen preparation with the brand name Levonelle which consists of one pill containing 1.5 mg of levonorgestrel and is available in many countries throughout the world. In the UK it is free from sexual health clinics, walk-in centres, some accident and emergency departments and GP practices. Many health centres and clinics provide EHC free of charge through selected pharmacies in an effort to reduce unwanted pregnancies. It can also be purchased over the counter from pharmacies.

This method works by delaying ovulation or preventing implantation of the fertilized oocyte, depending on the stage of ovulation. This method may be contraindicated if there has been more than one episode of unprotected sexual intercourse (UPSI) during the cycle, as the earlier sexual intercourse may already have resulted in a pregnancy. Very careful questioning by the practitioner needs to take place prior to supplying EHC to prevent an unfavourable outcome.

Nausea is uncommon with the progestogen-based pill but an additional pill may be required if the woman vomits within 2 hours of taking the medication. The next menstrual period may begin earlier or later than expected and it should be stressed that contraception must be used until the next period commences. If the woman receives the EHC in a contraception clinic in the UK, she is always given an appointment to return to the clinic if menstruation does not commence on time, or is shorter or lighter than usual. If menstruation is more than 7 days late, a pregnancy test will be offered. Any unusual lower abdominal pain must be investigated as this could be a sign of an ectopic pregnancy.

The efficacy of EHC depends on how quickly the emergency contraception is commenced. If taken within 24 hours of unprotected sexual intercourse, it will prevent

95% of pregnancies. This gradually decreases to 58% by 72 hours (FPA 2011c). There are very few contraindications to using this method but those health professionals administering Levonelle need to know about any other medication being used by the woman. Emergency hormonal contraception can be used more than once in each menstrual cycle, but it may disrupt the menstrual period pattern.

Selective progesterone receptor modulator (SPRM)

Ulipristal acetate with the brand name ellaOne is an emergency contraception that has been in use since 2009. In the UK ellaOne is free from sexual health clinics, walk-in centres, some accident and emergency departments and GP practices. It is given as a 30 mg oral dose which should be taken as soon as possible after UPSI or failed contraception. The action of SPRM is thought to be due to inhibition or delay in ovulation and alteration of the endometrium (Brache et al 2010). EllaOne is licensed for up to 120 hours following an exposure of risk to pregnancy. Only one dose of ellaOne can be taken per menstrual cycle. As with EHC, careful questioning within a consultation is required to ensure that there has been no previous risk of pregnancy either within a previous or the current menstrual cycle.

Randomized controlled trials (RCTs) have shown that ellaOne is at least as effective at preventing pregnancy as Levonelle, and pooled data demonstrate that ellaOne is more effective than EHC up to 120 hours following UPSI or failed contraception (FSRH 2011b).

Side-effects include abdominal pain, menstrual disorders such as irregular vaginal bleeding, disruption to the menstrual cycle with most women reporting lengthening of their cycle by 3 days; however, some women report a shortening of their cycle. Drug interactions can occur with liver enzyme-inducers such as carbemazepine and drugs that increase gastric pH, such as antacids. Ulipristal binds to progesterone receptors and therefore may reduce the efficacy of progesterone-containing contraceptives (FSRH 2011b).

Women may be asked to return to the clinic in 3-4 weeks to have a pregnancy test, or if menstruation is more that 7 days late.

The copper intrauterine device (IUCD)

The IUCD is the most effective method of emergency contraception, with a failure rate of less than 1%. Implantation of the fertilized oocyte is avoided if the IUCD is inserted within 5 days of UPSI or earliest estimated date of ovulation. This provides the clinician a much longer time range in which to offer emergency contraception. For example, in a regular 28-day cycle, the IUCD can be fitted up to day 19 of the cycle. It can then be left in place for use as a regular method of contraception, or removed during the next menstrual period.

COITUS INTERRUPTUS

Technically coitus interruptus should not be considered a form of contraception as it potentially has a high failure rate. It involves withdrawal of the penis from the vagina prior to ejaculation, and couples should be made aware of emergency contraception. Many euphemisms are used when referring to this, such as 'being careful' or the 'withdrawal method'. Andrews (2005) gives a rate of 90% effectiveness as a contraceptive. Failure is due to the small amount of semen that may leak from the penis prior to ejaculation with the potential of penetrating the ovum. The success of this method depends on the man exercising a great amount of self-control and is based on trust and honesty. This method is used widely throughout the world by different cultures and is the oldest form of contraception, being referred to in the Old Testament of the Bible.

FERTILITY AWARENESS (NATURAL FAMILY PLANNING)

The study of fertility awareness, previously (and sometimes still) referred to as *natural family planning*, is a fascinating observation of the way in which the female body works to produce the optimum conditions for conception.

According to UK Medical Eligibility Criteria for Contraceptive Use (FSRH 2009b), Natural Family Planning includes all the methods of contraception based on the identification of the fertile time in the menstrual cycle. The effectiveness of these methods depends on accurately identifying the fertile time and modifying sexual behaviour. To avoid pregnancy, the couple can either abstain from sexual intercourse or use a barrier method of contraception during the fertile time. Natural methods are attractive to couples who do not wish to use hormonal or mechanical methods of contraception. The midwife can provide the appropriate FPA leaflet, signpost the couple to the local contraception clinic or find local information on fertility awareness teachers and available education from the website: www.fertilityuk.com.

The method can also be used as a guide to women wishing to become pregnant, by concentrating sexual intercourse on the days they are most fertile. The fertile time lasts around 8–9 days of each menstrual cycle. The oocyte survives for up to 24 hours, however the FPA (2010b) suggest that a second oocyte could, occasionally, be released within 24 hours of the first. In addition, the FPA (2010b) state that as a sperm can live inside a female body for up to 7 days, this means that should sexual intercourse occur 7 days before ovulation, a pregnancy could result.

Fertility awareness methods

Physiological signs of fertility are:

- cervical secretions (Billings or ovulation method)
- basal body (waking) temperature
- cervical palpation
- calendar calculation.

Cervical secretions

Following menstruation the vagina will become dry. As oestrogen levels rise, the fluid and nutrient content of the secretions increases to facilitate sperm motility, consequently a sticky white, creamy or opaque secretion is noticed. As ovulation approaches the secretions become wetter, more transparent and slippery with the appearance of raw egg white that are capable of considerable stretching between the finger and thumb. The last day of the transparent slippery secretions is called the *peak day*, which coincides closely with ovulation. Following ovulation, the hormone progesterone causes the secretions to thicken forming a plug of mucus in the cervical canal, acting as a barrier to sperm. The secretions will then appear sticky and dry until the next menstrual period.

When practising this method of contraception, the cervical secretions are observed daily. The fertile time starts when secretions are first noticed following menstruation and ends on the third morning after the peak day. If the secretions are used as a single indicator of fertility, the presence of seminal fluid can make observation difficult. Changes in secretions will be affected by seminal fluid, menstrual blood, spermicidal products, vaginal infections and some medications (Guillebaud and MacGregor 2013).

Postpartum considerations

In the first 6 months following childbirth, the majority of women who are fully breastfeeding will be able to rely on the *lactational amenorrhoea method* (LAM) for contraception. Women who wish to continue using natural methods of contraception should begin observing cervical secretions for the last two weeks before the LAM criteria will no longer apply (i.e. 5 months and 2 weeks postpartum), in order to establish their basic infertile pattern.

Basal body temperature

A woman can calculate her ovulation by recording her temperature immediately on waking each day. Should the woman have arisen during the night, she must take at least

3 hours rest before recording her temperature. After ovulation, the hormone progesterone produced by the corpus luteum causes the temperature to rise by about 0.2 °C. The temperature remains at this higher level until the next menstrual period. The infertile phase of the menstrual cycle will begin on the third day after the temperature rise has been observed. Andrews (2005) points out that the temperature can be affected by infection, therefore care needs to be taken when interpreting temperature charts.

Postpartum considerations

A mother with the demands of a new baby may find difficulty in recording her temperature at the same time every day. Consequently many women prefer to rely on examining cervical secretions, or combine noting secretions with cervical changes at this time.

Cervical palpation

Changes in the cervix throughout the menstrual cycle can be detected by daily palpation of the cervix by the woman or her partner. After menstruation the cervix is low, easy to reach, feels firm and dry and the os is closed. As ovulation approaches, the cervix shortens, softens, sits higher in the vagina and the os dilates slightly under the influence of oestrogen.

Postpartum considerations

Hormonal changes in pregnancy take around 12 weeks to settle postpartum. The cervix will not revert completely to its pre-pregnant state as the os will remain slightly dilated even in the infertile time.

Calendar calculation

The calendar method (see Fig. 27.10) is based on observation of the woman's past menstrual cycles. When commencing to use this method, the specialist practitioner and the woman should examine the previous six menstrual cycles (Andrews 2005). The shortest and longest cycles

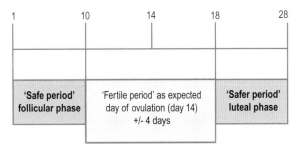

Fig. 27.10 Natural family planning: The fertility awareness (rhythm) method. Diagram to illustrate rhythm method of contraception in a 28-day menstrual cycle.

over the previous six months are used to identify the likely fertile time. The *first fertile day* is calculated by subtracting 21 days from the end of the shortest menstrual cycle. In a 28-day cycle, this would be day 7. The *last fertile day* is calculated by subtracting 11 days from the end of the longest menstrual cycle. In a 28-day cycle, this would be day 17. Cycle length is constantly reassessed and appropriate calculations made. Guillebaud and MacGregor (2013) indicate that the calendar method is not sufficiently reliable to be recommended as a single indicator of fertility, but is useful when combined with other indicators of fertility. Ovulation usually takes place 14 days before the first day of the next menstrual period. Therefore a woman who has a 28-day cycle would ovulate on approximately day 14 of her cycle and a woman who has a 30-day cycle would ovulate on approximately day 16 of her cycle.

Postpartum considerations

Calendar calculations must be recalculated once normal menstruation has recommenced.

Symptothermal method

This is a combination of temperature charting, observing cervical secretions and calendar calculation, with the option of observing cervical palpation in order to identify the most fertile time. Andrews (2005) also includes in this method the observation of *ovulation pain* or 'mittelschmerz' and cyclic changes such as breast tenderness. Use of more than one indicator increases the accuracy in identification of the fertile time. When combining indicators, a couple should avoid sexual intercourse from the first fertile day by calculation, or the first change in the cervix until the third day of elevated temperature, provided all elevated temperatures occur after the peak day.

Fertility monitoring device

These hand-held computerized devices monitor luteinizing hormone (LH) and oestrone-3-gluronide (a metabolite of oestradiol) through testing the urine. The most well known in the UK is the 'Persona' monitoring device which is about 94% effective and will detect from the urine test when a woman is fertile, indicating this through a series of lights. A green light indicates the infertile phase and a red light indicates the fertile phase, therefore barrier methods must be used should sexual intercourse be contemplated. A yellow light indicates that the database requires more information and a further urine test is required.

Postnatal considerations

The fertility monitor is not recommended as a method of contraception during lactation. The manufacturers of the Persona recommend that a woman has had two normal

menstruations with cycle lengths from 23 to 35 days before using the monitor at the beginning of the third period (Guillebaud and MacGregor 2013).

Lactational amenorrhoea method (LAM)

It is thought that the action of the infant suckling at the breast causes neural inputs to the hypothalamus. This results in the inhibition of gonadotrophin release from the anterior pituitary gland, leading to suppression of ovarian activity. The delay in return of postnatal fertility in lactating mothers varies greatly as it depends on patterns of breastfeeding, which are influenced by local culture and socioeconomic status. The time taken for the return of ovulation is directly related to sucking frequency and duration. The maintenance of night-feeds and the introduction of supplementary feeds also affects the return of ovulation.

The lactational amenorrhoea method (LAM) is a very effective method of contraception when used according to the Bellagio consensus statement (Guillebaud and MacGregor 2013). Research data concludes that there is over 98% protection against pregnancy during the first 6 months following birth if a woman is still amenorrhoeic and fully or almost fully breastfeeding her baby (FPA 2010b). In order to confirm that LAM remains effective as a contraceptive method, the woman should be asked if three questions (as indicated in Fig. 27.11) still apply. Mothers who work outside the home can still be considered to be nearly fully breastfeeding, provided they stimulate their breasts by expressing breastmilk several times a day.

The LAM is not recommended for use after 6 months following birth, because of the increased likelihood of ovulation. Studies throughout the world have been conducted on the effectiveness of LAM as a contraceptive,

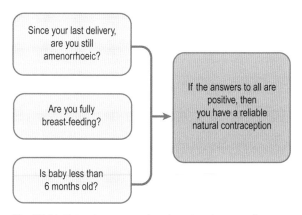

Fig. 27.11 Natural contraception: lactational amenorrhoea method (LAM).

confirming a rate of over 98% protection against pregnancy (Labbok 2012), suggesting it is a viable option for some postnatal breastfeeding women.

MALE AND FEMALE STERILIZATION

This is the choice of contraception for many couples once they have decided their family is complete. Sterilization should be viewed as permanent, although in a few cases reversal of the operation is requested. Couples requesting sterilization need thorough counselling to ensure that they have considered all eventualities, including possible changes in family circumstances. Although consent of a partner is not necessary, joint counselling of both partners is desirable. The procedure is available on the NHS for both sexes but waiting times can vary. There are no alterations to hormone production following sterilization in males or females and some couples find the freedom from fear of pregnancy very liberating.

Female sterilization

An estimated 600 million women worldwide have undergone female sterilization (Guillebaud and MacGregor 2013). During the procedure (Fig. 27.12), the uterine tube is occluded using division and ligation, application of clips or rings, diathermy or laser treatment.

The operation is performed under local or general anaesthetic. The procedure can be performed via a laparotomy, minilaparotomy or laparoscopy. It can also be performed vaginally using a hysteroscope. The procedure usually requires a day in hospital.

Women are advised to continue to use contraception for four weeks following the procedure, or in the case of hysteroscopic sterilization (Essure) contraception should continue for 3 months, after which successful tubal blockage is confirmed by hysterosalpingography (FPA 2010c). The couple should be advised to seek medical help urgently if they suspect pregnancy following sterilization because of the increased risk of ectopic pregnancy if the procedure is unsuccessful.

Postpartum considerations

Should sterilization occur around the time of birth, it is vital that the woman receives thorough counselling prior to the procedure to avoid any regret later on. Women are often advised to wait 6 weeks after the birth before undergoing the procedure. The FRSH (2009a) suggest that if sterilization is going to be undertaken at the same time as an elective caesarean operation, then one week or more should be provided for counselling and decision-making before the procedure finally takes place.

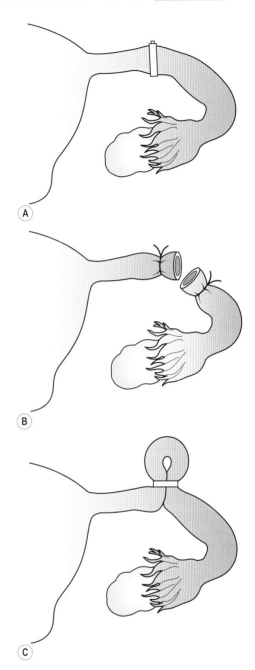

Fig. 27.12 Female sterilization.

Guillebaud and MacGregor (2013) suggest that a waiting period of 12 weeks is desirable to ensure that the couple will have no regrets over the sterilization.

The failure rate for female sterilization is 1 in 200 (FPA 2010c). Reversal of the sterilization is not usually available though the NHS in the UK and can be difficult and expensive to obtain privately. Women considering sterilization

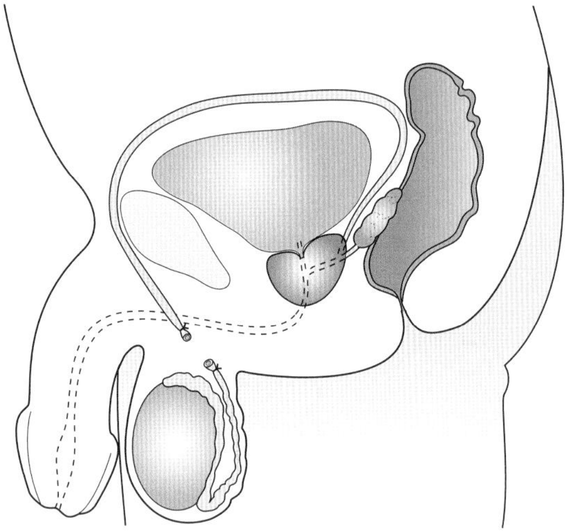

Fig. 27.13 Male sterilization (vasectomy).

should be made aware of the availability of LARC methods, which are highly effective but reversible.

Male sterilization (vasectomy)

The procedure of male sterilization involves excision or removal of part of the vas deferens, which is the tube that carries sperm from the testes to the penis (Fig. 27.13). A small cut or puncture to the skin of the scrotum is made to gain easier access to the vas deferens. The tubes are cut and the ends closed by tying them or sealing them with diathermy. The wound on the scrotum will be very small and stitches are not usually required. In the UK the operation is carried out in an outpatients department or clinic setting. It is usually completed under local anaesthetic and takes around 10–15 minutes. Men are advised to refrain from excessive physical activity for about one week and to avoid heavy lifting following the procedure (Andrews 2005).

It may take some time for sperm to be cleared from the vas deferens; it can take approximately 12 weeks after the operation for this to occur. Consequently, the semen must be tested to confirm that it no longer contains sperm and sometimes further tests are necessary to confirm the absence of sperm. Sexual intercourse can take place during this period but contraception must be used until a negative sperm result is confirmed.

The failure rate of male sterilization is 1 in 2000 (FPA 2010c). Careful counselling needs to take place before the procedure is carried out. Reversal of vasectomy is not usually available through the NHS and Andrews (2005) quotes around a 50% success rate in achieving a pregnancy following successful reversal within 10 years of the procedure being undertaken.

THE FUTURE OF CONTRACEPTION AND SEXUAL HEALTH SERVICES

In the UK the government remains committed to developing confidential, non-judgemental, integrated sexual health services, including STI screening and treatment, contraception, termination of pregnancy, health promotion and prevention (HM Government 2010). A recent Department of Health (DH) publication, 'A framework for sexual health improvement in England' (DH 2013), sets out a clear strategy for tackling sexual health issues such as STIs and teenage pregnancy. However, current financial challenges mean that the FSRH (2012) are concerned that budget cuts and changes to commissioning processes may compromise access to and quality of contraceptive and sexual health services for the forseeable future.

In response to the Social Exclusion Unit Report (DH 1999), many NHS Trusts now provide clinics and projects for young people, and improved access to contraceptive and sexual health services has led to a decrease in the conception rate of the under-18s. One of the specific targets of this report was to reduce the teenage pregnancy rate by 50% by 2010. The actual statistics showed a 13.3% decline in conceptions to the under-18s and 25% reduction in births in this same age group. Plans to decrease teenage conceptions further continue (DH 2010). With strict adherence to the Fraser guidelines (Guillebaud and MacGregor 2013), teenagers under the age of 16 can receive advice and treatment from a contraceptive and sexual health practitioner.

The NICE guidelines (2005) have emphasized the need to promote long acting reversible contraception (LARC). This recommendation will encourage more women to use a form of contraception that does not have to be remembered on a daily basis.

There is a trend in the UK for many women to have their children later in life and to have much smaller families. Throughout the world, couples will seek to find new ways to limit their family size as the need to reduce population growth continues (Guillebaud and MacGregor 2013).

ONGOING DEVELOPMENTS

An extended regimen of combined contraceptive pills for 84 days, e.g. Seasonale, has been confirmed to be safe. Seasonale is a COC pill that has the equivalent of Microgynon 30 but is packaged in four packets to be taken consecutively followed by a pre-determined pill-free interval (Guillebaud and MacGregor 2013). It is currently licensed in many countries, including the USA, and may be available in the UK soon. Other similar products include Seasonique. Alternative delivery systems reducing the need for daily pill-taking are being explored. Subcutaneous injections (depo-subQ) and chewable tablets are being developed for progestogens. Research into biodegradable implants (which would be particularly useful in low income countries) and the use of transdermal spray for the delivery of a potent progestogen is ongoing. The Population Council is considering research into proteomics and an immunological approach to contraception. Effective methods for men are still problematic and the long-awaited male pill is still not imminent (Guillebaud and MacGregor 2013). Gene blockers (reducing sperm mobility), the male patch and heat-based methods are amongst those being developed. Long acting testosterone injections with implanted progestogens or semen blocking methods may be available in the future (Dorman and Bishai 2012).

REFERENCES

Allan M, Koppula S 2012 Risk of venous thromboembolism with various hormonal contraceptives. Canadian Family Physician 58(10):1097

Andrews G (ed) 2005 Women's sexual health, 3rd edn. Elsevier, Edinburgh

Brache V, Cochon L, Jesam C et al 2010 Immediate pre-ovulatory administration of 30 mg ulipristal acetate significantly delays follicular rupture. Human Reproduction 25:2256–63

Brucker C, Karck U, Merkle E 2008 Cycle control, tolerability, efficacy and acceptability of the vaginal contraceptive ring, NuvaRing: results of clinical experience in Germany. European Journal of Contraception and Reproductive Health Care 13(1):31–8

DH (Department of Health) 1999 Teenage pregnancy. Report by the Social Exclusion Unit. TSO, London

DH (Department of Health) 2010 Teenage pregnancy strategy beyond 2010. DH, London

DH (Department of Health) 2013 A framework for sexual health improvement in England. DH, London

Dorman E, Bishai D 2012 Demand for male contraception. Expert Reviews in Pharmacoeconomics and Outcomes Research 12(5):605–13

FPA (Family Planning Association) 2010a Leaflet: Your guide to diaphragms and caps. FPA, London

FPA (Family Planning Association) 2010b Leaflet: Your guide to natural family planning. FPA, London

FPA (Family Planning Association) 2010c Leaflet: Your guide to male and female sterilization. FPA, London

FPA (Family Planning Association) 2011a Leaflet: Your guide to the contraceptive patch. FPA, London

FPA (Family Planning Association) 2011b Leaflet: Your guide to male and female condoms. FPA, London

FPA (Family Planning Association) 2011c Leaflet: Your guide to emergency contraception. FPA, London

FPA (Family Planning Association) 2012 Leaflet: Your guide to the combined pill. FPA, London

FSRH (Faculty of Sexual and Reproductive Healthcare) Clinical Effectiveness Unit 2008a (updated 2009) Progestogen-only pills. RCOG, London

FSRH (Faculty of Sexual and Reproductive Healthcare) Clinical Effectiveness Unit 2008b (updated 2009) Progestogen-only implants. RCOG, London

FSRH (Faculty of Sexual and Reproductive Healthcare) Clinical Effectiveness Unit 2009a Postnatal sexual and reproductive health. RCOG, London

FSRH (Faculty of Sexual and Reproductive Healthcare) Clinical Effectiveness Unit 2009b UK medical eligibility criteria for contraceptive use. RCOG, London

FSRH (Faculty of Sexual and Reproductive Healthcare) Clinical Effectiveness Unit 2011a (updated 2012) Combined hormonal contraception. RCOG, London

FSRH (Faculty of Sexual and Reproductive Healthcare) Clinical Effectiveness Unit 2011b (updated 2012) Emergency contraception. RCOG, London

FSRH (Faculty of Sexual and Reproductive Healthcare) 2012 FSRH response to the APPG SRH inquiry into restrictions in access to contraceptive services. RCOG, London

Guillebaud J, MacGregor A 2013 Contraception: your questions answered, 6th edn. Churchill Livingstone, Edinburgh

HM Government 2010 Healthy lives healthy people: our strategy for public health in England. TSO, London

Jogee, M 2004 Religions and cultures, 6th edn. R & C Publications, Edinburgh

Labbok M 2012 The lactational amenorrhoea method (LAM) for postnatal contraception. Australian Breastfeeding Association, Malvern East, VIC

McDonald E, Brown S 2013 Does method of birth make a difference to when women resume sex after childbirth? BJOG: An International Journal of Obstetrics and Gynaecology 120(7):823–30

NICE (National Institute for Health and Clinical Excellence) 2005 (modified 2013) Long acting reversible contraception. Department of Health, London

NICE (National Institute for Health and Clinical Excellence) 2006 Routine postnatal care for women and their babies. Department of Health, London

NMC (Nursing and Midwifery Council) 2012 Midwives rules and standards. NMC, London

Roumen F, op ten Berg M, Hoomans E 2006 The combined contraceptive vaginal ring (NuvaRing): first experience in daily clinical practice in The Netherlands. European Journal of Contraception and Reproductive Health Care 11:14–22

Scholes D, LaCroix A Z, Ichikawa L E et al 2005 Change in bone mineral density among adolescent women using and discontinuing depot medroxyprogesterone acetate contraception. Archives of Paediatric and Adolescent Medicine 159:139–44

FURTHER READING

Gebbie A, O'Connell White K 2009 Fast facts contraception. Health Press, Abingdon

This textbook covers the wide spectrum of contraception, in an easy to read and accessible format.

Guillebaud J, MacGregor A 2013 Contraception: your questions answered, 6th edn. Churchill Livingstone, Edinburgh

The latest edition of this book is extremely comprehensive and up-to-date, covering all available contraceptive methods not just available in the UK but worldwide. It is in a question and answer style regarding each particular contraceptive method and provides the best available evidence to guide and support clinical practice.

National Institute for Health and Clinical Excellence 2005 (modified 2013) Long acting reversible contraception. Department of Health, London

This document has been recently modified to reflect the replacement of Implanon with Nexplanon, and also includes guidance on the management of unscheduled bleeding in women with implants in situ. It is therefore still applicable to current contraceptive services, as it recognizes the value of encouraging the use of long acting reversible contraception in reducing unwanted pregnancies.

USEFUL WEBSITES/CONTACTS

Brook: www.brook.org.uk. UK tel: 0808 802 1234

Free and confidential information for under 25s

Faculty of Sexual and Reproductive Healthcare: www.fsrh.org.uk

Family Planning Association UK: www.fpa.org.uk. Northern Ireland: tel: 0845 122 8687. England tel: 0845 122 8690

Fertility UK: www.fertilityuk.org

Section | 6 |

The neonate

Chapter |28|

Recognizing the healthy baby at term through examination of the newborn screening

Carole England

This chapter will focus upon the characteristics of the healthy term baby. The midwife performs a systematic screening assessment of a baby's health and wellbeing on a regular basis. These include the first examination after birth, the ongoing daily examination and for those who have received specialist education and training, the Newborn and Infant Physical Examination (NIPE), performed within three days (72 hours) of birth. Each examination assesses the whole baby and builds on previous findings related to the pregnancy, birth and neonatal assessments. The midwife's role is *not to diagnose but to examine and distinguish the healthy baby from the one that requires referral to a medical practitioner.* To do this effectively the midwife must have a sound knowledge of abnormality to be able to make appropriate and timely referral, especially if the condition is immediately life-threatening.

THE CHAPTER AIMS TO:

- highlight the features of a healthy baby and know which baby needs referral to a medical practitioner
- emphasize the importance of reading the woman's records before any physical assessment of her baby is attempted
- recognize the vital importance of appropriate communication with the parents, especially when

obtaining consent, listening to the mother on her opinion of her baby's health and in reporting the findings of the examination

- provide the details of a top-to-toe examination of the newborn performed in the first 24 hours of life
- explore the assessment provided in the daily examination of the baby
- critically discuss the NIPE assessment
- discuss how each screening examination is an opportunity for health education/promotion and psychological empowerment of both parents in how to recognize health and wellbeing in their baby
- stress the importance of writing (and drawing if indicated) a clear detailed record of findings and communications that have taken place.

THE FIRST EXAMINATION AFTER BIRTH

The aim of the first examination performed within 24 hours of birth is to detect any observable congenital malformations and to assess initial adaptation to extrauterine life that could compromise health and wellbeing (Resuscitation Council 2011). The examination should be performed in the presence of the mother and partner (as appropriate). The ideal time is after the baby has had skin-to-skin contact and had its first feed, during which it maintained a body temperature within normal parameters. The midwife present at the birth often performs this examination and should ensure that the environment is warm and draught-free, with equipment ready for use. Diligent handwashing is essential. The baby should be at rest on a flat surface. The skills of observation, palpation and auscultation should be utilized. See Box 28.1 for screening principles that should be communicated when screening is undertaken.

Assessment of the neonatal skin

According to Baston and Durward (2010), the colour of the skin is generally considered a reflection of good health, but is most difficult to assess accurately in the first few hours of extrauterine life and the midwife needs to distinguish between different types and degrees of blue skin to know if the baby is well or whether to refer to the neonatal registrar.

A blue skin as a result of central cyanosis

To assess blueness due to accumulation of carbon dioxide and deprivation of oxygen is a difficult task in white ethnic groups and even more so in babies from black ethnic

---

> **Box 28.1 The principles of screening**
>
> The midwife should:
> - inform the mother exactly why the examination is being conducted
> - obtain informed consent from the mother to perform the examination on her baby
> - ensure the baby is wearing identification bracelets that correspond with the mother's identity and documentation
> - perform a thorough examination of the baby
> - provide full details of the findings of the examination
> - offer an action plan of care as required
> - document detailed findings and evidence of communication that arose between the midwife and mother/parents before, during and after the examination
>
> Source: UK National Screening Committee (2008)

---

groups who have a pigmented skin. The baby's oral mucus membranes and tongue are not pigmented and will provide the midwife with reliable evidence of central cyanosis. A dull blue skin may indicate poor perfusion and can be assessed by measuring capillary refill time (CRT) by blanching the baby's chest skin with a finger and, on release, seeing how long it takes for the capillaries to refill. Any time over 2 seconds indicates poor peripheral perfusion. Pallor of the skin is a result of peripheral shutdown and is always a serious sign as this could also indicate acute blood loss, anaemia, the processes involved in cooling or/and the presence of infection. Jaundice that develops from birth in the first 24 hours is considered pathological, is usually as a result of haemolysis (excessive breakdown of red blood cells) and should also be reported immediately (England 2010b) (see Chapter 33).

A blue skin as a result of other factors

Most babies will have peripheral shutdown (acrocyanosis) in hands and feet as blood is diverted to major organs. Occasionally babies will present with a blue face as a result of petechiae, which are pinpoint haemorrhagic spots on the skin, usually as a result of a tightening cord around the neck which constricts the jugular veins during fetal descent in the second stage of labour. The venous blood is trapped in the sinuses of the brain and will find an exit point into the skin, thus the facial tissues become bruised. The use of a pulse oximeter will indicate the amount of haemoglobin saturated with oxygen in the baby's blood and should be about 95% or above in the first 24 hours of life.

Common skin lesions found at birth

Skin lesions, as they are discovered either by the parents or midwife, need addressing immediately. There is no room for guesswork and the prudent midwife will ask for a second opinion should there be any doubt.

Cuts, abrasions and bruises

These are carefully assessed as they may serve as portals of entry for infection. Create a line drawing in documentation to illustrate size and complexity to avoid disputes regarding origin (iatrogenic lesions caused by treatment, e.g. use of forceps or ventouse; see Chapter 31, Figs 31.1, 31.2) or as a result of non-accidental injury. Extensive bruising may lead to clinical jaundice.

Vascular birth marks found at birth

Vascular proliferations (increase in growth) in the skin will resolve and involute in time:

- Salmon patch haemangioma or 'stork marks': occur in 50% of babies, are superficial capillaries that blanche on pressure, resolve spontaneously, commonly found on the nape of the neck, eyelids and glabella.
- Strawberry haemangioma: not always present at birth; occurs in 10% of babies by the age of one year; bright red in colour. Benign but can develop over orifices, e.g. anus, to cause obstruction and can leave scar tissue. Laser treatment is available but natural resolution offers a better cosmetic outcome.
- Cavernous haemangioma: similar to the strawberry haemangioma but invades deeper into the vascular tissues; leaves a blue discoloration to the skin and grows with the child.

Vasculature malformations that do not involute are permanent and always present at birth:

- Port wine stain: red, purple markings present in 0.3 % of neonates (Gordon and Lomax 2011) can be an isolated mark or associated with syndromes. Some lesions (Sturge–Weber syndrome) follow the trigeminal nerve (fifth cranial nerve); have a midline cut off and can infiltrate into the meninges and cerebral cortex on the affected side resulting in seizures and eye abnormalities. This condition can devastate parents and the midwife needs to provide empathic informed support.

Pigmented birthmarks

- Mongolian blue spots are produced by clusters of melanocytes in the dermis, are benign and have no clinical significance. Present in 90% African, 81% Asian and 9.6% white caucasian babies, they have a slate-grey to blue-black discoloration usually found over the buttocks, back and legs and fade by 7 years of age. They resemble bruising so a line drawing is

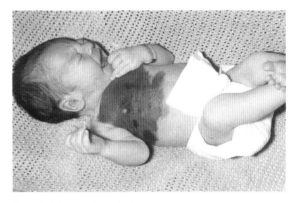

Fig. 28.1 Large pigmented naevus.
With thanks to Carl Kuschel 2007.

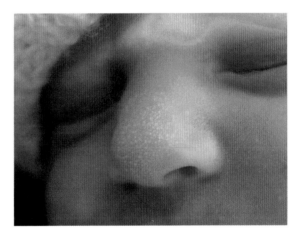

Fig. 28.2 Milia.

useful to distinguish from future non-accidental injury (Griffith 2009).
- Pigmented naevi affect 3% of babies, present at birth as a dark brown patch on the lower back or buttocks with speckles around the edge of the lesion, usually as a solitary patch (Fig. 28.1). Major concern is the development of malignancy over time and must be monitored closely for changes in size and shape (Gordon and Lomax 2011).
- Milia are small white follicular cysts commonly known as milk spots (Fig. 28.2). They normally appear on the cheeks forehead and nose and are thought to be retention of keratin and sebaceous secretions. They clear within 4 weeks of birth.

The head

According to Noonan et al (2011), the shape, size and symmetry of the head in relation to the face and rest of the body should be assessed. The head circumference measurement of the occipitofrontal diameter should be in the range of 32–36 cm for a term baby. Lumsden (2010) asserts that *macro*cephaly (greater than the 97th centile) or *micro*cephaly (below the 2nd centile) can be plotted on a head circumference growth chart in the Child Health Record. A head that is disproportionate to body size may indicate asymmetrical intrauterine growth restriction where the head has been spared disruption to its growth (see Chapter 30). Be aware that a stand-alone head measurement may appear perfectly normal but its relationship with the body may render it large. A large head is also associated with hydrocephaly and congenital syndromes. A small head is associated with poor brain development. Fetal alcohol spectrum disorders (FASD) and transplacental infections will deleteriously affect fetal brain growth. Observation and palpation of the scalp will indicate the presence and degree of caput succedaneum which will resolve in 2–3 days. The direction and degree of moulding can indicate the engaging diameter of the fetal skull involved in the process of labour. The bones, sutures and fontanelles can then be examined. The anterior fontanelle (bregma) closes at 18 months of age and if tense or bulging can indicate congenital hydrocephaly, intercranial haemorrhage or meningitis. A sunken bregma is associated with dehydration because as an extracellular fluid, cerebrospinal fluid is derived from venous blood. The posterior fontanelle (lambda) closes around 6 weeks. More than one lambda along the lamboidal suture lines often alongside a flat occiput can indicate trisomy 21, as can abnormal patterns of hair growth (low hair line, extra crowns) which are featured in a variety of syndromes (see Chapter 32).

The face

The midwife should endeavour to see both parents before expressing concern on an unusual-looking face, however an assumption should not be made that the male partner is the biological father of the baby. The face should be analysed as a whole. Individual features in isolation do not necessarily indicate a syndrome but in combination with other features they make a syndrome more likely. The baby's facial expression could indicate an underlying condition, e.g. pain, irritability, distress and is worthy of note. The symmetry of the face should be observed as this could indicate birth trauma in the form of facial paralysis where one side of the face appears to droop, especially around the eye and mouth on one side, when the baby is crying (Fig. 28.3). This is a result of damage to the seventh cranial nerve (facial), known as Bell's palsy, during the application of forceps or from head compression against the sacral promontory during birth. Any degree of recovery will depend upon the amount of damage to the myelin sheath that covers and feeds the nerve.

The ear position should be similar on both sides. The upper margin of the ear pinna should be on the level of

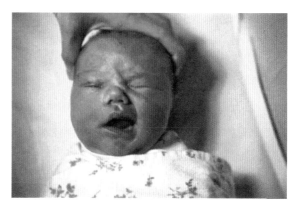

Fig. 28.3 Right-sided facial palsy. Note that the eye is open on the paralysed side and the mouth is drawn over to the non-paralysed side.
Reproduced from Thomas R, Harvey D 1997 Colour guide: neonatology, 2nd edn, Churchill Livingstone, Edinburgh, with permission of Elsevier.

the eyes. However, a finding of low set ears alone may be a normal variation. Malformed and/or low set ears are associated with chromosomal abnormalities or urogenital malformations and warrant referral. Roth et al (2008) argue that peri-auricular skin tags can indicate hearing impairment. The incidence of significant permanent congenital hearing impairment (PCHI) is 1 : 1000 births in developed countries. The NHS Newborn Hearing Screening Programme (UK National Screening Committee 2012) offers hearing screening in the first week of life and aims to provide high-quality detection care and support for babies and their families. A pre-auricular sinus may be blind-ending or connected to the inner ear. The latter condition will need referral to the Ear Nose and Throat (ENT) surgeon.

The nose shape will vary, but the two nares should be centrally placed and be patent. Most babies are obligatory nose-breathers and patency can be observed when the baby is breathing normally at rest. Nasal flaring may be indicative of respiratory distress. Choanal atresia is a condition in which one or both posterior nasal passages are blocked by either bone or soft tissue. In the bilateral condition the baby will be centrally cyanosed at rest but will become better perfused when crying. Urgent referral to an ENT surgeon will be required.

When a cleft lip is detected by antenatal screening, automatic referral is made to the local cleft lip and palate team (plastic surgeon, ENT surgeon, audiologist, orthodontic surgeon and speech therapist) before the baby is born. For those babies who have their condition detected after birth, the midwife should refer to the registrar who will make referral to the cleft lip and palate team. Cleft lip can be either unilateral or bilateral and can extend into the hard and soft palate. A cleft palate is not always obvious and requires thorough assessment in order to confirm its presence. A gloved finger should be inserted

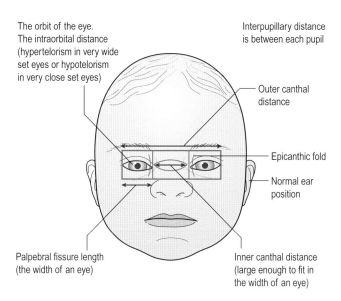

The orbit of the eye.
The intraorbital distance
(hypertelorism in very wide
set eyes or hypotelorism
in very close set eyes)

Interpupillary distance
is between each pupil

Outer canthal
distance

Epicanthic fold

Normal ear
position

Palpebral fissure length
(the width of an eye)

Inner canthal distance
(large enough to fit in
the width of an eye)

Fig. 28.4 Features of the baby's eyes in relation to the face.

into the mouth, eliciting a suck reflex. By palpating the hard palate it should be possible to feel if a cleft is present. Detection of clefts in the soft palate should involve visual inspection using a pen torch and tongue depressor. The palate should be high arched, intact with a central uvula. Cleft lip and/or palate may be familial or may be as a result of maternal medication (e.g. phenytoin) or chromosomal abnormality (e.g. Down and Patau's syndrome). Lumsden (2010) reports that clefting of the lip and palate affects 1:700 babies in the United Kingdom (UK), with 50% lip and palate together, 25% lip alone and 25% palate alone, so is a relatively common condition. A small jaw (micrognathia) may be familial or part of a syndrome like Pierre Robin, which comprises a midline cleft palate and protruding tongue (glossoptosis). The midwife must be aware that the main problem is of the tongue falling back and obstructing the oropharynx. The baby may also experience problems with feeding. Referral to the ENT and orthodontic surgeons will be made alongside the speech therapist.

Epstein's pearls are a cluster of several white spots in the mouth at the junction of the soft and hard palate in the midline. They are the same as milia, are of no significance and disappear spontaneously. Natal teeth are lower incisors that have small crowns with no roots and pose the risk of tongue ulceration and, if they become loose, inhalation into the trachea. Referral to the orthodontic team for elective removal is required. The tongue should also be examined for cysts and dimples. A tight frenulum that is attached too far forward to the floor of the mouth restricts mobility of the tongue to different degrees and will give the appearance of tongue-tie (ankyloglossia). Treatment for severe tongue-tie is frenulotomy (surgical division of the frenulum), especially when breastfeeding is being adversely affected.

The eyes should be symmetrically positioned on the face in relation to the other facial features such as eyelids, eyebrows and the slant of the palpebral fissures (see Fig. 28.4). The outer canthal distance can be divided equally into thirds, with one eye width fitting into the inner canthal space. Extremely wide (hypertelorism) or narrowly spaced eyes are abnormal and may indicate a syndrome, as may epicanthic folds, however the latter finding is a normal feature in some ethnic groups, so some caution is warranted. The sclera is normally white in colour; a yellow discoloration occurs with jaundice. Conjunctival haemorrhages may occur as a result of the birth, are insignificant and will take a few days to resolve but are, according to Griffith (2009), associated with non-accidental injury, so documentation of their appearance and size is vital. The iris of a baby is navy blue with fibres radiating from the centre. It should be perfectly circular with a round pupil in the centre. White specks on the iris called Bushfield spots are associated with Down syndrome. Opacity of the lens could indicate congenital cataract. Clouding of the cornea could be a sign of congenital glaucoma. Small eyes occur as a result of transplacental infection, e.g. rubella, cytomegalovirus. Any profuse or purulent discharge from the eyes (Fig. 28.5) should be swabbed and sent for culture and sensitivity. Eye drops/ointments to treat gonococcal infection, staphylococci and chlamydial conjunctivitis should be started while awaiting the results. Absence of one or both eyes may have an environmental or chromosomal cause and such a finding requires referral to the ophthalmologist.

The neck

This may be shortened or webbed with extra skin and is a sign of Turner's syndrome. The clavicles should be

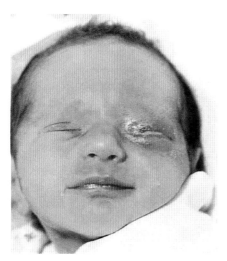

Fig. 28.5 Ophthalmia neonatorum.
Reproduced from Mitchell H 2004 Sexually transmitted infections in pregnancy. In: Adler M W, Cowen F, French P et al (eds) ABC of sexually transmitted infections, 5th edn, p 35, with permission from Blackwell Publishing.

examined for fractures, especially if there is any history of shoulder dystocia or any suggestions of Erb's palsy (see Chapter 31 and Fig. 31.5).

The chest and abdomen

Bedford and Lomax (2011) assert that the heart rate will vary in range from 100 to 160 beats per minute (bpm). The respiratory rate will be 30–40 breaths per minute (bpm), but not exceed 60 bpm and will vary in rhythm with small periods of apnoea (absence of breathing for 20 seconds or more). There should be no sternal or costal recession. The nipples should be lateral to the mid-clavicular line and should be normal in shape and form. The presence of abnormal or supernumerary (extra) nipples should be recorded as a line drawing on a body map with referral to the registrar.

Observation of respiratory movement should reveal that chest and abdominal movements are synchronous as the diaphragm is the major muscle of respiration. Asymmetrical chest movement may be caused by either unilateral pneumothorax or phrenic nerve damage on the side that isn't moving. Also consider the presence of a diaphragmatic hernia noted when the chest looks relatively big in comparison to a scaphoid (sunken) abdomen. Auscultation of ectopic bowel sounds in the chest may support this supposition (see Chapter 33).

The abdomen should look and feel soft and rounded. The cord should be checked for bleeding. The cord vessels should have two arteries and one vein. A single umbilical artery increases the chances of congenital abnormalities but further investigations are not justified on this finding

alone. Exomphalos is where the bowel, covered by a transparent sac composed of amnion and peritoneum, protrudes through the umbilical cord and is associated with Beckwith–Wiedemann syndrome (exomphalos, large for gestational age, abnormal glucose metabolism, characteristic skin creases to the ears). By comparison, gastroschisis is caused by a defect in the abdominal wall, which allows bowel to protrude through it. No sack covers the loops of bowel, so before birth the bowel has been in contact with the irritant properties of amniotic fluid, but there are no associations with other congenital abnormalities. Both conditions may be found on antenatal screening and at birth the protruding bowel is covered with film wrap to prevent fluid and heat loss in readiness for surgical repair.

The anus

Inspection for the presence and appearance of the anus is vital. *The presence of meconium does not always exclude imperforate anus (anal atresia).* In a perforate anus, the rectum and anal sphincter connect so that substantial amounts of meconium can be passed at any one time. If there is an underlying defect referred to as a high imperforate obstruction, there could be a rectal–vaginal fistula or a rectal–urethral fistula that may allow passage of small amounts of meconuim. A 'low' anomaly may merely consist of a membrane covering the anal sphincter, which, while in place, will impede the passage of all meconium. England (2010a) contends that anal abnormalities can indicate that other gastrointestinal malformations may be present, so caution with feeding is recommended. The passage of a nasogastric tube and withdrawal of hydrochloric acid can exclude oesophageal atresia but does not necessarily rule out tracheo-oesophageal fistula.

The genitalia

Male genitalia

The penis should be about 3 cm in length, straight, with no chordee (a bend in the shaft). According to Fox et al (2010), an apparently short penis is more common, usually buried in supra-pubic fat, but remains a finding that can cause real consternation to parents. True micropenis is rare and associated with hypopituitarism and referral to the paediatric endocrinologist may occasionally be warranted. The midwife should never attempt to withdraw the foreskin.

Observing the baby pass urine may help to detect a hypospadius where the urethral meatus opens on the ventral (under) side of the penis and an epispadius where the urethral meatus opens on the dorsal (upper) side. Parents should be advised not to have their baby circumcised for religious or cultural reasons, as the foreskin will be used to surgically repair the defect.

According to Gordon (2011), the scrotum should be examined to ensure symmetry on both sides as asymmetry may indicate a persistent connection between the abdominal cavity and scrotum, so that fluid (hydrocele) or loops of bowel (inguinal hernia) can escape and occupy the scrotal sac on the affected side. A dark discoloration of the scrotum, with or without swelling, is abnormal and may indicate testicular torsion. The testicle twists on itself, limits its own blood supply and the testicle dies from ischaemia. Torsion can occur at any age and requires immediate surgical review. The testicles should descend into the scrotal sac by term. Each testicle is 1–1.5 cm in size, palpable along the route from the posterior abdomen to the scrotal sac, often found in the groin. Undescended testicles (cryptorchidism) occurs in 2–4% of term babies. If not descended by one year, orchidopexy is performed to surgically place the testicle in the scrotal sac to prevent infertility and malignancy in later life.

Female genitalia

The examination will confirm that the general anatomy appears appropriate, with the labia majora covering the labia minora.

Disorders of sex development (ambiguous genitalia)

The midwife's communication skills will be of utmost importance as the parents ask 'What have we got and is it alright?' The stark but not recommended answer to these questions is, 'I don't know and no'. Honesty is the only way to effectively manage this situation, however, and the midwife's choice of words should be tactful but truthful, with an immediate response to the parents' queries. Recent practice of placing the newborn onto the mother's abdomen has enabled the parents to examine their baby and make their own discoveries, often before the midwife has had chance to see for her/himself. It is helpful to suggest to the parents that they initially give their baby a cross-gender name like Sam or Jo so that pronouns like he and she are avoided. This may also help as a temporary measure when informing family members of the birth and the baby's name.

According to Wassner and Spack (2012), there are many different causes of ambiguous genitalia: the most common is congenital adrenal hyperplasia, with an incidence of 1:15 000 babies. An XX female baby has an enlarged clitoris that appears like a penis and labia that may look more like a scrotum. This is an autosomal recessive condition where lack of an enzyme called 21 hydroxylase interferes with the cholesterol pathway in the production of progesterone (from which cortisol and aldosterone are formed), testosterone and oestradiol. In the absence of serum cortisol and aldosterone, the anterior pituitary hormone adrencorticotrophin (ACTH) stimulates the pathway but only testosterone is produced, which results in masculinized genitalia and life-threatening imbalances in sodium and cortisol levels. Referral to an endocrinologist and a paediatric surgeon will follow (see Chapters 32 and 33). The genitalia of male XY babies look within normal limits but these babies may present later with failure to thrive, vomiting and dehydration related to abnormal aldosterone and steroid physiology. The midwife should warn the parents of the likelihood that their baby may be transferred to the neonatal intensive care unit (NICU) for extra monitoring.

Limbs, hands and feet

The term baby will lie in a flexed position with the head in the midline or turned slightly to one side. The hands are flexed, with the thumb lying beneath the fingers in a fist. In addition to noting length and movement of the limbs and joints, it is essential that the digits are counted and separated to ensure that webbing (syndactyly) is not present on hands and feet. The hands should be opened fully as any extra digits (polydactyly) may be concealed in the clenched fist. X-ray assessment will determine whether the defect needs referral to either the plastic surgeon (skin only) or orthopaedic surgeon (bone and skin). A single palmar (Simian) crease is associated with Down syndrome, however 10% of the normal population have a single palmar crease on one hand and 5% have one on both hands.

Davis (2011) uses the word structural clubfoot to refer to the most common foot deformity (1 : 1000 births in the UK), known as congenital talipes equinovarus. The word talipes means ankle and foot. In this condition the foot is plantar-flexed (turned downwards like a horse's foot and inwards towards the midline of the baby). The ratio of boys to girls is 3 : 1 and in 50 % of cases, both feet are affected. The cause is unknown but is associated with Down syndrome and spina bifida. Referral to an orthopaedic surgeon is required. First line treatment is the Porseti method of gentle manipulation and serial casting in plaster of Paris at weekly intervals, which allows the foot to be gradually corrected over a period of 6 weeks.

Positional conditions of the foot are caused by intra-uterine overcrowding. These are:

- positional clubfoot/talipes equinovarus, which when gently manipulated will easily correct. Davis (2011) argues that a normal baby's foot can be turned outwards by 50–70° and upwards by 20°. If this can be achieved, a physiotherapist can advise the parents on gentle massage. Davis further argues that it is not uncommon for a child to have *a structural clubfoot on one side and a positional one on the other*, with no clear view if they are of the same entity. This notion does call for the midwife to check each foot individually and not

597

automatically assume that both feet are affected in the same way.

- talipes calcaneo-valgus, which is characterized by dorsiflexion where the foot is turned upwards and outwards and associated with the breech position and developmental dysplasia of the hip (DDH). Referral to an orthopaedic surgeon is required. Often gentle manipulation conducted by parents will bring about correct alignment, with occasional need for a plaster cast.

The spine

The best way to examine the spine is by holding the baby per chest/abdomen on one hand, and running the fingers of the other hand down the spinal processes. Any curvature of the spine can be noted. Spina bifida occulta (characterized by a missing vertebral process) *may* lie beneath a fat pad, swelling, dimple, tuft of hair or birthmark. For spina bifida cystica (mylomeningocele and meningocele), see Chapter 32. A sacral dimple should be carefully examined to make sure it is skin-lined with no sinus to the CSF pathway. If CSF is leaking it represents a portal for infection, so referral to both the plastic surgeon and neurosurgical teams will be made. In the interim, X-ray of the lumbosacral spine and an ultrasound scan of the lower spinal cord, kidneys and bladder will be arranged.

Communication and documentation

As soon as the examination is completed, the baby should be handed back to the mother and skin-to-skin contact re-established. *This first examination after birth is extremely important and needs to be done thoroughly.* According to England and Morgan (2012), parents are often taken aback by the course of events that unfolds if a malformation or problem is identified. This is often because they are not correctly prepared for the screening intervention. The words used to obtain consent from the mother set the scene on how she will perceive the importance of the examination. For example, if the midwife says 'I need to take a quick look over your baby to see if everything is alright', this could imply that the examination is being done quickly because it is not really necessary but is routine and has to be done. If the midwife says 'Will you please allow me to examine your baby in detail, so that if I find anything that I think will affect your baby's health, I can tell you about it and then, with your permission, ask for a second opinion?', this question offers a detailed explanation of the midwife's intention in gaining consent. What the midwife says should be documented alongside details of examination findings, parental reaction, referral details and support provided. The midwife should not be influenced by the limited space provided in the record being completed (England and Morgan 2012).

THE DAILY EXAMINATION SCREEN

This examination is usually performed daily while the baby remains in hospital and continues on a more intermittent basis once the baby is in community until discharge to the care of the health visitor. Health education stems from how the baby is behaving and its general appearance. A healthy term baby weighs approximately 3.5 kg, has a clear skin, good muscle tone, cries lustily, feeds well, keeps warm and sleeps. The midwife will continue the health screening process by always asking the mother how her baby is. Carefully listening to her answer is a crucial part of the examination and her response will often dictate in what order the midwife performs the examination, starting with any areas of concern. Recording what the mother has said (and how she said it) is helpful for other health care practitioners who will see the baby at a future time (England 2010c).

Breathing

The midwife should observe the baby's respiratory rate that involves the diaphragm, chest and abdomen rising and falling synchronously. It should be explained to the parents that babies have a periodic breathing pattern that is erratic, with respirations being shallow and irregular, interspersed with brief 10–15 second periods of apnoea. Given that babies are either obligatory (required) or preferential nose-breathers, it is important to check that their nostrils are clear of dried secretions. Tickling the edge of the nostrils with cotton wool can induce sneezing, which aids some clearance. An irritable baby with excessive snuffles and sneezing could indicate opiate withdrawal. In an assessment of health, the midwife must consider that respiratory difficulties can occur because of neurological, metabolic, circulatory or thermoregulatory dysfunction as well as infection, airway obstruction or abnormalities of the respiratory tract itself.

Thermoregulation – the importance of keeping warm

One of the midwife's priorities is to make sure the baby is maintaining a body temperature within normal parameters. According to Brown and Landers (2011), *a neutral thermal environment is one that is neither too hot nor too cold and enables the baby to use the minimal amount of energy to stay warm.* Babies are individuals, with each one having their own metabolic rate, so the clinical acceptable temperature range of 36.5–37.5 °C is wide. In the first week of life core temperature can be unstable as the heat-regulating centre in the hypothalamus and medulla oblongata is attempting to adapt from a hot water intrauterine environment to a cooler extrauterine air

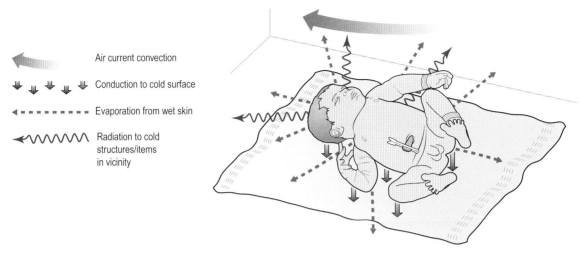

Air current convection

Conduction to cold surface

Evaporation from wet skin

Radiation to cold structures/items in vicinity

Fig. 28.6 Modes of heat loss in the neonate.

environment with concurrent threats of heat loss via radiation, conduction, evaporation and convection (Fig. 28.6). Cooling babies are unable to shiver and instead attempt to maintain body heat by a means of *non-shivering thermogenesis* whereby they utilize brown fat and simultaneously increase their metabolic rate by increasing glucose and oxygen consumption to make more energy, carbon dioxide and heat. For this process of *aerobic glycolysis* to function effectively, the baby needs available oxygen and glucose. As oxygen is consumed, energy can be made in the absence of, or with minimal amounts of oxygen, which is referred to as *anaerobic glycolysis*, however the amounts of glucose to maintain this form of energy production is more than 20 times greater to make the same amount of energy as in aerobic glycolysis. Hence the baby becomes hypoxic and may begin to show signs of respiratory distress. England (2010a) argues that a *transient* expiratory grunt may be one of the first respiratory signs of cooling. Nasal flaring, tachypnoea, sternal or subcostal recession, are all signs of respiratory distress that may follow. Hence the importance of *listening to how the mother or father describes the baby.* The baby will not grunt like a pig; one father described how his son made 'a strange noise on each breathe'. Subtle colour changes may accompany these fleeting episodes.

The first step is to observe the baby overall and feel the head and chest to gather a general sense of how warm the baby is. Follow this by the use of a thermometer via the axilla, tympanic membrane (ear), or in the groin. A clothed term baby should maintain its body temperature satisfactorily provided the environmental temperature is draught-free, sustained between 18 °C and 21 °C, nutrition is adequate and movements are not restricted by tight swaddling. Inadequate clothing or/and being inadvertently left exposed is a common cause of heat loss. If the baby is cooling, skin-to-skin contact with the mother

should be initiated immediately. The baby's temperature and general condition should be reviewed after 30 minutes.

Blackburn (2007) argues that pyrexia (37.7 °C and above) in a term baby may indicate infection; however, hyperthermia can occur if the baby is exposed to an inappropriate heat source (placed in a sunny window) or dressed inappropriately for the ambient temperature. Feet-to-foot placing of the baby in the cot in the supine position has contributed to the reduction in overheating and associated sudden infant death syndrome (Foundation for Sudden Infant Death 2013). Over-heating increases metabolic rate and can draw upon supplies of glucose and oxygen to maintain the required energy level. Respiratory distress may follow unless the baby is allowed to cool *slowly*.

Skin care

Although sterile at birth, the skin, when exposed to air is quickly colonized by microorganisms, which produce a pH of 4.9, creating an acid mantle that protects the skin from infection. Vernix caseosa should be allowed to absorb into the skin because it is a highly sophisticated mixture of proteins and fatty acids that produce an antibacterial and antifungal skin barrier. Gordon and Lomax (2011) assert that the midwife should not be tempted to apply anything to a post-term skin that is dry and cracked, because within a few days of peeling, perfect skin will be revealed beneath. Skin-to-skin contact just after birth and during subsequent feeding (to include formula-fed babies too) is an excellent way to colonize the baby's skin with friendly bacteria. Great care must be provided to maintain the integrity of the lipids (fats) that seal each skin cell. Chemicals used in manufactured baby skin products can irrevocably damage epidermal lipids and lead to trans-epidermal water loss. It is recommended by Trotter (2010) that for the first month of life it is safer to bath all babies in plain water once or twice a week only. Cotton wool balls should be used for baby cleansing (top and tail).

According to Gordon and Lomax (2011), the midwife should inspect the skin for rashes, septic spots, excoriation or abrasions. Seborrhoeic dermatitis (cradle cap) is commonly seen on the scalp of the newborn, but can occur in the axillae, groins and nappy area. It presents with scaly lesions that are greasy to the touch and thought to be as a response to irritants. Skin rashes such as erythema toxicum that occur within 72 hours of birth as a red blotchy rash, usually over the face and trunk, may be a sign of over-heating. Removing some of the baby's clothing/bedding will usually resolve it. This is in comparison to septic spots that will need swabbing for culture and sensitivity followed by topical or systemic antibiotic therapy as necessary. Similarly, paronychia, which is infection of the nail cuticle caused by ragged nails, will be treated in the same way. Parents should be advised to file their baby's nails and *not use scissors or bite them off to keep them short*. The umbilical stump is rapidly colonized, necroses and separates by a process of dry gangrene, which usually takes between 7 and 15 days. The cord represents a portal of entry for infection (especially *Escherichia coli* as a result of contamination from stools) and must be observed for any signs of redness in the surrounding abdominal skin, referred to as an umbilical flare. If the flare begins to spread and extend up the abdomen, this must be reported immediately as antibiotic therapy will be required.

Cardiovascular system and blood physiology

The Resuscitation Council (2011) recommends that the umbilical cord is not clamped for at least the first minute after birth, to allow oxygenated blood to be transferred from the placenta to the baby. As a result, the total circulating blood volume at birth may exceed 80–90 ml/kg and ward off neonatal iron-deficiency anaemia. The haemoglobin level may also be in excess of 18–22 g/l. The red cell count ($5-7 \times 10^{12}$/l) may contribute to the development of physiological jaundice (see Chapter 33). Blackburn (2007) believes that conversion from fetal to adult haemoglobin, which commences at 36 weeks gestation, is completed in the first 1–2 years of life. The white cell count is high initially (18.0×10^9/l) but decreases rapidly.

According to Lwaleed and Kazmi (2009), the blood clotting system is immature because there is no transplacental passage of coagulation proteins from the mother, so all levels of blood clotting reflect fetal synthesis which is completed before the 30th gestational week. Vitamin K is poorly transferred across the placenta, and due to the low amount in breast milk the incidence of classic haemorrhagic disease of the newborn (HDN) occurring within the first week of life is enhanced in babies who are exclusively breastfed, until the bowel becomes colonized by *E. coli* and the Vitamin K-dependent clotting factors II (prothrombin), VII, IX and X can be synthesized in the presence of bile salts. Vitamin K (intramuscular or oral suspension) is available to all babies in the UK as a prophylactic precaution against HDN. Early onset HDN (within first 24 hours) is *exclusively* caused by transplacental passage of anticoagulant medicines that inhibit Vitamin K activity. In this situation the baby will be prescribed a therapeutic dose of Vitamin K via intramuscular injection (Lwaleed and Kazmi 2009).

Renal system

About 20% of babies will pass urine in the birthing room and this should be noted. Ninety per cent will void by 24 hours of age and 99% by 48 hours. The rate of urine formation varies from 0.05 to 5.0 ml/kg/*hour* at all gestational ages with a range of 25–300 ml/kg/*day*. The commonest cause of initial delay or decreased urine production is inadequate perfusion of the kidney. Added to this, the kidneys are immature and the glomerular filtration rate is low, but mature within the first month of life. Tubular reabsorption capabilities are also limited, which renders the baby unable neither to concentrate or dilute urine adequately, nor to compensate for high or low levels of sodium, potassium and chloride in the blood. This results in a narrow margin between under- and over-hydration and, as Blackburn (2007) argues, the ability to excrete medicines is also restricted. The urine is dilute, straw-coloured and odourless. Urate crystals may cause red brick staining in the nappy, which is usually a sign of under-hydration but is largely insignificant. It is the midwife's responsibility to assess whether the urine output falls within acceptable parameters by asking the mother about the character of the baby's wet nappies given that delay in urine production/passage may be due to physiological stress, intrinsic renal abnormalities or obstruction of the urinary tract. The midwife should check the records for antenatal scan findings that may identify abnormality such as the presence of oligohydramnios, which may indicate problems with passing urine as a fetus. Many syndromes involve kidney function, especially those babies with low set ears, abnormal genitalia, anal atresia and lower spine anomalies. Fox et al (2010) argue that the baby should be assessed for signs of dehydration, infection and a palpable abdominal bladder with referral to the registrar for further investigations as necessary.

Gastrointestinal system

The gastrointestinal (GI) tract of the neonate is structurally complete, although functionally immature in comparison with that of the adult (Blackburn 2007). The mucous membrane of the mouth is pink and moist. The teeth are buried in the gums and ptyalin secretion is low. Sucking and swallowing reflexes are coordinated. The tongue may be coated with milk plaques, which should be distinguished from the fungus *Candida albicans*, which will need treatment. The stomach has a small capacity (15–30 ml), which increases rapidly in the first weeks of life. The cardiac sphincter is weak, predisposing to regurgitation of milk or posseting. Gastric acidity, equal to that of the adult within a few hours after birth, diminishes rapidly within the first few days and by the 10th day the baby is virtually achlorhydric (without acid), which increases the risk of infection from the mouth. Gastric emptying time is normally 2–3 hours. Enzymes are present, although there is a deficiency of amylase and lipase, which diminishes the baby's ability to digest compound carbohydrates and fat, therefore no sandwiches are allowed! When milk enters the stomach, a gastrocolic reflex results in the opening of the ileocaecal valve. The contents of the ileum pass into the large intestine and rapid peristalsis means that *feeding is often accompanied by reflex emptying of the bowel.*

Bowel sounds can be heard on auscultation within one hour of birth. Sterile meconium present in the large intestine from 16 weeks' gestation, is passed within the first 24 hours of life and should be totally excreted within 48–72 hours. As a result of air entering the gastrointestinal (GI) tract, *E. coli* colonizes the bowel and the stools become brownish-yellow in colour and odorous. Once feeding is established the faeces become yellow. The consistency and frequency of stools reflect the type of feeding. Digested breast milk produces loose, bright yellow and inoffensive acid stools. The baby may pass 8–10 stools a day. The stools of the formula-fed baby are paler in colour, semi-formed, less acidic and have a more offensive odour. A melaena stool contains digested blood from high in the GI tract, has a tar-like appearance and may be caused by blood swallowed at birth, bleeding maternal nipples or damage to the baby's GI tract itself. Low GI bleeding may result in frank blood, which is blood that can be seen in the stools with the naked eye and may be related to HDN (Lwaleed and Kazmi 2009).

Glycogen stores are rapidly depleted so early feeding is required to maintain normal blood glucose levels (2.6–4.4 mmol/l). Weight loss is normal in the first few days but more than 10% body weight loss is abnormal and requires investigation. Most babies regain their birth weight in 7–10 days, thereafter gaining weight at a rate of 150–200 g per week.

Immunity

According to Paterson (2010), neonates demonstrate a marked susceptibility to infections, particularly those gaining entry through the mucosa of the respiratory and gastrointestinal systems. Localization of infection is poor,

with minor infections having the potential to become generalized very easily. The baby has some immunoglobulins at birth but the sheltered intrauterine existence limits the need for learned immune responses to specific antigens. There are three main immunoglobulins: IgG, IgA and IgM.

Immunoglobulin G is small enough to cross the placental barrier. It affords immunity to specific viral infections and at birth the baby's level of IgG is equal to or slightly higher than those of the mother. This provides passive immunity during the first few months of life and by 2 months the baby is able to produce a good response to protein vaccines hence the timing for the commencement of routine childhood immunization programmes (Paterson 2010).

Immunoglobulin M (IgM) and A (IgA) can be manufactured by the fetus and raised blood levels of IgM at birth are suggestive of intrauterine infection. This relatively low level of IgM is thought to render the baby more susceptible to gastroenteritis. Levels of IgA are also low and increase slowly. Secretory salivary levels attain adult values within 2 months and protect against infection of the respiratory tract, gastrointestinal tract and eyes. Colostrum and breastmilk provide the baby with passive immunity in the form of *Lactobacillus bifidus*, lactoferrin, lysozyme and secretory IgA.

Reproductive system: genitalia and breasts

In both sexes, withdrawal of maternal oestrogens results in transient breast engorgement, sometimes accompanied by a milky secretion around the 5th day. Girls may develop pseudo-menstruation, a blood-stained discharge in the nappy, for the same reason. Both findings are insignificant but can be concerning for parents and an appropriate explanation should dispel any anxieties.

Skeleto-muscular system

The muscles are complete, subsequent growth occurring by hypertrophy rather than by hyperplasia. Palpation around the sternomastoid muscle can identify a developing haematoma that feels hard to the touch and is referred to as a tumour (congenital torticollis). The head may be held to one side and is the result of traction and tearing of the muscle. Physiotherapy referral will be made once diagnosed. The long bones are incompletely ossified to facilitate growth at the epiphyses.

THE NEONATAL AND INFANT PHYSICAL EXAMINATION (NIPE)

Performed within the first 72 hours of birth, this examination specifically screens for congenital heart disease

(CHD), congenital cataract, developmental dysplasia of the hip (DDH) and undescended testes, usually in that order. This is not a top-to-toe examination but more of an opportunistic approach when the baby is quiet enough to support auscultation of the chest and awake sufficiently to open its eyes.

Examination of the heart

The incidence of CHD is 8/1000 live births and is the most common group of structural anomalies, accounting for 30% of all congenital malformations (Horrox 2002). Sinha et al (2012) argue that the best time for the heart examination to be conducted is when the baby's major physiological adaptations are complete, so 48 hours post birth is ideal. Half of the known cases of congenital heart disease are detected by antenatal ultrasound scan so the postnatal physical examination is the only other means of early detection. Less than 50% of heart defects are actually detected because many heart conditions are asymptomatic and trivial. Blake (2008) recommends that reading the case notes for details of the present pregnancy, perinatal events and neonatal examinations already performed, is a necessary prerequisite.

Park (2008) reports that maternal congenital heart disease offers 15% prevalence to the woman's children compared to 1% in the general population. When one child is affected the sibling recurrence risk is 3%, especially for a high prevalence condition like Ventricular Septal Defect (VSD), which is the most common variety of CHD and accounts for one-third of all cases. Fox et al (2010) assert that maternal rubella infection in the first trimester commonly results in patent ductus arteriosus (PDA) and pulmonary artery stenosis. Other viral infections in late pregnancy may cause myocarditis. Maternal medications such as anticonvulsants (phenytoin) and amphetamines are highly suspected teratogens. Excessive maternal alcohol intake may cause fetal alcohol syndrome in which VSD, PDA and the tetralogy of Fallot are commonly seen. Maternal diabetes increases the prevalence of transposition of the great arteries (TGA), VSD, PDA and cardiomyopathy. Sinha et al (2012) report that heart defects are common in chromosomal disorders, to include trisomy 13,18, 21 and Turner's syndrome (XO).

The cardiovascular examination

Gill and O'Brien (2007) recommend that the heart itself should technically be left until last with auscultation as the final step, however auscultation is ineffectual if the baby starts to cry, so many examiners listen to the heart earlier in the examination. The mother's view is invaluable and is treated as significant unless proven otherwise. Using words to describe her baby as happy, cranky, responsive, sleepy, floppy can provide useful information on the baby's neurological and homeostatic state, especially how her baby responds physically to taking a feed.

Inspection

England (2010c) believes that inspection is the most important skill because it yields more information about the baby's cardiovascular behaviour and therefore should not be rushed. The examiner should look at the sleeping/resting baby's general appearance and compare gestational age with weight and size, as smallness could indicate growth disruption at the time when major organs were evolving. The examiner should question whether the baby has any dysmorphic features indicative of chromosomal abnormalities that are associated with heart defects. Once the baby's chest is undressed, breathing can be assessed. The rate should be counted for over a minute as breathing tends to be irregular. Central cyanosis needs urgent management. Pallor may precede respiratory distress, but again is difficult to assess, and as Bedford (2011) argues, an oxygen saturation of haemoglobin <95% is abnormal and merits cardiologist assessment. It is wise to always check saturation levels pre and post ductal so if the baby has a PDA, proximal (hand) saturations may be within normal limits and post-ductal levels (foot) will be much lower. England (2010a) believes that respiratory distress may be a sign of cardiac compensation so it is important to inspect for asymmetrical chest wall movements, a tachypnoea >60 breaths per minute, nasal flaring, sternal or costal recession, the use of respiratory accessory muscles, head bobbing and the presence of an expiratory grunt. Capillary refill greater than 2 seconds is abnormal but oxygen therapy should always be considered cautiously as it may close a PDA, which could be is acting as a life-saving conduit in certain heart conditions (Horrox 2002; Bedford 2011).

Palpation

Palpation of the peripheral pulses for rhythm, strength, volume and character then follows. The easiest pulse to feel is the brachial at the antecubital fossa. The rate should be counted over a period of 10 seconds. Palpation of the femoral pulses is a difficult task. Many examiners apply too much pressure to the artery and in effect they eradicate the pulse wave. Strong arm pulses and weak leg pulses suggests coarctation of the aorta (COA). If the right brachial artery pulse is stronger than the left brachial artery pulse, this could suggest a COA where the constriction is proximal to the left subclavian artery. Equal but bounding brachial pulses are found in PDA with a wide but diminishing pulse pressure in the lower limbs. A weak thready pulse is found in congestive heart failure (CHF) and in circulatory shock.

Rhythms originating in the sino-atrial node are called sinus rhythms. In a regular sinus rhythm, the rhythm and rate of the heartbeat are normal for the age of the baby. In sinus tachycardia, with beats above 160 per minute, first consider pyrexia. Gill and O'Brien (2007) contend that the pulse rate will accelerate approximately 10 beats per minute for every 1 °C rise in temperature. Hypoxia, circulatory shock, CHF and thyrotoxicosis are other possible causes. Sinus bradycardia is defined as beats below 80 per minute. Hypothermia, hypoxia, increased intercranial pressure and hypothyroidism may be causative factors.

The midwife can place their open hand onto the precordium, which is the area over the sternum and ribs to the left side of the chest. A palpable precordium murmur is referred to as a thrill, which can sometimes be seen with the naked eye, is characteristic of heart disease with a high volume overload such as a left-to-right shunt through the ductus arteriosus and is always of diagnostic value. Right ventricular enlargement is best sought with one's fingertips placed between the 2nd, 3rd and 4th ribs along the left sternal edge. The apex beat is found in the 4th intercostal space along the mid-clavicular or nipple line. A diffuse, forceful and *displaced* apex beat, usually caused by hypertrophied heart muscle is relatively rare and described as a *heave*. Palpation of the upper abdomen that reveals an enlarged liver (*greater* than 1 cm below the costal margin) may indicate heart failure as the liver acts as a reservoir of blood because the heart cannot cope with the required workload. An enlarged spleen, palpable in the left upper quadrant of the abdomen, complements this clinical picture.

Auscultation

By the time inspection and palpation have been performed much of the information the baby can supply has been obtained and auscultation is the last step. It is recommended that a paediatric stethoscope should be used and its diaphragm (the flat side) utilized at all auscultation sites to hear the high-pitched sounds of a systolic murmur.

The sternum, clavicles and ribs, to include the costal and intercostal spaces, are important landmarks as well as the heart structures. There are two upper landmarks each side of the upper sternum. The right sternal, 2nd intercostal space is the aortic area. This is referred to as the upper right sternal border (URSB). The left sternal 2nd intercostal space is the pulmonary area and is known as the upper left sternal border (ULSB). A further two landmarks are both located to the left of the lower sternum. The left sternal 5th intercostal space is the tricuspid area and may be called the lower left sternal border (LLSB) and the apex is found below the nipple on the mid-clavicular line, in the 4th or 5th intercostal spaces. This is the mitral area. The baby should then be turned onto its right side and the heart should be examined for murmurs along the route of the aorta on the left side of the spine from the scapular area to below the ribs. The examiner is listening

for turbulence of blood in the newly developed collateral circulation caused by COA.

Each cardiac cycle has two heart sounds that can be heard through a stethoscope when applied to the chest wall. The first heart sound (S1) is known as 'lub' and is described as long and booming and occurs when the atriventricular (AV) valves, the tricuspid and bicuspid (mitral) valves are closing at the beginning of ventricular contraction (systole). The second heart sound is 'dub'; it is short and sharp, and reflects closure of the semi lunar valves of the aorta and pulmonary artery, at the beginning of ventricular relaxation (diastole). The best place to hear the first heart sound (S1) is at the apex or the LLSB. Splitting of the heart sound where the tricuspid and mitral valves close slightly out of synchrony, is not usually heard in a normal baby.

The second heart sound (S2) is heard in the ULSB. Splitting of closure of the aortic and pulmonary artery valves is easily heard with the stethoscope and the degree of splitting normally varies with respiration, increasing on inspiration and decreasing or becoming a single sound on expiration. The third and fourth heart sounds are not normally heard but can be best auscultated at the apex or LLSB. The third heart sound (S3) represents ventricular filling that starts as soon as the mitral and tricuspid valves open, and the fourth heart sound represents ventricular filling that occurs in response to contraction of the atria. The fourth heart sound (S4) if heard at the apex is pathological and is seen in conditions with decreased ventricular compliance (flexibility) or CHF. Where there is a combination of a loud S3 or S4 with a tachycardia, common in CHF, this is referred to as a gallop rhythm. This information can only complement a clinical picture of a deteriorating neonate that has a respiratory distress and is not feeding.

A heart murmur is an additional noise heard during the cardiac cycle. *Absence of a murmur does not exclude congenital heart disease*. The location, timing in the cycle, grade, duration or rhythm, quality and radiation of the murmur should be assessed. It is usual to listen to the chest wall in four specific areas. A systolic murmur occurs between S1 and S2 and is classified as one of two types, either an ejection or regurgitant murmur. The examiner should pay particular attention to the timing of the onset of the murmur because the onset in relation to S1 is far more important than the duration of the murmur. In ejection systolic murmurs there is always an interval between S1 and the onset of the murmur. They are referred to as crescendo–decrescendo murmurs as the murmur is at its maximum, half-way between S1 and S2. A murmur may be short or long in duration and can be caused either by a large volume of blood passing through the semi-lunar valves or a normal flow of blood passing through stenosed or deformed semi-lunar valves.

By comparison, regurgitant systolic murmurs *begin with* S1 and usually last through systole (and even into diastole) and are referred to as pansystolic, meaning from start to finish. Park (2008) argues that these murmurs are always pathological and are associated with VSD and feature regurgitation of the mitral and tricuspid valves. Bedford (2011) believes that examiners should only be concerned with systolic murmurs in the neonate as the heart is beating too fast to pick up a diastolic murmur, which occurs when the heart is at rest between S2 and S1.

The intensity of the murmur is customarily graded from 1 to 6. Innocent murmurs are no louder than 2. Grade 3 murmurs are moderately loud. Palpable murmurs (thrill) are graded as 4, are loud and regarded as pathological. Grades 5 murmurs are very loud and audible with the stethoscope barely on the chest wall, whilst grade 6 is audible when standing at the end of the baby's cot.

Quality refers to how the examiner describes the sounds heard, e.g. systolic murmurs of VSD have a uniform high-pitched quality often described as blowing whereas an ejection systolic murmur where stenosis is featured, has a harsh grating quality. If a murmur radiates from one area to another it is usually pathological (Park 2008). *The things that matter most* are the presence of central cyanosis, poor perfusion, tachycardia, an abnormal precordium, a heart murmur with a gallop rhythm and hepatosplenomegaly. Thorough documentation should reflect inspection, palpation and auscultation findings. A cardiac murmur if present should include details of location, timing in the cycle, grade, character and be illustrated. If the baby looks and feels healthy but the midwife can hear extra heart sounds that warrant a second opinion, referral should be made to the registrar, with the parent's informed consent. As a result of the registrar's opinion, the parents should be informed that *at this moment in time* their baby's heart appears healthy or, alternatively, needs further investigation (see Box 28.2).

Box 28.2 Case vignette: Baby Joe

This vignette is to illustrate that significant cardiovascular disease may not be clinically apparent at the time of the NIPE and that consent information should highlight this fact to the parents.

Consider the case of baby Joe, born at term in good condition with no history of scan anomalies. His 36-hour NIPE reports him as a healthy baby in all aspects. At 52 hours of age he deteriorates quickly and presents with central cyanosis, poor perfusion and respiratory distress. His tone is poor. The precordium and pulses are normal. On auscultation there are no heart murmurs or extra sounds. Joe is extremely sick.

The care provided:

- emergency referral and admission to the NICU
- prostaglandin E prescribed to open the ductus arteriosus
- transposition of the great arteries diagnosed on echocardiograph
- transfer to cardiac surgical unit arranged.

The care provided to Joe's parents:

A NIPE midwife may be called upon to provide/contribute to information given to the parents about their sick baby. The parents will usually be upset, fearful, possibly angry and, as a result, not able to listen effectively (England and Morgan 2012). In this situation the most asked questions are:

- why didn't the anomaly scan and NIPE examination reveal the condition?
- what is the condition?
- what is happening to Joe now?
- will Joe die ... when can we see him?

Using language that will have to be personalized for both parents to understand, the following information may be given. Short explanations that answer parents' direct questions are required. Line drawings that are created alongside the verbal explanations may be helpful:

'Joe has a rare condition called transposition of the great arteries. This is where the aorta which transports blood to the body and the pulmonary artery which takes it to the lungs are in the wrong position. On a 20-week anomaly scan the four chambers of the heart can be seen but it is not always possible to see which major blood vessel arises from which ventricle. In Joe's case his pulmonary artery was coming from his left ventricle, blood was going to his lungs and then returning to the left side of his heart creating a mini circulation. On the right side, blood was returning to his heart but instead of going to his lungs, the blood was directed into the misplaced aorta, which took the blood back to his body. From birth, Joe appeared well because an extra vessel called the ductus arteriosus was open and able to shunt oxygen to Joe's body tissues, but as this vessel started to close (which is a normal occurrence), Joe started to deteriorate. This is why the midwife examiner emphasized to you at the end of Joe's examination "at this point in time ... on this occasion, Joe appears well", because at that time, he did appear well.'

England (2010c) believes there is an accepted given that *thorough* examiners will send home a baby that will be readmitted with a serious heart defect. This emphasizes the importance of ensuring that parents *really understand* that the assessment can only reflect the status of the baby *at the time of the examination*.

Examination of the eye

The neonatal eye is 75% of the adult size but the visual system is immature and neural connections from eye to brain are incomplete. Babies have no depth perception because this relies on both eyes working together and neonatal eyes resemble those of chameleons where one eye appears to be functioning independently from the other. During the first three months of life there is a need for both eyes to function well because reduced light stimulation to the eye causes the condition amblyopia where the brain fails to pay enough attention to the messages coming from each eye and as a result, the neural connections for each eye are not created. By 6 months of age, the eyes and brain become 'locked on' to each other and this then sets the stage for the baby's future visual acuity. Amblyopia can occur in one or both eyes and is usually caused by disruption of the light pathways to the retina when there is *corneal clouding or scarring, congenital cataract or clouding of the vitreous humour*. It is vital to screen for these media opacities within 72 hours of birth and later at 6 weeks of age.

The skills of examination start with inspection. Oedema of the eyelids is common and bruising may be present. The examiner should confirm that any trauma and bruising is commensurate with the birth history and ensure the bruising is not a birth mark. The ocular landmarks are the structures that surround the eye and how they appear as part of the face as a whole. With the ophthalmoscope ready for use, the examiner should be prepared to inspect the eyes should the baby open them. Prising eyelids open may add to any oedema and a ptosis (drooping of the eyelid) may go unnoticed. Reducing the room lighting, sitting the baby up or asking the mother to hold the baby over her shoulder with the examiner approaching from behind the mother, works well for some.

The red reflex should be elicited first. The retina is the nervous tissue of the eye, which is stimulated by light. Anteriorly, it is in contact with the vitreous humour and is avascular. Posteriorly it is supported by a vascular and lymphatic supply from the underlying choroid. When a light is shone into the eyes, the vascular retina *shines back* and is known on photographs as 'red eye'. *If the red reflex can be seen, this should indicate to the examiner that there are no media opacities present.* However the redness of the red reflex may be affected by the pigmentation of the baby's skin, and particularly in Asian, Afro-Caribbean, Chinese and Japanese babies they offer different hues of redness from brown to grey to purple, which is a reflection of their pigmented choroid and is a normal finding.

The ophthalmoscope dial should be turned to 0 and with the right hand the scope should be held to the examiner's right eye (or vice versa if left handed). Holding the scope close to the examiner's eye is important if one uses the analogy of a hole in a fence. To look through a hole in a fence, one needs to get up close to the hole to see through to the other side. Each eye of the baby is initially examined separately. Thus the examiner should shine a white light from the ophthalmoscope at the baby's eye from a distance of 5–10 cm and focus on the pupil margin. A red glow from the pupil will be silhouetted against the edge of the iris. To examine both eyes together, the examiner now holds the ophthalmoscope at a distance of 20 cm from the baby's eyes to simultaneously elicit the red reflex from each eye. If there is any asymmetry (inequality) of the colour and intensity of the red reflex, or a white papillary reflex (leucocuria) is seen, the possibility of a media opacity in one or both eyes should be considered and documented. A congenital cataract (2–3 per 10 000 births) is, according to Noonan et al (2011), the commonest cause of blindness and should be uppermost in the examiner's differential diagnosis, but retinoblastoma, a malignant tumour (44 per million births in Europe), represents the most common intraocular tumour of childhood. Congenital infection from toxoplasmosis and retinopathy of prematurity are less common causes.

The ophthalmoscope should then be set to +9 dioptres to conduct a detailed examination of the front of the eye to detect any abnormalities that are not available to the naked eye. The conjunctiva and sclera should be white. Sub-conjunctival haemorrhages are of no clinical significance (but their presence and size should be documented, as non-accidental injury cannot be ruled out). A blue sclera is worthy of note as it is indicative of collagen disease. The sclera looks blue because it is thin and not supported by collagen and is associated with the collagen disease osteogenesis imperfecta (brittle bone disease), which warrants referral.

The cornea should be clear and any lacerations or scarring should be noted. Clouding and/or bulging of the cornea could indicate congenital glaucoma, which needs *urgent* referral. Both pupils should equally respond to light. A coloboma is where the iris does not form a complete circle and may be associated with abnormalities that extend to include the ciliary body and choroid. Complete absence of the iris known as aniridia will also need referral. Different-coloured irises at this stage in life is also suspicious (Gill and O'Brien 2007).

Assessing whether the eye is infected should be no casual task and the examiner should always consider the gravity of ophthalmia neonatorum. According to Noonan et al (2011), a sticky eye demands microbiological investigation to rule out gonococcal and/or chlamydial infection, which if untreated can *rapidly* lead to corneal ulceration and blindness. Gonococcal conjunctivitis can present from 1 to 3 days with a profuse purulent discharge with swelling of the conjunctiva and lids. A swab must be taken for microscopy and culture followed by saline irrigation, topical and systemic antibiotics, usually penicillin. The mother and sexual contact(s) need referral to the genitourinary clinic. Likewise chlamydial conjunctivitis presents later, at 5–14 days, but is associated with neonatal pneumonia if the initial systemic antibiotic treatment has been inadequate.

Fox et al (2010) assert that specific chlamydial swabs should be used with erythromycin the choice of antibiotic. Noonan et al (2011) further contend that *herpes virus type II* and bacterial infections such as *Staphylococcus aureus, Streptococci* and *E. coli* need immediate treatment. Full documentation of what has been found should be detailed for *each eye* and the parents informed that *on this occasion,* the eyes appear healthy (or otherwise).

Examination of the hips

Developmental dysplasia of the hip (DDH) represents a spectrum of defects where the femoral head is not totally in the acetabulum, but possibly on its border and can only be diagnosed on ultrasound scan (Kasser 2012). Dislocation is when the femoral head is outside of the acetabulum. The femoral head continues to grow but if the femoral head is not in the acetabulum, *the acetabulum fails to grow.* Secondary adaptive changes occur so that ligaments and muscles shorten and tighten and the acetabulum fills with scar-like tissue. The incidence is 1 in 400 live births and there are two factors that relate to the natural history of DDH which makes screening difficult. Jones (1998) asserts that as many as 20 babies in every 1000 births have unstable hips but 90% of these will stabilize spontaneously. It is not possible to predict which 10% of these hips will remain unstable. *Stable hips at birth may later develop DDH.* The hip is at its most unstable at the time of term birth. In early gestation there is nearly total spherical enclosure of the femoral head by the acetabulum, but by term when the tightness of the uterus and the lack of leg and hip freedom is at its peak the femur is shallow, then deepens again in the postnatal period. The low incidence of DDH in preterm babies supports this notion. Paton (2011) argues that predominantly it is a disease of girls, with a 6 : 1 ratio with boys, and is more common on the left side (2 : 1). The ideal time for screening the newborn hip is 7 days. The NIPE screen is technically too early, is a compromise but should be followed by an examination at 4–8 weeks by the general practitioner or the health visitor.

The baby must be warm and comfortable, be on a firm flat surface and one of the parents must be present. The midwife must have enough room to gain access to the baby and be physically able and comfortable to perform the manoeuvres (Jones 1998). A general inspection followed by a detailed skeletal examination of the baby may reveal additional risk factors (see Box 28.3) that the history has not elicited. Oligohydramnios, postural foot deformities, plagiocephaly, scoliosis and a prominent sacral dimple are all associated with hip abnormalities. Babies that show the effects of intrauterine growth restriction (IUGR) and those with dysmorphic features are particularly at risk.

With the baby lying on its back and legs bent at the knee with feet on the surface, an initial inspection should look for any asymmetry in the appearance of the legs and groin skin folds. Examination of the knees may show uneven

---

> **Box 28.3 Predisposing factors to developmental dysplasia of the hip (DDH)**
>
> 1. Squashed hips *in utero*. The emphasis is breech birth to include vaginal and caesarean section and to include those babies when external cephalic version has been performed near to and at term for breech presentation. When oligohydramnios is featured, look for structural or positional talipes (equino-varus/calcaneo-valgus) or a combination of these two presentations
> 2. Genetic predisposition. There is a higher proportion of identical twins with DDH compared to non-identical twins
> 3. Family history of dislocation of the hip/DDH
> 4. Ligament hyperlaxity can lead to full abduction in the presence of a dislocated hip
> 5. Geographical variation where abduction of the child's hips is a strong cultural feature, with an incidence of 0.25 per 1000 live births; however, where swaddling the legs together (usually for warmth) is the cultural norm, the incidence rises to 10/1000.
>
> Source: Dove et al 2011

---

knee height. On the affected side, the knee is lower because the head of the femur has dropped into the soft tissues because it is not being held by the bony acetabulum. However, equal knee height could indicate either normality of both hips or bilateral dislocation of both hips. Pulling the legs straight to measure leg length, should be done *after* the hip examination as this manoeuvre stimulates flexor tone resistance, which is enough to upset a settled baby and render the examination less valid.

The modified Ortolani and Barlow manoeuvres are referred to as the *combined stress test* and are performed to diagnose the subluxatable (dislocatable) or dislocated hip and make it possible to notice the presence or absence of knee and hip clicks. The range of abduction in flexion is also a useful sign to indicate the degree (if any) of abnormality.

The Ortolani manoeuvre is described for examination of the left hip, using the examiner's right hand. The examiner steadies the pelvis between the thumb of the left hand on the baby's symphysis pubis and fingers under the sacrum. With the baby's left leg flexed in the palm of the right hand, the head of the femur is held between the examiner's right thumb on the inner side of the thigh opposite the lesser trochanter and the middle longest finger over the greater trochanter. In an attempt to relocate a posteriorly displaced head of the femur forwards into the acetabulum, the middle finger applies gentle pressure upon the greater trochanter. The baby's thighs are flexed forward (to the head of the baby) onto the abdomen and rotated and *abducted* through an angle of 70–90° towards the examining surface. If the hip is dislocated, a *clunk* will be felt (and sometimes heard) as the head of the femur slips *into* the acetabulum. A high-pitched click is probably a product of soft tissue structures moving over bony prominences. Remember Ortolani – Out to In (Baston and Durward 2010).

The Barlow manoeuvre is described for examination of the left hip and the examiner's right hand. From a position of abduction, the hip is *adducted* to 70° and gentle pressure is exerted by the examiner's right thumb on the lesser trochanter in a backward and lateral direction. If the thumb is felt to move backwards over the labrum (the fibro-cartilaginous rim of the acetabulum) onto the posterior aspect of the joint capsule, a clunk may be heard as the head of the femur dislocates *out* of the acetabulum. England (2010c) describes the noise as a deeper clunk with significant movement. The dislocatable hip can feel strangely soft with little or no resistance. The Ortolani manoeuvre will then be performed to return the head of femur to the acetabulum. To examine the right hip the role of the examiner's hands is reversed. Dove et al (2011) support the view that it is acceptable for the experienced examiner to undertake the Ortolani and Barlow manoeuvres sequentially on both hips simultaneously.

The Barlow and Ortolani tests involve gentle manoeuvres. The softer the touch, the more information is secured; indeed very little pressure is needed to dislocate the head of femur because the acetabulum is so shallow. A heavy-handed approach will often make the baby stiffen and resist being touched. In this circumstance the examiner needs to abandon the examination, talk to the baby (and parents) in an attempt to relax him (and them) and then attempt a further examination. A useful analogy is a gear stick in a car. Gentle manipulation of the baby's legs in a circular rotation helps to reduce muscle and nerve tension. Likewise, the lightest of touch can help guide that gear stick home.

Documentation of findings in the Personal Child Health record should offer details and be explained to the parents. Dove et al (2011) assert that it is not enough to place a tick against the word hips. When an abnormality is found an example of the record may be written thus: 'The right hip abducted fully in flexion; is stable and the combined stress test Ortolani/Barlow manoeuvre was negative with no shortening on knee height inspection. The left hip shows shortening on knee height inspection with resistance to abduction, which resulted in an Ortolani clunk as the head of femur returned to the acetabulum. The findings were confirmed by Dr Smith (neonatal registrar). Double nappies were applied. Referral arranged for a 2 week follow-up for ultrasound scan and appointment with orthopaedic consultant. Both parents were present at the examinations and have been informed of the clinical findings and referral arrangements.' An entry that communicates health must reflect that both hips abduct fully in flexion and there is no apparent shortening on knee height

inspection. It should be clear that both hips are stable and the combined stress test comprising the Ortolani and Barlow manoeuvres is negative for both hips. The parents should be told that *on this examination/occasion*, their baby's hips appear healthy.

Examination of the genitalia

This examination will repeat the previous examinations reported in this chapter and review any new developments.

Neurological examination

The neurological examination will be performed continuously throughout the examination, noting how the baby handles and behaviourly tolerates the examination. The healthy term baby will make eye-to-eye contact, fix and follow a face when held 30 centimetres from the examiner. There should be natural facial movements with blinking of the eyes. When lying supine the baby will be flexed at the knees with hips abducted; the head turned to one side. Movements are smooth, symmetric and varied. The baby should be able to demonstrate a rooting reflex. Coordinated movements of lip, tongue, palate and pharynx are required to suck and swallow successfully. Failure to suck when the stomach is empty is indicative of abnormal function and an important sign of brain stem damage.

Primary (primitive) reflexes (see Box 28.4) are best performed at the end of the NIPE screen as they will usually unsettle, even distress the baby. They provide information about lower motor neuron activity and muscle tone. Persistence beyond the normal age suggests that higher cortical centres are not gaining control of tone and movement as expected and can be an early sign of cerebral palsy. Extremes of tone (rag doll floppiness) or persistent extension of the back (opisthotonus) are both abnormal. Flexed arms and extended legs is also an abnormal posture. Jitteriness is a feature of the healthy baby and can be stopped by touching the affected area. Irritability in the form of repetitive movements, for example an eyelid or finger, could represent a convulsion in a baby and warrants referral.

At present NIPE training is largely regarded as an expanded role of the registered midwife. However the Midwifery 2020 report (Department of Health 2010) recommends that overall care of the neonate needs to be improved, and according to Lumsden (2012), NIPE training is now becoming part of pre-registration midwifery education. There is a requirement for all midwives to further develop their neonatal knowledge in recognizing health, by knowing and understanding the abnormal. This will involve enhancing their communication and examining skills in being able to conduct all three screening examinations discussed in this chapter, in order to provide truly holistic, individualized care that will place the midwife as the lead practitioner for the healthy baby.

Box 28.4 Neurological reflexes in the newborn

- **Placing reflex.** Whilst the baby is being held upright, the top of the foot is touched by the edge of a surface and the baby will lift and place its foot on the surface. Presents from 36 weeks' gestation and disappears at 3 months of age.
- **Palmar and plantar grasps.** Flexion of fingers/toes when an object is placed in the palm of the hand/on the ball of the foot. Presents at 28 weeks' gestation and disappears by 2–3 months.
- **Asymmetric tonic neck reflex** (the fencing sign). When the head is turned to one side, the arm and leg on that side extend, while the arm and leg on the other side remain flexed. Established from 36 weeks' gestation and disappears at 6 months.
- **Moro (startle) reflex.** On sudden head extension, symmetrical abduction and extension followed by

flexion and adduction of the arms, with accompanying cry. Present at 37 weeks' gestation and disappears around 4 months of age. Absent in heavy sedation or hypoxic, ischaemic encephalopathy. Unilateral presentation implies fractured clavicle, hemiplegia, brachial plexus palsy.
- **Rooting reflex.** Stroking the baby's cheek with a finger causes the head to turn towards the stimulation and the mouth will open. Established at 34 weeks' gestation and disappears at 4 months of age, when visual cues take over.
- **Sucking reflex.** Elicited to assess the strength and coordination of the sucking reflex by placing a clean finger in the mouth. Disappears by age of 12 months.

For visual display of reflexes go to www.youtube.com/watch?v=Sv5SsLH70mY

REFERENCES

Baston H, Durward H 2010 Examination of the newborn. A practical guide. Routledge, London

Bedford C D 2011 Cardiovascular and respiratory assessment of the baby. In: Lomax A (ed) Examination of the newborn. An evidence-based guide. Wiley–Blackwell, Chichester

Bedford C D, Lomax A 2011 Development of the heart and lungs and transition to extrauterine life. In: Lomax A (ed) Examination of the newborn. An evidence-based guide. Wiley–Blackwell, Chichester

Blackburn S T 2007 Maternal fetal and neonatal physiology. Saunders Elsevier, Philadelphia

Blake D 2008 Assessment of the neonate: involving the mother. British Journal of Midwifery 16(4):224–6

Brown V D, Landers S 2011 Heat balance. In: Gardner S L, Carter B S, Enzman-Hines M et al (eds) Neonatal intensive care. Mosby, St Louis

Davies N 2011 Abnormalities of the foot. In: Lomax A (ed) Examination of the newborn. An evidence-based guide. Wiley–Blackwell, Chichester

Department of Health 2010 Midwifery 2020: delivering expectations. www.midwifery2020.org.uk (accessed 4 March 2013)

Dove R, Hunter J, Wardle S 2011 Nottingham neonatal service clinical guidelines. Screening for developmental dysplasia of the hip. Nottingham University Hospital NHS Trust

England C 2010a Neonatal respiratory problems. In: Lumsden H, Holmes D (eds) Care of the newborn by ten teachers. Hodder Arnold, London

England C 2010b Care of the jaundiced baby. In: Lumsden H, Holmes D (eds) Care of the newborn by ten teachers. Hodder Arnold, London

England C 2010c Physical examination of the neonate. In: Marshall J E, Raynor M D (eds) Advancing skills in midwifery practice. Churchill Livingstone, London

England C, Morgan R 2012 Communication skills for midwives. Challenges in everyday practice. Open University Press/McGraw-Hill Education, Maidenhead

Foundation for Sudden Infant Death 2013 http://fsid.org.uk (accessed 2 April 2013)

Fox G, Hoque N, Watts T 2010 Oxford handbook of neonatology. Oxford University Press, Oxford

Gill D, O'Brien N 2007 Paediatric clinical examination made easy. Churchill Livingstone, London

Gordon M 2011 Examination of the newborn abdomen and genitalia. In: Lomax A (ed) Examination of the newborn. Wiley–Blackwell, Oxford

Gordon M, Lomax A 2011 The neonatal skin: examination of the jaundiced newborn and gestational age assessment. In: Lomax A (ed) Examination of the newborn. Wiley–Blackwell, Oxford

Griffith R (2009) Safeguarding children from significant harm. British Journal of Midwifery 17(1):58–9

Horrox F 2002 Manual of neonatal and paediatric heart disease. Whurr Publishers, London

Jones, A J 1998 Hip screening in the newborn. A practical guide. Butterworth–Heinemann, Oxford

Kasser J R 2012 Orthopaedic problems In: Cloherty J P, Eichenwald E C, Hansen A R et al (eds) Manual of neonatal care. Lippincott, Williams and Wilkins, Philadelphia

Lumsden H 2010 Examination of the newborn. In: Lumsden H, Holmes D (eds) Care of the newborn by ten teachers. Hodder Arnold, London

Lumsden H 2012 Embedding NIPE into the pre-registration midwifery programme. Midwives (1):42–3

Lwaleed B A, Kazmi R 2009 An overview of haemostasis. In: Hall M, Noble A,

Smith S (eds) A foundation for neonatal care. A multidisciplinary guide. Radcliffe, Oxford

Noonan C, Rowe F J, Lomax A 2011 Examination of the head, neck and eyes. In: Lomax A (ed) Examination of the newborn. Wiley–Blackwell, Oxford

Park M K 2008 Pediatric cardiology for practitioners. Mosby, Philadelphia

Paterson L 2010 Infections in the newborn period. In: Lumsden H, Holmes D (eds) Care of the newborn by ten teachers. Hodder Arnold, London

Paton R W 2011 Developmental dysplasia of the hip. In: Lomax A (ed) Examination of the newborn. Wiley–Blackwell, Oxford

Resuscitation Council UK 2011 Newborn life support, 3rd edn. London

Roth D A, Hildesheimer M, Bardenstein S et al 2008 Periauricular skin tags and ear pits are associated with permanent hearing impairment in newborns. Paediatrics 122:884–90

Sinha S, Miall L, Jardine L 2012 Essential neonatal medicine. Wiley–Blackwell, Chichester/Oxford

Trotter S 2010 Neonatal skincare. In: Lumsden H, Holmes D (eds) Care of the newborn by ten teachers. Hodder Arnold, London

UK National Screening Committee 2008 Newborn and infant physical examination: standards and competencies NHS. http://newbornphysical.screening.nhs.uk (accessed 3 February 2013)

UK National Screening Committee 2012 NSC policy database. Hearing (newborn). www.screening.nhs.uk/hearing-newborn (accessed 28 October 2012)

Wassner A J, Spack N P 2012 Disorders of sex development. In: Cloherty J P, Eichenwald E C, Hansen A R (eds) Manual of neonatal care. Lippincott, Williams and Wilkins, Philadelphia, p 791–807

FURTHER READING

Bedford C D, Lomax A 2011 Development of the heart and lungs and transition to extrauterine life. In: Lomax A (ed) Examination of the newborn. An evidence-based guide. Wiley–Blackwell, Chichester

This chapter provides a detailed exploration of the fetal circulation and the adaptations that occur with the first breath at birth. It also integrates the impact of hypoglycaemia, hypoxia and hypothermia on these transitional events and offers a useful discussion on the energy triangle.

McCallum L 2010 www.slideshare.net/Prezi22/physical-examination-of-the-newborndoc

This text offers useful information on examination of the newborn and could be used as a revision script.

Quarrell C 2011 Examining the neonate in the hospital and community: child protection issues. In: Lomax A (ed) Examination of the newborn: an evidence-based guide. Wiley–Blackwell, Chichester

This chapter asserts that the midwife is the baby's advocate and safeguarding considerations should be integral to the examination of the newborn by ensuring that the baby remains the focus of the examination. Does the evidence observed fit with the parent's account? Who is the midwife's designated referral professional in safeguarding situations? These questions are well addressed.

USEFUL WEBSITES

Resuscitation Council (UK): www.resus.org.uk

The Resuscitation Council in the definitive resource for keeping up to date on techniques and information about neonatal resuscitation.

The Auscultation Assistant: www.wilkes.med.uncla.edu/inex.htm

A good site to listen to and differentiate the different heart sounds and murmurs.

Chapter |29|

Resuscitation of the healthy baby at birth: the importance of drying, airway management and establishment of breathing

Carole England

CHAPTER CONTENTS

Midwives are the lead practitioners in normal birth and attend most births in the hospital and home setting. It is therefore important that they have applicable knowledge and skills of resuscitation to enable them to care for the newborn baby (and parents) in a competent supportive manner. The aim of this chapter is to uphold the principles of care offered by the Resuscitation Council United Kingdom [RCUK] (2011) and explore the specific role of the midwife in drying the baby and airway management. Noting the time of birth and starting the clock on the resuscitaire (if applicable) is always the starting point for care and documentation requirements. Requesting assistance from the multiprofessional team at any stage of the process is recognized as an essential component.

THE CHAPTER AIMS TO:

- emphasize the importance of thoroughly drying the baby to prevent heat loss
- support the principle of enabling the baby to resuscitate itself by placing its head in the neutral position
- detail how to open the airway by giving inflation breaths in order to clear the lung fluid
- reiterate the importance of starting and maintaining a record of the events of the resuscitation process
- highlight the need to ask for help from the multiprofessional team at any stage of the process.

DRYING THE BABY

Thoroughly drying of the baby is always the first step to management of resuscitation at birth. Taking the time to dry the baby's head, to include the face alongside the arm and leg creases, is sometimes not performed as thoroughly as it should be. According to Connolly (2010), heat loss and cooling of the baby is inevitable but failure to spend time doing this task meticulously can result in the baby using oxygen and glucose to maintain or raise its metabolic rate. Also, in order to place a baby in skin-to-skin contact with its mother, *the baby needs to be thoroughly dry*; furthermore, the mother needs to be dry so that the baby can benefit from *conductive heat* gains.

During this time of drying, which can take up to a minute, the midwife should assess the baby for its colour and muscle tone. The Apgar score is used as a communication tool to inform other team members should it be necessary. A score at 1, 5 and 10 minutes is entered into the record (Nursing and Midwifery Council [NMC] 2009). Most babies will be *blue* at birth, which indicates that there is accumulation of carbon dioxide (CO_2) in the blood and tissues. It is important to remember that CO_2 is a stimulant to the respiratory centre in the medulla oblongata, so blue skin is a *normal physiological* sign and most babies will not require resuscitating. However, too much CO_2 will depress respiration and this may account for why the baby may be showing little or no respiratory effort. *White or mottled grey skin* is an indication of peripheral shut down as the baby is responding to low oxygen levels and is conserving the available oxygen for the heart and brain by diverting blood away from the skin and other non-essential organs (Leone and Finer 2012). This is the baby that needs to be thoroughly dried as their reserves of oxygen cannot be wasted on attempting to keep warm. So, the rule of thumb must be *the poorer the colour, the more thorough the drying process should be*. The midwife should not let their own anxiety or that of others hurry them in this drying process. All wet towels should be discarded and the baby covered in warmed dry ones. Identification name bands should also be placed on the baby in the hospital setting, should there be need to separate the baby from the mother at any time.

According to Rennie and Kendall (2013), the assessment of muscle tone indicates to what degree the nerves are stimulating the skeletal muscles. When a baby is well toned for its gestational age, this signals that the baby is generally in good condition even though they may not be breathing. A baby that is both white and *floppy* reflects the possibility of long-term hypoxia as a result of the labour process or some other co-existing factor, for example, infection. The midwife should simultaneously assess whether the baby is breathing by assessing the presence or absence of chest movement and any other signs, such as gasping. *If the baby is crying, the baby has an open airway.* This assessment is followed by auscultation of the chest to assess the heart rate. Dawson et al (2010) argue that the midwife needs to establish whether there is a heart rate and, if so, if it is above or below 60 beats per minute (bpm). In the first minute, the average heart rate of a healthy term baby is below 100 bpm, however by the second minute it has usually risen to around 140 bpm and by 5 minutes to 160 bpm. Dawson et al (2010) consider that the heart rate is the most important indicator of health in newborn babies and this is why it is so important to make a regular assessment, hence the 1 and 5 minutes time-frame of the Apgar score (Apgar 1952). During this time of assessment, the umbilical cord can remain uncut so that extra red blood cells can be transported to the baby and enhance the baby's oxygen-carrying capacity. Even if the heart rate is really slow, opening the airway must be the first task to achieve. Without an open airway, the baby has no way of being oxygenated, as this is the only means of assisting the heart to function. Hence the midwife should note the **A**irway, **B**reathing and **C**irculation of resuscitation when **C** *must* follow **B** and **B** *must* follow **A**: *there is no room for any short cuts.*

AIRWAY MANAGEMENT AND BREATHING

If the baby is not breathing, *opening the airway is always the first step.* A flat surface is needed so the umbilical cord can be cut and secured. In the home setting, the floor is a tempting location to place the baby, especially if the room is cluttered. However, the floor is not ideal, as even in the summer it is often cold and draughty and therefore likely to cool the baby. *Furthermore, in any resuscitation situation, the first consideration is practitioner safety.* The midwife must always make sure the environment is safe for her to function, and bad posture in particular can contribute to poor performance and awkward communications. It is therefore better to clear a table or use the seat of a firm chair to place the baby on.

The prominence of the neonatal occipital protuberance can affect the natural position of the baby's head, when lying on its back, with the result of either the chin falling down to the chest in flexion or extending into the *chin-up* position. Both postures consequently close the airway. The head should be placed in the *neutral* position (Fig. 29.1) with the nose uppermost, the ideal situation being when another person can hold the baby's head for the midwife (Tracy et al 2011).

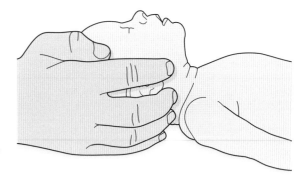

Fig. 29.1 Neutral position.

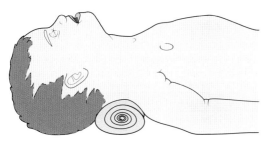

Fig. 29.2 Small towel under the neck (sniffing position).

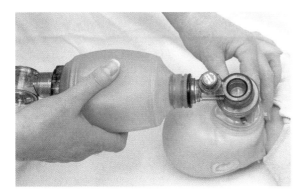

Fig. 29.3 Bagging demonstration.

Alternatively, a small sheet/towel or equivalent can be placed under the neck of the baby to secure the neutral position (*sniffing position*) (Fig. 29.2).

Intermittent positive pressure ventilation (IPPV) will then be commenced using a bag and mask if available or a T-piece, mask and resuscitaire in the hospital. The mask must be the correct size for the baby to prevent any leaks of air to occur on inflation of the bag. The mask should be rolled onto the face from the chin, using the stem of the mask (like a champagne glass) to hold it in position. The soft part of the mask should not be touched as this may distort its shape and lead to leakage of air (Fig. 29.3).

The bag when manually compressed will deliver positive pressure of air at 30 cmH$_2$O. Given that the alveoli are filled with lung fluid, this pressure should be applied for 3 seconds, which is the time it takes to steadily count '1–2–3', to begin the process of forcing the lung fluid into the lymphatic channels of the lungs. The bag should be allowed to refill before giving the second breath, '2–2–3', the third breath, '3–2–3', '4–2–3', and finally '5–2–3'. *Five inflation breaths should be sufficient to clear the lung fluid to make room for the air.* While these inflation breaths are being given, the baby should be covered but with the chest exposed so that any chest movement (which is the sign of an open airway) can be seen and noted. It must be appreciated that while there is an exchange of one substance with

another, i.e. lung fluid with air, there is no accumulation of air to lift the chest *until the 4th or 5th inflation breath.* This can be a nervous time for the midwife because it is natural to think that the chest will rise on the first inflation and it is easy for midwives to blame their own technique. Once chest movement has been seen, the facemask should be removed to assess if the baby is spontaneously breathing. The heart rate can also be assessed at this time to establish whether the rate has increased.

Babies that are blue with good muscle tone and a heart rate above 60 bpm often do not need any further assistance. As soon as normal respiratory effort is established and their heart rate is over 100 bpm, they can be given to their mother for skin-to-skin contact. However, some babies in this category may not be breathing spontaneously because there remains too much CO$_2$ in their blood and tissues (*hypercapnoea*) that is depressing their respiratory effort. *Ventilatory breaths* are then commenced to provide oxygen (21% in air) and blow off the excess CO$_2$. Given at a rate of 30 breaths per minute, these breaths are therefore 2 seconds in duration. It is important to assess the baby every 30 seconds to see if they are making spontaneous efforts to breathe. It is vital that the midwife does not over-ventilate the baby and reduce their CO$_2$ too much and cause apnoea. Babies should be allowed to resuscitate themselves, noting the time when the baby is breathing spontaneously. (See Box 29.1.)

DIFFICULTIES IN ESTABLISHING AN OPEN AIRWAY

If there is no chest movement after five inflation breaths, this indicates that the airway is not open, so the alveoli will remain filled with lung fluid. This is a good time to

---

Box 29.1 **Reflective question**

'If a baby is not breathing, is it acceptable to blow oxygen onto the baby's face instead of using IPPV with a bag and mask?'

This is totally *inappropriate* for two reasons:

1. You must first establish that the airway is open. The only way to do this is by giving five inflation breaths and seeing the chest rise by the fifth inflation breath. *The time you spend not giving IPPV is wasted and the baby is not receiving any benefit from you.*
2. Resuscitation gas now consists of air as standard *not* oxygen. Air is a *cold* gas and if you blow this onto the face of the baby, you will quickly cool the baby.

consider calling for medical assistance because failure of the following interventions may result in the need for tracheal intubation (RCUK 2011). In the home, paramedic support will take longer to arrive so early anticipation of problems is considered good practice. If the baby has a poor colour and muscle tone, this may indicate that the position of their head has not been maintained in the neutral position and there is a definite need for a second person's help both to hold the head and apply jaw thrust. The jaw of a floppy baby can fall backwards and as the tongue is attached to the jaw, the tongue falls back into the airway, blocking the airway. A second person, with their fingers on each side of the jaw, can push the jaw forwards and hold it in that position. This is an easily performed manoeuvre because the baby does not offer any muscle tone resistance. Five inflation breaths should then be given. If there is still no chest movement, suction to the oropharynx under direct vision using the light of a laryngoscope may be considered should there be an obstruction. Occasionally if there is maternal bleeding at the birth, some blood may have entered the baby's mouth, initially as fluid but then over time may have clotted. (*Please note: The management of meconium is not considered in this context, as the resuscitation would be approached in a different way:* Chapters 32 and 33). After this intervention five inflation breaths are given. If not successful, an oropharyngeal (Guedel) airway can be inserted to open the airway mechanically, especially in babies who may have congenital abnormalities such as *choanal atresia* and/ or *micrognathia*. The correct sizing of the airway is vital. When held along the line of the lower jaw with the flange at the level of the middle of the lips, the end of the airway should reach the angle of the jaw. The airway is slipped over the tongue in the same attitude that it will finally lie. The midwife should make sure that the tongue is not pushed back into the back of the mouth. Once *in situ* the mask can be placed over the airway (*both the mouth and nose*) and a further five inflation breaths should be given. If the chest fails to rise after these interventions, intubation of the trachea will be required and an experienced neonatal registrar will be needed to assist.

PARENTAL SUPPORT THROUGH EFFECTIVE COMMUNICATION

According to England and Morgan (2012) resuscitation of the baby occurs in the presence of the parents, so a clear, simple explanation in a calm tone should be given to inform and support them during the process. Parental stress and anxiety will affect how the couple are able to receive information and respond to it. Non-verbal communication is more influential in informing the parents of the midwife's state of mind. Documentation should always reflect obtained consent and specific aspects of the resuscitation, including any interactions between the parents and multiprofessional team that have occurred (NMC 2008, 2009, 2012). It is important to recognize that records should always be sequentially detailed enough, should they be required to support the midwife's actions at a later date and read out in court or at the NMC.

REFERENCES

Apgar V 1952 Proposal for a new method of evaluation of newborn infants. Anaesthesia and Analgesia 32: 260–7

Connolly G 2010 Resuscitation of the newborn. In: Boxwell G (ed) Neonatal intensive care nursing. Routledge, London, p 65–86

Dawson J A, Kamlin C O F, Wong C et al 2010 Changes in heart rate in the first minutes after birth. Archives of Disease in Childhood Fetal and Neonatal Edition 95(3): F177–81

England C, Morgan R 2012 Communication skills for midwives: challenges in everyday practice.

McGraw–Hill/Open University Press, Maidenhead

Leone T A, Finer N N (2012) Resuscitation in the delivery room. In: Gleason C A, Devaskar S U (eds) Avery's diseases of the newborn. Elsevier, Philadelphia, p 328–40

NMC (Nursing and Midwifery Council) 2008 The Code: standards of conduct, performance and ethics for nurses and midwives. NMC, London

NMC (Nursing and Midwifery Council) 2009 Record keeping. Guidance for nurses and midwives. NMC, London

NMC (Nursing and Midwifery Council) 2012 Midwives rules and standards. NMC, London

RCUK (Resuscitation Council UK) 2011 Newborn life support. RCUK, London

Rennie J M, Kendall G S 2013 A manual of neonatal intensive care. Taylor and Francis, London

Tracy M B, Klimek J, Coughtrey H et al 2011 Mask leak in one-person mask ventilation compared to two-person in a newborn infant manikin study. Archives of Disease in Childhood Fetal and Neonatal Edition 96(3):F195–200

FURTHER READING

England C, Morgan R 2012 Communication skills for midwives: challenges in everyday practice. McGraw–Hill/Open University Press, Maidenhead

Chapter 7 provides details regarding personal interactions in acute clinical situations and explores in depth how the midwife should communicate with parents and members of the multiprofessional team in the neonatal resuscitation situation.

Mosley C M J, Shaw B N J 2013 A longitudinal cohort study to investigate the retention of knowledge and skills following attendance on the Newborn Life Support course. Archives of Disease in Childhood 98(8):582–6

This article reports that practitioners following specialist training, over time experience deterioration in neonatal resuscitation ability and technique, especially if they are not exposed to clinical resuscitation situations on a regular basis. Practitioners failed on simple but essential interventions such as not removing the wet towel from the baby and not assessing the baby's heart beat. It is suggested that practitioners should attend resuscitation updates on a regular basis to maintain and hone their skills, which should improve confidence.

Chapter |30|

The healthy low birth weight baby

Carole England

CHAPTER CONTENTS

Between 6% and 7% of all babies born in the United Kingdom (UK) weigh <2500 g at birth. Preterm babies make up two-thirds of low birth weight (LBW) babies, with the other one-third being small for their gestational age (SGA), some of which will be born at term.

It is now common practice for healthy LBW babies from 32 weeks' gestation with a birth weight of 1.7–2.5 kg to be cared for on a postnatal ward with their mother. The majority of these babies remain well, will have minimal or no illness in the neonatal period and can be cared for by midwives as the lead practitioner (Department of Health [DH] 2010). This chapter will examine the role of the midwife in supporting parents to care for their healthy LBW baby and the specific knowledge and skills the midwife requires to fulfil this effectively.

THE CHAPTER AIMS TO:

- examine the terminology and classifications of babies in relation to gestational age and birth weight
- critically discuss the importance of skin-to-skin contact and early feeding in the prevention of cold stress and hypoglycaemia
- discuss the provision of an accommodating environment that supports the developing needs of the LBW baby on the postnatal ward.

CLASSIFICATION OF BABIES BY GESTATION AND WEIGHT

Definitions of gestational age disregard any considerations of birth weight and likewise definitions of LBW are based upon weight alone and do not consider the gestational age of the baby.

Gestational age

According to Smith (2012), babies should preferably be classified by gestational age, as this is a better physiological measure compared to birth weight. A preterm baby is born before completion of the 37th gestational week (259 days), which is calculated from the first day of the mother's last menstrual period (LMP) and has no relevance to the baby's weight, length, head circumference, or indeed any other measurement of fetal or neonatal size. Smith (2012) further asserts that gestational age estimates by first-trimester ultrasonography are accurate within 4 days, so that the combination of fetal crown–rump length and menstrual history are now considered more accurate indices for estimating gestational age.

Birth weight

The World Health Organization (WHO 1997a) recommend that babies who weigh <2500 g should be called low birth weight (LBW). As neonatal care has become more effective and babies are surviving at earlier gestations, new LBW categories are now recognized:

- very low birth weight (VLBW) babies are those weighing below 1500 g at birth
- extremely low birth weight (ELBW) babies are those who weigh below 1000 g at birth.

It is the *relationship* between weight (for assessment of *growth*) and gestational age (for assessment of *maturity*) that is of great importance. This relationship can be seen plotted on centile charts (Fig. 30.1) to visually demonstrate that growth is appropriate, excessive or diminished for gestational age and that the baby is either preterm, term or post-term. Growth charts, however, should be

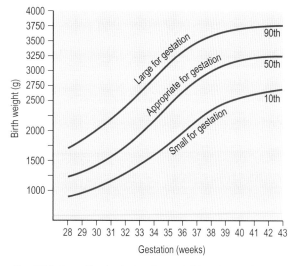

Fig. 30.1 A centile chart, showing weight and gestation.

derived from studies of local populations, because genetically derived growth differences exist between countries, cultures and lifestyles.

Various presentations of LBW babies can be described as follows:

1. Babies whose rate of intrauterine growth is normal at the moment of birth. They are small because labour began before the end of the 37th gestational week. These preterm babies are *appropriately grown* for their gestational age (*AGA*). Their weight is between the 90th and 10th centiles for their gestation age.
2. Babies whose rate of intrauterine growth has slowed down and who are born at, or later than, term. These term or post-term babies are *under-grown* for gestational age and are consequently small for their gestational age (*SGA*). Their weight is below the 10th centile for their gestational age.
3. Babies whose rate of intrauterine growth has slowed down and who are also born before term. These preterm babies are small by virtue of both their early birth and impaired intrauterine growth. They are both *pre-term* and *SGA* babies because their weight will be below the 10th centile for their reduced gestational age.

Babies are considered *large* for their gestational age (*LGA*) when their weight exceeds the 90th centile. Consequently, it should be recognized that both term and preterm babies can fall into the category of AGA, SGA, or LGA (Fig. 30.2).

SMALL FOR GESTATIONAL AGE (SGA)

Babies that are small for their gestational age are of a size that is smaller when compared to other babies. If a baby is under-grown and below the 10th centile for weight, historically there has been for some an *automatic assumption* that as a fetus the baby has experienced intrauterine growth restriction (IUGR). Wilkins-Haug and Heffner (2012) define IUGR as a rate of fetal growth that is less than the normal growth potential for a specific baby. However, this does not mean that all SGA babies are small as a result of IUGR. Some small babies are genetically small because they have small parents or grandparents and this familial factor determines their smallness. They are well, healthy babies who need to be treated accordingly.

Centile charts can act only as guides. Trotter (2009) states that maternal characteristics, obstetric history and birth details in addition to the appearance and behaviour of the baby should determine what care is required. Should a baby be born at 36 weeks' gestation with a birthweight of 2100 g, which according to weight, is well below the 50th centile, this baby would not fall below the 10th

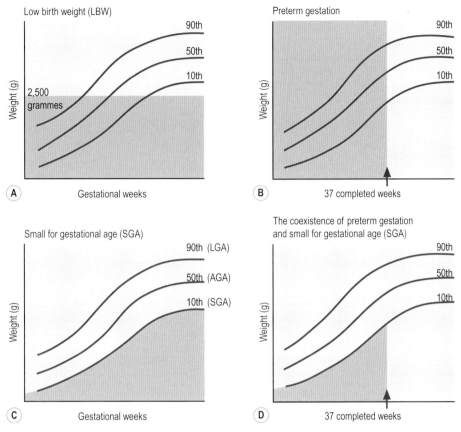

Fig. 30.2 Centile charts that illustrate how low birth weight babies are categorized by weight and gestation. (A) Low birth weight. (B) Preterm gestation. (C) Small for gestational age. (D) Co-existence of preterm gestation and small for gestational age.

centile line for weight, so should *not* be identified as SGA but may be under-grown. Similarly it should not be assumed that all infants of diabetic mothers (IDM) are macrosomic and only fall into the LGA category. Diabetes and obesity are conditions that deleteriously affect maternal circulation and perfusion, so some babies will suffer from IUGR and could be *small* for their gestational age.

Types of intrauterine growth restriction (IUGR)

There are two recognized types of IUGR. The causes and predisposing factors are seen as multi-factorial (Box 30.1).

IUGR that begins early in the first trimester caused by a combination of intrinsic and extrinsic factors, results in *symmetrical* fetal growth

In this scenario, the fetus suffers significant interruption to *hyperplastic* cell division (Fig. 30.3). As a result, the

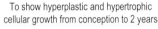

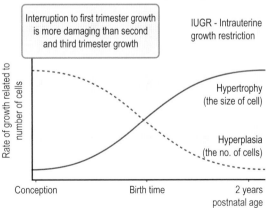

Fig. 30.3 Graph to show hyperplastic and hypertrophic cellular growth from conception to 2 years.

Box 30.1 Causes of intrauterine growth restriction (IUGR)

Fetal growth is regulated by maternal, placental and fetal factors and represents a mix of genetic mechanisms and environmental influences through which growth potential is expressed. The mechanisms that appear to limit fetal growth are multifactorial.

Maternal factors

- Pregnancy-induced hypertension, pre-eclampsia, to include HELLP syndrome
- Congenital and acquired heart disease, to include chronic hypertension
- Diabetes mellitus
- Undernutrition, to include obesity. Underweight mother/small stature. Eating disorders
- Smoking, alcohol misuse
- Drugs: therapeutic (anticancer, thyroid medication), recreational (narcotic, prescription)
- Renal disease, collagen disorders, anaemia, thyroid disorders and epilepsy
- Genetic diseases such as maternal phenylketonuria and cystic fibrosis

- Extremes in young and elderly mothers
- Poor obstetric history that includes preterm labour
- Respiratory disorders, to include asthma
- Maternal work and ability to rest

Fetal factors

- Multiple gestation
- Chromosomal/genetic abnormality (particularly trisomy conditions), including inborn errors of metabolism, dwarf syndromes
- Intrauterine infection: toxoplasmosis, rubella, cytomegalovirus, herpes simplex (ToRCH) and syphilis

Placental factors

- Abruptio placenta
- Placenta praevia
- Chorioamnionitis
- Abnormal cord insertion
- Oligohydramnios

Sources: Nodine et al 2011; Smith 2012

---

head circumference, length and weight are all proportionately reduced for gestational age. The main causes are referred to as *intrinsic factors* that operate from *within* the fetus and cause *symmetrical* growth restriction, often as a result of transplacental infections or chromosomal/genetic defects. In addition, the deleterious effects of maternal lifestyle where a poor quality diet may be in combination with smoking, drug and/or alcohol misuse, can impact on fetal growth and development. These examples are referred to as *extrinsic factors* that can act upon the fetal environment and contribute to congenital malformations that culminate in conditions such as fetal alcohol syndrome (FAS) or chronic hypoxia associated with maternal smoking. Affected babies suffer interruption to hyperplastic (new cell) division, therefore look small and do not have the potential for normal growth. Remember a small head equates to a small brain. These babies make up 10–30% of all SGA babies in Western societies (Sinha et al 2012).

IUGR that begins in the last trimester, caused by extrinsic factors, results in *asymmetrical* fetal growth

This type of fetus has been growing normally then starts to experience interruption to hypertrophic cell growth (Fig. 30.3). This is influenced by extrinsic factors in its *intrauterine environment* that cause disruption to placental

perfusion of oxygen and nutrients. When serial ultrasound scans of head and abdominal circumference in addition to Doppler measurements indicate poor and disproportionate growth, the birth of many affected fetuses are expedited early, usually by elective caesarean section. For those women where an early birth is not possible (the smaller twin or triplet; a concealed pregnancy or through failing to access antenatal care), their baby will to varying degrees have a characteristic brain-sparing appearance. The baby's head appears relatively large compared to the body (see Fig. 30.4); however, the head circumference is usually within normal parameters and brain growth is usually spared. The skull bones are within gestational norms for length and density but the anterior fontanelle may be larger than expected, owing to diminished bone formation. The abdomen appears sunken owing to shrinkage of the liver and spleen, which surrender their stores of glycogen and red blood cell mass respectively as the fetus adapts to the adverse conditions of the uterus. As subcutaneous fat is used as a source of glucose and ketones, the skin becomes loose, giving the baby a wizened, old appearance. Vernix caseosa is frequently reduced or absent as a result of diminished skin perfusion. In the absence of this protective covering, the skin is continuously exposed to amniotic fluid and its cells will begin to desquamate (shed) so that the skin appears pale, dry and coarse. If the baby is of a mature gestation and has passed meconium *in*

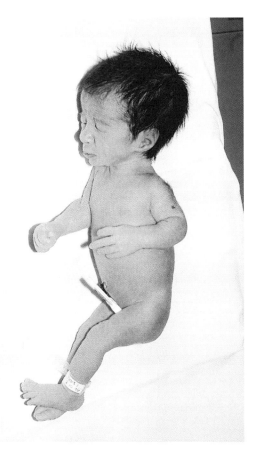

Fig. 30.4 Baby with asymmetrical growth restriction. Note the apparently large head compared with the undergrown body.

Box 30.2 **Causes of preterm labour**

Spontaneous causes

- 40% unknown
- Multiple gestation – the higher the multiple the greater the chance
- Hyperpyrexia as a result of viral or bacterial infection, often urinary tract infections
- Premature rupture of the membranes caused by maternal infection, especially chorioamnionitis. Also polyhydramnios
- Maternal short stature, age (<18 or > 35years) and parity
- Maternal uterine malformation; often bicornuate or significant fibroids
- Poor obstetric history; history of preterm labour
- Cervical incompetence, history of cone biopsy
- Maternal substance abuse, particularly alcohol and cigarette smoking

Elective causes

- Pregnancy-induced hypertension, pre-eclampsia, chronic hypertension
- Maternal disease: renal, heart
- Placenta praevia, abruptio placenta
- Rhesus incompatibility
- Congenital abnormality of the baby
- IUGR

Sources: Sinha et al 2012; Smith 2012

utero, the skin may be stained with meconium. Fetal distress in labour and hypoglycaemia are more likely to be seen in this group of babies. Unless severely affected, these babies appear hyperactive and hungry, with a lusty cry.

THE PRETERM BABY

The preterm baby is born before the end of the 37th gestational week, regardless of birth weight. Most of these babies are appropriately grown, some are SGA and a small number are LGA. The factors that play a role in the initiation of preterm labour are largely unknown and mainly overlay with factors that impair fetal growth. They are divided into those labours that commence spontaneously and those where a decision is made to terminate a viable pregnancy before term: referred to as *elective causes* (Box 30.2).

Characteristics of the preterm baby

The appearance of the preterm baby at birth will depend upon the gestational age. The following description will focus upon the baby *born from 32 weeks' gestation*. Preterm babies rarely grow large enough *in utero* to develop muscular flexion and fully adopt the fetal position. As a result their posture appears flattened, with hips abducted, knees and ankles flexed. Lissauer and Faranoff (2011) describe a generally hypotonic baby with a weak and feeble cry. The head is in proportion to the body, the skull bones are soft with large fontanelles and wide sutures. The chest is small and narrow and appears underdeveloped. The abdomen is prominent because the liver and spleen are large and abdominal muscle tone is poor (Fig. 30.5). The liver is large because it receives a good supply of oxygenated blood and is active in the production of red blood cells. The umbilicus appears low in the abdomen because linear growth is cephalo-caudal, being more apparent nearer to the head than rump, by virtue of fetal circulation

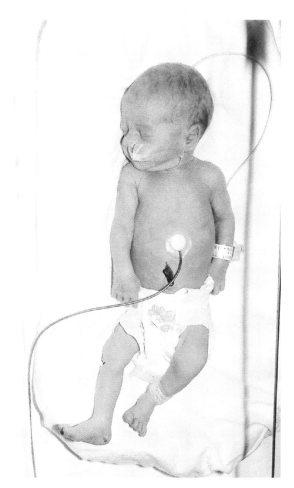

Fig. 30.5 Healthy preterm baby born at 32 weeks' gestation. Note the presence of a nasogastric tube. The thermocouple of the servo-mode is taped to the skin of the baby's upper abdomen.

oxygenation. Subcutaneous fat is laid down from 28 weeks' gestation, therefore its presence and amount will affect the redness and transparency of the skin. Vernix caseosa is abundant in the last trimester and tends to accumulate at sites of dense lanugo growth, such as the face, ears, shoulders and sacral region, protecting the skin from amniotic fluid maceration. The ear pinna is flat with little curve, the eyes bulge and the orbital ridges are prominent. The nipple areola is poorly developed and barely visible. The cord is white, fleshy and glistening. The plantar creases are absent before 36 weeks' gestation but soon begin to appear, as fluid loss occurs through the skin. In girls the labia majora fail to cover the labia minora and in boys the testes descend into the scrotal sac at about the 37th gestational week.

CARE OF THE HEALTHY LBW BABY

Many of the care issues relevant to the LBW baby apply to both the preterm and the SGA infant. Where differences do exist, these will receive further consideration.

Management at birth

Given the unpredictability of the birth process on growth and maturity, the role of the midwife in the birthing room is to prepare the environment, staff and parents for certain eventualities. This takes the form of informing members of the multiprofessional team such as a second midwife, neonatal practitioner and neonatal nurse, to be on standby for the birth. The incidence of perinatal asphyxia and congenital malformation is greater in SGA babies and the baby with a scaphoid abdomen could be physically normal, albeit thin, but could also deteriorate quickly if presenting with a diaphragmatic hernia. The midwife should be fully aware of the availability of cots in the neonatal intensive care unit (NICU), transitional care unit or postnatal ward according to the condition of the baby and their potential care demands following birth. The labour room ambient temperature should ideally be between 23 and 26 °C and the neonatal resuscitaire and accompanying equipment should be ready for use.

It is particularly important that the midwife attaches the correct labels to the baby at birth in case separation from the mother should occur at any time if the baby's condition becomes unstable. The midwife should cut the cord and leave an extra length to allow for easy access to the umbilical vessels in case they are needed at a later time. At birth, the midwife should ensure that the baby is thoroughly dried before skin-to-skin contact is attempted, in order to prevent evaporative heat losses. Skin-to-skin contact for a period of up to 50 minutes is recommended to secure the baby's conductive heat transfer gains and help the baby to become physically stabilized to feed. If the mother chooses not to engage in skin-to-skin contact, the father may wish to do so (Chin et al 2011) but if not, the baby can be dressed, wrapped and held by the parents. The baby's axilla temperature should be maintained between 36.5 °C and 37.5 °C. Early attempts at breastfeeding should be encouraged (Pollard 2012).

Assessment of gestational age

With developments of more accurate dating by antenatal ultrasound techniques, it is argued by Smith (2012) that there is less justification for a full assessment of gestational age in healthy LBW babies. The exception is applied when the mother deliberately conceals her pregnancy or has difficulty/is unable to communicate. The neonatal practitioner, with the view that no harm is caused as a result of the process, should carefully conduct any assessments that are carried out. Sasidharan et al (2009) considers that the Ballard Score (Ballard et al 1991) can give an accurate assessment of gestational age until at least 7 days of life and continues to be the most widely used tool.

The Department of Health (DH 2009) states that WHO has introduced growth charts based on *exclusively* breast-fed babies. A chart specifically for preterm babies 32–36 weeks has also been devised that has no centile lines between birth and the first two weeks of neonatal life and the 50th centile has been de-emphasized to better reflect the natural weight losses and gains of this category of baby. It is important that midwives are educated to use these specialized charts efficiently so that the baby's subsequent growth and development can be monitored effectively (DH 2009).

Thermoregulation

Thermoregulation is the balance between heat production and heat loss. The prevention of cold stress, which may lead to hypothermia – which is a body temperature below 35 °C – is critical for the intact survival of the LBW baby. Newborn babies are unable to shiver, move very much or seek extra warmth for themselves and therefore rely upon physical adaptations that generate heat by raising basal metabolic rate and utilize brown fat deposits. Thus, exposure to cool environments can result in multisystem changes. As body temperature falls, tissue oxygen consumption rises as the baby attempts to burn brown fat to generate energy and heat. Diversion of blood away from the gastrointestinal tract reduces all forms of digestion. *Attempting to warm a cold baby by feeding is ineffectual and carries the danger of milk inhalation.* Care measures should aim to provide an environment that supports the *neutral thermal environment.* This environment constitutes a range of ambient temperatures within which the metabolic rate is minimal, the baby is neither gaining nor losing heat, oxygen consumption is negligible and the core-to-skin temperature gradient is small (Blackburn 2007).

In the baby, the head accounts for at least one-fifth of the total body surface area and brain heat production is thought to be 55% of total metabolic heat production. Rapid heat loss due to the large head-to-body ratio and large surface area is exaggerated. Wide sutures and large fontanelles add to the heat-losing tendency. Once the baby is thoroughly dried, which includes the face, a pre-warmed hat will minimize heat loss from the head. Asymmetric SGA babies have increased skin maturity but often depleted stores of subcutaneous fat, which are used for insulation. Their raised basal metabolic rate helps them to produce heat but their high energy demands in the presence of poor glycogen stores and minimal fat deposition can soon lead to *hypoglycaemia* (<2.6 mmol/l) followed by physiological cooling (<36 °C) to reach a state of *hypothermia* (<35 °C) (Bedford and Lomax 2011).

All preterm babies are prone to heat loss because their ability to produce heat is compromised by their immaturity, so factors such as their large ratio of surface area to weight, their varying amounts of subcutaneous fat and their ability to mobilize brown fat stores will be affected by their gestational age (Blackburn 2007). During cooling, immaturity of the heat-regulating centres in the hypothalamus and medulla oblongata causes *failure to recognize the need to act.* In addition, preterm babies are unable to increase their oxygen consumption effectively through normal respiratory function and their calorific intake is often inadequate to meet increasing metabolic requirements. Furthermore, their open resting postures increase their surface area and, along with insensible water losses, these factors render the preterm baby more susceptible to evaporative heat losses. Fellows (2010) argues that when the baby is not receiving skin-to-skin contact with either parent and the baby is under 2 kg, the warm conditions in an incubator can be achieved either by heating the air to 30–32 °C (*air mode*) or by *servo-mode*: controlling the baby's body temperature at a desired set point (36 °C). In servo-mode, a *thermocouple* is taped to the upper abdomen and the incubator heater maintains the skin at that site at a preset constant temperature (Fig. 30.4). Within the incubator, the baby is clothed with bedding, in a room temperature of 26 °C. Most preterm babies between 2.0 kg and 2.5 kg will be cared for in a cot, in a room temperature of 24 °C.

Hypoglycaemia

The term *hypoglycaemia* refers to a low blood glucose concentration and is usually a feature of failure to adapt from the fetal state of continuous transplacental glucose consumption to the extrauterine pattern of intermittent milk supply (WHO 1997b). Within the first hour of life the blood glucose levels fall, which triggers the pancreas to stimulate the alpha cells of the Islets of Langerhans to produce glucagon, with the consequential effect of releasing glucose from glycogen stores in the liver to maintain the blood glucose levels within *safe* limits. However, it is generally questioned whether LBW babies are as effective in this metabolism compared to appropriately grown term babies and some caution is recommended (WHO 1997b). Asymmetrical SGA babies may have greater brain-to-body mass with a tendency towards *polycythaemia*, which increases their energy demands, and since both the brain and the red blood cells are obligatory glucose users, these factors can increase glucose requirements. Glycogen storage is initiated at the beginning of the third trimester of pregnancy but may be incomplete as a result of preterm birth or, in the asymmetrical SGA baby, may have been drawn upon before birth.

Hypoglycaemia in healthy LBW babies is more likely to occur in conditions where they become cold or where the initiation of early feeding (within the first hour) is delayed.

However, hypoglycaemia is associated with mild to moderate perinatal asphyxia and maternal history of beta-blocker use (e.g. labetolol) as it causes *hyperinsulinism* and interferes with glycogenolysis. The midwife should consider that there may be some underlying medical condition that may call for more thorough investigation (Chapter 33).

The signs of hypoglycaemia are varied and Wilker (2012) acknowledges that hypoglycaemia can present with no or few clinical signs. The clinical picture of tremor and irritability may occasionally lead to convulsion and decreased consciousness. A high-pitched cry, hypotonia, unexplained apnoea and bradycardia with central cyanosis are also recognized as serious signs of deterioration in the baby's health and need referral to a medical practitioner. Jitteriness is not a sign of hypoglycaemia (United Nations Childrens Fund [UNICEF] 2010). The aim of management is to maintain the true blood glucose level above 2.6 mmol/l, which is considered to be the lowest level of normal in the first few days of life (WHO 1997b; Lissauer and Fanaroff 2011).

Healthy LBW babies who show no clinical signs of hypoglycaemia, are demanding and taking nutritive feeds on a regular basis and maintaining their body temperature, do not need screening for hypoglycaemia. The emphasis of care is placed upon the concept of *adequate feeding* and the cornerstone of success is the midwife's ability to assess whether the baby is feeding sufficiently well to meet energy requirements. The preterm baby may be sleepy and attempts to take the first feed may reflect its gestational age. Midwives should be guided by the local policies within their employing organization regarding use of reagent strips to assess for hypoglycaemia, but prior to the baby's second feed is the best time to ascertain whether the first feed was effective in maintaining the capillary blood glucose level above 2 mmol/l. If a baby, despite being fed, presents with *clinical signs of hypoglycaemia*, a venous sample should be taken by the medical practitioner to assess the *true* blood glucose level which should be dispatched to the laboratory. A true blood glucose level that remains <2.6 mmol/dl, despite the baby's further attempts to feed by breast or take colostrum by cup, may warrant transfer to the NICU, because glucose by intravenous bolus may be necessary to correct the metabolic disturbance. Healthy mature SGA babies with an asymmetrical growth pattern will usually breastfeed within the first 30–60 minutes of birth and will demand feeds every 2–3 hours thereafter. For the majority of LBW babies, hypoglycaemia is relatively short-lived and limited to the first 48 hours following birth.

Feeding

According to Jones and Spencer (2008) both preterm and SGA babies benefit from human milk because it contains long chain polyunsaturated omega-3 fatty acids, which are thought to be essential for the myelination of neural membranes and for retinal development. Preterm breast milk has a higher concentration of lipids, protein, sodium, calcium and immunoglobulins, alongside lipases and enzymes that improve digestion and absorption. The uniqueness of the mother's milk for her own baby cannot be overstated but she needs to understand what her baby may be able to achieve related to the stage of their development, which is based upon the combined influences of their gestational age at birth and their neonatal age.

For a baby to feed for nutritive purposes, the coordination of breathing with suck and swallow reflexes reflects neurobehavioural maturation and organization, which is thought to occur between 32 and 36 weeks' gestation. Blackburn (2007) argues that preterm babies are limited in their ability to suck because they lack *cheek pads*, which leads to a weaker suck, coupled with weak musculature and flexor control, which are important for firm lip and jaw closure.

Als and Butler (2006) believe that parents should provide physical support for head, trunk and shoulders as sucking is part of the flexor pattern of development and may be enhanced by giving the baby something to grasp. The preterm baby's head is very heavy for the weak musculature of the neck and would, if not supported, result in considerable head lag, so correct positioning and attachment to the breast can be made much more difficult to achieve. Poor head alignment can result in airway collapse, which may lead to apnoea and bradycardia, therefore support from the midwife is essential when initiating breastfeeding.

If the baby requires feeding via a nasogastric tube, it is now common practice for parents to feed their own baby. Tube feeding has the advantage that the tube can be left in situ during a cup or breastfeed and has been shown to eliminate the need to introduce bottles into a breastfeeding regimen. However, babies are preferential nose breathers and the presence of a nasogastric tube will inevitably take up part of their available airway. Flint et al (2007) argue that the prolonged use of nasogastric tubes has been associated with delay in the development of a baby's sucking and swallowing reflexes simply because the mouth is bypassed. For these reasons, cup feeding has been used in addition or as an alternative to tube feeding, in order to provide the baby with a positive oral experience, to stimulate saliva and lingual lipases to aid digestion and to accelerate the transition from naso/oro-gastric feeding to breastfeeding. Oral gastric tubes have been associated with vagal stimulation and have resulted in bradycardia and apnoea.

Pollard (2012) reports that certain behaviours, such as licking and lapping, are well established *before* sucking and swallowing, and when babies are given the opportunity it is not unusual to see them as early as 28 and 29 weeks licking milk that has been expressed onto the nipple by their mother. Thus, babies between 30 and 32 weeks' gestation can be given expressed breastmilk (EBM) by cup. Pollard (2012) makes a further point that tongue movement is vital in the efficient stripping of the milk ducts, so cup-feeding can be seen as developmental preparation for breastfeeding. Between 32 and 34 weeks' gestation, cup-feeding can act as the main method of feeding, with the baby taking occasional complete breastfeeds. The baby uses less energy to take its feed by cup compared to bottle, which supports their general well-being and homeostasis.

A preterm baby of <35 weeks' gestation can be gently wrapped/swaddled prior to a feed and this is thought to provide reassurance and comfort, not unlike the unique close-fitting tactile stimulation of the uterus. McGrath (2004) argues that this approach supports development of flexion as well as decreasing disorganized behaviours that could detract from feeding success. A preterm baby may easily tire and the mother can be taught to start the flow of milk by hand expressing, before attempting to attach her baby to the breast. Long pauses between sucks are to be expected. This *burst–pause* pattern is a signal of normal development and seems to occur earlier with breastfeeding. The baby may appear to be asleep and a change in position may remind them of the task in hand, but it is thought to be a mistake to force a reluctant baby to feed. If it is obvious that the baby is more interested in sleeping, the mother can complete the feed by nasogastric tube. Feeding frequency can vary between 8 and 10 feeds per day. The baby should be left to establish their own volume requirements and feeding pattern. If necessary, the mother should use a breast pump to maintain her lactation to reflect her baby's feeding style.

OPTIMIZING THE CARE ENVIRONMENT FOR THE HEALTHY LBW BABY

The normal sensory requirements of the developing neonatal brain depend upon subtle influences, first from the uterus and then from the breast (Reid and Freer 2010). Any disruption to this natural arrangement renders the LBW baby vulnerable to influences in the care environment that can result in poor coordination as a result of delays in the development of different subsystems (autonomic, motor, sensory, etc.). Reid and Freer (2010) believe maternal role development depends upon the mother's self-esteem and her perception of mothering. By attempting to adapt the care environment to be more like the intrauterine environment, the midwife can help parents to become aware of their baby's behavioural and autonomic cues and utilize them in organizing care according to their baby's individual tolerance. The ethos

of care is for them to listen and learn from their baby, to come to know and see them as an individual, competent for their stage of development and not merely *a baby born too early*, or a *dysfunctional term baby*. They should be encouraged (but not cajoled) into taking a major role in their baby's emerging developmental agenda, enabling them to understand the situation in which they find themselves, so they are further able to reset their expectations and thus provide more baby-led support (Teti et al 2005; Reid and Freer 2010).

According to McGrath (2004), the emerging task of the term newborn baby is increasing alertness, with growing responsiveness to the outside world. By comparison, a preterm baby is at a stage of development that is more concerned with their internal world. Term babies have stable function of the autonomic and motor systems. Preterm babies will be at different stages of this development, depending on their gestational age and health status. They will spend more time in rapid eye movement (REM) sleep or drowsy states and have difficulty in achieving deep sleep. They are unable to shut out stimulation that prevents them from sleeping and resting, and sudden noise hazards provoke stress reactions, which can adversely affect respiratory, cardiovascular and digestive stability. The term baby is able to shut out such stimuli for rest and sleep purposes. The degree to which SGA term babies have been affected by their unique intrauterine experience is difficult to assess in the short term, but hyperactivity is seen as a feature of an adaptive stress reaction. These babies, like their preterm counterparts, need an environment that supports their level of robustness. Environmental disturbances, excessive or prolonged handling and even activities like feeding may add extra physiological burden to an already compromised state. Social contact is considered a vital element for the development of parent–baby interaction, yet stereotypical notions of social contact that revolve around practical caregiving and feeding may not be suitable for some babies and when these activities are pooled together, may draw too heavily on the baby's physical resources. When the baby is overstimulated and wishes to terminate the interaction, certain cues are known as *coping signals* and are recognized as *fist clenching, furrowing of the brow, gaze aversion, splayed fingers* and *yawning*. Should the baby wish to initiate or continue an interaction, they tend to demonstrate *approach signals* such as *raised eyebrows, head raising* and *engagement in different degrees of eye contact with their social partners*. The midwife can reassure parents that by paying attention to their baby's behaviour they can work *with* their baby's capabilities, which is crucial for maintaining the baby's healthy status (Als and Butler 2006).

Handling and touch

Kangaroo care (KC) is used to promote closeness between a baby and mother and involves placing the nappy-clad

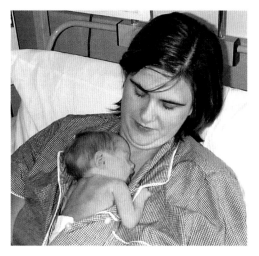

Fig. 30.6 Kangaroo care.

baby upright between the maternal breasts for skin-to-skin contact (Fig. 30.6). The LBW baby can remain beneath the mother's clothing for varying periods of time that suit the mother. Some mothers may have repeated contacts throughout the day, others may prefer specific periods around which they plan their daily activities. There are no rules or time limitations applied, but contact should be reviewed if there are any clinical signs of neonatal distress. Hake-Brooks and Anderson (2008) found that preterm babies of 32–36 weeks' gestation who had unlimited skin-to-skin contact, breast fed for longer compared to those who had traditional nursery care. Conde-Agudelo and Belizan (2009) support this view and also consider that the baby remained more physiologically stable, with less reported incidence of infection.

Noise and light hazards

The time spent in a postnatal ward should be a time of rest and recuperation for both the mother and her LBW baby. All extraneous noises should be eliminated from clinical areas, such as musical toys and mobiles, harsh clattering footwear, telephones, radios, intercom systems and raised voices. Clinicians should be aware of noise hazards, such as the closing of incubator portholes, use of peddle bins, ward doors and general equipment. Ward areas may be carpeted and *quiet signs* can be posted to remind visitors not to disrupt the peace. In dimmed lighting conditions preterm babies are more able to improve their quality of sleep and alert status. Reduced light levels at night will help to promote the development of circadian

rhythms and diurnal cycles. Light levels can be adjusted during the day with curtains or blinds to shade windows and protect the room from direct sunlight. Screens to shield adjacent babies from phototherapy lights are also essential.

Sleeping position

Hunter (2004) reports that preterm babies have reduced muscle power and bulk, with flaccid muscle tone, therefore their movements are erratic, weak or flailing. They exert energy to maintain their body position against the pull of gravity. Nesting preterm babies into soft bedding, in addition to the use of close flexible boundaries, helps to keep their limbs in midline flexion, however it is vital that they are nursed in a supine position to prevent asphyxia. The supine position is also thought to be effective in promoting engagement in self-regulatory behaviours such as exploration of the face and mouth, hand and foot clasping, boundary searching, flexion and extension of the limbs. Pressure on the occiput should, over time, ensure a more rounded head.

Placing healthy LBW babies to sleep in the prone position has been theoretically eradicated from neonatal practice and Warwood (2010) reiterates that all babies should be placed in the supine position, and it is incumbent upon midwives to accustom the baby and educate the parents in adopting this approach. Teaching resuscitation to parents is part of routine preparation for transfer home, although according to Younger et al (2007) this degree of preparedness can empower some parents but frighten others. The decision to receive training should be the parent's choice (Resuscitation Council United Kingdom 2011).

The importance of providing an appropriate environment for the healthy LBW baby cannot be overstressed and the ideal environment should resemble home, which provides a cycle of day and night, regular nourishment, rest, stimulation and loving attention. The midwife's role is to create such an environment, primarily for the physical development of the baby but at the same time to provide psychological support for the mother and her family. According to Fleury et al (2010) the mother should be encouraged to rely upon her own instincts and common sense so that the rhythm of total care she adopts in hospital will thoroughly prepare her for when she goes home. Gambini et al (2011) make the point that often the difference between early and late transfer home is more dependent upon the mother's positive attitude and skill development than the baby's maturity and inherent abilities.

REFERENCES

Als H, Butler S 2006 Neurobehavioural development of the pre-term infant In: Martin R J, Fanaroff A A, Walsh M C (eds) Faranoff and Martin's neonatal–perinatal medicine. Diseases of the fetus and infant, vol 2. Elsevier Mosby, London, p 1051–68

Ballard J L, Khoury C, Wedig K et al 1991 New Ballard Score expanded to include extremely premature infants. Journal of Paediatrics 119:417–23

Bedford C D, Lomax A 2011 Development of the heart and lungs and transition to extrauterine life. In: Lomax A (ed) Examination of the newborn: an evidence-based guide. Wiley–Blackwell, Chichester, p 47–58

Blackburn S T 2007 Maternal, fetal and neonatal physiology: a clinical perspective. Mosby Saunders, St Louis

Chin R, Hall P, Daiches A 2011 Father's experience of their transition to fatherhood: a metasynthesis. Journal of Reproductive and Infant Psychology 29(1):4–18

Conde-Agudelo A, Belizan J 2009 Kangaroo mother care to reduce morbidity and mortality in low birthweight infants. Cochrane Database of Systematic Reviews 2009, Issue 2. Art No. CD002771. doi:10:1002/14651858. CD002771

DH (Department of Health) 2009 Using the new UK–World Health Organization 0–4 years growth charts. DH, London. Available at www.dh.gov.uk/publications (accessed 11 April 2013)

DH (Department of Health) 2010 Midwifery 2020: delivering expectations. London, DH. Available from www.midwifery2020.org.uk (accessed 3 April 2013)

Fellows P 2010 Management of thermal stability. In: Boxwell G (ed) Neonatal intensive care nursing. Routledge, London

Fleury C, Parpinelly M, Makuch M Y 2010 Development of the mother–child relationship following pre-eclampsia. Journal of Reproductive and Infant Psychology 28(3):297–306

Flint A, New K, Davies M 2007 Cup feeding versus other forms of supplemental enteral feeding for newborn infants unable to fully breastfeed. Cochrane Database of Systematic Reviews 2007, Issue 2. Art. No. CD005092. doi: 10. 1002/14651858. CD005092.pub2

Gambini I, Soldera G, Benevento B et al 2011 Postpartum psychosocial distress and late preterm birth. Journal of Reproductive and Infant Psychology 29(5):472–9

Hake-Brooks S, Anderson G 2008 Kangaroo care and breastfeeding of mother–preterm infant dyads 0–18 months: a randomised controlled trial. Neonatal Network 27:151–9

Hunter J (2004) Positioning. In: Kenner C, McGrath J M (eds) Developmental care of newborns and infants: a guide for health care professionals. Mosby, St Louis, p 299–320

Jones E, Spencer A 2008 Optimising the provision of human milk in preterm infants. MIDIRS Midwifery Digest 18(1):118–21

Lissauer T, Fanaroff A A 2011 Neonatology at a glance. Wiley–Blackwell, Chichester

McGrath J M 2004 Feeding. In: Kenner C, McGrath J M (eds) Developmental care of newborns and infants: a guide for health care professionals. Mosby, St Louis, p 321–42

Nodine P M, Arrruda J, Hastings-Tolsma M 2011 Prenatal environment: effect on neonatal outcome. In: Gardner S L, Carter B S, Enzman-Hines M et al (eds) Merenstein and Gardner's handbook of neonatal intensive care. Mosby Elsevier, London, p 13–38

Pollard M 2012 Evidence-based care for breastfeeding mothers. Routledge, London

Reid T, Freer Y 2010 Developmentally focused nursing care. In: Boxwell G (ed) Neonatal intensive care nursing. Routledge, London, p 16–39

Resuscitation Council UK (RCUK) 2011 Newborn life support, 3rd edn. RCUK, London

Sasidharan K, Dutta S, Narang A 2009 Validity of New Ballard Score until 7th day of postnatal life in moderately preterm infants. Archives of Diseases in Childhood Fetal and Neonatal Edition 94: 39–44

Sinha S, Miall L, Jardine L 2012 Essential neonatal medicine, 5th edn. Wiley–Blackwell, Chichester

Smith V C 2012 The high-risk newborn: anticipation, evaluation, management and outcome. In: Cloherty J P, Eichenwald E C, Hansen A R et al (eds) Manual of neonatal care. Wolters Kluwer Lippincott Williams and Wilkins, London, p 74–90

Teti D M, Hess C R, O'Connell M 2005 Parental perceptions of infant vulnerability in a preterm sample: prediction from maternal adaptation to parenthood during the neonatal period. Journal of Development and Behavioral Paediatrics 26:283–92

Trotter C W 2009 Gestational age. In: Tappero E P, Honeyfield M E (eds) Physical assessment of the newborn. NICU INK California, p 21–40

UNICEF (United Nations Children's Fund) 2010 Guidance on the development of policies and guidelines for the prevention and management of hypoglycaemia of the newborn. Available at www.babyfriendly.org.uk (accessed 12 April 2013).

Warwood G 2010 Teaching resuscitation to parents. In: Lumsden H and Holmes D (eds) Care of the newborn by ten teachers. Hodder Arnold, London, p 168–77

Wilker R E 2012 Hypoglycaemia and hyperglycaemia. In: Cloherty J P, Eichenwald E C, Hansen A R et al (eds) Manual of neonatal care. Wolters Kluwer Lippincott Williams and Wilkins, London, p 284–96

Wilkins-Haug L E, Heffner L J 2012 Fetal assessment and prenatal diagnosis. In: Cloherty J P, Eichenwald E C, Hansen A R et al (eds) Manual of neonatal care. Wolters Kluwer Lippincott Williams and Wilkins, London, p 1–10

WHO (World Health Organization) 1997a Manual of international statistical classification of diseases, injuries and causes of death, vol 11. WHO, Geneva

WHO (World Health Organization) 1997b Hypoglycaemia of the newborn: review of the literature. WHO, Geneva

Younger J B, Kendell M J, Pickler R H 2007 Mastery of stress in mothers of preterm infants. Journal of Specialist Paediatric Nursing 2:29–35

FURTHER READING

McInnes R, Chambers J 2008 Supporting breastfeeding mothers: qualitative synthesis. Journal of Advanced Nursing 62(4):407–27 *These authors focus upon practices that support breastfeeding in neonatal and transitional care units. This article reflects the mothers' perspectives and can inform the midwife on whether the women felt supported.*

USEFUL WEBSITES

Ballard Score: www.ballardscore.com
The New Ballard Score assesses physical and neuromuscular maturity to assess gestational age.

Growth charts:
www.growthcharts.rcph.ac.uk
Materials for training on how to use the charts can be downloaded on this website.

Chapter |31|

Trauma during birth, haemorrhages and convulsions

Claire Greig

This chapter focuses on complications occurring in specifically vulnerable babies; the midwife's awareness of this vulnerability may prevent such complications. If a complication does occur, the midwife must report it to the baby's doctor and may work with that doctor and/or a wider multiprofessional team to diagnose it and implement effective treatment. Parents may be distressed when their baby suffers a complication and the midwife helps them to understand the complication, facilitating their discussions with the multiprofessional team members, and assisting them to care for their baby.

THE CHAPTER PRESENTS INFORMATION ON:

- trauma during birth to skin and superficial tissues, muscle, nerves and bones
- major types of neonatal haemorrhage due to trauma, disruptions in blood flow, coagulopathies and other causes
- neonatal convulsions
- specific interventions with parents.

TRAUMA DURING BIRTH

Despite skilled midwifery and obstetric care in developed, Western societies and a reduction in the incidence, birth trauma still occurs. Efforts continue to reduce the incidence even further.

Trauma during birth includes:

- trauma to skin and superficial tissues
- muscle trauma
- nerve trauma
- fractures.

Trauma to skin and superficial tissues

Skin

Skin damage is often iatrogenic, resulting from forceps blades (Fig. 31.1), vacuum extractor cups, scalp electrodes and scalpels. Poorly applied forceps blades or vacuum extractor cup may result in scalp abrasions (Fig. 31.2), although less so with softer vacuum extractor cups. Forceps

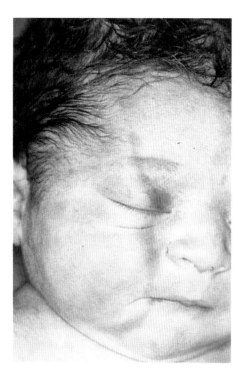

Fig. 31.1 Forceps abrasion on cheek.
Reproduced from Thomas and Harvey 1997, with permission of Elsevier.

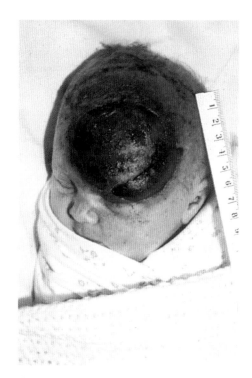

Fig. 31.2 Scalp abrasion during vacuum-assisted birth. Note the chignon.
Reproduced from Thomas and Harvey 1997, with permission of Elsevier.

blades may cause bruising, scalp electrodes cause puncture wounds, as do fetal blood sampling techniques. Occasionally laceration of the baby's skin may occur during uterine incision at caesarean section. While rare, subcutaneous fat necrosis may result from the pressure of forceps blades as well as following severe asphyxia/hypoxaemia, meconium aspiration syndrome and hypothermia (Pride 2012).

While superficial fat necrosis usually presents between days 1 and 28 with well-defined areas of induration (Pride 2012), all other skin injuries should be detected during the midwife's detailed examination of the baby immediately after birth (see Chapter 28). All trauma should be indicated to parents and reported to the paediatrician and General Practitioner (GP).

Abrasions and lacerations should be kept clean and dry. If there are signs of infection, further medical consultation should be sought by the midwife or parents. Antibiotics may be required. Deeper lacerations may require closure with butterfly strips or sutures. Healing is usually rapid with no residual scarring (Sorantin et al 2006). If related causes are successfully treated, fat necrosis should spontaneously resolve (Pride 2012).

Superficial tissues

This trauma involves oedematous swellings and/or bruising. During labour the fetal part overlying the cervical os

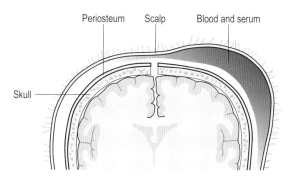

Fig. 31.3 Caput succedaneum.

may be subjected to pressure, a 'girdle of contact', with reduced venous return and resultant congestion and oedema.

Caput succedaneum

With cephalic presentation, there may be a diffuse oedematous swelling under the scalp but above the periosteum, called a caput succedaneum (Fig. 31.3). With an occipitoanterior position, one caput succedaneum may present. With an occipitoposterior position, a caput succedaneum may form, but if the occiput rotates anteriorly a second caput succedaneum may develop. If, during the second stage of labour, the birth of the head is delayed, the perineum may act as another 'girdle of contact' with a second caput succedaneum forming. A 'false' caput succedaneum can also occur if a vacuum extractor cup is used; because of its distinctive shape, the swelling is known as a 'chignon' (see Fig. 31.2).

A caput succedaneum is present at birth, thereafter decreasing in size. This swelling can 'pit' on pressure, can cross a suture line, may be discoloured or bruised, may be associated with increased moulding and the oedema may move to the dependent area of the scalp (Lee 2011). The baby may appear to experience discomfort and, although care continues as normal, gentle handling is appropriate. Abrasion of a chignon is possible.

The swelling is usually self-limiting, resolving within 36 hours, with no longer-term consequences (Sorantin et al 2006; Lee 2011). An abraded chignon usually heals rapidly if the area is kept clean, dry and is not irritated.

Other injuries

The cervical os may also restrict venous return when the fetal presentation is not cephalic. When the face presents, it becomes congested, bruised and the eyes and lips become oedematous. In a breech presentation bruised and oedematous genitalia and buttocks may develop. In both instances there may be discomfort and pain, therefore gentle handling is essential and mild analgesia may be required.

For babies with bruised or oedematous buttocks, maintaining nappy area hygiene is important and must be accomplished without inflicting further skin trauma. Barrier ointment or cream applications may be required if disposable nappies designed to limit the contact of urine and faecal fluid with the skin are not available. If skin excoriation does occur, the infection risk increases and consultation with a wound care specialist nurse may be required to ensure best skin care practice.

Uncomplicated oedema and bruising usually resolve within days. However, if the baby suffers significant trauma during a vaginal breech birth, resulting serious complications require specific treatment and take longer to resolve. These complications may include excessive haemolysis resulting in hyperbilirubinaemia; excessive blood loss resulting in hypovolaemia, shock, anaemia and disseminated intravascular coagulation (DIC); and damage to muscles resulting in difficulties with micturition and defecation.

Muscle trauma

Injuries to muscle result from tearing or when the blood supply is disrupted.

Torticollis

Torticollis is the result of tightness and shortening of one sternomastoid (sternocleidomastoid) muscle. The right and left sternomastoid muscles run from the respective side of the top of the sternum, along the right or left side of the neck and are inserted into the mastoid process of the right or left temporal bone. When contracted simultaneously, these muscles allow the head to flex. When contracted separately, each turns the head to the opposite side.

The aetiology of torticollis is not fully understood. One type may result when the muscle is torn due to excessive traction or twisting during the birth of the anterior shoulder of a fetus with a cephalic presentation, or during rotation of the shoulders when the fetus is being born by vaginal breech or caesarean section.

A 1–3 cm, apparently painless, hard lump of blood and fibrous tissue is felt on the affected sternomastoid muscle. The muscle length is shortened, therefore the neck is twisted to the affected side: a torticollis or wry neck. If the techniques for assisting at the above stages of birth are correctly applied, torticollis may be preventable (Saxena 2010).

Torticollis management involves carers and parents performing passive muscle-stretching exercises initially under the guidance of a physiotherapist, actively encouraging the baby to move the neck. The swelling usually resolves over several weeks to months with minimal sequelae. Surgical intervention is required if there is no resolution by one year. Follow-up to ensure achievement of normal movement is recommended (Saxena 2010).

Nerve trauma

The nerves most commonly traumatized are the facial and brachial plexus nerves. Spinal cord injury is very rare and is not discussed here; an excellent explanation is given in Brand (2006).

Facial nerve

The facial or seventh (VII) cranial nerve runs close to the skin surface and is vulnerable to compression resulting in unilateral facial palsy. Compression may occur in the uterus but is more likely during birth by the maternal sacral promontory or by a misapplied forceps blade, especially when the baby is macrosomic. On the affected side, the baby appears to have no nasolabial fold, the eyelid remains open and the mouth is drawn over to the unaffected side (Fig. 31.4). The baby will drool excessively, may be unable to form an effective seal on the breast or teat, resulting in initial feeding difficulties, and may also have difficulty swallowing (Bruns 2012).

There is no specific treatment. If the eyelid remains open, regular instillation of eye drops lubricate the eyeball. Feeding difficulties are usually overcome by the baby's

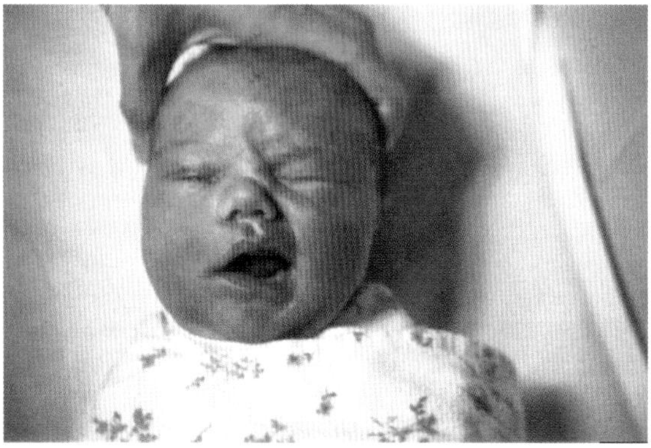

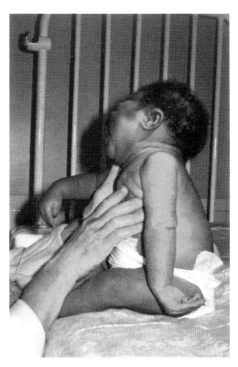

Fig. 31.4 Right-sided facial palsy. Note that the eye is open on the paralysed side and the mouth is drawn over to the non-paralysed side.
Reproduced from Thomas and Harvey 1997, with permission of Elsevier.

own adaptation, although alternative feeding positions may help. Spontaneous resolution is usual within weeks; this may extend to months or years if the damage is severe. Cosmetic surgical interventions for the most severely affected babies may be required (Bruns 2012).

Brachial plexus

Nerve roots exiting from the spine at the fifth to eighth cervical (C5–C8) and the first thoracic (T1) vertebrae form a matrix of nerves in the neck and shoulder: the brachial plexus. Brachial plexus trauma was thought to result from excessive lateral flexion, rotation or traction of the head and neck during vaginal breech birth or when shoulder dystocia occurred. However, the incidence of brachial plexus injury is relatively stable despite interventions such as elective caesarean section, less traction force and increased skill in the manoeuvers used to manage shoulder dystocia. Therefore it may be that brachial plexus trauma is related more to the force exerted by the uterus (Benjamin 2005; Sandmire and DeMott 2009).

The possible trauma to the brachial plexus ranges from oedema to haemorrhage to tearing of the nerves and occurs most commonly in babies born at term (Blackburn and Ditzenberger 2007). Foad et al (2009) explain four types of trauma using the Narakas classification. Trauma to C5–C6 results in Erb's (Erb–Duchenne/Duchenne–Erb) palsy where there is paralysis of the shoulder muscles, biceps, elbow flexor and forearm supinator muscles. The baby's affected arm is limp, inwardly rotated, the elbow extended and the wrist pronated. When C7 is also traumatized, an extended Erb's palsy presents in which the wrist and finger extensor muscles are affected, resulting in wrist and finger flexion – the 'waiter's tip position' (Fig. 31.5).

When there is trauma to C8–T1, Klumpke's palsy presents. The shoulder and upper arm are unaffected but

Fig. 31.5 Erb's palsy.
Reproduced from Thomas and Harvey 1997, with permission of Elsevier.

the lower arm, wrist and hand are paralysed, resulting in wrist drop, no grasp reflex and a claw-like appearance of the hand. If there is associated trauma to the cervical sympathetic nerves, Horner's syndrome may present with no sensation on the affected side, pupil constriction and eyelid ptosis.

If there is trauma to C5–T1, the result is total brachial plexus palsy (Erb–Klumpke) where there is complete paralysis of the shoulder, arm and hand, lack of sensation and circulatory problems. Horner's syndrome may also occur. If there is bilateral paralysis, spinal injury should be suspected (Benjamin 2005; Foad et al 2009; Semel-Concepcion 2012).

All types of brachial plexus trauma require further investigations, including X-ray and ultrasound scanning (USS) of the clavicle, arm, chest and cervical spine, and assessment of the joints. Magnetic resonance imaging (MRI) and electromyography may assist in definitive diagnosis. Unnecessary and extremes of movement of the affected arm should be avoided and care taken when holding or moving the baby to avoid the arm dangling. The baby should not be lifted by the arms or axilla and the affected arm should be dressed first and undressed last. After approximately 2 weeks, when any inflammation should have subsided, passive range of movement exercises are initiated under the direction of a physiotherapist.

Regular functional follow-up assessments are essential to gauge recovery. Most babies with brachial plexus trauma recover completely within 3 weeks. Babies with no recovery of biceps' function by 3 months and those with total brachial plexus injury with Horner's syndrome and no recovery by 1 month may be referred for surgical exploration and/or require microsurgical nerve repair. These babies are more likely to have ongoing functional deficits and may require further surgery (Benjamin 2005; Foad et al 2009; British Medical Journal [BMJ] Evidence Centre 2012).

Fractures

Fractures are rare but the most commonly affected bones are the clavicle, humerus, femur and those of the skull. With all such fractures, a 'crack' may be heard during the birth.

Clavicle

Clavicular fractures, the most common fractures, may occur with shoulder dystocia, vaginal breech birth, or if the baby is macrosomic. The affected clavicle is usually the one that was nearest the maternal symphysis pubis. Brachial plexus and phrenic nerve injuries should be excluded in the affected baby (Laroia 2010; Mavrogenis et al 2011; Vorvick and Kaneshiro 2011).

Humerus

Midshaft humeral fractures can occur with shoulder dystocia or during a vaginal breech birth if the extended arm is forced down and born (Laroia 2010).

Femur

Midshaft femoral fractures can occur during vaginal breech birth if the extended legs are forced down and born (Laroia 2010).

With most fractures, distortion, deformity, swelling or bruising are usually evident on examination; crepitus may be felt; the baby appears to be in pain and is reluctant to move the affected area. An X-ray examination may confirm the diagnosis.

The baby requires gentle handling to avoid further pain and a mild analgesic may be necessary. Fractures of the clavicle require no specific treatment. To immobilize a fractured humerus, place a pad in the axilla and firmly splint the arm with the elbow bent across the chest with a bandage, ensuring respirations are not embarrassed. Immobilize a fractured femur using a splint and bandage. Traction and plaster casting may be required. Stable union of a fractured clavicle usually occurs in 7–10 days, while the humerus and femur take 2–4 weeks (Laroia 2010).

Skull

Although rare, these fractures, linear or depressed, may occur during prolonged or difficult instrumental births. There may be no signs but an overlying swelling, cephalhaematoma, or signs of associated complications such as intracranial haemorrhage or neurological disturbances, may suggest the presence of a fracture.

X-ray examination may confirm the fracture. An ultrasound scan (USS) may help diagnose associated haemorrhage. A simple linear fracture usually requires no treatment and heals quickly with no sequelae. Treatment of a depressed fracture depends on the depth of the concavity. Shallow depressions in asymptomatic babies usually resolve spontaneously. With a deeper depression or where there are signs of complications, the fracture requires surgical repair. Contamination or evidence of cerebrospinal fluid (CSF) leakage via the ear or nose require antibiotic therapy. Treatment of associated complications is necessary. Babies who have a depressed skull fracture have an optimistic outcome except if complications occur, when permanent neurological damage is likely (Qureshi 2012).

HAEMORRHAGES

Blood volume in the term baby is approximately 80–100 ml/kg and in the preterm baby 90–105 ml/kg, therefore even a small haemorrhage may be potentially fatal. In this section, haemorrhages are discussed according to their principal cause, or in relation to other factors. Haemorrhages may be due to:

- trauma
- disruptions in blood flow

or can be related to:

- coagulopathies
- other causes.

Haemorrhages due to trauma

Cephalhaematoma

A cephalhaematoma (cephalohaematoma) is an effusion of blood under the periosteum that covers the skull bones (Fig. 31.6). During a vaginal birth if there is friction between the fetal skull and maternal pelvic bones, such as in cephalopelvic disproportion or precipitate labour, the periosteum may be torn from the bone, causing bleeding underneath. Cephalhaematomas may also occur during vacuum-assisted births. Because the fetal or newborn skull bones are not fused, and as the periosteum is adherent to the edges of the skull bones, a cephalhaematoma is confined to one bone. However, more than one bone may be affected; therefore multiple cephalhaematomas may

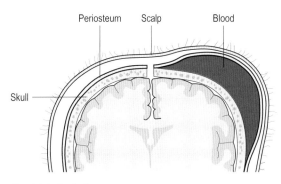

Fig. 31.6 Cephalhaematoma.

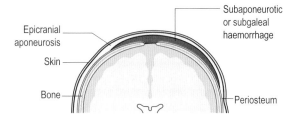

Fig. 31.8 Subaponeurotic haemorrhage.

Subaponeurotic haemorrhage

Subaponeurotic (subgaleal) haemorrhage is rare. Under the scalp, the epicranial aponeurosis, a sheet of fibrous tissue that covers the cranial vault allowing for muscles to attach to the bone, provides a potential space above the periosteum through which veins travel. Excessive traction on these veins results in haemorrhage, the epicranial aponeurosis is pulled away from the periosteum of the skull bones and swelling is evident (Fig. 31.8). Subaponeurotic haemorrhage may occur spontaneously with any type of birth but is more often associated with forceps and vacuum-assisted births, and severe dystocia (Reid 2007).

The swelling is present at birth, increases in size and is a firm, fluctuant mass. The scalp is movable rather than fixed. The swelling can cross sutures and extend into the subcutaneous tissue of neck and eyelids. The baby may appear pale, be hypotonic, tachycardic and tachypnoeic and demonstrate discomfort or pain with head movement or handling of the swelling. A caput succedaneum and/or a cephalhaematoma may co-exist with a subaponeurotic haemorrhage.

If the subaponeurotic haemorrhage is excessive, there is the potential for severe shock, disseminated intravascular coagulation (DIC) and death. This emergency situation requires immediate medical assistance, resuscitation, stabilization and full supportive care, including blood transfusion (Blackburn and Ditzenberger 2007).

With a smaller haemorrhage and in the babies who survive a larger haemorrhage, the blood is reabsorbed and the swelling and bruising resolve over 2–3 weeks. Hyperbilirubinaemia complicates recovery (Reid 2007; Schierholz and Walker 2010).

Subdural haemorrhage

A sickle-shaped, double fold of dura mater, the falx cerebri, dips into the fissure between the cerebral hemispheres. Attached at right angles to the falx cerebri, between the cerebrum and the cerebellum, is a horseshoe-shaped fold of dura mater – the tentorium cerebelli. In these folds of dura run large venous sinuses draining blood from the brain.

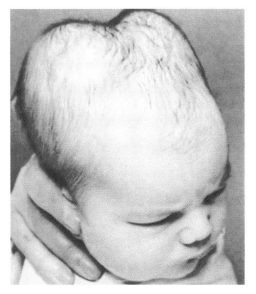

Fig. 31.7 Bilateral cephalhaematoma.

develop. A double cephalhaematoma is usually bilateral (Fig. 31.7). A caput succedaneum can co-exist with a cephalhaematoma.

Unlike caput succedaneum, a cephalhaematoma is not present at birth; the swelling appears after 12 hours, grows larger over subsequent days and can persist for weeks. The swelling is firm, does not pit on pressure, does not cross a suture and is fixed (Blackburn and Ditzenberger 2007).

No treatment is necessary and the swelling subsides when the blood is reabsorbed. Hyperbilirubinaemia may complicate recovery due to haemolysis of the extravasated blood. More rarely complications such as sepsis, osteomyelitis and meningitis may occur. As skull fractures may be associated with a cephalhaematoma, they should be excluded (Paul et al 2009; Laroia 2010).

Normally, moulding of the skull bones and stretching of the underlying structures during birth are well tolerated. Trauma to the fetal head, such as excessive compression or abnormal stretching, may tear the dura, particularly the tentorium cerebelli, rupturing venous sinuses and resulting in a subdural haemorrhage. Predisposing factors include rapid, abnormal or excessive moulding, such as in precipitate labour or rapid birth, malpositions, malpresentations, cephalopelvic disproportion, or undue compression during forceps manoeuvres (Barker 2007).

If the haemorrhage is excessive, there is the potential for severe shock, DIC and death. This emergency situation requires immediate medical assistance – resuscitation, stabilization and full supportive care, including blood transfusion (Blackburn and Ditzenberger 2007).

A baby with a small haemorrhage may demonstrate no signs and resolution is spontaneous. Alternatively, the haemorrhage may initially be small but if blood continues to leak, signs develop over several days. As blood accumulates, there is cerebral irritation, cerebral oedema and raised intracranial pressure. The baby is likely to vomit, be unresponsive and have a bulging anterior fontanelle, hypotonia, hyperthermia, apnoea, bradycardia and convulsions.

Blood in a non-traumatic lumbar puncture may assist in diagnosis as may cranial USS, computerized tomography (CT) or magnetic resonance imaging (MRI). Supportive treatment focuses on replacing blood volume and controlling the consequences of asphyxia and raised intracranial pressure. Surgery to relieve pressure or subdural taps or shunt placement to drain large collections of blood may be required. A shunt is a drainage tube surgically inserted and connected to a one-way valve placed subcutaneously behind the ear. The valve's outflow tube is attached to a catheter allowing drainage into a large vein in the neck, or into the peritoneum, allowing reabsorption and elimination (Blackburn and Ditzenberger 2007). The prognosis for all affected babies except those with massive haemorrhage is usually good (Barker 2007).

Haemorrhages due to disruptions in blood flow

Subarachnoid haemorrhage

A primary subarachnoid haemorrhage involves bleeding directly into the subarachnoid space. Preterm babies who suffer perinatal hypoxia resulting in disruption of cerebral blood flow are most often affected. A secondary haemorrhage involves leakage of blood into the subarachnoid space from an intraventricular haemorrhage. Although classified here as a haemorrhage due to a disruption in blood flow, a subarachnoid haemorrhage may also occur due to birth trauma similar to that which results in subdural haemorrhage.

Depending on extent of the haemorrhage, the affected baby may demonstrate no signs while others may have generalized convulsions from the second day of life and have apnoeic episodes. Although rare, a massive subarachnoid haemorrhage may occur and is usually fatal despite emergency resuscitation and stabilization efforts.

Blood in a non-traumatic lumbar puncture may assist in diagnosis, as may cranial USS, CT or MRI. Supportive treatment focuses on replacing blood volume and controlling the consequences of asphyxia and raised intracranial pressure. Surgery to relieve pressure or subdural taps or shunt placement to drain large collections of blood may be required (Barker 2007).

The condition is usually self-limiting. If post-haemorrhagic hydrocephalus occurs, drainage via a shunt may be required. The prognosis is usually very good for all affected babies except those with related damage due to hypoxia (Barker 2007).

Germinal matrix haemorrhage, intraventricular haemorrhage and periventricular haemorrhagic infarction (intraparenchymal lesion)

Germinal matrix haemorrhage (GMH), intraventricular haemorrhage (IVH) and periventricular haemorrhagic infarction (PHI), also known as intraparenchymal lesions (IPL), primarily affect babies born at less than 32 weeks' gestation and those weighing less than 1500 g at birth, although term babies may be affected. The incidence and severity of these haemorrhages/lesions are inversely correlated with gestational age.

There are three grades of GMH and IVH. A grade 1 haemorrhage into the germinal matrix is a germinal matrix, periventricular or subependymal haemorrhage. Extension of the haemorrhage into the lateral ventricle(s), results in an IVH or grade 2 haemorrhage. The choroid plexus of the lateral ventricles normally produces CSF. If a grade 2 haemorrhage is complicated by blockage to the outflow of CSF, post-haemorrhagic hydrocephalus develops and the ventricles dilate; a grade 3 haemorrhage (Annibale 2012).

Initially it was understood that a grade 3 haemorrhage may extend into the cerebral tissue, resulting in a parenchymal haemorrhage, known as a grade 4 haemorrhage (Papile et al 1978). Volpe (1997) proposed that the intraventricular clot in a grade 3 haemorrhage disrupts venous drainage, causing stasis and infarction. Reperfusion of the area causes haemorrhage into the infarcted area and necrotic damage of the white matter. Therefore a grade 4 haemorrhage was reclassified as a complication of a grade 3 IVH, referred to as a PHI with IPL used interchangeably.

The stage of brain development is a crucial factor in the aetiology of GMH, IVH and PHI/IPL. The two lateral ventricles are lined with ependymal tissue. Tissue lying immediately next to the ependyma is the germinal matrix, also known as the subependymal layer. From 8 to 32 weeks' gestation, neuroblasts and glioblasts are produced in the germinal matrix and migrate to the cerebral cortex. Neuronal migration is complete by 20 weeks' gestation but glial cell development and migration continues until approximately 32 weeks' gestation. During this period, a rich blood supply is provided to the germinal matrix through fragile immature capillaries that lack supporting muscle or collagen fibres. These vessels are particularly vulnerable to fluctuations in cerebral blood flow and pressure, rupturing easily causing haemorrhage. The ability of preterm babies to autoregulate cerebral blood flow and pressure is immature, resulting in an increased vulnerability to haemorrhage. After 32 weeks' gestation the germinal matrix becomes less active and by term has almost completely involuted; the capillaries become more stable and autoregulation becomes established; therefore GMH, IVH and PHI/IPL in more mature babies are less common than in those babies born at less than 32 weeks' gestation (Annibale 2012).

The venous drainage from white matter and the deep areas of the brain, including the lateral ventricles, involves a peculiar U-turn route in the area of the germinal matrix. Disruptions to venous flow lead to congestion, with a risk of venous infarctions and ischaemia. With reperfusion of these ischaemic areas, there may be haemorrhage demonstrated as PHI (Volpe 2008).

Multiple factors may compromise cerebral haemodynamics resulting in GMH, IVH and PHI/IPL. Early factors include obstetric haemorrhage, lack of antenatal steroids, low one minute Apgar score and low umbilical artery pH. Later risk factors include acidosis, hypotension, hypertension, mechanical ventilation, apnoea, rapid volume expansion, rapid administration of hyperosmolar solutions, pneumothorax and tracheal suctioning. Also implicated are excessive handling, exposure to light and noise, lateral flexion of the baby's head and crying (Annibale 2012; Blackburn 2013).

Most affected babies show no signs or signs that are non-specific therefore the haemorrhage/infarction/lesion is detectable only on USS. If the haemorrhage is larger or extends, the clinical features may gradually appear and worsen, including apnoeic episodes that become more frequent and severe, bradycardia, pallor, falling packed cell volume, tense anterior fontanelle, metabolic acidosis and convulsions. The baby may be limp or unresponsive. If the haemorrhage is large and sudden in onset, apnoea and circulatory collapse may present (Annibale 2012). At-risk babies should be screened by 7 days of life for GMH, IVH or PHI/IPL using cranial USS. Serial scanning may determine any increase, extension or complication.

Care of at-risk babies is focused on prevention (Blackburn and Ditzenberger 2007). The birth should be in a regional obstetric unit with neonatal intensive care facilities. Prenatal maternal steroids and postnatal surfactant replacement therapy should be administered. Postnatally, haemodynamic stability is essential, as is prevention of complications. Prevention of hypoxic events and blood flow and pressure fluctuations is essential. Care is focused on maintaining normothermia, normoglycaemia, oxygenation and comfort. Sophisticated monitoring equipment and the judicious use of analgesic, sedative and inotropic drugs may assist achieving and maintaining stability. The baby's developmental needs should be met, particularly in relation to supportive flexed positioning, reduction in bright lighting, a quiet, undisturbed environment and appropriate interaction with parents and others (Blackburn and Ditzenberger 2007).

Despite preventative measures, babies do develop GMH, IVH and PHI/IPL. The outcome depends on the nature of the haemorrhage/lesion and associated conditions/complications. The neurological prognosis for babies with a GMH or a small IVH is usually good. An IVH associated with ventricular dilatation may resolve spontaneously with no long-term consequences. However, with a large IVH and ventricular dilatation, the accumulating CSF may require temporary drainage using ventricular taps or external ventricular drainage. Some babies may require permanent CSF drainage via a shunt. Approximately 30–40% of these babies will have cognitive or motor disabilities. Approximately 50–80% of babies who have a large IVH with either PHI/IPL or periventricular leukomalacia will die; survival is usually complicated in the majority by significant cognitive and motor disabilities. Long-term follow-up is essential and parents need much support (Blackburn and Ditzenberger 2007; Annibale 2012).

Periventricular leucomalacia

Although not a haemorrhage, periventricular leucomalacia (PVL) is included here because of its association with GMH, IVH and PHI/IPL. Between 27 and 30 weeks' gestation, the area of white matter around the lateral ventricles and within the watershed area of the deep cerebral arteries is undergoing considerable development. It is sensitive to any insult that results in reduced cerebral perfusion, such as those associated with GMH, IVH, PHI/IPL and chorioamnionitis. The cerebral blood flow autoregulation ability in preterm babies is limited, increasing their risk of developing PVL. Reduced perfusion results in areas of ischaemia and degeneration of the nerve fibre tracts, disrupting nerve pathways between areas of the brain and between the brain and spinal cord. This softening and necrosis of the white matter is PVL; it may be a classic focal necrotic cystic type or a diffuse non-cystic type. Only the former is seen on USS but MRI may detect both types (Blackburn and Ditzenberger 2007; Volpe 2008; Zach 2012).

Similar pathogenesis is seen in the older preterm and term baby, but the lesion occurs in the subcortical region rather than the periventricular region. This is because the watershed moves away from the ventricles to the cortex once the germinal matrix involutes. These lesions are known as subcortical leucomalacia (Volpe 1997).

Care instituted to reduce the incidence of GMH, IVH and PHI/IPL may reduce the incidence of PVL or the severity of the related ischaemic damage. The prognosis is variable; some babies have little resulting impairment, others develop cognitive and neurodevelopmental impairment while the most severely affected babies may develop spastic diplegic cerebral palsy (Blackburn and Ditzenberger 2007; Zach 2012).

Haemorrhages related to coagulopathies

These haemorrhages occur due to disruption of the baby's blood-clotting abilities.

Vitamin K deficiency bleeding

Vitamin K deficiency bleeding (VKDB) may occur up to 6 months of age, although it more commonly occurs between birth and 8 weeks of life. It was previously known as haemorrhagic disease of the newborn (HDN). Several proteins, factor II (prothrombin), factor VII (proconvertin), factor IX (plasma thromboplastin component), factor X (thrombokinase) and proteins C and S, require vitamin K for their conversion to active clotting factors. A deficiency of vitamin K, as in VKDB, leads to a deficiency of these clotting factors and resultant bleeding.

Vitamin K_1 (phytomenadione/phytonadione/phylloquinone) is poorly transferred across the placenta and fetal liver stores are low. Any stores are quickly depleted after birth and for normal clotting to occur, the baby must receive dietary vitamin K_1, the absorption of which requires fat and bile salts. Vitamin K_2 (menaquinone) is synthesized by bowel flora and may assist in the conversion of proteins to active clotting factors. Because the neonate's bowel is sterile, vitamin K_2 production is restricted until colonization has occurred. Therefore all newborns are deficient in vitamin K and vulnerable to VKDB.

There are three forms of VKDB that were first described by Lane and Hathaway (1985):

- 'early' (0–24 hours)
- 'classical' (1–7 days)
- 'late' (1–6 months, although the peak onset is before 8 weeks).

Early VKDB is rare, principally affecting babies born to women who during pregnancy have taken anticonvulsants, e.g. phenytoin, barbiturates or carbamazepine; antitubercular drugs, e.g. rifampin, isoniazid; or vitamin K antagonists, e.g. warfarin (contraindicated during pregnancy) for treatment of their medical conditions. As these drugs interfere with vitamin K metabolism, avoidance during pregnancy reduces the risk of early VKDB. Taking

vitamin K_1 supplements during the last two weeks of pregnancy may prevent early VKDB (Nimavat 2012).

The babies most susceptible to developing classic VKDB are those with birth trauma, asphyxia, postnatal hypoxia and those who are preterm, or of low birth weight. They are more likely to spontaneously bleed or have invasive interventions resulting in bleeding that cannot be controlled. Disruptions to the colonization of the bowel due to antibiotic therapy, or lack of or poor enteral feeding, may also result in classic VKDB.

The bowel of a breastfed baby colonizes with lactobacilli that do not synthesize menaquinone. The amount of vitamin K_1 in breastmilk is naturally low, although colostrum and hindmilk do contain higher levels than foremilk. The vitamin K_1 in breastmilk is considered insufficient for the exclusively breastfed baby's needs. Artificial infant formulae are fortified with vitamin K_1, offering some prophylaxis against VKDB (Blackburn 2013). Therefore late VKDB occurs almost exclusively in breastfed babies. However, babies who have liver disease or a condition that disrupts vitamin K_1's absorption from the bowel, for example cystic fibrosis, may develop late VKDB (Blackburn 2013).

The baby who has VKDB may have bruising; or bleeding from the umbilicus, puncture sites, the nose or the scalp; or severe jaundice for more than one week and/or persistent jaundice for more than 2 weeks. Gastrointestinal bleeding manifests as melaena and haematemesis. In early and late VKDB, there may be extracranial and intracranial bleeding. With severe haemorrhage, circulatory collapse occurs. Late VKDB is associated with higher mortality and morbidity. Blood tests reveal prolonged prothrombin time (PT) and partial thromboplastin time (PTT), with a normal platelet count (Nimavat 2012).

Babies diagnosed with VKDB require investigation and monitoring to assess their need for treatment. With all forms of VKDB, the baby will require administration of vitamin K_1, 1–2 mg intramuscularly. In severe cases, when coagulation is grossly abnormal and there is severe bleeding, replacement of deficient clotting factors is essential. If circulatory collapse and severe anaemia occur, blood transfusion or exchange transfusion may be required. Affected babies usually require other supportive therapy to assist in their recovery.

As VKDB is a potentially fatal condition, prophylactic administration of vitamin K is recommended for all babies and is administered to all preterm and sick babies as part of their treatment regime (Nimavat 2012; Blackburn 2013). For otherwise healthy term babies the National Institute for Health and Clinical Excellence (NICE) (2006) recommends that vitamin K_1 1 mg given intramuscularly after birth is the most effective prophylaxis for prevention of early onset VKDB. Some vitamin K_1 remains within the muscle and acts as a slow release depot, providing prophylaxis for classic and probably also for late VKDB (Hey 2003).

While there are arguments against routine prophylaxis (Midwives Information and Resource Service [MIDIRS] Essence 2009), for healthy term babies whose parents decline a single intramuscular injection of vitamin K$_1$, an oral prophylaxis regimen is recommended (NICE 2006), although consensus on the most effective oral regime appears elusive. It is suggested that whatever oral regime is used, multiple doses are required in the first week of life and if the baby is breastfed, a further dosing regime is required until at least 12 weeks of age, if not longer. Such prophylaxis should reduce the risk of all forms of VKDB, however this is dependent on the involvement, motivation and compliance of healthcare professionals and parents. Medical advice should be sought if the baby vomits within one hour of oral administration or is too unwell to take the preparation orally.

All parents should be given the opportunity to discuss vitamin K$_1$ prophylaxis during pregnancy, understand the specific management of preterm, sick and 'at-risk' babies, and agree on their choice of prophylaxis. They should also understand the signs and treatment of VKDB, especially if their baby has one or more of the risk factors (NICE 2006; MIDIRS Essence 2009).

Thrombocytopenia

Thrombocytopenia results from a decreased rate of formation of platelets or an increased rate of consumption and is defined as a platelet count of less than 150×10^9/l, and severe thrombocytopenia is a platelet count of less than 50×10^9/l (Bagwell 2007; Roberts and Murray 2008).

Thrombocytopenia may be classified according to fetal, neonatal and late onset causes. Fetal causes include alloimmunity, congenital infection and trisomies. Early onset (less than 72 hours) neonatal causes include placental insufficiency, perinatal asphyxia, perinatal infection, DIC and alloimmunity. Late onset (after 72 hours) neonatal causes include late onset sepsis, necrotizing enterocolitis, congenital infection and autoimmunity.

The most at-risk babies are those with an older sibling who was diagnosed with thrombocytopenia, babies born preterm who have had chronic intrauterine hypoxia such as with pregnancy induced hypertension or diabetes and associated intrauterine growth restriction (Roberts and Murray 2008).

Neonatal alloimmune thrombocytopenia (NAIT) occurs when there is incompatibility between maternal and fetal platelets. Maternal antibodies cross the placenta destroying the fetal platelets – a mechanism similar to that of haemolytic disease of the newborn. If the fetus is severely affected, an intracranial haemorrhage may result in fetal death. If a previous sibling has developed NAIT, in subsequent pregnancies the fetus will be monitored using fetal blood sampling and/or USS to determine the need for maternal immunoglobulin administration and/or steroids and/or intrauterine platelet transfusions, and possibly

elective birth at 32–34 weeks' gestation (Roberts and Murray 2008). If diagnosed with NAIT postnatally, babies usually require platelet transfusions to achieve and maintain a platelet count within normal limits.

Neonatal autoimmune thrombocytopenia may occur in babies whose mothers have autoimmune conditions such as idiopathic thrombocytopenic purpura or systemic lupus erythematosis. The antibodies produced by the mother against her own platelets may cross the placenta, destroying the baby's platelets. The resultant thrombocytopenia is usually mild, but in severe cases, immunoglobulin administration is effective (Roberts and Murray 2008).

Thrombocytopenia may appear as a petechial rash, presenting in a mild case with a few localized petechiae. In a severe case there is widespread and serious haemorrhage from multiple sites. Intracranial haemorrhage may be fatal. Diagnosis is based on history, clinical examination and a reduced platelet count. It is differentiated from other haemorrhagic disorders because coagulation times, fibrin degradation products and red blood cell morphology are normal. Mild or moderate thrombocytopenia is usually self-limiting and requires no treatment. In severe cases, the treatment usually includes platelet concentrate transfusion/s, although the optimum regime is yet to be determined (Roberts and Murray 2008).

Disseminated intravascular coagulation (consumptive coagulopathy)

Disseminated intravascular coagulation (DIC), also known as consumptive coagulopathy, is an acquired coagulation disorder associated with the release of thromboplastin from damaged tissue, stimulating abnormal coagulation in the microcirculation as well as excess fibrinolysis. There is excessive consumption of clotting factors and platelets, predisposing the baby to haemorrhage. DIC is secondary to primary conditions. Maternal causes of neonatal DIC include pre-eclampsia, eclampsia and placental abruption. Fetal causes include severe fetal compromise, the presence of a dead twin in the uterus and traumatic birth. Neonatal causes include conditions resulting in hypoxia and acidosis, severe infections, hypothermia, hypotension and thrombocytopenia (Bagwell 2007; Levi 2012).

As clotting factors and platelets are depleted and fibrinolysis is stimulated, the baby will develop a generalized purpuric rash and bleed from multiple sites. With stimulation of the clotting cascade, multiple microthrombi may occlude vessels, with organ and tissue ischaemia, particularly affecting the kidneys, resulting in haematuria and reduced urine output. As the cycle of consumptive coagulopathy continues, multiorgan failure results (Bagwell 2007; Levi 2012). The diagnosis is made from clinical signs and laboratory findings that show a low platelet count, low fibrinogen level, distorted and fragmented red blood cells, low haemoglobin and raised fibrin degradation products (FDPs) with a prolonged PT and PTT (Bagwell 2007).

Treatment must focus on correction of the underlying cause if possible and full supportive care will be required. Control of DIC requires transfusions of fresh frozen plasma, concentrated clotting factors and platelets. Cryo-precipitate is an excellent source of fibrinogen. If anaemia is diagnosed, transfusions of whole blood or red cell concentrate are required. Occasionally an exchange transfusion of fresh heparinized blood may be performed, to remove FDPs while replacing the clotting factors. If treatment of the primary disorder and/or replacement of clotting factors is ineffective, the administration of heparin may reduce fibrin deposition (Levi 2012).

The prognosis depends on the severity of the primary condition, as well as of the DIC, and the baby's response to treatment.

Haemorrhages related to other causes

Umbilical haemorrhage

This usually occurs as a result of a poorly applied cord ligature. The use of plastic cord clamps has almost eliminated this type of haemorrhage, although it is essential to avoid catching or pulling the clamp. Tampering with partially separated cords before they are ready to separate is discouraged. Umbilical haemorrhage is a potential cause of death. A purse-string suture should be inserted if bleeding continues after 15 or 20 minutes of manual pressure.

Vaginal bleeding

A small temporary vaginal discharge of bloodstained mucus occurring in the first days of life, pseudomenstruation, is due to the withdrawal of maternal oestrogen. This is a normal expectation but is included here for completeness. Parents need to know that this is a possibility and is self-limiting. Continued or excessive vaginal bleeding warrants further investigation to exclude pathological causes.

Haematemesis and melaena

These signs may present when the baby has swallowed maternal blood during birth, or from cracked nipples during breastfeeding. The diagnosis must be differentiated from VKDB, from other causes of haematemesis that include oesophageal, gastric or duodenal ulceration, and from other causes of melaena, that include necrotizing enterocolitis and anal fissures. These causes need specific and usually urgent treatment.

If the cause is swallowed blood, the condition is self-limiting and requires no specific treatment. If the cause is cracked nipples, appropriate treatment for the mother must be implemented.

Haematuria

Haematuria may be associated with coagulopathies, urinary tract infections and structural abnormalities of the urinary tract. Birth trauma may cause renal contusion and haematuria. Occasionally, after suprapubic aspiration of urine, transient mild haematuria may be observed. Treatment of the primary cause should resolve the haematuria.

Bleeding associated with intravascular access

Some sick or preterm babies require the insertion of catheters, lines or cannulae into central or peripheral arteries or veins, or both, to provide routes for blood sampling, blood pressure monitoring or the infusion of fluids and drugs. However, there is a risk of severe external haemorrhage if there is dislodgement of these from the vessel or accidental disconnection from the sampling or infusion equipment, and of severe haemorrhage if a central vessel is punctured internally.

Skilled technique, close observation and careful handling of babies with intravascular access are imperative to prevent potentially fatal haemorrhage. If an external haemorrhage does occur, continuous pressure should be applied to the site until natural haemostasis occurs or until haemostatic sutures are inserted. If there is external bleeding from an umbilical vessel, the cord stump should be squeezed between the fingers until haemostasis occurs. A replacement transfusion of whole blood or packed red cells may be required. Internal haemorrhage may require surgical intervention.

CONVULSIONS

A convulsion (seizure/fit) is a sign of neurological disturbance, not a disease, and the occurrence of a convulsion is a medical emergency. Because the newborn brain is still developing, its function is immature and there is an imbalance between stimulation and inhibition of neural networks. Convulsions present quite differently in the neonate and may be more difficult to recognize than those of later infancy, childhood or adulthood (Volpe 2008).

Convulsive movements can be differentiated from jitteriness or tremors in that, with the latter two, the movements are rapid, rhythmic, equal, are often stimulated or made worse by disturbance and can be stopped by touching or flexing the affected limb. They are normal in an active, hungry baby and are of no consequence, although their occurrence should be documented. Convulsive movements tend to be slower, less equal, are not necessarily stimulated by disturbance, cannot be stopped by restraint, may be accompanied by abnormal eye movements and cardiorespiratory changes and are always pathological. Convulsive movements should also be differentiated from the benign bilateral or localized jerking that occurs normally in neonatal sleep, particularly rapid eye movement sleep (Prasad 2012).

Abnormal, sudden or repetitive movements of any part of the body that are not controlled by repositioning or containment holds require investigation. Volpe (2008) suggests that the type of movement can help classify the convulsion as subtle, tonic, clonic or myoclonic:

- *Subtle* convulsions include movements such as blinking or fluttering of the eyelids, chewing and cycling movements of the legs, and apnoea. There may or may not be associated abnormal electroencephalogram (EEG) activity.
- Focal *tonic* convulsions affect one extremity and abnormal brain electrical activity can be detected on EEG. With generalized tonic convulsions, that are more common than focal tonic convulsions, the baby sustains a rigid extended posture, similar to decerebrate posturing, that is not usually detected on EEG.
- Focal *clonic* convulsions are unilateral, affecting the face, neck or trunk or upper or lower extremity whereas multifocal clonic convulsions affect several areas of the body that jerk asynchronously and migrate. The movements are slow (one to three jerks per second), rhythmic and are most likely to be associated with EEG activity.
- *Myoclonic* convulsions differ from clonic convulsions in that they are faster and are not associated with EEG activity. Focal myoclonic convulsions affect the upper body flexor muscles. Multifocal myoclonic convulsions affect several parts of the body with asynchronous jerks. Generalized myoclonic convulsions affect the upper and sometimes lower extremities with jerking flexion movements.

During a convulsion the baby may have tachycardia, hypertension, raised cerebral blood flow and raised intracranial pressure, which predispose to serious complications.

As convulsions may be difficult to recognize, all at-risk babies must be continuously assessed. The underlying conditions that may result in a convulsion are classified as central nervous system, metabolic, other and idiopathic conditions (Table 31.1). Convulsions may be acute, recurrent or chronic (Blackburn and Ditzenberger 2007).

If a convulsion is suspected, a complete history and physical and laboratory investigations related to the possible cause would be undertaken. An EEG may help detect abnormal electrical brain activity and guide treatment. Immediate treatment necessitates obtaining assistance from a doctor while ensuring that the baby has a clear airway and adequate ventilation, either spontaneously or mechanically. The baby can be turned to the semi-prone position, with the head in a neutral position. Gentle oral

Table 31.1 Selected causes of neonatal convulsions

Category	Selected causes
Central nervous system	Intracranial haemorrhage Intracerebral haemorrhage Hypoxic-ischaemic encephalopathy Kernicterus Congenital abnormalities
Metabolic	Acquired disorders of metabolism Hypo- and hyperglycaemia Hypo- and hypercalcaemia Hypo- and hypernatraemia Inborn errors of metabolism
Other	Hypoxia Congenital infections Severe postnatally acquired infections Neonatal abstinence syndrome Hyperthermia
Idiopathic	Unknown

and nasal suction may be required to remove any milk or mucus. If the baby is breathing spontaneously but is cyanosed, facial oxygen is given. Active resuscitation may be required. The need for intravenous access should be assessed. Any necessary handling must be gentle and the baby is usually nursed in an incubator to allow for observation and temperature regulation.

It is important that the nature of the convulsion is documented, noting the type of movements, the areas affected, its length, the baby's state of consciousness, colour change, alteration in heart rate, respiratory rate or blood pressure and immediate sequelae (Blackburn and Ditzenberger 2007).

The aims of care are to treat the primary cause/s (details of which are not discussed in this chapter), and the pharmacologic control of the convulsions. The latter is controversial due to the potential for damage from the drugs versus the potential damage from the convulsion on the developing brain (Rennie and Boylan 2007; Volpe 2008). While there is little robust research evidence for the use of any anticonvulsants in neonates, there is consensus for the use of such drugs, particularly when the baby experiences prolonged or frequent convulsions (Volpe 2008; Jensen 2009).

If pharmacological treatment is prescribed, the drugs most commonly used are phenobarbital and phenytoin; less frequently benzodiazepines may be used. Newer anticonvulsants such as topiramate and levetiracetam are still being evaluated (Rennie and Boylan 2007; Volpe 2008; Jensen 2009). Anticonvulsant therapy may be discontinued when convulsions cease, preferably before the baby is transferred home.

The outcome for babies who have convulsions is likely to depend on the cause, onset, type of convulsion and frequency, whether it was demonstrated on EEG and whether the tracing became normal following treatment, what type of treatment was used and how long it was before any treatment was successful. A good prognosis is usual if convulsions were due to hypocalcaemia, hyponatraemia or an uncomplicated subarachnoid haemorrhage. Much poorer prognoses are associated with severe hypoxic ischaemia, severe IVH, severe infections and central nervous system congenital abnormalities (Blackburn and Ditzenberger 2007). Complications of neonatal seizures may include cerebral palsy, hydrocephalus, epilepsy and spasticity (Sheth 2011).

SUPPORT OF PARENTS

The care of parents is more comprehensively discussed elsewhere therefore in this section only specific aspects will be summarized. Trauma during birth, haemorrhages and convulsions are unexpected complications and parents may be shocked and anxious, and perhaps find themselves in a crisis situation. However, not all parents experience such feelings and some can adapt quickly to their baby's condition (Fowlie and McHaffie 2004; Carter et al 2005; McGrath 2007).

The extent of the midwife's and other professionals' contact with parents will depend on circumstances but the experiences parents have at this time have longer-term implications for them, their response to the situation, their relationships with the multiprofessional teams involved in their care as well as their interaction with and care of their baby (McGrath 2007).

One of the most important aspects of caring for the parents is in relation to communication. All parents are entitled to be given information about their baby's condition, treatment and care in ways that are considered

> **Box 31.1 Summary of key principles related to the baby, parents and family**
>
> The baby must be valued as a baby by:
> - using the baby's name
> - not predicting the future
> - when sharing information, keeping the baby with the parents if possible.
>
> The parents and family must be respected by:
> - facilitating parental support and empowerment
> - acknowledging cultural and religious differences
> - listening to their views and taking their concerns seriously
> - giving information honestly and sensitively using uncomplicated language
> - ensuring understanding and giving opportunities for questions
> - facilitating follow-up and providing further information when required.
>
> Source: Scope 2003

best practice. The 'Right from the Start template' (Scope 2003) provides an excellent guide, and the principles related to the baby, parents and family are summarized in Box 31.1.

Parental involvement in their baby's care is essential and the family-centered care/partnership with parents approach should now pervade all midwifery and neonatal settings. Midwives and neonatal nurses have an important role in promoting adaptive coping mechanisms and guiding parents to appropriate resources and support services (POPPY Steering Group 2009). The baby charity BLISS offers helpful information for parents and its website includes a parent message board. Additional support and information is available from specialized outside agencies and the charity Contact a Family is a useful resource in the longer term. (See Useful Websites, below.)

REFERENCES

Annibale D J 2012 Periventricular hemorrhage–intraventricular hemorrhage. http://emedicine.medscape.com/article/976654 (accessed June 2013)

Bagwell G A 2007 Haematological system. In: Kenner C, Lott J W (eds) Comprehensive neonatal care: an interdisciplinary approach, 4th edn.

Saunders/Elsevier, Philadelphia, ch 10, p 245–51

Barker S 2007 Subdural and primary subarachnoid haemorrhages: a case study. Neonatal Network 26(3):143–51

Benjamin K 2005 Part 2: Distinguishing physical characteristics and management of brachial plexus

injuries. Advances in Neonatal Care 5(5):240–51

Blackburn S T 2013 Maternal, fetal and neonatal physiology: a clinical perspective, 4th edn. Elsevier, Philadelphia, ch 8, p 239–40, ch 15, p 546–51

Blackburn S T, Ditzenberger G R 2007 Neurologic system. In: Kenner C,

Lott J W (eds) Comprehensive neonatal care: an interdisciplinary approach, 4th edn. Saunders/Elsevier, Philadelphia, ch 12, p 277–94

BMJ (British Medical Journal) Evidence Centre (2012) Erb's palsy. http://bestpractice.bmj.com/best-practice/monograph/746 (accessed January 2013)

Brand M C 2006 Part 1: Recognizing neonatal spinal cord injury. Advances in Neonatal Care 6(1):15–24

Bruns A D 2012 Congenital facial paralysis. http://emedicine.medscape.com/article/878464 (accessed June 2013)

Carter J D, Mulder R T, Bartram A F et al 2005 Infants in a neonatal intensive care unit: parental response. Archives of Disease in Childhood, Fetal and Neonatal edition 90(2): F109–F113

Foad S L, Mehiman C T, Foad M B et al 2009 Prognosis following neonatal brachial plexus palsy: an evidence-based review. Journal of Children's Orthopedics 3(6):459–63

Fowlie P W, McHaffie H 2004 Supporting parents in the neonatal unit. British Medical Journal 329:1336–8

Hey E 2003 Vitamin K – what, why and when. Archives of Disease in Childhood Fetal and Neonatal edition 88(2):F80–F83

Jensen F E 2009 Neonatal seizures: an update on mechanisms and management. Clinics in Perinatology 36(4):881.

Lane P A, Hathaway W E 1985 Vitamin K in infancy. Journal of Pediatrics 106:351–9

Laroia N 2010 Pediatric cardiac birth trauma. http://emedicine.medscape.com/article/980112 (accessed June 2013)

Lee K G 2011 Caput succedaneum. www.nlm.nih.gov/medlineplus/ency/article/001587.htm (accessed June 2013)

Levi M M 2012 Disseminated intravascular coagulation. http://emedicine.medscape.com/article/199627 (accessed June 2013)

Mavrogenis A F, Mitsiokapa E A, Kanellopoulos A D et al 2011 Birth fractures of the clavicle. Advances in Neonatal Care 11(5):328–31

McGrath J M 2007 Family: essential partner in care. In: Kenner C, Lott J W (eds) Comprehensive neonatal care: an interdisciplinary approach, 4th edn, Saunders/Elsevier, Philadelphia, ch 25, p 491–506

MIDIRS (Midwives Information and Resource Service) Essence 2009 Vitamin K – the debate and the evidence. www.midirs.org/development/MIDIRSEssence.nsf/articles/336837BED2143BE5802575D60044F8E9 (accessed June 2013)

NICE (National Institute for Health and Clinical Excellence) 2006 Routine postnatal care of women and their babies. NICE, London. Available at www.nice.org.uk/nicemedia/pdf/CG37NICEguideline.pdf (accessed June 2013)

Nimavat E J 2012 Hemorrhagic disease of the newborn. http://emedicine.medscape.com/article/974489 (accessed June 2013)

Papile L A, Burnstein J, Burnstein R et al 1978 Incidence and evolution of subependymal and intraventricular hemorrhage: a study of infants with birth weights less than 1500 g. Journal of Pediatrics 92(4):529–34

Paul S P, Edate S, Taylor T M 2009 Cephalhaematoma – a benign condition with serious complications: case report and literature review. Infant 5(5):146–8

POPPY Steering Group 2009 Family-centred care in neonatal units. A summary of research results and recommendations from the POPPY project. National Childbirth Trust, London

Prasad M 2012 Neonatal seizure: what is the cause? www.bmj.com/content/345/bmj.e6003 (accessed June 2013)

Pride H 2012 Superficial fat necrosis of the newborn. http://emedicine.medscape.com/article/1081910 (accessed June 2013)

Qureshi N H 2012 Skull fracture. http://emedicine.medscape.com/article/248108 (accessed June 2013)

Reid J 2007 Neonatal subgaleal haemorrhage. Neonatal Network 26(4):219–27

Rennie J M, Boylan G 2007 Treatment of neonatal seizures. Archives of Disease in Childhood, Fetal and Neonatal edition 92(2):F148–F150

Roberts I, Murray N A 2008 Neonatal thrombocytopenia. Seminars in Fetal and Neonatal Medicine 13(4):256–64

Sandmire H F, DeMott R K 2009 Controversies surrounding the causes of brachial plexus injury. International Journal of Gynecology and Obstetrics 104(1):9–13

Saxena A K 2010 Paediatric torticollis surgery. http://emedicine.medscape.com/article/939858 (accessed June 2013)

Schierholz E, Walker S R 2010 Responding to traumatic birth. Advances in Neonatal Care 10(6):311–15

Scope (2003) Right from the start template. www.scope.org.uk/help-and-information/publications/right-start-template (accessed June 2013)

Semel-Concepcion J 2012 Neonatal brachial plexus palsies. http://emedicine.medscape.com/article/317057 (accessed June 2013)

Sheth R D 2011 Neonatal seizures. http://emedicine.medscape.com/article/1177069 (accessed June 2013)

Sorantin E, Brader P, Thimary F 2006 Neonatal trauma. European Journal of Radiology 60(2): 199–207

Thomas R, Harvey D 1997 Colour guide: neonatology, 2nd edn, Churchill Livingstone, Edinburgh

Volpe J J 1997 Brain injury in the premature infant. Clinics in Perinatology 24(3):567–87

Volpe J J 2008 Neurology of the newborn, 5th edn. Elsevier Health Sciences, Philadelphia, ch 5, p 203–44 and ch 11, p 517–88

Vorvick L J, Kaneshiro N K 2011 Fractured clavicle in the newborn. www.nlm.nih.gov/medlineplus/ency/article/001588.htm (accessed June 2013)

Zach T 2012 Pediatric periventricular leukomalacia. http://emedicine.medscape.com/article/975728 (accessed June 2013)

FURTHER READING

Boxwell G (ed) 2010 Neonatal intensive care nursing, 2nd edn. Routledge, London

This book is primarily written for neonatal nurses and teachers. Student midwives and midwives would benefit from the additional more detailed information about many of the conditions addressed in this present chapter. Chapters 3, 8, 9 and 18 are recommended.

Meeks M, Hallsworth M, Yeo H (eds) (2010) Nursing the neonate, 2nd edn. Wiley–Blackwell, Malaysia

Written primarily for neonatal nurses and midwives, it provides a resource for other professionals working in neonatal care. Chapters 4, 14 and 17 are recommended.

Rennie J M 2012 Rennie and Roberton's Textbook of neonatology, 5th edn. Elsevier, London

A classic textbook that gives excellent explanations of physiology and discusses the management of neonatal complications, albeit from a mainly medical perspective.

USEFUL WEBSITES

Advances in Neonatal Care (journal): http://journals.lww.com/advancesinneonatalcare

Archives of Disease in Childhood (journal): http://adc.bmj.com

BLISS: (premature and sick baby charity): www.bliss.org.uk

Contact a Family: www.cafamily.org.uk

Infant (journal for neonatal nursing and paediatric healthcare professionals): www.infantgrapevine.co.uk

Medscape: http://emedicine.medscape.com

Chapter |32|

Congenital malformations

Judith Simpson, Kathleen O'Reilly

CHAPTER CONTENTS

The incidence of major congenital malformations is 2–3% of all births, although this figure is subject to familial, cultural and geographic variations. It is therefore likely that every practising midwife will at some time in their career be confronted with the challenge of providing appropriate care and support for such babies and their families.

THE CHAPTER AIMS TO:

- address issues such as who should tell the parents and how and when they should be told
- describe and explain specific congenital anomalies
- consider the psychological impact on staff and the strategies that could be put in place to minimize the accompanying stress.

COMMUNICATING THE NEWS

Improved prenatal screening and diagnostic techniques (see Chapter 11) have led to the increased recognition of malformations, particularly in early pregnancy. As a result some women may make the decision to have their pregnancy terminated, whilst for others it provides time to adjust to and begin to come to terms with the news that their baby will be born with a particular problem. One advantage of prenatal diagnosis is that, if necessary, arrangements can be made for the mother to give birth in a unit where appropriate specialist neonatal services are available. The disadvantage of such a transfer is that the mother may then be separated from family, friends and the support of the midwives she knows best. This makes it all the more imperative that the staff in these units are sensitive to the needs of such women.

However, even with universal fetal screening not all malformations will be identified prenatally and in this situation it is often the midwife who first notices an anomaly either at birth or on routine newborn examination. Whilst all anomalies should be notified to medical staff there is sometimes uncertainty as to who should communicate the news to the parents.

There is a very strong argument for suggesting that this should be done by the midwife present at the birth. The midwife–mother relationship is, or ought to be, one of mutual trust and respect. Honesty is an implicit tenet of such a relationship. It is well recognized that one of the first questions a mother will ask the midwife after the birth is 'is the baby all right?' For the midwife to be non-committal or economical with the truth is to betray that trust. It is preferable that the midwife tells both parents sensitively but honestly that she has concerns, and shows them any obvious anomaly in the baby.

Where there is doubt in the midwife's mind, for example in cases of suspected chromosomal disorders, it could be argued that the issue is less clear cut. Discretion could therefore be exercised in the precise form of words used, but the intention of inviting a second opinion should be made clear to the parents. It is advisable that both the parents and the midwife are present when an experienced paediatrician examines the baby and that the midwife is present during any dialogue between the parents and medical staff so that she is aware of exactly what has been said. She is then in a position to clarify or repeat any points that were not fully understood. Opportunities for follow-up consultation with the paediatrician should be offered as and when the parents desire. Patience, tact and understanding are prerequisites for midwives caring for these families.

Some malformations may appear minor to staff; however, it is important to appreciate that parental perceptions may be quite different and that the degree of distress can be unrelated to the apparent severity of the anomaly. The psychological impact on parents of being told or shown, or both, that their baby has a congenital malformation has been likened to the grieving process discussed in Chapter 26. Great sensitivity is therefore required on the part of the midwife when communicating with the parents for the first time.

Whatever the anomaly, it is essential that families receive accurate, consistent and appropriate information about their baby's condition. Since a comprehensive discussion of every malformation is clearly not possible, selection has therefore been made of those the midwife is most likely to encounter.

PALLIATIVE CARE

There are a number of severe congenital malformations which are incompatible with sustained life, such as anencephaly. Many of these conditions are diagnosed antenatally and, whereas some parents opt for termination of the pregnancy, others choose palliative care after birth. It is important that parents feel supported in the choices they make. When parents opt to continue with the pregnancy, where possible, a plan should be made antenatally with the parents for care of the baby when he or she is born. Discussion with the parents should explore any anxieties they may have, e.g. pain relief for the baby. It should also include factual information about the likely clinical course including how long the baby may survive and a gentle explanation of the process of death. It is important to be honest in cases where there is uncertainty. It may also be appropriate at this time to explore any specific wishes the parents may have, regarding religious ceremonies for example.

After birth priority should be given to ensuring the comfort of the baby whilst at the same time supporting the parents. In cases where the baby survives for longer than expected the specific aspects of the care plan may need to be reviewed and discussed with parents (e.g. feeding). It is important to treat the parents and the baby with kindness and dignity at all times and to remember that the life of the baby is precious to the parents no matter how short that life is.

Providing end of life care for infants with severe congenital malformations can be difficult and emotionally draining for staff. It is essential that staff caring for the baby feel comfortable with clinical decisions and able to discuss any concerns they have. A formal debrief within the multi-professional team may be useful.

DEFINITION AND CAUSES

By definition, a congenital malformation is any defect in form, structure or function. Identifiable defects can be categorized as follows (Fig. 32.1):

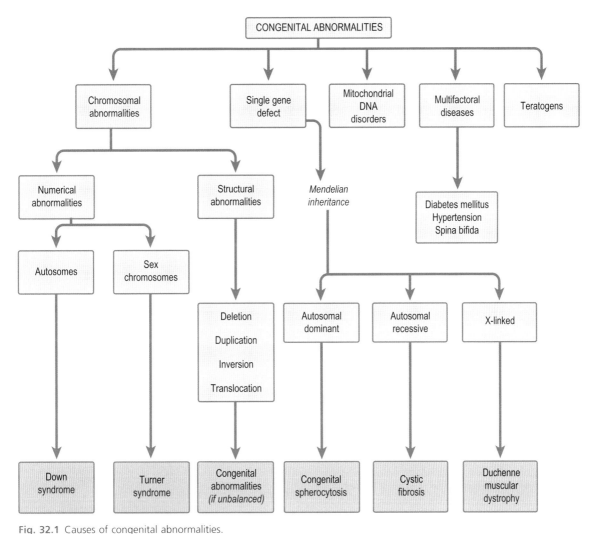

Fig. 32.1 Causes of congenital abnormalities.
Adapted from Beattie J, Carachi R (eds) 2005 Practical paediatric problems: a textbook for MRCPCH. Hodder Education, London.

- chromosomal abnormalities
- single gene defects
- mitochondrial deoxyribonucleic acid (DNA) disorders
- teratogenic causes
- multifactorial causes
- unknown causes.

Chromosomal abnormalities

Definitions of terms used in this and subsequent sections are provided in the Glossary at the end of the book.

Every human cell carries a blueprint for reproduction in the form of 44 chromosomes (autosomes) and two sex chromosomes. Each chromosome comprises a number of genes, which are specific sequences of DNA coding for particular proteins. The zygote should have 22 autosomes and one sex chromosome from each parent. Should a fault occur in either the formation of the gametes or following fertilization (see Chapter 5), abnormalities in chromosome number (aneuploidies) or structure (deletions, duplications, inversions, translocations) may occur. Each abnormal chromosomal pattern has a characteristic clinical presentation, the most common of which will be discussed further.

Gene defects (Mendelian inheritance)

Genes are composed of DNA and each is concerned with the transmission of one specific hereditary factor. Genetically inherited factors may be dominant or recessive.

A dominant gene will produce its effect even if present in only one chromosome of a pair. An autosomal dominant condition can usually be traced through several generations although the severity of clinical expression may vary from generation to generation. Congenital spherocytosis, achondroplasia, osteogenesis imperfecta, adult polycystic kidney disease and Huntington's chorea are examples of dominant conditions.

A recessive gene needs to be present in both chromosomes before producing its effect. An individual who is carrying only one abnormal copy of the gene (a heterozygote) is unaffected. Examples of autosomal recessive conditions are cystic fibrosis or phenylketonuria.

Some congenital malformations are a consequence of single gene defects. In a dominantly inherited disorder the risk of an affected fetus is 1 : 2 (50%) for each and every pregnancy. In a recessive disorder, the risk is 1 : 4 (25%) for each and every pregnancy. In an X-linked recessive inheritance the condition affects almost exclusively males, although females can be carriers. X-linked recessive inheritance is responsible for conditions such as haemophilia A and B and Duchenne muscular dystrophy. Spontaneous mutations commonly arise in X-linked recessive disorders. When a woman is a carrier of an

X-linked condition, there is a 50% chance of each of her sons being affected and an equal chance that each of her daughters will be carriers.

Work on the human genome continues to identify gene defects; for example, polycystic kidney disease (see p. 663) arises from a mutation on chromosome 6 and cystic fibrosis is due to a defect on chromosome 7. Recent advancements in our understanding of inherited conditions have focused on epigenetics. This is the study of factors other than DNA structure which can alter gene expression. Epigenetics is involved in genomic imprinting and X-chromosome inactivation in humans. Epigenetic factors influencing early development may be responsible for specific congenital syndromes. Continuing research may offer further diagnostic and treatment options in the future.

Mitochondrial inheritance

Mitochondria are cellular structures responsible for energy production. Mitochondria are always inherited from the mother. Symptoms and signs of mitochondrial disorders can be diverse but tend to occur in tissues that have high energy requirements such as the brain and muscles. Examples are very rare but include, *m*itochondrial *e*ncephalomyopathy with *l*actic *a*cidosis and *s*troke-like episodes (MELAS) and *m*yoclonic *e*pilepsy with *r*agged *r*ed *f*ibres myopathy (MERRF) (Chinnery et al 1998).

Teratogenic causes

A teratogen is any agent that raises the incidence of congenital malformation. The list of known and suspected teratogens is continually growing but includes: prescribed drugs (e.g. anticonvulsants, anticoagulants and preparations containing large concentrations of vitamin A such as those prescribed for the treatment of acne), drugs used in substance abuse (e.g. heroin, alcohol and nicotine), environmental factors such as radiation and chemicals (e.g. dioxins, pesticides), infective agents (e.g. rubella, cytomegalovirus) and maternal disease (e.g. diabetes). It should be borne in mind that several factors influence the effect(s) produced by any one teratogen, such as gestational age of the embryo or fetus at the time of exposure, length of exposure and toxicity of the teratogen. Direct cause and effect is sometimes difficult to establish. Accurate recording of all congenital malformations on central registers, such as those included in the British Isles Network of Congenital Anomaly Registers (BINOCAR; www .binocar.org), facilitates the early recognition of new teratogens.

Multifactorial causes

These are due to interactions between specific genes (genetic susceptibility) and environmental influences (teratogens).

Unknown causes

In spite of a growing body of knowledge, the specific cause of many congenital anomalies remains unspecified and they occur sporadically in families.

CHROMOSOMAL ABNORMALITIES

Trisomy 21 (Down syndrome)

The classic features of what is now known as Down (ubiquitously referred to as Down's) syndrome were first described in 1866 by physician John Langdon Down (Fig. 32.2). He recognized a commonly occurring combination of facial features among individuals with low intelligence. Characteristic features of Down syndrome include: upslanting palpebral fissures, a small head with flat occiput, small nose, small mouth with relatively large tongue, short broad hands with an incurving little finger (clinodactyly), a single palmar (simian) crease, a wide space between the great toe and second toe (sandal gap), Brushfield spots in the eyes and generalized hypotonia.

Not all of these manifestations need be present and any of them can occur alone without implying chromosomal aberration. Babies born with Down syndrome also have a higher incidence of cardiac anomalies, cataracts, hearing loss, leukaemia and hypothyroidism. Intelligence quotient is below average, at 40–80.

Down syndrome arising sporadically as a result of a non-disjunction process occurs in 95% of cases. Unbalanced translocation occurs in 2.5% of cases, usually between chromosomes 14 and 21. Mosaic forms also occur. There is no difference between the types in clinical appearance. Parents who have a baby with Down syndrome, therefore, should be offered genetic counselling to establish the risk of recurrence. The overall incidence of Down syndrome is 1 in 700.

Although there may be little doubt in the midwife's mind that a baby has Down syndrome, she should be careful not to make any definitive statements. Family likeness alone may explain some babies' appearance. Parents themselves may voice their suspicions. If they do not, a sensitive but honest approach should be made by either the midwife or paediatrician to alert them to the possibility and to request permission to conduct further

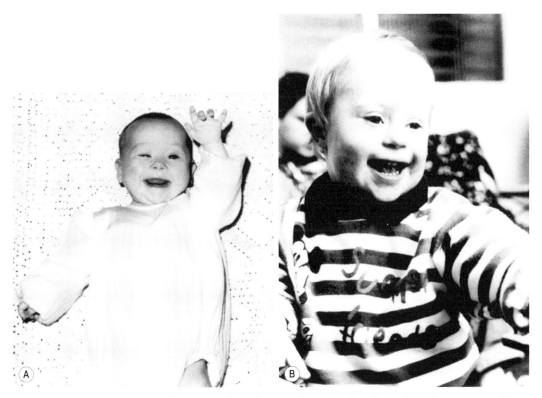

Fig. 32.2 (A) Baby with Down syndrome: note slant of eyes and incurving little finger. (B) With good parental involvement and stimulus these infants can reach maximum potential.
Photographs courtesy of Scottish Down's Syndrome Association.

investigations. It is inappropriate to transfer the baby to the special care baby unit in order to carry out these investigations under the guise of the baby being cold or sleepy. Investigations indicated include chromosome analysis and echocardiography, because of the increased risk of congenital heart disease. Some centers offer rapid genetic diagnosis (see Chapter 11).

An individual baby's needs will vary depending on whether there are any co-existing anomalies. Although initial feeding problems are common owing to generalized hypotonia, breastfeeding should be encouraged if that is what the mother had planned. The parents are likely to require a great deal of emotional support in the first few days following diagnosis. Providing audiovisual or reading material about Down syndrome for the parents may be helpful, or the address of the local branch of the Down Syndrome Association (see Useful Websites).

Trisomy 18 (Edwards syndrome)

This condition is found in about 1 in 5000 births. An extra 18th chromosome is responsible for the characteristic features. Facial features include a small head with a flattened forehead, a receding chin and frequently a cleft palate. The ears are low set and maldeveloped. The sternum tends to be short, the fingers often overlap each other and the feet have a characteristic rocker-bottom appearance. Malformations of the cardiovascular and gastrointestinal systems are common. The lifespan for these children is short and the majority die during their first year.

Trisomy 13 (Patau syndrome)

An extra copy of the 13th chromosome leads to multiple abnormalities. These children have a short life. Only 5% live beyond 3 years. Affected infants are small and are microcephalic. Midline facial abnormalities such as cleft lip and palate are common and limb abnormalities are frequently seen. Brain, cardiac and renal abnormalities may co-exist with this trisomy.

Turner syndrome (XO)

In this monosomal condition, only one sex chromosome exists: an X. The absent chromosome is indicated by 'O'. The child is a girl with a short, webbed neck, widely spaced nipples and oedematous feet. The genitalia tend to be underdeveloped and the internal reproductive organs do not mature. The condition may not be diagnosed until puberty fails to occur. Congenital cardiac defects may also be found. Mental development is usually normal.

GASTROINTESTINAL MALFORMATIONS

Most of the malformations affecting this system call for prompt surgical involvement, for example atresias, gastroschisis and exomphalos. With increasing access to fetal anomaly ultrasound screening at 18–20 weeks' gestation, many are likely to be diagnosed prenatally (Haddock et al 1996). If prenatal diagnosis has been made, the parents will be at least partially prepared. They should have had the opportunity to meet with the paediatric surgeon who will explain the probable sequence of events. They should also have had the opportunity to visit the specialist neonatal unit in which their baby will be cared for. Once the baby is born, prior to obtaining their consent for surgery, the paediatric surgeon will have a further discussion with the parents. If the baby's condition allows, the parents should be encouraged to hold the baby and take photographs.

Gastroschisis and exomphalos

Gastroschisis (Fig. 32.3) is a paramedian defect of the abdominal wall with extrusion of bowel that is not covered by peritoneum. Closure of the defect is usually possible; the size of the defect will determine whether early primary closure is possible or whether a temporary silo made from synthetic materials (e.g. Silastic) is necessary until the abdominal cavity is able to contain all the abdominal organs (Schlatter et al 2003).

Exomphalos or omphalocele (Fig. 32.4) is a defect in which the bowel or other viscera protrude through the umbilicus. Very often these babies have other anomalies, for example heart defects, which require evaluation prior to surgery. The timing of surgical closure is again determined by the size of the defect; small defects (exomphalos minor) undergo early primary closure whilst a large defect (exomphalos major) is encouraged to granulate over, prior to delayed closure at 6–12 months (Lee et al 2006).

The immediate management of both the above conditions is to cover the herniated abdominal contents with clean cellophane wrap (e.g. Clingfilm) or warm sterile saline swabs to reduce fluid and heat losses and to give a degree of protection. An orogastric or nasogastric tube should be passed and stomach contents aspirated. Transfer of the baby to a surgical unit is then expedited.

Atresias

Oesophageal atresia

Oesophageal atresia occurs when there is incomplete canalization of the oesophagus in early intrauterine development. It is commonly combined with a tracheo-oesophageal fistula, which connects the trachea to the

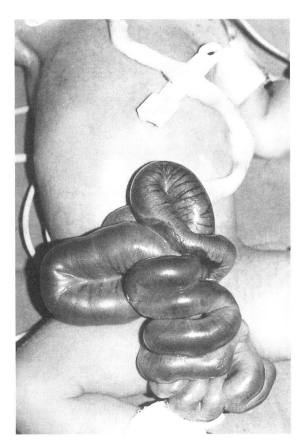

Fig. 32.3 Gastroschisis showing prolapsed intestine to the right of umbilical cord.
From Rennie J M, Roberton N R C (eds) 1999 Textbook of neonatology, 3rd edn, with permission of Churchill Livingstone.

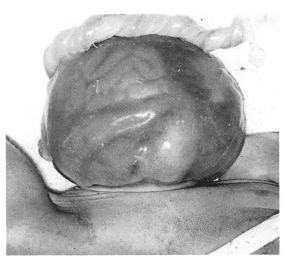

Fig. 32.4 Omphalocele defect with bowel visible through sac in the lower part and abnormally lobulated liver in the sac in the upper part.
From Rennie J M, Roberton N R C (eds) 1999 Textbook of neonatology, 3rd edn, with permission of Churchill Livingstone.

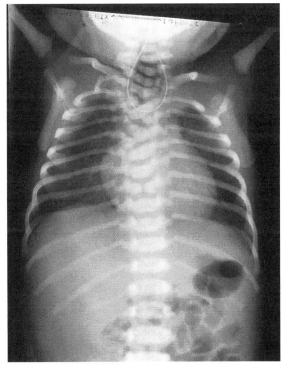

Fig. 32.5 Oesophageal atresia. Coiled feeding tube in proximal pouch. Note vertebral and rib abnormalities. Distal gas confirms a tracheo-oesophageal fistula.
From Rennie J M, Roberton N R C (eds) 1999 Textbook of neonatology, 3rd edn, with permission of Churchill Livingstone.

upper or lower oesophagus, or both. The commonest type of malformation is where the upper oesophagus terminates in a blind upper pouch and the lower oesophagus connects to the trachea. Around 50% of cases are associated with other malformations either as part of a chromosomal disorder or a syndrome such as the VACTERL spectrum (*v*ertebral anomalies, *a*nal anomalies, *c*ardiac, *t*racheo*e*sophageal, *r*adial aplasia, renal and *l*imb anomalies). Further evaluation, particularly of the heart, is required prior to surgery (Pedersen et al 2012).

Oesophageal atresia should be suspected in the presence of maternal polyhydramnios and should be screened for after birth in all such affected pregnancies. At birth the baby may be described as 'mucousy' or may have 'colour changes' associated with copious secretions. The midwife should attempt to pass a wide bore orogastric tube but it may travel less than 10–12 cm. Radiography will confirm the diagnosis (Fig. 32.5). The baby must be given no oral fluid but a wide bore oesophageal tube should be passed into the upper pouch and connected to gentle continuous suction apparatus. Ideally a double lumen (Replogle) tube is used. The baby should be transferred promptly to a surgical unit, ensuring that continuous suction is available throughout the transfer. It is usually possible to anastomose the blind ends of the oesophagus. If the gap in the oesophagus is too large a series of bouginages can be carried out in an attempt to stretch the ends of the oesophagus, stimulate growth and thereby eventually facilitate repair by end-to-end anastomosis. Very rarely, if the repair is delayed, cervical oesophagostomy may be performed to allow drainage of secretions. Meanwhile the baby will need to be fed via a gastrostomy tube. This method of feeding obviously deprives the baby of oral stimuli. Such a baby may be given 'sham' feeds to allow him/her to taste the milk and to promote sucking, swallowing and normal development of the mandible.

Duodenal atresia

Atresia can occur at any level of the bowel but the duodenum is the most common site. If this has not already been diagnosed in the prenatal period, persistent vomiting within 24–36 hours of birth will be the first feature encountered. The vomit may contain bile unless the obstruction is proximal to the entrance of the common bile duct, in which case it will be non-bilious. Abdominal distension is not necessarily present and the baby may pass meconium. A characteristic double bubble of gas is seen on radiological examination (Fig. 32.6). Treatment is by surgical repair. This anomaly is commonly associated with chromosomal disorders, in particular trisomy 21, which accounts for 30% of cases of duodenal atresia.

Anorectal malformations

Careful examination of the perineum is an important aspect of any newborn examination. An imperforate anus should be obvious on examination at birth, but a rectal atresia might not become apparent until it is noted that the baby has not passed meconium. However, it is important to remember that a history of passing meconium does not exclude a diagnosis of an anorectal malformation. Occasionally meconium is passed through a fistulous connection to the vagina, bladder or urethra and this may mask an imperforate anus (Figs 32.7–32.9). Whatever the anatomical arrangement, all babies should be referred for surgery.

Malrotation/volvulus

This is a developmental abnormality where incomplete rotation (malrotation) of the small bowel has taken place. This predisposes the bowel to intermittent episodes of twisting (volvulus) and obstruction. A baby with a malrotation may be entirely asymptomatic in the neonatal period, however episodes of obstruction can lead to bilious vomiting and abdominal distension. Due to the risks of severe, irreversible bowel damage secondary to

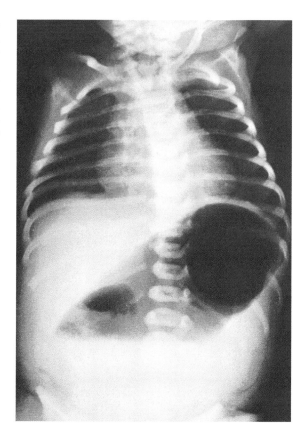

Fig. 32.6 Double bubble of duodenal atresia. The stomach is overlapping the duodenum with the second bubble being seen through the stomach.
From Rennie J M, Roberton N R C (eds) 1999 Textbook of neonatology, 3rd edn, with permission of Churchill Livingstone.

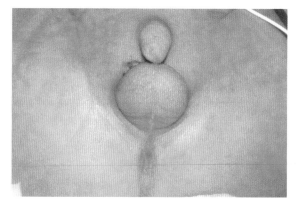

Fig. 32.7 Imperforate anus with recto-vesical fistula (1).
Reproduced with permission of Donna Bain.

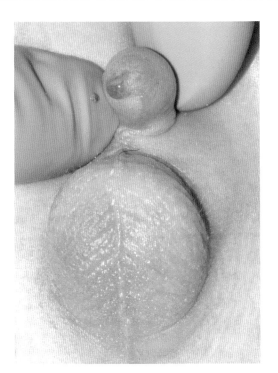

Fig. 32.8 Imperforate anus with recto-vesical fistula (2).
Reproduced with permission of Donna Bain.

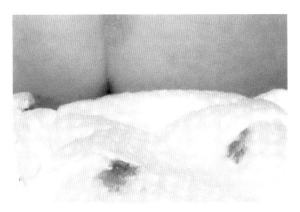

Fig. 32.9 Imperforate anus with recto-vesical fistula and napkin containing meconium stained urine.
Reproduced with permission of Donna Bain.

the obstruction of blood flow in the mesentery in unrecognized volvulus, any newborn infant with bile-stained vomiting requires urgent assessment. Surgical correction is necessary if a malrotation is confirmed.

Meconium ileus (cystic fibrosis)

Some 15% of children with cystic fibrosis present with meconium ileus in the neonatal period. This occurs because the meconium is particularly viscous and causes intestinal obstruction. There is accompanying abdominal distension and bile-stained vomiting. Intravenous fluids and a Gastrografin enema may relieve the obstruction but sometimes surgery is required. Histology of any resected bowel may indicate the likelihood of cystic fibrosis, but genetic mutation analysis is required to confirm the diagnosis. Subsequent treatment of cystic fibrosis is supportive rather than curative and involves optimized nutrition, administration of pancreatic enzymes and a rigorous programme of chest physiotherapy and antibiotics.

Hirschsprung's disease

In this disease, which has an incidence of 1 in 5000 live births, an aganglionic section of the bowel is present. This means that peristalsis does not occur and the bowel therefore becomes obstructed. The baby will present with any combination of delayed (>24 hours) passage of meconium, abdominal distension and bile-stained vomiting. Hirschsprung's disease is often suspected from radiography and contrast enema, however a rectal biopsy is required to confirm the diagnosis. Surgical resection of the aganglionic segment of bowel is indicated.

Cleft lip and cleft palate

The incidence of cleft lip occurring as a single malformation is 1.3 per 1000 live births. This anomaly may be unilateral or bilateral. Since it is very often accompanied by cleft palate, both will be considered together.

Clefts in the palate may affect the hard palate, soft palate, or both. Some defects will include alveolar margins and some the uvula. The greatest problem for these babies initially is feeding. If the defect is limited to unilateral cleft lip, mothers who had intended to breastfeed should be encouraged to do so. Where there is the additional problem of cleft palate, arranging for the baby to be fitted with an orthodontic plate may facilitate breastfeeding but this obviously does not afford the same stimulus as nipple-to-palate contact. Expressed breast milk via a cup is an alternative method but for those who wish to bottle-feed there is a wide variety of specially shaped teats available to accommodate the different sizes and positions of palate defects. Above all else, an unending supply of patience and reassurance is required. The midwife should encourage the mother and father to find the most successful technique rather than 'taking over' since this may compound any feelings of guilt or inadequacy the parents feel. Early referral to the cleft palate team of paediatric or plastic surgeon and orthodontists should be arranged. These teams will also include specialist nursing staff, speech and language therapists and audiologists.

Corrective surgery will be carried out at some stage, however agreement regarding optimal timing remains elusive (Manna et al 2009). To some extent a compromise

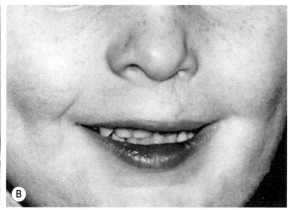

Fig. 32.10 (A) Cleft lip and palate. (B) The repaired cleft.
From Raine P 1994 Cleft lip and palate, in Freeman N V et al, Surgery of the newborn, ch 34, p 375, with permission of Churchill Livingstone.

must always be made regarding the balance of risk from surgery, the psychological impact of the malformation, the effect on speech and language acquisition and future facial growth. In general, lips are repaired between 10 and 12 weeks and palates between 6 and 18 months. It can be helpful for the midwife to show families 'before and after' photographs of babies for whom surgery has been a success (Fig. 32.10).

Clearly, although the midwife may offer valuable support in these early days, she is limited in the length of time she has available to help these families. Giving the parents the address of a support group such as the Cleft Lip and Palate Association (CLAPA) is useful (see Useful Websites).

Pierre Robin sequence

Pierre Robin sequence is characterized by micrognathia (hypoplasia of the lower jaw), posterior displacement of the tongue, which allows it to fall backward and occlude the airway, and a central cleft palate. This triad of anomalies presents challenges for nursing care, notably airway obstruction and feeding difficulties. Airway obstruction can often be managed with fairly straightforward interventions, such as prone positioning or the use of a nasopharyngeal airway. In a minority of situations the anatomical anomaly is so severe that surgery, for example jaw distraction or tracheostomy is required (Bacher et al 2010). Feeding can be problematic with a high risk of aspiration occurring. Some of these babies may be fitted with an orthodontic plate to facilitate feeding. The action of sucking will encourage development of the mandible. Parents will need considerable support during what may for some babies be a protracted period of hospitalization.

MALFORMATIONS RELATING TO RESPIRATION

Making a successful transition from fetus to neonate includes being able to establish regular respiration. Any malformation of the respiratory tract or accessory respiratory muscles is likely to hamper this process.

Diaphragmatic hernia

This malformation occurs in 1 in 2000 live births and consists of a defect in the diaphragm that allows herniation of abdominal contents into the thoracic cavity (Fig. 32.11). The extent to which lung development is compromised as a result depends on the size of the defect and the gestational age at which herniation first occurred. The condition is increasingly diagnosed antenatally by ultrasound; where there is prenatal diagnosis, birth in a specialist unit is advisable. At birth, the condition may be suspected if the baby is cyanosed and unexpected difficulty is experienced in resuscitation. In addition, since the majority of such defects are left-sided, heart sounds will be displaced to the right. The abdomen may have a flat or scaphoid appearance. Chest X-ray will confirm the diagnosis. Babies with this condition usually have significant respiratory distress and require intubation and mechanical ventilation. A large bore nasogastric tube on free drainage should be used to minimize gaseous distension of the displaced abdominal viscera. Surgical repair of the defect is necessary, but this is not urgent. It is more important to stabilize the baby's general condition before surgery. It is especially critical to deal with the problem of persistent pulmonary hypertension and right-to-left shunting of blood within

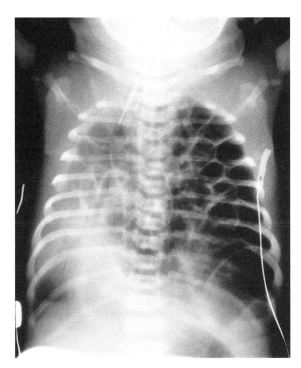

Fig. 32.11 Chest radiograph of infant at 1 hour of life, showing left diaphragmatic hernia, displacement of air-filled viscera into the hemithorax and a marked shift of mediastinum and heart.
From Rennie J M, Roberton N R C (eds) 1999 Textbook of neonatology, 3rd edn, with permission of Churchill Livingstone.

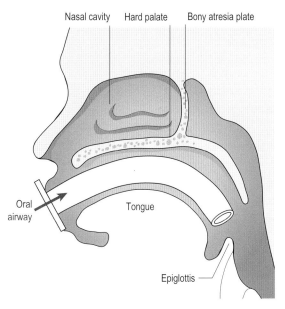

Fig. 32.12 Choanal atresia. A bony plate blocks the nose.
From Rennie J M, Roberton N R C (eds) 1999 Textbook of neonatology, 3rd edn, with permission of Churchill Livingstone.

the heart. This may necessitate the use of newer ventilation techniques and pharmacological agents such as nitric oxide. Prognosis relates to the degree of pulmonary hypoplasia and reversibility of the pulmonary hypertension. There is also the possibility of co-existent problems such as cardiac defects or skeletal anomalies.

Congenital pulmonary airway malformations (CPAM)

These include lesions formally known as congenital adenomatous malformation (CCAM), bronchopulmonary sequestration (BPS) and congenital lobar emphysema. The incidence is thought to be around 1 in 2000 live births although an increasing number are being detected prenatally by ultrasound scanning. Antenatal complications may include mediastinal shift and the development of hydrops, although many lesions seem to regress during the third trimester. Although most lesions are asymptomatic in the neonatal period, some lesions may expand rapidly after birth leading to air trapping, over-inflation and respiratory compromise. In such cases urgent surgical removal of the abnormal lung tissue is necessary. Babies known

prenatally to have a CPAM should be monitored closely after birth for signs of respiratory distress.

Some CPAM have been reported to be associated with lung infection and malignant change in later life. The true incidence of such complications is unknown but is likely to be low. However, even in asymptomatic patients, surgical removal may be undertaken in infancy in order to prevent long-term complications.

Choanal atresia

Choanal atresia describes a unilateral or bilateral narrowing of the nasal passage(s) with a web of tissue or bone occluding the nasopharynx (Fig. 32.12). The incidence is 1 in 8000 live births. Tachypnoea and dyspnoea are cardinal features, particularly when a bilateral lesion is present. The diagnosis is made relatively easily by noting that the baby mouth-breathes and finds feeding impossible without cyanosis. In addition, nasal catheters cannot be passed into the pharynx and if a mirror or cold metal spoon is held under the nose no vapour will collect. A helpful diagnostic aid is that the baby's colour will improve with crying. A unilateral defect may not be noticed until the baby feeds for the first time. The midwife should therefore bear in mind the possibility of this problem if respiratory difficulty and cyanosis occur at this time. Maintaining a clear airway is obviously essential and an oral airway may have to be used to affect this. Surgery will be required to remove the obstructing tissue.

Occasionally choanal atresia is associated with other anomalies such as CHARGE syndrome, a condition in which there are defects found in the eye (coloboma), the heart, occasionally oesophageal atresia, usually growth restriction, plus genital and ear abnormality.

Laryngeal stridor

This is a noise made by the baby, usually on inspiration and exacerbated by crying. Most commonly the cause is laryngomalacia. This is due to laxity of the laryngeal cartilage which collapses inwards during inspiration. Although it sounds distressing, the baby generally is not at all upset. Laryngomalacia usually resolves over time and intervention is only required in the most severe cases.

There are a number of other causes of stridor in the neonate which should be considered, particularly if the stridor is accompanied by signs of respiratory distress or feeding problems. Other causes include subglottic stenosis, laryngeal web, laryngeal cleft, vocal cord paralysis and extrinsic compression by a vascular ring. Investigations including laryngoscopy, bronchoscopy and barium swallow may be necessary in order to establish the diagnosis in cases not typical of mild laryngogomalacia.

CONGENITAL CARDIAC DEFECTS

Babies born with congenital heart defects comprise the second largest group of babies born with malformations. Approximately 8 per 1000 live births have some degree of congenital heart disease and about one-third of these babies will be symptomatic in early infancy.

Causes

Approximately 90% of cardiac defects cannot be attributed to a single cause. Chromosomal and genetic factors account for 8%, and a further 2% are thought to be caused by teratogens. The critical period of exposure to teratogens in respect of embryological development of cardiac tissue is from the 3rd to the 6th week of gestation.

Prenatal detection

An increasing number of cardiac problems are being identified by means of detailed prenatal ultrasound scanning (see Chapter 11). For babies with complex congenital heart disease this enables a multidisciplinary plan for birth and immediate neonatal care, to be made well in advance of delivery. However, the detection of many defects is still dependent upon accurate observations and examination during the neonatal period.

Postnatal recognition

Babies with congenital heart disease can present in a number of ways: heart murmur, cyanosis, tachypnoea, weak or absent femoral pulses. Those babies in whom the pulmonary or systemic blood flow is dependent upon the arterial duct may present with severe cyanosis or shock when the duct closes.

It is obviously important to try to identify those infants with life-threatening cardiac malformations prior to transfer home. Additionally, early identification and referral of babies with significant cardiac malformations is desirable. Whilst it must be remembered that not all babies with heart murmurs have an underlying cardiac malformation, it should also be noted that some babies with significant congenital heart disease may have no abnormal findings at the time of their routine newborn examination. As an adjunct to routine newborn examination some units therefore also measure oxygen saturations. This has been shown to improve the detection of some duct dependent heart lesions (Ewer et al 2011).

Ideally, every baby should be examined by a competent practitioner before going home. Although changing patterns of postnatal care often mean early transfer home, a baby with suspected congenital heart disease should not be sent home until he/she has been reviewed by an experienced paediatrician or a definitive diagnosis has been made. As some babies with significant congenital heart disease may have no clinical signs prior to transfer, there is a need for community midwives to be observant and to communicate effectively with parents. Parents who report any changes in the baby's behaviour such as breathlessness or cyanosis should never be ignored, but rather encouraged to seek medical advice promptly.

Traditionally, babies with cardiac anomalies have been divided into two groups: those with central cyanosis and those without, i.e. cyanotic and acyanotic congenital heart disease.

Cardiac defects presenting with cyanosis

Defects included in this group are:

- transposition of the great arteries
- pulmonary atresia
- tetralogy of Fallot
- tricuspid atresia
- total anomalous pulmonary venous drainage
- univentricular/complex heart.

Although cyanosis can be a presenting feature of a number of non-cardiac conditions (e.g. respiratory disease, persistent pulmonary hypertension of the newborn, sepsis), congenital heart disease should always be considered as a possible explanation. Administration of oxygen to babies with cyanotic heart disease may have little effect on their oxygen saturation levels. This observation, along with other routine investigations excluding other causes of cyanosis, may suggest a diagnosis of cyanotic heart disease. The definitive diagnostic investigation is echocardiography.

Cyanosis occurs when there is more than 5 g/dl of circulating deoxygenated haemoglobin. In congenital cyanotic heart disease, abnormal anatomy leads to mixing of oxygenated and deoxygenated blood ± inadequate pulmonary blood flow or, in the case of transposition of the great arteries, complete separation of the pulmonary and systemic circulations. In cases where there is severe obstruction to pulmonary blood flow, e.g. pulmonary atresia, there is often early presentation with marked cyanosis.

The most common cyanotic heart conditions are transposition of the great arteries and tetralogy of Fallot. Transposition of the great arteries is the most common cyanotic heart condition presenting in the neonatal period. This is a condition wherein the aorta arises from the right ventricle and the pulmonary artery from the left ventricle (Fig. 32.13). Consequently, oxygenated blood is circulated back through the lungs and deoxygenated blood back into the systemic circulation. It is apparent therefore that, unless there is an opportunity for oxygenated blood to access the systemic circulation, either by means of a patent arterial duct or through an accompanying septal defect, such a baby will die. In congenital cardiac defects such as this where the patency of the arterial duct is essential for survival ('duct-dependent' lesions), a prostaglandin infusion should be commenced in order to maintain ductal patency pending more definitive management. For babies with transposition of the great arteries a balloon septostomy is often performed to enlarge the foramen ovale and allow mixing of oxygenated and deoxygenated blood at atrial level. Corrective surgery (arterial switch operation) is then carried out, usually within a few weeks of birth.

Tetralogy of Fallot has four anatomical components; pulmonary outflow tract obstruction, a ventricular septal defect, right ventricular hypertrophy and an overriding aorta (Fig. 32.14). It seldom presents with cyanosis in the immediate newborn period, but this may become apparent within a few weeks of birth. Increasingly, the diagnosis is made prenatally. Most babies with this condition remain well in the neonatal period. Surgical treatment options include a Blalock Taussig shunt for cases where it is necessary to increase pulmonary blood flow, and corrective repair, usually within the first year of life.

Although prostaglandin infusion is life-saving for duct-dependent heart conditions it should be noted that it may lead to apnoea, particularly when higher doses are required. It is essential that there are facilities to provide respiratory support available for any baby on an infusion of prostaglandin.

'Acyanotic' cardiac defects

These congenital cardiac conditions include left-to-right shunt lesions and obstructive lesions.

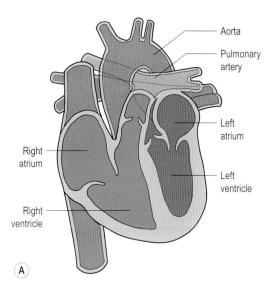

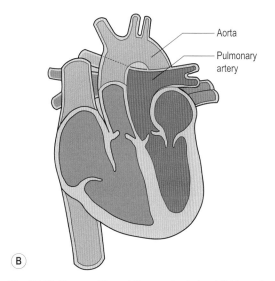

Fig. 32.13 Transposition of the great arteries. (A) Normal. (B) Transposition.

Left-to-right shunts

* Persistent arterial duct (also known as persistent ductus arteriosus)
* Ventricular or atrial septal defects.

These lesions may present with a murmur or, if the shunt is large, with symptoms and signs of heart failure: tachypnea, poor feeding, sweating, precordial heave, gallop rhythm or hepatomegaly.

A persistent arterial duct is more common in preterm infants and surgical closure is sometimes necessary if

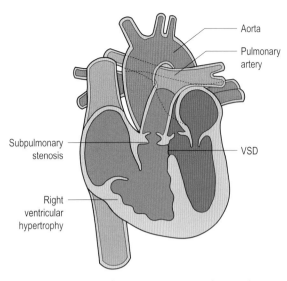

Fig. 32.14 Tetralogy of Fallot (VSD = ventricular septal defect).

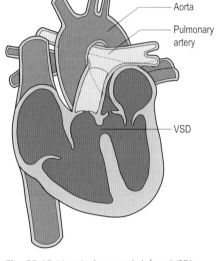

Fig. 32.15 Ventricular septal defect (VSD).

medical treatment with ibuprofen or indomethacin is ineffective. Term infants with a persistent arterial duct more usually undergo cardiac catheterization with device closure in childhood.

Ventricular septal defects are a common cause of murmurs in the term infant. Many of these defects are small, of no haemodynamic consequence and close spontaneously. Larger defects may lead to heart failure and surgical closure may be necessary although not usually in the neonatal period. (See Fig. 32.15.)

Obstructive lesions

- Coarctation of the aorta
- Pulmonary stenosis
- Aortic stenosis
- Hypoplastic left heart syndrome.

Some of these lesions may be difficult to pick up clinically and a proportion of serious left heart obstructive lesions are not diagnosed before transfer home. Such lesions should always be considered in the baby with poor volume femoral pulses or unexplained tachypnoea, remembering that even severe lesions may have no associated murmur. If the obstruction is severe, e.g. critical aortic stenosis, then the systemic blood flow is often dependent upon the arterial duct and the baby will become very unwell when this closes. As in the duct-dependent cyanotic heart conditions, a prostaglandin infusion may be required whilst further investigations and discussions regarding the possibility of surgical correction take place.

Coarctation of the aorta and aortic stenosis are usually amenable to surgical correction. Hypoplastic left heart syndrome remains a major surgical challenge, requiring a number of surgical procedures in childhood, with a poor long-term outcome. Because of this, some parents opt for a palliative approach with no surgical intervention. Death usually occurs within a few days, although it may take substantially longer in some cases, particularly if the baby is preterm. If palliation is the chosen care path, then the priorities are to ensure the comfort of the baby and to support the family. Whatever treatment decisions they make, following confirmation of such a diagnosis there is a substantial psychological impact on the parents, which calls for particularly supportive management.

CENTRAL NERVOUS SYSTEM MALFORMATIONS

Neural tube defects are the commonest malformations of the central nervous system. They arise from abnormalities during formation and closure of the neural tube, the embryonic precursor of the central nervous system. Ingestion of folic acid supplements prior to conception and during the early stages of pregnancy has helped to reduce the incidence of such anomalies (Medical Research Council [MRC] Vitamin Study Research Group 1991), however they have not provided the hoped-for panacea. Prenatal screening is very effective at identifying these malformations (see Chapter 11) and some parents choose selective termination of pregnancies where severe neural tube defects are found. Many parents elect to continue with their pregnancy and data from Wales suggest a rise in live births with spina bifida over the last decade (Czapran et al 2011).

Anencephaly

This major anomaly describes the absence of the forebrain and vault of the skull. It is a condition that is incompatible with sustained life but occasionally such a baby is born alive. The midwife should wrap the baby carefully before showing him/her to the parents. It is recognized that seeing and holding the baby will facilitate the grieving process (Chapter 26). It may be beneficial for the parents then to see the full extent of the malformation, unpleasant though it is. Seeing the whole baby will help them to accept the reality of the situation and prevent imagination of an even more gruesome picture.

Spina bifida

Spina bifida results from failure of fusion of the vertebral column. If there is no skin covering the defect, there is protrusion of the meninges, hence the term meningocele (Fig. 32.16). The meningeal membrane may be flat or appear as a membranous sac, with or without

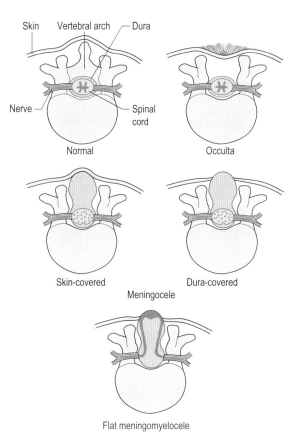

Fig. 32.16 Various forms of spina bifida.
After Wallis S, Harvey D 1979 Disorders in the newborn, Nursing Times 75: 1315–27, with permission of Nursing Times.

cerebrospinal fluid, but it does not contain neural tissue. A meningomyelocele, on the other hand, does involve the spinal cord (Fig. 32.17). This lesion may be enclosed, or the meningocele may rupture and expose the neural tissue. A meningomyelocele usually gives rise to neurological damage, producing paralysis distal to the defect, and impaired bladder and bowel function. The lumbosacral area is the most common site for these to present, but they may appear at any point in the vertebral column. When the defect is at base of skull level it is known as an encephalocele. The added complication here is that the sac may contain varying amounts of brain tissue. Normal progression of labour may be impeded by a large lesion of this type.

Immediate management involves covering open lesions with a non-adherent dressing. Babies with enclosed lesions should be handled with the utmost care in an attempt to preserve the integrity of the sac. This will limit the risk of meningitis occurring. A paediatric surgeon or neurosurgeon should be contacted. Surgical intervention for myelomeningocele carries a high rate of success of skin closure, but has no impact on any damage already present in the cord or more distally. There is associated hydrocephalus (see below) in up to 90% of cases, with the majority requiring surgical shunting to prevent a rapid increase in the intracranial pressure. It is seldom necessary to close the back within 24 hours of birth and priority should be given to stabilization of the baby and assessment of the defect (Jensen 2012). Following examination of the baby, discussion with the parents will allow them to make an informed choice about whether or not they wish their baby to have surgery.

Recent advances in the management of myelomeningocele include prenatal surgery performed at around 26 weeks' gestation (Adzick et al 2011). Clearly this option is not without risk to both mother and fetus and evidence of long-term benefit is yet to be established.

Spina bifida occulta

Spina bifida occulta (see Fig. 32.16) is the most minor type of defect where the vertebra is bifid. There is usually no spinal cord involvement. A tuft of hair or sinus at the

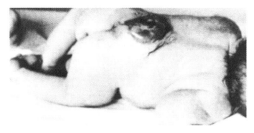

Fig. 32.17 Baby with meningomyelocele.
Reproduced with permission from Professor Robert Carachi.

base of the spine may be noted on first examination of the baby. Ultrasound investigation will confirm the diagnosis and rule out any associated spinal cord involvement.

Parents who have a baby with a neural tube defect should be offered genetic counselling since there is a 50-fold increased risk of recurrence in future pregnancies (Saleem et al 2009).

Hydrocephalus

This condition arises from a blockage in the circulation and absorption of cerebrospinal fluid, which is produced from the choroid plexuses within the lateral ventricles of the brain. The large lateral ventricles increase in size and eventually compress the surrounding brain tissue. It is a common accompaniment to the more severe spina bifida lesions because of a structural defect around the area of the foramen magnum known as the Arnold–Chiari malformation. Consequently, hydrocephalus may either be present at birth or develop following surgical closure of a myelomeningocele. In the absence of a myelomeningocele, congenital aqueduct stenosis is the commonest cause of hydrocephalus. The risk of cerebral damage may be minimized by the insertion of a ventriculoperitoneal shunt. As the baby grows, this will need to be replaced. Attendant risks with these devices are that the line blocks and that the shunt is a source for infection leading to meningitis. The midwife must be alert for the signs of increased intracranial pressure:

- large tense anterior fontanelle
- splayed skull sutures
- inappropriate increase in occipitofrontal circumference
- sun-setting appearance to the eyes
- irritability or abnormal movements.

Microcephaly

This is where the occipitofrontal circumference is more than two standard deviations below normal for gestational age. The disproportionately small head may reflect a familial pattern of head growth, however it may also be a manifestation of abnormal brain development. Underlying aetiologies include conditions that adversely affect the early fetal brain, e.g. intrauterine infection, fetal alcohol exposure, or chromosomal disorders. The longer-term neurodevelopmental sequelae are determined by the underlying cause but may include learning difficulties, cerebral palsy and seizures.

MUSCULOSKELETAL DEFORMITIES

These range from relatively minor anomalies, for example an extra digit, to major deficits such as absence of a limb.

Polydactyly and syndactyly

Careful examination, including separation and counting of the baby's fingers and toes during the initial examination, is important otherwise anomalies such as syndactyly (webbing) and polydactyly (extra digits) may go unnoticed.

Syndactyly more commonly affects the hands. It can appear as an independent anomaly or as a feature of a syndrome such as Apert's syndrome; this is a genetically inherited condition in which there is premature fusion of the sutures of the vault of the skull, cleft palate and complete syndactyly of both hands and feet. Whether or not any surgical division needs to be carried out depends on the degree of webbing or fusion.

In polydactyly the extra digit(s) may be fully formed or simply extra tissue attached by a pedicle. Even where there is only a rudimentary digit without bone involvement, better cosmetic results are obtained if the digit is surgically excised rather than 'tied off'. Surgical excision is mandatory in more complex cases.

A family history of either of these defects is common, and in this situation the mother is often anxious to examine the baby for herself.

Limb reduction deficiencies

Limb reduction deficiencies describe the congenital absence or hypoplasia of a long bone and/or digits. The prevalence is around 0.7 per 1000 live births and the most common identifiable cause, present in a third of cases, is a vascular disruption defect (Gold et al 2011). An example of this is an amniotic band-elated deficiency where the amnion is believed to wrap itself around a developing limb causing strangulation and necrosis. Other identifiable causes include teratogens (such as thalidomide), genetic mutations, chromosomal disorders or as part of a syndrome such as the VACTERL spectrum described earlier in the chapter (see page 651) (McGuirk et al 2001).

Limb reduction deficiencies may also be classified by site (upper versus lower limb), or by type (transverse versus longitudinal). In a transverse defect the limb has developed normally to a particular level beyond which no skeletal elements exist (Fig. 32.18), whilst in a longitudinal defect there is a reduction or absence of an element(s) within the long axis of the limb (Gold et al 2011).

Specific management plans are often reached only after detailed assessment by an orthopaedic surgeon with a special interest in limb malformations. For those who require them, different types of prostheses are available and can be fitted as early as 3 months of age. Innovative surgical techniques such as limb lengthening or the transferring of toe(s) to hand to serve as substitute finger(s) are proving successful for some children. Once again one of the most helpful things the midwife can do in these early days of parental adjustment is to offer the address of a

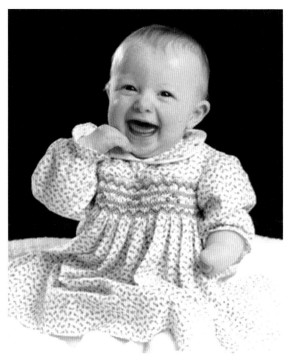

Fig. 32.18 A baby with a limb reduction defect quickly learns to adapt.
Photograph courtesy of Reach.

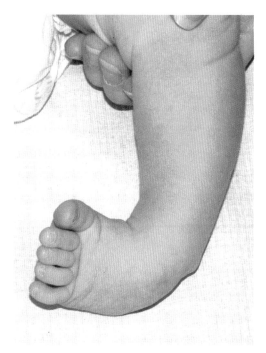

Fig. 32.19 Congenital talipes equinovarus.

support group such as Reach (see Useful Websites). This appropriately named support group for parents of children with upper limb deformities has branches throughout the United Kingdom (UK).

Talipes

Talipes equinovarus (TEV, club foot) (Fig. 32.19) is the descriptive term for a deformity of the foot where the ankle is bent downwards (plantar flexed) and the front part of the foot is turned inwards (inverted). Talipes calcaneovalgus describes the opposite position where the foot is dorsiflexed and everted. TEV is a relatively common malformation, occurring in 1 in every 1000 live births. It is bilateral in 50% of cases and occurs in males more commonly than females, with a ratio of 2 : 1. Historically it was thought that these deformities were more likely to occur when intrauterine space was restricted, for example in multiple pregnancy or oligohydramnios. It is now recognized that there is an important genetic element involved in their causation and parents who have had a baby with TEV have a 1 in 30 risk of recurrence in future pregnancies. TEV is also more likely to occur in conjunction with neuromuscular disorders such as spina bifida. In the mildest form, postural TEV, the foot may be easily returned to the

correct position. The midwife should encourage the mother to exercise the baby's foot in this way several times a day. More severe forms will require one or more of manipulation, splinting, or surgical correction. The advice of an orthopaedic surgeon should be sought as soon as possible after birth as early treatment with manipulation or splinting may enhance results and minimize the need for surgery. Care should be taken to ensure that, for babies who have splints applied, the strapping is not too tight and that the baby's toes are well perfused.

Developmental dysplasia of the hip

Congenital hip dysplasia is an abnormality more commonly found where there has been a breech presentation at term, oligohydramnios, a foot deformity or a family history in a first-degree relative. It most often occurs in primigravida pregnancies and is commoner in girls than boys. The left hip is more often affected than the right. The dysplastic hip may present in one of three ways: dislocated, dislocatable or with subluxation of the joint. Prenatal diagnosis by ultrasound is possible; most, however, are diagnosed incidentally during the routine newborn examination. Any abnormal findings should be reported and the baby referred for an orthopaedic opinion, ultrasound scan of the hips, or both. Where the diagnosis is confirmed it is usual for the baby to have a splint or harness such as

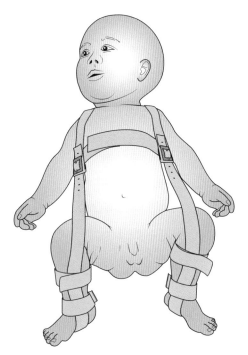

Fig. 32.20 Pavlik harness for congenital dislocation of hip. *From Barr D G D et al 1998 Disorders of bone, joints and connective tissue, in Campbell A G M, McIntosh N (eds) Forfar and Arneil's textbook of pediatrics, ch 23, p 1628, with permission of Churchill Livingstone.*

the Pavlik harness (Fig. 32.20) applied, which will keep the hips in a flexed and abducted position of about 60%. The splint should not be removed for napkin changing or bathing. Parents will require additional support in learning how to handle and care for their baby. Particular attention should be paid to skin care and checking for signs of rubbing or excoriation.

Achondroplasia

Achondroplasia is an autosomal dominant condition where the baby is generally small with a disproportionately large head and short limbs. Some 80% of cases are due to new mutations of fibroblast growth factor receptor genes and hence these families may have no anticipation of the disorder unless an antenatal diagnosis has been made.

Osteogenesis imperfecta

Osteogenesis imperfecta (OI) is sometimes referred to as brittle bone disease. It is due to a disorder of collagen production that can result in multiple fractures either *in utero* or at birth. There are eight different types and the

severity of symptoms varies between types. Inheritance was originally believed to be autosomal dominant; however it is now recognized that autosomal recessive forms exist as well as new mutations arising in a third of cases (Basel and Steiner 2009). Recognition and genetic counselling are therefore important for future pregnancies.

ABNORMALITIES OF THE SKIN

Vascular naevi

These anomalies in the development of the skin can be divided into two main types, which commonly overlap.

Capillary malformations

These are due to defects in the dermal capillaries. The most commonly observed are 'stork marks'. These are usually found on the nape of the neck. They are generally small and will fade. No treatment is necessary.

Port wine stain

This is a purple–blue capillary malformation affecting the face. It occurs in approximately 1 in 3000 live births. It is generally fully formed at birth and does not regress with time. However, laser treatment and the skilful use of cosmetics will help to disguise the problem. The parents, and later the child, may need substantial psychological support.

Should the malformation mimic the distribution of the ophthalmic branch of the trigeminal nerve, further malformations in the eyes (glaucoma), meninges or brain (epilepsy) may be suspected. This is known as the Sturge–Weber syndrome.

Capillary haemangiomata ('strawberry marks')

Capillary haemangiomata are not usually noticeable at birth but appear as red, raised lesions in the first few weeks of life (Fig. 32.21). These common lesions affect up to 10% of the population by the age of 1 year. They are five times more common in girls than boys and are also commoner in preterm infants. They can appear anywhere in the body but cause particular distress to the parents when they appear on the face. However, parents may be reassured that, although the lesion will grow bigger for the first few months it will then regress with associated central pallor (Fig. 32.22) and usually disappears completely by the age of 5–6 years. No treatment is normally required unless the haemangioma is situated in an awkward area where it is

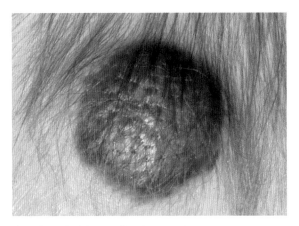

Fig. 32.21 Evolving capillary haemangioma.
Reproduced with permission of Sharon Murphy.

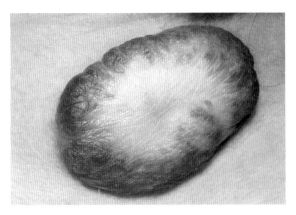

Fig. 32.22 Regressing capillary haemangioma with typical pallor.
Reproduced with permission of Sharon Murphy.

likely to be subject to abrasion, such as on the lip or around the eye where it may interfere with vision. Treatment with propranolol, steroids or pulsed laser therapy is possible.

Pigmented (melanocytic) naevi

These are brown, sometimes hairy, marks on the skin that vary in size and may be flat or raised. A minority of this type of birthmark can become malignant. Surgical excision may be recommended to pre-empt this.

It is unlikely that treatment for any of these birthmarks will be carried out in the immediate neonatal period except in the case of larger pigmented naevi. The midwife's responsibilities are therefore to notify appropriate medical staff and offer parents general emotional support.

GENITOURINARY SYSTEM

Improved prenatal screening and diagnostic techniques (see Chapter 11) mean that information regarding urinary tract architecture is often available at birth. In addition, knowledge of liquor volume provides reassurance that fetal renal function is adequate. If an anomaly has been prenatally identified a plan regarding the timing of postnatal investigation(s) and subsequent management should be available at birth. Occasionally renal tract malformations may be undiagnosed at birth, in which case the absence of urine for 24 hours or a poor urinary stream may indicate underlying problems.

Potter syndrome

The impact of fetal renal agenesis or severe hypoplasia was first described in a series of stillborn infants by Edith Potter, a perinatal pathologist, in 1946. A characteristic facial appearance due to the compressive effects of long-standing oligohydramnios is seen in association with limb contractures. The presence of adequate liquor volume is critical to the development of normal lungs and babies with renal agenesis will all die at or shortly after birth as a consequence of lung hypoplasia.

Posterior urethral valve(s)

This is a malformation affecting boys where the presence of valves in the posterior urethra obstructs the normal outflow of urine. As a result, the bladder distends, causing back pressure on the ureters and kidneys. This will ultimately cause bilateral hydronephrosis and renal parenchymal damage. Prenatal diagnosis is common and *in utero* intervention with the insertion of a shunt from the bladder to the amniotic fluid is possible. Improved long-term renal function following prenatal treatment is not guaranteed and postnatal valve ablation remains the mainstay of treatment (Salam 2006). Unfortunately even with early identification and management many of these boys will have life-long renal impairment.

Cystic kidneys

Cystic changes within the kidney(s) are often identified prenatally. Extensive bilateral changes are likely to be associated with impaired renal function and oligohydramnios. Unfortunately the prognosis in this situation is poor, with some babies dying at birth and others developing renal failure. The severest forms of polycystic kidney disease are usually linked to an autosomal recessive inheritance, but an autosomal dominant variety also occurs with a less gloomy prognosis. Unilateral cystic changes, e.g. multicystic dysplastic kidney, have a good prognosis assuming that the contralateral kidney is normal. Postnatal renal imaging and follow-up is required but the baby is usually well at birth.

Hypospadias

Examination of a baby boy may reveal that the urethral meatus opens on to the undersurface of the penis. The meatus can be placed at any point along the length of the penis and in some cases will open onto the perineum. This abnormality often co-exists with chordee, in which the penis is short and bent and the foreskin is present only on the dorsal side of the penis. It is important that the parents are made aware that circumcision should be deferred until consultation with the paediatric surgeon is completed.

Cryptorchidism

Undescended testes may be unilateral or bilateral and occur in 1–2% of male infants. If on examination of the baby after birth the scrotum is empty, the undescended testes may be found in the inguinal pouch. Sometimes the testis in this position can be manipulated into the scrotal pouch. If neither testis is palpable further investigation to exclude endocrine or chromosomal causes is required. In unilateral undescended testis parents should be encouraged to have the baby examined at regular intervals. If descent of the testis has not occurred by the time the child is one year old, arrangements for orchidopexy may be made.

DISORDERS OF SEX DEVELOPMENT (DSD)

DSD are a group of conditions in which the external genitalia and the reproductive organs do not develop normally. They may present at birth when the baby's external appearance is neither definitely male nor female. In this very challenging situation it is vital that the midwife is positive, honest and does not assign a gender to the baby. Examination of the baby may reveal any of the following: a small hypoplastic penis, chordee, bifid scrotum, undescended testes (careful examination should be made to detect undescended testes in the inguinal canal) or enlarged clitoris and incompletely separated or poorly differentiated labia. It can be impossible to differentiate by clinical examination alone between female masculinization, male under-virilization or mixed gender and expert clarification is always needed. The decision of gender attribution is made following chromosomal studies to determine genetic make-up, hormone assays and consideration of the potential surgical options. In the longer term specialist multi-disciplinary support, including clinical psychologists, is essential for these children and their families.

Congenital adrenal hyperplasia

This is the commonest cause of female masculinization (i.e. genetically female with male-looking genitalia). In this inherited condition the adrenal gland is stimulated to overproduce androgens because of a deficiency of an enzyme called 21-hydroxylase, which is necessary for normal production of steroid from cholesterol. If aldosterone production is also reduced then these babies will rapidly lose salt and may present collapsed and dehydrated. Urea and electrolyte levels, blood glucose and 17-hydroxy progesterone concentrations should be measured and appropriate fluid replacement given. Prenatal diagnosis by genetic mutation analysis is possible and facilitates prenatal steroid treatment to minimize virilization in affected females (Forest 2004).

Androgen insensitivity syndrome

This is one of several causes of male under-virilization (genetically male with female-looking genitalia). In this condition cells are unresponsive to the effects of androgenic hormones. In the fetus this prevents normal masculinization of the external genitalia despite the presence of a Y chromosome.

TERATOGENIC CAUSES

Fetal alcohol syndrome/spectrum

Fetal alcohol exposure remains a leading cause of intellectual impairment despite Department of Health recommendations to drink no alcohol at all during pregnancy. This reflects the difficulties of translating health promotion objectives into successful outcomes, particularly in an environment where the alcohol consumption of young women is constantly increasing.

The teratogenic effects of alcohol include growth restriction, distortion of craniofacial features and brain damage (De Sanctis et al 2011). The midwife may be alerted to the possibility of a baby being born with this syndrome if there have been concerns about *in utero* growth, particularly in the context of excess alcohol consumption. Postnatally the following characteristics may be recognizable: a small for gestational age infant with microcephaly, small palpebral fissures, a smooth philtrum and a thin upper lip. These facial features may become less pronounced as the child grows, however microcephaly, small stature and behavioural problems remain. The midwife will need to exercise excellent counselling skills to provide much-needed support for the mother. Collaboration with social services is usually called for to ensure that the care options decided are in the best interests of the infant and family.

Establishing such a direct link between a teratogen and a complex clinical pattern remains the exception rather than the rule although as mentioned earlier accurate recording of all congenital malformations on a central register can aid early recognition of potential new teratogens.

SUPPORT FOR THE MIDWIFE

Caring for a mother whose baby has some major congenital malformation places extra demands on the midwife. This stress is compounded if the anomaly was not anticipated prior to birth or if the midwife has not previously encountered the particular problem. The exercising of effective counselling and communication skills is invaluable in helping the family to adjust and in facilitating appropriate lines of support. The extra effort expended can be costly in terms not only of time but of the emotional stress the midwife may experience.

It is important that support is available for midwives in these situations and an opportunity to debrief with a senior colleague(s) or named supervisor of midwives can be helpful. Preparatory courses on grief and bereavement counselling are also of some benefit as many parents with affected babies will experience many of these emotions (Chapter 26). Midwives who have acquired experience in this realm should not, however, automatically be targeted as the experts and always be called upon to fulfil this role. Conversely, student midwives ought not to be deliberately shielded from being involved in caring for such families. The provision of quality care for parents who have a child with a congenital malformation is contingent upon meeting the needs of the carers.

Midwives may also find information available via the Internet, however, they should be aware of the dubious quality of some of this information. They should therefore exercise caution in how they utilize it. It might also be wise to caution parents, who often search the Internet for further information, of this potential risk.

REFERENCES

Adzick N S, Thom E, Spong C et al 2011 A randomized trial of prenatal versus postnatal repair of myelomeningocele. New England Journal of Medicine 364(11):993–1004

Bacher M, Linz A, Buchenau W et al 2010 Treatment of infants with Pierre Robin sequence. Laryngorhinootologie 89(10): 621–9

Basel D, Steiner R D 2009 Osteogenesis imperfecta: recent findings shed new light on this once well understood condition. Genetic Medicine 11(6):375–85

Chinnery P F, Howell N, Lightowlers R N et al 1998 MELAS and MERRF: The relationship between maternal mutation load and the frequency of clinically affected offspring. Brain 121:1889–94

Czapran P, Gibbon F, Beattie B et al 2011 Neural tube defects in Wales: changing demographics from 1998 to 2009. British Journal of Neurosurgery 26:456–9

De Sanctis L, Memo L, Pichini S et al 2011 Fetal alcohol syndrome: new perspectives for an ancient and underestimated problem. Journal of Maternal Fetal and Neonatal Medicine 24(1): 34–7

Ewer A K, Middleton L J, Furmston A T et al 2011 Pulse oximetry screening for congenital heart defects in newborn infants (Pulse Ox): a test accuracy study. Lancet 378:785–94

Forest M G 2004 Recent advances in the diagnosis and management of congenital adrenal hyperplasia due to 21-hydroxylase deficiency. Human Reproduction Update 10(6):469–85

Gold N B, Westgate M N, Holmes L B 2011 Anatomic and etiological classification of congenital limb deficiencias. American Journal of Medical Genetics 155A(6):1225–35

Haddock G, Davis C F, Raine P A M 1996 Gastroschisis in the decade of prenatal diagnosis. European Journal of Paediatric Surgery 6:18–24

Jensen A 2012 Nursing care and surgical correction of neonatal myelomeningocele. Infant 8(5):142–6

Lee S L, Beter T D, Kim S S et al 2006 Initial nonoperative management and delayed closure for the treatment of giant omphaloceles. Journal of Pediatric Surgery 41(11):1846–9

Manna F, Pensiero S, Clarich G et al 2009 Cleft lip and palate: current status from the literature and our experience. Journal of Craniofacial Surgery 20(5):1383–7

McGuirk C K, Westgate M N, Holmes L B 2001 Limb deficiencies in newborn infants. Pediatrics 108(4):E64

Medical Research Council Vitamin Study Research Group 1991 Prevention of neural tube defects: results of the Medical Research Council Vitamin Study. Lancet 338:131–7

Pedersen R N, Calzolari E, Husby S et al. EUROCAT Working Group 2012 Oesophageal atresia: prevalence, prenatal diagnosis and associated anomalies in 23 European regions. Archives of Disease in Childhood 97(3):227–32

Salam M A 2006 Posterior urethral valves: outcome of antenatal intervention. International Journal of Urology 13(10):1317–22

Saleem S N, Said A H, Abdel-Raouf M et al 2009 MRI in the evaluation of fetuses referred for sonographically suspected neural tube defects: impact on diagnosis and management decisions. Neuroradiology 51(11):761–72

Schlatter M, Norris K, Uitvlugt N et al 2003 Improved outcomes in the treatment of gastroschisis using a preformed silo and delayed repair approach. Journal of Pediatric Surgery 38(3):459–64

FURTHER READING

Jones K L (ed) 2006 Smith's recognizable patterns of human malformation, 6th edn. Saunders/ Elsevier, Philadelphia

This book provides a comprehensive and systematic approach to dysmorphic syndromes.

USEFUL WEBSITES

Antenatal Results and Choices (ARC): www.arc-uk.org

This website provides non-directive support and advice to parents throughout the antenatal testing process and when a malformation has been diagnosed

Association for Spina Bifida and Hydrocephalus (ASBAH): www.asbah.org

Children's Heart Federation: www.chfed.org.uk

Cleft Lip and Palate Association (CLAPA): www.clapa.com

Contact a Family: www.cafamily.org.uk

This website provides information and support for families with disabled children.

Cystic Fibrosis Trust (CF): www.cftrust.org.uk

Down's Syndrome Association: www.downs-syndrome.org.uk

Genetic Alliance UK: www.geneticalliance.org.uk

This is a national alliance of organizations which support children and families affected by genetic disorders.

On-line Mendelian Inheritance in Man (OMIM): www.ncbi.nlm.nih.gov/omim

Detailed information about clinical features and genetics of inherited diseases

Reach: The Association for Children with Upper Limb Deficiencies: www.reach.org.uk

Scottish Down's Syndrome Association (SDSA): www.dsscotland.org.uk

SOFT (Support Organization for Trisomy 13/18): www.soft.org.uk

STEPS (National Association for Children with Lower Limb Deficiencies): www.steps-charity.org.uk

Chapter |33|

Significant problems in the newborn baby

Stephen P Wardle, Carole England

A wide variety of conditions may present in the newborn baby that warrant early referral to the neonatal multiprofessional team. The midwife needs to be able to recognize and assess problems that distinguish healthy babies from those that are ill/sick. Some problems will be life-threatening and will require urgent assistance; others will be more subtle in their presentation, but nevertheless remain important. Knowledge of the signs, characteristics and features of the conditions presented will enable the midwife to make well-informed and appropriate referrals, while also providing valuable support for the parents before, during and after the neonatologist has examined their baby.

THE CHAPTER AIMS TO:

- assist the midwife in the assessment and identification of the sick newborn baby
- summarize possible problems that may be identified in a newborn baby and offer an approach to dealing with them.

INTRODUCTION

The majority of newborn babies are born in good condition and require no intervention after birth except to be dried with a warm towel and then to have skin-to-skin contact with their mother (Chapter 29). Labour and birth may have been straightforward but the baby may still need to be observed at this time to ensure a healthy transition from uterine to postnatal life. Approximately 5–10% of babies will require admission to a neonatal unit. Many of these are preterm babies or those with antenatally detected problems; however 6–9% of term babies will also require some type of neonatal care (Tracy et al 2007). The length of time a mother spends in hospital with her newborn baby has decreased significantly in recent years and many babies may be born outside the hospital setting, at home or in a midwifery-led unit. Context may impact on early recognition and management of problems in the early newborn period. The focus of this chapter is to aid the early detection of problems to enable the midwife to

distinguish the ill from the well baby and to decide when intervention is required and what that initial action should be. The aim is not to give detailed management about conditions that will clearly need the involvement of the neonatal specialists, but to summarize those conditions that may first be recognized or come to the attention of midwives and require their involvement.

INITIAL EXAMINATION AND RECOGNITION OF PROBLEMS

Most of the information the midwife requires for the assessment of a baby's wellbeing comes from observation. The normal term baby will lie with their limbs partially flexed and active, the skin colour should be centrally perfused, indicating adequate oxygenation, and there should be no rashes or skin lesions. After the initial observation there should follow a more systematic examination to ensure the newborn baby is well (Chapter 28). The following areas should be examined carefully.

The skin

The skin of a neonate varies in its appearance and can often be the cause of unnecessary anxiety in the mother, midwife and medical staff. It is, however, often the first sign that there may be an underlying problem in the baby. The presence of meconium on the skin, which is usually seen in the nail beds and around the umbilicus, in a baby with respiratory problems may indicate meconium aspiration as a factor. More generally, the skin of all babies should be examined for pallor, plethora, cyanosis, jaundice and skin rashes.

Pallor

A pale, mottled baby may be an indication of poor peripheral perfusion, however the hands and feet are often blue soon after birth (acrocyanosis) and this does not indicate an underlying problem. Always examine the baby's face and chest when assessing colour. The anaemic baby's appearance is usually pale pink, white or, in severe cases where there is vascular collapse, grey. Other presenting signs are tachycardia, tachypnoea and poor capillary refill (CR) (press the skin briefly on the forehead or chest and observe how long it takes for the colour to return; this should be less than 2 seconds). The most likely causes of anaemia immediately after birth are:

- a history in the baby of haemolytic disease of the newborn (HDN)
- twin-to-twin transfusions *in utero* (which can cause one baby to be anaemic and the other polycythaemic)

- feto-maternal haemorrhage
- fetal haemorrhage from vasa praevia or bleeding from the umbilical cord.

Pallor can also be observed in babies who are hypothermic or hypoglycaemic. Significant pallor can be associated with:

- anaemia and shock
- respiratory disorders
- cardiac anomalies
- sepsis.

Plethora

Babies who are very red in colour may be described as plethoric. Their colour may indicate a high level of circulating red blood cells (polycythaemia). Newborn babies can become polycythaemic if they are recipients of:

- twin-to-twin transfusion *in utero*
- a large placental transfusion.

Contributing factors may include deferred clamping of the umbilical cord or holding the baby below the level of the placenta, thereby allowing blood to flow into the baby and giving a greater circulating blood volume (can occur in unassisted births). Other babies at risk are:

- those that are small for their gestational age (SGA) as a means to increase oxygen carrying capacity in the hypoxic situation (Chapter 30)
- infants of diabetic mothers (IDM) as a result of increased levels of growth hormone and an overactive metabolism.

The diagnosis of polycythaemia is based upon levels of haemoglobin and haematocrit (the relationship between red blood cells and plasma in the blood) and how they compare with normal values, based on gestational age. Some poor outcomes have been associated with polycythaemia, however according to (Özek et al 2010) there is no evidence that a particular level of haematocrit requires treatment nor that treatment is of any benefit.

Cyanosis

Peripheral cyanosis of the hands and feet is common during the first 24 hours of life and is of no significance. Central cyanosis should always be taken seriously. The tongue and mucous membranes are the most reliable indicators of central colour in all babies and if they appear blue this indicates low oxygen saturation levels in the blood, usually of respiratory or cardiac origin. Episodic central cyanosis may be an indication that the baby is having convulsions. Central cyanosis always demands urgent attention (see later sections on respiratory problems and assessment of the cyanosed baby).

Other factors that affect the appearance of the skin

Preterm babies have thinner skin that is redder in appearance than that of term infants. In post-term babies, the skin is often dry and cracked. The skin is a good indicator of the nutritional status of the baby. The SGA baby may look malnourished and have folds of loose skin over the joints, owing to the lack or loss of subcutaneous fat. This can predispose the baby to hypoglycaemia due to poor glycogen stores in the liver and can also cause problems with hypothermia. If the baby is dehydrated, the skin looks dry and pale and is often cool to the touch. If gently pinched, the skin will be slow to retract. Other signs of dehydration are tachycardia, pallor or mottled skin, sunken eyes and anterior fontanelle. The best clinical indicator of dehydration is the baby's reduced weight.

Skin rashes

Skin rashes are quite common in newborn babies but most are benign and self-limiting. There are some rashes, however, which may indicate significant illness and should not be ignored:

- Petechiae or purpura rash over the upper part of the body, particularly the face and chest, may occur due to venous obstruction after normal or prolonged birth. Petechiae can occur when there is a low platelet count (thrombocytopenia as discussed later in the chapter) and this may present with a petechial rash over the whole body with prolonged bleeding from puncture sites and/or the umbilicus and bleeding into the intestinal system.
- Bruising can occur following breech extractions, forceps and ventouse-assisted births. A sub-aponeurotic haemorrhage (Chapter 31) can cause a decrease in circulating blood volume, which can result in anaemia and, if severe, hypotension.
- Vesicular rash is where small fluid-filled raised lumps occur on the skin associated with some congenital viral infections, in particular herpes simplex or congenital chicken pox (Varicella). *These can be very serious infections in the newborn and should always be carefully assessed.* The midwife should enquire about a history of maternal genital herpes infection although it can occur without any known history of infection. Referral for neonatal medical assessment is essential and a diagnosis should be confirmed before commencing treatment.
- Blistering rash is where areas of skin are raised and are fluid-filled. The surface of the skin may also slough off, leaving red raw areas. This can occur in bacterial infections, in particular *Staphylococcus aureus*, and in some rare but important skin diseases, e.g. epidermolysis bullosa (EB), part of a group of inherited skin conditions some of which are very

serious and associated with significant morbidity and mortality. There may be a family history. It presents as widespread tender erythema, followed by blisters, which break leaving raw areas of skin or sometimes yellow-filled bullae. This is particularly noticeable around the napkin area but can also cause umbilical sepsis, breast abscesses, conjunctivitis and, in systemic infections, there may also be involvement of the bones and joints. Babies with this condition are likely to be very unwell and require admission to a neonatal intensive care unit (NICU). A blistering skin rash should always be treated with broad spectrum intravenous (IV) antibiotics that particularly cover S. aureus.

The respiratory system

Healthy babies should establish normal regular respiration within minutes of birth. Many babies may display a slightly irregular breathing pattern for a few minutes after birth but should have regular respiration with a respiratory rate of 40–60 by approximately 2 minutes. The baby's breathing pattern will alter depending on his/her level of activity but a respiratory rate consistently above 60 breaths per minute is considered as tachypnoea.

Cardiorespiratory adaptations at birth

- Before birth the lungs are fluid-filled. At birth the newborn must clear this fluid in order to breathe successfully. Some fluid is removed by physical means during normal labour (Stephens et al 1998) but most is absorbed into the pulmonary lymphatics and capillaries.
- The lungs inflate and remain inflated as a result of the presence of surfactant. In some preterm babies, IDM and sick term babies, surfactant production may be decreased, resulting in respiratory distress.
- Newborn babies are obligate nasal breathers. Obstruction to the nares (nostrils) can therefore result in serious respiratory distress.
- The shape of the newborn thorax and the rib orientation tend to mean that the expansion potential of the thorax is limited. The baby's soft and flexible ribs also make the chest wall subject to collapse during increased respiratory efforts. To compensate for this the baby tends to elevate lung volume at end expiration by a rapid respiratory rate, intercostal activity and grunting.

Because of the factors described above the clinical signs of respiratory distress in the newborn are different from other patient groups. The following features may be seen:

- Expiratory grunting is a characteristic noise and occurs due to partial closure of the glottis during expiration. The baby is attempting to preserve some internal lung pressure and prevent the airways from collapsing completely at the end of the breath.
- Intercostal recession uses the intercostal muscles more effectively, but as a result the spaces between the ribs and the sternum are sucked in during each breath.
- Tachypnoea is an increased respiratory rate that occurs as the baby attempts to compensate for an increased carbon dioxide concentration in the blood and extracellular fluids. A normal respiratory rate in the newborn is 40–60 breaths per minute.
- Nasal flaring is an attempt to minimize the effect of the airways resistance by maximizing the diameter of the upper airways. The nares are seen to flare open with each breath.
- Apnoea is an absence of breathing for more than 20 seconds and may occur as a result of increasing respiratory fatigue in the term baby. The preterm baby may also experience apnoea of prematurity due to immaturity of the respiratory centre and/or obstructive apnoea from occluded airways.

A baby with significant signs of respiratory distress should be reviewed by the neonatal team and should be admitted to the NICU for further investigation and observation. Occasionally in the first few minutes after birth, particularly following a caesarean section, a baby may have mild respiratory abnormalities that settle quickly, but babies with abnormal signs should always remain under observation as deterioration can occur rapidly in some cases. On initial assessment it may not be easy to distinguish the cause of the respiratory distress and further evaluation, including a chest X-ray, may be required (the initial assessment and treatment is described later in the chapter).

The importance of body temperature control

A neutral thermal environment is defined as the ambient air temperature at which oxygen consumption or heat production is minimal, with body temperature in the normal range (Lissauer and Faranoff 2006). The normal body temperature range for term babies is 36.5–37.3 °C. Merenstein and Gardner (2011) assert the importance of the neutral thermal environment and how everyone caring for babies should understand the need for maintenance of normal body temperature. Mothers are often hot during labour and measures may be taken to produce a cooler environment for the mother's comfort. It is important to always consider this effect and maintain a suitable environmental temperature for the newborn baby. In addition to skin-to-skin contact, this may require extra measures like use of a radiant heater or cot warmer, in some circumstances. Environments that are outside the neutral thermal environment may result in babies who are too cold or too warm, who will attempt to regulate their temperature, and this can destabilize more vulnerable babies such as those of low birth weight (preterm and SGA). An abnormal temperature, either high or low, can be an early sign of an underlying problem such as an infection, a respiratory or cardiac problem, a metabolic abnormality or encephalopathy.

Hypothermia is defined as a core body temperature below 36 °C (Jain 2012). When the body temperature is below this level the baby is at risk from cold stress. This can cause complications such as increased oxygen consumption, lactic acid production, apnoea and hypoglycaemia. In preterm babies cold stress may also cause a decrease in surfactant production, which is associated with increased mortality (Costeloe et al 2000; Confidential Enquiries into Stillbirths and Deaths in Infancy [CESDI] 2003). The hypothermic baby often looks pale or mottled and may be uninterested in feeding.

Hyperthermia is defined as a core temperature above 38.0 °C (Jain 2012). The usual cause of hyperthermia is overheating of the environment, but it can also be an important clinical sign of sepsis as the baby will attempt to regulate its temperature by increasing his/her respiratory rate leading to an increased fluid loss by evaporation through the airways. Other problems caused by hyperthermia are hypernatraemia, jaundice and apnoea.

Central nervous system

Assessment of a baby's neurological status is usually carried out on a baby who is awake but not crying. Important signs are the tone and quality of a baby's movements, level of activity, posture and presence of normal newborn reflexes. An abnormal posture such as neck retraction, frog-like posture, hyperextension or hyperflexion of the limbs, jittery or abnormal involuntary movements and a high-pitched or weak cry, could be indicative of neurological impairment and a need for investigation (Lawn and Alton 2012).

Terminology that describes abnormal movement in babies is very variable and includes fits, convulsions, seizures, twitching, jumpy and jittery. In contrast, a baby with poor muscle tone is described as hypotonic or floppy. It is often very difficult to distinguish a seizure from jitteriness or irritability. The jittery baby has tremors, rapid movement of the extremities or fingers that are stopped when the limb is held or flexed. Jitteriness can be normal but is sometimes seen in babies who are affected by drug withdrawal or in babies with hypoglycaemia (see section on seizures, p 674).

Hypotonia

Hypotonia describes the loss of muscle tension and tone. As a result, the baby adopts an abnormal posture that is noticeable on handling. If hypotonia and a lack of movement have been significant features before birth then limb contractures may also be seen. Preterm babies below 30 weeks' gestation have a resting position that is usually characterized as hypotonic. By 34 weeks their thighs and hips are flexed and they lie in a frog-like position, usually with their arms extended. At 36–38 weeks' gestation the resting position of a healthy newborn baby is one of total flexion with immediate recoil. Hypotonia in a term baby is not normal and requires investigation. It is also important to determine whether the hypotonia is associated with weakness or normal power in the limbs, i.e. are there spontaneous movements? Can the baby make normal movements against gravity? There are several causes of hypotonia in the newborn.

Systemic causes

- maternal sedation or drugs (in particular some antidepressants)
- prematurity
- infection
- Down syndrome
- endocrine (e.g. hypothyroidism)
- metabolic problems (e.g. hypoglycaemia, hyponatraemia, inborn errors of metabolism)

Central (brain) causes

- perinatal hypoxia-ischaemia or neonatal encephalopathy (see p 672 below)
- traumatic brain injury
- structural brain abnormality, e.g. holoprosencephaly

Peripheral nervous system causes

- neurological problems (e.g. spinal cord injuries sustained by difficult breech or forceps assisted birth)
- neuromuscular disorders (e.g. spinal muscular atrophy, myasthenia gravis related to maternal disease, myotonic dystrophy etc.)

The renal and genitourinary system

Documentation of the passage of urine after birth is important as it provides a record that may help if later concerns arise. The genitourinary tract has the highest percentage of anomalies, congenital or genetic, of all the organ systems. Prenatal diagnosis is possible with ultrasound and aids the early assessment and intervention that is essential if kidney damage is to be prevented. Urine that only dribbles out, rather than being passed with a good stream, may be an indication of a problem with posterior urethral valves. Other renal problems may present as a failure to pass urine. The healthy baby usually passes urine within 4–10 hours after birth. Urinalysis using reagent strips will give information that may be helpful in diagnosis. Urinary infections in the newborn period are uncommon. The signs of urinary tract infection are often vague and can be mistaken for other problems. The baby typically presents with lethargy, poor feeding, increasing jaundice and vomiting. Urine infections when present are important, however, because renal scarring can result. Reduced urine output is usually due to low fluid intake, often in breast-fed babies, but also consider:

- increased fluid loss due to hyperthermia, use of radiant heaters and phototherapy units
- perinatal hypoxia-ischaemia
- congenital abnormalities
- infection.

The gastrointestinal tract

Assess the baby's abdomen, looking for signs of distension, discoloration or tenderness. Most babies should feed early and pass meconium within the first 8–12 hours of birth. Healthy babies should be able to feed within 30 minutes of birth. Vomiting can be a sign of a problem but the midwife should distinguish between possetting, which occurs with winding and over-handling after feeding, and vomiting due to overfeeding, infection or intestinal abnormalities. Whilst possetting small amounts of milk is common, babies with large vomits should be evaluated, as should babies with blood in their vomit. Vomit containing green material can occasionally be due to swallowed meconium but green bile is usually unmistakable.

Bile-stained vomiting

There should never be green bile in the vomit of a newborn baby and this **always** requires prompt investigation. It may indicate bowel obstruction and in the newborn one of the possible causes is malrotation and volvulus, which could lead to bowel damage and bowel loss if not promptly investigated. If bile-stained vomiting is seen or reported, check the baby carefully looking for abdominal distension or tenderness. Check that the anus is patent. An X-ray and contrast study is usually required to rule out bowel obstruction and malrotation. Other possible causes include infection, bowel atresias, meconium ileus, anorectal malformations or necrotizing enterocolitis (NEC).

NEC is generally a problem in premature babies but may also occur in term babies, particularly those who have risk factors such as perinatal hypoxia, polycythaemia and hypothermia. It is an acquired disease of the small and large intestine caused by ischaemia of the intestinal mucosa. NEC may present with vomiting and this may be bile-stained. The abdomen becomes distended, stools may be loose and may have blood in them or the baby may not open its bowels. In the early stages of NEC, the baby can display non-specific signs of temperature instability, unstable glucose levels, lethargy and poor peripheral circulation. As the illness progresses, the baby may become apnoeic and bradycardic and may need respiratory support.

Passage of meconium

According to Metaj et al (2003), 97% of babies will pass meconium by 24 hours of age, an event that should be documented. If a baby has not passed meconium then examine the abdomen to look for signs of distension or tenderness. Check that the anus is patent. Possible causes of delayed passage of meconium include bowel atresia, meconium ileus and imperforate anus. Hirschsprung's disease should be suspected in term babies with failure to pass meconium in the first 48 hours after birth. Passage of first meconium occurs later with earlier gestational age (Kumar and Dhanireddy 1995).

The normal term baby usually passes about eight stools a day. Breastfed babies' stools are looser and more frequent than those of bottle-fed babies, and the colour varies more and sometimes appears greenish. The baby who has a systemic infection can often display signs of gastrointestinal problems, usually poor feeding and vomiting. Diarrhoea may be a feature of this or may indicate a more serious gastrointestinal disorder such as NEC. Diarrhoea caused by gastroenteritis is unusual in the newborn although it may be seen after the first week. Outbreaks of viral diarrhoea due to Rotavirus have been reported. Babies with this condition must be isolated and scrupulous handwashing must be adhered to (Isaacs and Moxon 1999). Loose stools can also be a feature of babies receiving phototherapy.

RECOGNITION OF PROBLEMS AT THE TIME OF RESUSCITATION, INCLUDING NEONATAL ENCEPHALOPATHY

Aspects of resuscitation of the newborn are covered in Chapter 29, but problems that might be encountered, or may present during or immediately after resuscitation, will be covered here. It is important to recognize promptly those babies who have adapted poorly to extrauterine life and are in poor condition at birth because of hypoxia-ischaemia, or have tolerated the birth process poorly as a result of pre-existing problems.

Neonatal encephalopathy

Neonatal encephalopathy is a clinical syndrome of abnormal levels of consciousness, tone, primitive reflexes, autonomic function and sometimes seizures in newborn babies.

Which babies get encephalopathy?

The commonest cause is hypoxia-ischaemia, termed hypoxic ischaemic encephalopathy (HIE), but it is important to remember that not all encephalopathy is due to hypoxia-ischaemia.

Encephalopathy can be due to:

- cord obstruction (prolapse or compression)
- placental abruption
- breech
- shoulder dystocia etc.

In addition, other causes such as metabolic, infective, malformation or trauma should also be considered. The term neonatal HIE should be used only when there is clear evidence of hypoxia and ischaemia. Globally, neonatal HIE is a very large problem, with a high morbidity and mortality in developing countries (Vannucci 1990). In the United Kingdom (UK) and other developed countries the incidence varies depending on the definition used but is approximately 0.5/1000 live births (Levene et al 1986). No specific treatment, other than general supportive treatment, has been available for these babies but the advent of whole body cooling following the publication of randomized controlled trials of this intervention in 2005–9, has improved the outcome for some babies and has increased the need for prompt early identification and treatment (Shankaran et al 2005; Azzopardi et al 2009; Jacobs et al 2013). Midwives play a vital role in this new approach.

Features suggestive of hypoxia-ischaemia are detailed in Box 33.1.

Neonatal encephalopathy is often classified according to a grading system (modified by Sarnat and Sarnat 1976; see Table 33.1). In general, a neonatologist should be asked to review any baby when:

- the heart rate remains <100 for more than 1 minute
- normal respiration is not established by 5 minutes of age

- the Apgar score is <5 at 5 minutes
- gasping respiration is seen
- cord pH <7.0.

In these babies whole body cooling may be considered. This treatment requires 72 hours of cooling of core body temperature to 33–34 °C. Several studies have shown that this treatment reduces the risk of cerebral palsy and increases the likelihood of survival without significant disability by 50% (Shankaran et al 2005; Azzopardi et al 2009; Jacobs et al 2013). If cooling is being considered, the neonatal team may commence 'passive' cooling before

---

Box 33.1 Features suggestive of hypoxia-ischaemia

(A) Before birth:
  - evidence of antenatal compromise
  - decreased fetal movements
  - abnormal fetal heart rate patterns
  - low fetal pH
  - meconium-stained amniotic fluid
(B) Poor condition at birth:
  - low heart rate
  - failure to establish normal respiration soon after birth (apnoea or gasping respiration)
  - acidotic cord pH
  - cyanosis or pallor
(C) Abnormal neonatal neurology:
  - decreased consciousness
  - decreased tone
  - poor suck and other primitive reflexes

Table 33.1 Grading criteria for neonatal encephalopathy

	Grade 1 (mild)	Grade 2 (moderate)	Grade 3 (severe)
Clinical features	Hyper-alert, staring	Lethargy, hypotonia	Decreased consciousness
	Mild decreased tone/activity	Seizures	Hypotonia
	Poor feeding for up to 24 hours	Poor suck/feeding for >24 hours	Frequent prolonged seizures
			Multi-organ involvement – breathing, kidneys, blood pressure affected
			Absent gag/sucking reflexes
Management	May be able to stay with mother on postnatal ward but needs observation/feeding support	Will need neonatal admission. May require cooling	Intensive care, cooling
Outcome (Jacobs et al 2013)	Complete recovery, normal outcome	Most recover well but up to 25% may have long-term neurological problems. Cooling has significant benefits	Generally poor. Death or significant neurodisability likely, but with cooling approximately 70% die or have major disability

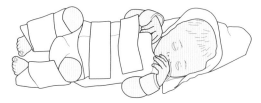

Fig. 33.1 Cooling jacket.

a firm decision is made. This means active warming of the baby is stopped and the baby's body temperature is allowed to fall passively towards the levels required. This is only a temporary measure though while a decision is being made, equipment is being prepared or transfer is being organized. Active cooling requires the use of a cooling jacket or mattress (see Fig. 33.1) to cool the whole body, or sometimes a cap to cool the head. The treatment is started as soon as possible after diagnosis (maximum within 6 hours) and then continued for 72 hours, after which the baby is gradually warmed. A systematic review of 10 randomized controlled trials (RCTs) (1320 babies in total) by Jacobs et al (2013) reported a lower risk of death in cooled babies (whole body or head) in the first 18 months of life than in babies treated by standard care. In three of these studies with 18-month follow-up (767 babies in total) the combined risk of death and severe disability was significantly lower in cooled babies compared with those treated by standard care, and cooling increased survival with normal neurological function compared with standard care at 18-month follow-up. In summary therefore, using cooling decreases the risks of death by more than 20% and increases the chance of survival without disability by 50%.

Babies with less severe problems

Some babies with neonatal encephalopathy may not have clinically obvious signs immediately and repeated assessment is necessary in babies who have risk factors such as those listed above. In some of these babies there will be poor feeding and low tone for the first 24 hours after birth. These babies need careful observation and may need additional feeding support but they are often well enough to remain with their mother rather than being admitted to the NICU. Babies with this pattern of encephalopathy should improve after 24 hours and should not have any long-term consequences of their encephalopathy. Babies with a mild encephalopathy like this have not been shown to benefit from whole body cooling.

Seizures and abnormal movements

Seizures in the newborn period can be difficult to recognize; however, they are an important indicator of potentially serious problems and their recognition is therefore important. The most common cause is neonatal encephalopathy, most commonly HIE, but readily treatable causes such as hypoglycaemia must not be missed. Seizures in newborns differ from those in later life. They are often subtle and difficult to differentiate from other normal behaviour. Different types of seizures may be seen and include tonic seizures (sustained posturing of the limbs or trunk or deviation of the head), clonic (usually involves one limb or one side of the body jerking rhythmically at 1–4 times per second) or myoclonic (rapid isolated jerking of muscles). Subtle seizures may include behaviours such as repetitive lip smacking, staring, blinking or repetitive movements of the limbs such as cycling movements.

Causes of seizures

Seizures in the newborn almost always have an identifiable cause, e.g.

- HIE (49%)
- cerebral infarction (neonatal stroke) (12%)
- cerebral trauma (7%)
- infections (meningitis or encephalitis) (5%)
- metabolic abnormalities, including hypoglycaemia (3%)
- narcotic drug withdrawal (4%).

It is important to distinguish seizures from jitteriness and neonatal sleep myoclonus, both of which are benign. Jitteriness is symmetrical rapid movements of the hands and feet. It is often stimulus-sensitive and may be initiated by sudden movement or noise and there are no associated eye movements. Benign sleep myoclonus involves bilateral or unilateral jerking during sleep. It occurs during active sleep, is not stimulus-sensitive and tends to be seen in upper limbs more than lower limbs. It is important to ensure that the newborn is not at risk from the seizure, so ensure that the airway is clear and the baby is breathing. Ensure that readily treatable causes are identified and treated. In particular check the blood sugar to exclude hypoglycaemia, and electrolytes to include calcium and sodium; also consider infection. Hypocalcaemia can be a readily treatable cause of seizures in women with vitamin D deficiency.

INFECTION IN THE NEWBORN

Infection in the newborn contributes significantly to morbidity and mortality and possible infection is one of the commonest reasons for newborn babies becoming unwell and requiring admission to a neonatal unit. Newborn babies may acquire infections antenatally (transplacental infection), during birth, or after birth.

Umbilical cord

Until its separation, the umbilical cord can be a focus for infection by bacteria that colonize the skin of the newborn. The umbilical stump should be dry. If peri-umbilical redness occurs or a discharge is noted, infection should be considered and it may be necessary to commence antibiotic therapy in order to prevent an ascending infection. Babies are protected from infection by the passive transfer of antibodies from their mother. The major advantage of this is that they receive passive immunity for those infections they are most likely to come into contact with. The immune system is functional at birth and newborn babies can also mount their own humeral (antibody) response to new infections; however, preterm babies are particularly vulnerable to infection as placental transfer of IgG mainly occurs after 32 weeks' gestation and their own antibody response is immature.

Bacterial infection in the newborn

Early signs of infection may be subtle and difficult to distinguish from other problems. The mother or midwife may simply feel the baby is 'off colour' or not right. The physical signs that may be apparent are:

- Temperature instability. This may be a low temperature just as much as an increased temperature. Always take seriously and carefully assess any normally grown baby who is unable to maintain a temperature of 37 °C with a normal room temperature and normal wrapping/clothing.
- Lethargy or poor feeding. In general, babies, particularly those who are breastfeeding, will not get very large volumes of colostrum in the first 24 hours after birth, however they should show an interest in feeding, be able to attach to the breast and have a sucking reflex.
- Unexplained bradycardia (heart rate <100/min) or tachycardia (heart rate >180/bpm) and any apnoea or episodes of cyanosis.
- Increased respiratory rate or signs of respiratory distress.
- Irritability, abnormal movements.
- Skin mottling, rashes, prolonged capillary refill time.

If bacterial infection is suspected then antibiotics should be commenced and investigations performed (often referred to by neonatologists as a 'septic screen'). Antibiotics are generally given until blood and cerebrospinal fluid (CSF) cultures have confirmed no growth of pathogenic organisms (usually 36–48 hours). The investigations performed are usually:

- blood culture
- full blood cell count and blood film
- C-reactive protein measurement
- lumbar puncture for examination and culture of CSF.

Treatment of infection and management of babies with risk of infection

The overall aim is to reduce the risk of septicaemia and life-threatening septic shock in this vulnerable group. Bacterial infections are an important cause of neonatal morbidity and mortality. The two commonest organisms in the newborn are group B streptococcus (GBS) and *Escherichia* (*E.*) *coli*, which are both organisms the baby may come into contact with via the maternal birth canal. Risk factors for early onset neonatal infection include the following (Oddie and Embleton 2002; Ungerer et al 2004; Royal College of Obstetricians and Gynaecologists [RCOG] 2012):

- maternal intrapartum fever
- prolonged rupture of membranes greater than 18 hours
- prematurity less than 37 weeks
- maternal genital tract colonization with GBS
- previous baby with GBS disease.

These factors are therefore used in the UK to decide which babies should receive antibiotics based on a risk-based approach. In high-risk pregnancies, early onset neonatal GBS infection can be reduced with antibiotics during labour (Law et al 2005). Similarly, antibiotic use for preterm rupture of membranes is associated with reduced neonatal morbidity (Kenyon et al 2010). Generally therefore risk factors should be identified before labour so that, if possible, intrapartum antibiotics should be given at least 4 hours prior to birth to obtain maximal antibiotic concentration in the amniotic fluid (Pylipow et al 1994). There is, however, also some evidence that suggests 2 hours may be adequate (de Cueto et al 1998). In babies with more than one risk factor, observation or treatment with antibiotics after birth can be considered.

The age of presentation of early onset GBS varies between studies. In a prospective UK study, when intrapartum antibiotics were not given, 50% of babies with early onset GBS presented by 1 hour of age, 72% by 24 hours and 92% by 48 hours (Oddie and Embleton 2002). Bromberger et al (2000), in a retrospective study, found that 95% of term babies with early onset GBS presented within the first 24 hours of life. Additionally, intrapartum antibiotics did not alter the constellation and timing of onset of clinical signs of early onset GBS. Therefore if babies are well by 12 hours of age they are unlikely to develop early onset disease.

Group B streptococcus (GBS) infection

It is estimated that about one in 2000 babies born in the UK and Ireland develop early onset GBS infection. This means that every year in the UK (with 680 000 births a year) around 340 babies will develop early onset GBS infection. GBS is recognized as the most frequent cause of sepsis in the newborn (Oddie and Embleton 2002; Heath et al 2004). A survey by the Public Health Laboratory Service (PHLS) GBS Working Group during a 13-month period in 2000 and 2001 identified a total of 568 cases of invasive GBS disease (early and late onset) in the UK and Republic of Ireland (Heath et al 2004). This is equivalent to a total incidence of 0.72 per 1000 live births; the incidence for early onset disease (n=377) was 0.48 per 1000 live births and for late onset disease (n=191) was 0.24 per 1000 live births. Overall mortality of the disease was 9.7% (n=53): 10.6% (n=38) early onset and 8% (n=15) late onset.

One-third of the population carry GBS in the gut and over 20% of women have vaginal colonization (Barcaite et al 2008). In the United States of America (USA), Australia and several European countries, screening of pregnant women is used with treatment with antibiotics during labour, which is effective at reducing the incidence of early onset GBS. This approach, however, has not been shown in trials to reduce the risk of death or long-term harm from GBS; its introduction in the UK has been hotly debated but the introduction of screening has not been recommended (United Kingdom National Screening Committee [UKNSC], 2012). The current UK recommendations (RCOG 2012; UKNSC 2012) are therefore based on a risk factor approach described above, whereby intrapartum antibiotic prophylaxis (IAP) is offered to all women with recognized risk factors for early onset GBS disease. Mathematical modelling in the USA suggests that this approach will result in approximately 25% of women being offered IAP with a decrease in the incidence of early onset GBS disease of 50.0–68.8% (RCOG 2012). UK data suggest that approximately 16% of pregnancies will have one or more risk factors for early onset GBS disease and approximately 60% of early onset GBS cases will have a risk factor (Oddie and Embleton 2002; RCOG 2012).

Meningitis

Neonatal meningitis is an inflammation of the membranes covering the brain and spinal column caused by such organisms as GBS, *E. coli*, *Listeria monocytogenes* and, less often, *Candida* and herpes. In the UK, neonatal meningitis is most often caused by GBS (Law et al 2005). In Australia and New Zealand, the incidence of GBS early onset neonatal bacterial meningitis decreased significantly between 1993 and 2002, while the incidence of *E. coli* meningitis remained the same (May et al 2005).

Very early signs are often non-specific, followed by those of meningeal irritation and raised intracranial pressure such as crying, irritability, bulging anterior fontanelle, increasing lethargy, tremors, twitching, severe vomiting, diminished muscle tone and alterations in consciousness. Babies may also present with abnormal neurological signs. Early diagnosis and treatment are critical to prevent collapse and death. Diagnosis may be confirmed by examination of CSF. Very ill babies require intensive care,

intravenous fluids and antibiotic therapy. Although acute phase mortality has declined in recent years, long-term neurological complications still occur in many surviving babies. De Louvois et al (2005) report that in one group aged 5 years, 23% had a serious disability, with isolation of bacteria from CSF the best single predictor. For such babies, long-term comprehensive developmental assessment is essential, including audiometry and vision testing.

Viral infections acquired before or during birth

Rubella and varicella (chickenpox) can be major causes of fetal morbidity and mortality, as can the protozoa toxoplasmosis. Infections may be acquired through the placenta, from amniotic fluid, or the birth canal. For management of sexually transmissible and reproductive tract infections see Chapter 13. The acronym TORCH is often used for congenital infections:

- Toxoplasmosis
- Other (includes syphilis)
- Rubella
- Cytomegalovirus
- Hepatitis/HIV

All of these may cause significant illness in the newborn.

Rubella

For most immunocompetent children and adults (including pregnant women), the rubella virus causes a mild, insignificant illness spread by droplet infection. Congenital rubella syndrome (CRS) in the newborn however remains a major cause of developmental anomalies that include blindness and deafness (Banatvala and Brown 2004). Maternal rubella is now rare in many countries as a result of successful rubella vaccination programmes (Robinson et al 2006). In most industrialized countries the measles, mumps and rubella (MMR) vaccine has significantly reduced the incidence of rubella (Wright and Polack 2006), although in recent years in the UK and some other countries, vaccination rates have declined due to press scare stories that have resulted in a lower uptake of the vaccine. It is feared this may result in a rise in the incidence. Countries without routine MMR programmes report rates similar to those of industrialized countries before vaccination became available (Banatvala and Brown 2004). Midwives need to emphasize the importance of avoiding contact with rubella during pregnancy, as reinfection has been reported despite previous vaccination. As part of their extended public health role, midwives can encourage vaccination for seronegative women before and after – but *not* during – pregnancy, and also discuss the importance of vaccinating their child. Generally individuals will only be infected with rubella once during their lifetime as they then develop an antibody response.

Primary rubella infection is most likely to cause problems if it is acquired in the first 12 weeks of pregnancy and in this situation maternal–fetal transmission rates are as high as 85%. Intrauterine infection is unlikely when the mother's rash appears before, or within 11 days after the last menstrual period, and with proven infection later than the 16th week, the risk of severe fetal sequelae is much lower (Enders et al 1988). First trimester infection can result in spontaneous abortion and in surviving babies, a number of serious and permanent consequences. These include cataracts, sensorineural deafness, congenital heart defects, microcephaly, meningoencephalitis, dermal erythropoiesis, thrombocytopenia and significant developmental delay (Banatvala and Brown 2004; Bedford and Tookey 2006).

Diagnosis and treatment

Congenital rubella can be recognized when there has been a maternal history of infection during pregnancy, or as a result of anomalies detected in the fetus or the newborn. All women have screening for rubella titres at booking in the UK. Those with negative titres cannot be offered immunization during pregnancy but can be offered it after pregnancy. They should also avoid contact with anyone known to have the illness during pregnancy. If there is any contact then rubella titres should be measured with increased surveillance of the fetus. Most women with first trimester infection may request termination of pregnancy. Babies with CRS are highly infectious and should be isolated from other babies and pregnant women (but not their own mothers). Long-term follow-up is essential, as some problems may not become apparent until the baby is older.

Varicella zoster

Varicella zoster virus (VZV) is a highly contagious virus of the herpes family that causes varicella (chickenpox). Transmitted by respiratory droplets and contact with vesicle fluid, it has an incubation period of 10–20 days and is infectious for 48 hours before the rash appears until vesicles crust over. After primary infection the virus remains dormant in the sensory nerve root ganglia and with any recurrent infection can result in herpes zoster (shingles). Primary infection during pregnancy can result in serious adverse outcomes (Meyberg-Solomayer et al 2006).

Incidence and effects during pregnancy

Fetal effects vary with gestation at the time of maternal infection. During the first 20 weeks of pregnancy the baby has about a 2% risk of fetal varicella syndrome (FVS). Signs can include skin lesions and scarring, eye problems, such as chorioretinitis and cataracts. Skeletal anomalies include limb hypoplasia. Severe neurological problems may include encephalitis, microcephaly and significant developmental delay. About 30% of babies born with skin lesions die in the first months of life. From 20 weeks' gestation up to almost the time of birth, infection can result in milder forms of neonatal varicella that do not result in negative sequelae for the neonate. The child may have shingles during the first few years of life. Maternal infection after 36 weeks, and particularly in the week before the birth (when cord blood VZV IgG is low) to 2 days after, can result in infection rates of up to 50%. About 25% of those infected will develop neonatal clinical varicella. Most affected babies will develop a vesicular rash and about 30% will die. Other complications of neonatal varicella include pneumonia, pyoderma and hepatitis.

Diagnosis and treatment

Diagnosis can be made if there has been a recent history of maternal chickenpox, and polymerase chain reaction (PCR) to identify VZV in amniotic fluid. Antenatal ultrasound may confirm the effects of fetal varicella syndrome, e.g. limb contractures and deformities, cerebral anomalies, borderline ventriculomegaly, intracerebral, intrahepatic and myocardial calcifications, articular effusions and intrauterine growth restriction (IUGR) (Degani 2006; Meyberg-Solomayer et al 2006).

Most pregnant women with chickenpox will need a great deal of information and support. Women infected during the first 20 weeks may request termination of pregnancy. Although mother and baby should be isolated from others, they should always be kept together. Varicella zoster immune globulin (VZIG) can be offered to seronegative pregnant women who are exposed to chickenpox, within 72 hours of contact, and always within 10 days. VZIG should also be offered to a baby whose mother develops chickenpox between 7 days before and 28 days after the birth, or whose siblings at home have chickenpox (if the mother is seronegative). Although no clinical trials have shown that antiviral chemotherapy prevents fetal infection, the antiviral drug acyclovir may reduce the mortality and risk of severe disease in some groups, particularly if VZIG is not available. These include pregnant women with severe complications, and newborns if they are unwell or have added risk factors such as prematurity or corticosteroid therapy (Sauerbrei & Wutzler 2000; Hayakawa et al 2003).

Toxoplasmosis

Toxoplasmosis is caused by *Toxoplasma gondii* (*T. gondii*), a protozoan parasite infecting up to a third of the world's population. It is found in uncooked meat, cat and dog faeces. Primary infection can be asymptomatic, or characterized by malaise, lymphadenopathy and ocular disease. Primary infection during pregnancy can cause severe damage to the fetus (Montoya and Liesenfeld 2004). Childhood-acquired infection also causes half of toxoplasma ocular disease in UK and Irish children (Gilbert et al 2006).

Incidence and effects during pregnancy

Risks for the infected fetus can include intrauterine death, low birth weight, enlarged liver and spleen, jaundice, anaemia, intracranial calcifications, hydrocephalus, retinochoroidal and macular lesions. Infected neonates may be asymptomatic at birth, but can develop retinal and neurological disease. Those with subclinical disease at birth can develop seizures, cognitive and motor problems and reduced cognitive function over time (Gilbert et al 2006; Schmidt et al 2006; Systematic Review on Congenital Toxoplasmosis [SYROCOT] Group 2007). In one group of 38 children with confirmed toxoplasma infection, 58% had congenital infection. Of these, 9% were stillborn while 32% of the live births had intracranial abnormalities and/or developmental delay, and 45% had retinochoroiditis with no other abnormalities. Of the 42% of children infected after birth, all had retinochoroiditis (Gilbert et al 2006).

The effectiveness of antenatal treatment in reducing the congenital transmission of *T. gondii* is not proven. A meta-analysis of 1438 treated mothers (26 cohorts) also found no evidence that antenatal treatment significantly reduced the risk of clinical signs (SYROCOT 2007). Babies with congenital toxoplasmosis are usually treated with pyrimethamine, sulfadiazine and folinic acid for an extended period (Montoya and Liesenfeld 2004; Schmidt et al 2006).

Prevention

Midwives have an essential role in prevention as health education can result in a 92% reduction in pregnancy seroconversion. Breugelmans et al (2004) found the most effective strategy was a leaflet explaining toxoplasmosis and how to avoid the condition during pregnancy, with this information reinforced in antenatal classes. In the UK, NHS Choices (2013) website provides useful information, as well as the Toxoplasmosis Trust for women, their families and healthcare professionals. Appropriate information includes advising women about washing kitchen surfaces following contact with uncooked meats, stringent handwashing and avoiding cat and dog faeces.

Candida

Candida is a Gram-positive yeast fungus with a number of strains (see Chapter 13). *Candida* (C.) *albicans* is responsible for most fungal infections, including thrush in babies. Infection can affect the mouth (oral candidiasis), skin (cutaneous candidiasis) particularly the nappy area and internal organs (systemic candidiasis). Oral candidiasis is a common mild illness that may present as white patches on the baby's gums, palate or tongue. It can be acquired during birth or from caregivers' hands or feeding equipment. Raw areas (removed by sucking) on the edge of the baby's tongue can assist diagnosis. Risk factors for thrush include bottle use during the first 2 weeks, the presence of siblings (Morrill et al 2005) and antibiotic exposure (Dinsmoor et al 2005). Breastfeeding women may also have infected breasts, with flaky or shiny skin of the nipple/areola, sore, red nipples and persistent burning, itching or stabbing pain in the breasts (Chapter 34). Risk factors for maternal thrush include bottle use in the first 2 weeks after the birth, pregnancy duration of >40 weeks (Morrill et al 2005), and intrapartum antibiotic use (Dinsmoor et al 2005).

Accurate diagnosis and treatment of thrush is important for continued breastfeeding. Morrill et al (2005) found only 43% of women with thrush 2 weeks after the birth were breastfeeding at 9 weeks, compared with 69% of women without.

Cutaneous candidiasis often co-exists with oral thrush and presents as a moist papular or vesicular skin rash, usually in the region of the axillae, neck, perineum or umbilicus. Although it is usually benign, recognition and treatment is important in preventing problems (Smolinski et al 2005). Management includes keeping the area dry and applying topical nystatin. In preterm babies the thin cutaneous barrier, invasive procedures and immune system immaturity may contribute to the early onset of systemic *Candida* infection. Antifungal prophylaxis may be used to prevent systemic *Candida* colonization. Systemic candidiasis in a preterm baby is a serious problem and requires a prolonged course of treatment with intravenous antifungal medication. It is associated with significant morbidity and mortality.

Significant eye infections

Eye infection caused by *Chlamydia* or *Gonococcus* will present with a red sore eye with a large amount of purulent discharge, usually after the first week after birth. Ophthalmia neonatorum is defined in England as any purulent eye discharge within 21 days of birth, and in Scotland as eye inflammation within 21 days of birth accompanied by a discharge. A swab must be taken for culture and sensitivity testing, with immediate medical referral. Identification of the organism responsible is essential as chlamydial and gonococcal infections can cause conjunctival scarring, corneal infiltration, blindness and systemic spread. Treatment includes local cleaning and care of the eyes with normal saline, and appropriate drug therapy for the baby and mother if required.

RESPIRATORY PROBLEMS

There are several important causes of respiratory distress in the newborn, which are not always easy to distinguish. The commonest are infection, transient tachypnoea of the newborn (TTN) and surfactant-deficient lung disease of prematurity. The latter (also named hyaline membrane disease in the past) is confusingly called respiratory distress syndrome (RDS), but this is just one possible cause of respiratory distress in newborn babies.

Initial management of babies presenting with respiratory distress

Babies who are unwell should be assessed in a good light, ideally on a resuscitaire if available so that oxygen and airway support can be given if necessary. If a baby shows any of the signs of respiratory distress after birth he/she should be closely observed. In general any baby who has a respiratory rate >80/min and central cyanosis should be reviewed urgently. In distinguishing the cause and importance of clinical signs, the history of the pregnancy and birth are clearly important. Relevant factors are:

- gestation
- meconium in amniotic fluid
- mode of birth (caesarean section vs vaginal)
- high vaginal swabs during pregnancy
- antenatal scans.

Observe for:

- the respiratory rate, heart rate, work of breathing, colour
- the colour for cyanosis and skin perfusion, pallor, mottled or white
- the baby's level of activity and tone
- whether the baby has been able to feed – babies with significant respiratory distress will not feed and should not be allowed to feed
- apnoea, and listen for heart rate. Proceed as for resuscitation at birth (see Chapter 29).

If the baby is breathing:

- position the airway with the head in a neutral position and if necessary use a jaw thrust to help keep the airway patent
- avoid suction unless the baby clearly has fluid (blood/vomit) obstructing the upper airway
- give air/oxygen via a face mask if the baby is initially cyanosed
- liaise with the neonatal medical team with regard to further intervention
- consider admission to a NICU for further investigations and intervention if a significant respiratory distress persists.

Possible causes of respiratory distress in the newborn

Infection (particularly GBS)

All newborn babies presenting with features of respiratory distress should be treated with IV antibiotics until infection is excluded as this may be the only presenting feature

and it can be very difficult to distinguish from other causes of respiratory distress. A number of infectious disease processes present with signs of respiratory distress in the newborn. All babies presenting with respiratory distress need to be treated for infection until there is proof to the contrary.

Meconium aspiration syndrome

Meconium in the amniotic fluid is common and usually does not require treatment or intervention if the baby is in good condition at birth and shows no signs of respiratory distress. Meconium aspiration occurs because hypoxia-ischaemia causes the fetus to pass meconium into the amniotic fluid. This meconium is generally unproblematic unless the baby gasps or breathes in the meconium. Gasping respiration may also occur as a result of hypoxia-ischaemia. *Consequently, it is the baby showing signs of fetal hypoxia which develops meconium aspiration syndrome.* Greenough and Milner (2012) report the incidence for meconium aspiration syndrome in one UK hospital as 0.2/1000 live births; however, this incidence is low and other countries, such as the USA, have higher disease rates of 2–5/1000 (Greenough and Milner 2012). The initial respiratory distress may be mild, moderate or severe with a gradual deterioration over the first 12–24 hours in moderate or severe cases. The baby may present with cyanosis, increased work of breathing and a barrel-shaped chest. This chest appearance occurs as a result of air trapping, leading to hyperexpansion of the lungs. The meconium can become trapped in the airways and cause a ball-valve effect: air can enter the lung during inhalation, the meconium then blocks the airway during expiration so that air accumulates behind the blockage. This accumulation can then lead to the rupture of the alveoli and cause the baby to develop a pneumothorax. Where the meconium has contact with the lung tissue a chemical pneumonitis occurs and there is a risk of super-added infection. Endogenous surfactant is also broken down in the presence of meconium.

These babies may need intensive care and ventilation to prevent further deterioration. Modalities such as nitric oxide (Finer and Barrington 2006) are of benefit in reducing death or the need for extracorporeal membrane oxygenation (ECMO) in some babies. ECMO has been shown to increase survival by 50% (UK Collaborative ECMO Trial Group 1996). A number of the most severely affected babies will have signs of respiratory distress for some months, with ongoing residual respiratory problems during early childhood.

Transient tachypnoea of the newborn (TTN)

The recorded incidence of TTN varies widely, partly as a result of the variety of recording methods, differences in radiological interpretation and clear diagnostic features. It is frequently seen as a diagnosis of exclusion of other possible respiratory causes. Nevertheless, babies present with mild to moderate signs of respiratory distress and usually require admission to the NICU for further observation. Supplemental oxygen may be required, however the condition gradually resolves during the 24 hours following birth. The chest X-ray may show a streaky appearance with fluid in the horizontal fissure of the right lung that confirms the diagnosis, but sometimes it is only the clinical course that distinguishes between this, respiratory distress syndrome (RDS) and infection. The lungs are completely fluid-filled before birth and most of this is squeezed out through chest compression, the rest is absorbed via the lymphatic system. Babies born by elective caesarean section are at increased risk because the thorax has not been squeezed while the baby descends into the vagina. Being born this way appears to increase the risk of respiratory morbidity by approximately six times. In addition, birth at each week below 39 weeks approximately doubles the risk (Morrison et al 1995). Although these babies tend to require initial care on a NICU, their stay is usually of a short duration with the provision of oxygen and observation.

Respiratory distress syndrome (RDS)

RDS is generally a condition that affects preterm babies, however it can also occur in those born at term as other disorders like maternal diabetes can also inhibit surfactant production. Approximately 50% of babies born before 30 weeks' gestation develop RDS while 1% of all newborn babies may develop the condition (Greenough and Milner 2012). Surfactant is made up of phospholipids and proteins and is produced by the type II pneumocytes to reduce the surface tension within the alveoli, preventing their collapse at the end of exhalation. Collapsed alveoli require much greater pressures and exertion to re-inflate them compared to partially collapsed alveoli. The introduction of surfactant therapy into neonatal care during the 1980s and 1990s, combined with much wider use of antenatal steroids in the 1990s, significantly decreased the mortality and morbidity previously seen in RDS.

In preterm babies with RDS the clinical picture is of a baby with progressive respiratory distress developing over the first hours. The X-ray typically has a homogenous ground-glass appearance (indicating poorly aerated alveoli) with air bronchograms (black air-filled bronchi seen against white airless alveoli), although this may be less obvious if the baby has already received exogenous surfactant. Babies with RDS experience increasing respiratory distress and work of breathing. It may take 48–72 hours to reach the peak of the disease without the administration of exogenous surfactant. Resolution of the associated inflammation and the hyaline membrane formation may take up to 7 days in the unsupported baby. In extremely preterm babies surfactant is often given on the

labour suite at birth, although alternative approaches using continuous positive airways pressure (CPAP) can also be used (Morley et al 2008; SUPPORT 2010). Exogenous surfactant can be given as 'rescue treatment' if the baby develops significant early signs.

Pneumothorax

Pneumothoraces may occur spontaneously in 1% of the newborn population either during or after birth; however, only one-tenth will be seen (Steele et al 1971). A pneumothorax at birth may be caused by the large pressures generated by the baby's first breaths, which may be in the range of 40–80 cmH$_2$O. This can lead to alveoli distension and rupture that allows air to leak to a number of sites, most notably the potential space between the lung pleura. Babies receiving any assisted ventilation have an increased susceptibility to a pneumothorax. This could be due to either maldistribution of the ventilated gas in the lungs, high ventilation settings or baby-ventilator breathing interactions. Spontaneous pneumothorax can occur in otherwise healthy term babies. They may present with signs of respiratory distress on the postnatal ward. Although it is difficult to diagnose a pneumothorax in the absence of a chest X-ray, there may be reduced breath sounds on the affected side, displaced heart sounds and a distorted chest/diaphragm movement. A baby with a suspected pneumothorax will need closer observation and may need intervention with a chest drain, although many spontaneously breathing term babies can be managed without a chest drain as long as they are closely observed. Most pneumothoraces will resolve spontaneously.

Congenital diaphragmatic hernia (CDH)

CDH has an incidence of 3.5/1000 live births. It is an important condition because despite improvements in neonatal care reported, mortality rates remain high (Wright et al 2010). Most babies with a diaphragmatic hernia have a prenatal diagnosis, usually made at the 20th week anomaly scan; in some babies, however, the diagnosis is not made until after birth. In babies where there is a prenatal diagnosis most neonatologists manage these babies with immediate intubation, insertion of a large bore nasogastric (NG) tube to decompress the stomach and bowel and early sedation/muscle relaxation. This allows optimal ventilation as early as possible to try to allow the underdeveloped lungs to expand and to try to prevent significant problems with persistent pulmonary hypertension and continual right-to-left shunting of blood through the foramen ovale and ductus arteriosus. Intensive care is difficult in these babies and the priorities are to maintain good ventilation and perfusion to avoid hypoxia. A surgical repair of the diaphragm will usually be performed at 2–7 days after birth. In all babies presenting with respiratory distress a chest X-ray is important to look for the cause, and one of the possibilities that can be recognized is a CDH. Babies with this condition typically have unilateral chest movement, heart sounds and an apex beat on the right side (in the case of left-sided CDH, which is more common) and a scaphoid abdomen. Babies with a postnatal diagnosis of CDH have a much better prognosis, with greater expected survival rates (van den Hout et al 2010).

Upper airway obstruction and stridor

Upper airway obstruction in the newborn is uncommon but is characterized by noisy breathing on inspiration, different to grunting, which is an expiratory noise. The importance is that obstruction to the upper airway significantly increases the work of breathing for a newborn, and in the short term, in the most severe cases, this could lead to respiratory arrest. Babies with stridor therefore always need neonatal medical assessment. It is important to assess the degree of respiratory distress and assess whether the baby is managing to breathe comfortably despite the stridor. There are many possible causes, the commonest being laryngomalacia, which tends not to cause significant respiratory distress but the work of breathing may increase when the baby is placed on his/her back. External compression of the trachea is a serious condition, so any baby with stridor must always be carefully assessed by a neonatologist.

CONGENITAL HEART DISEASE (CHD)

CHD (moderate or severe) occurs in 6/1000 live births but only 25% show signs in the neonatal period (Fyler 1980). Early diagnosis is extremely important for some conditions and it is vital that newborn babies are examined carefully to look for signs of CHD (see Chapter 28). There are a number of ways that CHD may present in the newborn period and these give some clues as to the underlying anatomical diagnosis:

- prenatal diagnosis on antenatal scan
- associated with a syndrome or other congenital problems, e.g. Down syndrome
- asymptomatic murmur
- cyanosis
- sudden collapse
- heart failure.

Management of a baby with an antenatal diagnosis of CHD

In a baby where an antenatal diagnosis of CHD has been made, early intervention may be required depending on the type of lesion. Usually an antenatal plan of postnatal care will have been made and should be available to those providing postnatal care. For some types of serious congenital malformations (transposition of the great arteries, pulmonary atresia [with or without VSD], Fallot's tetralogy, coarctation of the aorta, hypoplastic left heart syndrome) these will involve giving a prostaglandin infusion to maintain patency of the ductus arteriosus. Wherever the baby is born, immediate stabilization and transfer to a cardiology centre will be required. Some types of CHD do not need intervention, but the baby will need follow-up with a cardiologist.

Care of a baby with a murmur

Babies who are detected to have an asymptomatic heart murmur on their newborn check (see Chapter 28) should be carefully evaluated by having a careful examination to look for other signs of cardiac disease. Oxygen saturation measurement using a pulse oximeter shows normal values >96%. *Be aware that babies with a saturation of 85% often do not look cyanosed on visual inspection*, so measuring the saturation of oxygen on haemoglobin is an effective way of assessing the baby's respiratory and cardiac status and represents good practice. Measuring pre- and post-ductal saturations can be useful alongside measuring the blood pressure in all four limbs to look for signs of coarctation of the aorta (lower pressures in lower limbs). All babies with a cardiac murmur should be evaluated by a neonatologist and local guidelines are usually in place for appropriate cardiac referral.

JAUNDICE

Jaundice is one of the most common conditions needing medical attention in newborn babies. Jaundice refers to the yellow coloration of the skin and the sclera caused by a raised level of bilirubin in the circulation (hyperbilirubinaemia). Approximately 60% of term and 80% of preterm babies develop jaundice in the first week after birth, and about 10% of exclusively breastfed babies are still jaundiced at one month of age. In most babies early jaundice is harmless. However, a few babies will develop very high levels of bilirubin, which can be harmful if not treated. Clinical recognition and assessment of jaundice can be difficult, particularly in babies with dark skin tones. Once jaundice is recognized, there is uncertainty about when to treat, and there is widespread variation in the use of phototherapy and exchange transfusion. In the UK a national guideline produced by the National Institute for Health and Clinical Excellence (NICE 2010) has tried to standardize monitoring and treatment and similar guidelines exist in other countries (American Academy of Paediatrics [AAP] 2004).

Bilirubin physiology

In order to understand when jaundice is important and why the fat soluble, unconjugated bilirubin concentration might be raised, it is important to understand its metabolism. Bilirubin is produced as one of the breakdown products of haemoglobin (Fig. 33.2A,B). Ageing, immature or malformed red cells are removed from the circulation and broken down in the reticuloendothelial system (liver, spleen and macrophages). Haemoglobin from these cells is broken down into the byproducts of haem, globin and iron. Haem is converted to biliverdin and then to unconjugated bilirubin. Globin is broken down into amino acids, which are used by the body to make proteins. Iron is stored in the body or used for new red blood cells. The unconjugated bilirubin is then transported to the liver. Once in the liver, unconjugated bilirubin is detached from albumin, combined with glucose and glucuronic acid and *conjugation* occurs using the enzyme uridine diphosphoglucuronyl transferase (UDP-GT). The conjugated bilirubin is now water-soluble and available for excretion. Conjugated bilirubin is excreted via the biliary system into the small intestine where normal bacteria change the conjugated bilirubin into urobilinogen. This is then oxidized into orange-coloured urobilin. Most is excreted in the faeces, with a small amount excreted in urine (Ahlfors and Wennberg 2004; Kaplan et al 2005).

Physiological jaundice

All newborn babies have a rise in unconjugated bilirubin during the first few days after birth. This occurs for several reasons:

- The turnover of haemoglobin is high in the fetus and newborn but before birth the bilirubin from the fetus is removed via the placenta.
- At birth, as the more efficient lungs increase oxygen levels, there is haemolysis of excessive RBCs that are now not needed.
- At birth the newborn liver enzymes systems may be immature and not as effective.

As a result of these factors there is a rise in serum unconjugated bilirubin in healthy babies during the first few days after birth and this physiological jaundice follows a characteristic pattern (see Fig. 33.3). Typically, babies on the first day after birth will not appear jaundiced but most babies will look yellow by day 3–4. As unconjugated bilirubin levels rise, the serum albumin becomes saturated and then any excesses spills over into the blood plasma. Unconjugated bilirubin is fat-soluble and will deposit in

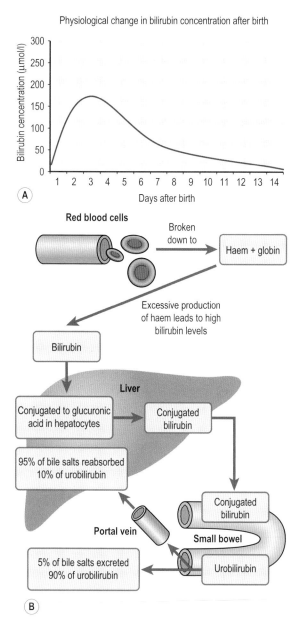

Fig. 33.2 **Bilirubin pathway.** (A) Physiological change in bilirubin concentration after birth. (B) Production and circulation of bilirubin.

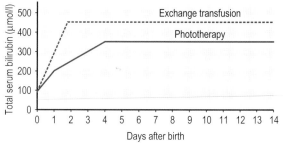

Fig. 33.3 Bilirubin chart.

subcutaneous fat, which makes the skin look yellow. Once these sites are saturated, the brain is the next target, particularly the basal ganglia. High levels of unconjugated bilirubin can potentially be a serious problem because it can cross the blood–brain barrier and be deposited in the basal ganglia in the brain. This can cause a bilirubin encephalopathy and in the longer term can result in cerebral palsy and learning difficulties. The cerebral palsy is typically an athetoid type due to the site of the damage in the brain. Kernicterus is the pathological (post mortem) finding of bilirubin encephalopathy. Whilst bilirubin encepalopathy is a serious complication it is rare because of the decrease in incidence of Rhesus haemolytic disease since the introduction of anti-D prophylaxis (Chapter 11) and the use of other interventions to control high unconjugated bilirubin levels in babies. In recent years, however, there have been concerns that the incidence is increasing again (Manning et al 2007) and midwives can play a pivotal role in trying to prevent this devastating complication.

Causes of concern in physiological jaundice

There are several situations where a midwife should be concerned about jaundice in the newborn:

- Jaundice in the first 24 hours after birth.
- History of antibodies (which may cause RBC haemolysis) identified on the maternal antibody screen.
- Any baby who is visibly jaundiced. The serum bilirubin (SBR) level should be checked as the visual assessment of jaundice is not sufficiently accurate (NICE 2010).
- Any baby who remains jaundiced beyond 14 days of age.

Early physiological jaundice (within first 5 days after birth)

Possible causes include:

- physiological jaundice
- haemolysis (Rhesus isoimmunization, ABO incompatibility, other blood group antigen problems)
- infection
- bruising
- polycythaemia
- dehydration (unlikely in the first 48 hours but must be considered in babies presenting between 2–7 days after birth, particularly those who are breast fed).

This is not an exhaustive list but these are the causes that midwives will encounter on a daily basis. As a general rule, haemolysis must always be considered when a baby is jaundiced in the first 24 hours after birth.

Assessment and diagnosis of physiological jaundice

Two initial important questions are:

- Is the jaundice physiological due to the normal process of breakdown of bilirubin or the presence of another pathological process?
- Is the baby at risk of bilirubin encephalopathy?

Individual risk factors

The initial assessment of a baby should include identifying risk factors for jaundice. These include any disease or disorder that increases bilirubin production, or alters the transport or excretion of bilirubin. For example:

- birth trauma or evident bruising (increased production of unconjugated bilirubin)
- family history of significant haemolytic disease or jaundiced siblings
- maternal antibodies at booking
- evidence of infection
- prematurity
- timing of jaundice, for example, within the first 24 hours (suggesting haemolysis). Jaundice at 3–6 days of age could be related to dehydration, particularly in a breast-fed baby. Always take a feeding history and check the baby's weight when presenting at this age to check hydration status. Even with significant weight loss, exclude other causes too.

Physical assessment includes observation of the extent of changes in skin and scleral colour, skin bruising or cephalhaematoma (Chapter 31) and other clinical signs such as lethargy and decreased eagerness to feed with accompanying dehydration. Consider signs of infection (temperature, vomiting, irritability or high-pitched cry). Also observe for dark urine and light stools, which could indicate intrahepatic or extrahepatic obstructive disease.

Laboratory investigations will always include SBR. If the bilirubin level is high then the following investigations should also be carried out:

- direct Coomb's test (DCT) to detect presence of maternal antibodies on baby's red blood cells
- blood groups (baby and mother) and Rh type for possible incompatibility
- haemoglobin concentration to assess anaemia/polycythaemia
- conjugated bilirubin if there are any factors to suggest conjugated hyperbilirubinaemia.

Management of physiological jaundice

If maternal antibodies were present on the booking screen, the neonatal team should be informed and regular SBR concentrations should be checked. These babies may need early phototherapy. In the case of Rh-D antibodies and some other blood group antigens with a high likelihood of causing haemolysis, other interventions such as the use of immunoglobulin or exchange transfusion are likely to be needed, so many of these babies may need admission to a NICU. Plotting the SBR concentration on a chart is always useful to see how the level compares with phototherapy intervention and/or exchange transfusion interventions. An example of a bilirubin chart is shown in Fig. 33.3. The trend or change in bilirubin can also be assessed from the chart as a guide to whether the level is rising too quickly or is following a normal physiological pattern. Treatment strategies for physiological jaundice include phototherapy, immunoglobulin therapy and occasionally exchange transfusion.

Phototherapy

The use of light therapy was first discovered by the observation in the 1950s at Rochford Hospital, Essex, that babies cared for in sunlight became less jaundiced, as was described by Dobbs and Cremer (1975). It works because ultraviolent blue light (wavelength 420–448 nm) catalyses the conversion of transbilirubin into the water-soluble cis-bilirubin isomer. This can then be excreted via the kidneys. Its use is based on SBR levels and the individual condition of each baby and standardized charts are used to guide treatment (NICE 2010). Commercially available phototherapy systems include those delivering light via fluorescent bulbs, halogen quartz lamps, light-emitting diodes and fibreoptic mattresses (Stokowski 2006). Conventional phototherapy systems use high intensity light from conventional white and/or blue, blue–green and turquoise fluorescent phototherapy lamps. Fibreoptic light systems use a woven fibreoptic pad that delivers high intensity light with no ultraviolet or infrared irradiation. They can be used as bilibeds in especially adapted cots or fitted around the chest and abdomen of the baby. These systems may be more comfortable for babies and allow easier accessibility and handling for parents.

Phototherapy is a very safe and effective treatment. Side-effects are mild but can include hyperthermia because of increased fluid loss and dehydration, damage to the retina from the high intensity light, lethargy or irritability, decreased eagerness to feed, loose stools, skin rashes and skin burns and alterations in a baby's state and neurobehavioural organization. Phototherapy may be intermittent or continuous (Lau and Fung 1984) with mild/moderate jaundice and has been described as being delivered at home (Walls et al 2004), although babies need to be carefully selected for this approach and it is not suitable for all. Babies receiving phototherapy should be nursed naked in an incubator or cot with lid, a minimum of 40 cm from the light. In addition phototherapy equipment should be routinely checked for safety. The baby's temperature should be measured and recorded at least 4-hourly, more frequently if unstable, and the baby should be turned regularly to maximize exposed areas of skin. For overhead fluorescent therapy the baby's eyes should be shielded using Posey eye shields. If eye shields are used, these should not be applied too tightly to avoid constriction to the scalp and excessive pressure over eyes and they should be removed regularly and the baby's eyes inspected for signs of infection. Application of topical creams or lotions should be avoided as there is a risk of burns and blistering. Particular attention should be paid to careful cleaning and drying of the skin, especially if the stools are loose. The baby should be assessed regularly for signs of dehydration using as a measure urine output or frequency of wet nappies. Consider not nursing babies on a white sheet because of reflective glare. Parents should be informed of the need for phototherapy and normal parental consent obtained and contact encouraged for routine care. The baby may not always have to receive continuous phototherapy and the phototherapy unit can be removed/switched off during cares and feeds (for up to 30 minutes in every 3 hour period is acceptable while on single phototherapy). However, if the baby is requiring multiple phototherapy this should not be interrupted.

Stopping phototherapy

The SBR should be measured at least every 6–12 hours whilst phototherapy continues. It should be monitored more frequently when the rate of rise is rapid. Phototherapy may be safely discontinued when the bilirubin is 50 μmol/l below the threshold. Repeat SBR measurement is necessary 12–18 hours after ceasing phototherapy to check for rebound hyperbilirubinaemia.

Immunoglobulin

Infusion of a set volume of pooled human immunoglobulin is an effective treatment which may help to prevent the need for an exchange transfusion (Gottstein and Cooke 2003). It is used with isoimmune haemolysis and may help to mop up excessive antibodies, preventing a rapid rise in bilirubin. It may help to prevent exchange transfusions but may slightly increase the risk of needing a later top-up transfusion but these are safer and less invasive.

Exchange transfusion

If the bilirubin level cannot be controlled with phototherapy and good hydration and the level exceeds recommended limits (NICE 2010) an exchange transfusion is performed to prevent the bilirubin level reaching levels known to be linked to bilirubin encephalopathy. Exchange transfusion carries significant risks and should always be carried out in a neonatal intensive care unit (refer to individual hospital guideline) with experienced operators. Complications can result from the procedure and from blood products. Babies with other medical problems are more likely to have severe complications, such as hypocalcaemia and thrombocytopenia. It involves transfusing a large volume of blood to the baby (double the baby's blood volume or 160 ml/kg) whilst removing blood from the baby, usually via an umbilical venous catheter. This process removes excess bilirubin and, if the cause is isoimmunization, antibodies that may be causing the RBC haemolysis. With haemolytic disease of the newborn sensitized erythrocytes are replaced with blood that is compatible with both the mother's and the baby's serum.

Pathological jaundice

Haemolytic jaundice

As described above, jaundice within the first 24 hours after birth is assumed to be due to haemolysis until proven otherwise. Haemolysis is increased haemoglobin destruction in the fetus or newborn and has several causes, the most important being blood group incompatibility. This can occur due to various antibodies, but the most important is caused by Rhesus (Rh-D) isoimmunization/incompatibility. This occurs if blood cells from a Rhesus-positive baby enter a Rhesus-negative mother's bloodstream. Her blood treats the D antigen on positive blood cells as a foreign substance and produces antibodies. These antibodies can then cross the placenta and destroy fetal red blood cells (see Figs 33.4–33.9).

While other causes of increased haemolysis are important, this condition is emphasized because of the midwife's critical role in the injection of anti-D immunoglobulin (anti-D Ig). Without this anti-D prophylaxis, Rh-D isoimmunization can cause severe haemolytic disease of the newborn (HDN) with significant mortality and morbidity (NICE 2010). With the effectiveness of anti-D prophylaxis, antibodies against other blood groups are now more common than anti-D (e.g. anti-A, anti-B and anti-Kell). Although few antibodies to blood group antigens other than those in the Rh system cause such severe haemolytic disease of the newborn, some report mortality and morbidity with antibodies other than anti-D. These include anti-E haemolytic disease of the fetus or newborn (Joy

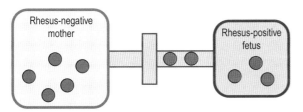

Fig. 33.4 Normal placenta with no communication between maternal and fetal blood.

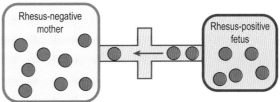

Fig. 33.5 Fetal cells enter maternal circulation through 'break' in 'placental barrier', e.g. at placental separation.

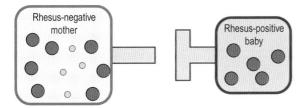

Fig. 33.6 Maternal production of Rhesus antibodies following introduction of Rhesus-positive blood.

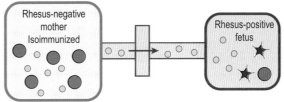

Fig. 33.7 In a subsequent pregnancy maternal Rhesus antibodies cross the placenta, resulting in haemolytic disease of the newborn.

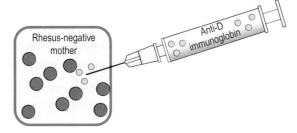

Fig. 33.8 Anti-D immunoglobulin administered within 72 hours of birth or other sensitizing event.

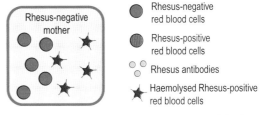

Fig. 33.9 Anti-D immunoglobulin has destroyed fetal Rhesus-positive red cells and prevented isoimmunization.

Figs 33.4–33.9 Isoimmunization and its prevention.

et al 2005), and anti-Kell (van Dongen et al 2005). ABO incompatibility can also occur and is the most frequent cause of mild to moderate haemolysis in neonates.

Rh-D isoimmunization

Rh-D isoimmunization is commonest among Caucasians, about 15% of whom are Rh-negative, compared with 3–5% of African and about 1% of Asian populations (Bianchi et al 2005). Before the introduction of anti-D Ig in 1969, Rh-D isoimmunization was a major cause of perinatal mortality and morbidity. In England and Wales, about 500 cases of Rh-D haemolytic disease of the fetus and newborn still occur each year, resulting in 25–30 deaths and 15 children with major permanent developmental problems (NICE 2010).

Causes of Rh-D isoimmunization

The placenta usually acts as a barrier to fetal blood entering the maternal circulation (Fig. 33.4). However, during pregnancy or birth, fetomaternal haemorrhage (FMH) can occur, when small amounts of fetal Rh-positive blood can cross the placenta and enter the Rh-negative mother's blood (Fig. 33.5). The woman's immune system produces anti-D antibodies (Fig. 33.6). In subsequent pregnancies these maternal antibodies can cross the placenta and destroy the red cells of any Rh-positive fetus (Fig. 33.7). Rh-D isoimmunization can result from any procedure or incident where positive blood leaks across the placenta, or from any other transfusion of Rh-positive blood (e.g. blood or platelet transfusion or drug use). Haemolytic disease of the fetus and newborn caused by Rh-D isoimmunization can occur during the first pregnancy. However, in most cases sensitization during the first pregnancy or birth leads to extensive destruction of fetal red blood cells during subsequent pregnancies (Finning et al 2004; Bianchi et al 2005; Geifman-Holtzman et al 2006; NICE 2010).

Prevention of Rh-D isoimmunization

Most cases of Rh-D isoimmunization can be prevented by injecting anti-D Ig within 72 hours of birth or any other sensitizing event (Fig. 33.8). Anti-D Ig is a human plasma-based product that is used to prevent women producing anti-D antibodies. Anti-D Ig is of value to women with non-sensitized Rh-negative blood who have a baby with Rh-positive blood type (Fig. 33.9). *It is not used when anti-D antibodies are already present in maternal blood.* As well, anti-D Ig does not protect against the development of other antibodies that cause haemolytic disease of the newborn.

Routine prophylaxis

In the UK since 2002 (and some other countries), routine antenatal anti-D prophylaxis at 28 and 34 weeks' gestation is recommended for all non-sensitized Rh-negative women (NICE 2008). With postnatal anti-D Ig prophylaxis, about 1.5% of Rh-negative women still develop anti-D antibodies following a first Rh-positive pregnancy. A meta-analysis (Allaby et al 1999) and Cochrane Review (Crowther et al 2013) suggest the antenatal sensitization rate is further reduced by routine antenatal prophylaxis. Antenatal prophylaxis should always be given following possible sensitization events such as spontaneous miscarriage before 12 weeks, any threatened, complete, incomplete or missed abortion *after* 12 weeks of pregnancy, termination of pregnancy by surgical or medical methods regardless of gestational age, fetal death *in utero* or stillbirth, ectopic pregnancy or amniocentesis, cordocentesis, chorionic villus sampling, fetal blood sampling or other invasive intrauterine procedure such as shunt insertion. In addition, postnatal prophylaxis should be given. A systematic review of six eligible trials of more than 10 000 women found when given within 72 hours of birth (and other antenatal sensitizing events), anti-D Ig lowered the incidence of Rh isoimmunization 6 months after birth and in a subsequent pregnancy, regardless of the ABO status of the mother and baby (Crowther and Middleton 1997).

Management of Rh-D isoimmunization

Destruction of fetal RBCs results in fetal anaemia and less oxygen reaches fetal tissue, and oedema and congestive cardiac failure can develop. Lesser degrees of red cell destruction may result in fetal anaemia only, while extensive haemolysis can cause hydrops fetalis and fetal death. Mortality rates are higher for those with hydrops fetalis (van Kamp et al 2005). Early referral to specialist care for women with Rh-D antibodies detected at booking is essential. While early specialist care influences fetal outcome (Ghi et al 2004; Craparo et al 2005; van Kamp et al 2005), ongoing midwifery information and support are also important. Treatment aims to reduce the effects of haemolysis. Intensive fetal monitoring is usually required, and often a high level of intervention throughout the pregnancy. Monitoring and treatment can include the principles outlined in Box 33.2.

Postnatal treatment of isoimmunization

Management aims to monitor the SBR level so that early intervention can be made if the level is high or increasing rapidly to try to prevent levels reaching those that might be harmful. The following factors are worthy of consideration:

- Using phototherapy from birth helps to prevent a rapid rise in some babies.
- Regular SBR measurements from birth every 4 hours.
- A low haemoglobin concentration at birth may indicate the need for early intervention with an exchange transfusion.
- If the SBR level is increasing too rapidly or is too high then intervention is required.

- In early pregnancy maternal blood is grouped for Rh type, and women who are Rh-negative are screened for antibodies (indirect Coombs' test). A positive test indicates the *presence* of antibodies, or sensitization.
- Maternal blood is re-tested frequently to monitor any increase in antibody titres. Even with low anti-D levels, sudden and unexpected rises in serum anti-D levels can result in hydrops fetalis.
- Red blood cells obtained by chorionic villus sampling can be Rh-phenotyped as early as 9–11 weeks' gestation.
- If antibody titres remain stable, ongoing monitoring is continued.
- If antibody titres increase, Doppler ultrasonography of the middle cerebral artery peak systolic velocity is used for non-invasive diagnosis of fetal anaemia. This procedure is as sensitive as amniocentesis in predicting anaemia and bilirubin breakdown products, has less associated risk and can safely replace invasive testing in the management of isoimmunized pregnancies (Joy et al 2005; Mari et al 2005; van Dongen et al 2005; Oepkes et al 2006).
- Intravenous immunoglobulin (IVIG) blocks fetal red cell destruction, reducing maternal antibody levels, and may be used to maintain the fetus until intrauterine fetal transfusion can be performed (see below).
- Intrauterine intravascular transfusion can be used to treat fetal anaemia until the fetus is capable of survival outside the uterus (Craparo et al 2005; van Kamp et al 2005).
- Detailed fetal neuroimaging using multiplanar sonography and/or magnetic resonance imaging may be used to assess brain anatomy in fetuses with severe anaemia (Ghi et al 2004).
- The ongoing severity of the haemolysis and the condition of the fetus will influence the duration of the pregnancy. In general, a gestational age greater than 34 weeks is aimed for to minimize the complications of prematurity.

Treatment depends upon the baby's condition. Careful monitoring but less aggressive management may be adequate, with mild to moderate haemolytic anaemia and hyperbilirubinaemia. Severely affected babies often require early admission to the NICU. Babies with hydrops fetalis are pale, have oedema and ascites. In some cases phototherapy alone can be effective and is very useful to help to prevent the need for exchange transfusion, which carries many more risks. Despite this, exchange transfusion is often required, and later packed cell transfusion may be needed to increase haemoglobin levels as babies are at risk of ongoing haemolytic anaemia and this may occur up to 6–8 weeks of age. Treatment with IVIG can be effective at blocking ongoing haemolysis, with shorter duration of phototherapy and fewer exchange transfusions although this may also increase the likelihood of a later 'top-up' blood transfusion (Gottstein and Cooke 2003).

ABO isoimmunization

ABO isoimmunization usually occurs when the mother is blood group O and the baby is group A, or sometimes group B. Individuals with type O blood develop antibodies throughout life from exposure to antigens in food, Gram-negative bacteria or blood transfusion and by the first pregnancy may already have high serum anti-A and anti-B antibody titres. Some women produce IgG antibodies that can cross the placenta and attack to fetal red cells and destroy them (see effects of isoimmunization in the discussion below referring to Rhesus disease). ABO incompatibility is also thought to protect the fetus from Rh incompatibility as the mother's anti-A and anti-B antibodies destroy any fetal cells that leak into the maternal circulation. Although first and subsequent babies are at risk, destruction is usually much less severe than with Rh incompatibility. In most cases haemolysis is fairly mild but can be more severe. ABO isoimmunization can, rarely, cause severe fetal anaemia and hydrops fetalis.

Antibodies are not often detected in pregnancy and it is usually a diagnosis made in a baby with an unexpectedly high SBR level. Postnatal management depends on the severity of haemolysis and, as with isoimmunization, aims to prevent bilirubin levels that may be harmful. The diagnosis is usually made after birth in an unexpectedly jaundiced baby. The direct Coombs' test is positive and the maternal and baby's blood groups are consistent with ABO incompatibility (i.e. maternal group O and baby A or B or AB). As with other causes of haemolysis, if babies require phototherapy it is usually commenced at a lower serum bilirubin level (140–165 µmol/l or 8–10 mg/dl). In rare cases, babies with high SBR levels require exchange transfusion. IVIG administration to newborns with significant hyperbilirubinaemia due to ABO haemolytic disease (with a positive direct Coombs' test) has reduced the need for exchange transfusion (Miqdad et al 2004).

Late neonatal jaundice

This is generally defined as a bilirubin concentration that remains raised beyond 14 days of age. There are a number of causes and investigation is important because, whilst uncommon, some of the causes are conditions that have significant long-term implications if not treated and treatments are available which are effective if used early enough.

Causes of late neonatal jaundice

Any disease or disorder that increases bilirubin production or alters transport or metabolism of bilirubin is superimposed upon normal physiological jaundice. It is best to divide the causes into those conditions that cause a raised unconjugated bilirubin (fat soluble) and those that cause a raised conjugated bilirubin (water soluble).

Late neonatal (>14 days) unconjugated hyperbilirubinaemia

Increased red cell destruction or haemolysis causes raised SBR levels and blood type/group incompatibility, including Rhesus (Rh-D) and ABO incompatibility, anti-E and anti-Kell. Other factors include sepsis, particularly urinary tract infection, hypothyroidism and galactosaemia. Non-immune haemolysis features spherocytosis (fragile red cell membranes) and enzyme deficiencies. Glucose-6-phosphate dehydrogenase (G6PD) is an enzyme that maintains the integrity of the cell membrane of RBCs and deficiency results in increased haemolysis. G6PD deficiency is an X-linked genetic disorder carried by females that can affect male babies of African, Asian and Mediterranean descent.

Late neonatal (>14 days) conjugated hyperbilirubinaemia

Always consider this when there are pale stools and dark urine. Important causes can include:

- biliary atresia
- dehydration, starvation, hypoxia and sepsis (oxygen and glucose are required for conjugation)
- TORCH infections (toxoplasmosis, others, rubella, cytomegalovirus, herpes)
- other viral infections (e.g. neonatal viral hepatitis)
- other bacterial infections, particularly those caused by E. coli
- metabolic and endocrine disorders that alter uridine diphosphoglucuronyl transferase (UDPGT) enzyme activity (e.g. Crigler–Najjar disease and Gilbert's syndrome)
- other metabolic disorders such as hypothyroidism and galactosaemia.

HAEMATOLOGICAL PROBLEMS

Bleeding

Bleeding is generally rare in the newborn, however there are a small number of significant conditions that can result in bleeding of which the midwife should be aware. Blood from the gastrointestinal tract (vomiting or passed per rectum as malaena) is sometimes seen and the commonest cause is swallowed maternal blood. This is supported if there is a clear history of maternal bleeding and bloodstained amniotic fluid. The baby should be carefully evaluated and the possibility of bleeding from the gastrointestinal tract considered. This could occur if there was a clotting or platelet abnormality, or occasionally with some serious gastrointestinal disorders such as NEC.

Possible causes of bleeding abnormalities

Vitamin K-deficient bleeding (VKDB)

Early VKDB, occurring in the first 48 hours, is rare and usually occurs to babies born to mothers who have received medications that interfere with vitamin K metabolism. These include the anticonvulsants phenytoin, barbiturates or carbamazepine, the antitubercular drugs rifampicin or isoniazid and the vitamin K antagonists warfarin and phenprocoumarin. It is prevented by giving vitamin K to the mother (except those that require ongoing anticoagulation) in the last weeks of pregnancy and ensuring a dose of intramuscular (IM) vitamin K is given to the baby. Vitamin K is given to all newborn babies by virtue of their mother's consent, usually as an IM injection to prevent VKDB. If there is unexplained bruising or bleeding it is important to check that vitamin K has been given as some mothers will decline from giving consent. Classic VKDB occurs in the first week of life, often in sick babies or those slow to establish feeds. Gastrointestinal bleeding is common and may be severe, epistaxis or unexplained bruising or oozing from the umbilical cord are common features. Bleeding into the brain is uncommon. It is prevented by ensuring that an early first dose of vitamin K is given by any route.

Late VKDB occurs from the first week up to 6 months, usually between 4 and 12 weeks. This form is more commonly associated with intracranial bleeds (30–50%) than classic VKDB, and this can be fatal or leave permanent disability. It is almost completely confined to fully breast-fed babies. About half will have an underlying liver disease or other malabsorptive state. Late VKDB can be optimally prevented by 1 mg vitamin K IM at birth or significantly reduced by repeated doses of oral vitamin K.

Thrombocytopenia

A low platelet count may present with bleeding or a petechial rash. It may be due to:

- maternal idiopathic thrombocytopenic purpura (ITP), where autoimmune maternal antibodies destroy maternal and fetal platelets
- isoimmune thrombocytopenia, where maternal antiplatelet antibodies destroy fetal platelets of a different group
- congenital infections, both viral and bacterial
- drugs, administered to mother or baby
- severe Rhesus haemolytic disease.

Haemophilia and other inherited problems

Haemophilia A is an X-linked recessive disorder, which therefore affects only boys. Females may be carriers. The diagnosis is often known or suspected antenatally because of a family history. In these cases investigation should occur after birth and IM injections and invasive procedures should be avoided. The diagnosis can be made by checking a clotting profile and should always be considered in a male baby who has unexpected bleeding.

METABOLIC PROBLEMS

Many metabolic abnormalities can occur in the newborn, particularly in preterm or IUGR babies. By far the most common problem is hypoglycaemia.

Glucose homeostasis

The fetus has a constant supply of glucose via the placenta. Following birth, this supply of nutrients ceases and there is a fall in glucose concentration (Srinivasan et al 1986). At the same time, however, endocrine changes (decrease in insulin and a surge of catecholamines and release of glucagon) result in an increase in glycogenolysis (breakdown of glycogen stores to provide glucose), gluconeogenesis (glucose production from the liver), ketogenesis (producing ketones, an alternative fuel) and lipolysis (release of fatty acids from adipose) bringing about an increase in glucose and other metabolic fuel. Problems arise in the newborn when there is either a lack of glycogen stores to mobilize (preterm and IUGR babies) or excessive insulin production (infants of diabetic mothers) or when the babies are sick and have a poor supply of energy and increased requirements.

Low glucose concentrations are a potential problem in the newborn because if there is a lack of fuel or nutrients available for the brain, cerebral dysfunction and potentially brain injury may occur. The problem for those caring for newborn babies is not only to identify those who are at risk and treat them appropriately, but also to avoid excessive treatment and investigation in babies where intervention is not required.

Hypoglycaemia

The definition of hypoglycaemia is controversial and many different definitions can be found in the literature (Koh et al 1988b). The problem is that defining a specific level of blood glucose is unhelpful because a baby's ability to compensate and use alternative fuels may be as important as the specific glucose concentration. Pragmatically, however, a specific level is helpful for management purposes. The consensus appears to favour a cut-off value in the newborn of 2.6 mmol/l although the evidence for the use of this level is not strong. This figure comes mainly from two studies (Koh et al 1988a; Lucas et al 1988). Koh et al (1988a) demonstrated abnormal sensory-evoked brain stem potentials in a small number of term babies. This did not occur in any infants where the blood glucose was above 2.6 mmol/l, whether or not signs were present (Koh et al 1988a). In addition, and perhaps more importantly, in a retrospective study of preterm infants the neurological outcome was less favourable if the blood glucose concentration had been <2.6 mmol/l on ≥5 days during the neonatal period (Lucas et al 1988). These studies suggest that levels of blood glucose concentration above 2.6 mmol/l are likely to be safe but they do not take into account the baby's ability to compensate for low glucose concentrations. Lower values may be safe in some babies.

Signs of hypoglycaemia

A baby who has signs of hypoglycaemia has a glucose concentration that is too low and this should be treated whatever the exact glucose level. The signs of hypoglycaemia are lethargy, poor feeding, seizures and decreased consciousness level. Jitteriness is commonly ascribed to hypoglycaemia but is a common feature in the newborn and *alone should not be used as an indication for measuring blood glucose concentration.*

Healthy term babies

It is likely that healthy term babies are able to tolerate low blood glucose concentrations using compensatory mechanisms and use alternative fuels such as ketone bodies, lactate or fatty acids (Hawdon et al 1992). These babies may have blood glucose concentrations as low as 2.0 mmol/l without any ill-effects because, if responding normally, they are likely to have increased ketone body concentrations so that fuel is available for the brain (Hawdon et al 1992). Term babies who are breastfed are particularly likely to have low blood glucose concentrations, probably because of the low energy content of breastmilk in the first few postnatal days. However, these babies have higher ketone body concentrations to compensate (Hawdon et al 1992) and they are unlikely, therefore, to suffer any ill-effects. Unfortunately, however, routine measurements of ketone body concentrations are not readily available and when glucose measurements are made in these babies it becomes difficult for practitioners to resist giving treatment that may involve supplementary formula feeding or even IV dextrose at the expense of breastfeeding. This should obviously be avoided unless there are other clinical indications for intervention. Because of their ability to counter-regulate, clinically well, appropriately grown, full-term babies who are feeding do not require monitoring of their glucose concentration. Doing so would result in many babies being inappropriately treated.

Babies at risk of neurological sequelae of hypoglycaemia

Babies where monitoring and treatment should be considered are those in whom counter-regulation may be impaired. Preterm babies (<37 completed weeks) and IUGR babies (<3rd centile for gestation) have lower glycogen stores and cannot therefore mobilize glucose as rapidly during the immediate postnatal period. In addition they also have immature hormone and enzyme responses and are less likely to be enterally fed at an early stage. Infants of diabetic mothers (IDM) frequently have low blood glucose concentrations because of an excess of insulin production. This is produced by the fetal pancreatic gland as a result of stimulation by increased maternal glucose concentrations. This excess of insulin also acts as a growth factor and brings about excessive fat and glycogen deposition. This is why these infants have a characteristic appearance and are relatively macrosomic (Fig. 33.10; note macrosomic appearance with increased adiposity). A study by the Confidential Enquiry into Maternal and Child Health (CEMACH 2005) demonstrated that practice across the UK varies with regard to the management of IDM and many babies appear to be inappropriately admitted to NICU. This should be avoided where possible but it requires the ability to monitor these babies on routine postnatal wards. In sick babies following perinatal hypoxia-ischaemia or sepsis there may also be low substrate stores compounded by feeding difficulties that add to the problem. Also consider babies with inborn errors of metabolism (discussed later in this chapter).

Diagnosis, prevention and management of hypoglycaemia

Term babies who are admitted to the postnatal ward and are feeding should not have blood glucose measured unless they are symptomatic. In particular, breastfeeding information and intervention should not be based on blood glucose concentrations. Prevention is important in at-risk babies and they should therefore have:

- adequate temperature control – keep warm
- early breastfeeding within 1 hour of birth (100 ml/kg per day if formula feeding)
- frequent feeding (≤3 hourly)
- a blood glucose check immediately before the second feed and then 4–6 hourly thereafter.

There is no advantage in checking the blood glucose concentration earlier than this providing there are no clinical signs as it is likely to be low and the appropriate treatment at this stage is to feed the baby. If there are signs of hypoglycaemia, the glucose should be checked and treatment given immediately. Breastfed babies are particularly difficult to manage in this situation as it is important to avoid supplemental feeding with formula to promote successful breastfeeding but the risks associated with significant hypoglycaemia in at risk-babies outweigh this advantage. If the blood glucose concentration is <2.6 mmol/l then a feed should be given at an increased volume and decreased frequency (2 hourly or even hourly). This may require supplementary feeding with colostrum or formula milk for those who are being breastfed and the use of a nasogastric tube should always be considered.

If the blood glucose concentration remains low despite these measures and there is an adequate feed volume intake, then IV treatment with dextrose is required. It is important in this situation that enteral feeding is continued as colostrum/milk contains much more energy than 10% dextrose and promotes ketone body production and metabolic adaptation. If the blood glucose concentration is >2.6 mmol/l before the second and third feed then glucose monitoring can be discontinued but feeding should continue at 3-hourly intervals. In babies where enteral feeding is contraindicated for some reason, IV 10% dextrose at least 60 ml/kg on the first day should commence.

Hyperglycaemia

Hyperglycaemia is much less of a clinical problem than hypoglycaemia and occurs predominantly in preterm and severely affected IUGR babies. It is also seen in term babies in response to stress, especially following perinatal hypoxia-ischaemia, surgery or drugs (especially corticosteroids). In general no treatment is required. In preterm babies it is usually a transient phenomenon related to the immature autoregulation or inability to deal with excessive glucose intakes. In general, treatment is not required unless there is significant loss of glucose in the urine that may cause an osmotic diuresis. If treatment is required the rate of glucose infusion can be decreased, but there may

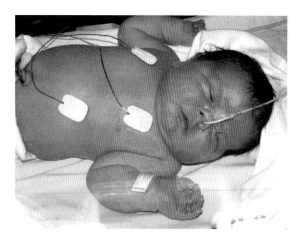

Fig. 33.10 Macrosomic infant.

be some advantages in this situation of giving an IV insulin infusion. This allows glucose input to continue and sufficient calories to continue to be given and may result in better weight gain (Collins et al 1991).

ELECTROLYTE IMBALANCES IN THE NEWBORN

In the first few days after birth all babies lose weight due to a loss of extracellular fluid. This diuresis and loss of weight is associated with cardiopulmonary adaptation; it occurs rapidly in healthy babies but may be delayed in those with RDS. As extracellular fluid is lost there is a net loss of both water and sodium over these first few days after birth, although the baby's serum sodium should remain within the normal range. The healthy baby should lose up to 10% of its birth weight. This weight loss is physiological and should be expected.

Sodium

Sodium is normally excreted via the kidney, controlled by the renin–angiotensin system. This control mechanism is functional in the preterm baby but loss of sodium may occur in these babies because of renal tubule unresponsiveness. Term breastmilk has relatively little sodium (<1 mmol/kg per day), showing that the healthy newborn can preserve sodium via the kidney in order to maintain growth. Normal sodium requirements are 1–2 mmol/kg per day in term babies and 3–4 mmol/kg per day in preterm babies. Changes in serum sodium reflect changes in sodium and water balance. In order to assess changes in sodium concentration it is important to know a baby's weight as hypernatraemia in the presence of a loss of weight suggests dehydration whereas when there is weight gain it is due to fluid and sodium overload. Hyponatraemia in the presence of weight gain represents fluid overload whereas a reduced sodium with inappropriate weight loss represents sodium depletion. The normal serum sodium concentration is 133–146 mmol/l (Ayling and Bowron 2012).

Hyponatraemia

Hyponatraemia is due either to fluid overload or sodium depletion. The latter may be due to inadequate intake or excessive losses.

Fluid overload

In the first few days after birth this is the commonest cause of a low sodium concentration. It is commonly seen in babies receiving IV fluids or in babies with oliguric renal failure or those on medication, e.g. indomethacin given to preterm babies. Appropriate treatment is to limit the fluid

intake whilst maintaining normal sodium intake with appropriate intravenous fluids.

Sodium depletion

The causes include renal loss in preterm babies, which is treated by increasing sodium intake to compensate for the losses. Some preterm babies may require a very large daily intake of IV sodium with their IV fluids when losses are high. Also consider loss of sodium into the bowel due to ileus (intestinal obstruction, sepsis or prematurity) or severe vomiting. Diuretics can affect the loss and occasionally adrenocortical failure. This is rare but may be due to congenital adrenal hyperplasia or hypoplasia, or adrenal haemorrhage in a sick baby.

Hypernatraemia

Increased sodium concentration is almost always due to water depletion and loss of extracellular fluid but can also rarely be due to an excessive sodium intake. These causes can again be easily differentiated, by weighing the baby to assess the change since birth.

Water depletion

This is rare in term babies but does occur occasionally in babies with an inadequate intake of breastmilk. It is more common in preterm babies. The causes include:

- transepidermal water loss in preterm babies – this occurs particularly in babies <28 weeks' gestation and can be prevented by adequate environmental humidity and regular weighing to gauge fluid loss to predict fluid requirements
- excessive urine output in preterm babies during recovery from RDS
- high rates of fluid loss during vomiting, diarrhoea or bowel obstruction
- inadequate lactation.

Water depletion is perhaps the most important cause of hypernatraemia. The incidence has been estimated as 2.5/10 000 live births and it typically occurs in term babies of breastfeeding primiparous mothers (Oddie et al 2001). It can be associated with significant morbidity and even mortality (Edmondson et al 1997), however, it can be prevented with sufficient assistance and supervision of feeding. Babies typically present at 5–9 days of age with lethargy and poor feeding. They have lost >15% of their birthweight and are usually significantly jaundiced. The serum sodium concentration can be between 150 and 200 mmol/l.

In general, many babies are not weighed during this period. Mothers who are breastfeeding can be discouraged by the fact that their baby has lost weight despite a good technique and this can serve to undermine breastfeeding no matter how carefully the physiology of the phenomenon is explained. Additionally (particularly in primiparous mothers) lactogenesis is only just starting at between 48 and 72 hours. Thus the volume of milk transferred to the baby is still rising sharply between 72 and 96 hours of age. However, weighing babies during this period can be very useful when a baby is unwell or if there are concerns about intake and fluid and electrolyte balance. It has been suggested that routine weighing of babies may be useful to prevent dehydration and hypernatraemia in breastfed babies with referral to hospital if weight loss exceeds 10% (van Dommelen et al 2007). The baby's fluid deficit can be calculated from the loss in weight and this is then replaced by gradual rehydration over 24–48 hours. Feeding can continue but IV treatment is often required with normal saline and dextrose. Assistance with lactation can then be given to continue to promote breastfeeding.

Excessive sodium intake

In general this is rare in term babies, although it may be seen in sick preterm babies due to excessive bicarbonate and other sodium-containing fluids. Causes are:

- incorrect fluid prescription
- excessive administration of sodium bicarbonate
- incorrectly formulated powdered feeds
- Münchausen's syndrome by proxy – intentional administration of salt to a baby.

Potassium

Potassium is the major intracellular cation. A low serum concentration therefore implies significant potassium depletion. Abnormalities in serum potassium concentration are important because they can cause significant arrhythmias. Potassium concentrations can be severely affected by measurement technique, and any haemolysis of the blood sample, especially from capillary sampling, is likely to lead to a falsely high value.

Hyperkalaemia

Causes include:

- acidosis
- acute renal failure
- congenital adrenal hyperplasia.

Treatment is to remove all potassium supplements from IV fluids, and to consider giving calcium resonium rectally, calcium gluconate IV, sodium bicarbonate to increase pH and IV glucose and insulin. In general these measures will be required only where there is a serum potassium that is very high (>8 mmol/l) and/or evidence of an abnormal electrocardiogram (ECG) or arrhythmia.

Hypokalaemia

Causes include:

- inadequate intake of potassium
- bowel losses (vomiting or diarrhoea)

- diuretic therapy
- hyperaldosteronism.

Hypokalaemia is treated by adding potassium to IV infusion fluids or orally. The normal daily requirement of potassium is 2 mmol/kg per day.

Calcium

Calcium metabolism is closely linked to phosphate metabolism and these are very important minerals in relation to bone development. This is of particular importance in preterm infants as they need much higher concentrations of phosphate and calcium. These are given as IV supplements, by supplementing breastmilk with fortifier (Lucas et al 1996) or by giving specific preterm milk formula rather than term formula. High serum calcium concentrations are unusual but there are rare but important causes of low serum calcium. The normal serum concentration is 2.2–2.7 mmol/l but this must be interpreted with the serum albumin concentration as serum calcium is bound to albumin therefore a low albumin concentration will lead to a falsely low serum value. Calcium concentrations fall within 18–24 hours of birth as the baby's supply of placental calcium ceases but accretion into bone continues. In the past, hypocalcaemia during the first week after birth used to be caused by giving unmodified cow's milk. This has a high phosphate concentration and a relatively low calcium concentration that depressed the serum calcium concentration and caused seizures. This is now rare with modern formula feeds.

Hypocalcaemia can cause seizures, tremors, jitteriness, lethargy, poor feeding and vomiting. Severe signs can be treated by IV replacement of calcium. Longer-term management depends on the cause. Hypocalcaemia can be caused by:

- prematurity
- significant hypoxia-ischaemia
- renal failure
- hypoparathyroidism including DiGeorge syndrome (see later)
- maternal diabetes mellitus.

INBORN ERRORS OF METABOLISM IN THE NEWBORN

Inborn errors of metabolism (IEM) are rare inherited disorders occurring in approximately 1 in 5000 births. They result mainly from enzyme deficiencies in metabolic pathways leading to an accumulation of substrate, leading to toxicity. *In utero*, the placenta provides an effective dialysis system for most disorders, removing toxic metabolites. Most affected babies are therefore initially born in good condition with normal birth weight. A high index of

Box 33.3 Clinical features associated with many diagnoses – a combination of these features could be indicative of an IEM

- Septicaemia
- Hypoglycaemia
- Metabolic acidosis
- Convulsions
- Coma
- Cataracts
- Cardiomegaly
- Jaundice/liver disease
- Severe hypotonia
- Unusual body odour
- Dysmorphic features
- Abnormal hair
- Hydrops fetalis
- Diarrhoea

suspicion is needed when evaluating an acutely sick neonate, as many disorders are treatable and early diagnosis and treatment can reduce morbidity. It has been estimated that 20% of babies presenting with sepsis in the absence of risk factors have an inborn error of metabolism.

The mode of inheritance is usually autosomal recessive, therefore family history is crucial and the following information should be sought:

- any affected siblings
- previous stillbirth/neonatal death
- parental consanguinity
- features associated with feeding, fasting or a surgical procedure
- improvement when feeds are stopped and relapse on restarting.

A clinical examination often reveals little specific evidence and the baby can appear healthy. The features in Box 33.3 may be seen in isolation with many diagnoses, however multiple features indicate that an underlying IEM should be seriously considered

The following laboratory tests are a basic first step in the investigation process:

- full blood count
- septic screen
- creatinine, urea and electrolytes (including chloride)
- liver enzymes
- blood gas
- blood glucose and lactate concentration
- urine reducing substances (sugar)
- urine ketones (dipstick)

- plasma ammonia concentration
- coagulation tests.

Many other investigations may be necessary and useful, but in general, investigations need to be discussed with a consultant biochemist or paediatrician with an interest in metabolic disorders. Principles of emergency management are to reduce any abnormal load on affected pathways by removing toxic metabolites and stimulating residual enzyme activity. Hypoglycaemia is corrected, adequate ventilatory support and hydration are maintained, convulsions are treated and significant metabolic acidosis is treated with IV sodium bicarbonate, and electrolyte abnormalities are corrected. In general, antibiotics are frequently given as infection may have precipitated metabolic decompensation and occasionally dialysis may also be required (Wraith and Walker 1996).

Phenylketonuria

Phenylketonuria (PKU) is important, first because it is a treatable cause of brain injury and second because it is possible to successfully screen for it during the first week of life in order to identify affected individuals and treat them appropriately to produce a favourable outcome.

PKU is an autosomal recessive disorder of protein metabolism that has an incidence of approximately 1 in 10 000 in the UK. Babies with PKU are born in good condition but begin to be affected by their condition during the first few weeks/months after birth. Untreated it leads to severe learning difficulties/disability (IQ <30). However, if it is identified early (within the first 3 weeks), it can be treated by a diet specifically restricted in phenylalanine. The common type is caused by the absence of or reduction in an enzyme called phenylalanine hydroxylase which, in the liver, converts the essential amino acid phenylalanine to another essential amino acid, tyrosine. The toxic accumulation of phenylalanine and the deprivation of tyrosine leads to brain damage.

PKU is particularly suitable for mass screening because there is a simple widely available diagnostic test and because treatment is effective. Midwives collect the blood sample for PKU screening in the UK between days 5 and 8 after birth with the knowledge that the baby has been taking milk feeds. The level of phenylalanine is analysed and babies with increased levels need to be prescribed a low phenylalanine diet and have further assessment to determine whether they are affected by the 'classic' type of the disease or other variants. If it is treated early, the prognosis for PKU is good and normal intelligence can result. Affected people will have to stay on a low phenylalanine diet for life and women who wish to conceive need to pre-conceptionally have their diet reviewed to prevent congenital abnormalities like microcephaly in their developing fetus. This is because fetal brain injury may result from exposure to high concentrations of phenylalanine and its metabolites in the mother.

Galactosaemia

Galactosaemia is a disorder of carbohydrate metabolism that is autosomal recessive in inheritance and has an incidence of 1 in 60 000. It is caused by an absence or severe deficiency of the enzyme galactose-1-phosphate uridyltransferase (often referred to as Gal-I-P UT). This enzyme is important for converting galactose to glucose and since milk's main sugar lactose is a disaccharide containing glucose and galactose, babies with this condition rapidly become affected when fed either human breastmilk or cow's milk formulae. The metabolite that builds up and is harmful is galactose-1-phosphate.

The clinical signs of the disorder are those of liver failure and renal impairment. Affected babies tend to present with vomiting, hypoglycaemia, jaundice, bleeding, acidosis, failure to gain weight and hypotonia during the first few days after birth. Another important clinical feature is congenital cataract. Affected babies may also present with septicaemia (particularly *E. coli*) due to damage to intestinal mucosa by high levels of galactose in the bowel. Galactosaemia is an important differential diagnosis to consider when dealing with a baby with unresponsive hypoglycaemia and prolonged or severe jaundice. Babies with galactosaemia will have galactose but not glucose in their urine. The diagnosis therefore can be made by looking for urine-reducing substances (galactose) using a Clinitest, whereas a urine test for glucose will be negative. Confirmation of the diagnosis is by assay of the enzyme level (Gal-I-P UT) within red blood cells.

Treatment is with a lactose-free milk formula, commenced as soon as the diagnosis is suspected. This results in a rapid correction of the abnormalities. However, cataracts and mild brain injury have occurred even when galactosaemic babies have been fed lactose-free milk from birth. Screening for this disorder is possible but many babies will have presented before the screening test is available and there is little evidence to suggest that diagnosis at or soon after birth gives a better long-term outlook than diagnosis by rapid screening of the deteriorating sick baby.

ENDOCRINE PROBLEMS

Endocrine problems in the newborn are relatively rare but may be serious, even life-threatening, but are nearly always treatable so identification and diagnosis is important. Disorders of blood glucose homeostasis have already been described so this section will concentrate on other endocrine abnormalities that may present in the newborn.

Thyroid disorders

The thyroid gland produces hormones that have an effect on the metabolic rate in most tissues. They are also essential for normal neurological development. Thyroid stimulating hormone (TSH) is produced by the anterior pituitary gland and this stimulates production of T3 and T4 by the thyroid gland with a feedback mechanism to the anterior pituitary.

Hypothyroidism

The incidence of hypothyroidism in the newborn is 1 in 3500. There are several possible causes for hypothyroidism in the newborn, including abnormalities in gland formation (thyroid dysgenesis), defects in hormone synthesis (dyshormonogenesis) and rarely secondary pituitary causes. The latter causes a decrease or lack of TSH, whereas primary (thyroid) causes result in very high TSH values. The presentation is, however, the same, although this has implications for screening. Babies with hypothyroidism tend to be large, post term and have a large posterior fontanelle. They have coarse features and often have an umbilical hernia. These features are often missed, which is why screening for this disorder is so important. Untreated babies develop impaired motor development with growth failure, a low IQ, impaired hearing and language problems. With treatment the physical signs of hypothyroidism do not appear but the intellectual and neurological prognosis is poor unless treatment is started within the first few weeks of life and this should always occur when affected babies are detected by screening. Screening for hypothyroidism involves measuring thyroid stimulating hormone (TSH) on a blood spot taken at 5–8 days of age. This method detects almost all cases, however it cannot detect cases caused by secondary (pituitary) hypothyroidism that will have a low TSH. This condition is, however, much less common, with an incidence of 1 in 60 000 to 1 in 100 000 (Fisher et al 1979).

Hyperthyroidism

Graves' disease is an autoimmune disorder that causes hyperthyroidism. Neonatal hyperthyroidism occurs relatively rarely but is possible when the mother has or has had Graves' disease. It occurs not because of neonatal autoantibodies but as a result of the transfer of maternal thyroid stimulating immunoglobulins. These are autoantibodies that are produced and act in the same way as TSH. This can occur when a mother has active, inactive or treated Graves' disease (Teng et al 1980). Thyrotoxicosis in the fetus can lead to preterm labour, low birth weight, stillbirth and fetal death, but only a small percentage of babies of mothers with Graves' disease show signs of thyrotoxicosis. In the baby the signs are irritability, jitteriness, tachycardia, prominent eyes, sweating, excessive appetite and weight loss. These may be present immediately after birth or presentation may be delayed for as long as 4–6 weeks (Skuza et al 1996). The baby therefore needs to be observed for this period and treatment will be required with anti-thyroid medication if any signs appear.

Adrenal disorders

The adrenal glands are vital for the normal function of many systems within the body. They are divided into a medulla and a cortex. The medulla produces catecholamines, which help to maintain blood pressure and are produced at times of stress. Abnormalities of function of the adrenal medulla are not described in the newborn. The adrenal cortex produces three groups of hormones – glucocorticoids, mineralocorticoids and sex hormones – that have distinct functions. Glucocorticoids regulate the general metabolism of carbohydrates, proteins and fats on a long-term basis. They have a particular role in modifying the metabolism in times of stress. Mineralocorticoids regulate sodium, potassium and water balance. The sex hormones are responsible for normal development of the genitalia and reproductive organs. Abnormalities in function of the glands represent the functions of these different groups of hormones.

Adrenocortical insufficiency

This is caused by congenital hypoplasia, adrenal haemorrhage, enzyme defects or can be secondary to pituitary problems. It generally presents with the signs of hypoglycaemia, vomiting, poor feeding and weight gain with prolonged jaundice. The baby may have hyponatraemia, hypoglycaemia, hyperkalaemia and acidosis. Treatment is by IV therapy with glucose and electrolytes followed by replacement of corticosteroid and mineralocorticoid hormones.

Adrenocortical hyperfunction

This may occur in the form of congenital adrenal hyperplasia (CAH). This is the name given to a group of inherited disorders that are due to deficiency of enzymes responsible for hormone production within the adrenal gland. The most common enzyme deficiency results in an excess of androgenic hormones but a deficiency of glucocorticoid and mineralocorticoids often also occurs. These disorders can cause abnormalities in the formation of the genitalia leading to ambiguous genitalia (virilization of females or inadequate virilization of males) (see Fig. 33.11) and features of adrenal insufficiency (vomiting, diarrhoea, vascular collapse, hypoglycaemia, hyponatraemia, hyperkalaemia). The classification of disorders of sexual differentiation has been revised in recent years. For more information see the consensus statement by Hughes et al (2006).

It is important to make a prompt diagnosis. The genetic sex must be determined (chromosome analysis) and it is important not to assign a sex until the diagnosis has been

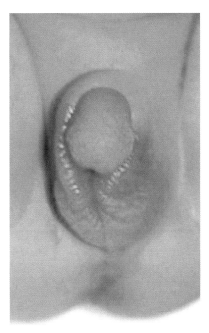

Fig. 33.11 Female infant with ambiguous genitalia due to congenital adrenal hyperplasia.

established (see Chapter 28). The biochemical diagnosis is made by analysing urine and plasma for steroid hormone metabolites. Treatment is as for adrenocortical insufficiency by replacement of glucocorticoid and mineralocorticoid hormones. Virilized girls may also require surgical intervention to correct the genital abnormalities.

Pituitary disorders

Pituitary insufficiency is rare in the newborn. It may occur in association with other abnormalities, particularly midline developmental defects. Presentation is with signs of glucocorticoid deficiency (hypoglycaemia), prolonged jaundice or signs of hypothyroidism. Growth hormone deficiency generally causes hypoglycaemia but no other signs in the newborn. When it is recognized, treatment is with replacement of the missing hormones.

Parathyroid disorders

The parathyroid glands are responsible for control of calcium metabolism but abnormalities of the parathyroid glands are rare causes of hypocalcaemia and hypercalcaemia in the newborn. When hypoparathyroidism does occur it may be familial or may occur in association with deletions of chromosome 22 (22q11 deletion or DiGeorge syndrome). The signs associated with hypocalcaemia are detailed above.

EFFECTS ON THE NEWBORN OF MATERNAL DRUG ABUSE/USE DURING PREGNANCY

The incidence of drug use within the UK population has a large geographical variation. As a result the incidence of drug withdrawal amongst babies also has a markedly varying incidence. Inner city areas are more likely to be affected but even within cities large variation is seen in the incidence of problems.

Opiates and other drugs cross the placenta and the fetus during pregnancy is likely to be exposed to the same peaks and troughs of drug exposure as the mother. Withdrawal may be manifested before birth. The increased incidence of fetal distress may be related in part to drug withdrawal during labour but the effects of drugs and withdrawal on the fetus and newborn are related to the timing of drug doses. Babies born to mothers who have used illicit drugs during pregnancy are at risk of withdrawal effects. Other problems that are more common in these pregnancies are:

- obstetric complications of pregnancy including placental abruption, IUGR, signs of fetal compromise during labour, stillbirth
- poor attendance for antenatal care
- non-disclosure of information regarding drugs taken during pregnancy
- risk of infectious disease (hepatitis B and C, and HIV)
- social problems such as poor housing, chaotic lifestyle, care of other children
- poor attendance for neonatal follow-up.

Attendance for antenatal care and supervision during pregnancy may be improved by midwifery support and community liaison. It is important to identify these women during pregnancy in order to try to prevent some of the above problems and offer appropriate support. Identification during pregnancy also allows screening for infectious diseases and this is particularly important for hepatitis B and HIV where treatments are available to decrease the chance of the newborn being affected.

Signs of withdrawal

Many drugs have been reported to cause problems of withdrawal in the newborn. The most common seen in the UK are opiates in the form of heroin and methadone but barbiturates, benzodiazepines, cocaine and amphetamines are also frequently seen. Multidrug use is common and usually leads to prolonged difficult withdrawal. Each drug has a different half-life and this leads to different patterns of withdrawal behaviour. In general methadone produces effects for longer periods than heroin (Herzlinger et al 1977) but benzodiazepines may also contribute to this (Sutton and Hinderliter 1990).

The signs most frequently seen are jitteriness, irritability and constant high-pitched crying. Babies often fail to settle between feeds and are hyperactive. When feeds are offered they often feed voraciously although some have a poor suck. Vomiting is common. Diarrhoea and an irritant nappy rash are also often seen. Sneezing and yawning are also seen alongside episodes of high temperature in the absence of infection. In rare circumstances babies may also have seizures.

Several scoring systems have been developed to help to guide when to give pharmacological treatment (Finnegan et al 1975). These scoring systems aim to make the assessment more objective, however most of the features and their severity are difficult to quantify. Babies assessed for signs of drug withdrawal by a scoring system are less likely to be inappropriately treated and may have a shorter hospital stay. It is important not to over-treat them with drugs as the long-term effects are not clear and the treatment may then be difficult to withdraw. Also treatment in many maternity hospitals means admitting the baby to the NICU therefore possibly separating mother and baby. On the other hand babies who are withdrawing appear to be in discomfort, which arguably warrants management, but the long-term effects of withdrawal are also unclear. From experience the most useful feature is whether the baby settles and sleeps between feeding. If the baby does, then pharmacological treatment may be unnecessary.

Treatment

Treatment can be divided into general care given to these babies and pharmacological treatment. It is important, if at all possible, to keep mother and baby together. Bonding with and care of these babies by their mother should be positively encouraged. The mother is likely to be feeling upset and guilty because of the baby's appearance/behaviour and the co-existing social problems involved with these families makes for a challenging time for all involved. Breastfeeding can be encouraged as long as there is no evidence of HIV or ongoing drug use (heroin and cocaine) that precludes this. Some recommend limiting this to mothers who are taking methadone on a dose that is less than 20 mg/day (Committee on Drugs, American Academy of Pediatrics 1989). A quiet environment with reduced light and noise is helpful in keeping stimuli to a minimum. Swaddling is useful and feeds may need to be given frequently. These babies will often take large volumes of milk, which is acceptable as long as vomiting is not a problem. Rocking or cradling are also useful interventions.

Pharmacological treatment

Several different treatments have been recommended in the past. Previously, the four drugs recommended for use were paregoric (a mixture of alcohol and opiate), phenobarbitone, diazepam and chlorpromazine (Committee on Drugs, American Academy of Pediatrics 1998). A number of randomized trials have been performed attempting to assess the use of various drugs in the treatment of neonatal abstinence syndrome (NAS) (Theis et al 1997). It seems logical to treat opiate withdrawal with opiates and now the two most commonly used treatments are oral methadone and oral morphine. These appear to control withdrawal seizures much more effectively (Lawn and Alton 2012). They can be given in increasing doses if necessary until the features are controlled and then the dose gradually reduced. A possible dosing regimen for oral morphine is shown below:

- initially 0.04 mg/kg morphine sulphate oral 4-hourly
- then 0.03 mg/kg morphine sulphate oral 4-hourly
- then 0.02 mg/kg morphine sulphate oral 4-hourly
- then 0.01 mg/kg morphine sulphate oral 4-hourly.

The dose is reduced every 24 hours if the baby is feeding well and settling better between feeds. If the feeding and settling does not improve or profuse watery stools and excessive vomiting continue, other treatment needs to be considered. Other medication may sometimes be useful, e.g. clonazepam for benzodiazepine use or chloral hydrate as a general sedative.

Cocaine

Cocaine deserves special mention because its effects on the newborn are different. It is a larger problem in the USA than in the UK but the incidence of its use during pregnancy is unknown. It is only present in maternal urine for 24 hours after exposure therefore detection is difficult (Zuckerman et al 1989). It can produce significant withdrawal signs although these are often less severe and less troublesome than with other drugs, but it is associated with many other harmful effects on the fetus (Fulroth et al 1989). These include significant fetal IUGR, brain injury due to haemorrhage or infarction (Hadeed and Siegel 1989), abnormalities of brain development, limb reduction defects and atresias of the gastrointestinal system. Correlation between cocaine exposure, small head size and developmental scores has been reported (Chasnoff et al 1992).

Discharge and long-term effects

Discharge must be planned with the involvement of other support agencies. This may include a planning meeting involving all agencies concerned with the care of the mother and baby. Although it seems intuitive that exposure to drugs *in utero* would cause neurodevelopmental impairment, this is not borne out by carefully controlled studies (Lifschitz et al 1985). This implies that impairment in intellectual outcome in these children relates to other adverse prenatal and postnatal factors. Babies born to these mothers are smaller and have smaller head circumferences (Kandall et al 1976). However, it is difficult to be certain about the exact causes of any long-term harmful effects because so many factors are involved, all of which are interlinked. These include:

- the effects of the drugs themselves on the developing fetus
- the use of other harmful substances by mothers who use drugs (e.g. cigarettes and alcohol)
- the effect of pregnancy complications
- the effect of the withdrawal syndrome on the developing neonate
- the effect of treatment to prevent withdrawal behaviours
- the effect of the home environment of the chaotic drug-user for the developing child
- genetic effects
- reporting bias means that negative associations with drug-taking are more likely to be reported (Koren et al 1989).

REFERENCES

AAP (American Academy of Pediatrics) 2004 Clinical Practice Guideline: Management of hyperbilirubinemia in the newborn infant >35 weeks of gestation. Pediatrics 114(1):297–316

Ahlfors C E, Wennberg R P 2004 Bilirubin-albumin binding and neonatal jaundice. Seminars in Perinatology 28(5):334–9

Allaby M, Forman K, Touch S et al 1999 The use of routine anti-D prophylaxis antenatally to Rhesus negative women. Trent Institute for Health Services Research, Universities of Leicester, Nottingham and Sheffield, ref 99/04

Ayling R M, Bowron A 2012 Neonatal biochemical reference ranges. In: Rennie J M (ed), Rennie and Roberton's textbook of neonatology, 5th edn. Churchill Livingstone, Edinburgh, A6: p 1309–18

Azzopardi D V, Strohm B, Edwards A D et al. 2009 Moderate hypothermia to treat perinatal asphyxial encephalopathy. New England Journal of Medicine 361(14):1349–58

Banatvala J E, Brown D W G 2004 Rubella. Lancet 363 (9415): 1127–37

Barcaite E, Bartusevicius A, Tameliene R et al 2008 Prevalence of maternal group B streptococcal colonisation in European countries. Acta Obstetrica et Gynecologica Scandinavica 87(3):260–71

Bedford H, Tookey P 2006 Rubella and the MMR vaccine. Nursing Times 102(5):55–7

Bianchi D W, Avent N D, Costa J M et al 2005 Noninvasive prenatal diagnosis of fetal rhesus D. Ready for prime(r) time. Obstetrics and Gynecology 106(4):841–4

Breugelmans M, Naessens A, Foulou W 2004 Prevention of toxoplasmosis during pregnancy – an epidemiologic survey over 22 consecutive years. Journal of Perinatal Medicine 32(3):211–14

Bromberger P, Lawrence J M, Braun D et al 2000 The influence of intrapartum antibiotics on the clinical spectrum of early-onset group B streptococcal infection in term infants. Pediatrics 106 (Pt 1):244–50

CEMACH (Confidential Enquiry into Maternal and Child Health) 2005 Pregnancy in women with type 1 and type 2 diabetes in 2002–2003, England, Wales and Northern Ireland. CEMACH, London

CESDI (Confidential Enquiries into Stillbirths and Deaths in Infancy) Project 27/28. 2003 An enquiry into quality of care and its effect on the survival of babies born at 27–28 weeks (ed Mary Macintosh). TSO, Norwich

Chasnoff I J, Griffith D R, Freier C et al 1992 Cocaine/polydrug use in pregnancy: two year follow-up. Pediatrics; 89(2):284–9

Collins J W Jr, Hoppe M, Brown K et al 1991 A controlled trial of insulin infusion and parenteral nutrition in extremely low birth weight infants with glucose intolerance. Journal of Pediatrics 118(6):921–7

Committee on Drugs, American Academy of Pediatrics 1989 Transfer of drugs and other chemicals into human milk. Pediatrics 84:924–36

Committee on Drugs, American Academy of Pediatrics 1998 Neonatal drug withdrawal. Pediatrics 101(6):1079–88

Costeloe K, Hennessy E, Gibson A T et al. 2000 The EPIcure study: outcomes to discharge from hospital for infants born at the threshold of viability. Pediatrics 106(4):659–71

Craparo F J, Bonati F, Gementi P et al 2005 The effects of serial intravascular transfusions in ascitic/hydropic-alloimmunized fetuses. Ultrasound in Obstetrics and Gynecology 25(2):144–8

Crowther C A, Middleton P 1997 Anti-D administration after childbirth for preventing Rhesus

alloimmunisation. Cochrane Database of Systematic Reviews 1997, Issue 2. Art. No. CD000021. doi: 10.1002/14651858.CD000021

Crowther C A, Middleton P, McBain R D 2013 Anti-D administration during pregnancy for preventing Rhesus alloimmunization. Cochrane Database of Systematic Reviews 2013, Issue 2. Art. No. CD000020. doi: 10.1002/14651858.CD000020. pub2

de Cueto M, Sanchez M J, Sampedro A et al 1998 Timing of intrapartum ampicillin and prevention of vertical transmission of group B streptococcus. Obstetrics and Gynecology 91(1):112–14

de Louvois J, Halket S, Harvey D 2005 Neonatal meningitis in England and Wales: sequelae at 5 years of age. European Journal of Pediatrics 164(12):730–4

Degani S 2006 Sonographic findings in fetal viral infections: a systematic review. Obstetrical and Gynecological Survey 61(5):329–36

Dinsmoor M J, Viloria R, Lief L et al 2005 Use of intrapartum antibiotics and the incidence of postnatal maternal and neonatal yeast infections. Obstetrics and Gynecology 106 (1):19–22

Dobbs R H, Cremer R J 1975 Phototherapy. Archives of Disease in Childhood 50(11):833–6

Edmondson M B, Stoddard J J, Owens L M 1997 Hospital admission with feeding-related-problems after early postpartum discharge of normal newborns. Journal of the American Medical Association 278(4):299–303

Enders G, Pacher U N, Miller E et al 1988 Outcome of confirmed periconceptional maternal rubella. Lancet 1(8600):1445–6

Finer N, Barrington K J. 2006 Nitric oxide for respiratory failure in infants born at or near term. Cochrane Database of Systematic Reviews 2006, Issue 4. Art. No. CD000399. doi: 10.1002/14651858. CD000399.pub2

Finnegan L P, Kron R E, Connaughton J F et al 1975 Assessment and treatment of abstinence in the infant of the drug dependent mother. International Journal of Clinical Pharmacology and Biopharmacy 12(1-2):19–32

Finning K, Martin P, Daniels G 2004 A clinical service in the UK to predict fetal Rh (Rhesus) D blood group using free fetal DNA in maternal plasma. Annals of the New York Academy of Sciences 1022:119–23

Fisher D A, Dussault J H, Foley T P et al 1979 Screening for congenital hypothyroidism: results of screening one million North American infants. Journal of Pediatrics 94(5):700–5

Fulroth R, Phillips B, Durand D 1989 Perinatal outcome of infants exposed to cocaine and/or heroin in utero. American Journal of Diseases of Children 143(8):905–10

Fyler D C 1980 Congenital heart disease (CHD) in the newborn: presentation and screening for critical CHD. Report of the New England Regional Infant Cardiac Program. Pediatrics 65(Suppl):375–461

Geifman-Holtzman O, Grotegut C A, Gaughan J P 2006 Diagnostic accuracy of noninvasive fetal Rh genotyping from maternal blood – a meta-analysis. American Journal of Obstetrics and Gynecology 195(4):1163–73

Ghi T, Brondelli L, Simonazzi G et al 2004 Sonographic demonstration of brain injury in fetuses with severe red blood cell alloimmunization undergoing intrauterine transfusions. Ultrasound in Obstetrics and Gynecology 23(5):428–31

Gilbert R, Tan H K, Cliffe S et al 2006 Symptomatic toxoplasma infection due to congenital and postnatally acquired infection. Archives of Disease in Childhood 91(6):495–8

Gottstein R, Cooke R W I 2003 Systematic review of intravenous immunoglobulin in haemolytic disease of the newborn. Archives of Disease in Childhood Fetal and Neonatal Edition 88(1):F6–F10

Greenough A, Milner A D 2012 Acute respiratory disease. In: Rennie J M (ed), Rennie and Roberton's textbook of neonatology, 5th edn. Churchill Livingstone, Edinburgh, ch27.2, p 468–551

Hadeed A J, Siegel S R 1989 Maternal cocaine use during pregnancy: effect on the newborn infant. Pediatrics 84(2):205–10

Hawdon J M, Ward Platt M P, Aynsley-Green A 1992 Patterns of metabolic adaptation for pre-term and term infants in the first neonatal week. Archives of Disease in Childhood 67(4):357–65

Hayakawa M, Kimura H, Ohshiro M et al 2003 Varicella exposure in a neonatal medical centre: successful prophylaxis with oral acyclovir. Journal of Hospital Infection 54(3):212–15

Heath P T, Balfour G, Weisner A M et al. 2004 Group B streptococcal disease in UK and Irish infants younger than 90 days. Lancet 363 (9405):292–4

Herzlinger R A, Kandall S R, Vaughan H G 1977 Neonatal seizures associated with narcotic withdrawal. Journal of Pediatrics 91(4):638–41

Hughes I A, Houk C, Ahmed S F et al 2006 LWPES/ESPE Consensus Group Consensus statement on management of inter-sex disorders. Archives of Disease in Childhood 91(7):554–63

Isaacs D, Moxon R 1999 Handbook of neonatal infections: a practical guide. W B Saunders, London, p 423–34

Jacobs S E, Berg M, Hunt R et al 2013 Cooling for newborns with hypoxic ischaemic encephalopathy. Cochrane Database of Systematic Reviews 2013, Issue 1. Art. No. CD003311. doi: 10.1002/14651858.CD003311. pub3

Jain A 2012 Temperature control and disorders. In: Rennie J M (ed), Rennie and Roberton's textbook of neonatology, 5th edn. Churchill Livingstone, Edinburgh, ch 15, p 263–76

Joy S D, Rossi K Q, Krugh D et al 2005 Management of pregnancies complicated by anti-E alloimmunization. Obstetrics and Gynecology 105(1):24–8

Kandall S R, Albin S, Lowinson J et al 1976 Differential effects of maternal heroin and methadone use on birthweight. Pediatrics 58(5):681–5

Kaplan M, Muraca M, Vreman H J et al 2005 Neonatal bilirubin production-conjugation imbalance: effect of glucose-6-phosphate dehydrogenase deficiency and borderline prematurity. Archives of Disease in Childhood: Fetal and Neonatal Edition 90(2):F123–7

Kenyon S, Boulvain M, Neilson J 2010 Antibiotics for preterm rupture of membranes (Cochrane Review). Cochrane Database of Systematic

Reviews 2010, Issue 2. Art. No. CD001058. doi: 10.1002/14651858. CD001058.pub2

Koh T H H G, Aynsley-Green A, Tarbit M et al 1988a Neural dysfunction during hypoglycaemia. Archives of Disease in Childhood 63(11):1353–8

Koh T H H G, Eyre J A, Aynsley-Green A 1988b Neonatal hypoglycaemia – the controversy regarding definition. Archives of Disease in Childhood 63(11):1386–8

Koren G, Shear H, Graham K et al 1989 Bias against the null hypothesis: the reproductive hazards of cocaine. Lancet 334(8677):1440–2

Kumar S L, Dhanireddy R. 1995 Time to first stool in premature infants: effect of gestational age and illness severity. Journal of Pediatrics 127(6):971–4

Lau S P, Fung K P 1984 Serum bilirubin kinetics in intermittent phototherapy of physiological jaundice. Archives of Disease in Childhood 59:892–4

Law M R, Palomaki G, Alfirevic Z et al 2005 The prevention of neonatal group B streptococcal disease: a report by a working group of the Medical Screening Society. Journal of Medical Screening 12(2):60–8

Lawn C, Alton N 2012 The baby of the substance abusing mother. In: Rennie J M (ed) Rennie and Roberton's textbook of neonatology, 5th edn. Churchill Livingstone, Edinburgh, ch 26, p 431–42

Levene M I, Sands C, Grindulis H et al 1986 Comparison of two methods of predicting outcome in perinatal asphyxia. Lancet 1(8472):67–9

Lifschitz M H, Wilson G H, Smith E O et al 1985 Factors affecting head growth and intellectual function in children of drug addicts. Pediatrics 75(2):269–74

Lissauer T, Faranoff A A 2006 Neonatology at a glance, 2nd edn. Blackwell Science, London

Lucas A, Fewtrell M S, Morley R et al 1996 Randomized outcome trial of human milk fortification and developmental outcome in preterm infants. American Journal of Clinical Nutrition 64(2):142–51

Lucas A, Morley R, Cole T J 1988 Adverse neurodevelopmental outcome of moderate neonatal hypoglycaemia. British Medical Journal 297(6659):1304–8

Manning D, Todd P, Maxwell M et al 2007 Prospective surveillance study of severe hyperbilirubinaemia in the newborn in the UK and Ireland. Archives of Disease in Childhood Fetal and Neonatal Edition 92(5):342–6

Mari G, Zimmermann R, Moise K J et al 2005 Correlation between middle cerebral artery peak systolic velocity and fetal hemoglobin after 2 previous intrauterine transfusions. American Journal of Obstetrics and Gynecology 193(3):1117–20

May M, Daley A J, Donath S et al 2005 Early onset neonatal meningitis in Australia and New Zealand, 1992–2002. Archives of Disease in Childhood 90(4):F324–7

Merenstein G V, Gardner S L 2011 Merenstein & Gardner's handbook of neonatal intensive care, 7th edn. Mosby, St Louis

Metaj M, Laroia N, Lawrence R A et al 2003 Comparison of breast- and formula-fed normal newborns in time to first stool and urine. Journal of Perinatology 23: 624–8.

Meyberg-Solomayer G C, Fehm T, Muller-Hansen I et al 2006 Prenatal ultrasound diagnosis, follow-up, and outcome of congenital varicella syndrome. Fetal Diagnosis and Therapy 21(3):296–301

Miqdad A M, Abdelbasit O B, Shaheed M M et al 2004 Intravenous immunoglobulin G (IVIG) therapy for significant hyperbilirubinemia in ABO hemolytic disease of the newborn. Journal of Maternal-Fetal and Neonatal Medicine 16(3):163–6

Montoya J G, Liesenfeld O 2004 Toxoplasmosis. Lancet 363(9425):1965–76

Morley C J, Davis P G, Doyle L W et al 2008 Nasal CPAP or intubation at birth for very preterm infants. New England Journal of Medicine 358(7):700–8

Morrill J F, Heinig M J, Pappagianis D et al 2005 Risk factors for mammary candidosis among lactating women. Journal of Obstetric, Gynecologic and Neonatal Nursing 34(1):37–45

Morrison J J, Rennie J M, Milton P J 1995 Neonatal respiratory morbidity and mode of delivery at term: influence of timing of elective caesarian section. British Journal of

Section | 6 | The Neonate

Obstetrics and Gynaecology
102(2):101–6

NICE (National Institute for Clinical
Excellence) 2008 Routine antenatal
anti-D prophylaxis for women who
are rhesus D negative. Review of
NICE technology appraisal guidance
41. www.nice.org.uk (accessed 10
August 2013)

NICE (National Institute for Clinical
Excellence) 2010 Neonatal jaundice.
CG 98. www.nice.org.uk/guidance/
CG98 (accessed 10 August 2013)

NHS Choices 2013 Toxoplasmosis www
.nhs.uk/conditions/Toxoplasmosis/
Pages/Introduction.aspx (accessed 10
August 2013)

Oddie S, Embleton N D, 2002 On
behalf of the Northern Neonatal
Network. Risk factors for early onset
neonatal group B streptococcal
sepsis: case-control study. British
Medical Journal 325:308

Oddie S, Richmond S, Coulthard M
2001 Hypernatraemic dehydration
and breast feeding: a population
study. Archives of Disease in
Childhood 85(4):318–20

Oepkes D, Seaward G, Vandenbussche F
P H A et al 2006 Doppler
ultrasonography versus
amniocentesis to predict fetal
anemia. New England Journal of
Medicine 355(2):156–64

Özek E, Soll R, Schimmel M S 2010
Partial exchange transfusion to
prevent neurodevelopmental
disability in infants with
polycythemia. Cochrane Database
of Systematic Reviews 2010, Issue 1.
Art. No. CD005089. doi:
10.1002/14651858.CD005089.pub2

Pylipow M, Gaddis M, Kinney J S 1994
Selective intrapartum prophylaxis for
group B streptococcus colonization:
management and outcome of
newborns. Pediatrics 93(4):631–5

RCOG (Royal College of Obstetricians
and Gynaecologists) 2012 Prevention
of early-onset neonatal group B
streptococcal disease. Green-top
Guideline No. 36, 2nd edn. www
.rcog.org.uk/files/rcog-corp/GTG36
_GBS.pdf (accessed 10 August
2013)

Robinson J L, Lee B E, Preiksaitis J K
et al 2006 Prevention of congenital
rubella syndrome – what makes
sense in 2006? Epidemiologic
Reviews 28(1):81–7

Sarnat H B, Sarnat M S 1976 Neonatal
encephalopathy following fetal
distress: a clinical and
electroencephalographic study.
Archives of Neurology
33(10):696–705

Sauerbrei A, Wutzler P 2000 The
congenital varicella syndrome.
Journal of Perinatology
20(8):548–54

Schmidt D R, Hogh B, Andersen O
et al 2006 The national neonatal
screening programme for congenital
toxoplasmosis in Denmark: results
from the initial four years, 1999–
2002. Archives of Disease in
Childhood 91(8):661–5

Shankaran S, Laptook A R, Ehrenkranz
R A et al 2005 Whole-body
hypothermia for neonates with
hypoxic-ischemic encephalopathy.
New England Journal of Medicine
353(15):1574–84

Skuza K A, Sills I N, Rapaport R
1996 Prediction of neonatal
hyperthyroidism in infants born to
mothers with Graves' disease. Journal
of Pediatrics 128(2):264–8

Smolinski K N, Shah S S, Honig P J
et al 2005 Neonatal cutaneous
fungal infections. Current Opinion
in Pediatrics 17(4):486–93

Srinivasan G, Pildes R S, Cattamanchi G
et al 1986 Plasma glucose values in
normal neonates: a new look.
Journal of Pediatrics 109:114–17

Steele R W, Metz J R, Bass J W et al
1971 Pneumothorax and
pneumomediastinum in the
newborn. Radiology 98:629–32

Stephens R H, Benjammin A R, Walters
D V 1998 The regulation of lung
liquid absorption by endogenous
cAMP in postnatal sheep lungs
perfused in situ http://dx.doi
.org/10.1111%2Fj.1469-7793
.1998.587bh.x (accessed 10
August 2013)

Stokowski L A 2006 Fundamentals of
phototherapy for neonatal jaundice.
Advances in Neonatal Care
6(6):303–12

SUPPORT Study (2010) Group of the
Eunice Kennedy Shriver NICHD
Neonatal Research Network. Early
CPAP versus surfactant in extremely
preterm infants. New England
Journal of Medicine 362(21):1970–9

Sutton L R, Hinderliter S A 1990
Diazepam abuse in pregnant women

on methadone maintenance.
Implications for the neonate.
Clinical Pediatrics 29(2):108–11

SYROCOT (Systematic Review on
Congenital Toxoplasmosis) Study
Group 2007 Effectiveness of prenatal
treatment for congenital
toxoplasmosis: a meta-analysis of
individual patients' data. Lancet
369(9556):115–22

Teng C S, Tong T C, Hutchinson J H
et al 1980 Thyroid stimulating
immunoglobulins in neonatal
Graves' disease. Archives of Disease
in Childhood 55:894–5

Theis J G W, Selby P, Ikizler Y et al 1997
Current management of the neonatal
abstinence syndrome: a critical
analysis of the evidence. Biology of
the Neonate 71(6):345–56

Tracy S K, Tracy M B, Sullivan E 2007
Admissions of term infants to
neonatal intensive care: a population
based study. Birth 34(4):301–7

UK Collaborative ECMO Trial Group
1996 UK collaborative randomized
trial of neonatal extracorporeal
membrane oxygenation. Lancet
348(9020):75–82

UKNSC (United Kingdom National
Screening Committee) 2012
Screening for group B streptococcal
infection in pregnancy. External
review against programme appraisal
criteria for the UK National
Screening Committee (UK NSC)
Version: 3. www.screening.nhs.uk/
groupbstreptococcus (accessed 10
August 2013)

Ungerer R L S, Lincetto O, Gulmezoglu
A M et al 2004 Prophylactic versus
selective antibiotics for term
newborn infants of mothers with
risk factors for neonatal infection.
Cochrane Database of Systematic
Reviews 2004, Issue 2. Art. No.
CD003957. doi: 10.1002/14651858.
CD003957

van den Hout L, Reiss I, Felix J F et al
2010 Congenital Diaphragmatic
Hernia Study Group. Risk factors for
chronic lung disease and mortality
in newborns with congenital
diaphragmatic hernia. Neonatology
98(4):370–80

van Dommelen P, van Wouwe J P,
Breuning-Boers J M et al 2007
Reference chart for relative weight
change to detect hypernatraemic
dehydration. Archives of Disease in
Childhood 92 (6):490–4

700

van Dongen H, Klumper F J C M, Sikkel E et al 2005 Non-invasive tests to predict fetal anemia in Kell-alloimmunized pregnancies. Ultrasound in Obstetrics and Gynecology 25(4):341–5

van Kamp I L, Klumper F J C M, Oepkes D et al 2005 Complications of intrauterine intravascular transfusion for fetal anemia due to maternal red-cell alloimmunization. American Journal of Obstetrics and Gynecology 192 (1):165–70

Vannucci R C 1990 Current and potentially new management strategies for perinatal hypoxic-ischemic encephalopathy. Pediatrics 85(6):961–8

Walls M, Wright A, Fowlie P et al 2004 Home phototherapy: a feasible, safe and acceptable practice. Journal of Neonatal Nursing 10(3):92–4

Wraith J E, Walker J H 1996 Inherited metabolic disorders diagnosis and initial management. Willink Biochemical Genetics Unit, Royal Manchester Children's Hospital, Manchester

Wright J C E, Budd J L S, Field D J et al 2010 Epidemiology and outcome of congenital diaphragmatic hernia: a 9-year experience. Paediatric and Perinatal Epidemiology 25(2):144–9

Wright J A, Polack C 2006 Understanding variation in measles–mumps–rubella immunization coverage – a population-based study. European Journal of Public Health 16(2):137–42

Zuckerman B, Frank D A, Hingson R et al 1989 Effects of maternal marijuana and cocaine use on fetal growth. New England Journal of Medicine 320:762–8

FURTHER READING

Wylie L 2010 Newborn screening and immunization. In: Lumsden H, Holmes D (eds), Care of the newborn by ten teachers. Hodder Arnold, London, p 51–64

This chapter provides further information on all conditions that are screened by blood spot at present, to include medium-chain *acyl CoA dehydrogenase deficiency (MCADD), cystic fibrosis and sickle cell disease.*

WEBSITES

GBS Support: www.gbss.org.uk

National Society for Phenylketonuria: www.nspku.org

Chapter |34|

Infant feeding

Sally Inch

Midwives have a key role in supporting mothers to breastfeed successfully. It is strongly in the interest of both individual mothers and the community as a whole that those who chose to breastfeed are enabled to do so for as long as they want. The reasons women give for discontinuation are consistent over time and internationally: they think they do not have enough milk, breastfeeding is painful and they have problems getting the baby to feed. Preventing these distressing problems requires a multifaceted approach that has to start with effective, practical and evidence-based training of all those who offer help and support to

Author's note: In this chapter, where the masculine pronoun has been used to refer to a baby this is simply to avoid the cumbersome 'he or she' and to more clearly distinguish the baby from the mother.

breastfeeding mothers, especially in the first week of their baby's life.

For those mothers who cannot, or choose not to breastfeed, the midwife has an equally important role in ensuring that the baby is fed safely and appropriately.

THE CHAPTER AIMS TO:

- explain the structure and function of the female breast
- describe the properties and components of breastmilk
- emphasize the role of the midwife in ensuring breastfeeding success for both mother and baby
- discuss the role of breastmilk expression and human milk banking
- describe the different causes of difficulty with breastfeeding
- discuss the use of formula feeding and the various products available
- outline the requirements and recommendations of the International Code of Marketing of Breastmilk Substitutes and the Baby Friendly Hospital Initiative

INTRODUCTION

Breastfeeding for the first 6 months of life is the ideal start for babies. Breastfeeding improves infant and maternal health and cognitive development in both developed and developing countries, and it is the single most important preventive approach for saving children's lives (Renfrew and Hall 2008). Low breastfeeding rates in the United Kingdom (UK) have led to a progressive increase in the incidence of illness that has a significant cost to the National Health Service (NHS). Recent calculations from a mere handful of illnesses (where breastfeeding is thought to have a protective effect and enough data existed to determine total cost of care expected for each episode of a particular disease) revealed potential annual savings to the NHS from a moderate increase in breastfeeding rates of about £40 million per year (Renfrew et al 2012). The true cost savings are likely to be much higher (UNICEF–UK 2012a).

The problems that deter women from breastfeeding can mostly be prevented (Renfrew and Hall 2008). This requires a multi-faceted approach, with implementation of the UNICEF–UK Baby Friendly Initiative at its core (NICE 2008).

THE BREAST AND BREASTMILK

Anatomy and physiology of the breast (Fig. 34.1)

The breasts are compound secreting glands, composed of varying proportions of fat, glandular and connective tissue, and arranged in lobes. Each lobe is divided into lobules consisting of alveoli and ducts.

Because of the intimate and congruous connection between fat and glandular tissue within the breast (Nickell

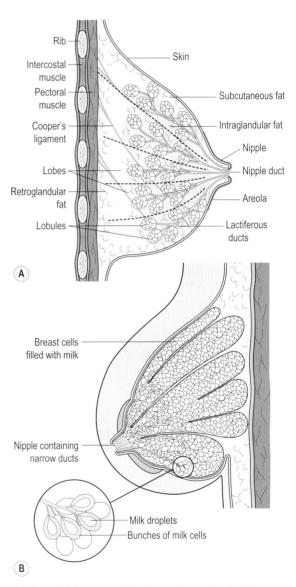

Fig. 34.1 (A) Anatomy of the breast (reproduced with permission of Liz Ellis). (B) Cross-section of the breast.

and Skelton 2005), the relative proportion of fat to glandular tissue is difficult to calculate non-invasively. However, analysis of 21 non-lactating breasts (surgically removed for carcinoma in situ) (Vandeweyer and Hertens 2002) revealed that the percentage weight of fat per breast varied from 3.6 to 37.6. Mammographic studies of non-lactating breasts have reported breast glandularity decreasing with age (Jamal et al 2004).

Investigations carried out on 25 sections of central breast tissue removed during breast reduction operations performed on women with an average body mass index (BMI) of 28, found a mean of 61% fat (Cruz-Korchin et al 2002). On average, the women's central breast area contained only 7% glandular tissue and 29% connective tissue. This finding, that larger breasts contain relatively more fat, is supported by an observational study of 136 patients with an average BMI of 32, undergoing breast reduction surgery (Nickell and Skelton 2005).

Research on the volumes of 20 complete duct systems (*lobes*) in an autopsied breast, found considerable variation in the proportion of breast tissue serviced by each duct. The largest lobe drained 23% of breast volume, 50% of the breast was drained by three ducts and 75% by the largest six. Conversely, eight small duct systems together accounted for only 1.6% of breast volume (Going and Moffat 2004).

Ultrasound investigations of the *lactating* breasts of 21 subjects (Ramsay et al 2005) identified nine or so milk ducts per breast (range being 4–18), fewer than previously believed but commensurate with the investigations conducted by Love and Barsky (2004). Taneri et al (2006) examined 226 mastectomy specimens and found the mean number of ducts in the nipple duct bundle was 17.5. This is significantly higher than the number reported to open on the nipple surface. They reflected that this discrepancy could be due to duct branching within the nipple or the presence of some ducts that do not reach the nipple surface.

Taken together, the intimate and inseparable relationship between fat and glandular tissue, the uneven distribution of milk glands and the high variability in the number of milk ducts, have implications for those women who require breast surgery. This is especially the case with women who have breast reduction surgery, as the loss of only a few ducts may inadvertently compromise a woman's future ability to breastfeed (see below).

The *alveoli* contain milk-producing *acini cells*, surrounded by myoepithelial cells, which contract and propel the milk out (Fig. 34.2). Small lactiferous ducts, carrying milk from the alveoli, unite to form larger ducts. Several large ducts (lactiferous tubules) conveying milk from one or more lobes emerge on the surface of the nipple. Myoepithelial cells are oriented longitudinally along the ducts and, under the influence of oxytocin, these smooth muscle cells contract and the tubule becomes shorter and wider (Woolridge 1986; Ramsay et al 2004). The tubule distends during active milk flow, while the myoepithelial cells are

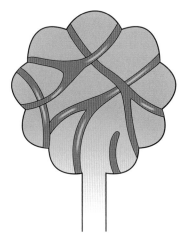

Fig. 34.2 Alveoli surrounded by myoepithelial cells, which propel the milk out of the lobule.

maintained in a state of contraction by circulating oxytocin for about 2–3 minutes. The fuller the breast when let-down occurs, the greater the degree of ductal distension (Ramsay et al 2004).

The human *nipple*, in common with other mammalian nipples, is covered with epithelium and contains cylindrically arranged smooth muscle and elastic fibres. When this contracts and the nipple becomes erect, a tight sphincter is formed at the end of the teat (Cross 1977) to prevent unwanted loss of milk from the mammary gland when it is not being suckled.

Surrounding the nipple is an area of pigmented skin called the *areola*, which contains Montgomery's glands. These produce a sebum-like substance, which acts as a lubricant during pregnancy and throughout breastfeeding. Breasts, nipples and areolae vary considerably in size from one woman to another.

The breast is supplied with blood from the internal and external mammary arteries and branches from the intercostal arteries. The veins are arranged in a circular fashion around the nipple. Lymph drains freely from the two breasts into lymph nodes in the axillae and the mediastinum.

During pregnancy, oestrogens and progesterone induce alveolar and ductal growth, and stimulate the secretion of colostrum. Other hormones (such as growth hormone, prolactin, epidermal growth factor, fibroblast growth factor, human placental lactogen, parathyroid hormone-related protein and insulin-like growth factor) are involved, governing a complex sequence of events that prepares the breast for lactation (Neville et al 2002).

Lactogenesis

Once the alveolar epithelial cells have developed into lactocytes, around mid pregnancy (Lactogenesis I), they are able to produce small quantities of secretion: colostrum. Although some women may produce as much as 30 ml per day in late pregnancy (Cox et al 1999), the production of milk is held in abeyance until after 30–40 hours following the birth, when levels of placental hormones have fallen sufficiently to allow the already high levels of prolactin to initiate milk production (Lactogenesis II). Continued production of prolactin is caused by touch, as the baby feeds at the breast, with concentrations highest during night feeds. Prolactin is involved in the suppression of ovulation, and some women may remain anovular until lactation ceases, although for others the effect is not so prolonged (Kennedy et al 1989; Ramos et al 1996) (see Chapter 27).

Maternal nutritional intake and nutritional status are known to affect birth outcome, and the fetus *in utero*. The mother's diet during pregnancy may also *programme* the fetus, affecting health in adult life (Hall Moran 2012), but the effects of maternal nutrition on the development of the mammary gland in pregnancy are less well known. Evidence from rats (Kim and Parks 2004) suggests that undernutrition may actually enhance cell growth and milk production. Torgersen et al (2010) found no differences in the risk of cessation of exclusive breastfeeding in mothers with and without eating disorders. Overnutrition (*obesity*), however, has been shown to adversely affect lactogenesis II (Rasmussen 2007).

If breastfeeding (or expressing) is delayed for a few days, lactation can still be initiated because prolactin levels remain high, even in the absence of breast use, for at least the first week (Kochenour 1980). However, the establishment of lactation is more secure if breastfeeding or expressing begins as soon after birth as possible.

Prolactin seems to be much more important to the initiation of lactation than to its continuation. As lactation progresses, the prolactin response to suckling diminishes and milk removal becomes the driving force behind milk production. This is known to be due to the presence in secreted milk of a whey protein that is able to inhibit the synthesis of milk constituents (Prentice et al 1989; Daly 1993; Wilde et al 1995).

The protein collects in the breast as the milk accumulates, exerting negative feedback control on the continued production of milk. Removal of this autocrine inhibitory factor (sometimes referred to as *Feedback Inhibitor of Lactation: FIL*) by extracting the milk, allows milk production to accelerate.

Because this mechanism acts locally within the breast, each breast can function independently of the other. It is also the reason that milk production slows as the baby is gradually weaned from the breast. If necessary, it can be increased again if the baby is put back to the breast more often, perhaps because of illness.

Milk is synthesized continuously into the alveolar lumen, where it is stored until milk removal from the breast is initiated. Only when oxytocin is released, and the myoepithelial cells contract, is milk made available to the suckling baby. Milk release is under neuroendocrine control. Tactile stimulation of the breast also stimulates the oxytocin, causing contraction of the myoepithelial cells. This process is known as the *let-down* or *milk-ejection* reflex and makes the milk available to the baby. This occurs in discrete pulses throughout the feed and may trigger bursts of active feeding.

In the early days of lactation, this reflex is unconditioned. Later, as it becomes a conditioned reflex, the mother may find her breasts responding to the baby's cry or other circumstances associated with the baby or feeding. In one small study, psychological stress (mental arithmetic or noise) was found to reduce the frequency of the oxytocin pulses without affecting the amplitude of the pulse. Neither was there any effect on either prolactin levels or the amount of milk the baby received (Ueda et al 1994).

Milk production and the mother

The human mother manages the process of lactation in an entirely different way from her non-primate counterpart. Much of the mis-information to which women are subjected derives from extrapolation from veterinary and dairy science (Woolridge 1995). Adequate milk production is largely independent of the mother's nutritional status and BMI (Prentice et al 1994).

Dietary surveys in developed countries have consistently found calorie intake to be less than the recommended amount (Whitehead et al 1981; Butte et al 1984). Controlled trials conducted in developing countries have demonstrated that giving extra food to mothers, even those who were poorly nourished, did not increase the rate of growth of their babies (Prentice et al 1980, 1983). It has been suggested that metabolic efficiency is enhanced in lactating women, thus enabling them to conserve energy and subsidize the cost of their milk production (Illingworth et al 1986).

The lactational performance of the human female is compromised when undernutrition is sufficiently severe, but it appears that this occurs only in famine or near-famine conditions. As milk production appears to drive appetite, rather than the reverse, hunger effectively regulates the calorie intake of a breastfeeding woman, and the practice of encouraging breastfeeding mothers to eat excessively should be abandoned. Similarly, if healthy breastfeeding women wish to undertake strenuous exercise from 6–8 weeks after birth, or to lose weight (500–1000 g/week), they can be assured that neither the quality nor the quantity of their milk will be affected (Dewey et al 1994; Dusdieker et al 1994). Exclusive breastfeeding combined with low fat diet and exercise will result in more effective weight loss than diet and exercise alone (Hammer et al 1996; Dewey 1998).

Milk production is similarly unaffected by fluctuations in the woman's fluid intake. It has been repeatedly demonstrated that neither a significant decrease (Dearlove and Dearlove 1981) nor a significant increase (Morse et al 1992) in maternal fluid intake has any effect on milk production or the baby's weight.

Properties and components of breastmilk

Human milk varies in its composition:

- with the time of day (e.g. fat content is lowest in the morning and highest in the afternoon)
- with the stage of lactation (e.g. the fat and protein content of colostrum is higher than in mature milk)
- in response to maternal nutrition (e.g. although the *total amount* of fat is not influenced by diet, the *type* of fat that appears in the milk will be influenced by what the mother eats)
- because of individual variations.

The most dramatic change in the composition of milk occurs during the course of a feed (Hall 1979). At the beginning of the feed the baby receives a high volume of relatively low fat milk (the foremilk). As the feed progresses, the volume of milk decreases but the proportion of fat in the milk increases, sometimes to as much as five times the initial value (the hindmilk) (Jackson et al 1987). The baby's ability to obtain this fat-rich milk is not determined by the length of time he spent sucking at the breast, but by the quality of the attachment to the breast. The baby needs to be well attached so that the tongue can be used to maximum effect, stripping the milk from the breast, rather than relying solely on the mother's milk ejection reflex. A poorly attached baby may have difficulty in obtaining enough fat to meet their needs, resorting to very frequent feeds to obtain sufficient calories from low-fat feeds. A well-attached baby may, however, obtain all he requires in a very short time.

The length of the feed, provided that the baby is well attached, is thus determined by the rate of milk transfer from mother to baby. If milk transfer occurs at a high rate, feeds will be relatively short; if it occurs slowly, feeds will be longer (Woolridge et al 1982) (Fig. 34.3). Milk transfer seems to be more efficient (and thus feeds are shorter) in a second lactation than in a first (Ingram et al 2001).

Fats and fatty acids

For the human baby, with its unique and rapidly growing brain, fat, not protein, in human milk has particular significance. Some 98% of the lipid in human milk is in the form of triglycerides: three fatty acids linked to a single molecule of glycerol. More than 100 fatty acids have so far been identified, about 46% being saturated fat and 54% unsaturated fat. Over the past decade, there has been an explosion of interest in the unsaturated fatty acid content of human milk, particularly in the long chain

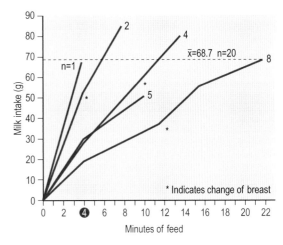

Fig. 34.3 Pattern of milk intake at a feed for 20 6-day-old babies.
From Woolridge et al 1982, with permission.

polyunsaturated variety (LC-PUFAs), because of their role in brain growth and myelination (Fernstrom 1999). Two of them, arachidonic acid (AA) and docosahexanoic acid (DHA) appear to play an important role in the development of the retina and visual cortex of the newborn. Fat also provides babies with >50% of their calorific requirements (Picciano 2001). Fat is utilized very rapidly because the milk itself contains the enzyme bile-salt-stimulated lipase, needed for fat digestion, but in a form that becomes active only when it reaches the baby's intestine. Pancreatic lipase is not plentiful in the newborn, so a baby who is not fed human milk is less able to digest fat.

Cholesterol, a risk factor for coronary heart disease (CHD) in adults, occurs in human milk at higher levels than are currently present in infant formulae (Kamelska et al 2012). However, these high levels not only play an important role in brain growth and development (Scholtz et al 2013), but also paradoxically lower the cholesterol concentration in blood in later life (Owen et al 2008).

Carbohydrate

The carbohydrate component of human milk is provided chiefly by lactose, providing the baby with about 40% of calorific requirements. Lactose is converted into galactose and glucose by the action of the enzyme lactase in order to be more readily metabolized and absorbed. These sugars provide energy to the rapidly growing brain. Lactose enhances the absorption of calcium, promoting the growth of lactobacilli, which increase intestinal acidity thus reducing the growth of pathogenic organisms in the baby.

Protein

Human milk contains less protein than any other mammalian milk (Akre 1989a). This accounts in part for its more transparent appearance. Human milk is whey-dominant, which is mainly α-lactalbumin, and forms soft, flocculent curds when acidified in the stomach.

Allergies occur less frequently in breastfed babies than in those fed with formula milk. This may be because the infant's intestinal mucosa is permeable to proteins before the age of 6–9 months and proteins in cow's milk can act as allergens. In particular, bovine β-lactoglobulin, which has no human milk protein counterpart, is capable of producing antigenic responses in atopic infants (Bahna 1987; Adler and Warner 1991).

Occasionally a baby may react adversely to substances in their mother's milk that come from her diet. However, this is rare and can usually be resolved by the mother identifying and avoiding the foods that cause the adverse reaction so that she may continue to breastfeed. Another bovine whey protein, bovine serum albumin, has been implicated as the trigger for the development of insulin-dependent diabetes mellitus (Vaarala et al 1999; Paronen et al 2000).

Vitamins

All the vitamins required for good nutrition and health are supplied in breastmilk, and although the actual amounts vary from mother to mother, none of the normal variations poses any risk to the infant (Hopkinson 2007).

Fat-soluble vitamins

Vitamin A

Vitamin A is present in human milk as retinol, retinyl esters and beta carotene. Colostrum contains twice the amount present in mature human milk, giving colostrum its yellow colour. Bile-salt-stimulated lipase (present in human milk: see Fatty acids, above) assists the hydrolysation of the retinyl esters and may account for the rarity of vitamin A deficiency in breastfed babies in affluent societies (Fredrikzon et al 1978; Leaf 2007).

Vitamin D

Vitamin D plays an essential role in the metabolism of calcium and phosphorus in the body, preventing osteomalacia in adults and rickets in children. It is not strictly a vitamin, but a hormone triggered by ultraviolet light. The principal unfortified dietary source of vitamin D is fish liver oils, with butter, eggs and cheese contributing much smaller amounts. In the UK, only margarine fortification with 2800–3520 IU/kg of vitamin D is compulsory. In other countries, vitamin D fortification of various other foods is either compulsory or permitted.

Vitamin D is the name given to two fat-soluble compounds: *calciferol* (vitamin D_2) and *cholecalciferol* (vitamin D_3). A plentiful supply of *7-dehydrocholesterol*, the precursor of vitamin D_3, exists in human skin, and needs only to be activated by sufficient ultraviolet light (<30 min of summer sunlight a day) to become fully potent.

For light-skinned babies, exposure to sunlight for 30 minutes per week wearing only a nappy, or 2 hours per week fully clothed but without a hat, keeps vitamin D requirements within the lower limits of the normal range (Specker et al 1985). However, latitude and strength of the sunlight is important. In Scandinavia, photo-conversion of 7-dehydrocholesterol has been found to occur only between March and October, with a maximum in June and July (Moan et al 2008). In the UK, reseachers in Aberdeen found that sunlight exposure in summer and spring provided 80% of the baby's total annual intake of vitamin D (Macdonald et al 2011). Those living in regions where exposure to the sun is low have always been at risk for vitamin D deficiency (Garza and Rasmussen 2000).

In order to ensure adequate stores in the baby's liver at birth, pregnant women would need to maintain own their vitamin D levels at a high enough level to supply sufficient amounts via the placenta, as the concentration of vitamin D in human milk is low. However, social mobility, cultural considerations and concerns over skin cancer from sunlight have increased the risk of vitamin D deficiency by reducing the skin's exposure to sunlight. In the UK this is of particular concern in women and infants of Asian and Afro-Caribbean ethnic origin (Gregory et al 2000; Leaf 2007).

Maternal vitamin D deficiency during pregnancy has been implicated as a risk factor for diabetes, ischaemic heart disease and tuberculosis. In addition to the previously known paediatric problems of hypocalcaemic convulsions, dental enamel hypoplasia, infantile rickets and congenital cataracts in early life, vitamin D deficiency has been shown to affect neonatal head and linear growth and may adversely affect the developing fetal brain (Shaw and Pal 2002).

The National Institute for Health and Clinical Excellence (NICE) (2008) published specific recommendations to guide health professionals in advising women about the benefits of taking a vitamin D supplement of 10 μg per day during pregnancy and while breastfeeding. Such advice is also supported by the Department of Health (DH) (2009). In addition, healthy breastfed babies should receive a vitamin D supplement from 6 months of age as part of a multivitamin supplement. Unless a baby who is being fed on formula milk is considered to be at risk, they would not routinely require any vitamin D supplementation as this will already be contained within the formula milk.

Vitamin E

Although vitamin E is present in human milk, its role is uncertain. It appears to prevent the oxidization of poly-unsaturated fatty acids and may prevent certain types of anaemia to which preterm infants are susceptible.

Vitamin K

Vitamin K is the generic name for a group of structurally similar, fat-soluble vitamins. The two naturally occurring forms of this vitamin are vitamin K1 (phytonadione) found in green leafy vegetables, and K2 (menaquinone), which is synthesized by gut flora. It has been suggested that, by 2 weeks of age, the breastfed baby's gut flora should be synthesizing adequate amounts of vitamin K2 (Akre 1989b).

Vitamin K is essential for the synthesis of blood-clotting factors II, VII, IX and X. It is present in human milk and absorbed efficiently. Because it is fat-soluble, it is present in greater concentrations in colostrum and in the high-fat hindmilk (Kries et al 1987). The increased volume of milk as lactation progresses means that the baby obtains twice as much vitamin K from mature milk than from colostrum (Canfield et al 1991). Greer (1997) found that marked increases in breastmilk concentrations of vitamin K, with corresponding increases in babies' blood levels, can be obtained by giving mothers oral vitamin K, although this subsequently received little attention.

Vitamin K deficiency bleeding (VKDB), formerly called haemorrhagic disease of the newborn, is a coagulation disturbance in newborns due to vitamin K deficiency. The incidence of classic VKDB, occurring between 1 and 7 days of life, ranges from 0.25 to 1.7 cases per 100 births (Willacy 2010). However, those instances where VKDB occurs in the first 24 hours of life are largely confined to the babies of mothers who were taking medications such as isoniazid, rifampicin, anticoagulants and anticonvulsant agents in pregnancy. Late VKDB occurs between 2 weeks and 12 weeks of life and occurs predominantly in exclusively breastfed babies as vitamin K is added to infant formula milks, but may also occur in any baby who is unable to absorb the fat-soluble vitamin K (see Chapter 31).

There has been much debate over which babies are at risk of VKDB, and if supplements should be given after birth and how these should be given. Puckett and Offringa (2000) found that a single intramuscular (IM) dose (1 mg) was more effective than a single oral dose at achieving appropriate plasma vitamin K levels at 2 weeks and 1 month, but achieved lower plasma vitamin K levels than a 3-dose oral schedule at 2 weeks and at 2 months. It was recommended by NICE (2006a) that *all* babies should be offered intramuscular vitamin K within the first 24 hours of birth. However, where parents declined to give consent to the injection, they should be offered an oral form of the vitamin, with the further explanation that this would need to be given several times in the first few weeks to be effective.

In the two years following the issuing of this guidance, Busfield et al (2013) found that all (236) of the consultant maternity units they surveyed were offering vitamin K routinely at birth. In 72% of units it was offered intramuscularly, 20% offered parents a choice and the remaining 8% offered an oral, multidose regime. They identified 11 babies as suffering from VKDB after birth, of these, six had received no prophylaxis (five because the parents withheld consent) and two had received incomplete oral prophylaxis. The remaining three developed VKDB despite intramuscular prophylaxis.

Water-soluble vitamins

Unless the mother's diet is seriously deficient, breastmilk will contain adequate levels of the water-soluble vitamins, B and C. Since they are fairly widely distributed in foods (vitamin C in most fruit and vegetables), a diet significantly deficient in one vitamin will be deficient in others as well. Thus, an improved diet will be more beneficial than artificial supplements. Water-soluble vitamins are actively transported across the placenta throughout pregancy.

Vitamin B complex

Vitamin B complex consists of eight water-soluble vitamins: thiamine (B1), riboflavin (B2), niacin (B3), pantotenic acid (B5), pyridoxine (B6), biotin (B7), folic acid (B9) and cyanocobalamin (B12). All play an important role in metabolism in the body.

Vitamin C

Vitamin C (L-ascorbic acid) is an antioxidant that helps protect cells from free radical damage. It is necessary to form collagen, and thus plays a role in growth and repair of bone, skin and connective tissue. It also assists the body to absorb iron. With some vitamins, e.g. vitamin C and thiamine, a plateau may be reached where increased maternal intake has no further impact on breastmilk

Minerals and trace elements

Iron

Healthy term babies are usually born with a high haemoglobin level (16–22 g/dl), which decreases rapidly after birth. The iron recovered from haemoglobin breakdown is re-utilized. Babies also have ample iron stores, sufficient for at least 4–6 months. Although the amounts of iron are less than those found in formula milks, the bioavailability of iron in breastmilk is very much higher: 70% of the iron in breastmilk is absorbed, against 10% from formula milk (Saarinen and Siimes 1979). The difference is due to a complex series of interactions taking place within the gut. Babies receiving fresh cow's milk or formula may become anaemic because the cow's milk protein, especially if unmodified, can irritate the lining of the stomach and intestine, leading to loss of blood into the stools (Ziegler 2011).

Zinc

A deficiency of this essential trace mineral may result in the baby's failure to thrive and development of typical skin lesions. Although there is more zinc present in formula milk than in human milk, the bioavailability is greater in human milk. Breastfed babies maintain high plasma zinc values compared with formula-fed babies, even when the concentration of zinc is three times that of human milk (Sandstrom et al 1983; Khaghani et al 2010) as zinc is actively transported from the maternal circulation to the mammary gland (Krebs 1999). Preterm babies may need zinc supplements.

Calcium

Calcium is more efficiently absorbed from human milk than from breastmilk substitutes because of the higher calcium : phosphorus ratio of human milk. Formula milks based on cow's milk inevitably have higher phosphorus content than human milk.

Other minerals

Human milk has significantly lower levels of calcium, phosphorus, sodium and potassium than formula milk. Copper, cobalt and selenium, however, are present at higher levels. The higher bioavailability of these minerals and trace elements ensures that the baby's needs are met while also imposing a lower solute load on the neonatal kidney than do breastmilk substitutes.

Anti-infective factors

Leucocytes

During the first 10 days following birth, there are more white cells/ml in breastmilk than there are in blood. Macrophages and neutrophils are among the most common leucocytes in human milk and they surround and destroy harmful bacteria by their phagocytic activity.

Immunoglobulins

Five types of immunoglobulin have been identified in human milk: IgA, IgG, IgE, IgM and IgD. Of these the most important is IgA, which appears to be synthesized and stored in the breast. Although some IgA is absorbed by the baby, the majority is not. Instead, it coats the intestinal epithelium and protects the mucosal surfaces against entry of pathogenic bacteria and enteroviruses. It affords protection against *Escherichia coli*, salmonellae, shigellae, streptococci, staphylococci, pneumococci, poliovirus and the rotaviruses.

The mother's body is also able to monitor and respond to potential pathogens in her infant's environment from moment to moment via an elegant system known as GALT and BALT (*gut-associated lymphoid tissue* and *bronchus-associated lymphoid tissue*) or the broncho-mammary and entero-mammary circulation. Pathogens that enter the mother's respiratory or gastrointestinal tract stimulate pre-committed lymphocytes in the bronchial submucosa or in the Peyer's patches of the small intestine. The activated Beta cells migrate via the blood to the mammary (and salivary) glands where they become transformed into

plasma cells that start secreting large quantities of the appropriate neutralizing antibody into the milk.

Lysozyme

Lysozyme kills bacteria by disrupting their cell walls. The concentration of lysosyme increases with prolonged lactation (Hamosh 1998; Montagne et al 2001).

Lactoferrin

Lactoferrin binds to enteric iron, thus preventing potentially pathogenic E. coli from obtaining the iron they need for survival. It also has antiviral activity against human immunodeficeincy virus (HIV), cytomegalovirus (CMV) and herpes simplex virus (HSV), by interfering with virus absorption or penetration (Liu and Newberg 2013).

Bifidus factor

Bifidus factor in human milk promotes the growth of Gram-positive bacilli in the gut flora, particularly Lactobacillus bifidus, which discourages the multiplication of pathogens. Babies fed on cow's-milk-based formulae, however, have more potentially pathogenic bacilli present in the flora of their gut.

Hormones and growth factors

Epidermal growth factor and insulin-like growth factor stimulate the baby's digestive tract to mature more quickly and strengthen the barrier properties of the gastrointestinal epithelium. Once the initially leaky membrane lining the gut matures, it is less likely to allow the passage of large molecules, and becomes less vulnerable to microorganisms. The timing of the first feed has a significant effect on gut permeability, which decreases markedly if the first feed takes place soon after birth.

MANAGEMENT OF BREASTFEEDING

Exclusive breastfeeding for the first 6 months of life

Human milk is species-specific. In 2003, the Global Strategy for Infant and Young Child Feeding called for all mothers to have access to skilled support to initiate and sustain exclusive breastfeeding for 6 months and ensure the timely introduction of adequate and safe complementary foods with continued breastfeeding up to 2 years or beyond (World Health Organization [WHO]/UNICEF 2003). This was echoed in the same year by the Department of Health and is still current policy (DH 2011).

It has been known for some time that exclusively breastfed babies who consume enough breastmilk to satisfy their energy needs will easily meet their fluid requirements, even in hot dry climates (Sachdev et al 1991; Ashraf et al 1993). Extra water does nothing to speed the resolution of physiological jaundice, should it occur (Carvahlo et al 1981; Nicoll et al 1982). The only consistent effect of giving additional fluids to breastfed infants is to reduce the time for which they are breastfed (Fenstein et al 1986; White et al 1992).

Antenatal preparation

Breasts and nipples are altered by pregnancy (Chapter 9). Increased sebum secretion obviates the need for cream to lubricate the nipple. Women who have inverted and non-protractile (flat) nipples often find that they improve spontaneously during pregnancy (Hytten and Baird 1958). If not, help given with attaching the baby to the breast after birth often results in successful breastfeeding. Neither the wearing of Woolwich shells nor Hoffmann's exercises are of any value (Main Trial Collaborative Group 1994) and should not be recommended, nor should any other unevaluated commercially available device. Education of the mother is likely to be more effective than any physical exercises.

The first feed

The mother should have her baby with her immediately after birth. Early and extended skin contact ensures the cues that indicate that the baby is ready to feed will not be missed. Early feeding contributes to the success of breastfeeding, but the time of the first feed should, to a large extent, depend on the needs of the baby. Some may demonstrate a desire to feed almost as soon as they are born; others show no interest until they are an hour or so old (Widström et al 1987; Righard and Alade 1990). Babies of mothers who have received narcotics in labour may be sleepy and thus require additional support to breastfeed so they do not lose an excess of weight in the first week (Dewey et al 2003).

The first feed should be supervised by the midwife. If it proceeds without pain and the baby is allowed to end the feed spontaneously, both mother and baby will have been helped to begin the learning process necessary for effective breastfeeding in a happy and positive way.

The next feed

All mothers should be offered help with the next feed, within approximately 6 hours of birth or earlier if desired. Once the baby is feeding satisfactorily the mother should be told about the cause and prevention of sore nipples, being advised to seek help if any problems arise. She should also be informed about the changes that will take place in her breasts during the following few days. Helping mothers to understand that breastfeeding is a learned, not an instinctive, skill enables them to be patient with themselves and their babies during this time (Royal College of

Midwives [RCM] 2002). Mothers who receive the right help and education at the start will require less support and remedial intervention later.

Effective positioning for the mother

A comfortable position is a prerequisite of comfortable breastfeeding. A woman who has recently given birth, especially one new to breastfeeding, may need some help with this.

After a caesarean section, or where the perineum is very painful, *lying on her side* may be the only position a woman can tolerate in the first few days after birth, as shown in Fig. 34.4. It is likely that she will need assistance in placing the baby at the breast in this position, because she has only one free hand. When feeding from the lower breast it may be helpful to raise her body slightly by tucking the end of a pillow under her ribs. Once the woman can do this unaided, she may find this a comfortable and convenient position for night feeds, enabling her to get more sleep.

If the woman shares her bed with her baby in hospital, the hospital's guidelines on bed-sharing should be followed. All mothers, whether they intend to bed-share at home or not, should receive guidance on the subject from the midwife (NICE 2013). Guidance on this complex and sometimes emotive issue is available for both parents and health professionals (UNICEF 2011a; UNICEF 2011b).

Alternatively, the mother may prefer to *sit up* to feed her baby, as in Fig. 34.5. In the early days following the birth,

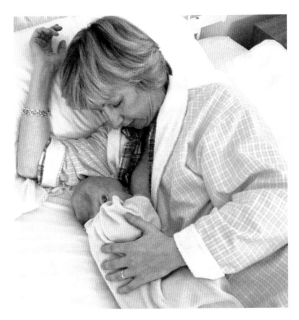

Fig. 34.4 Mother lying on her side.
Reproduced with kind permission from the Health Education Board for Scotland.

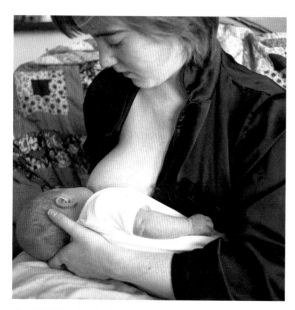

Fig. 34.5 Mother feeding sitting up.
Reproduced with kind permission from the Health Education Board for Scotland.

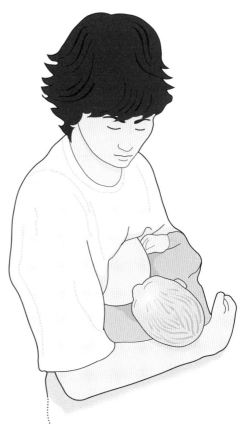

Fig. 34.6 Baby turned towards the mother's body.
From an original drawing by Hilary English.

it is particularly important that the mother's back is upright at a right-angle to her lap. This is not possible if she is sitting in bed with her legs stretched out in front of her, or sitting in a chair with a deep backward-sloping seat and a sloping back. Both lying on her side and sitting correctly in a chair with her back and feet supported enhance the shape of the breast and allow ample room in which to manoeuvre the baby.

Effective positioning for the baby

The baby's body should be turned towards the mother's body (Fig. 34.6) so that the baby is coming up to her breast at the same angle as her breast is coming down to the baby.

The more the mother's breast points down, the more the baby needs to be on his back (Fig. 34.7). The advice to have the baby *tummy to tummy* may be mistakenly taken to imply that the baby should always be lying on his side. However, taking account of the *angle of the dangle* might be more useful.

If the baby's nose is opposite his mother's nipple, being brought to the breast with the neck slightly extended, the baby's mouth will be in the correct relationship to the nipple (Fig. 34.8).

Attaching the baby to the breast

The baby should be supported across the shoulders, so that slight extension of the neck can be maintained. The

baby's head may be supported by the extended fingers of the mother's supporting hand (Fig. 34.9) or on the mother's forearm (Fig. 34.10). It may be helpful to wrap the baby in a small sheet (Vancouver wrap), as shown in Fig. 34.11, so that his hands are by his side.

Healthy term babies are equipped with a number of primitive reflexes that enable them to obtain the nourishment they require. At birth, all reflexes are of brainstem origin, with minimal cortical control. As the baby matures, higher, cortical pathways develop and the reflexes disappear sequentially: rooting at about 4 months of age and tongue protrusion by about 6 months of age (Bagnall 2005).

If the newborn baby's mouth is moved gently against the mother's nipple, the baby will open his mouth wide, as shown in Fig. 34.12. As the baby drops his lower jaw and darts his tongue down and forward, he should be moved quickly to the breast. The intention of the mother should be to aim the baby's bottom lip as far away from the base of the nipple as is possible. This allows the baby to draw breast tissue as well as the nipple into his mouth with his tongue. If correctly attached, the baby will have

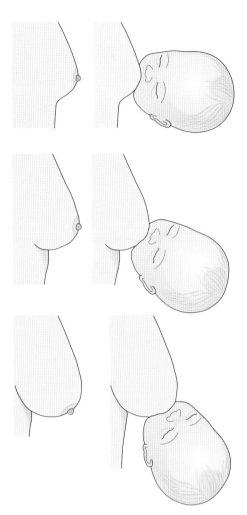

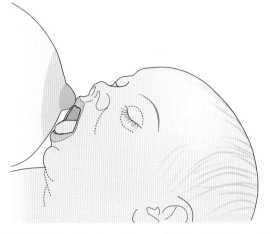

Fig. 34.8 The baby's mouth opposite the nipple, the neck slightly extended.
From an original drawing by Jenny Inch.

Fig. 34.7 Baby's body in relation to the mother's body, depending on the angle of the breast.
From an original drawing by Hilary English.

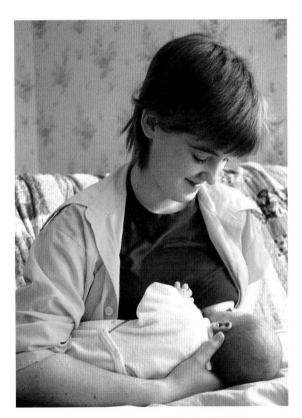

Fig. 34.9 Mother supporting the baby's head with her fingers.
Reproduced with kind permission from the Health Education Board for Scotland.

formed a *teat* from the breast and the nipple (Fig. 34.13) (Woolridge 1986, 2011).

The nipple should extend almost as far as the junction of the hard and soft palate. Contact with the hard palate triggers the sucking reflex. The baby's lower jaw moves up and down, following the action of the tongue. Although the mother may be startled by the physical sensation, she should not experience pain. If the baby is well attached, minimal suction is required to hold the *teat* within the oral cavity. The tongue can then apply rhythmical cycles of compression and relaxation so that milk is removed from the ducts. This view of the main mechanism a baby uses to remove milk from the breast has been recently challenged (Geddes et al 2008), but even more recently confirmed by further ultrasound studies (Monaci and

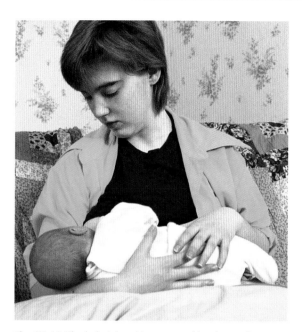

Fig. 34.10 The baby's head is supported by the mother's forearm.
Reproduced with kind permission from the Health Education Board for Scotland.

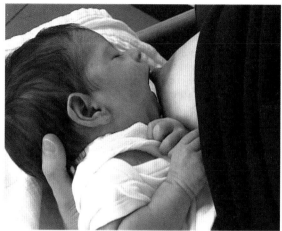

Fig. 34.12 A wide gape.
Photo courtesy of the Health Education Board for Scotland and Mark-it TV www.markittelevision.com.

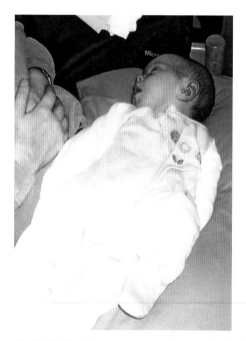

Fig. 34.11 The Vancouver wrap to keep the baby's hands by his side.

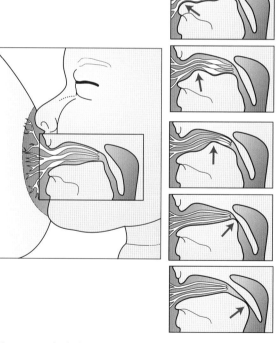

Fig. 34.13 The baby has formed a 'teat' from the breast and the nipple, which causes the nipple to extend back as far as the junction of the hard and soft palates. The lactiferous ducts are within the baby's mouth. A generous portion of areola is covered by the bottom lip.
Reproduced from Woolridge 1986, with permission.

Woolridge 2011). Although the tongue is used from time to time to generate increased suction pressure aiding milk removal, this is superimposed on the peristaltic action and does not occur in isolation (Woolridge 2011).

The baby feeds from the breast rather than from the nipple, and the mother should guide her baby towards her breast without distorting its shape. The baby's neck should be slightly extended and the chin in contact with the breast. If the baby approaches the breast as illustrated in Fig. 34.8, a generous portion of areola will be taken in by the lower jaw, but it is positively unhelpful to urge the mother to try to get the whole of the areola in the baby's mouth (see Fig. 34.14).

The role of the midwife

The midwife's role during the first few feeds is twofold. First, she must ensure that the baby is adequately fed at the breast. Secondly her role is to support the mother in developing the necessary practical positioning and attachment skills so that she is able to feed her baby independently. Whilst the baby is reflexly equipped for breastfeeding, mothers are not. For all primate mothers breastfeeding is a learned/socially acquired skill. A common pitfall is the assumption that breastfeeding is instinctive for the mother. All new mothers, but particularly those who have never experienced breastfeeding before, require encouragement and reassurance (emotional support), advice and guidance on the fundamentals of effective attachment so that feeding is pain free (practical support), and factual information about breastfeeding (informational support) in small, manageable quantities. Some mothers will need more help and support than others.

Many mothers who have had babies before require as much support with breastfeeding as those who have given birth to their first baby. Reasons for this include:

- Previous unsuccessful breastfeeding.
- Breastfeeding may have gone well last time by chance rather than knowledge.
- The new baby may behave very differently, or have different needs, from the mother's previous baby/babies.
- The mother may have recently fed (or still be feeding) a toddler and has forgotten quite how much help a new baby requires to breastfeed.
- Their previous baby may have been born at a time when underpinning information now known to be outdated was thought to be correct.

Hands-on help from the midwife

Where possible, breastfeeding support from the midwife should always be hands off, but pragmatically, it may be necessary for the midwife to help the mother attach the baby to the breast for the first few feeds. In this case, the midwife should think of her own comfort, as well as that of the mother and the baby. The midwife will put less strain on her own back if she kneels on a foam mat beside the mother, rather than bending over her (see Fig. 34.15).

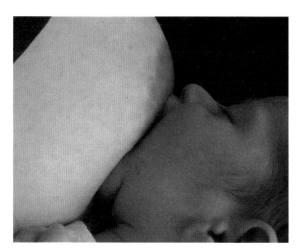

Fig. 34.14 The baby's lower jaw takes in a generous amount of the areola.
Photo courtesy of the Health Education Board for Scotland and Mark-it TV www.markittelevision.com.

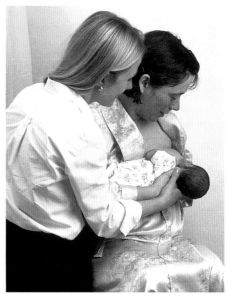

Fig. 34.15 The midwife is kneeling by the mother to assist her with attaching the baby to the breast.
Reproduced with kind permission of Nancy Durrel-McKenna.

The midwife should also consider which hand guides the baby most skilfully. For example, a right-handed midwife helping a mother who is lying on her left side will attach the baby to the left breast with her right hand. Instead of asking the mother to turn on her right side so that she can feed from the right breast, the midwife could raise the baby on a pillow and attach him to the right breast, again using her right hand. Alternatively, if the mother is sitting up, she could consider placing the baby under the mother's arm on the right side, so that she can again use her right hand.

Once a baby has fed efficiently he is more likely to do so again and from this point the mother can begin to learn how to feed her baby independently. If the midwife needs to give hands-on help to the mother, she should also explain what she is doing, and the reason, so that the mother learns from the encounter. The importance of observing babies as they go to the breast and feed cannot be overemphasized. The midwife cannot be confident the baby has attached correctly and feeds effectively if she does not see it happen.

Feeding behaviour

A breastfeeding baby typically performs one of three activities (Monaci and Woolridge 2011):

1. Doing nothing.
2. Stimulating the mother's nipple, without swallowing milk (*non-nutritive sucking/simply sucking*).
3. Sucking and swallowing milk (*nutritive sucking/ swallowing*).

After an initial burst of nipple stimulation that is short frequent sucking, two sucks per second, the baby begins swallowing – slow, deep, one suck per second (*nutritive*) sucking – and feeds vigorously with few pauses (Bosma et al 1990). As the feed progresses, pausing occurs more frequently and lasts longer. Pausing is an integral part of the baby's feeding rhythm and should not be interrupted. The midwife should simply encourage the mother to allow the baby to pace the feed. The change in the pattern generally relates to milk flow.

The foremilk is more generous in quantity but lower in fat than the hindmilk delivered at the end, which is thus higher in calories (Woolridge and Fisher 1988). If the baby receives an excessive quantity of foremilk as a result of either poor attachment or premature breast switching (see below), it may result in increased gut fermentation causing colic, flatus and explosive stools (Woolridge and Fisher 1988; Evans et al 1995). This is the commonest cause of *colic* in breastfed babies (see Fig. 34.16) and is resolved in this case by improving attachment. Neither simeticone preparations, which are often prescribed for this condition, nor commonly used complementary medicines, have been shown to be of value (Metcalf et al 1994; Perry et al 2011; Cohen and Albertini 2012).

Finishing the first breast and finishing a feed

The baby will release the breast when he has had sufficient milk from it. His ability to know this may be controlled either by the calories he has received or by the change in the volume available. He should be offered the second breast after he has had the opportunity to expel any wind, which he may take according to appetite.

The baby should not be deliberately removed from the breast before he releases it spontaneously, unless the mother is experiencing pain, in which case the baby should be reattached, if still willing to feed. Taking the baby off the first breast before he has finished may cause two problems. First, the baby is deprived of the high calorie hindmilk; second, if adequate milk removal has not taken place, milk stasis may occur ultimately leading to the mother developing mastitis or experiencing reduced milk production, or both. Provided that the baby starts each feed on alternate sides, both breasts should be used equally. If a baby does not release the breast or will not settle after a feed, the most likely reason is that he has not been correctly attached to the breast and was therefore unable to remove the milk efficiently.

Other reasons for babies withdrawing from the breast are:

* incorrect attachment
* the milk flow is very fast and the baby needs to let go and pause
* the baby has swallowed air with the generous flow of milk that occurs at the beginning of a feed and requires an opportunity to expel wind.

There is no justification for imposing either one breast per feed or alternatively both breasts per feed as a feeding regimen.

Timing and frequency of feeds

A healthy term baby knows better than anyone else how often and for how long he needs to be fed. This is now being described as responsive feeding, superseding the terms baby-led feeding and demand feeding (UNICEF–UK 2012b). The baby who remains close to his mother can signal his need to feed so that the feed can begin while he is still calm. When the baby wakes up he will start to move about, beginning with movement of the head and mouth, including licking his lips. Finally the baby finds something to suck, which is usually his fingers. If the mother misses these feeding cues the baby may then start to cry. Crying is a sign of distress, which is a late sign of hunger, and as a result, the baby will need to be calmed before he can feed effectively.

It is not unusual in the first day or so for the baby to feed infrequently, and have 6–8 hour gaps between effective feeds, each of which may be quite long (Inch and Garforth 1989; Waldenström and Swensen 1991). This is

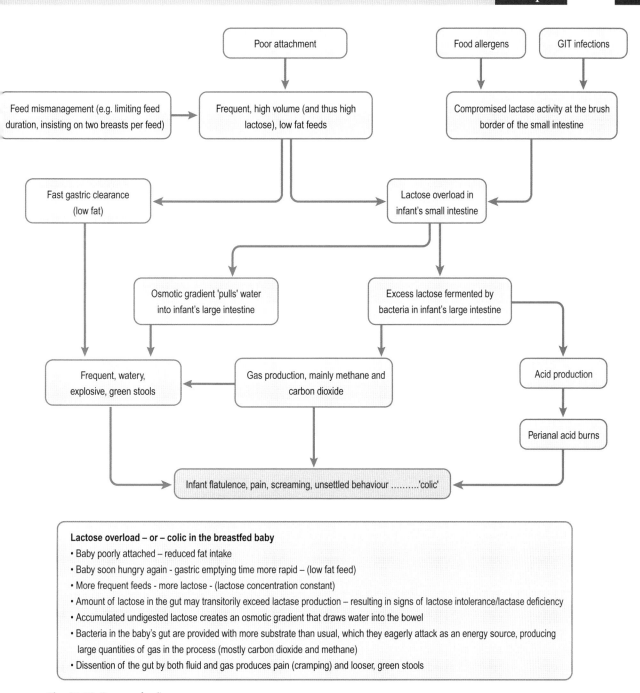

Fig. 34.16 Causes of colic.

normal, providing the mother with the opportunity to sleep if she needs to. As milk volume increases, the feeds tend to become more frequent and a little shorter. It is unusual for a baby to feed less often than six times in 24 hours from the 3rd day and most babies are taking at least six feeds every 24 hours by the time they are one week old.

Babies who feed infrequently may be consuming less milk than they need, or they may be unwell, or both, whereas babies who feed frequently (10–12 feeds in 24 hours after they are a week old) may be poorly attached to the breast. The feeding technique and the baby's weight should be monitored. However, individual mother–baby pairs develop their own unique pattern of feeding and, providing the baby is thriving and the mother is happy, there is no need to change it.

Volume of the feed

Well-grown term babies are born with good glycogen reserves and high levels of antidiuretic hormone (ADH). Consequently babies do not need large volumes of milk or colostrum before they become available physiologically. In the first 24 hours, the baby takes an average of 7 ml per feed and by the second 24 hours, this has increased to 14 ml per feed (RCM 2002; Santoro et al 2010). No precise information is available on the actual volume of breastmilk an individual baby requires in order to grow satisfactorily. Previous recommendations (150 ml/kg) were based on the requirements of formula fed babies, and these can therefore be used only as a guideline (Davies et al 1972).

Weight loss and weight gain

Most newborn babies lose some weight during their first week of life. There is a general expectation that the baby will regain their birthweight by 10–14 days. There is less agreement about how great a weight loss is normal or acceptable. Although the figure of 10% is often cited as the upper limit of normal, there is little evidence to support a figure as high as this. Data from nine studies conducted between 1986 and 1999 suggest a normal range of 3–7%; and normative data on 435 breastfed babies born in a Scottish *Baby Friendly* Hospital, reported median maximum weight loss of 6.6% (Macdonald et al 2003).

Monitoring milk transfer

A noticeable change in the baby's sucking/swallowing pattern is the most consistent sign of milk transfer. Soft but audible swallows may also be heard at the beginning of the feed. Most mothers are aware that their breast feels softer after the baby has fed well. A well-fed baby will release the breast spontaneously, appear satisfied and remain content.

Over the first four days of life, the baby's stools change from black meconium to the characteristic yellow stool, typical of a baby fed on breastmilk. A stool that is still *changing* at 96 hours of life could indicate that further attention needs to be paid to the way the mother is feeding her baby. Similarly, urine output should increase from one or more wet nappies per day in the first two days of life, to three or more over the next two days. From the end of the first week onwards, the baby's urine output should have increased such that there are around six or more wet nappies evident.

An assessment of milk transfer should be made at each postnatal contact. This should ideally be done daily for the first week, to reduce the risk of babies losing an unacceptable amount of weight. An assessment tool, suitable for use by face-to-face or telephone contact, has been developed by UNICEF–UK for this purpose (UNICEF–UK 2010a).

Difficulty with attachment is the commonest reason for babies failing to obtain enough milk. If the baby is difficult to attach, because he is sleepy or because the breast tissue is inelastic, the same principles should apply in this situation as when the baby and mother are separated by illness or prematurity: namely, to support the mother in hand expression to encourage the establishment of lactation. If this is not accomplished, the mother's lactation will be in arrears of her baby's requirements by the time he is in need of larger volumes around the 3rd/4th day.

If the mother is still not able to feed effectively by the end of the first week, it is important that she expresses her milk, using either her hands or an effective breast pump, so that her lactation is maintained and her baby is fed. Ongoing help from the midwife to improve breastfeeding is essential.

Expressing breastmilk

Although all women who choose to breastfeed their babies should know how to hand express milk, *routine* expression of the breasts should not be part of the normal management of lactation, even for mothers who have given birth by caesarean section (Chapman et al 2001). Provided no limitation is placed on either feed frequency or duration, and the baby is attached effectively, the volume of milk produced will be in accordance with the requirements of the baby. This should prevent the occurrence of problems such as breast engorgement requiring removal of milk by hand/pump.

Expression *is* appropriate in the following situations, if:

- there is concern about the interval between feeds in the early perinatal period (expressed colostrum should always be given in preference to formula milk to healthy term babies)
- there are difficulties in attaching the baby to the breast
- the baby is separated from the mother, due to prematurity or illness
- there is concern about the baby's rate of growth, or the mother's milk supply (expressing to top up with the mother's own milk may be necessary in the short term while the cause of the problem is resolved)
- the mother needs to be separated from her baby for periods (occasionally or regularly), as the baby gets older.

Manual expression of milk

Manual expression has several advantages over mechanical pumping and should be taught to all mothers. It is usually the most efficient method of obtaining colostrum. Some mothers will find hand expressing superior to any breast pump.

Expressing with a breast pump

If it is possible and practical, the mother should be able to experiment with a variety of breast pumps to discover what will suit her best (Auerbach and Walker 1994) as not all pumps work well for every woman.

Manually operated pumps

Most manually operated pumps are not efficient enough to allow initiation of full lactation but they can be useful when expressing is required once lactation is established. It is helpful for midwives to explain to mothers that these pumps function most efficiently if the vacuum phase is considerably longer than the release phase.

Electrically controlled pumps

Some electrically controlled pumps provide a regular vacuum and release cycle, with variability in the strength of the suction and others also vary the frequency of the cycle. *Double pumping* is possible with most models, and this has repeatedly been shown to be of benefit, either reducing the time for which the mother needs to use the pump at each session to obtain the available milk (Groh-Wargo et al 1995; Hill et al 1999), or increasing the volume of milk obtained for term babies (Auerbach 1990) and preterm babies (Jones et al 2001).

How much and how often?

Mothers of preterm babies who begin expressing milk by a pump as soon as possible after birth and use the pump a *minimum* of six times per 24 hours, are more likely to sustain lactation at adequate levels than those who delay expressing or express less frequently. In a *Baby Friendly* hospital the mother will be advised to express her milk at least 8 times in 24 hours, including once at night. The earlier the mother is able to express good volumes of milk in a 24 hours period, the better the outlook for sustaining adequate milk production for her baby. Breast massage (Jones et al 2001) and *kangaroo care* (see Fig. 30.6, p 626): holding the baby in skin to skin contact between the mother's breasts (Hill et al 1999) have also been positively associated with enhanced milk production.

No time limit should be set for the length of each expressing session. The mother should be guided by the milk flow, not the clock. Expressing should continue until milk flow slows, followed by a short break, and each breast should be expressed twice, either separately (*sequential pumping*) or together (*double pumping*). When milk flow slows for the second time, the session should end. Fre-quent expressing sessions are more likely to have the desired effect than lengthy, infrequent sessions.

Inadequate milk volume, followed by declining production, is a common problem for mothers who are expressing their milk for their preterm baby. In order to *prevent* this from happening, the midwife should discuss with the mother the value of early initiation of expressing, the appropriate use and correct size of equipment and the importance of the frequency of expression, rather than trying to rescue failing lactation pharmacologically. It may also be helpful to show the mother how to express *hands free*, using an expressing brassiere to hold the breast shields securely in place. For examples of hands-free expressing please go to http://www.phdinparenting .com/blog/2010/9/13/hands-free-pumping-options-for -breastfeeding-moms.html.

Storage of breastmilk

NICE (2008) advises that expressed milk can be stored for up to:

- 5 days in the main part of a fridge, at 4 °C or lower
- 2 weeks in the freezer compartment of a refrigerator
- 6 months in a domestic freezer, at −18 °C or lower.

Care of the breasts

Daily washing is all that is necessary for breast hygiene. Brassieres may be worn in order to provide comfortable support and are useful if the breasts leak and breast pads (or breast shells) are used.

Breast problems

Sore and damaged nipples

The cause is almost always trauma from the baby's mouth and tongue, which results from incorrect attachment of the baby to the breast. Correcting this will provide immediate relief from pain and allow rapid healing to take place. Epithelial growth factor, contained in fresh human milk and saliva, may aid this process.

Resting the nipple enables healing to take place but makes the continuation of lactation much more complicated because it is necessary to express the milk and to use some other means of feeding it to the baby. Nipple shields should be used with caution, and never before the mother has begun to lactate, as the baby is unlikely to extract colostrum via a shield. They may make feeding less painful, but often they do not. Their use does not enable the mother to learn how to feed her baby correctly, and their longer-term use may result in reduced milk transfer from mother to baby. This in turn may result in mastitis in the mother (reduced milk removal), slow weight gain or prolonged feeds in the baby (reduced milk transfer), or both. If mothers choose to use them, they should be advised to seek help with learning to attach the baby comfortably without a nipple shield as soon as practicable (McKechnie and Eglash 2010).

Other causes of soreness

Infection with *Candida albicans* (thrush) can occur, although it is not common during the first week following the baby's birth. Sudden development of pain after a period of trouble-free feeding is suggestive of thrush. The nipple and areola are inflamed and shiny, and pain typically persists throughout the feed. The baby may show signs of oral or anal thrush. Both mother and baby should receive concurrent fungicidal treatment, such as miconazole, and it may take several days for the pain in the nipple to disappear.

Dermatitis

Sensitivity may develop to topical applications such as creams, ointments or sprays, including those used to treat thrush.

Anatomical variations

Short nipples

Short nipples should not cause problems as the baby is able to form a teat from both the breast and nipple.

Long nipples

Long nipples can lead to poor feeding because although the baby is able to latch on to the nipple, he is unable to draw any breast tissue into his mouth, due to the length of the nipple.

Abnormally large nipples

If the baby is small, his mouth may not be able to get beyond the nipple and onto the breast. Lactation can be initiated by expressing, by hand or by pump, provided the nipple fits into the breastshield. As the baby grows and the breast and nipple become more protractile, breastfeeding may become possible.

Inverted and flat nipples

If the nipple is deeply inverted it may be necessary to initiate lactation by expressing and delay attempting to attach the baby to the breast until lactation is established and the breasts have become soft and the breast tissue more elastic.

Difficulties with breastfeeding

Engorgement

This condition occurs around the 3rd or 4th day following the baby's birth. The breasts become hard, often oedema-

---

> ### Box 34.1 **Babies who are difficult to attach**
>
> Inelastic breast tissue, overfull or engorged breasts or deeply inverted nipples may present the baby with more of a challenge.
> - If the breast is engorged, pushing away the oedema by gently manipulating the tissue that lies under the areola may be all that is required.
> - Hand expression, or the use of a breast pump, may relieve fullness to the point where the baby can draw in the inner tissue to create the necessary teat from the breast.
> - If attachment is still difficult, try asking the mother to lie on her side with the short edge of a pillow under her ribs to raise the breast off the bed. The midwife may need to assist the baby in attaching.
> - If the midwife is unable to attach the baby to the breast, the mother should be shown how to hand express and how to give her colostrum to her baby.
> - It may also be necessary to show the mother how to use a breast pump (hand or electric). However, in the first 24–48 hours colostrum is usually best expressed by hand.
>
> When attachment is difficult, the priorities should be to ensure that the baby is adequately fed on his mother's milk, and to work on making the breast tissue more elastic (both of which can be facilitated by hand or electrical expressing). Attaching the baby to the breast directly can come later.

---

tous, painful and sometimes appear flushed. The mother may be pyrexial. Engorgement is usually an indication that the baby is not keeping pace with the stage of lactation. Engorgement may occur if feeds are delayed or restricted or if the baby is unable to feed efficiently because he is not correctly attached to the breast.

Management should be aimed at enabling the baby to feed well (Box 34.1). In severe cases the only solution will be the gentle use of a pump. This will reduce the tension in the breast and *will not* cause excessive milk production. The mother's fluid intake should not be restricted, as this has no effect on milk production.

Deep breast pain

In most cases, deep breast pain responds to improvement in breastfeeding technique and is likely to be due to raised intraductal pressure caused by inefficient milk removal. Although it may occur during the feed, it typically occurs afterwards. This distinguishes it from the sensation of the *let-down reflex*, which some mothers experience as a fleeting pain. Very rarely, deep breast pain may be the result of ductal thrush infection.

Mastitis

In the majority of cases, mastitis, an inflammation of the breast, is the result of milk stasis, not infection, although infection may supervene (Thomsen et al 1984). Typically, one or more adjacent segments of breast tissue are inflamed through milk being forced into the connective tissue of the breast, and appear as wedge-shaped areas of redness and swelling. If milk is forced back into the bloodstream, the woman's pulse and temperature may rise and in some cases flu-like symptoms, including shivering attacks or rigors, may occur. The presence or absence of systemic symptoms does not help to distinguish infectious from non-infectious mastitis (WHO 2000).

Non-infective (acute intramammary) mastitis

Non-infective (acute intramammary) mastitis results from milk stasis and may occur during the early days of breastfeeding as the result of unresolved engorgement or at any time due to poor feeding technique when milk from one or more segments of the breast is not being efficiently drained by the baby. It occurs much more frequently in the breast that is opposite the mother's dominant side for holding her baby (Inch and Fisher 1995). Pressure from fingers or clothing has been blamed for causing the condition, without any supporting evidence. It is extremely important that breastfeeding from the affected breast continues, otherwise milk stasis will increase further, providing ideal conditions for pathogenic bacteria to replicate. An infective condition could then arise, leading to abscess formation if left untreated.

Where supervision is available from the midwife, 12–24 hours could elapse to ascertain whether the mastitis can be resolved by helping the mother to improve her feeding technique and encouraging her to allow the baby to complete the first breast initially. If supervision is not available or if there is no improvement during the 24 hours period, antibiotics such as cephalexin, flucloxacillin or erythromycin, should be given prophylactically (WHO 2000; RCM 2002).

Infective mastitis

The main cause of superficial breast infection is damage to the epithelium, allowing bacteria to enter the underlying tissues. The damage usually results from incorrect attachment of the baby to the breast, which has caused trauma to the nipple. The mother therefore requires urgent assistance to improve her feeding technique, as well as appropriate antibiotics. Multiplication of bacteria may be enhanced by the use of breast pads or shells. In spite of antibiotic therapy, abscess formation may occur. Infection may also enter the breast via the milk ducts if milk stasis remains unresolved (WHO 2000).

Breast abscess

A fluctuant swelling develops in a previously inflamed area: namely a *breast abscess*. Pus may be discharged from the nipple. Simple needle aspiration may be effective, or incision and drainage may be necessary (Dixon 1988). It may not be possible for the baby to feed from the affected breast for a few days, however milk removal should continue by expression with breastfeeding recommencing as soon as practicable as this would reduce the chances of further abscess formation (WHO 2000). A sinus that drains milk may form, but it is likely to heal in time.

Blocked ducts

Lumpy areas in the breast are not uncommon, due to distended glandular tissue. If such lumps become very firm and tender and sometimes flushed, they are often described as *blocked ducts*. This description carries with it the image of a physical obstruction within the lumen of the duct. However, this is very rarely the cause of the symptoms. It is much more likely that milk drainage has been somewhat uneven due to less than optimal attachment and that secreted milk is trying to occupy more space than is actually available, causing the alveoli to distend. Milk may subsequently be forced out into the connective tissue of the breast where it causes inflammation. The inflammatory process narrows the lumen of the duct by exerting pressure on it from the outside as the tissue swells, resulting in *mastitis* or *incipient mastitis*. Consequently, the solution is to improve milk drainage by improved attachment, with possibly milk expression, and to treat the accompanying pain and inflammation. Massage, often advocated to clear the imagined blockage, may make matters worse, as all it does is force more milk into the surrounding tissue.

White spots/epithelial overgrowth

Very occasionally, a ductal opening in the tip of the nipple may become obstructed by epithelial overgrowth. A white blister is evident on the surface of the nipple, effectively causing a physical obstruction closing off the exit points from one or more milk-producing sections of the breast. This may sometimes be resolved by the baby feeding. Alternatively, after the baby has fed and the skin is softened, the blister may be removed with a clean fingernail, a rough flannel, or a sterile needle. True blockages of this sort tend to recur, but once the woman understands how to deal with them, the progression to mastitis can be avoided.

Feeding difficulties due to the baby

Colic in the breastfed baby

Figure 34.16 represents diagrammatically the causes and effects of secondary lactose intolerance – or 'colic' – in the breastfed baby.

Although not all abdominal discomfort is due to poor attachment, symptoms of 'colic' in a breastfed baby, such as abdominal discomfort, excessive flatus/wind, explosive stools, light green stools, may often be explained in terms of the foremilk/hindmilk mixture that the baby receives during the course of the feed/day.

If the baby is not well attached, he may not be able to access the fat-rich milk as the feed volume diminishes. Since it is the fat that provides most of the calories, as well as slowing gastric emptying time, the poorly attached baby will be hungry again sooner than he would be if he had been well attached. Once again (unless the mother makes changes to the attachment) the baby will receive another 'low fat' feed.

Over 24 hours the baby will have consumed a much greater volume of milk than he would have done if he had been better attached. *Since the concentration of lactose in milk is fairly constant*, he will have also received much more lactose than otherwise. This excess lactose in the gut may transitorily exceed the amount of the enzyme lactase which the baby's intestinal brush border is able to generate. The baby thus exhibits the signs of lactose intolerance/lactase deficiency. The accumulated undigested lactose creates an osmotic gradient that draws water into the bowel. Added to which the bacteria in the baby's gut are provided with more substrate than usual, which they eagerly attack as an energy source, producing large quantities of gas in the process (mostly carbon dioxide and methane). Distension of the gut by both fluid and gas produces pain (cramping) and looser stools. These are often green in colour due to the presence of bile that has not been re-absorbed. Depending on the extent of the lactase deficiency and the quantity of lactose ingested, symptoms can range from mild abdominal discomfort to severe dehydrating diarrhoea.

(Among the pharmaceutical industry's responses has been the production of 'over the counter' simethicone and lactase, which distraught mothers can buy. Not only are there no good quality trials demonstrating their effectiveness in breastfed babies, there is a much simpler solution than trying to fix the symptoms – which is to address the cause – and improve attachment.)

If the baby who is not well attached can consume sufficient milk in each 24-hour period to get the calories he needs, he will grow. But he may have to feed very frequently to achieve this. Frequent feeds may in turn increase his mother's milk supply, giving rise to the frustrating scenario of a mother with an abundant supply, yet a baby who is feeding 'round the clock'. If the baby simply cannot hold enough milk, the situation above will be compounded by a baby who is also failing to grow well.

Cleft lip

Provided that the palate is intact, the presence of a cleft in the lip should not interfere with breastfeeding because the vacuum that is necessary to enable the baby to attach to the breast is created between the tongue and the hard palate, not the breast and the lips.

Cleft palate

Because of the cleft, the baby is unable to create a vacuum and form a teat out of the breast and nipple. There is no reason why the mother should be discouraged from putting the baby to the breast, for comfort, pleasure or food, provided that she is aware of the above and appreciates that it is likely that she will need to give her baby her expressed milk as well. A variety of measures are available to support feeding in infants thus affected until surgery can take place (around 6 months of age) but little to suggest that many of these babies will successfully breastfeed (Reid 2004; Garcez and Guigliani 2005).

Tongue tie (Ankyloglossia)

If the baby cannot extend his tongue over his lower gum he is unlikely to be able to draw the breast deeply into his mouth to feed effectively (Johnson 2006). This may be due to the tongue being short or because the frenulum, which is the whitish strip of tissue attaching the tongue to the floor of the mouth, is too tight or not stretchy enough. As the baby tries to lifts his tongue, the tip may sometimes become heart-shaped as the frenulum pulls on it.

Increasingly it is argued that more emphasis should be placed on tongue function rather than simply its appearance as tongue movement is more complex than simply the ability to protrude it beyond the gum ridge. Many practitioners maintain that when attention to attachment does not resolve a breastfeeding problem, a full assessment should be carried out, observing any impairment of activities that require a functional tongue (Hazelbaker 2010).

The National Institute for Health and Clinical Excellence recommended that the surgical release of the frenulum (*frenotomy*) was safe, only taking a few seconds to perform in a young baby (NICE 2005). The procedure is usually bloodless and painless and its practice is further supported by evidence from clinical trials (Dollberg et al 2006; Hogan et al 2005) and ultrasound studies (Ramsay 2005; Geddes et al 2008).

Blocked nose

Babies normally breathe through their noses. Obstruction causes great difficulty with feeding because they have to interrupt the process in order to breathe. Blockages caused by mucus may be relieved with a twist of damp cotton wool, or by instilling drops of normal saline before a feed (Bollag et al 1984).

Down syndrome

Babies who have Down syndrome can be successfully breastfed, although extra help and encouragement may be necessary initially (Chapter 32).

Prematurity

Preterm infants who have developed sucking and swallowing reflexes may successfully breastfeed, which is considered to be less tiring than taking a feed by bottle (Meier and Cranston-Anderson 1987). However, if the reflexes are not strongly developed, the baby may tire before the feed is complete and complementary feeding by nasogastric tube may be necessary.

Babies who are too immature to breastfeed may be able to cup-feed, as an alternative to being tube-fed (Lang et al 1994). Less mature babies who are unable to suck or swallow will be dependent on receiving nutrition via artificial methods such as tube-feeding and intravenous alimentation.

Illness or surgery

In general, babies recover quickly following illness or surgery, but if they have never been to the breast, or if feeding has been interrupted for a long period, the mother will require skilled help from the midwife to initiate or re-establish feeding.

Contraindications to breastfeeding

Breastfeeding may have to be suspended temporarily following the administration of certain drugs, e.g. chloramphenicol, or following diagnostic techniques using radiopharmaceuticals. Most regions have drug centres/ hospital pharmacy information services where advice may be sought about the safety of drugs for lactating women.

Carcinoma

If the mother has carcinoma, the cytotoxic treatment she receives will make it impossible to breastfeed without causing harm to the baby. However, if she wishes to, she could express and discard her milk for the duration of the treatment and resume breastfeeding later. If she has had a mastectomy, she may feed successfully from the other breast. The woman may also be able to breastfeed following a lumpectomy for carcinoma, but it is advisable to seek advice from her surgeon.

Breast surgery

Neither breast reduction nor augmentation is an inevitable contraindication to breastfeeding, but much depends on the techniques used. Where possible, advice should be sought from the surgeon. If the nipple has been displaced, the duct system may not be patent. Nickell and Skelton (2005) recommend that if surgery is proposed for a woman who wishes to breastfeed in the future, it may be possible to alter the surgery to preserve the ductal system. Ultimately, the only way to determine if the breast will function effectively is to test it by encouraging the baby to go to the breast.

Breast injury

Injuries caused by scalding to the chest in childhood may cause such severe scarring that breastfeeding is impossible. Burns or other accidents may also cause serious damage.

One breast only

It is perfectly possible to feed a baby effectively using just one breast. If the mother has only one functioning breast, she should be reassured that each breast works independently of the other. If the baby is offered only one breast, that breast will make enough milk to feed that individual baby. There are documented cases of women feeding two babies with just one breast (Nicolls 1997).

Human immunodeficiency virus (HIV) infection

Human immunodeficiency virus (HIV) may be transmitted in breastmilk. In developed countries, where formula milk feeding is relatively safe, the mother may be advised not to breastfeed if she is HIV-positive (Chapter 13). In countries where formula feeding is a significant cause of infant mortality, exclusive breastfeeding for the first 6 months may be the safer option (Coutsoudis et al 1999; Coovadia et al 2007; WHO et al 2010).

Cessation of lactation

Suppression of lactation

If a mother chooses not to breastfeed, or if she has a late miscarriage or stillbirth, lactation will still commence. The woman may experience discomfort for a day or two, but if unstimulated the breasts will naturally cease to produce milk. Very rarely, severe discomfort with engorgement occurs. Expressing small amounts of milk once or twice can afford great relief without interfering with the rapid regression of the condition. The mother will be more comfortable if her breasts are supported, but it is doubtful if binding the breasts contributes anything towards suppression (Swift and Janke 2003).

There is no basis on which to advise the mother to restrict her fluid intake or to seek a prescription for a diuretic, which will be equally ineffective (Hodge 1967).

These measures merely add to the woman's discomfort by making her thirsty. Pharmacological suppression of lactation with dopamine receptor agonists such as bromocriptine and cabergoline is effective but is not recommended for routine use. Bromocriptine and cabergoline are currently licensed in the UK, although bromocriptine had its licence withdrawn in the United States of America (USA) some time ago.

Discontinuation of breastfeeding

Discontinuing lactation abruptly once breastfeeding has become established may cause serious problems for the woman, leading to engorgement, mastitis or even a breast abscess. The woman should be encouraged to mimic normal weaning by expressing her breasts, reducing the frequency over several days or possibly weeks. The gradual reduction in the volume of milk removed from the breasts results in a corresponding diminution in the production of milk. Eventually the woman should be encouraged to express only if she feels uncomfortable. Pharmacological suppression using cabergoline might be appropriate following the death of a baby.

Returning to work

If the breastfeeding mother returns to work, her baby will require feeding in her absence. If the woman wishes her baby to continue taking breastmilk, she will need to express her milk in advance. However, if the woman finds it difficult to express her milk at work, her baby could receive a formula feed (or *solid* food, if over 6 months), while she is away, but continue breastfeeding at all other times. Returning to work does not mean that breastfeeding has to be terminated.

Weaning from the breast

When the mother or the baby decides to stop breastfeeding, feeds should be tailed off gradually. Breastfeeds may be omitted, one at a time, and spaced further apart. Adding supplementary foods should not begin until about 6 months of age. If the mother uses solid food to give the baby *tasters* and the experience of different textures before weaning, these should be given *after* the breastfeed. Solid foods given to the baby before the breastfeed (weaning) will result in them taking less milk from the breast and less milk being produced. Allowing the baby to lead the process of weaning (Rapley 2012) may make the transition much easier.

Complementary and supplementary feeds

Complementary feeds or *top-ups* are feeds given to the baby *after* a breastfeed. Complementary feeds of breastmilk substitutes (formula milk) should be given as a last resort, not

as an alternative to helping the mother with breastfeeding or expressing milk. Exposure to non-human milk proteins has been implicated in the development of type 1 diabetes, eczema and wheeze/asthma (Renfrew et al 2012). Even a single exposure can sensitize susceptible infants (Host 1991).

The 2010 Infant Feeding Survey (McAndrew et al 2012) found that 31% of babies born in UK hospitals received breastmilk substitutes while in hospital. The mothers of these babies were three times more likely to have given up breastfeeding by the time their baby was a week old, in comparison with mothers whose babies received only breastmilk.

About 10% of newborns are at risk of hypoglycaemia (Chapter 33), and may thus need a higher calorific intake straight from birth than their mothers can provide. Where possible this should be the mother's expressed colostrum or human milk obtained from a human milk bank.

Babies who are well but sleepy (Box 34.2), jaundiced (Chapter 33), unsettled (Box 34.3), or difficult to attach (see Box 34.1 above), should be given their mother's own expressed milk if necessary, in addition to being offered the breast.

If complementary feeds are clinically indicated and the mother cannot express sufficiently, donor milk from a human milk bank could be used. Donors are serologically tested for HIV and other conditions.

If the baby is very young, additional feeds should be given by oral syringe or cup, rather than by bottle. An oral syringe (or dropper) will reduce wastage and the use of a cup would allow the baby to remain more in control of their intake. If the difficulty persists, for example with attachment, the mother may find it quicker and more

---

Box 34.2 'Sleepy' babies

Provided that the baby is otherwise well, which will be determined by examining the baby from time to time, there is no evidence that long intervals between feeds have any adverse affect. As few as three feeds in the first 24 hours of life is within the normal range.

- The baby should remain close to the mother, in accordance with UNICEF–UK (2012b guidelines). The mother will thus be able to respond immediately to her baby's feeding cues.
- The baby could be roused at intervals, possibly by changing the nappy, and being offered the breast.
- The baby could be undressed down to the nappy and placed in skin contact with the mother and offered the breast.
- The mother could be shown how to hand express some colostrum, and how to give this to the baby.
- It is unnecessary to measure the baby's blood glucose levels (see Chapter 33).

Box 34.3 If the baby is unsettled

An unsettled baby of any age that is crying again soon after he has been fed may not have been well attached.

- Observe what the mother is doing and, if necessary, guide her or help her directly.
- If the attachment is good, then the baby may be reacting to being removed from the closeness of the mother's body. If the mother needs to sleep, suggest that she feeds lying down and help her if necessary. However, it is imperative that the baby's safety is maintained should the feed take place in the bed.
- The mother might try to express some colostrum/milk to give to the baby if she is concerned that the baby has not received all that he can from the breast
- Some babies will appear unsettled even if they have fed well at the breast. The baby may be uncomfortable. The act of changing the nappy may help; so may wrapping the baby comfortably but securely and providing rhythmic motion, such as walking or holding the baby over the shoulder or over the forearm, both of which apply gentle pressure to the baby's abdomen to help settle him down
- Show the mother what you are doing, so that she learns appropriate coping strategies from you.
- If *you* give the baby formula or a dummy to settle him, that is what the mother will do when she goes home
- *Do not offer* to remove the baby. Separating mother and baby, particularly removing the baby at night in the mistaken belief that the mother will benefit if she does not wake to breastfeed her baby at night, is strongly correlated with reduced breastfeeding success (WHO, 1998).
- If the mother *asks* you to, and you agree to take the baby away to settle, return the baby to her when he wakes again to be fed.

Box 34.4 Donated breastmilk

If you are offering a mother donated human milk for her baby for any reason, she might find the information below helpful in deciding whether to accept it.

- All human milk donors meet the same criteria as blood donors; they are in a low risk group to start with and give consent to an HIV blood test
- All human milk donors sign a form to that effect and all have their blood tested.
- Almost all donors are currently feeding their own baby while donating.
- No donated milk is used for any baby until the results of the donor's blood test have been received.
- All donated milk is collected in sterilized bottles, kept in the fridge and frozen within 24 hours of expression.
- When it arrives, still frozen, at the milk bank, it is thawed, a small sample taken for bacteriological screening and the rest is pasteurized.
- After pasteurization another small sample is taken (for post-pasteurization bacteriological screening) and the rest refrozen in a holding freezer.
- Only when the results of both samples have been received is the milk transferred to the freezer from which it can be used for preterm and term babies.
- Donors are not paid for the milk they donate: it is freely given! Quite often, mothers choose to donate milk because their own babies were themselves helped in this way by the generosity of other mothers.

---

efficient to give her expressed milk to the baby by bottle. There is no evidence that the baby will subsequently refuse the breast in these circumstances (Brown et al 1999; Howard et al 2003; Flint et al 2007).

Supplementary feeds are feeds given *in place of* a breastfeed. There is no justification for their use except in exceptional circumstances, such as severe illness or unconsciousness. This is because each breastfeed that is missed by the baby interferes with the establishment of lactation and affects the mother's confidence in being able to successfully breastfeed her baby.

Human milk banking

Research over the past couple of decades has demonstrated the effectiveness of pasteurization as a means of destroying

HIV (Eglin and Wilkinson 1987) and the importance of human milk in preventing necrotizing enterocolitis (NEC) (Quigley et al 2008). This resulted in the formation of the UK Association for Milk Banking (UKAMB) in 1998 and re-establishing human milk banks.

Banked human milk is used predominantly for preterm and sick babies. Occasionally, if there is sufficient, it is used for term babies whose mothers are temporarily unable to meet their babies' needs with their own expressed milk. Mothers who are offered donated milk for their babies must have sufficient information about the collection and screening of human milk to enable them to make an informed choice whether or not to accept it (see Box 34.4).

CHOOSING BREAST OR FORMULA MILK

Although the majority of women who choose to breastfeed have made this decision very early on, some may not make a final decision until after giving birth. The subject of infant feeding should be part of an ongoing conversation that the woman has with her midwife as her pregancy progresses. During these conversations the midwife should share the value of skin contact for all mothers and babies, explore what parents already know about breastfeeding and help them to appreciate the value of breastfeeding as protection, comfort and food so they can make an informed choice (UNICEF–UK 2012b).

Observing a baby being breastfed can strongly influence the decision to breastfeed either positively or negatively, depending on the context (Hoddinott and Pill 1999). This is of particular relevance for women for whom theoretical knowledge may have less power than embodied knowledge. Peer group support can influence both initiation and continuation of breastfeeding (Fairbank et al 2000) and introducing pregnant women to other mothers who are breastfeeding young babies may also be helpful. This is now done in many 'Baby Cafés' throughout the UK.

Time should be taken during the antenatal period to talk briefly about the day-to-day progress and management of early breastfeeding. The woman should be aware that:

- Breastfeeding is a learned skill.
- It should not hurt.
- She does not need to be taught the major details of management until after the baby is born.

The midwife's responsibility to the woman is to ensure that her choice is fully informed, rather than to persuade her to breastfeed. This cannot be achieved if the midwife withholds information from her. The nutritional and immunological consequences of not breastfeeding are seen in population studies, and are to do with relative risks. It is not possible to narrow the risk down to the individual. Nevertheless, all pregnant women should be made aware that, compared with a fully breastfed baby, a baby fed on formula milk from birth is:

- five times more likely to be hospitalized with gastroenteritis (within the first 3 months of life)
- five times more likely to suffer from urine infections (within the first 6 months of life)
- twice as likely to suffer from chest infections (within the first 7 years of life)
- twice as likely to suffer from ear infections (within the 1st year of life)
- twice as likely to develop atopic disease where there is a family history
- up to 20 times more likely to develop necrotizing enterocolitis if born prematurely.

Additionally, the pregnant woman should know that she may increase her own risk of postnatal depression, premenopausal breast cancer, ovarian cancer and osteoporosis if she does not breastfeed (UNICEF and Department of Health 2012).

FEEDING WITH FORMULA MILK

Most breastmilk substitutes (infant formulae) are modified cow's milk. The minimum and maximum permitted levels of named ingredients, and named prohibited ingredients in all cow's milk-based (and soya infant) formulae have to meet strict criteria (Infant Formula and Follow-on Formula Regulations 2007). However, considerable variations in composition exist within the legally permitted ranges.

The two main components are *skimmed milk*, which is a by-product of butter manufacture, and *whey*, which is a by-product of cheese manufacture. Breastmilk substitutes may contain fats from any source, animal or vegetable, except from sesame and cotton, provided that they do not contain >8% trans isomers of fatty acids. The fat source may not always be apparent from reading the label: for example *oleo* is beef fat and would be unacceptable to Hindus and vegetarians, and *oils of vegetable origin* may have come from marine algae. Formula milks may also contain soya protein, maltodextrin, dried glucose syrup and gelatinized and pre-cooked starch.

Types of formula milk

There are two main types of formula milk: *whey-dominant* and *casein-dominant*. Both can be used from birth. There is a comprehensive and quarterly updated report for health professionals called *Infant Milks in the UK* (Crawley and Westland 2013) produced by an independent charity, *First Steps Nutrition Trust*.

Whey-dominant formulae

In these, a small amount of skimmed milk is combined with demineralized whey. The ratio of proteins in the formulae approximates to the ratio of whey to casein found in human milk (60 : 40). These feeds are more easily digested than the casein-dominant formulae, which have an effect on gastric emptying times, with feeding patterns that more closely resemble those of breastfed babies.

Casein-dominant formulae

Although these formulae are also promoted as suitable for use from birth and are aimed at mothers whose babies are *hungrier*, their use is not recommended for young babies. Whilst the macronutrient proportions (fat, carbohydrate, protein, etc.) are the same as in whey-dominant formulae, more of the protein is in the form of casein (20 : 80). The higher casein content causes large, relatively indigestible curds to form in the baby's stomach, intending to make them *feel full* for longer. There is no evidence that babies settle better or sleep longer if given these milks (Taitz and Scholey 1989; Thorkelsson et al 1994).

Milks for babies intolerant of standard formulae

Predicting which babies will be prone to allergies is an inexact science. It is estimated that the likelihood of a baby being predisposed to allergy is about 20–35% if one parent is affected, 40–60% if both parents are affected and 50–70% if both parents have the same allergy (Brostoff and Gamlin 1998).

Hydrolysate formula

Hydrolysate formula is made of cow's milk, cornstarch and other foods, treated with digestive enzymes so that the milk proteins are partially broken down. It has been thought in the past that these alternatives carry less risk of allergy than standard formulae.

Some of these (prescription-only) hydrolysates are intended to *treat* an existing allergy, and others are designed for *preventative* use in babies who are at high risk of developing cow's milk protein allergy and who are not breastfeeding (Brostoff and Gamlin 1998). Not only are these substances considerably more expensive than either standard or soya-based formula, NICE (2008) guidance now maintains that there is insufficient evidence that infant formula based on partially or extensively hydrolysed cow's milk protein helps prevent allergies.

Whey hydrolysates

These formulae are made from the whey of cow's milk (rather than from whole milk) and have been thought to be potentially more useful for highly allergenic babies.

Amino-acid-based formula, or elemental formula

Amino-acid-based formula, or elemental formula has a completely synthetic protein base, providing essential and non-essential amino acids, together with fat, maltodextrin, vitamins, minerals and trace elements. This type of formula milk is very expensive.

Soya-based formula

Soya-based formula was developed as a response to the emergence of cow's milk protein intolerance in babies fed on formula milk. However, there has been mounting evidence that soya-based formula's high phytoestrogen content could pose a risk to the long-term reproductive health of infants (Martyn 1999; Minchin 2001). Consequently soya-based formula milk should be used only in exceptional circumstances to ensure adequate nutrition, for example with babies of vegan parents who are not breastfeeding or babies who are unable to tolerate alternatives, such as amino-acid formulae (Crawley and Westland 2013).

Many babies who are intolerant of cow's milk are also intolerant of soya. Early soya formula feeding runs the risk of inducing soya protein intolerance in the child and soya protein is much harder to avoid in the weaning diet than dairy products.

Goat's milk formula

The European Food Standards Agency (EFSA) (2006) concluded that there were insufficient data to establish the suitability of goat's milk protein as a protein source in infant formula, and since March 2007 infant milks based on goat's milk were no longer sold in the UK. However, in 2012, EFSA revised their conclusion on the suitability of goat's milk as a protein source for infant and follow-on formula milks and the expectation was that the Infant Formula and Follow-on Formula (England) Regulations (2007) would be changed sometime in 2013 to allow goat's milk-based infant milks (Crawley and Westland 2013). However, at the time of going to press these changes have yet to be made.

Choosing a breastmilk substitute

Although not always enforced, it is an offence under UK law to sell any infant formula as being suitable from birth unless it meets the criteria set out in the Infant Formula and Follow-on Formula Regulations (2007). Despite claims made by formula manufacturers, there is no obvious scientific basis on which to recommend one brand over another.

It is not necessary for the mother to stick to one brand, and if she finds that one formula milk does not suit her baby she could try an alternative brand. This has been made easier by the availability of ready-to-feed sachets or cartons, with which mothers can experiment without having to buy large quantities of formula milk. Babies with underlying metabolic disorders, such as galactosaemia or phenylketonuria, however, require the appropriate, prescribable breastmilk substitute.

As formula milks are highly processed, factory-produced products, there inevitably can arise inadvertent errors, such as too much or too little of an ingredient, accidental contamination, incorrect labelling and foreign bodies. It is therefore imperative that mothers are advised to inspect the contents of the tin or packet before use and if it looks or smells strange, return it to the seller.

Preparation of an artificial feed

The introduction of ready-to-feed formula in hospital may save staff time, but it reduces the likelihood that the mother who chooses to feed her baby with formula milk will have been shown how to prepare a bottle feed safely before she goes home (Kaufmann 1999). It is now required, in Baby Friendly-accredited hospitals that all mothers intending to formula-feed their baby are given the information they need to do so in a way that reduces the risk to the baby (UNICEF–UK 2012b).

All powdered formula feed available in the UK is now reconstituted using one scoopful (the scoop being provided with the powder) to 30 ml of cooled boiled water. Clear instructions about the volumes of powder and water are also printed on the container. Many of the major UK manufacturers of formula milk now produce ready-to-feed cartons, reducing the risk of over- or under-concentration, but precluding universal use through higher cost. Another advantage of ready-to-feed formula is that the contents are sterile whereas powdered milk, in tins or packets, is not.

In response to growing concerns about bacterial contaminants in these powders, the WHO produced guidelines on the safe preparation, storage and handling of powdered infant formula (WHO 2007), and the Food Standards Agency (FSA) and Department of Health subsequently changed their recommendations in relation to reconstitution. Anyone making up feeds from powder is advised to make each feed just before it is needed, using water that has boiled and cooled to 70 °C, adding the powder, allowing the milk to cool and giving the feed straight away. Any remaining milk should be discarded (DH 2012).

The water supply

It is essential that the water used is free from bacterial contamination and any harmful chemicals. It is generally assumed in the UK that boiled tap water will meet these criteria, but from time to time this is shown not to be the case. If bottled water is used, a still, non-mineralized variety suitable for babies must be chosen and it should be boiled as usual. Softened water is usually unsuitable.

Feeding equipment

Concern over the nitrosamine content of rubber teats and dummies was addressed in the EU in 1993, and since 1995, teats and dummies that do not comply with the 1993 directive (EFSA 1993) have been prohibited. However teats that are frequently boiled can quickly become spongy and swollen. The alternative, silicone teats, have been known to split with repeated use. Mothers should be advised to check teats regularly for signs of damage and discard them if in doubt.

No bottle teat is like a breast. Real-time ultrasound measurements of infants during sucking using different types of teats were made by researchers (Nowak et al 1994) to determine the percentage of lengthening, lateral compression and flattening of the teats. Comparison with data obtained from studies using breastfed infants showed none of the teats lengthened like the human nipple. Scheel et al (2005) investigated the relative merits of three different types of teats. The rate of milk transfer for the preterm babies studied was the primary outcome measure. Suction amplitude and duration of the generated negative intraoral suction pressure were also measured. No type of teat had any advantage over any other. The mother should feel free to experiment, and use the type of teat that seems to suit her baby. It may be easier for the baby to use a simple soft long teat than industry-labelled orthodontic teats (Kassing 2002).

Feeding bottles must also meet the UK standard. This means they will be made of food-grade plastic and have relatively smooth interiors. Crevices and grooves in a bottle make cleaning difficult. Patterned or decorated bottles make it less easy to see whether the bottle is clean.

Sterilization of feeding equipment

Effective cleaning of all utensils used should be demonstrated to the mother and methods of sterilization discussed. The most important prerequisite is that all equipment is thoroughly washed in hot, soapy water and well rinsed before proceeding further. If boiling is to be used, full immersion is essential and the contents must be boiled for 10 minutes. If cold sterilization using a hypochlorite solution is the method of choice, the utensils must be fully immersed in the solution for the recommended time. The manufacturer's advice must be followed when rinsing items removed from the solution. If the item is to be rinsed, previously boiled water should be used and not water directly from the tap. Steam and microwave sterilization are also possible, but the mother should check that her equipment can withstand such methods.

Bottle teats

The size of the hole in the teat causes much anxiety to mothers. It is probably a good idea to have several teats with holes of different sizes so that the mother can experiment as necessary. *To test the hole size, turn the bottle upside down and the milk should drip at a rate of about one drop per second.*

Feeding the baby with the bottle

The baby must never be left unattended while feeding from a bottle and mothers should be warned about the dangers of *bottle propping*. The mother should try to simulate breastfeeding conditions for the baby by holding the baby close, maintaining eye-to-eye contact and allowing the baby to determine his intake. The baby should be held fairly upright, with his head supported in a comfortable, neutral position.

The innate skills a baby has for breastfeeding should also be used when feeding from a bottle. The baby's lips should be touched to elicit the mouth to open wide and the teat should follow the line of the baby's tongue, so that the baby uses the teat effectively. The bottle should be held horizontal to the ground, tilted just enough to ensure the baby is taking milk, not air, through the teat (UNICEF–UK 2010b).

When correctly prepared, modern formula milks do not cause hypernatraemia as did the older types. There is therefore no need to give the baby extra water.

The stools and vomit of a baby fed on formula milk have an unpleasant sour smell. The stools tend to be more formed than those of a breastfed baby and, unlike a breastfed baby, there is a real risk that the artificially fed baby may become constipated.

Healthy Start (and the Welfare Food Scheme)

In 1940 the Welfare Food Scheme was established in the UK, providing tokens to families on low incomes to be exchanged for liquid milk or breastmilk substitutes. This scheme was replaced, in November 2006, by the *Healthy Start Initiative*. This scheme broadened the nutritional base of the Welfare Food Scheme to allow fruit and vegetables as well as liquid milk or breastmilk substitutes to be obtained through the exchange of fixed value vouchers at a range of food and supermarket outlets. Those eligible to receive the vouchers include:

- Pregnant women and families with children under the age of 4 years who receive:
  - Income Support
  - Income-based Jobseeker's Allowance or
  - Child Tax Credit (but not Working Tax Credit), with an annual family income of ≤£16 190 a year 2013/2014)
- All pregnant women under the age of 18, whether or not they are receiving benefits or tax credits.

Those eligible for vouchers are also entitled to free vitamin supplements for themselves, and for their children from 6 months until their 4th birthday.

Midwives and the International Code of Marketing of Breastmilk Substitutes

In 1981, the combined forces of WHO and UNICEF produced a marketing code (WHO 1981), which was adopted at the 34th World Health Assembly. The code has major implications for the work of midwives. Although it is at present a voluntary code in most countries, some countries now have the code enshrined in law. Recommendations include:

- No advertising or promotion in hospitals, shops or to the general public (this includes posters and advertisements in mother-and-baby books).
- Not giving free samples of breastmilk substitutes to mothers.
- No free gifts relating to products within the scope of the code to be given to mothers (including discount coupons or special offers).

- No financial or material gifts to health workers for the purpose of promoting products, nor free or subsidized supplies to hospitals or maternity wards.
- Information provided by manufacturers to health workers should include only scientific and factual material, and not create or imply a belief that bottle-feeding is equivalent or superior to breastfeeding.
- Health workers should encourage and protect breastfeeding.

The code does not prevent mothers from feeding their babies with infant formula, but rather seeks to contribute to safe, adequate nutrition for babies and to promote and protect breastfeeding.

THE BABY FRIENDLY HOSPITAL INITIATIVE

The Baby Friendly Hospital Initiative (BFI) was an initiative launched worldwide in 1991 (and in the UK in 1994) by WHO and UNICEF to encourage hospitals to promote practices supportive of breastfeeding. It was focused around the 10 steps to successful breastfeeding (Box 34.5), with which all hospitals who wish to achieve *Baby Friendly* status must comply (WHO/UNICEF 1989). Evidence for

---

Box 34.5 **The 10 steps to successful breastfeeding**

1. Have a written breastfeeding policy that is routinely communicated to all healthcare staff.
2. Train all healthcare staff in skills necessary to implement this policy.
3. Inform all pregnant women about the benefits and management of breastfeeding.
4. Help mothers initiate breastfeeding soon after birth.
5. Show mothers how to breastfeed and how to maintain lactation even if they should be separated from their infants.
6. Give newborn infants no food or drink other than breastmilk, unless medically indicated.
7. Practice rooming-in: allow mothers and infants to remain together 24 hours a day.
8. Encourage breastfeeding on demand.
9. Give no artificial teats or dummies to breastfeeding infants.
10. Foster the establishment of breastfeeding support groups and refer mothers to them on discharge from hospital or clinic.

WHO/UNICEF 1989

---

the 10 steps is contained in the WHO/UNICEF document of the same name (Vallenas and Savage 1998). This has subsequently been extended to community-based facilities, neonatal units and university training programmes for midwifery and health visiting, all of which can be BFI-accredited in their own right. In addition, all accredited Baby Friendly facilities must fully implement the International Code on the Marketing of Breastmilk Substitutes.

Mothers should expect a certain standard of care from a Baby Friendly hospital (UNICEF–UK 2011c):

When pregnant:
- To have a full discussion about caring for and feeding their baby, including the benefits of breastfeeding, so that they have all the facts to make an informed choice.

When the baby is born:
- To be given their baby to hold against their skin straight after they are born, for as long as they want
- To have a midwife offer them help to start breastfeeding as soon as possible after the baby is born
- To have their baby stay with them at all times.

If they decide to breastfeed:
- To be shown how to hold the baby and how to help him latch on – making sure the baby gets enough milk and feeding is not painful

- To be given accurate and consistent advice about how to breastfeed and to make enough milk for the baby
- To be shown how to express milk by hand
- To receive information about how to get more support for breastfeeding, should they need it, once they leave hospital
- That the baby will *not* be given water or artificial baby milk, unless this is needed for a medical reason.

A mother can expect that staff will support her if she decides that she wants to care for her baby differently or she does not want the information offered. If she decides to feed her baby with formula milk, she can expect to be asked if she wants to be shown how to make up a bottle feed safely and correctly.

The National Institute for Health and Clinical Excellence (NICE 2006a) recommended that all maternity care providers should implement an externally evaluated, structured programme encouraging breastfeeding, using the BFI as a minimum standard. Thus all such healthcare providers should either implement NICE guidance or perform a risk assessment if they reject it (that is, placed on a risk register). Rejection on the grounds of cost, which has often been cited as a reason for not implementing BFI in the past, is unlikely to be acceptable, as NICE economists have documented the fact that implementation would be cost-effective (NICE 2006b; UNICEF–UK 2012a).

REFERENCES

Adler B R, Warner J O 1991 Food intolerance in children. Royal College of General Practitioners members reference book. Camden Publishing, London

Akre J 1989a Infant feeding: the physiological basis. Bulletin of the World Health Organization 67 (Suppl 1):25

Akre J 1989b Infant feeding: the physiological basis. Bulletin of the World Health Organization 67(Suppl 1):79

Ashraf R N, Jalil F, Aperia A et al 1993 Additional water is not needed for healthy babies in a hot climate. Acta Paediatrica 82: 1007–11

Auerbach K G 1990 Sequential and simultaneous breast pumping: a comparison. International Journal of Nursing Studies 27(3):257–65

Auerbach K G, Walker M 1994 When the mother of a premature infant

uses a pump: what every NICU nurse needs to know. Neonatal Network 13(4):23–9

Bagnall A. 2005 Feeding development. In: Jones E, King C (eds) Feeding and nutrition in the pre-term infant. Elsevier/Churchill Livingstone, Edinburgh

Bahna S L 1987 Milk allergy in infancy. Annals of Allergy 59:131–6

Bollag U, Albrecht E, Wingert W 1984 Medicated versus saline nose drops in the management of upper respiratory infection. Helvetica Paediatrica Acta 39(4):341–5

Bosma J F, Hepburn L G, Josell S D et al 1990 Ultrasound demonstration of tongue motions during suckle feeding. Developmental Medicine and Child Neurology 32(3):223–9

Brostoff J, Gamlin L 1998 The complete guide to allergy and food intolerance. Bloomsbury Publishing, London

Brown S J, Alexander J, Thomas P 1999 Feeding outcome in breast-fed term babies supplemented by cup or bottle. Midwifery 15:92–6

Busfield A, Samuel R, McNinch A et al 2013 Vitamin K deficiency bleeding after NICE guidance and withdrawal of Konakion Neonatal: British Paediatric Surveillance Unit study, 2006–2008. Archives of Disease in Childhood 98:41–7.

Butte N F, Garza C, Stuff J E et al 1984 Effect of maternal diet and body composition on lactational performance. American Journal of Clinical Nutrition 39:296–306

Canfield L M, Hopkinson J M, Lima A F et al 1991 Vitamin K in colostrum and mature human milk over the lactation period – a cross-sectional study. American Journal of Clinical Nutrition 53(3):730–5

Carvahlo M, Hall M, Harvey D 1981 Effects of water supplementation on physiological jaundice in breast-fed babies. Archives of Disease in Childhood 56:568–9

Chapman D J, Young S, Ferris A M et al 2001 Impact of breast pumping on lactogenesis stage II after caesarean delivery: a randomized clinical trial. Pediatrics 107(6):E94

Cohen G M, Albertini W 2012 Colic. Pediatrics in Review 33:332. Available at: http//:pedsinreview .aappublications.org/ content/33/7/332 (accessed 5 August 2013)

Coovadia H M, Rollins N C, Bland R M et al 2007 Mother-to-child transmission of HIV-1 infection during exclusive breastfeeding in the first 6 months of life: an intervention cohort study. Lancet 369(9567):1107–16

Coutsoudis A, Pillay K, Spooner E et al 1999 Influence of infant-feeding patterns on early mother-to-child transmission of HIV-1 in Durban, South Africa: a prospective cohort study. South African Vitamin A Study Group. Lancet 354(9177):471–6

Cox D B, Kent J C, Casey T M et al 1999 Breast growth and the urinary excretion of lactose during human pregnancy and early lactation: endocrine relationships. Experimental Physiology 84(2):421–34

Crawley H, Westland S 2013 Infant milks in the UK: a practical guide for health professionals – June 2013. Available at: www.firststepsnutrition .org/newpages/Infants/infant _feeding_infant_milks_UK.html (accessed 5 August 2013)

Cross B A 1977 Comparative physiology of milk removal. Symposium of the Zoological Society of London No. 41, p 193–210. In: Peaker M (ed) Comparative aspects of lactation. Academic Press, London. Available at: http://catalogue.nla.gov.au/ Record/993562 (accessed 5 August 2013)

Cruz-Korchin N, Korchin L, Gonzalez-Keelan C et al 2002 Macromastia: how much of it is fat? Plastic Reconstruction Surgery 109(1): 64–8

Daly S 1993 The short term synthesis and infant regulated removal of milk in lactating women. Experimental Physiology 78:209–20

Davies P A, Robinson R J, Scopes J W et al 1972 Medical care of newborn babies. Clinics in Developmental Medicine Nos 44/45. Spastics International Medical Publications/ William Heinemann Medical Books, London, p 204

Dearlove J C, Dearlove B M 1981 Prolactin, fluid balance and lactation. British Journal of Obstetrics and Gynecology 123:845–6

Dewey K G 1998 Effects of maternal caloric restriction and exercise during lactation. Journal of Nutrition 128 (2 Suppl):386S–9

Dewey K G, Lovelady C A, Nommsen-Rivers L A et al 1994 A randomized study of the effects of aerobic exercise by lactating women on breast-milk volume and composition. New England Journal of Medicine 330(7):449–53

Dewey K G, Nommsen-Rivers L A, Heinig M J et al 2003 Risk factors for suboptimal infant breastfeeding behavior, delayed onset of lactation, and excess neonatal weight loss. Pediatrics 112(3 Pt 1):607–19

DH (Department of Health) 2009 Vitamin D – an essential nutrient for all … but who is at risk of vitamin D deficiency? Important information for healthcare professionals. DH, London

DH (Department of Health) 2011 Introducing solid foods – giving your baby a better start in life. C4L175 (February 2011) Brochure 750K. Available at: www.gov.uk/ government/publications/ introducing-solid-foods-giving-your -baby-a-better-start-in-life (accessed 5 August 2013)

DH (Department of Health) 2012 Guide to bottle feeding (302064) Available at: www.gov.uk/ government/publications/start4life -updated-guide-to-bottle-feeding (accessed 5 August 2013)

Dixon J M 1988 Repeated aspiration of breast abscess in lactating women. British Medical Journal 297:1517–18

Dollberg S, Botzer E, Grunis E et al 2006 Immediate nipple pain relief after frenotomy in breast-fed infants with ankyloglossia: a randomized, prospective study. Journal of Pediatric Surgery 41(9):1598–600

Dusdieker L B, Hemingway D L, Stumbo P J 1994 Is milk production impaired by dieting during lactation? American Journal of Clinical Nutrition 59:833–40

EFSA (European Food Standards Agency) 1993 Commission Directive 93/11/EEC of 15 March 1993 concerning the release of N-nitrosamines and N-nitrosatable substances from elastomer or rubber teats and soothers. Available at: http://europa.eu/legislation _summaries/food_safety/ contamination_environmental _factors/l21088_en.htm (accessed 5 August 2013)

Eglin R P, Wilkinson A R 1987 HIV infection and pasteurization of breast milk. Lancet i:1093

European Food Standards Agency 2006 Statement replying to applicant's comment on the Panel's Opinion relating to the evaluation of goat's milk protein as a protein source for infant formulae and follow-on formulae by the Scientific Panel on Dietetic Products, Nutrition and Allergies (NDA). Available at: www .efsa.europa.eu/en/efsajournal/ pub/30a.htm (accessed 5 September 2013)

Evans K, Evans R, Simmer K 1995 Effect of the method of breast feeding on breast engorgement, mastitis and infantile colic. Acta Paediatrica 84(8):849–52

Fairbank L, Woolridge M J, Renfrew M J et al 2000 Effective healthcare: promoting the initiation of breast-feeding. NHS Centre for Reviews and Dissemination/ University of York, 6(2):1–185

Fenstein J, Berkelhamer J, Gruszka M et al 1986 Factors related to early termination of breast-feeding in an urban population. Pediatrics 78(2):210–15

Fernstrom J D 1999 Effects of dietary polyunsaturated fatty acids on neuronal function. Lipids 34(2):161–9

Flint A, New K, Davies M W 2007 Cup feeding versus other forms of supplemental enteral feeding for newborn infants unable to fully breastfeed. Cochrane Intervention Review. Available at: http:// onlinelibrary.wiley.com/ doi/10.1002/14651858.CD005092 .pub2/abstract (accessed 5 August 2013)

Fredrikzon B, Hernell O, Blackberg L et al 1978 Bile salt-stimulated lipase in human milk: evidence of activity in vivo and of a role in the digestion of milk retinol esters. Pediatric Research 12(11):1048–52

Garcez L W, Giugliani E R J 2005 Population-based study on the practice of breastfeeding in children born with cleft lip and palate. The Cleft Palate-Craniofacial Journal 42(6):687–93

Garza C, Rasmussen K M 2000 Pregnancy and lactation. In: Garrow J S, James W P T, Ralph Alan (eds) Human nutrition and dietetics, 10th edn. Harcourt Medical, Edinburgh, p 437–48

Geddes D T, Kent J C, Mitoulas L R et al 2008 Tongue movement and intra-oral vacuum in breastfeeding infants. Early Human Development 84(7):471–7

Going J J, Moffat D F 2004 Escaping from Flatland: clinical and biological aspects of human mammary duct anatomy in three dimensions. Journal of Pathology 203(1): 538–44

Greer F R 1997 Vitamin K status of lactating mothers and their infants. Acta Paediatrica 88(430):95–103

Gregory J 2000 National diet and nutrition survey young people aged 4–18 years, volume 1. Report of the diet and nutrition survey. Great Britain Office for National Statistics Social Survey Division. TSO, London

Groh-Wargo S, Toth A, Mahoney K et al 1995 The utility of a bilateral breast pumping system for mothers of premature infants. Neonatal Network 14(8):31–6

Hall B 1979 Changing content of human milk and early development of appetite control. Keeping Abreast, April/June: 139

Hall Moran V 2012 Nutrition in pregnant and breastfeeding adolescents: a biopsychosocial perspective. In: Hall Moran V (ed) Maternal and infant nutrition and nurture: controversies and challenges, 2nd edn. Quay Books, London, p 45–88

Hammer R L, Babcock G, Fisher A G 1996 Low-fat diet and exercise in obese lactating women. Breast-feeding Review 4(1):29–34

Hamosh M 1998 Protective functions of proteins and lipids in human milk. Biology of the Neonate 74:163

Hazelbaker A K 2010 Tongue-tie: morphgenesis, impact, assessment and treatment. Aidan and Eva Press, Ohio

Hill P, Aldag J, Chatterton R 1999 Effect of pumping style on milk production in mothers of non-nursing preterm infants. Journal of Human Lactation 15(3):209–16

Hoddinott P, Pill R 1999 Qualitative study of decisions about infant feeding among women in the East End of London. British Medical Journal 318(7175):30–4

Hodge C 1967 Suppression of lactation by stilboestrol. Lancet ii(7510):286–7

Hogan M, Westcott C, Griffiths M 2005 Randomized, controlled trial of division of tongue-tie in infants with feeding problems. Journal of Paediatrics and Child Health 41(5–6):246–50

Hopkinson J 2007 Nutrition in lactation. In: Hale T V, Harmann P F (eds) Textbook of human lactation. Hale Publishing, Amarillo, TX, p 379–81

Host A 1991 Importance of the first meal on the development of cow's milk allergy and intolerance. Allergy Proceedings 12:227–32

Howard C R, Howard F M, Lanphear B et al 2003 Randomized clinical trial of pacifier use and bottle-feeding or cupfeeding and their effect on breast-feeding. Pediatrics 111(3):511–18

Hytten F E, Baird D 1958 The development of the nipple in pregnancy. Lancet i:1201–4

Illingworth P J, Jong R T, Howie P W et al 1986 Diminution in energy expenditure during lactation. British Medical Journal 292:437–41

Inch S, Fisher C 1995 Mastitis in lactating women. The Practitioner 239:472–6

Inch S, Garforth S 1989 Establishing and maintaining breastfeeding. In: Chalmers I, Enkin M, Keirse M (eds) Effective care in pregnancy and childbirth. Oxford University Press, Oxford, p 1359–70

Infant Formula and Follow-on Formula Regulations 2007 Statutory

Instrument first introduced 1995; updated 2007. HMSO, London

Ingram J, Woolridge M, Greenwood R 2001 Breast-feeding: it is worth trying with the second baby. Lancet 358(9286):986–7

Jackson D A, Woolridge M W, Imong S M et al 1987 The automatic sampling shield: a device for sampling suckled breast milk. Early Human Development 15(5):295–306

Jamal N, Ng K H, McLean D et al 2004 Mammographic breast glandularity in Malaysian women: data derived from radiography. American Journal of Roentgenology 182(3):713–17

Johnson P R 2006 Tongue-tie – exploding the myths. Infant 2(3):96–9. Available at: www .neonatal-nursing.co.uk/pdf/ inf_009_exm.pdf (accessed 5 August 2013)

Jones E, Dimmock P, Spencer S A 2001 A randomised controlled trial to compare methods of milk expression after preterm delivery. Archives of Disease in Childhood Fetal and Neonatal Edition 85:F91–5

Kamelska A M, Pietrzak-Fiećko R, Bryl K 2012 Variation of the cholesterol content in breast milk during 10 days collection at early stages of lactation. Acta Biochimica Polonica 59(2):243–7

Kassing D 2002 Bottle-feeding as a tool to reinforce breastfeeding. Journal of Human Lactation 18(1):56–60

Kaufmann T 1999 Infant feeding: politics vs pragmatism? RCM Midwives Journal 2(8):244

Kennedy K I, Rivera R, McNeilly A S 1989 Consensus statement on the use of breast-feeding as a family planning method. Contraception 439:477

Khaghani S, Ezzatpanah H, Mazhari N et al 2010 Zinc and copper concentrations in human milk and infant formulas. Iranian Journal of Pediatrics 20(1):53–7

Kim H H, Park C S 2004 A compensatory nutrition regimen during gestation stimulates mammary development and lactation potential in rats. Journal of Nutrition 134(4):756–61

Kochenour N K 1980 Lactation suppression. Clinical Obstetrics and Gynecology 23:1052–9

Krebs N F 1999 Zinc transfer to the breastfed infant. Journal of Mammary Gland Biology and Neoplasia 4(3):259–68

Kries R V, Shearer M, McCarthy P T et al 1987 Vitamin K1 content of maternal milk: influence of the stage of lactation, lipid composition, and vitamin K1 supplements given to the mother. Pediatric Research 22(5): 513–17

Lang S, Lawrence C, Orme R L 1994 Cup feeding: an alternative method of infant feeding. Archives of Disease in Childhood 71:365–9

Leaf A A 2007 Vitamins for babies and young children: RCPCH Standing Committee on Nutrition. Archives of Disease in Childhood 92(2): 160–4

Liu B, Newburg D S 2013 Human milk glycoproteins protect infants against human pathogens. Breastfeeding Medicine 8(4):354–62

Love S M, Barsky S H 2004 Anatomy of the nipple and breast ducts revisited. Cancer 101(9):1947–57

Macdonald H M, Mavroeidi A, Fraser W D et al 2011 Sunlight and dietary contributions to the seasonal vitamin D status of cohorts of healthy postmenopausal women living at northerly latitudes: a major cause for concern? Osteoporosis International 22(9):2461–72

Macdonald P D, Ross S R, Grant L et al 2003 Neonatal weight loss in breast and formula fed infants. Archives of Disease in Childhood Fetal and Neonatal Edition 88: F472–6

Main Trial Collaborative Group 1994 Preparing for breastfeeding: treatment of inverted and non-protractile nipples in pregnancy. Midwifery 10:200–14

Martyn T 1999 Soya in artificial baby milks. Practising Midwife 2(6): 17–19

McAndrew F, Thompson J, Fellows L et al 2012 Infant Feeding Survey 2010. A survey carried out on behalf of Health and Social Care Information Centre by IFF Research in partnership with Professor Mary Renfrew, Professor of Mother and Infant Health, College of Medicine, Dentistry and Nursing, University of Dundee. Available at: www.hscic.gov .uk/ (accessed 5 August 2013)

McKechnie A C, Eglash A 2010 Nipple shields: a review of the literature. Breastfeeding Medicine 5(6):309–14

Meier P, Cranston-Anderson J 1987 Responses of small pre-term infants to bottle and breast-feeding. Maternal–Child Nursing Journal 12:97–105

Metcalf I J, Irons T G, Lawrence D S et al 1994 Simethicone in the treatment of infant colic: a randomized placebo-controlled multicentre trial. Pediatrics 94:29–34

Minchin M 2001 Towards safer artificial feeding (booklet). Alma Publications, St Kilda South, Australia

Moan J, Porojnicu A C, Dahlback A et al 2008 Addressing the health benefits and risks, involving vitamin D or skin cancer, of increased sun exposure. Proceedings of the National Academy of Science 105 (2): 668–73

Monaci G, Woolridge M 2011 Ultrasound video analysis for understanding infant breastfeeding. Proceedings of the 18th Institut d'Economia Ecològica i Ecologia Política International (IEEEP) Conference on Image Processing (ICIP), 1765–8. doi: 10.1109/ ICIP.2011.6115802

Montagne P, Cuillière M L, Molé C et al 2001 Changes in lactoferrin and lysozyme levels in human milk during the first twelve weeks of lactation. Advances in Experimental and Medical Biology 501:241–7

Morse J M, Ewing G, Gamble D et al 1992 The effect of maternal fluid intake on breast milk supply: a pilot study. Canadian Journal of Public Health 83(3):213–16

Neville M C, McFadden T B, Forsyth I 2002 Hormonal regulation of mammary differentiation and milk secretion. Journal of Mammary Gland Biology and Neoplasia 7(1):49–66

NICE (National Institute for Health and Clinical Excellence) 2005 Division of ankyloglossia (tongue tie) for breastfeeding – information for the public. IPG 149. Available at: www .nice.org.uk/page.aspx?o=284318 (accessed 5 August 2013)

NICE (National Institute for Health and Clinical Excellence) 2006a Postnatal care: Routine postnatal care of

women and their babies – full guideline. CG 37. NICE, London. Available at: http://guidance.nice.org .uk/CG37/guidance/pdf/English (accessed 5 August 2013)

NICE (National Institute for Health and Clinical Excellence) 2006b Postnatal care: national cost impact report. Available at www.nice.org.uk/ nicemedia/live/10988/30155/30155 .doc (accessed 23 October 2013)

NICE (National Institute for Health and Clinical Excellence) 2008 (Reviewed and re-issued unchanged 2011) Improving the nutrition of pregnant and breast-feeding mothers and children in low-income households. PH 11. Available at: www.nice.org .uk/guidance/index.jsp? action=byID&o=11943 (accessed 5 August 2013)

NICE (National Institute for Health and Care Excellence) 2013 Postnatal care: Quality Statement 4: Infant health – safer infant sleeping. Available at: http://publications.nice.org.uk/ postnatal-care-qs37/quality -statement-4-infant-health-safer -infant-sleeping (accessed 5 August 2013)

Nickell W B, Skelton J 2005 Breast fat and fallacies: more than 100 years of anatomical fantasy. Journal of Human Lactation 21(2):126–30

Nicoll A, Ginsburg R, Tripp J 1982 Supplementary feeding and jaundice in newborns. Acta Paediatrica Scandinavica 71:759–61

Nicolls H 1997 Two on to one will go. Midwifery Matters 73:6–7

Nowak A J, Smith W L, Erenberg A 1994 Imaging evaluation of artificial nipples during bottle feeding. Archives of Pediatrics and Adolescent Medicine 148(1):40–2

Owen C G, Whincup P H, Kaye S J et al 2008 Does initial breastfeeding lead to lower blood cholesterol in adult life? A quantitative review of the evidence. American Journal of Clinical Nutrition 88:305–14

Paronen J, Knip M, Savilahti E et al. 2000 Effect of cow's milk exposure and maternal type 1 diabetes on cellular and humeral immunization to dietary insulin in infants at genetic risk for type 1 diabetes. Finnish Trial to Reduce IDDM in the Genetically at Risk Study Group. Diabetes 49(10):1657–65

733

Perry R, Hunt K, Ernst E 2011 Nutritional supplements and other complementary medicines for infantile colic: a systematic review. Pediatrics 127:720–33

Picciano M F 2001 Nutrient composition of human milk. Pediatric Clinics of North America 48(1):53–67

Prentice A M, Addey C V P, Wilde C J 1989 Evidence for local feedback control of human milk secretion. Biochemical Society Transactions 17(122):489–92

Prentice A M, Goldberg G R, Prentice A 1994 Body mass index and lactational performance. European Journal of Clinical Nutrition 48(Suppl 3):S78–89

Prentice A M, Lunn P G, Watkinson M et al 1983 Dietary supplementation of lactating Gambian women II. Effect on maternal health, nutritional status and biochemistry. Human Nutrition and Clinical Nutrition 37(1):65–74

Prentice A M, Roberts S B, Whitehead R G 1980 Dietary supplementation of Gambian nursing mothers and lactational performance. Lancet ii:886–8

Puckett R M, Offringa M 2000 Prophylactic vitamin K for vitamin K deficiency bleeding in neonates. Cochrane Database Systematic Review 2000, Issue 4. Art. No. CD002776. doi:10.1002/14651858 .CD002776

Quigley M, Henderson G, Anthony M Y et al 2008 Formula milk versus donor breast milk for feeding preterm or low birth weight infants. Cochrane Intervention Review. Available at: http://onlinelibrary .wiley.com/doi/10.1002/14651858 .CD002971.pub2/abstract (accessed 5 August 2013)

Ramos R, Kennedy K I, Visness C M 1996 Effectiveness of lactational amenorrhoea in prevention of pregnancy in Manila, the Philippines: non-comparative prospective trial. British Medical Journal 313:909–12

Ramsay D 2005 Investigation of the sucking dynamics of the breast-feeding term infant: ultrasound and intraoral vacuum research. Presented at the ILCA Conference: Breaking the Barriers to Breast-feeding: Research, Policy and Practice, Chicago, USA

Ramsay D T, Kent J C, Hartmann R A et al 2005 Anatomy of the lactating human breast redefined with ultrasound imaging. Journal of Anatomy 206(6):525–34

Ramsay D T, Kent J C, Owens R A et al 2004 Ultrasound imaging of milk ejection in the breast of lactating women. Pediatrics 113:361–7

Rapley G 2012 Baby-led weaning. In: Hall Moran V (eds) Maternal and infant nutrition and nurture: controversies and challenges, 2nd edn. Quay Books, London, p 261–84

Rasmussen K M 2007 Maternal obesity and the outcome of breastfeeding. In: Hale T W, Hartmann P E, eds. Hale and Hartmann's textbook on human lactation. Hale Publishing, Amarillo, TX, p 387–402

RCM (Royal College of Midwives) 2002 Successful breastfeeding, 3rd edn. Churchill Livingstone, Edinburgh

Reid J 2004 A review of feeding interventions for infants with cleft palate. Cleft Palate–Craniofacial Journal 41(3):268–78

Renfrew M J, Hall D. 2008. Enabling women to breast feed. Editorial. British Medical Journal 337:a1570

Renfrew M J, Pokhrel S, Quigley M et al 2012 Preventing disease and saving resources: the potential contribution of increasing breastfeeding rates in the UK. Available at: www.unicef.org .uk/breastfeeding (accessed 5 August 2013)

Righard L, Alade M O 1990 Effect of delivery room routines on success of first breast-feed. Lancet 336:1105–7

Saarinen U M, Siimes M A 1979 Iron absorption from breast milk, cow's milk and iron supplemented formula: an opportunistic use of changes in total body iron determined by hemoglobin, ferritin and body weight in 132 infants. Pediatric Research 13:143–7

Sachdev H P S, Krishna J, Puri R K 1991 Water supplementation in exclusively breast-fed infants during the summer in the tropics. Lancet 337: 929–33

Sandstrom B, Cederblad A, Lonnerdal B 1983 Zinc absorption from human, cows' milk and infant formula. American Journal of Diseases of Childhood 137:726–9

Santoro W Jr, Martinez F E, Ricco R G et al 2010 Colostrum ingested during the first day of life by exclusively breastfed healthy newborn infants. Journal of Pediatrics 156(1):29–32

Scheel C E, Schanler R J, Lau C 2005 Does the choice of bottle nipple affect the oral feeding performance of very-low-birth weight (VLBW) infants? Acta Paediatrica 94(9):1266–72

Scholtz S A, Gottipati B S, Gajewski B J et al 2013 Dietary sialic acid and cholesterol influence cortical composition in developing rats. Journal of Nutrition 143(2): 132–5

Shaw N J, Pal B R 2002 Vitamin D deficiency in UK Asian families: activating a new concern. Archives of Disease in Childhood 86:147–9

Specker B L, Valanis B, Hertzberg V R et al 1985 Sunshine exposure and serum 25-hydroxyvitamin D concentrations in exclusively breast-fed infants. Journal of Pediatrics 107 (3):372–6

Swift K, Janke J 2003 Breast binding … is it all that it's wrapped up to be? Journal of Obstetrics, Gynecology and Neonatal Nursing 32(3):332–9

Taitz L S, Scholey E 1989 Are babies more satisfied by casein based formulas? Archives of Disease in Childhood 64(4):619–21

Taneri F, Kurukahvecioglu O, Akyurek N et al 2006 Micro-anatomy of milk ducts in the nipple. European Surgery Research 38(6):545–9

Thomsen A C, Espersen M D, Maigaard S 1984 Course and treatment of milk stasis, non-infectious inflammation of the breast, and infectious mastitis in nursing women. American Journal of Obstetrics and Gynecology 149:492–5

Thorkelsson T, Mimouni F, Namgung R et al 1994 Similar gastric emptying rates for casein- and whey-predominant formulas in preterm infants. Pediatric Research 36(3):329–33

Torgersen T, Ystrom E, Haugen M et al 2010 Breastfeeding practice in mothers with eating disorders. Maternal Child Nutrition 6(3):243–52

Ueda T, Yokoyama Y, Irahara M et al 1994 Influence of psychological stress on suckling-induced pulsatile oxytocin release. Obstetrics and Gynecology 84:259–62

UNICEF and Department of Health 2012 Off to the best start. Available at: www.unicef.org.uk/BabyFriendly/Parents/Resources/Resources-for-parents/Off-to-the-best-start/ (accessed 5 August 2013)

UNICEF–UK 2010a Breastfeeding assessment tool. Available at: www.unicef.org.uk/Documents/Baby_Friendly/Guidance/bf_assessment_tool.pdf?epslanguage=en (accessed 5 August 2013)

UNICEF–UK 2010b A guide to infant formula for parents who are bottle feeding. Available at: www.unicef.org.uk/BabyFriendly/Resources/Resources-for-parents/A-guide-to-infant-formula-for-parents-who-are-bottle-feeding/ (accessed 5 August 2013)

UNICEF–UK 2011a Caring for your baby at night – a parents' guide. www.unicef.org.uk/BabyFriendly/Resources/Resources-for-parents/Caring-for-your-baby-at-night/ (accessed 5 August 2013)

UNICEF–UK 2011b Caring for your baby at night. A health professional's guide to 'Caring for your baby at night' Available at: www.unicef.org.uk/Documents/Baby_Friendly/Leaflets/HPs_Guide_to_Coping_At_Night_Final.pdf (accessed 5 August 2013)

UNICEF–UK 2011c How to implement Baby Friendly standards – a guide for maternity setting Available at: www.unicef.org.uk/Documents/Baby_Friendly/Guidance/Implementation%20Guidance/Implementation_guidance_maternity_web.pdf (accessed 5 August 2013)

UNICEF–UK 2012a Preventing disease and saving resources: the potential contribution of increasing breastfeeding rates in the UK. Available at: www.unicef.org.uk/Documents/Baby_Friendly/Research/Preventing_disease_saving_resources.pdf?epslanguage=en (accessed 5 August 2013)

UNICEF–UK 2012b Guide to the Baby Friendly Initiative standards. Available at: www.unicef.org.uk/BabyFriendly/Health-Professionals/New-Baby-Friendly-Standards/ (accessed 5 August 2013)

Vaarala O, Knip M, Paronen J et al 1999 Cow's milk formula feeding induces primary immunization to insulin in infants at genetic risk for type 1 diabetes. Diabetes 48(7): 1389–94

Vallenas C, Savage F 1998 Evidence for the ten steps to successful breastfeeding. Division of Child Health and Development, WHO, Geneva

Vandeweyer E, Hertens D 2002 Quantification of glands and fat in breast tissue: an experimental determination. Annals of Anatomy 184(2):181–4

Waldenström U, Swensen Å 1991 Rooming-in at night in the postpartum ward. Midwifery 7: 82–9

White A, Freith S, O'Brien M 1992 Infant feeding 1990. Survey carried out for the Department of Health by the Office of Population Censuses and Surveys. HMSO, London

Whitehead R G, Paul A A, Black A E et al 1981 Recommended dietary amounts of energy for pregnancy or lactation in the UK. In: Torun B, Young V R, Rang W M (eds) Protein energy requirements of developing countries: evaluation of new data. United Nations University, Tokyo, p 259–65

WHO (World Health Organization) 1981 International code of marketing of breast-milk substitutes. WHO, Geneva

WHO (World Health Organization) 1998 Evidence for the ten steps to successful breastfeeding. WHO, Geneva, p 627

WHO (World Health Organization) 2000 Mastitis: causes and management (WHO/RCH/CAH/00.13). Department of Child and Adolescent Health and Development, WHO, Geneva

WHO (World Health Organisation) 2007 Guidelines for the safe preparation, storage and handling of powdered infant formula. WHO Geneva. Available at: www.who.int/foodsafety/publications/micro/pif2007/en/ (accessed 5 August 2013)

WHO (World Health Organization)/UNICEF 1989 Joint statement – protecting, promoting and supporting breastfeeding. WHO, Geneva

WHO (World Health Organization)/UNICEF 2003 Global strategy on infant and young child feeding. Available at: www.who.int/nutrition/topics/global_strategy/en/ and www.who.int/nutrition/publications/infantfeeding/9241562218/en/index.html (accessed 5 August 2013)

WHO (World Health Organisation)/UNICEF/UNAIDS 2010 Guidelines on HIV and infant feeding. Available at: http://whqlibdoc.who.int/publications/2010/9789241599535_eng.pdf (accessed 5 August 2013)

Widström A M, Ransjo-Arvidson A B, Christensson K et al 1987 Gastric suction in healthy newborn infants. Acta Paediatrica Scandinavica 76:566–78

Wilde C J, Addey C V P, Boddy L M et al 1995 Autocrine regulation of milk secretion by a protein in milk. Biochemical Journal 305: 51–8

Willacy H 2010 Vitamin K deficiency bleeding. Review article for EMIS (Egton Medical Information Systems) Document ID: 2224, Version: 23. Available at: www.patient.co.uk/doctor/Haemorrhagic-Disease-of-Newborn.htm#ref-2 (accessed 5 August 2013)

Woolridge M W 1986 The 'anatomy' of sucking. Midwifery 2:164–71

Woolridge M W 1995 Breast-feeding: physiology into practice. In: Davis D P (ed) Nutrition in child health. Royal College of Physicians, London, p 13–31

Woolridge M 2011 The mechanisms of breastfeeding revised – new insights into how babies feed provided by fresh ultrasound studies of breastfeeding. Evidence-Based Child Health (A Cochrane Review Journal) 6(Suppl 1):46

Woolridge M W, Baum J D, Drewett R F 1982 Individual patterns of milk intake during breast-feeding. Early Human Development 7: 265–72

Woolridge M W, Fisher C 1988 Overfeeding and symptoms of malabsorption in the breast-fed baby: a possible artefact of feed management? Lancet ii:382–4

Ziegler E E 2011 Consumption of cow's milk as a cause of iron deficiency in infants and toddlers. Nutritional Review 69 (Suppl 1):S37–42

FURTHER READING

Hale T, Hartmann P 2007 Hale and Hartmann's textbook of human lactation. Hale Publishing, Amarillo TX

A multi-author textbook, in six sections: anatomy and biochemistry, immunobiology, management of the infant, management of the mother, maternal and infant nutrition and medications.

Hall Moran V (ed) 2012 Maternal and infant nutrition and nurture: controversies and challenges, 2nd edn. Quay Books, London

This multi-author book uses a sociobiological perspective to examine the complex interaction between political, sociocultural and biological factors in food and health in relation to maternal and infant nutrition.

Inch S, Fisher C 1999 Breast-feeding: into the 21st century. NT clinical monographs, No. 32. Emap Healthcare, London. Available at www.amazon.ca/dp/190249976X

A concise but wide-ranging review of the importance of breastfeeding, the difficulties facing midwives who want to help breastfeeding women and the ways in which these might be overcome.

Infant Formula and Follow-on Formula Regulations 1995; updated 2007 Stationery Office, London. Online. Available at: www.legislation.gov.uk/ uksi/2007/3521/contents/made

This is the UK government's response to the European Directive 1991 (91/321/EEC OJ No. L175, 4.7.91), which sought to persuade all EU countries to adopt the International Code of Marketing of Breastmilk Substitutes. It still falls short of the code in several important respects, notably in relation to advertising.

Palmer G 2009 The politics of breast-feeding, 3rd edn. Pinter and Martin, London

This book links biology and politics (sexual, economic and environmental) in an exploration of the consequences of women's changing role in society and the acceleration of the Industrial Revolution, which created the demand for 'artificial milks'.

Renfrew M J, Fisher C, Arms S 2004 Breastfeeding: how to breastfeed your baby, 3rd edn. Celestial Arts, Berkeley, CA

Taking up where texts addressed primarily to health workers leave off, the authors blend wisdom, experience, idealism and learning to produce a clear, basic breastfeeding guide that is focused primarily at mothers.

World Health Organization (WHO)/ UNICEF 1981 International Code of Marketing of Breast Milk Substitutes. Online. Available at: www .babymilkaction.org/regs/thecode .html

This was adopted by a resolution (WHA34.22) of the World Health Assembly in 1981. A copy of the code can also be obtained from Baby Milk Action (see Useful Websites and Contact Details, below).

World Health Organization (WHO) 1989 Protecting, promoting and supporting breast-feeding: the special role of maternity services. A Joint WHO/UNICEF Statement. WHO, Geneva

This is the document that first set out the 10 steps for successful breastfeeding, which formed the basis of the global Baby Friendly Hospital Initiative, and makes recommendations concerning the structure and function of (maternity) healthcare services.

USEFUL WEBSITES AND CONTACT DETAILS

Association of Breastfeeding Mothers: www.abm.me.uk
Helpline: tel 0300 330 5453
Baby Milk Action: www.babymilkaction.org
34 Trumpington Street, Cambridge CB2 1QY. Tel 01223 464420
Baby Feeding Law Group: www.babyfeedinglawgroup.org.uk/

The Baby Feeding Law Group is made up of leading UK health professional and mother support organizations working to strengthen UK baby feeding laws in line with UN recommendations.

Breastfeeding Network: www.breastfeedingnetwork .org.uk
BfN Supporterline: tel 0300 100 0210
CLAPA (Cleft Lip And Palate Association): www.clapa.com
235–237 Finchley Road, London NW3 6LS. Tel 020 7431 0033
Healthy Start Initiative: www.healthystart.nhs.uk
La Leche League: www.laleche.org.uk
Helpline: tel 0845 120 2918

National Childbirth Trust: www.nct.org.uk
Tel: 0870 444 8708; enquiry line: 0870 444 8707
UNICEF UK Baby Friendly Initiative: www.babyfriendly.org.uk
Africa House, 64–78 Kingsway, London WC2B 6NB. Tel: 0300 330 0700
A short video *How to hand express* is available at: www.unicef.org.uk/ BabyFriendly/Resources/AudioVideo/ Hand-expression/

Glossary of terms and acronyms

Abruptio placenta: Premature separation of a normally situated placenta. This term is commonly used from viability (24 weeks).

Acridine orange: A stain used in fluorescence microscopy; it that causes bacteria to fluoresce green to red.

Aetiology: The science of the cause of disease.

Affective awareness: An awareness of feelings and ability to express them.

Affective neutrality: Known as professional detachment.

Alveoli: Terminal sacs at the end of the bronchial tree where gaseous exchange takes place.

Anhedonia: The loss of pleasure.

Amenorrhoea: Absence of menstrual periods.

Amniotic fluid embolism (AFE): The escape of amniotic fluid through the wall of the uterus or placental site into the maternal circulation, triggering life-threatening anaphylactic shock in the mother. (*The word 'embolism', denoting a clot, is a misnomer.*)

Amniotomy: Artificial rupture of the amniotic sac.

Anteflexion: The uterus bends forwards upon itself.

Anterior obliquity of the uterus: Altered uterine axis. The uterus leans forward due to poor maternal abdominal muscles and a pendulous abdomen.

Anteversion: The uterus leans forward.

Antigen: A substance that stimulates the production of an antibody.

Anuria: Lack of urine production.

Apnoea: An absence of breathing for more than 20 seconds.

Asynclitism: The presentation of the fetal head at an oblique angle between the axis of the presenting part of the fetus and the pelvic planes during labour/childbirth (also known as obliquity).

Atresia: Closure or absence of an usual opening or canal.

Augmentation of labour: Intervention to correct slow progress in labour.

Bandl's ring: An exaggerated retraction ring seen as an oblique ridge above the symphysis pubis between the upper and lower uterine segments, which is a sign of obstructed labour.

Basal body temperature: The temperature of the body when at rest. In natural family planning, it is taken as soon as the woman wakes from sleep and before any activity occurs or after a period of at least 1 hour's rest.

Basal plate: The maternal side of the placenta.

Beneficence: To do good.

Bicornuate uterus: A structural congenital malformation of the uterus that results in two horns; commonly referred to as a 'heart-shaped' uterus.

Bioavailability: The degree to which or rate at which a drug or other substance becomes available to the target tissue after administration.

Bioequivalent: Acting on the body with the same strength and similar bioavailability as the same dosage of a sample of a given substance.

Bipolar disorder: A mental illness or mood disorder where the individual experiences periods of depression and elevated mood (mania). (*Previously known as manic depression.*)

Birth centres: These may be freestanding (*away from hospital*) or in hospital grounds or in the hospital. The emphasis is on providing a less medical environment and supporting normal birth.

Bishop's Score: Rating system to assess suitability of cervix for induction of labour.

Bregma: Anterior fontanelle.

Burns–Marshall manoeuvre: A method of breech birth involving traction to prevent the fetal neck from bending backwards.

Caput succedaneum: A diffuse oedematous swelling under the scalp but above the periosteum.

Cardiotocogram/graphy (CTG): Measurement of the fetal heart rate and uterine contractions on a machine that is able to provide a paper printout of the information it records.

Care of the Next Infant (CONI): A programme of support facilitated by The Lullaby Trust (previously known as the Foundation for the Study of Infant Deaths [FSID]).

Caseload practice: A personal caseload where named midwives care for individual women.

Central venous pressure (CVP) line: An intravenous (IV) tube that measures the pressure in the right atrium or superior vena cava, indicating the volume of blood returning to the heart and by implication, hypovolaemia.

Cephalhaematoma (cephalohaematoma): An effusion of blood under the periosteum that covers the skull bones.

Cephalopelvic disproportion (CPD): Disparity between the size of the woman's pelvis and the fetal head.

Cerclage: Non-absorbable suture inserted to keep cervix closed.

Cervical eversion: Physiological response by cervical cells to hormonal changes in pregnancy. Cells proliferate and cause the cervix to appear eroded.

Cervical intra-epithelial neoplasm (CIN): Progressive and abnormal growth of cervical cells.

Cervical ripening: Process by which the cervix changes and becomes more susceptible to the effect of uterine contractions. Can be physiological or artificially produced.

Cervicitis: Inflammation of the cervix.

Choanal atresia: (Bilateral) membranous or bony obstruction of the nares; the baby appears

Glossary of terms and acronyms

blue when sleeping and pink when crying.

Chorionic plate: The fetal side of the placenta.

Choroid plexus cyst: Collection of cerebrospinal fluid within the choroid plexi, from where cerebrospinal fluid is derived.

Chromosome: An organized structure of DNA and organized proteins that carries genes.

Coloboma: A malformation characterized by the absence of or a defect in the tissue of the eye; the pupil can appear keyhole-shaped. It may be associated with other anomalies.

Colposcopy: Visualization of the cervix using a colposcope.

Commensal: Micro-organisms adapted to grow on the skin or mucous surfaces of the host, forming part of the normal flora.

Conjoined twins: Identical twins where separation is incomplete so their bodies are partly joined together and vital organs may be shared.

Coronal suture: Membranous tissue separating the frontal bones from the parietal bones.

Couvelaire uterus (uterine apoplexy): Bruising and oedema of uterine tissue seen in placental abruption when leaking blood is forced between muscle fibres because the margins of the placenta are still attached to the uterus.

Cricoid pressure: A technique whereby pressure is exerted on the cartilaginous ring below the larynx (the cricoid) to occlude the oesophagus and prevent reflux. Cricoid pressure is employed during the induction of a general anaesthetic to prevent acid aspiration syndrome.

Cryotherapy: Use of cold or freezing to destroy or remove tissue.

Cryptorchidism: Undescended testes, which may be unilateral or bilateral.

Decidualization: The structural changes that occur in the endometrium in preparation for implantation.

De-infibulation: Being opened.

Delusion: A false fixed belief that is impenetrable to reason.

Deontology: Duty-based theory.

Deoxyribonucleic acid (DNA): The substance containing genes. DNA can store and transmit information, can copy itself accurately and can occasionally mutate.

Diastasis symphysis pubis: A painful condition in which there is an abnormal relaxation of the ligaments supporting the pubic joint; also referred to as pelvic girdle pain.

Dichorionic twins: Two individuals who have developed in their own separate chorionic sacs.

Diploid: Containing two sets of chromosomes.

Disseminated intravascular coagulation/coagulopathy (DIC): A condition secondary to a primary complication where there is inappropriate blood clotting in the blood vessels, followed by an inability of the blood to clot appropriately when all the clotting factors have been used up.

Dizygotic (binovular): Formed from two separate zygotes.

Ductus arteriosus: A temporary fetal structure which leads from the bifurcation of the pulmonary artery to the descending aorta.

Ductus venosus: A temporary fetal structure which connects the umbilical vein to the inferior vena cava.

Dyspareunia: Painful or difficult intercourse experienced by the woman.

Ectoderm: The outermost layer of three primary germ cell layers present in the early embryo.

Ectopic pregnancy: An abnormally situated pregnancy, most commonly in a uterine tube.

Endocervical: Relating to the internal canal of the cervix.

Endoderm: The innermost layer of three primary germ cell layers present in the early embryo.

Epicanthic folds: A vertical fold of skin on either side of the nose which covers the lacrimal caruncle. They may be common in Asian babies, but may indicate Down syndrome in other ethnic groups.

Episiotomy: A surgical incision made to enlarge the vaginal orifice during childbirth.

Erb's palsy: Paralysis of the arm due to the damage to cervical nerve roots 5 and 6 of the brachial plexus.

Erythematous: Reddening of the skin.

Erythropoiesis: The process by which erythrocytes (red blood cells) are formed. After the 10th week of gestation, erythropoiesis production rises and seems to be involved in red cell production in the bone marrow during the third trimester.

Exomphalos (omphalocele): A defect in which the bowel or other viscera protrude through the umbilicus.

External cephalic version (ECV): The use of external manipulation on the pregnant woman's abdomen to convert a breech to a cephalic presentation.

False-negative rate: The proportion of affected pregnancies that would not be identified as high risk. Tests with a high false-negative rate have low sensitivity.

False-positive rate: The proportion of unaffected pregnancies with a high-risk classification. Tests with a high false-positive rate have low specificity.

Female genital mutilation (FGM): Also known as **female circumcision**. Any procedure that intentionally alter or cause injury to the external female genital organs for non-medical reasons. Four main types are reported.

Ferguson reflex: Surge of oxytocin, resulting in increased contractions, due to stimulation of the cervix, and upper portion of the vagina.

Fetal reduction: The reduction in the number of viable fetuses/embryos in a multiple (usually higher multiple) pregnancy by medical intervention.

Feto-fetal transfusion syndrome: Also known as **twin-to-twin transfusion syndrome (TTTS)**. Condition in which blood from one monozygotic twin fetus transfuses into the other fetus via blood vessels in the placenta.

Fetus-in-fetu: Parts of a fetus may be lodged within another fetus. This can only happen in monozygotic twins.

Fibroid (fibromyoma): Firm, benign tumour of muscular and fibrous tissue.

Foramen magnum: A large opening in the occipital bone of the skull through which the spinal cord exits.

Foramen ovale: A temporary structure of the fetal circulation allowing blood to be shunted from the right to left atrium in utero.

Fossa ovalis: Oval shaped depression in the intra-atrial septum. Formed following the closure of the foramen ovale at birth.

Framing effect: A means of cognitive bias insofar that individuals react differently to a particular choice such as antenatal screening tests, based on the manner in which the information is presented, i.e. whether they perceive the risk of screening as a loss or a gain.

Fraternal twins: Dizygotic *(non-identical)*.

Fundal height: The distance between the upper part of the uterus (*the fundus*) and the upper part of the symphysis pubis (*the junction between the pubic bones*). This assessment is undertaken to assess the increasing size of the uterus antenatally and decreasing size postnatally.

Funis: The umbilical cord.

Gastroschisis: A paramedian defect of the abdominal wall with extrusion of bowel that is not covered by peritoneum.

Glabella: The area between the eyebrows.

Globalization: The increased interconnectedness and interdependence of people and countries.

Grande multipara: A woman who has given birth five times or more.

Greater vestibular glands (Bartholin's glands): Two small glands that open on either side of the vaginal orifice, located in the posterior part of the labia majora.

Group practice: A small group of midwives who provide care for a group of women.

Haematuria: Blood in the urine.

Haemostasis: The arrest of bleeding.

Hallucinations: A sensory perception in the absence of any stimulus. Any of the five sensory modality can be affected.

Haploid: Containing only one set of chromosomes.

HELLP syndrome: A condition of pregnancy characterized by haemolysis, elevated liver enzymes and low platelets.

Herpes gestationis: An autoimmune disease precipitated by pregnancy and characterized by an erythematous rash and blisters.

Homan's sign: Pain is felt in the calf when the foot is pulled upwards *(dorsiflexion)*. This is indicative of a venous thrombosis and further investigations should be undertaken to exclude or confirm this.

Homeostasis: The condition in which the body's internal environment remains relatively constant within physiological limits.

Hydatidiform mole: A gross malformation of the trophoblast in which the chorionic villi proliferate and become avascular.

Hydropic vesicles: Fluid-filled sacs, or blisters.

Hypercapnia: An abnormal increase in the amount of carbon dioxide in the blood.

Hyperemesis gravidarum: Protracted or excessive vomiting in pregnancy.

Hypertrophy: Overgrowth of tissue.

Hypogastric arteries: Temporary fetal structures that branch off from the internal iliac arteries and become the umbilical arteries when they enter the umbilical cord.

Hypospadias: A condition where the urethral meatus opens on to the undersurface of the penis.

Hypothermia: A core body temperature below 36 °C.

Hypotonia: The loss of muscle tension and tone.

Hypovolaemia: Reduced circulating blood volume due to external loss of body fluids or to loss of fluid into the tissues.

Hypoxia: Lack of oxygen.

Hypoxic ischaemic encephalopathy (HIE): Condition where there is evidence of hypoxia and ischaemia.

Hysteroscope: An instrument used to access the uterus via the vagina.

Immunoglobulins: Antibodies.

Induction of labour: Intervention to stimulate uterine contractions before the onset of spontaneous labour.

Intermittent positive pressure ventilation (IPPV): Inflation breaths are given to clear lung fluid and ventilatory breaths are given to remove excess CO_2 and provide oxygen.

Internationalization: Has no agreed definition but best describes the process of harmonizing relationships from a cross-cultural or international perspective.

Intervillous spaces: The spaces between the chorionic villi that fill with maternal blood.

Intraepithelial: Within the epithelium, or among epithelial cells.

Intrahepatic cholestasis of pregnancy (ICP): An idiopathic condition of abnormal liver function.

Jaundice: Yellow coloration of the skin and the sclera caused by a raised level of bilirubin in the circulation *(hyperbilirubinaemia)*.

Kleihauer test: A standard blood test used to quantitatively assess or measure the degree of feto-maternal haemorrhage.

Glossary of terms and acronyms

LAM: A method of contraception based upon an algorithm of lactation and amenorrhoea over a 6-month time period.

Lamda: Posterior fontanelle.

Lamdoidal suture: Membranous tissue separating the occipital bone from the two parietal bones of the fetal skull.

Lanugo: Soft downy hair that covers the fetus *in utero* and occasionally the neonate. It appears at around 20 weeks' gestation and covers the face and most of the body. It disappears by 40 weeks' gestation.

Layer of Nitabusch: A collaginous layer between the endometrium and myometrium.

Ligamentum arteriosum: Permanent ligament formed from the ductus arteriosus following birth.

Ligamentum teres: Permanent ligament formed from the umbilical vein following birth.

Ligamentum venosum: Permanenet ligament formed from the ductus venosus following birth.

Linea nigra: A common dark line of pigmentation running longitudinally in the centre of the abdomen below and sometimes above the umbilicus.

Lochia: A Latin word traditionally used to describe the vaginal loss a woman experiences following the birth of a baby.

Løvset manoeuvre: A manoeuvre for the birth of the fetal shoulders and extended arms in a breech presentation.

Macrosomia: Large baby weighing 4–4.5 kg or greater.

Malposition: A cephalic presentation other than normal well-flexed anterior position of the fetal head, e.g. occipitoposterior.

Malpresentation: A presentation other than the vertex, i.e. face, brow, compound or shoulder.

Mauriceau–Smellie–Veit manoeuvre: A manoeuvre to assist the birth of the fetal head in a breech presentation that involves jaw flexion and shoulder traction.

McRoberts manoeuvre: A manoeuvre to rotate the angle of the symphysis pubis superiorly and release the impaction of the anterior shoulder of the fetus when there is shoulder dystocia. The woman brings her knees up to her chest.

Mendelson's syndrome: A chemical pneumonitis caused by the reflux of gastric contents into the maternal lungs during a general anaesthetic.

Meningitis: Inflammation of the membranes covering the brain and spinal column.

Mentum: Chin.

Mesenchyme: A mesh of embryonic connective tissue.

Mesoderm: The middle layer of three primary germ cell layers present in the early embryo.

Microchimerism: The presence of a small number of cells in one individual that originated in a different individual.

Midwife-led care: Midwives or a midwife take the lead role in care of a woman or group of women.

Miscarriage: Spontaneous loss of pregnancy before viability.

Modified Early Obstetric Warning Score (MEOWS): A chart or track and trigger system used to record maternal observations or physiological vital signs antenatally and postnatally for all mothers who are hospitalized in the maternity service.

Monoamniotic twins: Two individuals who have developed in the same amniotic sac.

Monochorionic twins: Two identical individuals who have developed in the same chorionic sac.

Monozygotic (monozygous): Formed from one zygote (identical twins).

Moulding: The change in shape of the fetal head that takes place during its passage through the birth canal.

Multifetal reduction: see Fetal reduction.

Naegele's rule: A method of calculating the expected date of birth.

Natural family planning (NFP): Methods of contraception based on observations of naturally occurring signs and symptoms of the fertile and infertile phases of the menstrual cycle.

Necrotizing enterocolitis (NEC): An acquired disease of the small and large intestine caused by ischaemia of the intestinal mucosa.

Neonatal encephalopathy: A clinical syndrome of abnormal levels of consciousness, tone, primitive reflexes, autonomic function and sometimes seizures in newborn babies.

Neoplasia: Growth of new tissue.

Neurulation: The formation of the neural plate and its transformation in to the neural tube.

Nerve innervation: Nerve supply.

Neutral thermal environment (NTE): The range of environmental temperature over which heat production, oxygen consumption and nutritional requirements for growth are minimal, provided the body temperature is normal.

Non-maleficence: Do no harm.

Oedema: The effusion of body fluid into the tissues.

Oligohydramnios: Abnormally small amount of amniotic fluid in pregnancy.

Oliguria: The production of an abnormally small amount of urine.

One-to-one midwifery: One midwife takes responsibility for individual women with a partner backing up the named midwife. Such a system integrates a high level of continuity of caregiver and midwifery-led care. It is geographically based and includes women who are both 'high risk' and 'low risk'.

Paco$_2$: Carbon dioxide partial pressure. Measures the partial pressure of dissolved carbon dioxide. This dissolved CO_2 has moved out of the cell and into the bloodstream. The measure of a Paco$_2$ accurately reflects the alveolar ventilation.

Pao₂: Arterial oxygen partial pressure. Measures the partial pressure of oxygen in the arterial blood. It reflects how the lung is functioning but does not measure tissue oxygenation.

Paronychia: An inflamed swelling of the nail folds; acute paronychia is usually caused by infection with *Staphylococcus aureus.*

Partnership: A relationship of trust and equity through which both partners are strengthened and power is diffused.

Peak mucus day: A retrospective assessment of the last day of highly fertile mucus which is observed vaginally or felt around ovulation.

Pedunculated: Stem or stalk.

Pemphigoid gestationis: see Herpes gestationis.

Perinatal: Events surrounding labour and the first 7 days of life.

Perinatal mental illness: A term used both nationally and internationally to emphasize the importance of psychiatric disorder in pregnancy as well as following childbirth and the variety of psychiatric disorders that can occur at this time, in addition to postnatal depression.

pH: A solution's acidity or alkalinity is expressed on the pH scale, which runs from 0 to 14. This scale is based on the concentration of hydronium (H^+) ions in a solution expressed in chemical units called moles per litre (mol/l). Solutions with a pH less than 7 are said to be *acidic* and solutions with a pH greater than 7 are *basic* or *alkaline*. Pure water has a pH very close to 7. When the fetus is hypoxic the increased acid produced raises the acidity of the blood and the pH falls.

Phenylketonuria (PKU): An autosomal recessive disorder of protein metabolism.

Pill-free interval: The 7 days when no pills are taken during combined oral contraceptive regimen.

Placenta accreta: Abnormally adherent placenta into the muscle layer of the uterus.

Placenta increta: Abnormally adherent placenta into the perimetrium of the uterus.

Placenta percreta: Abnormally adherent placenta through the muscle layer of the uterus.

Placenta praevia: A condition in which some or all of the placenta is attached in the lower segment of the uterus.

Placental abruption: see Abruptio placenta.

Placentation: The forming of the placenta.

Polyhydramnios: An excessive amount of amniotic fluid in pregnancy. Also referred to as *hydramnios.*

Polyp: Small growth.

Porphyria: An inherited condition of abnormal red blood cell formation.

Postnatal blues: A transitory emotional or mood state, experienced by 50–80% of women depending on parity.

Postnatal period: The period after the end of labour during which the attendance of a midwife upon the woman and baby is required, being not less than 10 days and for such longer period as the midwife considers necessary.

Postpartum: After labour.

Precipitate labour: The expulsion of the fetus within 3 hours of commencement of contractions.

Pre-eclampsia: A condition peculiar to pregnancy, which is characterized by hypertension, proteinuria and systemic dysfunction.

Primary postpartum haemorrhage (PPH): A blood loss in excess of 500 ml or any amount that adversely affects the condition of the mother within the first 24 hours of birth.

Progestogen: Synthetic progesterone used in hormonal contraception.

Prostaglandins: Locally acting chemical compounds derived from fatty acids within cells. They ripen the cervix and cause the uterus to contract.

Proteinuria: Protein in the urine.

Proteolytic enzymes: Enzymes that break down proteins.

Pruritus: Itching.

Psychosis: A disorder of the mental state that affects mood and cognitive processes which may cause the individual to lose touch with reality (i.e. hallucinations and delusional thoughts are usually present).

Ptyalism: Excessive salivation.

Pudendal block: This is the procedure where local anaesthetic is infiltrated into the tissue around the pudendal nerve within the pelvis; employed for some operative procedures during vaginal births.

Puerperal psychosis: Describes a rare but serious psychiatric emergency and the most severe form of postpartum affective (mood) disorder.

Puerperal sepsis: Infection of the genital tract following childbirth; still a major cause of maternal death where it is undetected and/ or untreated.

Puerperium: A period after childbirth where the uterus and other organs and structures that have been affected by the pregnancy are physiologically returning to their non-gravid state, lactation is establishing and the woman is adjusting socially and psychologically to motherhood. Usually described as a period of up to 6–8 weeks.

Quickening: The first point at which the woman recognizes fetal movements in early pregnancy.

Reciprocity: A mutual relationship between two individuals where there is an exchange of positive regard for each other.

Regional anaesthesia: More commonly are epidural and intrathecal (spinal) anaesthetic.

Retraction: The process by which the uterine muscle fibres shorten after a contraction. This is unique to uterine muscle.

Glossary of terms and acronyms

Rubin's manoeuvre: A rotational manoeuvre to relieve shoulder dystocia. Pressure is exerted over the fetal back to adduct and rotate the shoulders.

Sandal gap: Exaggerated gap between the first and second toes.

Secondary postpartum haemorrhage: Any abnormal or excessive bleeding from the genital tract occurring between 24 hours and 12 weeks postnatally.

Selective fetocide: The medical destruction of a malformed twin fetus in a continuing pregnancy.

Sinciput: The forehead.

Sheehan's syndrome: A condition where sudden or prolonged shock leads to irreversible pituitary necrosis characterized by amenorrhoea, genital atrophy and premature senility.

Short femur: Shorter than the average thigh bone, when compared with other fetal measurements.

Shoulder dystocia: Failure of the shoulders to spontaneously traverse the pelvis after birth of the fetal head.

Speculum (vaginal): An instrument used to open the vagina.

Subinvolution: The uterine size appears larger than anticipated for the number of days postpartum, and may feel not well contracted. Uterine tenderness may be present.

Succenturiate lobe: A small extra lobe of placenta separate from the main placenta.

Surfactant: Complex mixture of phospholipids and lipoproteins produced by type 2 alveolar cells in the lungs that decreases surface tension and prevents alveolar collapse at end expiration.

Symphysiotomy: A surgical incision to separate the symphysis pubis and enlarge the pelvis to aid birth of the baby.

Symphysis pubis dysfunction: see Diastasis symphysis pubis.

Tachypnoea: Increased respiratory rate that occurs as the baby attempts to compensate for an increased carbon dioxide concentration in the blood and extracellular fluids.

Talipes: A complex foot deformity, affecting 1/1000 live births and more common in males. The affected foot is held in a fixed flexion (*equinus*) and in-turned (*varus*) position. It can be differentiated from positional talipes because the deformity in true talipes cannot be passively corrected.

Team midwifery: Midwives are team-based rather than on a ward or within a community base. The team takes responsibility for a number of women. Teams may be restricted to hospital or community, or cover both.

Tentorium cerebelli: An arched fold of the dura mater, covering the upper surface of the cerebellum.

Teratogen: An agent believed to cause congenital malformations, e.g. thalidomide.

Tocophobia: A fear of childbirth.

Torsion: Twisting.

Torticollis: The result of tightness and shortening of one sternomastoid muscle.

Tregs: Adapted T regulator cells that play a part in immunity.

Trizygotic: Formed from three separate zygotes.

Trophoblasts: Peripheral cells surrounding the blastocyst.

Twin-to-twin transfusion syndrome: see Feto-fetal transfusion syndrome.

Uniovular: Monozygotic.

Unstable lie: After 36 weeks' gestation, a lie that varies between longitudinal and oblique or transverse is said to be unstable.

Uterine involution: The physiological process that starts from the end of labour and results in a gradual reduction in the size of the uterus until it returns to its non-pregnant size and location in the pelvis.

Uterotonics: Also known as **oxytocics** or **ecbolics**. Pharmacological agents/drugs (e.g. syntometrine, syntocinon, ergometrine and prostaglandins) that are used in the active management of the third stage of labour to stimulate the smooth muscle of the uterus to contract.

Utilitarianism: Providing the greatest good for greatest number.

Vanishing twin syndrome: The reabsorption of one twin fetus early in pregnancy (usually before 12 weeks).

Vasa praevia: A rare occurrence in which umbilical cord vessels pass through the placental membranes and lie across the cervical os.

Vasculogenesis: The formation of new blood vessels.

Vernix caseosa: White creamy substance protecting the fetus from dessication and present from 18 weeks gestation.

Wharton's jelly: Gelatinous substance surrounding the umbilical cord.

Withdrawal bleed: Vaginal bleeding due to withdrawal of hormones.

Wood's manoeuvre: A rotational or screw manoeuvre to relieve shoulder dystocia. Pressure is exerted on the fetal chest to rotate and abduct the shoulders.

Zavanelli manoeuvre: Last choice of manoeuvre for shoulder dystocia. The head is returned to its pre-restitution position, then the head is flexed back into the vagina. Birth is by caesarean section.

Zygosity: Describing the genetic make-up of children in a multiple birth.

Acronyms

ABPM: ambulatory blood pressure monitoring

ACE: angiotensin converting enzyme

ACTH: adrenocorticotrophic hormone

ADH: anti-diuretic hormone

AED: antiepileptic drug

AFLD: acute fatty liver disease

AGA: appropriate for gestational age

AIDS: acquired immunodeficiency syndrome

ALT: Alanine Transaminase

ANP: atrial natriuretic peptide

Anti HBe: hepatitis B e-antibodies

APEC: Action on Pre-Eclampsia

APH: Antepartum Haemorrhage

APS: antiphospholipid syndrome

ARB: angiotensin receptor blocker

ARM: artificial rupture of the membranes/Association of Radical Midwives

ART: antiretroviral therapy

ASD: atrial septal defect

ATP: adenosine triphosphate

BALT: bronchus-associated lymphoid tissue

BFI: Baby Friendly Initiative

BMI: body mass index

BMR: basal metabolic rate

BNF: British National Formulary

BNP: brain natriuretic peptide

BOC: British Oxygen Company

BP: blood pressure

BTS: British Thoracic Society

CCG: Clinical Commissioning Group

C. Diff: *Clostridium difficile*

CHD: congenital heart disease

CHRE: Council for Healthcare Regulatory Excellence (now **PSA** Professional Standards Authority)

CIN: cervical intraepithelial neoplasia

CINORIS: Clinical Negligence and Other Risks Indemnity Scheme

CMACE: Centre for Maternal and Child Enquiries

CMB: Central Midwives Board

CEMACH: Confidential Enquiry into Maternal and Child Health.

CESDI: Confidential Enquiries into Stillbirths and Deaths in Infancy

CMV: cytomegalovirus

CNS: central nervous system

CNST: Clinical Negligence Scheme for Trusts

COC: combined oral contraceptive

COMET: The Comparative Obstetric Mobile Epidural Trial

CQC: Care Quality Commission

CRH: corticotrophin-releasing hormone

CRT: capillary refill time

CSF: cerebral spinal fluid

CSII: continuous subcutaneous insulin infusion

CT: computerized tomography

CTG: cardiotograph/cardiotocogram

CVA: cerebral vascular accident

CVS: chorionic villus sampling

DCSF: Department for Children, Schools and Families (until 2010; now DfE)

DDH: developmental dysplasia of the hip

DfE: Department for Education

DH/DoH: Department of Health

DHA: docosahexanoic acid

DMPA: depot medroxyprogesterone acetate

DVT: deep vein thrombosis

EBM: expressed breast milk

ECG: electrocardiogram/graphy

E. Coli: *Escherichia coli*

ECM: extracellular matrix

EFM: electronic fetal monitoring

EFSA: European Food Standards Agency

eGFR: epidermal growth factor receptor

EHC: emergency hormonal contraception

ELBW: extremely low birth weight (below 1000 g)

ENB: English National Board for Nursing, Midwifery and Health Visiting

ENT: ear, nose and throat

ERPC: evacuation of retained products of conception

ESC: Essential Skills Clusters

EU: European Union

FASD: fetal alcohol spectrum disorders

FBC: full blood count

FIL: feedback inhibitor of lactation

FPA: Family Planning Association

FSA: Food Standards Agency

FSH: follicle stimulating hormone

FSRH: Faculty of Sexual and Reproductive Health

GALT: gut-associated lymphoid tissue

GAS: Group A streptococcus

GBS: Group B streptococcus

GDM: gestational diabetes mellitus

GF: glomerular filtrate

GFR: glomerular filtration rate

GNC: General Nursing Council

GnRH: gonadotrophic-releasing hormone

GP: General Practitioner

GTD: gestational trophoblastic disease

GTI: genital tract infection

GTN: gestational trophoblastic neoplasia

GTT: glucose tolerance test

HAART: highly active antiretroviral therapy

Hb: haemoglobin

HbA: adult haemoglobin

HbAS: sickle cell trait (heterozygous)

HbA1c: glucated/glycosylated haemoglobin

HBeAg: hepatitis B e-antigen

HbF: fetal haemoglobin

HbH: haemoglobin H disease

HbSS: sickle cell anaemia/disease (homozygous)

HBV: hepatitis B virus

HCAI: healthcare-acquired infection

hCG: human chorionic gonadotrophin

hCG-H: hyperglycosylated human chorionic gonadotrophin

hCS: human chorionic somatomammotropin hormone

HDCU: high dependency care unit

HDL: high-density lipoprotein

HDN: haemorrhagic disease of the newborn

HEI: Higher Education Institution

HIV: Human Immunodeficiency Virus

hPGL: human placental growth hormone

hPL: human placental lactogen

HPT: home pregnancy test

HPV: human papilloma virus

HSCIC: Health and Social Care Information Centre

HSE: Health Survey for England

HSV: herpes simplex virus

HVS: high vaginal swab

ICM: International Confederation of Midwives

ICU: intensive care unit

IFCC: International Federation of Clinical Chemistry

IHD: ischaemic heart disease

IOM: Institute of Medicine

IM: intramuscular

IQ: intelligence quotient

ITP: Intention to Practice

IUCD: intrauterine contraceptive device

Glossary of terms and acronyms

IUFD: intrauterine fetal death

IUGR: intrauterine growth restriction

IUS: intrauterine system

IV/IVI: intravenous/intravenous infusion

IVF: in vitro fertilization

JEC: Joint Epilepsy Council

L3: third lumbar vertebra

LA: Local Authority

LARC: long-acting reversible contraceptive

LBW: low birth weight (below 2500 g)

LC-PUFA: long chain poyunsaturated fatty acids

LFT: liver function test

LGA: large for gestational age

LH: luteinizing hormone

LMP: last menstrual period

LMWH: low molecular weight heparin

LSA: Local Supervising Authority

LSAMO: Local Supervising Authority Midwifery Officer

MA: mentoanterior

MCH: mean cell/corpuscular haemoglobin

MCV: mean cell/corpuscular volume

MH(P)RA: Medicines and Healthcare Products Regulatory Agency

MI: myocardial infarction

MIDIRS: Midwives Information Resource Service

MODY: mature onset diabetes of the young

MOH: Medical Officer of Health

MPV: mean platelet volume

MRI: magnetic resonance imaging

MRSA: methicillin-resistant *Staphylococcus aureus*

MSU/MSSU: mid-stream specimen of urine

MSW: Maternity Support Worker

NCT: National Childbirth Trust

NET-EN: norethisterone enanthate

NHS: National Health Service

NHSLA: National Health Service Litigation Authority

NICE: National Institute for Health and Clinical Excellence/National Institute for Health and Care Excellence (from 2013)

NICU/NNICU: neonatal intensive care unit

NIPE: neonatal and infant physical examination

NMC: Nursing and Midwifery Council

NOP: Notification of Practice

NPEU: National Perinatal Epidemiology Unit

NPSA: National Patient Safety Agency

NTD: neural tube defect

OA: occipitoanterior

OC: obstetric cholestasis

OF: cccipitofrontal

OP: occipitoposterior

PAP: pulmonary artery pressure

PCA: patient-controlled analgesia

PCT: Primary Care Trust

PDA: patent ductus arteriosus

PE: pulmonary embolism/embolus

PET: pre-eclampsia toxaemia

PGP: pelvic girdle pain

PID: pelvic inflammatory disease

PIH: pregnancy-induced hypertension

PND: postnatal depression

POC: point of care

POP: progesterone-only pill

PPI: proton pump inhibitor

PPROM: preterm prelabour rupture of the membranes

PREP: Post-Registration Education and Practice

PROM: prelabour rupture of membranes

PSA: Professional Standards Authority

PTH: parathyroid hormone

RAAS: renin–angiotensin–aldosterone system

RCoA: Royal College of Anaesthetists

RCM: Royal College of Midwives

RCOG: Royal College of Obstetricians and Gynaecologists

RCPCH: Royal College of Paediatrics and Child Health

RCT: randomizd controlled trial

RCUK: Resuscitation Council of the United Kingdom

RHA: Regional Health Authority

RNA: ribonucleic acid

RPF: renal plasma flow

SACN: Scientific Advisory Committee on Nutrition

SANDS: Stillbirth and Neonatal Death Society

SBAR: situation, background, assessment and recommendation

SFH: symphysis fundal height

SGA: small for gestational age

SHA: Strategic Health Authority

SI: Statutory Instrument

SIGN: Scottish Intercollegiate Guidelines Network

SLE: systemic lupus erythematosus

SPRM: selective progesterone receptor modulator

STI: sexually transmitted infection

SUDEP: sudden unexpected death in epilepsy

SUI: stress urinary incontinence

T11: eleventh thoracic vertebra

TBG: thyroxine-binding globulin

TBV: total blood volume

TED: thromboembolism deterrent

TENS: transcutaneous electrical nerve stimulation

TRH: thyrotropin-releasing hormone

TSH: thyroid-stimulating hormone

UK: United Kingdom

UKAMB: United Kingdom Association for Milk Banking

UKCC: United Kingdom Central Council for Nursing, Midwifery and Health Visiting

UKOSS: United Kingdom Obstetric Surveillance System

UNAIDS: United Nations Programme on HIV/AIDS

UNICEF: United Nations International Children' Fund

UPSI: unprotected sexual intercourse

USA: United States of America

US(S): ultrasound (scan)

UTI: urinary tract uifection

VE: vaginal examination

VKDB: vitamin K deficiency bleeding

VLBW: very low birth weight (below 1500 g)

VSD: ventricular septal defect

VTE: venous thromboembolism

WHO: World Health Organization

Index

Illustrations are comprehensively referred to from the text. Therefore, significant items in illustrations (figures and tables) have only been given a page reference in the absence of their concomitant mention in the text referring to that illustration.

A

Index

Index

Index